Contributors

Karen Bawel-Brinkley, RN, PhD
Associate Professor
San Jose State University School of Nursing
San Jose, California
Test Questions

Diane M. Billings, EdD, RN, FAAN
Chancellor's Professor Emeritus
Indiana University School of Nursing
Indianapolis, Indiana
Managing Client Care Delivery
Managing Client Safety
Managing Emergencies, Crises, and Disasters
Test Questions

Lori Bork, RN, MS, CCRN
Assistant Professor of Nursing
Dakota Wesleyan University
Mitchell, South Dakota
Test Questions

Linda Carman Copel, PhD, APRN, BC, CNE, DAPA
Associate Professor
Villanova University College of Nursing
Villanova, Pennsylvania
Test Questions

Linda R. Delunas, PhD, RN, CNE
Associate Professor
Indiana University Northwest School of Nursing
Gary, Indiana
Test Questions

Margie A. Hull, MEd, MSN, CNS-BC, CDE, RN
Formerly, Visiting Lecturer
Indiana University School of Nursing
Indianapolis, Indiana
Diabetes CNS, CDE
Department of Clinical Education
Wishard Health Services
Indianapolis, Indiana
The Client With Upper Gastrointestinal Tract Health Problems
The Client with Lower Gastrointestinal Tract Health Problems
The Client With Endocrine Health Problems
The Client With Urinary Tract Health Problems
The Client With Musculoskeletal Health Problems
The Client Having Surgery
Managing Client Care Delivery
Test Questions

Juanita Johnson, PhD, RN
Adjunct Professor
Oklahoma Baptist University
Shawnee, Oklahoma
Test Questions

Susan C. Johnston, MSN, RN
Instructor
Chippewa Valley Technical College
Eau Claire, Wisconsin
Introduction to Nursing Care of the Adult Client
The Client With Reproductive Health Problems
The Client With Health Problems of the Integumentary and Sensory Systems

Kathy Jorgensen, RN, MA, MSN
Associate Professor
Department of Nursing
The University of South Dakota
Vermillion, South Dakota
The Client With Mood and Anxiety Disorders and the Client at Risk for Suicide
The Client With Schizophrenia and Related Psychotic Disorders, Cognitive Disorders, Psychosexual Disorders, and Mental Health Disorders in Children and Adolescents
The Client With Personality Disorders, Substance Abuse and Addiction, and Eating Disorders
Abuse and Mental Health Crises
Test Questions

Cindy Kohtz, EdD, RN, CNE
Associate Professor of Nursing
Saint Francis Medical Center College of Nursing
Peoria, Illinois
Test Questions

Cheryl Laskowski, DNS, APRN-BC
Adjunct Faculty
University of Vermont
Burlington, Vermont
Clinical Practice, FAHC for Pain Medicine
South Burlington, Vermont
Test Questions

Ann Lowenkron, DNS, RN
Associate Professor, Emeritus
Indiana University School of Nursing
Indianapolis, Indiana
Test Questions

Lesley Milgrom, MSN, RN
Clinical Assistant Professor
Indiana University School of Nursing
Indianapolis, Indiana
The Client With Cardiac Health Problems
The Client With Vascular Disease
The Client With Respiratory Health Problems
The Client With Biliary Tract Disorders
The Client With Neurologic Health Problems
Test Questions

Lynn M. Murphy, RN, MSN, CPNP
Assistant Professor
Bellin College of Nursing
Green Bay, Wisconsin
Test Questions

Susie Oliver, MSN, RNC, NP
Assistant Professor of Nursing
University of Indianapolis
Indianapolis, Indiana
Test Questions

Wendy R. Ostendorf, RN, EdD
Associate Professor
Neumann College
Aston, Pennsylvania
Introduction to Nursing Care of Children
The Child With Common Health Problems
The Child With Respiratory Health Problems
The Child With Cardiovascular Health Problems
The Child With Hematologic Health Problems
The Child With Health Problems of the Gastrointestinal Tract
The Child With Health Problems Involving Ingestion, Nutrition, or Diet
The Child With Health Problems of the Genitourinary System
The Child With Neurologic Health Problems
The Child With Musculoskeletal Health Problems

Jacquelyn Reid, EdD, CNM, CNE
Associate Professor of Nursing
Indiana University Southeast
New Albany, Indiana
Test Questions

Virginia Richardson, RN, DNS, CPNP
Associate Professor
Coordinator of Pediatric Nurse Practitioner Program
Indiana University School of Nursing
Indianapolis, Indiana
Test Questions

Gayle Roux, PhD, RN, NP-C
Associate Professor and Associate Dean for Faculty
Loyola University
Chicago, Illinois
Test Questions

Kay Scharn, RN, MSN, EdS
Nursing Faculty
Chippewa Valley Technical College
Eau Claire, Wisconsin
Test Questions

Emily Karwacki Sheff, MS, CMSRN, FNP-BC
Lecturer/Clinical Instructor
Massachusetts General Hospital Institute of Health Professions/Boston College
Boston, Massachusetts/Chestnut Hill, Massachusetts
The Client With Hematologic Health Problems
The Client With Cancer

Evelyn Stephenson, MSN, RNC
Clinical Assistant Professor
Indiana University School of Nursing
Indianapolis, Indiana
Introduction to Nursing Care of the Childbearing Family and Neonate
The Neonatal Client
Test Questions

Sharon A. Vinten, MSN, RNC, WHNP
Associate Professor Emeritus
Indiana University School of Nursing
Indianapolis, Indiana
Staff Nurse
Carolinas Healthcare System
Charlotte, North Carolina
Introduction to Nursing Care of the Childbearing Family and Neonate
Antepartal Care
Complications of Pregnancy
The Birth Experience
Postpartum Care

Mary Ann Wehmer, MSN, RN, CNOR
Nursing Faculty
University of Southern Indiana
Evansville, Indiana
Test Questions

Shirley Woolf, RN, MSN, MA, CNRN, CNE
Clinical Assistant Professor
Indiana University School of Nursing
Indianapolis, Indiana
The Client With Cardiac Health Problems
The Client With Respiratory Health Problems
The Client With Neurologic Health Problems
Test Questions

K. L. Jean Yockey, MSN, FNP, CNE, RN
Assistant Professor
University of South Dakota
Vermillion, South Dakota
Introduction to Nursing Care of Clients With Psychiatric Disorders and Mental Health Problems
The Client With Mood and Anxiety Disorders and the Client at Risk for Suicide
Test Questions

Reviewers

Deborah Adelman, PhD, RN, CAN, BC, CNS
Associate Professor
State University of New York at Delhi
Delhi, New York

Peggy Baikie, DNP, RN, PNP-BC, NNP-BC
Clinical Coordinator/Nurse Practitioner; Adjunct Professor
St. Anthony Hospitals; Metropolitan State College of Denver
Denver, Colorado

Jennifer Beck, PhD(c), MS, RN
Chair, Undergraduate Studies; ASN Program Director, Associate Professor
Our Lady of the Lake College
Baton Rouge, Louisiana

Leona Beezley, RN, MS, MSN
Assistant Professor
Cox College of Nursing and Health Sciences
Springfield, Missouri

Judy A. Bourrand, RN, MSN
Assistant Professor
Ida V. Moffett School of Nursing; Samford University
Birmingham, Alabama

Margaret Brady, PhD, RN, CPNP
Professor of Nursing
Department of Nursing, California State University Long Beach
Long Beach, California

Michele Brimeyer, MSN, ARNP, WHNP-BC
Assistant Professor
University of Florida College of Nursing
Gainesville, Florida

Marietta Brooks, RN, BSN, CRRN
Nurse Case Manager—Practice Management Support Services
University of Michigan Health Systems
Ann Arbor, Michigan

Marie Cobb, RNC, MSN, IBCLC
Instructor
The University of Akron
Akron, Ohio

Kathy Dewan, RN, MN, PNP
Professor, Nursing Program; Assistant Program Director
Ohlone College
Fremont, California

Leslie Folds, EdD, APRN, BC
Assistant Professor of Nursing
Belmont University
Nashville, Tennessee

Vivian Gamblian, RN, MSN
Nursing Faculty
Baylor University, Louise Herrington School of Nursing
Dallas, Texas

Donna Glanker, MSN, RN
Assistant Professor
College of Mount St. Joseph
Cincinnati, Ohio

Susan Golden, MSN, RN
Nursing Faculty
Eastern New Mexico University–Roswell
Roswell, New Mexico

Debbie Green, MSN, RN, BC
Clinical Education Coordinator
Clarian North Medical Center
Indianapolis, Indiana

Betsy Gulledge, RN, MSN
Instructor of Nursing
Jacksonville State University
Jacksonville, Alabama

Marlene Huff, PhD, MSN, RNC
Associate Professor
The University of Akron College of Nursing
Akron, Ohio

Sonya Jakubec, RN, BHScN, MN, PhD(c)
Faculty, School of Nursing
Mount Royal College
Calgary, Alberta

Dena Jarog, RN, MSN, CCNS
Pediatric Critical Care Clinical Nurse Specialist
Saint Joseph's Children's Hospital of Marshfield
Marshfield, Wisconsin

Cindy Kohtz, EdD, RN, CNE
Associate Professor of Nursing
Saint Francis Medical Center College of Nursing
Peoria, Illinois

Mary Kozy, MSN, APRN, BC
Assistant Professor
University of Toledo, College of Nursing
Toledo, Ohio

Timothy Legg, PhD, CRNP, APRN-BC
Faculty
State University of New York at Delhi
Delhi, New York

Barb Leon, RN, MSN, CMSRN
Med-Surg Clinical Instructor
Washington State University, Intercollegiate College of Nursing
Spokane, Washington

Janet Massoglia, RN, MSN, FNP-BC
Nursing Faculty—Instructor
Delta College
University Center, Michigan

Bonnie Nelson, MSN, RN
Director, Instructional Services (ret.)
University of Toledo, College of Nursing
Toledo, Ohio

Karen Rich, PhD, RN
Assistant Professor
The University of Southern Mississippi, Gulf Coast Campus
Gulfport, Mississippi

Ora Robinson, RN, PhD
Assistant Professor
California State University San Bernardino
San Bernardino, California

Linda Rodenbaugh, EdD, MSN, RN
Associate Professor of Nursing
University of Indianapolis
Indianapolis, Indiana

Iris Rudnisky, RN, BScN, Med(Psychology)
Faculty Lecturer
University of Alberta
Edmonton, Alberta

Kay Scharn, RN, MSN, EdS
Nursing Faculty
Chippewa Valley Technical College
Eau Claire, Wisconsin

Judy Scott, MSN, RN
Professor of Nursing
The College of Southern Nevada
Las Vegas, Nevada

Susan Seibolt, MSN, RN, CNE
Assistant Professor; Associate Degree Program
Carl Sandburg College
Galesburg, Illinois

Suzan Shane, RN, APN-P, EdD
Associate Professor
OSF St. Francis College of Nursing
Peoria, Illinois

Pamela Spencer, BA, RN, BSN, FNP
Family Nurse Practitioner, Palliative Care and Surgery
Veterans Medical Center
Saginaw, Michigan

Ralph Vogel, RN, PhD, CPNP
Pediatric Specialty Coordinator (Graduate)
University of Arkansas for Medical Sciences, College of Nursing
Little Rock, Arkansas

Julie Will, RN, MSN
Chair, School of Health Sciences
Ivy Tech Community College of Indiana
Terre Haute, Indiana

K.L. Jean Yockey, MSN, RN, FNP, CNE
Assistant Professor
University of South Dakota
Vermillion, South Dakota

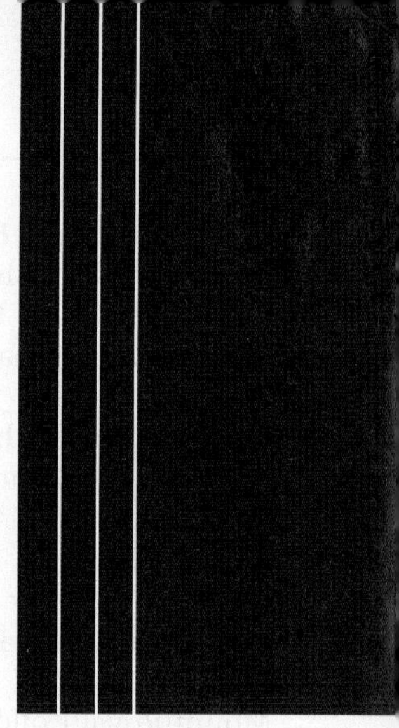

Preface

Today's fast-paced, complex, and technology-driven health care environment requires nurses who can critically synthesize information to provide safe nursing care. Clients and their families are assured that they will receive competent care when nurses demonstrate they have met graduation requirements of schools of nursing and pass licensing exams. *Lippincott's Content Review for NCLEX-RN®* (National Council Licensure Examination for Registered Nurses) is designed to assist students and graduate nurses review requisite nursing knowledge and skills and provides practice for taking exams similar to the ones used to assess competency for nursing practice.

Organization of the Book

Lippincott's Content Review for NCLEX-RN® is organized in three parts to help readers understand the format of the NCLEX-RN® licensing exam, review essential nursing content, and practice taking exams.

Part One explains the test plan for the NCLEX-RN licensing exam and types of questions used on this exam. It also gives information about how to develop a study plan and strategies for successful test taking.

Part Two presents, in outline format, content review of four major nursing subjects—Nursing Care of the Childbearing Family and Neonate, Nursing Care of Children, Nursing Care of Adults With Medical–Surgical Health Problems, and Nursing Care of Clients With Psychiatric Disorders and Mental Health Problems—as well as an entire section on Management of Care. Health problems in each chapter are organized around the nursing process and client needs as tested on the NCLEX-RN test plan. Each chapter is followed by a 20-item practice test that allows readers to validate their understanding of chapter content. Each section within Part Two concludes with an integrated test to confirm the reader's ability to apply, synthesize, and evaluate all of the content within the unit in a nursing care context.

Part Three provides three comprehensive postreview tests. Each of these 100-item exams is designed to simulate the licensing exam. The tests include content from all five section topics. Users of this book can take these exams to estimate the time it takes to answer 100 randomly generated questions.

This book is also accompanied by a CD-ROM, as well as online student and faculty resources that can be found at thePoint* (http://thepoint.lww.com), Lippincott Williams & Wilkins' online course and content manager. Resources include **1,500 *additional* questions** to provide an experience of taking computer-administered tests; 300 questions available **for use with an iPod;** student **study tips** and **study plan;** and an **NCLEX alternate-item format tutorial.** Instructors can access student resources as well as **faculty question writing tips!**

Features

This book has been designed to facilitate learning, provide opportunities for practice test taking, and prepare readers for taking exams.

Facilitates Learning

- Organizes content around **client needs**—the framework for the National Council of State Boards of Nursing Test Plan.
- Includes hundreds of **alternate format questions** (drag and drop/ordered response; hot spot; multiple response; fill-in-the blank; chart/exhibit) to promote full preparation for actual NCLEX-RN examination.
- Uses **clinical framework** to highlight nursing care by four major nursing subject areas: obstetrics, pediatrics, medical–surgical, and psychiatric and mental health problems.

*thePoint is a trademark of Wolters Kluwer Health | Lippincott Williams & Wilkins.

- Provides a specific unit on **management of care,** including managing care delivery; managing client safety; and managing emergencies, crises, and disasters.
- Emphasizes nursing care for **common health problems** as tested on the licensing exam.
- Provides charts, tables, and figures to clarify difficult-to-learn content, including **drug tables** that present specific drugs with expected outcomes, reduction of risk potential, and management of care.

Provides Opportunity for Practice Test Taking

- Includes **more than 3,000 NCLEX-RN-style questions** written at higher levels of cognitive domain to:
  - Assist with higher-order learning.
  - Develop skills of "thinking like a nurse."
- Includes **test questions written in all the exam formats** used on the NCLEX-RN licensing exam:
  - Multiple choice
  - Multiple response multiple choice
  - Hot spot
  - Fill-in-the-blank
  - Chart/exhibit
  - Drag and drop/ordered response
- Provides a **rationale for *each* answer,** for both correct and incorrect responses.
- Includes **codes for the eight general client needs** within each answer.
- Focuses questions on the National Council of State Boards of Nursing (NCSBN) Practice Analysis, with **emphasis on common nursing care.**
- Presents questions in text, CD, and iPod formats for flexible practice:
  - **40 content-focused chapter tests,** each with 20 test questions
  - **Five section practice tests** to review overall chapter content within each section
  - **Three comprehensive postreview tests** with questions in random order to simulate the licensing exam format
  - **1,500 test questions** on CD-ROM for practice taking computer-administered examinations
  - **300 questions available for download to iPod**
- Follows **course and curriculum sequences** used in nursing schools.
- **Prepares students for end-of-course, end-of-semester, and end-of-program competency exams.**

Prepares Readers for Taking Exams

- Explains the NCLEX-RN Test Plan.
- Provides strategies for taking tests.
- Explains how to manage test anxiety.
- Gives suggestions on how to prepare for the day of the actual test.
- Includes a template for developing a Personal Study Plan.
- Provides study tips from students who have passed the licensing exam.
- Lists address, phone number, and Web site for the National Council of State Boards of Nursing and each state and jurisdiction.

Acknowledgments

Preparing the first edition of a book requires a special team who can expertly guide the book's development. It is my pleasure to acknowledge the team at Lippincott Williams & Wilkins. *Margaret Zuccarini,* identified the need for the book and provided the guiding vision, which was then carried through by *Elizabeth Nieginski,* Executive Acquisitions Editor. *Helene Caprari,* Developmental Editor, patiently and persistently organized the content outlines and test questions for clarity and completeness; because of her work, no client need goes unmet! *Audrey Alt,* Senior Ancillary Editor, prepared the CD-ROM and iPod tests. And thanks to *Kathy Lane,* my assistant, for coordinating the project, the contributors, the reviewers, and me.

It is also a pleasure to recognize the team of chapter contributors, test item writers, and reviewers. Because of their understanding of how students learn, judicious choice of content, and ability to write high-level test questions, this book will prepare students to give competent and safe nursing care and be successful test-takers. Please note their names within the front matter of this book.

We hope you enjoy the first edition of this book. We offer best wishes as you take—and pass—the many exams you will face throughout your career.

Diane M. Billings, EdD, RN, FAAN

Contents

PART ONE

Introduction to the NCLEX-RN® Licensing Examination

chapter 1

Introduction to the NCLEX-RN® Licensing Examination

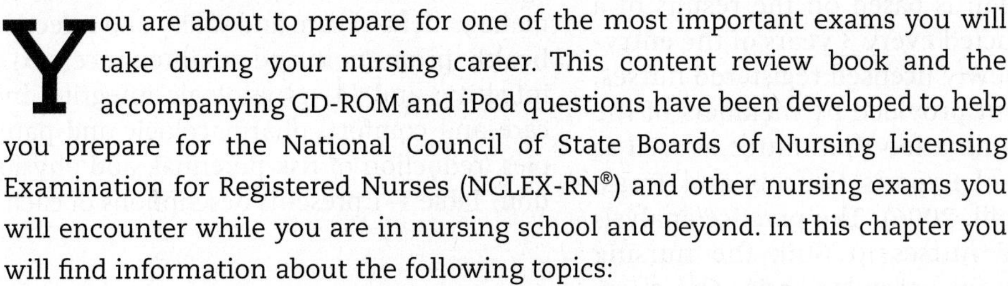

You are about to prepare for one of the most important exams you will take during your nursing career. This content review book and the accompanying CD-ROM and iPod questions have been developed to help you prepare for the National Council of State Boards of Nursing Licensing Examination for Registered Nurses (NCLEX-RN®) and other nursing exams you will encounter while you are in nursing school and beyond. In this chapter you will find information about the following topics:

- Overview: The NCLEX-RN® Licensing Examination
- The Test Plan
- The Test Questions
- Examination Format
- How to Use this Book to Prepare for the NCLEX-RN®

Overview: The NCLEX-RN® Licensing Examination

The NCLEX-RN® is administered to graduates of nursing schools to test the knowledge, abilities, and skills necessary for entry-level safe and effective nursing practice. The exam is developed by the National Council of State Boards of Nursing, Inc., an organization with representation from all state boards of nursing (information available at http://www.ncsbn.org). The same exam is used in all 50 states, the District of Columbia, and United States possessions, as well as at international testing sites around the world. Students who have graduated from baccalaureate, diploma, associate-degree, or other generic RN entry programs in nursing must pass this exam to meet licensing requirements in the United States.

The Test Plan

The National Council of State Boards of Nursing, Inc., prepares the test plan used to develop the licensing exam. The test plan is based on an analysis of current nursing practice and the skills, abilities, and processes nurses use to provide nursing care.

Practice Analysis: The Foundation of the Test Plan

The NCLEX-RN test plan is based on the results of a practice analysis conducted every 3 years of the entry-level performance of newly licensed registered nurses, and on expert judgment provided by members of the National Council's Examination Committee as well as a Job Analysis Panel of Experts (Aucoin and Treas, 2005; Wendt and O'Neill, 2006). The practice analysis asks newly graduated nurses to rank the nursing activities they perform on a regular basis. The questions used on the test plan therefore include those activities that nurses commonly perform. For example, the 2005 RN practice analysis revealed that nursing practice commonly involved assessing and evaluating clients' physical status, treatments, outcomes of interventions, and lab results; administering medication and assessing incompatibilities, side effects, and outcomes; applying principles of infection control; ensuring proper identification of the client; and managing care, including supervising, communication, teaching staff, and discharge planning. Less common activities involved performing microdermabrasion, leading group therapy sessions, and implementing phototherapy (Wendt and O'Neill, 2006). This information is helpful to you in anticipating the content emphasis for the questions that will appear on the NCLEX-RN exam.

Test Item Writers

Writers of the test question for the NCLEX-RN exam include nurse clinicians and nurse educators who are nominated by the Council of State Boards of Nursing. Because the item writers come from a variety of geographical areas and practice settings, the test items reflect nursing practice in all parts of the country.

Test Plan Details

Test plans, or test blueprints, are developed to indicate the components and the relative weights of the components that will be tested on an exam. Because exams test both content (knowledge) and process (critical thinking, synthesis of information, and clinical decision making), test plans usually have two or three dimensions. The test plan for the NCLEX-RN addresses two components of nursing care; the first involves Client Needs categories and the second integrates methods such as the nursing process, caring, communication and documentation, and teaching and learning (Box 1-1). Representative items test knowledge of these components as they relate to specific health care situations in all of the four major areas of Client Needs. The questions developed for the test plan are written to test nursing knowledge and the ability to apply nursing knowledge to client situations.

Client Needs

Health needs of clients are grouped under four broad categories: (1) safe, effective care environment, including management of care and safety and infection control; (2) health promotion and maintenance; (3) psychosocial integrity; and (4) physiologic integrity, including basic care and comfort, pharmacologic and parenteral therapies, reduction of risk potential, and physiologic adaptation. Table 1-1 presents descriptions of each category and

Box 1-1. NCLEX-RN® Test Plan Structure

Client Needs

Safe, effective care environment
1. Management of care
2. Safety and infection control

Health promotion and maintenance
Psychosocial integrity
Physiologic integrity
3. Basic care and comfort
4. Pharmacologic and parenteral therapies
5. Reduction of risk potential
6. Physiologic adaptation

Integrated Concepts and Processes

Nursing process
Caring
Communication and documentation
Teaching/learning

Table 1-1 Categories and Subcategories of Client Needs

A. Safe, Effective Care Environment

1. *Management of Care*—providing integrated, cost-effective care to clients by coordinating, supervising, and/or collaborating with members of the multidisciplinary health care team. Related content includes but is not limited to:
   - Advance Directives
   - Advocacy
   - Case Management
   - Client Rights
   - Collaboration with Multidisciplinary Team
   - Concepts of Management
   - Confidentiality
   - Consultation
   - Continuity of Care
   - Delegation
   - Establishing Priorities
   - Ethical Practice
   - Incident/Irregular Occurrence/Variance Reports
   - Informed Consent
   - Legal Rights and Responsibilities
   - Organ Donation
   - Performance Improvement (Quality Assurance)
   - Referrals
   - Resource Management
   - Staff Education
   - Supervision
2. *Safety and Infection Control*—protecting clients and health care personnel from environmental hazards. Related content includes but is not limited to:
   - Accident Prevention
   - Disaster Planning
   - Emergency Response Plan
   - Error Prevention
   - Handling Hazardous and Infectious Materials
   - Home Safety
   - Injury Prevention
   - Medical and Surgical Asepsis
   - Reporting of Incident/Event/Irregular Occurrence/Variance
   - Safe Use of Equipment
   - Security Plan
   - Standard/Transmission-Based/Other Precautions
   - Use of Restraints/Safety Devices

B. Health Promotion and Maintenance

The nurse provides and directs nursing care of the client and family/significant others that incorporates expected growth and development principles, prevention and early detection of health problems, and strategies to achieve optimal health. Related content includes but is not limited to:

- Aging Process
- Ante/Intra/Postpartum and Newborn Care
- Developmental Stages and Transitions
- Disease Prevention
- Expected Body Image Changes
- Family Planning
- Family Systems
- Growth and Development
- Health and Wellness
- Health Promotion Programs
- Health Screening
- High Risk Behaviors
- Human Sexuality
- Immunizations
- Lifestyle Choices
- Principles of Teaching and Learning
- Self-care
- Techniques of Physical Assessment

C. Psychosocial Integrity

The nurse provides and directs nursing care that promotes and supports the emotional, mental, and social well-being of the client and family/significant others experiencing stressful events, as well as clients with acute and chronic mental illness. Related content includes but is not limited to:

- Abuse/Neglect
- Behavioral Interventions
- Chemical Dependency
- Coping Mechanisms
- Crisis Intervention
- Cultural Diversity
- End of Life
- Family Dynamics
- Grief and Loss
- Mental Health Concepts
- Psychopathology
- Religious and Spiritual Influences on Health
- Sensory/Perceptual Alterations
- Situational Role Changes
- Stress Management
- Support Systems
- Therapeutic Communication
- Therapeutic Environment
- Unexpected Body Image Changes

D. Physiologic Integrity

The nurse promotes physical health and well-being by providing care and comfort, reducing client risk potential, and managing the client's health alterations.

3. *Basic Care and Comfort*—providing comfort and assistance in the performance of activities of daily living. Related content includes but is not limited to:
   - Alternative and Complementary Therapies
   - Assistive Devices
   - Elimination
   - Mobility/Immobility
   - Nonpharmacologic Comfort Interventions
   - Nutrition and Oral Hydration
   - Palliative/Comfort Care
   - Personal Hygiene
   - Rest and Sleep

(Continued)

Table 1-1 Categories and Subcategories of Client Needs (Continued)

4. *Pharmacologic and Parenteral Therapies*—managing and providing care related to the administration of medications and parenteral therapies. Related content includes but is not limited to:
   - Adverse Effects/Contraindications and Side Effects
   - Blood and Blood Products
   - Central Venous Access Devices
   - Dosage Calculations
   - Expected Outcomes/Effects
   - Intravenous Therapy
   - Medication Administration
   - Parenteral Fluids
   - Pharmacologic Agents/Actions
   - Pharmacologic Interactions
   - Pharmacologic Pain Management
   - Total Parenteral Nutrition
5. *Reduction of Risk Potential*—reducing the likelihood that clients will develop complications or health problems related to existing conditions, treatments, or procedures. Related content includes but is not limited to:
   - Diagnostic Tests
   - Laboratory Values
   - Monitoring Conscious Sedation
   - Potential for Alterations in Body Systems
   - Potential for Complications of Diagnostic Tests/Treatments/Procedures
   - Potential for Complications from Surgical Procedures and Health Alterations
   - System Specific Assessments
   - Therapeutic Procedures
   - Vital Signs
6. *Physiologic Adaptation*—managing and providing care for clients with acute, chronic, or life-threatening physical health conditions. Related content includes but is not limited to:
   - Alterations in Body Systems
   - Fluid and Electrolyte Imbalances
   - Hemodynamics
   - Illness Management
   - Infectious Diseases
   - Medical Emergencies
   - Pathophysiology
   - Radiation Therapy
   - Unexpected Response to Therapies

Used by permission of the National Council of State Boards of Nursing, Inc., Chicago. IL.

subcategories of Client Needs. The current percentage of test items in each subcategory on the NCLEX-RN exam is shown in Figure 1-1.

Integrated Processes

The NCLEX-RN test plan is organized according to four integrated processes. These include the nursing process, caring, communication and documentation, and teaching and learning (Box 1-1).

The Nursing Process

The NCLEX-RN test plan includes questions from all five steps of the nursing process, including assessment, analysis, planning, implementation, and evaluation. Each of the five phases is equally important; therefore, each is represented by an equal number of items on the NCLEX-RN and integrated throughout the exam. In this book you will have opportunities to respond to questions using all five steps of the nursing process.

Assessment. Assessment involves establishing a database. The nurse gathers objective and subjective information about the client, then verifies the data and communicates information gained from the assessment.

Analysis. Analysis involves identifying actual or potential health care needs or problems based on assessment data. The nurse interprets the data, collects additional data as indicated, and identifies and communicates the client's nursing diagnoses. The nurse also determines the congruency between the client's needs and the ability of the health care team members to meet those needs.

Planning. Planning involves setting outcomes and goals for meeting the client's needs and designing strategies to attain them. The nurse determines the goals of care, develops and modifies the plan, collaborates with other health team members for delivery of the client's care, and formulates expected outcomes of nursing interventions.

Implementation. Implementation involves initiating and completing actions necessary to accomplish defined goals. The nurse organizes and manages the client's care; performs or assists the client in performing activities of daily living; counsels and teaches the client, significant others, and health care team members; and provides care to attain established client goals. The nurse also provides care to optimize the achievement of the client's health care goals, including supervising, coordinating, and evaluating delivery of the client's care as provided by nursing staff; and recording information on the client's health record and exchanging information with health team members, the client, and the client's family.

Evaluation. Evaluation determines goal achievement. The nurse compares actual outcomes of therapy with expected outcomes, evaluates compliance with prescribed or proscribed therapy, and records and

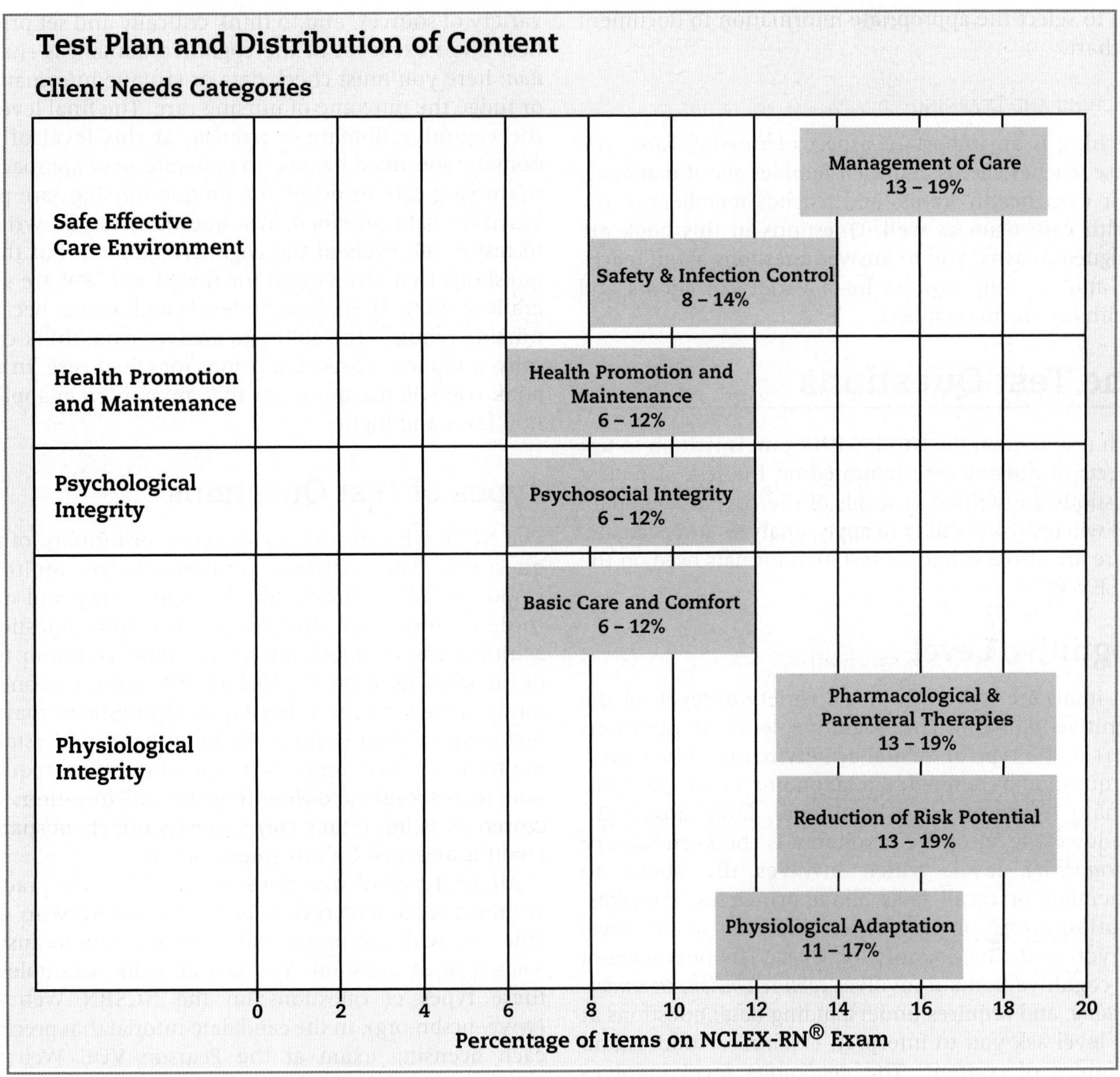

Figure 1-1. Reprinted with permission from the National Council of State Boards of Nursing, Inc., Chicago, IL.

describes the client's response to therapy or care. The nurse also modifies the plan, as indicated, and reorders priorities.

Caring

The caring process refers to the interaction between the nurse, client, and family in a way that conveys mutual respect and trust. The nurse offers encouragement and hope to clients and their families while providing nursing care. Questions about the caring process are threaded throughout the licensing exam to test the candidate's attitudes and values for caring for and about clients. In this book you will have the opportunity to respond to questions that test your ability to apply the caring process in a variety of situations.

Communication and Documentation

Additional elements of the licesning exam include questions that test the nurse's ability to communicate with clients, families, and health team members, and questions about documenting nursing care according to standards of nursing practice. In this book you will be presented with questions that ask you to determine the most effective way to communicate with clients, families, and other health professionals. You will also have the opportunity to respond to questions that require you to select the appropriate information to document or chart.

TEACHING AND LEARNING

Teaching is an important aspect of nursing care. The nurse teaches clients and their families about managing their own health status, and teaches members of the health care team as well. Questions in this book are designed to assist you to answer questions about teaching and learning process for a variety of clients and health care team members.

The Test Questions

Each test item on the NCLEX-RN exam is written to test aspects of nursing care indicated on the test plan. Test questions are written at levels of the cognitive domain that will test your ability to apply, analyze, and evaluate. There are also a variety of test item formats used on the NCLEX-RN.

Cognitive Level

Test items are written to test a variety of levels of the cognitive domain. The cognitive level of questions refers to the type of mental activity required to answer the question as defined in a taxonomy of the cognitive domain (Anderson and Krathwohl, 2001; Box 1-2). The lowest level of the taxonomy is the *knowledge,* or *remembering,* level, which involves the ability to remember or recall facts about principles, concepts, theories, terms, or procedures; questions at this level ask you to define, identify, or select. The next level of the cognitive domain involves *comprehension,* or *understanding,* and requires understanding data; questions at this level ask you to interpret, explain, or understand examples of content. The *application* level involves using information in new situations; questions at this level promote problem-solving and ability to develop or modify nursing care plans, manipulate data, and demonstrate appropriate use of information. *Analysis* requires recognizing and differentiating relationships between parts; questions at this level test your ability to analyze, select, differentiate, or interpret data from a variety of sources, and to think critically and set priorities. The next level of the cognitive domain is *evaluation;* here you must check data or critique information, or judge the outcome of nursing care. The final level of the cognitive domain is *creation;* at this level of the domain you must be able to generate new approaches to nursing care or develop a unique nursing care plan based on data provided. Test questions can be written to test at all levels of the cognitive domain, but those questions that are written for the NCLEX-RN are generally written at application levels and above, because nursing requires the ability to analyze data, think critically, and make clinical decisions for client care. In this book you will use questions that are written at application level and higher.

Box 1-2. Levels of the Cognitive Domain

Knowledge/Remembering: Recognizing, recalling
Comprehension/Understanding: Interpreting, exemplifying, classifying, summarizing, inferring, comparing, explaining
Application: Executing, implementing
Analysis: Differentiating, organizing, attributing
Evaluation: Checking, critiquing
Creation: Generating, planning, producing

Types of Test Questions

The NCLEX-RN exam uses six types, or formats, of test questions. These include multiple-choice, multiple-response, fill-in-the-blank, hot-spot, drag-and-drop (ordered response), and chart and exhibit questions. Multiple-choice questions are the most common type of question used on the NCLEX-RN exam, but one or more of each of the other types of questions may be included. While questions aim to test your understanding of nursing content, each type of question requires you to respond in different ways. All questions are scored as being either correct or incorrect; no partial credit is awarded for any question type.

All six types of questions are available for practice within this content review book and CD-ROM to provide you with the opportunity to learn how to answer each type of question. You can also find examples of these types of questions on the NCSBN Web site (www.ncsbn.org), in the candidate tutorial that precedes each licensing exam at the Pearson VUE Web site (www.pearsonvue.com/nclex), and in the candidates' bulletin that you will receive prior to taking the licensing exam.

Multiple-Choice Questions

Multiple-choice questions include a situation or scenario, a question, and four answers, only one of which is correct. The situation is a client-based scenario presenting information about the client or care management. The question that follows is based on information given in the situation (Fig. 1-2). As you answer the question, relate the answer to background information. Pay particular attention to information about the client's age, family status, health status, ethnicity, or point in the care plan (e.g., early admission versus preparation for discharge).

The question (stem) poses the problem to solve. The question may be written as a direct question, such as "What should the nurse do first?" or as an incomplete sentence such as "The nurse should. . . ."

Sample Single-Response Multiple-Choice Question

26. The charge nurse is making assignments on the acute psychiatric care unit. Which of the following clients should be assigned to an RN?

- ☐ 1. Client with schizophrenia who is experiencing a fever of 103.6°F, blood pressure of 180/100, diaphoresis, and pallor.
- ☐ 2. Client with schizophrenia who has delusions that his food is being poisoned.
- ☐ 3. Client with depression who wants to spend the entire day in his room.
- ☐ 4. Client with mania who has not slept for three nights and spends much of the day pacing in the dayroom.

Figure 1-2.

Sample Hot-Spot Question

AF **48.** The nurse is assessing the anterior fontanelle of a 2 month old. Select the area where the nurse should place the fingers to palpate the anterior fontanelle.

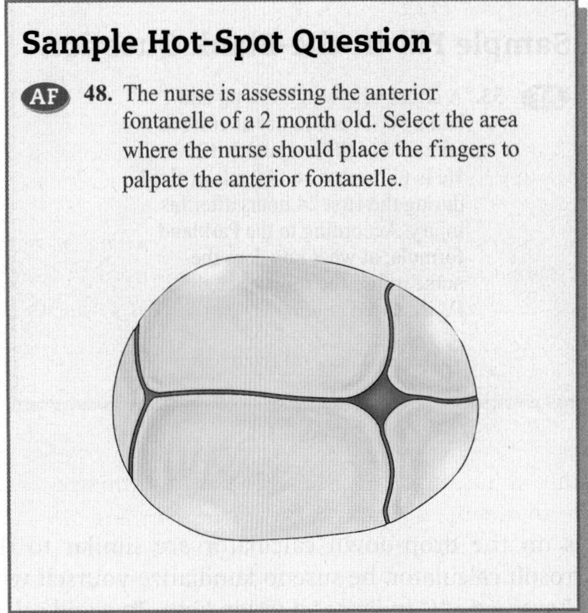

Figure 1-4.

The answers (options) are possible responses to the stem. Each stem has one correct option and three incorrect options. The options may be written as complete sentences or may complete the sentence stated as a question.

Multiple-Response Questions

Multiple-response questions are similar to multiple-choice questions, but may include more than four answers, and more than one answer may be correct. The question asks you to "select all that apply" in order to identify all of the answers that are correct (Fig. 1-3).

Sample Multiple-Response Question

AF **50.** A client is admitted to the hospital with an exacerbation of multiple sclerosis. Which of the following symptoms indicates the client is at risk for impaired gas exchange? Select all that apply.

- ☐ 1. Blurred vision
- ☐ 2. Muscle weakness
- ☐ 3. Slurred speech
- ☐ 4. Loss of sensation
- ☐ 5. Numbness
- ☐ 6. Partial paralysis

Figure 1-3.

Hot-Spot Questions

Hot-spot questions involve identifying the location of a specific item, such as an appropriate injection site, assessment area, or correct part of a waveform. The question is phrased "identify the location," or "select the area." During the computer exam, and on the NCLEX-RN CD-ROM accompanying this book, you will select an answer by moving the cursor over the area until an "x" appears over the site you wish to select for your answer. The answer is selected with a left mouse click; if you make an error, you can move the cursor to the part of the figure that is the answer you wish to enter. Hot-spot questions appear in this book as shown in Figure 1-4. Correct answers determining the specific site in question are located as appropriate within the correct answer and rationale section for that test and are indicated by a red "x."

Fill-in-the-Blank Questions

Fill-in-the-blank questions involve calculations such as determining a drug dose, calculating an IV drip rate, or adding intake-output records. These questions require a numeric answer. When an answer includes a measurement amount such as milliliter, gram, or inches, the measurement unit will be stated in the stem of the question and supplied in the answer box. The question indicates if you are to "round" your answer, and if so, to how many decimal places. An example of fill-in-the-blank questions as they appear in the book can be seen in Figure 1-5. The computer-administered NCLEX-RN exam includes a drop-down calculator to assist you in calculating your answers. Because the mathematical function

Sample Fill-in-the-Blank Question

AF 53. A client who weighs 90 kg and had a 50% burn injury at 1000 is admitted to the hospital at 1200. He is to receive 18,000 mL of fluid during the first 24 hours after his injury. According to the Parkland formula, at what rate does the nurse infuse the fluid when the IV is started at noon?

__________ mL/hour

Figure 1-5.

keys on the drop-down calculator are similar to the Microsoft calculator, be sure to familiarize yourself with the keys (e.g., "/" indicates division key). To avoid calculation errors, it is important that you take your time to enter numbers into the calculator.

Chart and Exhibit Questions

Chart and exhibit questions present data from a chart. The data are presented from one or more chart "tabs," labeled as prescriptions, history and physical, laboratory results, miscellaneous reports, imaging results, flow sheets, intake and output, medication administration record, progress notes, or vital signs. The question asks that you use the data to make a nursing decision. You are to observe and interpret the data, validate if the data are correct or sufficient, and then respond to a question based on the data. When these types of questions are administered by the computer (as in the NCLEX-RN exam), you may be asked to determine which tab to use to locate the information that is required to answer the question. Chart and exhibit questions are presented in this book on a particular tab and followed by a question that asks you to use the data to respond to the question (Fig. 1-6).

Drag-and-Drop Questions

Drag-and-drop questions, or ordered-response questions, require you to place information in a specified order. For example, the question may ask you to put steps of a procedure in order, the question may provide information about several clients and ask you to determine their priorities for nursing care, or the question may ask you to select the order in which to teach a client about a procedure or self-care. For the licensing exam and the CD-ROM accompanying this book, you are asked to drag each response from the answers column and drop it into the correct order on the corresponding column. You can move the items around until you have them in the correct order and submit your final answer

Sample Chart/Exhibit Question

AF 16. A child who is 15 years of age is hospitalized with bacterial meningitis. At 17:30 PM, the client's mother reports her child is "burning up." The nurse is reviewing the client's medication administration records below.

NURSE'S FULL SIGNATURE, STATUS AND INITIALS

	INIT.		INIT.
Linda Roberts, RN	LR		
Rick Jones, RN	RJ		

DIAGNOSIS: Bacterial meningitis

ALLERGIES: None DIET: Regular

ROUTINE/DAILY ORDERS/ FINGERSTICKS/ INSULIN COVERAGE — DATE: 4/21/09

ORDER DATE	MEDICATIONS, DOSE, ROUTE, FREQUENCY	TIME	SITE	INIT.
4/21/09	Aspirin 325mg for temperature over 99°F. every 3 to 4 hours as needed	0910		LR T = 100°F
		1315		LR T = 99.5°F
		1610		RJ T = 101°F

The physician has ordered aspirin 325 mg every 3 to 4 hours for temperature over 99°F. The child's temperature at 5:30 is 102.5°F. The nurse should do which of the following first?

☐ 1. Notify the physician.
☐ 2. Initiate tepid sponge baths.
☐ 3. Institute seizure precautions.
☐ 4. Administer another dose of aspirin.

Figure 1-6.

by clicking the "submit" option. Drag-and-drop practice questions appear in this book as shown in Figure 1-7.

Examination Format

Unlike most paper-and-pencil tests administered in the classroom, or most computer-generated tests that you may have completed in which all test takers receive the same questions, the National Council of State Boards of Nursing uses computer-adaptive testing and administers

Sample Drag-and-Drop/Ordered-Response Question

AF 15. A child is hospitalized with a seizure disorder. The child, who is in a bed with padded side rails, has a tonic-clonic seizure. The nurse should do which of the following in priority order? Place the nursing actions in order of first to last.

___ 1. Loosen clothing around the neck.
___ 2. Turn the child on the side.
___ 3. Clear the area around the child.
___ 4. Suction the airway.

Figure 1-7.

the exam at specified locations with a greater level of security than you may have experienced in the past. This section includes general information to help you prepare for this type of testing format.

Computer-Adaptive Testing

The NCLEX-RN is administered using computer-adaptive testing (CAT) procedures. CAT uses a computer to randomly generate questions from an item pool in order to administer individually tailored exams. CAT has several advantages. For example, an exam can be given in less time because there are potentially fewer questions for each candidate. CAT exams also can be administered frequently, allowing a graduate of a nursing program to take the exam following graduation, receive the results quickly, and enter the work force as a registered nurse in less time than is possible with paper-and-pencil exams. Study results also show that because CAT is self-paced, there is less stress on the candidate. CAT uses the memory and speed of the computer to administer a test for each candidate. The test is generated from a large pool of questions (a test item bank) based on the NCLEX-RN test plan. The test item bank will include all types of questions, but an individual candidate may or may not receive each type of question (multiple-response, fill-in-the-blank), depending on the questions generated from the item bank for each candidate.

The exam begins as the computer randomly selects a question of medium difficulty for each candidate. The next question is based on the response to the previous question. If the question is answered correctly, an item of similar or greater difficulty is generated; if it is answered incorrectly, a less-difficult item is selected. Thus, the test is adapted for each candidate. Once competence has been determined, the exam is completed at a passing level.

The exams for all candidates are derived from the same large pool of test items and contain comparable questions for each component of the test plan. Although the questions are not exactly the same, they test the same knowledge, skills, and abilities from the test plan. All candidates must meet the requirements of the test plan and achieve the same passing score. Each candidate, therefore, has the same opportunity to demonstrate competence. Although one candidate may answer fewer questions, all candidates have the opportunity to answer a sufficient number of questions to demonstrate competence until the stability of passing or failing is established or the time limit expires.

All candidates must answer at least 75 test questions; the maximum number of questions is 265. Each exam also includes 15 "pretest" questions that are being tested for validity and reliability for use on exams to be given to other candidates after review and consideration by the test item writers. You will not be able to differentiate which items are pretest items or the operational items for the exam you are taking.

Six hours are available to each candidate for completing the test. This time includes opportunity to review the online candidate tutorial about the test and to take rest breaks. Although some candidates may finish in a shorter time, others will use the entire 6 hours. The amount of time used during testing is not an indication of passing or failing the exam, but rather, reflects the time required to establish competence for each candidate.

Exam Locations

The Council of State Boards of Nursing contracts with vendors in each state and international location to serve as exam sites. Your school of nursing can inform you of the location nearest you. You can also contact your state board of nursing for information (see Appendix A for addresses). You can also find updated information from the National Council of State Boards of Nursing, Inc., at its Web site: http://www.ncsbn.org.

Scheduling the Examination

The first step is to apply to the state board of nursing in the state or location in which you plan to take the exam. You will then receive the Authorization to Test (ATT). Registration for the exam can be done by mail, telephone, or online, and confirmation of registration will occur within several days, or immediately if done online. At this point, you can schedule an appointment to take the exam. Check for current information at the National Council of State Boards of Nursing Web site and the Web site of your state board of nursing (Appendix A).

Computer Use and Screen Design

Test questions are presented on the computer screen (monitor); you select your answer and use the keyboard or a mouse to enter your answer. The CD-ROM included with this book provides you with an opportunity to simulate taking computer-generated exams. At every testing site, written directions are provided at each computer exam station. There are also tutorials and practice questions on the computer that you can complete to be sure you understand how to use the computer before you begin the exam.

Exam Security

Each testing site maintains a high level of security for the exam and for the candidate. The exam is administered on a secured file server and uses password security and host site authentication. All exam sites use proctors and video/audio monitoring. Candidates are required to show their ATT and specified identification, which may include showing a photo ID, fingerprint testing, and providing a digital signature. Check with your state board of nursing and the National Council of State Boards of Nursing for details about exam security in the jurisdiction in which you are taking the exam.

Special Accommodations

Special accommodations for ADA candidates can be made with authorization from the individual state board of nursing and the National Council of State Boards of Nursing. If approved, the accommodations will be noted on the Authorization to Test and the accommodations made at the testing center. Check with your state board of nursing for additional information.

Results Reporting

Computerized testing allows timely reporting of exam results. The results of the exam are first reviewed at the testing site and then forwarded to the state board of nursing within 8 hours. Results are reported to the candidate within 2 weeks. Some jurisdictions have "quick results" services; for a fee, the candidate can obtain "unofficial" results by Internet or a 900 number telephone call. The exam can be retaken within 45 days. Check with your state board of nursing for details.

When to Take the NCLEX-RN®

Recent research indicates that better results are attained on the licensing exam if the candidate takes the exam within 6 months of graduating (National Council of State Boards of Nursing, 2002). You should, therefore, plan your own schedule to be prepared to take the NCLEX-RN exam as soon after graduation as is possible. Suggestions for developing a study plan are discussed in Chapter 2 of this book.

Additional Information

For further information about the NCLEX-RN, the test plan, test questions, or exam format, visit the Council's Web site at http://www.ncsbn.org, or write to the National Council of State Boards of Nursing, Inc. For information about the dates, requirements, and specifics of writing the exam in your state, contact your state board of nursing. The addresses and telephone numbers of the National Council of State Boards of Nursing, Inc., and each state board of nursing are provided in the Appendix. Information can also be obtained from the vendor who has contracted to provide the testing center for the NLCEX-RN exam. The current vendor is Pearson VUE, and information can be found at their Web site: http://www.pearsonvue/nclex.

How to Use This Book to Prepare for the NCLEX-RN®

Lippincott's Content Review for NCLEX-RN® is organized to provide opportunity for review and practice; this section provides suggestions for using this book for effective and efficient study. The step-by-step approach is designed to build confidence as you complete practice tests, unit tests, and comprehensive review tests.

Organization

This book is organized in three parts. *Part One* provides an introduction to the NCLEX-RN licensing exam and how to study for the exam. *Part Two* presents content review and practice questions for nursing care throughout the lifespan, including care of OB, pediatric, and medical-surgical clients, as well as clients with psychiatric disorders and mental health problems. The final section of part two is unique in that it is devoted to management of care, an area of increasing emphasis in nursing and in competency testing. Each of the five sections includes detailed content review organized to help you study and think in the way you will be tested on the NCLEX-RN exam, with an emphasis on nursing process and the Client Needs framework of the test plan. Each chapter ends with a *chapter* practice test including 20 questions with rationale. Each section ends with a *section* practice test of 30 to 150 test items with rationale covering all of the content in that section. *Part Three* includes three postreview tests, each with 100 questions and rationales presented in random order, to test all of the content you have studied. This book also has a CD-ROM with 1,500 additional questions and 300 questions for use with an iPOD, both of which include rationales to provide you with ample opportunity to experience test-taking using computer-administered questions.

Box 1-3. Codes Referencing Client Needs

Management of care = M
Safety and infection control = S
Health promotion and maintenance = H
Psychological integrity = P
Basic care and comfort = C
Pharmacologic and parenteral therapies = D
Reduction of risk potential = R
Physiologic adaptation = A

Codes Referencing Client Needs

All questions in this book and on the CD-ROM include a content code that refers to the specific client need that is being tested (Box 1-3). A code is presented along with the answer/rationale for each question; using this code will help you diagnose which of the client needs requires additional study and preparation.

Study Tips and Recommendations

Although you will develop your own approach to prepare for the NCLEX-RN exam, the following steps present study tips and recommendations for the sequence to best use this book and the accompanying CD-ROM.

Step 1: Read the Content Outline in Each Chapter

Content outlines serve as quick summaries of important information relating to specific topics or health problems. The content is organized to guide your review according to the NCLEX-RN test plan, beginning with the definition of the topic or health problem and nursing process, and placing special emphasis on client needs. As you read the content outline, pay particular attention to identifying client needs. Underline or highlight content that you do not know, or did not easily recall or understand. Refer to these highlighted areas for further review. If you study best by writing or reorganizing the content, take notes or make concept maps. If you study best by listening, consider making an audiotape of these highlighted areas so you can listen to content that is important for you to review. Do not continue to review content that you already know; focus on content that is new or difficult to learn.

Step 2: Take Each Chapter Practice Test

Each test has 20 questions, organized by health problems. These questions focus only on the content of that chapter and they use all of the test item formats. Each test question has a detailed rationale for each option in the question. Read the rationale carefully to reinforce your understanding and determine what about the distracters is incorrect. Score the test and note which items you have missed based on content (see Learning From Your Test Results).

Step 3: Take Each Section Test

When you have read all of the content outlines in the unit and taken each chapter practice test, take the section practice test. These tests include content from all chapters in that unit. The tests do not have content "headings" and the questions are placed in random order. The questions in these tests are designed to require you to synthesize information, understand growth and development needs of the clients, set priorities, and manage care for groups of clients. These questions also test your understanding of related skills and procedures—you may be asked to perform drug-dose calculation and intravenous fluid infusion-rate calculation. If you miss ANY of these questions, be sure to review the mathematical formulas used to perform the calculation; you MUST be able to answer these questions successfully. Score the test and note which items you have missed based on content (see Learning From Your Test Results).

Step 4: Take Each Postreview Test

After reading all of the chapters and taking all of the chapter and unit tests, then take the postreview tests. These tests contain questions from all five sections. The questions are placed in random order and require you to integrate content across all age groups and health problems. These tests have 100 questions and give you an opportunity to practice answering questions in the same way you will be receiving the questions on the licensing exam. As you take the postreview tests, time yourself. Can you answer 100 questions in 100 to 130 minutes? Can you maintain your concentration for this period of time? Score the test and note which items you have missed based on content (see Learning From Your Test Results).

Step 5: Use the CD-ROM and iPod

Finally, when you have completed your reading and have practiced taking a variety of test questions, use the CD-ROM. The CD-ROM more closely simulates taking computer-administered exams. Be sure to use your computer's calculator as you will encounter a similar calculator on the licensing exam. You can also use the iPod questions for practice on the go.

Learning From Your Test Results

After you complete a test, score the test as noted in the next paragraph. The final step in learning from your results is to reflect on the implications of your test score and take the necessary steps to be fully prepared to take the licensing exam.

Score Your Test

Score the test and note which items you missed. To evaluate your results after completing each test, divide the number of your correct responses by the total number of questions in the test and multiply by 100. If you answered more than 75% of the items correctly, you are most likely prepared to answer questions in that area on the NCLEX-RN. If you answered fewer than 75% of the questions correctly, try to determine why. Did you answer incorrectly because of lack of content knowledge or because you did not read carefully? Use this information to guide your study. If you are studying with a group, discuss the questions and answers. Clarify any points you missed; expand the discussion to related topics or develop additional questions for your group to discuss. As you review your score for these tests, for each question you missed, identify the *content focus* of the question as well as the *process of the question*, for example, setting priorities, making clinical decisions, or managing care. As with the chapter tests, read the teaching rationale and score the test. Discuss with your study group if you are working with a group.

Reflect

The last step is to reflect. What content areas are not clear to you? Where should you set priorities for your study? Do you understand how the questions relate to the National Council of State Boards of Nursing test plan? Do you know how to respond to each of the test question formats? Use your reflections to guide the rest of your preparation for the licensing exam.

Bibliography

Anderson, L.W., & Krathwohl, D. (Eds.). (2001). *A taxonomy for learning, teaching, and assessing: A revision of Bloom's taxonomy of educational objectives*. New York: Longman.

Aucoin, J., & Treas, L. (2005). Assumptions and realities of NCLEX-RN. *Nursing Education Perspectives, 26*(5), 268–271.

National Council of State Boards of Nursing. (2002). The NCLEX delay pass rate study. Retrieved January 5, 2007, from www.ncsbn.org/pdfs/recentNCLEXResearch_web_testing017B02.pdf

Wendt, A., & O'Neill, T. (2006). *Report of findings from the 2005 RN practice analysis: Linking the NCLEX-RN to examination and practice*. Chicago, IL: National Council of State Boards of Nursing.

chapter 2

Preparing to Take the Licensing Examination

Studying for the NCLEX-RN® or other similar nursing exams requires careful planning and preparation. You can make the best use of your time by developing a systematic approach to study. In order to help you develop a study plan, topics in this chapter include:

- Assessing Study Needs
- Developing a Study Plan
- Refining Test-Taking Strategies
- Strategies for Managing Test Anxiety
- Evaluating Progress
- Exam-Taking "Tips"

Assessing Study Needs

The first step toward test success is to determine your strengths and limitations. Even students who have been successful throughout their academic life, and nurses who are excellent caregivers have areas in which they need improvement. Be honest with yourself as you assess your own study needs. Use the Personal Study Plan (Box 2-1) to help develop your own study plan. Use these five steps as you take your first test in nursing school. Refine your test-taking strategies as you evaluate your progress at each step of the way so that when you are ready to take the licensing exam you will be an experienced and successful test-taker.

Review Your Success in Nursing School

Review your record of achievement in courses in the nursing curriculum. Success on the NCLEX-RN tends to correlate with grades (grade point average) achieved in nursing school. Subjects in which you received high grades, that you found easy to learn, or in which you have had additional clinical practice or work experience are likely to be areas of strength. On the other hand, subjects you found difficult to learn or in which you did not achieve high grades should be areas for concentrated review. Also consider content areas that you have not studied for a while. Recent course work will be the most familiar and therefore

Box 2-1. Personal Study Plan

Assess Study Needs

1. Review your success in nursing school.

☐ I did best in these courses:

____

____

☐ I needed to study harder in these courses:

____

____

☐ I took these courses near the beginning of the curriculum:

____

____

☐ I scored best on these practice exams in this book:

____

____

☐ I am not satisfied with my scores on these practice exams in this book:

____

____

☐ I need further study in these content areas:

____

____

☐ I need further study in these areas of the nursing process:

____

____

☐ I need further study in these areas of Client Needs:

____

____

2. Review your test-taking skills.

☐ I can identify the components of a test question.
☐ I read questions carefully before answering.
☐ I can make reasonable guesses if I am not certain of the correct answer.

3. Review your test-anxiety management skills.

☐ I can do relaxation and deep-breathing exercises.
☐ I can visualize success.
☐ I can give myself positive feedback.
☐ I can concentrate for extended periods of time.

4. Review your computer skills.

☐ I am able to use a computer to read and answer test questions.
☐ I have used the CD-ROM accompanying this book.

Develop a Study Plan

☐ I will study in this location:

____

____

☐ I will study at these times and dates:

____

____

☐ I have assembled all of the materials I need to study:

____

____

☐ I will study with this study group:

____

____

Evaluate Progress

☐ I have completed the practice tests in this book.
☐ I have completed the comprehensive tests in this book.
☐ I need to improve my scores in these areas:

____

____

☐ I am prepared to take the NCLEX-RN examination.

Strategies for Taking Tests

- Read the question carefully.
- Anticipate the correct answer.
- Read for key words.
- Base answers on nursing knowledge.
- Identify the components of the test item.

Strategies for Managing Test Anxiety

- Mental rehearsal
- Relaxation
- Deep breathing
- Positive self-talk
- Distraction
- Concentration

may require the least amount of study. All students, even students who have achieved success in nursing courses, benefit from identifying areas requiring study and spending time practicing test-taking skills. You also can use the practice tests in this book to identify areas needing further study. Begin with the subjects you find most difficult or in which you have the least confidence.

Assess Your Test-Taking Skills

Using effective test-taking skills contributes to exam success. What have you done in the past to make you confident about taking a test? How do you feel when you are in the exam situation? What has worked in the past to help you be successful? Review these strategies to build on past successes and work on problem areas. Consider additional strategies suggested in the following section, Refining Test-Taking Strategies. You can practice these skills by simulating the testing situation using the practice tests and comprehensive exams in this review book.

Understand the Levels of the Cognitive Domain and Question Formats

Effective test-taking involves application, analysis, and evaluation. Test questions used on the licensing exam are written at higher levels of the cognitive domain. Many candidates' experiences with taking tests have come from taking "teacher-made" tests—tests developed by the faculty at your school of nursing. Often these tests are written to test students' knowledge and understanding of course content and do not include questions that require application, analysis, or evaluation of course material. Additionally, several of the newer "alternative format" types of questions used on the NCLEX-RN exam have only been added within the past few years, and nursing faculty may not yet be designing their own test questions to use these formats.

Finally, some students are able to "second-guess" the teacher and use this ability to their advantage when taking teacher-made classroom tests. However, it is not as easy to anticipate test questions on standardized and licensing exams, and you will need to develop skills that help you think critically when presented with an unfamiliar situation. As you prepare to take the licensing exam, spend time on questions for which you need to "figure out" the best approach to answering the question. Use the questions in this book and CD-ROM to be sure you understand the difference in questions that require only recall and understanding and those that require you to apply information to client care, make clinical judgments, and initiate nursing actions.

Estimate the Time You Need to Complete the Test

Are you always the last one to finish a test? Do you request additional time to complete a test? If so, you will want to practice taking timed tests and doing your best, while completing as many questions as possible. The licensing exam is designed to be completed in 6 hours, and your score will depend on the number of answers to test questions submitted within that time period. As you use the practice questions and tests in this book and CD-ROM, time yourself and, if needed, determine ways that you can increase your speed without sacrificing accuracy.

Assess Your Skills for Taking Computer-Administered Exams

Although previous computer experience is not necessary to take the NCLEX-RN, you should familiarize yourself with the differences between taking a paper-and-pencil exam and taking exams administered by the computer, and practice taking computer-administered test questions. The CD-ROM accompanying this content review book will help simulate the experience of taking questions using a computer. Practice reading questions from the computer screen. If you are accustomed to underlining key words or making notes in the margins of paper-and-pencil tests, adapt these strategies to reading and answering the questions on the computer screen. Also, be sure that you can use a drop-down calculator to answer questions requiring the use of math skills. If you have not used a computer before, find a learning resource center at your college, university, library, or hospital where you can become familiar with basic computer keyboard skills.

Assess Your English Language Skills

Persons for whom English is a second language or who do not have well-developed reading and comprehension skills may require additional practice in reading and answering NCLEX-RN style test questions. If you are one of these persons, be sure to plan for additional time in practicing reading and answering questions, timing yourself when answering the questions, and validating that you understand the question correctly. If necessary, seek assistance.

Developing a Study Plan

Once you have identified areas of strength and areas needing further study, develop a specific plan and begin to study regularly (see Box 2-1). Students who study a small amount of content over a longer period of time tend to have higher success rates than students who wait until the last few weeks before the exam and then "cram." Consider the following suggestions.

Identify a Place for Study

The area you select for study should be quiet and include space for your books and papers. This area might be in your home, at your nursing school, at your workplace, or in a library. Be sure your friends and family understand the importance of not interrupting you when you are studying.

Obtain All Necessary Resources

As you begin to study, it is helpful to have easy access to textbooks, notes, and study guides. It is helpful to consider the sources presented in the bibliography included at the end of each chapter within this book.

Establish Regular Study Times

Make appointments with yourself to ensure a commitment to study. Frequent, short study periods (1 or 2 hours) are preferable to sporadic, extended study periods. Plan to finish your studying 1 week before the NCLEX-RN; last-minute cramming tends to increase anxiety.

Make the Best Use of Your Time

Make review cards that you can carry with you to study during free moments throughout the day. Some students tape record review notes and listen to the tapes or Podcasts while driving or exercising.

Reduce or Eliminate Stressful Situations

Students who are living in stressful situations such as working, managing a family, taking courses, planning a wedding, or caring for elderly parents may find it difficult to find time to study, and to concentrate when studying. Managing a variety of stressful situations puts students at risk factor for passing exams. Although easier to say than to do, if possible, reduce the number of stressful situations you are involved in during the time you are preparing to take the NCLEX-RN exam.

Practice Effective Study Skills

Study skills enable you to acquire, organize, remember, and use the information you need to take the NCLEX-RN. These skills include outlining, summarizing, applying, synthesizing, reviewing, and practicing test-taking. Use these study skills each time you prepare for an exam. The following are some student-tested study skills:

Use Familiar Study Skills

Use study skills with which you are familiar and that have worked well for you in the past. Recall effective study behaviors that you used in nursing school, such as reviewing highlighted text, outlines, or content maps.

Study to Learn, Not to Memorize

The NCLEX-RN tests application and analysis of knowledge. When reviewing content, continually ask yourself, "How is this information used in client care?" "What clinical decision-making will be required of this information?" "What is the role of the nurse in using this information?" Being able to use information, rather than just being able to list or recognize information, is one of the most important of your study skills.

Identify Learning Style and Study Preferences

Each student has a preferred way of learning. For example, some students prefer learning material by listening; they are considered *auditory* learners. If this describes your preference you will benefit from taping your notes or, if possible, taping class lectures. Some students learn best in a visual mode, and learn by reading, reviewing PowerPoint slides, or looking at illustrations. For *visual* learners, reading and looking at images is helpful. Some learners benefit from making concept maps or drawing relationships of concepts as a way to focus their learning. *Kinesthetic* learners, those who like to touch and manipulate to learn, benefit from working with models and manikins to reinforce their learning. Although you likely have one learning style and study preference, using a variety of styles will enhance the study experience.

Form a Study Group

Some students prefer to study alone, while others benefit from study groups. Know which approach works best for you and develop your study plan accordingly. If you do form or participate in a study group, limit the group to four to six members. Develop norms for working together and focus on understanding and applying nursing content, rather than memorizing facts. Enforce that every member comes prepared to contribute.

Anticipate Questions

As you study, formulate questions around the content. Practice giving a rationale for your answer to these questions. If you work in a study group, have each member contribute questions that the entire group answers.

Study Common Nursing Care Situations

Study common, not unique, nursing care situations. The NCLEX-RN tests minimum competence for nursing practice; therefore, focus on common health problems and client needs. Review the *RN Practice Analysis* published by the National Council of State Boards of Nursing and the current Licensing Exam Test Plan to determine common nursing care activities.

Simulate Test-Taking

The comprehensive postreview tests in section three of this book are designed to simulate the random order in which questions appear in the NCLEX-RN. Use these tests to focus on areas of common concern in nursing care rather than on the traditional content delineation of adult, pediatric, psychiatric, and childbearing clients. Make additional copies of answer sheets and retake the exams on which you had low scores.

Refining Test-Taking Strategies

Knowing how to take a test is as important as knowing the content being tested. Strategies for taking tests can be learned and used to improve test scores. The following are some suggestions for building a repertoire of effective test-taking strategies.

Understand the Question

Understand the type of test question and the components of the test item. See Chapter 1 for examples of the test question formats used in the NCLEX-RN. Refer to Box 2-2 for keys to answering NCLEX-RN test questions.

Understand Which Integrated Process Is Being Used

Integrated process refers to steps of the nursing process: caring, communication, documentation, teaching, and learning. For example, as you read the question, determine whether the question is asking you to set priorities (planning) or judge outcomes (evaluation).

Understand Client Needs

As you read the question, consider the question in the context of Client Needs (see Box 1-3). Be sure to understand if the question is asking you to determine what to do "first" or to select the nursing action that is "best."

Understand Client Age

Understand the age of the client noted in the test question. If the age of the client is specified, consider what information about that age group is important to answering the question. If the age of the client is not specified, assume that the age of the client is not a factor in answering the question.

Read Questions Carefully

This is one of the most important aspects of effective test-taking. Do not rush. Ask yourself, "What is this question asking?" and "What is the expected response?" If necessary, rephrase the question in your own words. Do not read meaning into a question that is not intended, and do not make a question more difficult than it is. If you do not understand the question, try to figure it out. If, for example, the question is asking about the fluid balance needs of a client with pheochromocytoma and you do not remember what pheochromocytoma is, then try to answer the question based on your knowledge of principles of fluid balance. The exam questions reflect national nursing practice standards and are not written to test knowledge of procedures or practices at specific health care agencies. Thus, it is important to answer the question from the framework of best nursing practice, not unique practices.

Determine What the Question Is Asking

Determine if the question is asking you to set priorities or place steps of a procedure in a particular order. Read the stem of the question carefully and be clear about the priority (first, last) or order (first, last) in which you are to answer the question. Questions that ask you to set priorities or use a procedure are written to assume that you have all of the resources necessary, including an order from the health care provider, to make the decision. While in "real life" you may be able to delegate, do several tasks at once, or have others working with you, when answering the test question you can base your response only to the situation using the options provided in the question! Do not try to imagine other situations; base your answer on the concept that is being tested and the answers from which you can choose.

Look for Key Words

Look for key words that provide clues to the correct answer. For instance, words such as *except, not,* or *but* can change the meaning of a question; words such as *first, next,* and *most* ask you to establish a priority or use an order or sequence of steps. When the question indicates "select all that apply," be sure you are considering each option as having the possibility of being correct. Be certain you understand the meaning of all words in the question. If you see a word you do not know, try to determine its meaning from a familiar base of the word or from the context of the question.

Use Nursing Knowledge

Base answers on nursing knowledge. Remember that the NCLEX-RN is used to test for safe practice and that you have learned the information needed to answer the question.

Box 2-2. Keys to Answering NCLEX-RN® Test Questions

Questions About Communication

A. Communications with the client
- Focus on Client Needs
- Establish trust
- Ask questions to clarify needs
- Use open-ended questions
- Do not offer an opinion
- Do not ask the client to respond to a "why"
- Use active listening
- Provide honest information
- Include family

B. Communications with other nurses
- Maintain collegiality
- Maintain lines of communication
- Follow organization structure
- Report important information about the client: shift report, transfer report, medication reconciliation, and client safety protocols
- Consider ethics of reporting or not reporting nurse's behavior or actions
- Observe a culture of client safety

C. Communications with the health care provider (HCP)
- Notify HCP of change in client status
- Contact HCP to write order for client; use S-BAR to explain the **S**ituation, provide **B**ackground information, report **A**ssessments, and **R**ecommend the next steps such as ordering a medication, clarifying an order
- Do not notify if action is within scope of nursing practice
- Do not notify if standing orders are available to guide decisions

Questions About Steps of a Procedure
- Know when it is appropriate to use or not use a procedure
- Know the sequence of steps of the procedure being used
- Know the nurses' role in the procedure (prepare the client vs. perform the procedure)

Questions Requiring Use of Math Skills
- Know how to use a formula to calculate drug dosages
- Know how to use a formula to calculate intravenous infusion drip rates
- Know how to calculate intake and output
- Understand implications of the calculations; make decisions as needed

Questions About Clinical Judgment
- Be able to interpret laboratory results and understand nursing implications
- Be able to gather, assess, and analyze data and make a decision about the appropriate nursing care
- Determine when the status of a client has changed and what to do next
- Be able to explain tests, procedures, self-care to client and family
- Provide age-appropriate nursing care

Questions About Management of Care and Setting Priorities

A. For individuals
- Set priorities based on airway, breathing, circulation, damage
- Set priorities using Maslow's hierarchy of need
- Set priorities based on time frame of the problem, for example, immediately after surgery, during stage 2 of labor, 3 weeks after being on a medication

B. For groups of clients
- Set priority based on client who is least stable
- Set priority based on client who requires care based on individual priorities as noted above
- Set priority based on time frame of when client needs care; for example, giving a timed medication versus a client who is being discharged later in the day
- Set priority based on the client about whom the nurse has the least information
- Set priority based on the client who is at greatest risk
- Set priority based on the client who has the least predictable outcomes

C. Delegate care to appropriate persons
- Priority goals are accomplished by delegating to others
- Priority goals are accomplished by having client or family assume responsibility
- Follow up after delegation

Questions About Client Teaching
- Assess client and family needs prior to developing a teaching plan
- Use appropriate methods of instruction for the client
- Adapt instruction for client's age and health status
- Evaluate outcome of teaching

Questions About Client Safety and Risk Management
- Follow safety standards set by national organizations and the clinical agency
- Identify clients at risk for falls, pressure ulcers, infection, and other high-risk situations, and take measures to prevent risk
- Establish culture of safety
- Prevent and report errors according to agency policy and procedure

Anticipate Answers

Attempt to answer the question yourself before looking at the answers that are provided, then look for the answer(s) that is/are similar to the one(s) you generated. If you do not know the answer, make a reasonable guess. Hunches and intuition are often correct. If you do not know the answer, do not waste time and energy; move on to the next question. In CAT, you must answer each question before the next item is administered, and because the level of difficulty will be adjusted as you answer each question, it is likely that you will know the answer to one of the next questions.

Strategies for Managing Test Anxiety

All test-takers experience some anxiety. A certain amount of anxiety is motivating, but be prepared to control unwanted anxiety. Anxiety can be managed by both physical and mental activities. Practice, choose, and then use any of the following anxiety-management strategies. Practice those strategies while you are taking the comprehensive exams in this book and use them with *each* exam you take in school or elsewhere. Practicing managing test anxiety when taking "low stakes" tests such as classroom tests will make managing test anxiety that much easier when you are taking the "high stakes" tests such as course or program final exams and, of course, the licensing exam.

Mental Rehearsal

Mental rehearsal involves reviewing the events and environment during the exam. Anticipate how you will feel, what the setting will be like, how you will take the exam, what the computer screen will look like, and how you will talk to yourself during the exam. Visualize your success. Rehearse what you will do if you have test anxiety.

Relaxation Exercises

Relaxation exercises involve tensing and relaxing various muscle groups to relieve the physical effects of anxiety. Practice systematically contracting and relaxing muscle groups from your toes to your neck to release energy for concentration. You can do these exercises during the exam to promote relaxation. Smile! Smiling relaxes tense facial muscles and reminds you to maintain a positive attitude.

Deep Breathing

Take deep breaths by inhaling slowly while counting to 5, and then exhale slowly while counting to 10 to increase oxygen flow to the lungs and brain. Deep breathing also decreases tension and helps manage anxiety by focusing your thoughts on the breathing and away from worries.

Positive Self-Talk

Talking to yourself in a positive way serves to correct negative thoughts (e.g., "I can't pass this test" and "I don't know the answers to any of these questions") and reinforces a positive self-concept. Replace negative thoughts with positive ones, telling yourself, "I can do this" and "I studied well and am prepared," or "I can figure this out."

Distraction

Thinking about something else can clear your mind of negative or unwanted thoughts. Think of something fun, something you enjoy. Plan now what you will think about to distract yourself during the exam.

Concentration

During the exam, be prepared to concentrate. Have tunnel vision. Do not worry if others finish the test before you. Remember that everyone has his or her own speed for taking tests and that each test is individualized. Do not rush; you will have plenty of time. Focus, and do not let noises from the keyboard next to you divert your attention. Do not become overwhelmed by the testing environment. Use positive self-talk as you begin the exam. Some students become bored during the exam, and then become careless as they answer questions toward the end of the exam. Practice taking tests of at least 265 questions and discover how long you can focus your attention on the test questions. Practice taking breaks if you begin to loose your concentration.

Evaluating Progress

The last step of your study plan is to check your progress. Note if your scores on the practice and comprehensive tests improve. Do not spend time on content you have mastered, on areas in which you obtained high scores on the practice exam, or on areas with which you feel confident. Use the results of your evaluation to set priorities for study on areas needing additional review. As previously noted, evaluate your study skills, your test-taking abilities, and the use of test anxiety-management strategies as you take *each* test throughout your academic program. Doing so now will prepare you to test for success.

Exam-Taking "Tips"

Schedule to take the exam when YOU are ready, but as soon after graduation as is feasible. Candidates who take the exam before they are prepared are not as successful. You are in control of when you take the exam. Students who have successfully passed the NCLEX-RN offer these additional tips for preparing for and taking the exam.

Physical Preparation

In addition to studying for several months before the exam, make sure you are physically prepared. Get enough rest before the exam; fatigue can impair concentration. Eat regular meals before the exam. Remember that high-carbohydrate foods provide energy, but excessive sugar and caffeine can cause hyperactivity. Do not use any drugs you usually do not use (including caffeine and nicotine) and do not consume alcohol for 2 days before the exam. Dress comfortably, in layers that can be added or removed according to your comfort level. If you are working, it may be advisable not to work the day before the exam; if you are working on a shift that is different from the time of the exam, adjust your work schedule several days ahead of time. Avoid planning time-consuming activities (e.g., weddings, vacation trips) immediately before the exam. Also, make sure you know the date, time, and place the exam will be given; how to get to the exam site; how long it takes to drive there; and where you can park. It may be helpful to visit the exam site and see the room where the exam will be given. Organize the information you will need to bring to the testing center the night before the exam. You will need to present your Authorization to Test (ATT). You will also need to provide required identification.

Practice Tests

Practice taking randomly generated test questions. Most students are accustomed to taking teacher-made exams that cover several topics in the same content area. When taking the NCLEX-RN exam, however, each question comes from a different topic or content area and you will need to be prepared to shift your focus to a different practice area for each question. Use practice questions until you can score at least 75% on the exam. Use at least 2,000 practice questions so you test yourself with a wide range of content and types of questions.

Time Management

Use a timer to determine how many questions you can answer in a specified amount of time. Use the timer to be sure you are keeping a steady pace, but not rushing through the test. Visualize yourself in the room, taking the test. Use mental rehearsal to practice anxiety-managing strategies.

PART TWO

Content Review and Practice Questions

SECTION 1

Nursing Care of the Childbearing Family and Neonate

chapter 3

Introduction to Nursing Care of the Childbearing Family and Neonate

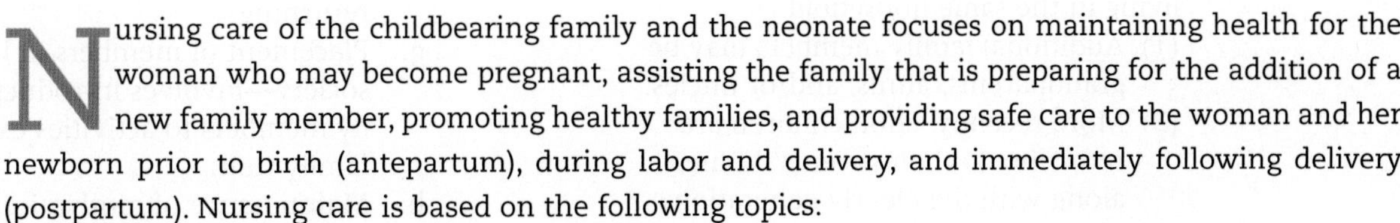

Nursing care of the childbearing family and the neonate focuses on maintaining health for the woman who may become pregnant, assisting the family that is preparing for the addition of a new family member, promoting healthy families, and providing safe care to the woman and her newborn prior to birth (antepartum), during labor and delivery, and immediately following delivery (postpartum). Nursing care is based on the following topics:

- Background Information: Growth and Development
- Health Assessment
- Health Promotion
- Principles of Nursing Care Management

Background Information: Growth and Development

I. Definition: The topic of growth and development concerns the woman prior to conception and the childbearing family.

A. Growth and development of the woman prior to conception: See Chapter 19 for general information about adult growth and development.

B. Family growth and development: Family can be described narrowly as individuals who live together or, more broadly, as a group of people who share bonds, emotions, and societal tasks. The family strongly influences the perception of health, practices of health promotion, and treatment of illness. Childbearing profoundly influences all aspects of family. Nurses provide care to families at all stages of the life cycle in every setting in which health care is needed. There are several types of family compositions to consider, as well as tasks and life cycles within each type of family:

1. Composition
   a. Dyad family—includes two individuals sharing a living area.
      (1) Couple may be early or late in the life cycle (see later description).
      (2) Couple may be together based on love, desire for companionship, or financial need.
   b. Nuclear family—includes a man, woman, and children in a shared living area.
      (1) Structure currently includes about 50% of all families, a decline in the last 50 years.
      (2) Bonding and cohesion between members of the family and a strong family unit serve as the foundation for a healthy society.
   c. Extended family—includes the nuclear family with additional family members living in the same household.
      (1) Additional family members may be grandparents, aunts, and/or uncles.
      (2) More recently, adult children are returning to their parents' home, along with the elderly generation.
   d. Single-parent family—includes one adult member with children.
      (1) This group is most frequently seen as a result of current divorce rates, and women bearing and raising children without an adult partner.
      (2) Common problems within this structure include poverty and lack of support when conflicts arise.
   e. Communal family—includes a group of individuals living together based on values shared by the members; this family unit is similar to "communes" prominent in the 1960s.
   f. Gay or lesbian families—includes adults of the same gender living together based on factors such as sexual orientation, companionship, love, or financial security.
   g. Foster or adoptive families—includes adults living together who bring children other than their own into their home to raise for a short time or until adulthood.
   h. Blended family—includes adults with children from previous marriages who are living together with some or all of the children from the previous marriages.
2. Tasks
   a. Physical maintenance—involves resources such as food, clothing, and shelter provided by the adult members of the family.
   b. Socialization of members—involves preparing children to be members of a larger culture and society.
   c. Distribution of resources—involves allocation of resources accrued by family to members.
   d. Order—promotes communication that leads to stable relationships among members, and common rules with respect and adherence to established guidelines.
   e. Division of labor—promotes responsibilities for each member of the household.
   f. Maintenance of family—promotes intactness of family unit in spite of changes such as birth, death, and various members leaving and/or returning.
   g. Placement of members in larger society—involves introduction of family members to activities external to the family unit.
   h. Maintenance of motivation and morale—involves maintaining family pride.
3. Life cycle
   a. Marriage—establishment of relationship between two individuals who are learning how to relate to and work with one another and their families.
   b. Early childbearing—time period during which there is an integration of new

members into the family; focus is on learning the physical and emotional skills of parenting.

c. Preschool children—a physically demanding period of life involving development of emotional stability, maintaining safety, and fostering growth of children.

d. School-aged children—time period involving tremendous responsibilities in physical care and emotional nurturing of children while maintaining and further developing adult relationships. With both adults working in many families, this is an intense, busy period.

e. Adolescence—time period accompanied by new activities involving risks not experienced prior to this time (e.g., sexual freedom, violence); children begin to move in their own directions, want more freedom, and often experience a strain in relationships with parents.

f. Launching children—time period when children begin leaving home and establishing their own households; indicates goal achievement: a family with members who have grown to become independent adult members of society.

g. Middle years—family returns to consist of two adults.

h. Retirement or older age—family of older individuals who may be parenting, experiencing physical and cognitive decline, or chronic illness; this family provides support and advises activities for younger members new to parenting.

Health Assessment

I. Definition: The health of the woman and the family dynamics change during pregnancy, and the nurse must assess these changes in order to develop a care plan with the client and family.

II. Nursing process

A. Assessment

1. Assess the woman prior to pregnancy (see health assessment skills of the adult client in Chapter 19 for general information about adult growth and development; also note the following information about health assessment and promotion).
2. Assess family structure, development, and function of unit as a whole, as well as individual members; assess for states of health/illness as a unit and as part of cultural or religious group and as members of society.

B. Analysis

1. Risk for Injury related to deficient knowledge of problem
2. Interrupted Family Processes related to inability to access health care, lack of financial resources for health care, and inability to physically or psychosocially care for other members of family
3. Ineffective Health Maintenance related to lack of knowledge of health care needs, inability to access health care system, and conflict with religious, family, or personal values
4. Impaired Parenting related to lack of knowledge of needs, lack of knowledge of development of family members, and lack of financial resources or access to care

C. Planning

1. Assess family and individual members.
2. Develop plan of care based on needs considered from nursing and family perspectives.
3. Evaluate plan of care.

D. Implementation

1. Assist family to adapt to pregnancy as needed.
2. Refer client and/or family to health care resources as needed.
3. Assure client is receiving adequate prenatal care.

E. Evaluation

1. Family continues to develop despite illness or dysfunction.
2. Family understands health problems. among members and how to care for them.
3. Family understands where to find health care assistance, knows how to seek professional services, and has resources to access care.
4. Family alters individual behaviors, leading to healthy outcomes for members.
5. Family is satisfied with state of health of individual members.

Health Promotion

I. Definition: Health promotion for a pregnant woman involves assisting the client to maintain a healthy lifestyle prior to pregnancy, make choices about family planning, and adapt to changes brought about by the pregnancy.

A. Preconception care is the act of developing and maintaining optimal health styles and habits prior to time of conception. This act includes:

1. Identify medical conditions client has or is at risk for; treat as needed to provide optimal environment for future pregnancy.
   a. Interview to determine over-the-counter medications, prescription medications, and recreational drugs being used, status of medical conditions.
   b. Obtain reproductive history and diseases (sexually transmitted infections [STIs], abnormal pap smears), family history, genetic concerns (thalassemia, sickle cell, etc.), and contraceptive history.
2. Develop healthy habits including rest, stress reduction, and a positive work environment; eliminate habits that diminish opportunities for healthy pregnancy outcome such as smoking, drugs, and alcohol; keep immunizations up to date, develop a nutrition plan, and assure adequate exercise.
3. Identify potential perinatal health care providers (HCPs) who support client's ways of thinking concerning childbearing.
4. Prepare client psychologically for changes in family composition and responsibilities.
5. Initiate genetic testing or counseling if medically indicated.

B. Contraception is a procedure or medication to prevent conception of a child. The following are characteristics of the ideal contraceptive: affordable; easily obtained, reversed, and used; acceptable and safe for both participants; and effective. Categories of contraceptives include:

1. Natural family planning—requires no chemical or physical barriers to prevent pregnancy.
2. Basal body temperature method—abstinence from intercourse 4 days before ovulation to 3 to 4 days after ovulation.
3. Symptothermal—basal body temperatures with observation of changes in cervical mucus that signal ovulation.
4. Calendar method—abstaining from intercourse during ovulation, using a calendar to predict the appropriate time based on prior cycles.
5. Abstinence—refraining from sexual activity.
6. Withdrawal—removal of penis from vagina prior to ejaculation.
7. Mechanical contraceptives
   a. Male condom: Sheath placed over penis after erection is achieved to collect ejaculate, and removed before erection is lost; also assists in preventing STIs.
   b. Female condom: Latex sheath placed inside vagina to collect sperm. A flexible ring is at each end of the condom, one placed high in the vagina (closed) and the other remaining outside the vagina (open). Also acts as physical barrier to reduce STIs.
   c. Diaphragm: Nondisposable rubber cap fitted to cover cervix. Used with spermicide and left in place 6 hr after intercourse. Requires prescription and fitting by HCP.
8. Chemical barriers/spermicides—physical and chemical barrier to sperm.
9. Intrauterine device (IUD)—device placed inside uterus, preventing pregnancy by altering cervical mucus and sperm and preventing implantation. IUDs may be implanted with progesterone or copper to enhance safety rates.
10. Hormonal contraceptives
    a. Depo-Provera: 150 mg of synthetic progesterone given IM once every 3 months to suppress ovulation. Return of fertility may be delayed with this method; bleeding is often irregular after the first injection and is suppressed after the second injection.
    b. Patch: Estrogen and progesterone implanted in a patch placed on skin and changed each week. Effects, side effects, and cautions similar to those of oral contraceptives.
    c. Oral contraceptives ("The Pill"): Composed of progesterone ("minipill") or estrogen and progesterone as a pill taken on a daily basis.
    d. Emergency contraception: Postcoital oral contraceptive taken as soon after unprotected intercourse as possible. Composed of estrogen and progesterone.
    e. Vaginal ring: Estrogen and progesterone in a ring placed in vagina for 3 weeks.
11. Sterilization
    a. Vas deferens is severed or banded to prevent passage of sperm
    b. Bilateral tubal ligation: Interruption of fallopian tubes to block movement of fertilized ovum to the uterus
    c. Hysterectomy: Surgical removal of uterus, eliminating implantation of fertilized ovum
    d. Oophorectomy: Surgical removal of ovaries to prevent production of ovum

12. Abortion
    a. First trimester: Abortion is safest and easiest during this time.
        (1) Dilation and suction (D and S)
        (2) Dilation and curettage (D and C)
        (3) Vacuum curettage
        (4) Mifepristone (Mifeprex): Used during first 7 weeks of pregnancy to alter endometrium; followed by misoprostol PO to contract uterus
    b. Second trimester: Dilation and evacuation with use of hypertonic saline or prostaglandins by various routes.

II. Nursing process

A. Assessment
1. Obtain a complete health history to determine safety for client (hypertension, diabetes, infection, thrombophlebitis); perform a comprehensive physical examination, as needed for method.
2. Assess birth control needs and prior contraceptive use—assess factors that may affect decision, including cost; cultural preferences; physical limitations, needs, and contraindications; and comfort and commitment of couple with method.

B. Analysis
1. Deficient Knowledge of Birth Control Options related to lack of exposure to method, no prior need for method, and desire to change methods.
2. Interrupted Family Processes related to differing opinions concerning birth control.

C. Planning
1. Provide individual or client education.
2. Demonstrate use of method as needed and appropriate.
3. Discuss availability of HCP to respond to client concerns.

D. Implementation
1. Analyze client health history to determine contraindications for a particular method.
2. Provide client education concerning normal menstrual cycle and how contraceptive prevents conception.
3. Provide client or couple education concerning available contraceptive methods including cost, side effects, and how to use; as well as a contraceptive back-up plan.
4. Fit diaphragm and request return demonstration.
5. Discuss proper timing of IUD insertion.
6. Instruct client on potential complications of contraceptive method.

E. Evaluation
1. Client states understanding of effects and side effects of contraceptive method and how to correctly use method.
2. Client states understanding of need for consistent use of method.
3. Client verbalizes advantages and disadvantages of method of choice.

CN

III. Client needs

A. Physiologic adaptation: Methods to prevent pregnancy include the following:
1. Hormonal contraceptives (Depo-Provera, estrogen patch, oral contraceptives, and vaginal ring)—Prevent release of luteinizing hormone and follicle-stimulating hormone, which cause ovulation; alters mucus in cervix, uterus, and fallopian tubes.
    a. If used postpartum and during breastfeeding, wait 4 to 6 weeks for lactation to be established before beginning use.
    b. Side effects include vaginal bleeding between periods and weight gain.
2. IUDs—Alter transportation and implantation of fertilized ovum, and change cervical mucus.
3. Sterilization—Prevents transportation of sperm and ovum but does not alter production unless ovaries are removed.

B. Management of care: Care of the childbearing family and neonate requires critical thinking skills and knowledge of assessment, and teaching and evaluation methods unique to the RN role. These skills cannot be delegated to an LPN or UAP.
1. Educate client concerning normal menstrual cycle and how contraceptives prevent conception.
2. Assess client needs, health history, comfort level, financial and insurance status, and religious beliefs to determine methods appropriate for client.
3. Provide information concerning motivation and proper use of methods.
4. Consider client and partner developmental level and culture to provide clues to needs of couple.
5. Follow up with client to reduce pregnancy risk by determining satisfaction and compliance.

C. Safety and infection control
1. Instruct client about need to remain free of STIs with IUD use.
2. Instruct client on potential complications of selected method.

3. Instruct client how to "catch up" when oral contraceptives have been missed; discuss use of "back-up" methods.
4. Review plan of care to determine if care is consistent with best practices of the profession and if it provides optimal outcomes for client based on the situation.

D. Health promotion and maintenance: Provide client education regarding access to information about family planning and assistance.

E. Psychologic integrity
1. Analyze impact of culture and religion on family planning decisions, and provide care accordingly.
2. Analyze verbal and nonverbal messages between partners concerning birth control methods, and plan care accordingly.

F. Basic care and comfort: Prevent side effects from contraceptives for client or partner, including rash, irritation, allergy, and blood-clotting problems.

G. Reduction of risk potential
1. Review client health history to determine contraindications for a particular method.
   a. Hormonal contraceptives
      (1) Relative contraindications: diabetes, migraine headaches, hypertension, age greater than 35 years
      (2) Absolute contraindications: thromboembolic disease, liver disease, cancer, smoking, pregnancy
   b. IUDs: Contraindicated for client with prior pelvic inflammatory disease, vaginal bleeding of unknown origin, abnormal uterine contour.
2. Provide client education concerning consistent and correct use of method.
3. Discuss need for back-up contraception if primary method has not been used correctly.

H. Pharmacologic and parenteral therapies: Client will state the purpose, usage, and associated side effects of all medications, including foam, creams, and gels, as well as oral contraceptives, patches, IM injections, vaginal rings, IUDs, mifepristone, and misoprostol.

Principles of Nursing Care Management

I. Background information: Trends in maternal/infant/family care include the following:
A. More than 50% of all households have a single parent.
B. The number of mothers working outside the home has increased.
C. Abuse is increasing and involves more than the physical maltreatment.
D. Families are increasingly mobile.
E. Families are having fewer children than in prior decades.
F. Deaths as a result of childbearing are being reduced, yet the United States continues to have the highest infant mortality rates of developed countries.
G. Preterm delivery is the leading cause of infant mortality.
H. Fetal alcohol syndrome is the leading cause of mental retardation in the United States and is entirely preventable.

II. Role of nurse
A. Coordinate access to care, and act as a liaison to facilitate care among agencies.
B. Implement and supervise care of members.
C. Assist client to navigate through health care system.
D. Center care around family and validate that it is desired by majority of members.
E. Advocate, clarify, and interpret for infant and family.
F. Act as educator to client, both formally and informally; take on role as researcher.
G. Ensure that health care and specifically perinatal care is on a continuum rather than being episodic.
H. Embrace role as counselor to client.

III. Nursing care standards
A. Safety and infection control: Document, report, and follow up on partner and neonatal abuse.
B. Client rights
1. Provide all clients with information concerning pregnant patient rights and responsibilities.
2. Facilitate access to care for all pregnant clients.
3. Participate in and advocate for research providing evidence-based information regarding maternity and neonatal care.
4. Arrange/advocate for appointments for care prior to and after working hours and on weekends.
5. Educate and emphasize health promotion and disease prevention.
6. Lobby for access to and health care for all categories of clients.
7. Consider family as a unit and part of a community when developing care.

E. Standards of care
1. Implement standards of care developed by Nurse Practice Act.
2. Advocate for national health care database to assure access to health care records of all individuals.

3. Anticipate situations creating ethical dilemmas in the childbearing setting.
4. Implement standards of care determined by the specialty organization, Association of Women's Health, Obstetric and Neonatal Nurses.
5. Review literature about current trends in ethical decision making and compare with current practice.

F. Ethical and legal considerations: Parents are considered decision makers for their infants, who are not capable. Uncertainty arises when parents ask about ability of infant to be "OK" as an adult. Medicine can give a statistical answer but cannot determine the outcome for a particular infant. The manner in which this is communicated may influence parental decision. Parents have the right to be fully informed concerning risks and benefits, outcomes, and current status prior to decision making, determining treatment or no treatment for their fetus or neonate.
   1. Influences on decision making in obstetric/neonatal setting involve:
      a. Ethics
      b. Law
      c. Spirituality
      d. Culture
      e. Male/female perspective
      f. Client/family perspectives
      g. Nursing/medicine perspective
   2. Clinical issues and dilemmas in childbearing setting include:
      a. United States is the only developed country that does not guarantee access to maternity care.
      b. The second client (fetus/neonate) and consumer of care in obstetrics is unseen and unable to determine need for medical procedures or to give consent.
      c. Children who determine they have been wrongfully treated can sue when they reach the legal age of 21 years.
      d. Hospital stays are shorter than in the past.
      e. Families are asking for alternatives to hospital births; more acute care is occurring in the home setting.
      f. Assistive reproduction technology is increasing availability for clients who are unable to bear children.
      g. Decisions to bear child or terminate pregnancy (including partial birth abortion) require careful consideration.
      h. Availability of prenatal testing, diagnosis, and genetic counseling is increasing.
      i. Issues concerning length of time to continue resuscitation efforts are made in various clinical settings.
      j. Additional clinical issues and dilemmas involve decisions regarding pain and pain management for those who cannot respond or who respond minimally, transferring neonates to a neonatal intensive care setting, use of fetal tissue for research, and issues related to determining "What is quality of life for a neonate?"

Bibliography

Developmental Tasks for the Individual and Family. Retrieved from http://faculty.ccri.edu/rarchambault/DevelopmentalTasksfortheIndividualandtheFamily.rtf. Retrieved May 5, 2008.

Duvall, E. M. (1977). *Marriage and family development.* Philadelphia: Lippincott.

Hogan, M. A., Glazebrook, R., Brancato, V., & Rodgers, J. (2007). *Maternal-newborn nursing reviews and rationales.* Philadelphia: Pearson Prentice Hall.

Klossner, N. J., & Hatfield, N. (2005). *Introduction to maternity and pediatric nursing.* Philadelphia: Lippincott Williams & Wilkins.

Pillitteri, A. (2006). *Maternal and child health nursing: Care of the childbearing and childrearing family* (5th ed.). Philadelphia: Lippincott Williams & Wilkins.

Ricci, S. S. (2006). *Essentials of maternity, newborn and women's health nursing.* Philadelphia: Lippincott, Williams & Wilkins.

Simpson, K. R., & Creehan, P. A. (2007). *AWHONN's perinatal nursing* (3rd ed.). Philadelphia: Lippincott Williams & Wilkins.

Witt, C. (2007). *Advances in neontal care.* Philadelphia: Lipincott Williams & Wilkins.

CHAPTER 3
Practice Test

Background Information: Growth and Development

1. On assessing the family, the nurse notices the following interactions. Which observation suggests the family is not functioning in a healthy way?

□ 1. The father comforts his crying daughter.
□ 2. The mother states, "This family couldn't function without me."
□ 3. The family pays cash for health care.
□ 4. The father doesn't share his financial concerns so his wife won't worry about them.

2. Which behavior suggests that a family is a healthy one?

□ 1. A brother is so jealous of his new sister that he hits her.
□ 2. A mother states she has grown up since giving birth to her children.
□ 3. A mother is angry that the father never helps with housework.
□ 4. A father wishes the family had more time together.

3. Which of the following may occur in the blended type of family at a greater level than in other types of families?

□ 1. Disagreement about childrearing practices.
□ 2. One of the children doesn't like to do homework.
□ 3. One of the children has frequent illness.
□ 4. Formation of a strong relationship with a parent.

4. An adolescent tells the nurse that it is taboo in his family to use credit cards. The nurse should interpret this to mean which of the following?

□ 1. His parents do not believe in the use of credit cards.
□ 2. His parents probably have few credit cards.
□ 3. The family is wealthy.
□ 4. The adolescent is too young to apply for a credit card.

Health Assessment

5. AF The nurse is assessing the nutrition status of a client who is 22 years of age and planning to become pregnant. The nurse reviews the following 24-hr dietary history:

HISTORY AND PHYSICAL

Breakfast	Lunch	Dinner
Breakfast bar	2 Bean burritos with shredded lettuce	Lettuce salad, 1/2 cup
Whole wheat toast, 1 slice	Iced tea	Baked chicken thigh
Peanut butter, 2 tbsp		Broccoli
Orange juice, 3/4 cup		Rice, 1/2 cup
		Dinner roll with butter
		Baked apple in crust

The nurse encourages the client to obtain more food from which of the following food groups?

□ 1. Fruits.
□ 2. Vegetables.
□ 3. Grains.
□ 4. Dairy.

6. A client seeking preconception counseling tells the nurse that her husband's family has a history of cystic fibrosis (CF). She asks the nurse what the risk to her planned child will be. The nurse should inform the client:

□ 1. If the father has CF, male children have a 100% risk of having CF.
□ 2. Only the mother can pass CF to a child; there is no risk.
□ 3. If both parents have the CF gene, each child has a 25% risk of having CF.
□ 4. If one parent has CF, each child has a 50% risk of having CF.

7. A woman is the carrier of a sex-linked recessive disease, hemophilia A; her husband is free of the disease. What frequency of hemophilia A could the woman expect to see in her children?

□ 1. All male children inherit the disease.
□ 2. All female children will be carriers, like herself.
□ 3. One half of male children inherit the disease.
□ 4. One half of female children inherit the disease.

8. A woman has requested genetic screening to determine the risk for having a child with

Huntington chorea. The nurse should do which of the following?

- ☐ 1. Avoid revealing a finding that would be detrimental to the woman's self-esteem.
- ☐ 2. Notify all family members of the finding as soon as possible.
- ☐ 3. Report findings to the health department.
- ☐ 4. Give the woman the findings as soon as possible.

9. A woman carries a recessive gene for sickle cell anemia. If her sexual partner also has this recessive gene, the chance that her first child will develop sickle cell anemia is:

- ☐ 1. 1 in 4.
- ☐ 2. 2 in 4.
- ☐ 3. 3 in 4.
- ☐ 4. 0 in 4.

10. The nurse is assessing a teenager who tells the nurse she wants to become pregnant. Which of the following puts this client at high risk for a safe pregnancy?

- ☐ 1. Client is 5 ft 3 in. tall.
- ☐ 2. Client is 16 years of age.
- ☐ 3. Client has had a miscarriage.
- ☐ 4. Client is not married.

11. The nurse is assessing a woman with diabetes mellitus who is planning to become pregnant. The woman has two stepchildren for whom she provides full-time care. The woman is considered to be at high risk for pregnancy. A high-risk pregnancy may affect roles within a family because

- ☐ 1. The mother may not be able to assume her normal role.
- ☐ 2. Support systems may falter if the mother needs to be on bed rest or hospitalized.
- ☐ 3. The husband may not be able to deal with the stress.
- ☐ 4. Changes in body image may produce negative responses for the client as the pregnancy progresses.

Health Promotion

12. The nurse is teaching a client who smokes and is considering becoming pregnant about the effects of smoking on pregnancy. Additional teaching is needed if the client makes which of the following comments?

- ☐ 1. "Smoking may cause prolonged length of pregnancy."
- ☐ 2. "Smoking may cause the placenta to separate from the uterine wall."
- ☐ 3. "Smoking may cause the placenta to implant low in the uterus or over the cervix."
- ☐ 4. "Smoking may cause stillbirth."

13. AF The nurse is instructing a client who is 20 years of age about healthy nutrition prior to becoming pregnant. The nurse advises the client to include adequate amounts of which of the following nutrients at this time? Select all that apply.

- ☐ 1. Fluids.
- ☐ 2. Folic acid.
- ☐ 3. Iron.
- ☐ 4. Vitamin A.
- ☐ 5. Antioxidants.

14. The nurse is instructing a client about the use of an emergency contraceptive. The client needs further education if she makes which of the following statements?

- ☐ 1. "I will take the emergency contraceptive within 12 hr of unprotected intercourse."
- ☐ 2. "I will take an over-the-counter antinausea medication 1 hr before taking the pills."
- ☐ 3. "I will have a pregnancy test if my period does not start in 21 days."
- ☐ 4. "I will use a barrier contraceptive method until my period starts."

15. A young married woman tells the nurse that she is going to have a tubal ligation because there are two people with mental retardation in her husband's family and she is afraid this problem will surface in her children. The nurse should:

- ☐ 1. Help the woman reject the idea of sterilization.
- ☐ 2. Strengthen the couple's resolve to remain childless.
- ☐ 3. Help the couple decide to have children.
- ☐ 4. Increase the couple's knowledge about genetic inheritance.

16. When counseling potential parents about genetic disorders, which of the following statements would be appropriate?

- ☐ 1. All genetic disorders follow Mendelian laws of inheritance.
- ☐ 2. Environmental influences may affect multifactorial inheritance.
- ☐ 3. All genetic disorders involve a similar number of abnormal chromosomes.
- ☐ 4. The absence of genetic disorders in both families eliminates the possibility of having a child with a genetic disorder.

Principles of Nursing Care Management

17. Infant mortality is a standard measurement of the quality of health care. What does this measure?

- ☐ 1. The number of babies who die at birth each year.
- ☐ 2. The number of deaths per 1,000 live births.

- □ 3. The number of deaths per 1,000 live births each year in children under age 12 months.
- □ 4. The number of babies who die of communicable diseases each year.

18. Infant mortality is higher in the United States than in other developed countries. Which of the following factors best explains the difference?

- □ 1. Most parents in the United States do not believe in immunizations, so infections occur.
- □ 2. The proportion of adolescents giving birth is greater in the United States than it is in other countries.
- □ 3. A larger portion of the United States is cold in the winter, so pneumonia occurs readily.
- □ 4. Infants in the United States have many milk allergies, so vomiting and aspiration occur easily.

19. A program designed to decrease the infant mortality rate in the Untied States would probably make the greatest impact if it focused on:

- □ 1. Providing free genetic counseling.
- □ 2. Reducing the number of home births.
- □ 3. Increasing the education level of parents.
- □ 4. Increasing the number of women receiving prenatal care.

20. A couple has given birth to an infant diagnosed with Down syndrome. The mother asks what the infant will be like when he reaches adulthood. The nurse should tell the parents that:

- □ 1. Most children with Down syndrome have an IQ of 70.
- □ 2. The child will have several other congenital defects that will require care.
- □ 3. Many infants with Down syndrome live to adulthood and can function in supported employment environments.
- □ 4. It is too soon to predict what their child will be like.

Answers and Rationales

1. 4 Effective families exhibit a great deal of open communication among family members. Protecting a spouse from concerns does not keep the communication open. It is appropriate for a father to comfort his daughter. In option 2 the mother is stating her belief in an open way. Paying cash is an appropriate way to manage finances. (P)

2. 2 Growing up with children is a mark of a healthy family. Lack of communication or time spent together leads to less than optimal families. It is normal for a sibling to be jealous of a new child in the family but not to the extent of physical abuse; the parents can intervene to help this child understand and cope with being jealous. (P)

3. 1 Because blended families merge two families, traditions and family patterns may not merge smoothly and there may be disagreement about childrearing practices. Additionally, as evidence about best practices for childrearing emerge, practices can change. The other options are not grounded in evidence. (P)

4. 1 A cultural taboo refers to an action that is disapproved. The nurse does not attribute other meaning to the communication. (P)

5. 4 The recommended daily dietary allowances for healthy nutrition are: Fruit: 2 to 4 servings; vegetables: 3 to 5 servings; grains: 6 to 11 servings; protein: 3 to 4 servings; dairy products: 2 to 3 servings. This client's diet is deficient in dairy products; therefore, the nurse discusses with the client ways she can increase her intake to meet the recommended allowance. (H)

6. 3 Cystic fibrosis is an autosomal recessive genetic disorder. Both genes of a pair must be abnormal for the disorder to be expressed. Persons who are heterozygous for the gene will be carriers. Two-carrier parents pass the gene to the child. The risk of cystic fibrosis for each child is 25%. (H)

7. 3 With X-linked inheritance, no female children will demonstrate the disease; 50% of male children will demonstrate the disease. (R)

8. 4 Genetic analysis information is shared only with the person requesting the analysis. Analysis is conducted voluntarily. It is not required to report findings to the health department. Relating the findings promptly increases client satisfaction. (R)

9. 1 Autosomal recessive inherited diseases occur at a 1 in 4 incidence in offspring. The other options are not accurate. (R)

10. 2 Because this client is only 16 years of age, she is at risk for many physical and psychosocial problems during pregnancy. A height of 5 ft 3 in. is within normal limits. Having a miscarriage does not place the client at risk for a term pregnancy. Not being married potentially decreases the client's support system, but is not a risk for a successful pregnancy. The nurse advises the client of those factors that put her at high risk for pregnancy and assists her in making decisions about her health. (H)

11. 1 Roles in the family are altered when the mother is not able to assume her normal role because of limits imposed by a high-risk pregnancy. Someone else is required to assume roles the mother usually performs for the family. Support systems for individual families vary widely, and others may be able to fulfill the mother's role. There are no data to indicate how the husband will be able to deal with the stress of his wife's pregnancy. Body image may or may not be a factor for the pregnant woman experiencing a high-risk pregnancy. The nurse assists the client and her family to anticipate changes in family dynamics if the client becomes pregnant. (P)

12. 1 Smoking is documented to be associated with placenta previa, placenta abruptio, premature birth, premature rupture of membranes, intrauterine fetal death, and fetal growth restriction. Smoking does not cause prolongation of the pregnancy. The nurse assists the woman to develop plans to stop smoking as soon as possible. (H)

13. 2,3 The nurse encourages the woman who is attempting to become pregnant to obtain adequate amounts of folic acid and iron in the diet. Folic acid is essential to preventing neural tube defects in the developing fetus and it is important for the woman to have adequate intake prior to conception and during the first 6 weeks of the pregnancy. Iron is necessary to maintain iron stores during pregnancy. Fluid intake is important to general health, but does not affect conception. Vitamin A is also important to general health, but does not affect fetal development in the way that folic acid and iron do. Antioxidants are associated with preventing cancer. (H)

14. 1 The client takes an emergency contraceptive within 72 hr of unprotected intercourse. The client can use antiemetics before taking the pill. If the client does not have a menstrual period within 3 weeks, the client may have become pregnant and is instructed to have a pregnancy test. The nurse advises the client to use barrier contraception until she is certain she is not pregnant. (A)

15. 4 Education about genetic patterns allows people to make informed decisions. The goal of genetic counseling is to provide information, not advice; in the other options the nurse is giving advice. (R)

16. 2 It is difficult to predict with certainty the incidence of genetic disorders because in some disorders more than one gene is involved and environmental insults may play a role (e.g., cleft palate). (R)

17. 3 The infant year is birth to 12 months; mortality refers to deaths. The mortality rate is not related to deaths from specific diseases. The mortality rate is an indicator of child health and health care services for children because most infant deaths can be prevented if identified and treated early. (M)

18. 2 Adolescents have higher risk factors than other groups because of psychologic and physiologic immaturity; therefore infant deaths are higher in this group. Most adolescents do not have health care insurance and may not be covered by family health care insurance policies, and therefore often do not seek health care services when they are pregnant. The other options are not based in fact. (M)

19. 4 Attending prenatal care has proven to be a major strategy for reducing infant mortality. Although genetic counseling may be helpful to prevent birth of infants with the likelihood of having genetically transmitted diseases, reduced infant deaths are not an outcome of genetic counseling. Home births can be managed safely and are not the sole cause of infant mortality. Clients with higher education levels tend to seek health care, but this strategy will not be effective in the short term. (M)

20. 3 The parents of children born with health problems often ask questions about the future life of their child. The nurse tells the parents that many children with Down syndrome live to adulthood and can function in supported environments. Giving information about a specific IQ is not appropriate as the exact IQ of this child will not be known at this time. It is also not appropriate to tell parents about other defects that are not known at this time. Although many aspects of the newborn's life are not known at this time, the parents are requesting information; the nurse responds with information that is based on current and documented health care outcomes. (M)

chapter 4

Preconception and Antepartal Care

The antepartal period encompasses the time from conception until labor begins. Providing safe nursing care to the woman who is pregnant as well as her developing fetus is an essential component of nursing care during the childbearing process. This chapter includes information about client needs during the antepartum stage of childbearing, including:

- Embryonic and Fetal Development
- Antepartal Care

Embryonic and Fetal Development

I. Definition: Embryonic and fetal development begins with conception (see Table 4-1). Conception occurs in outer third of fallopian tube, and fertilized ovum takes 10 days to migrate to and implant in uterus.

A. Periods of development

1. Pre-embryonic: Conception through first 2 weeks' gestation; initial development involves: fertilization → zygote → morula → blastocyst and trophoblast
   a. Ovum fertile for 24 hr; sperm fertile for 24 hr and viable for 72 hr.
   b. After fertilization, zygote contains 22 pair of autosomes and one pair of sex chromosomes (XY, male; XX, female).
2. Embryonic: 2 though 8 weeks' gestation; involves differentiation of cells with development of embryo, placenta, amniotic and yolk sacs.
   a. Amnion: Inner fluid filled membrane surrounding embryo and amniotic fluid
   b. Chorion: Outer membrane covering amnion and inside of uterus
   c. Chorionic villus: Vascular protrusions from the chorion into the uterine blood sinuses
   d. Placenta: Site of exchange between maternal and fetal systems; serves as GI tract, respiratory system, and kidneys for developing embryo and as endocrine organ during pregnancy
      (1) Produces human choriogonadotropin hormone (hCG), estrogen, progesterone, and human placental lactogen (HPL) during pregnancy
      (2) Transfers oxygen, nutrients, and immunoglobulins to fetus
   e. Amniotic fluid: Fluid cushion surrounding fetus during pregnancy; regulates fetal temperature, facilitates movement and muscle development, and provides protection for the fetus

Table 4-1 Fetal Development From Date of Last Menstrual Period

End of 4 Weeks' Gestation	End of 8 Weeks' Gestation	End of 12 Weeks' Gestation	End of 16 Weeks' Gestation	End of 20 Weeks' Gestation
• Rudimentary heart • Arms and legs are buds • Rudimentary eyes, ears, and nose	• Length, 1 in. • Weight, 2 g • Heart beating • Organ development complete • Blood forming • Testes, ovaries becoming distinguishable • Tail almost disappeared • Eyes, ears recognizable • Major blood vessels in position	• Length, 8 cm CR; 11.5 cm CH • Weight, 45 g • Large head • Bones outlined • Lungs take shape • Kidneys begin to secrete urine • External genitalia recognizable • Nails present	• Length, 13–15 cm • Weigh, 200 g • Face appears human with eyes, ears, nose typical shape • Bones identifiable • Teeth forming • Kidneys in position • Muscles move • Lung tissue becoming elastic • Sex determination possible	• Length, 25 cm • Weigh, 435 g • Meconium in gut • Vernix begins to form • Lanugo covers body • Sleep and wake patterns establishing • Sternum ossifies • Enamel and teeth begin to form
End of 24 Weeks' Gestation	**End of 28 Weeks' Gestation**	**End of 32 Weeks' Gestation**	**End of 36 Weeks' Gestation**	**End of 40 Weeks' Gestation**
• Length, 23–28 cm • Weight, 780 g • Lung surfactant being produced • Eyebrows and eyelashes seen • Eyes no longer fused • Responds to sound • Brain looks like mature brain	• Length, 35 cm • Weigh, 1,200 g • Surfactant in amniotic fluid • Lecithin being produced in lungs • Testes begin to descend	• Length, 38 cm • Weight, 2,000 g • SC fat begins to be deposited • Moro reflex present • Begins storing iron	• Length, 42 cm • Weight, 5–6 lb • Lanugo begins to decrease in amount; sole creases begin • Assumes vertex position • Stores glucose, iron, calcium well	• Length, 48 cm • Weight, 7 lb • Nails extend to fingertips • Creases over 2/3 of foot • Converts fetal hemoglobin to adult hemoglobin

Fetus swallows, breathes, and urinates into amniotic fluid. Normal amount is 800 to 1,200 ml, consisting mainly of fetal urine; terms for amount of amniotic fluid include:
(1) Polyhydramnios/hydramnios: 2,000 ml of amniotic fluid or less
(2) Oligohydramnios: 300 ml of amniotic fluid or less

f. Umbilical cord: Connects fetus to placenta, transports oxygen and nutrients to fetus, and returns wastes to maternal system. Composed of two arteries (carry deoxygenated blood away from fetus) and one vein (carries oxygenated blood to fetus)

3. Fetal: From 9 weeks' gestation to birth. All systems are present, and remainder of pregnancy is maturation and growth.

B. Terms associated with pregnancy
1. Nagele's rule: Determination of due date by acknowledging the first day of the last menstrual period, and then subtracting three months; adding 7 days; and, if necessary, adding 1 year.
2. Gravida: Pregnant woman
3. Gravidity: Number of times a woman has been pregnant
4. Nulligravida: Woman who has never been pregnant
5. Primigravida: Woman who is pregnant for the first time
6. Multigravida: Woman who is pregnant for at least the second time
7. Parity: Number of deliveries after 20 weeks' gestation whether the infant is born dead or alive; does not refer to number of fetuses in each pregnancy (e.g., twins, triplets)
8. Nullipara: Woman who has not delivered an infant past 20 weeks' gestation
9. Primipara: Woman who has delivered one infant past 20 weeks' gestation
10. Multipara: Woman who has delivered more than one infant past 20 weeks' gestation
11. Noting the obstetric history: Two methods:
a. GTPALM
(1) G, Gravida: Number of pregnancies
(2) T, Term: Number of fetuses delivered between completion of 37 and 42 weeks' gestation
(3) P, Preterm: Number of fetuses delivered between 20 and 37 weeks' gestation (full term)
(4) Ab, Abortion: Number of fetuses delivered before 20 weeks' gestation
(5) L, Living: Number of living children the client currently has, taking into account children who may have died after birth as a result of accident or diseases
b. TPAL
(1) T, Full term deliveries (37 weeks' gestation)
(2) P, Preterm deliveries (20–36 weeks' gestation)
(3) A, Abortions (elective or spontaneous)
(4) L, Living children
12. Quickening: First time a mother feels the fetus move in utero. In a primiparous woman, that occurs at 18 to 20 weeks' gestation. In a multiparous woman, that occurs from 14 to 16 weeks' gestation. Initially feels like gas moving in abdomen. Used as a parameter to validate the infant is either 14 to16 (multiparous) or 18 to 20 (primiparous) weeks' gestation and is part of the medical record.
13. Ballottement: Movement of the fetus in response to pressure from the examiner's hands.
14. Postterm pregnancy: Pregnancy lasting longer than 42 weeks' gestation.
15. Fetus: Infant in utero from 9 weeks' gestation through delivery.
16. Newborn/Neonate: Product of human birth from time of delivery to 28 days of life.
17. Embryo: Product of human conception through 8 weeks' gestation.

Antepartal Care

I. Definition: The antepartal period encompasses the time from conception until labor begins. A full-term pregnancy begins at 38 weeks' gestation and ends with the completion of 42 weeks' gestation.

II. Nursing process
A. Assessment
1. Perform the following assessments during initial prenatal visit:
a. Obtain a detailed health history including gynecologic, medical, surgical, family, psychosocial, nutritional, genetic and obstetric.
b. Perform a comprehensive physical examination, including both a focused medical surgical physical exam and a gynecologic examination (pelvic measurements):
(1) Pelvic inlet-obstetric conjugate
(2) Midpelvis
(3) Pelvic outlet-ischial tuberosity diameter
(4) Type of pelvis

(a) Gynecoid (female—favorable for vaginal delivery)
(b) Anthropoid (favorable)
(c) Android (male—not favorable)
(d) Platypelloid (flat—not favorable)

c. Assess for risk factors, including presence of extremes of childbearing ages (less than 19 years of age or greater than 35 years of age).
(1) Adolescents: Evaluate for developmental level (concrete versus abstract thinking), acceptance of own body image, personal values, productivity, acceptance of pregnancy, support systems, sense of independence, and plans to continue or terminate pregnancy.
(2) Advanced maternal age: Priority of career, presence of chronic diseases (e.g., diabetes, hypertension), plans to continue or terminate pregnancy.

d. Assess prenatal visit schedule (for uncomplicated pregnancy).
(1) Visits every 4 weeks until beginning of seventh month.
(2) Visits every 2 weeks until beginning of ninth month.
(3) Visits every 1 week from beginning of ninth month until delivery.

e. Obtain diagnostic tests.
(1) CBC; Rh factor; rubella titer; blood type; HbsAg titer; Pap smear; syphilis; gonorrhea; chlamydia; and HIV screening; also, urine testing for protein and glucose
(2) Testing specific to other disease processes, culturally based diseases (e.g., sickle cell screen for African Americans, Tay-Sachs for mothers of Jewish descent), amniocentesis, and chorionic villus sampling for client over 35 years of age, history of Down syndrome

2. Perform the following assessments during each visit:
a. Assess BP, weight, fetal heart tones (FHTs), location of FHTs, fetal movement.
b. Assess client education needs for changes related to next prenatal visit.
c. Perform urine testing for protein, glucose, nitrites, and ketones.

3. Obtain diagnostic studies during pregnancy (see Table 4-2): The nurse explains to the client the purpose of the diagnostic study and significance of the results, and assists in preparing the client for the study.
a. Initial laboratory findings
(1) CBC
(2) Rubella
(3) Blood type, Rh factor
(4) Pap smear
(5) Hepatitis B surface antigen
(6) Blood glucose
(7) Cultures for sexually transmitted diseases such as gonorrhea and chlamydia
(8) Syphilis screening
(9) Urine testing for protein, glucose
b. Laboratory findings later in pregnancy

Table 4-2 Fetal Assessment Tests

Daily Fetal Movement Counts (Kick Counts)	
General information	Tests that fetal movement (FM) is occurring.
Procedure	Client counts number of times she feels infant kick and move in 1 hr. One way to do the count is to record the amount of time it takes the infant to make 10 movements or "kicks." The movements can be flutters or rolling movements. If the woman does not feel any movements within 1 hr, the woman should eat or drink and count again. If no movements occur after 2 hr, the woman is instructed to call HCP.
Interpretation/results	Absence of FM requires additional testing to determine cause.
Ultrasound (U/S)	
General information	Level 1, Basic: Identifies viability, number of fetuses, placental location, amniotic fluid volume, presence of fetal organs.

(Continued)

Table 4-2 Fetal Assessment Tests (*Continued*)

Ultrasound (U/S) (continued)	
General information (continued)	Extensive Level 2, Targeted: Detects anatomically or physiologically abnormal fetus (increased AFP, poly-oligohydramnios, etc.); the earilier an abnormality is detected, the worse it is. As trimesters progress, additional information available. Also used to determine FHT, gestational age, fetal growth, placental location, position, fetal well-being, amniotic fluid volume, and blood flow.
Indications	Used to confirm pregnancy and estimated date of confinement and to follow fetal growth and development throughout the pregnancy.
Procedure (two methods)	Vaginal method: Client empties bladder; condom-covered probe inserted into vagina. Client experiences no pain, and slight pressure. Good for heavy women or when infant is low in pelvis. Abdominal method: Client drinks 24 oz H_2O 30 min prior to examination to move fetus up in pelvis. Warm jelly is placed on abdomen and probe is moved over abdomen. Client experiences no pain. Procedure lasts 5–30 min.
Risks	No evidence of harm in 25 years at particular ultrasonic intensity levels. Will continue to monitor.
Interpretation/results	Identifies fetal well-being or fetal defects. Specific information sought depends on rationale for testing and number of weeks' gestation.
Biophysical Profile-Examination of Fetus In Utero	
General information	Evaluates current fetal status to estimate risk of fetal death in immediate future.
Procedure	Infant placed on fetal monitor for NST for 0.5 hr, then complete US for evaluation of five characteristics of infant in utero: fetal breathing movements, FM, fetal tone, FHR, and amniotic fluid volume.
Risks	Same as for US and NST.
Interpretation/results	Current fetal status scored from 0–10 for each criterion. Score of 8–10 indicates fetal well-being. Score less than 8 indicates potential fetal compromise and further testing indicated. Use first biophysical profile (BPP)as baseline to evaluate against later. If score is low, may attempt to deliver.
Amniocentesis	
General information	Performed from 14 weeks of pregnancy until delivery (enough amniotic fluid present at that time). Obtains amniotic fluid from fetal cells to diagnose: • Genetic disorders (client with prior Down Syndrome child, family history of chromosomal abnormalities) • Lung maturation (L/S ratio of 2:1 or greater indicates adequate lung maturity, or phosphatidylglycerol presence indicates lung maturity) and the risk of respiratory distress syndrome in the neonate is low • Fetal hemolytic disease (identification and follow-up) • Physiologic abnormality (AFP: looks at enzymes produced by cells to confirm NTD)
Procedure	Client drinks water to fill bladder then US is completed to locate pockets of fluid, identify infant and placental location, and to guide needle. Abdomen prepared, needle guided by US to fluid area, and 20–40 ml of amniotic fluid is removed. Client is monitored briefly after the procedure, and educated concerning potential problems as result of test.
Risks	Mother: Hemorrhage, Rh isoimmunization, infection, labor, abruption, preterm labor, rupture of membranes Infant: Death, hemorrhage, infection, abortion
Interpretation/results	Genetic information available in 3–4 weeks; several hours for remainder of test results

Chorionic Villus Sampling	
General information	Performs genetic testing in first trimester by aspirating fetal cells.
Procedure	Completed at less than 10 weeks' gestation; guided by US picture; a catheter inserted to remove tissue from fetal side of placenta.
Risks	Mother: Hemorrhage, abortion, infection Infant: If completed less than 10 weeks' gestation, increased risk of fetal limb anomalies
Interpretation/results	Information about genetic disorders is available in several days.
Nonstress Test	
General information	Noninvasive outpatient procedure to measure accelerations in FHR in response to FM; however, has high false-positive (nonreactive) ratings. Hypoxia, acidosis, drugs, sleep, and congenital anomalies may blunt this response
Procedure	Client helped into semi-Fowler position and placed on fetal monitor, which monitors contractions, FM, and FHR; infant movement indicated on monitor strip. Goal is increase in FHR as response to fetal movement
Interpretation/results	Reactive tracing (desired outcome): Healthy fetuses produces two or more accelerations of 15 BPM lasting 15 s over a 20-min time frame, normal baseline, LTV greater than 10 BPM. If infant asleep, may use fetal acoustic stimulation, and prolong test by 10 min. Nonreactive tracing: Does not meet criteria for reactive strip in 40 min and further assessment indicated (BPP or contraction stress test).
Contraction Stress Test	
General information	Goal is to identify fetal response to stress of contractions for early warning signs of fetal compromise, and less false-positive results. Contractions are stress (less uterine blood flow with less placental perfusion, which may produce hypoxia; then deceleration in FHR as response).
Procedure	RN places client on FM in labor and delivery setting and baseline strip obtained. Client may have contractions without use of oxytocin (Pitocin) and three contractions of moderate intensity in 10 min without late decelerations are wanted. If adequate contractions are not spontaneous, use one of two methods: • **NSST** (nipple stimulation stress test): Natural form of oxytocin challenge test (OCT); cycles of nipple stimulation to release oxytocin from posterior pituitary gland. Difficult to regulate number of contractions • **OCT** (completed by RN): IV mainline begun, IV Pitocin piggybacked to primary IV to produce three contractions lasting 40–50 s in 10 min FR to contractions interpreted when appropriate number of contractions achieved.
Risks	Invasive, more expensive, time-consuming, may cause over stimulation
Interpretation/results	**Negative OCT:** Reassuring and desired outcome determining healthy fetus, indicated by three contractions of moderate intensity in 10 min without decelerations **Positive OCT:** Nonreassuring, late decelerations with 50% of contractions; may indicate potentially compromised fetus **Equivocal or suspicious results:** Significant variable decelerations or nonrepetitive late decelerations with less than half the contractions
Metabolic Screening	
General information	Screening 48° after infant birth for group of six metabolic disorders: PKU, maple sugar urine disease, homocystinuria, sickle cell, galactosemia, and hypothyroidism; early diagnosis of any of six metabolic disorders promotes early treatment.
Procedure	RN performs heel stick prior to hospital discharge if less than 48 hours and then again at 2–5 days of age after the infant has had breast milk or formula.
Risks	Infection at site
Interpretation/results	Results interpreted through state board of health and are available within a few days.

(Continued)

Table 4-2 Fetal Assessment Tests (*Continued*)

Triple Marker	
General information	Blood test at 16–18 weeks' gestation to evaluate level of MSAFP, uncongugated estriol and hCG.
Procedure	This test requires a blood sample.
Interpretation/results	High or low levels of these substances are associated with neural tube defects, Down syndrome, trisomy 18, 21 syndromes; results are available within several days to a week.
Alpha-Fetoprotein	
General information	Blood screening at 16–18 weeks' gestation for maternal blood levels of AFP with results referenced against values for a particular week of gestation
Procedure	Blood draw intravenously
Interpretation/results	High values: Correlate with neural tube defects Low values: Correlated with Down Syndrome

(1) Alpha-fetoprotein (AFP) screening for neural tube defects at 16 weeks' gestation
(2) 50-g glucola for gestational diabetes at 24 to 28 weeks' gestation
(3) Urine, vaginal, or rectal screening for group B streptococcal (GBS) infection at 36 weeks' gestation
(4) Ultrasound for pregnancy dating, problem identification
(5) Triple marker at 16 to 18 weeks' gestation measures levels of AFP, hCG, and unconjugated estriol to calculate risk for Down syndrome.
(6) Amniocentesis from 14 weeks' gestation or chorionic villus sampling from 10 to 12 weeks' gestation to determine genetic makeup of client only if indicated
  (a) Amniocentesis can be completed from 13 weeks' gestation. Reasons for amniocentesis varies with gestation (Rh sensitization, chromosomal studies, fetal lung maturity).
  (b) Choronic villus sampling is used for chromosomal studies from 8 to 12 weeks' gestation.

B. Analysis
1. Disturbed Body Image related to physical changes of pregnancy
2. Imbalanced Nutrition: Less than Body Requirements related to minimal needs in first trimester, nausea and vomiting, and fetal growth during second and third trimesters
3. Imbalanced Nutrition: Greater than Body Requirements related to obesity, fetal growth
4. Deficient Knowledge related to pregnancy and care of the newborn
5. Ineffective Coping related to pregnancy
6. Anxiety related to potential abnormality of fetus
7. Risk for Altered Parenting related to potential for new member(s) of the family

C. Planning
1. Review client pregnancy history.
2. Validate presence of pregnancy and determine presence of presumptive, probable, and positive signs of pregnancy.
3. Introduce client to available resources, such as childbirth education classes.
4. Educate client regarding the frequently prescribed antenatal medications (see pharmacologic and parenteral therapies).
5. Evaluate client for factors placing pregnancy at risk.
6. Evaluate client educational needs.

D. Implementation (see management of care)

E. Evaluation
1. Client gains 25 to 35 pounds in appropriate increments throughout the pregnancy.
2. Client verbalizes need for 2,500 calorie balanced diet with 60 g of protein, 30 g of fat, 1,200 mg calcium, and 600 mg folic acid.
3. Client relates normal physical and emotional changes associated with pregnancy.
4. Client identifies signs and symptoms of problems to be reported to the HCP during pregnancy (see reduction of risk potential under client needs).

5. Fetus grows according to pre-established standards for dates/age of pregnancy.
6. Client participates in childbirth education classes.
7. Client implements interventions for common discomforts of pregnancy.
8. Client seeks assistance of HCPs if problems or questions arise.
9. Client and partner accept pregnancy.

CN

III. Client needs
A. Physiologic adaptation
1. Skeletal
a. Softening of joints and ligaments as result of estrogen and relaxin
b. Increased swayback—center of gravity shifts, waddling gait appears
2. Integumentary
a. Melanin effect—darkening around areola and on face
b. Linea nigra—dark line between symphysis and fundus
c. Striae gravidarum—stretch marks on skin areas that stretch during pregnancy, such as the abdomen, breasts, and thighs
3. Psychosocial
a. First trimester—ambivalent, introverted, emotionally labile
b. Second trimester—increased sexual interest, fantasizing about fetus, incorporating infant into self, acceptance of pregnancy
c. Third trimester—birth preparation, concerned with ability to accomplish labor and delivery, and feelings of vulnerability
d. All trimesters—maternal role tasks of pregnancy Rubin (1984):
(1) Client ensures safe passage through pregnancy, labor, and delivery.
(2) Client seeks acceptance of child by others.
(3) Client commits herself to the child.
(4) Client learns to give of self for child.
4. Endocrine
a. Hormones
(1) hCG—indicator of pregnancy; maintains corpus luteum until placenta is functioning; may be the cause of morning sickness.
(2) Estrogen—maintains secondary sex characteristics; secreted by placenta during pregnancy.
(3) Progesterone—inhibits contractions, relaxes smooth muscles, resulting in constipation, heartburn, and urinary stasis.
(4) HPL—causes decreased ability to use insulin well (diabetogenic effect); prepares body for breastfeeding.
(5) Oxytocin—stimulates contractions from posterior pituitary; contracts uterus after delivery to prevent hemorrhage; stimulates milk ejection in lactation.
(6) Relaxin—works synergistically with progesterone to soften and lengthen the cervix; increases flexibility of joints.
(7) Thyroid—increase thyroid hormones, which are necessary in pregnancy for fetal growth.
5. Reproductive
a. Cells become hypertrophic and hyperplastic.
b. Uterine changes: term weight, 1,000 g; nonpregnant weight, 80 g.
(1) Goodell's sign—softening of cervix at 4 weeks' gestation.
(2) Hegar's sign—softening of lower uterine segment at 6 weeks' gestation.
(3) Chadwick's sign—blue-purple color of cervix due to increased vascularity of cervix and vaginal mucosa.
c. Breasts become larger, tender, and vascular; colostrum is secreted by third trimester.
6. Circulatory
a. 40% to 50% increase in blood volume to meet pregnancy needs, peaking at 28 weeks' gestation. Greatest increase is in plasma volume, resulting in physiologic anemia/reduced hematocrit due to hemodilution.
b. Cardiac output increases, peaking at 28 weeks' gestation.
c. Heart rate increases 10 to 15 beats per minute.
d. BP decreases slightly in second trimester.
e. Blood changes include increased clotting factors and WBCs.
f. Varicosities of legs and vulva; hemorrhoids develop as result of increased pressure in pelvis.
g. Edema in last 2 months of pregnancy may result from increased pelvic pressure.
h. Supine hypotensive syndrome: Pressure of fetus on vena cava while lying flat on back causes headache, hypotension, and faintness.

7. Gastrointestinal
   a. Nausea and vomiting in first trimester due to hCG.
   b. Constipation results from increased progesterone and smooth muscle relaxation.
   c. Heartburn due to reflux of acid, pressure of fetus, decreased gastric-emptying time, and progesterone effect.
   d. Gallstones may occur related to slower emptying time.
   e. Pica: Eating of unusual, nonnutritive substances such as starch, freezer frost, dirt, clay, and chalk.
   f. Ptyalism: Excessive salivation (estrogen effect).
8. Urinary
   a. Progesterone relaxes bladder, increasing capacity, delaying need to empty.
   b. Dilatation of renal pelvises, ureters from enlarging uterus, progesterone.
   c. Uterus as pelvic organ creates pressure on bladder in first and third trimesters, causing frequent need to void.
   d. Right ureter dilates more than left because of uterine positioning to right.
   e. Increased glomerular filtration rate during pregnancy as result of 30% to 50% increase in blood flow to kidneys.
   f. Kidneys most efficient when client is lying on left side, with optimal venous return, cardiac output, and perfusion in that position.
9. Respiratory
   a. Estrogen increase and increased perfusion causes nosebleeds and nasal congestion.
   b. Increase in respiratory rate as diaphragm moves upward in chest.
10. Common discomforts of pregnancy (see Box 4-1)

B. Management of care: Care of the client receiving antepartal care requires critical thinking skills and knowledge of assessment, and teaching and evaluation methods unique to the RN role. These skills cannot be delegated to an LPN or UAP.

Box 4-1. Managing Common Discomforts of Pregnancy

While you are pregnant, use these suggestions to help deal with some of the more common discomforts of pregnancy.

Urinary frequency or incontinence
- Try Kegel exercises to increase control over leakage.
- Empty your bladder when you first feel a full sensation.
- Avoid caffeine drinks, which stimulate voiding patterns.
- Reduce your fluid intake after dinner to reduce night-time urination.

Fatigue
- Attempt to get a full night's sleep, without interruptions.
- Eat a healthy balanced diet.
- Schedule a nap in the early afternoon daily.
- When you are feeling tired, rest.

Nausea and vomiting
- Avoid an empty stomach at all times.
- Munch on dry crackers/toast in bed before arising.
- Eat several small meals throughout the day.
- Drink fluids between meals rather than with meals.
- Avoid greasy, fried foods or ones with a strong odor, such as cabbage or Brussels sprouts.

Backache
- Avoid standing or sitting in one position for long periods.
- Apply heating pad (low setting) to small of your back.
- Support your lower back with pillows when sitting.
- Stand with your shoulders back to maintain correct posture.

Leg Cramps
- Elevate legs above the heart level frequently throughout the day.
- If you get a cramp, straighten both legs and flex your feet toward your body.
- Ask your health care provider about taking additional calcium supplements, which may be helpful to reduce leg spasms.

Varicosities
- Walk daily to improve circulation to extremities.
- Elevate both legs above heart level while resting.
- Avoid standing in one position for long periods of time.
- Don't wear constrictive stockings or socks.
- Don't cross your legs when sitting for long periods.
- Wear support stockings to promote better circulation.

Hemorrhoids
- Establish a regular time for daily bowel elimination.
- Prevent straining by drinking plenty of fluids, eating fiber-rich foods, and exercising daily.
- Use warm sitz baths and cool witch hazel compresses for comfort.

Constipation
- Increase your intake of foods high in fiber and drink at least eight 8-ounce glasses of fluid daily.
- Exercise each day (brisk walking) to promote movement through the intestine.
- Reduce the amount of cheese you eat.

Heartburn/indigestion
- Avoid spicy or greasy foods and eat small, frequent meals.
- Sleep on several pillows so that your head is elevated.
- Quit smoking and stop drinking caffeinated beverages.
- Avoid lying down for at least two hours after meals.
- Try drinking sips of water to reduce burning sensation.
- Take antacids *sparingly* if burning sensation is severe.

Braxton Hicks contractions
- Keep in mind that these contractions are a normal sensation.
- Try changing your position or engaging in mild exercise to help reduce the sensation.
- Drink more fluids if possible.

Adapted from Ricci, S. S. (2006). *Essentials of maternity, newborn, and women's health nursing.* Philadelphia: Lippincott Williams & Wilkins.

1. Review history of pregnancy.
2. Determine presence of presumptive, probable, and positive signs of pregnancy in client.
   a. Presumptive (subjective) signs may include amenorrhea, breast tenderness, urinary frequency, fatigue, nausea and vomiting—no reliable indicators; may be caused by other conditions.
   b. Probable signs (seen by HCP, but not diagnostic)
      (1) Goodell sign
      (2) Hegar sign
      (3) Chadwick sign
      (4) Abdominal enlargement
      (5) Braxton Hicks contractions
      (6) Pregnancy tests
   c. Positive signs (diagnostic of pregnancy)
      (1) Ultrasound visualization of fetus
      (2) Hearing FHTs
      (3) Palpating fetus
3. Evaluate height of fundus (top of uterus) and correlate with number of weeks' gestation to validate appropriate growth and accuracy of due date.
   a. 10 to 12 weeks' gestation: Fundus is at top of symphysis pubis.
   b. 16 weeks' gestation: Fundus is midway between symphysis and umbilicus.
   c. 20 weeks' gestation: Fundus is at umbilicus (approximately 20 cm) plus or minus 2 cm (some sources say 3 cm).
   d. Between 20 and 32 weeks' gestation: Fundal height in centimeters correlates with number of weeks' gestation. If client is 30 weeks' pregnant, fundal height is approximately 30 cm.
   e. 36 weeks' gestation: Fundus is at the xyphoid process.

C. Safety and infection control: Provide client and family teaching regarding the following:
   1. Expected weight gain and pattern of weight gain (usually 25 to 35 lb total weight gain: 3 to 5 lb during first trimester and 1 lb per week after first trimester until delivery)
   2. Nutritional needs through the trimesters
   3. Normal physical and emotional changes occurring during the pregnancy (nausea and vomiting, fatigue, and normal discomforts)
   4. Warning signs of potential complications during pregnancy
   5. Avoidance of drugs, alcohol, smoking, herbal products, and use of over-the-counter medication
   6. Options for childbirth preparation classes
   7. Options for location and type of birthing experiences

D. Health promotion and maintenance
   1. Educate client and family concerning client's nutritional needs. Basis of nutritional needs will depend on client age, weight, and any medical conditions influencing nutrition. Client should avoid dieting and maintain the following:
      a. Prescribed prenatal vitamins and iron
      b. 2,500 calories per day distributed in three balanced meals and two snacks per day
      c. Vitamins, minerals, and iron in diet as indicated by pica
      d. Cultural dietary variations and variations required by disease processes as appropriate
      e. Adequate sodium intake
      f. Increased protein (60 g, for maternal and fetal growth); folic acid (600 mcg, to prevent anemia), iron (to prevent anemia), and calcium (1,200 mg, to maintain maternal bone mass and fetal bone and tooth growth)
   2. Assist client to participate in childbirth education classes.
      a. Principles of childbirth education
         (1) Minimize pain caused by labor through client and partner or support person working together.
         (2) Decrease maternal discomfort during labor by developing and practicing a conditioned response to pain of contractions.
         (3) Obtain knowledge to diminish pain and fear and to facilitate better personal management during labor.
         (4) Become informed decision makers.
      b. Types of classes available
         (1) Lamaze: Relaxation and breathing techniques to reduce pain of contractions. Uses various types of breathing to focus attention during contractions; encourages control of body, focused relaxation, and minimal need for medications.
         (2) Bradley: Partner coached in use of exercises, comfort measures (e.g., massage), and controlled abdominal breathing to relax client.
         (3) Dick-Read: Focuses on eliminating fear through fear, tension, and pain cycle; which is seen as basis for pain. Encourages knowledge of labor, delivery process, and breathing as methods to eliminate pain.
         (4) Other classes: Base content on exercise; breathing; relaxation; knowledge

of labor and delivery process, anesthesia, cesarean sections, infant care, and breast and bottle feeding.

3. Provide teaching or resources for education to client and family concerning:
   a. Choice of breast- or bottle-feeding
   b. Birth control options with breast- and bottle-feeding after delivery

E. Psychological integrity: Incorporate significant other, family member, or husband into educational process.

F. Basic care and comfort: Educate client and family concerning common discomforts during pregnancy (e.g., urinary frequency, nausea and vomiting, fatigue, constipation, hemorrhoids, varicosities, indigestion, leg cramps, and Braxton Hicks contractions) and interventions to alleviate discomforts.

G. Reduction of risk potential
1. Educate the client and family to monitor for danger signs during pregnancy that indicate a need to notify HCP:
   a. Headache, dizziness, epigastric pain, seizures (pre-eclampsia)
   b. Continuous vomiting (hyperemesis, hydatidiform mole, dehydration)
   c. Decrease in or lack of fetal movement (fetal demise)
   d. Vaginal discharge that is bloody, or a change from prior discharge (rupture of membranes, sexually transmitted infection [STI] placenta previa)
   e. Temperature greater than 100.4°F (infection, influenza)
   f. Burning on urination, costrovertebral angle (CVA) pain (bladder, kidney infection)
   g. Regular uterine contractions (signs of preterm labor)
   h. Decrease in voiding, no voiding (pre-eclampsia)
   i. Facial edema (pre-eclampsia)
2. Wedge mother to side when lying in bed to prevent vena cava syndrome or supine hypotensive syndrome.
3. Encourage client to report consumption of unusual substances such as clay, starch, ice, or chalk (pica).
4. Provide client teaching about the following:
   a. Wear shoes that support feet and walking, and allow for shifting center of gravity.
   b. Drink six to eight glasses of fluid daily.
   c. Continue to wear seat belts, placed appropriately over abdomen.
   d. When traveling, get out of car to walk for approximately 10 minutes each hour.
   e. Avoid use of spas and saunas that may increase maternal temperature.
   f. Avoid activities that potentially cause trauma or excessive jarring of fetus.

H. Pharmacologic and parenteral therapies: Client will state the purpose for and associated side effects of all medications. Avoid use of drugs that cause risk to mother or fetus (FDA Pregnancy Risk Classification of Drugs; see Table 4-3). Assist client to understand use of

Table 4-3 Pregnancy Risk Categories of Drugs

Category	Description	Example
A	Adequate studies in pregnant women have failed to show a risk to the fetus in the first trimester of pregnancy; there is no evidence of risk in later trimesters.	Thyroid hormone
B	Animal studies have not shown an adverse effect on the fetus, but there are no adequate clinical studies in pregnant women.	Insulin
C	Animal studies have shown an adverse effect on the fetus, but there are no adequate studies on humans, or there are no adequate studies in animals or humans. Pregnancy risk is unknown.	Docusate sodium (Colace)
D	There is evidence of risk to the human fetus, but the potential benefits of use in pregnant women may be acceptable despite potential risks.	Lithium citrate
X	Studies in animals or humans show fetal abnormalities, or adverse reaction reports indicate evidence of fetal risk. The risks involved clearly outweigh potential benefits.	Isotretinoin (Accutane)

From Karch, A. M. (2007). *Lippincott's nursing drug guide*. Philadelphia: Lippincott Williams & Wilkins.

frequently prescribed antenatal medications, including:
1. Prenatal vitamins, one daily
2. Ferrous sulfate, 325 mg twice daily
3. Docusate sodium, 100 mg PO, twice daily

Bibliography

Klossner, N. J. & Hatfield, N. (2005). *Introduction to maternity and pediatric nursing*. Philadelphia: Lippincott Williams & Wilkins.

Pillitteri, A. (2006). *Maternal & child health nursing: Care of the childbearing and childrearing family* (5th ed.). Philadelphia: Lippincott Williams & Wilkins.

Rubin, R. (1984). *Maternal identity and the maternal experience*. New York: Springer

Simpson, K. R., & Creehan, P. A. (2007). *AWHONN's perinatal nursing* (3rd ed.). Philadelphia: Lippincott Williams & Wilkins.

Witt, C. (2007). *Advances in neontal care*. Philadelphia: Lippincott Williams & Wilkins.

CHAPTER 4

Practice Test

Embryonic and Fetal Development

1. A client is pregnant and expecting the birth of her infant any day. She had twin boys 7 years ago and a girl 4 years ago. Both of these pregnancies were carried to term. However, 2 years ago she delivered a stillborn infant at 7 months' gestation. Using the acronym GTPAL, which notation reflects this mother's obstetric history?

□ 1. G4-T3-P1-A0-L3.
□ 2. G4-T2-P1-A0-L3.
□ 3. G5-T3-P0-A0-L2.
□ 4. G3-T2-P1-A0-L3.

2. A client requests instructions about how to do a home pregnancy test. The nurse should tell her:

□ 1. "Hormone levels are stable throughout the pregnancy."
□ 2. "Be sure to drink plenty of fluids before doing the test."
□ 3. "Test the first voided specimen in the morning."
□ 4. "Wait 4 weeks after you missed your menstrual period."

3. A client reported to the nurse that her last menstrual period started on July 10. She asks the nurse when her estimated date of delivery will be. Using Nagele's rule, the nurse calculates the date to be:

□ 1. May 15.
□ 2. March 30.
□ 3. April 3.
□ 4. April 17.

4. A primigravida visits the prenatal clinic for the first time. The client asks the nurse why her BP, weight and urine are checked at each visit. The nurse instructs the client that these assessments:

□ 1. Diagnose problems with uterine growth during the pregnancy.
□ 2. Assist in identifying the onset of complications associated with pregnancy.
□ 3. Alert the HCP that the client needs assistance with diet modification.
□ 4. Are performed routinely on all pregnant clients during the prenatal period.

5. During a health history interview with a primigravida at her first prenatal visit, the nurse collects data related to the woman's menstrual history in order to determine her:

□ 1. Use of contraception.
□ 2. Potential for early delivery.
□ 3. Expected date of delivery.
□ 4. Likelihood of a twin pregnancy.

6. The term *gestational age* is used to describe the:

□ 1. Time fertilization took place.
□ 2. Completed weeks of fetal development.
□ 3. Mother's age when she became pregnant.
□ 4. Time when pregnancy can be confirmed.

Antepartal Care

7. At the first prenatal visit the nurse measures the height of the uterus of a primigravida. The fundal height is at the level of the umbilicus. The nurse estimates that the client is:

□ 1. 7 to 8 weeks pregnant.
□ 2. 12 to 14 weeks pregnant.
□ 3. 20 to 22 weeks pregnant.
□ 4. 30 to 32 weeks pregnant.

8. A newly pregnant client who appears to be quite anxious is experiencing morning sickness. The nurse advises the woman that:

□ 1. Eating small amounts more frequently throughout the day may be better tolerated.
□ 2. Eating carbohydrates with each meal may eliminate morning sickness.
□ 3. This is a common problem that usually lasts throughout the pregnancy in most women.
□ 4. Controlling your anxiety will prevent harm to the infant.

9. A pregnant woman is constipated. The nurse can advise the woman to:

□ 1. Use mineral oil and over-the-counter laxatives as needed.
□ 2. Stop taking prenatal vitamins with iron.
□ 3. Increase fluid intake, exercise more, and eat foods high in fiber.
□ 4. Avoid green vegetables, meats, and foods high in protein.

10. A woman who is 4 months pregnant complains of leg cramps.The nurse teaches the client that leg cramps during pregnancy can be managed by:

□ 1. Extending the knee and dorsiflexing the toe.
□ 2. Increasing the intake of iron and vitamin C.
□ 3. Rubbing the leg when cramps occur.
□ 4. Applying a cold pack to the sore muscle.

11. Which of the following is considered a warning sign of a problem that needs immediate attention during the first trimester?

□ 1. Absence of fetal movement.
□ 2. Nausea after meals.
□ 3. Urinary frequency.
□ 4. Vaginal bleeding.

12. The nurse teaches a pregnant woman about the presumptive, probable, and positive signs of pregnancy. The woman demonstrates understanding of the nurse's instructions if she states that a positive sign of pregnancy is:

□ 1. A positive home pregnancy test.
□ 2. Fetal movement palpated by a health care professional.
□ 3. Braxton Hicks contractions.
□ 4. Two missed menstrual periods.

13. A pregnant client at 36 weeks' gestation reveals that she prefers to sleep on her back. The nurse should encourage the client to lie on her left side because sleeping on her back will contribute to which of the following?

□ 1. Backaches during the day.
□ 2. Alteration in blood flow to the kidneys and the uterus.
□ 3. Increased nocturia.
□ 4. Increased intensity of Braxton Hicks contractions and potential for premature labor.

14. The nurse is teaching a pregnant client about taking iron (ferrous sulfate). The teaching is successful if the client says, "I will take the iron before breakfast with:

□ 1. Ice tea."
□ 2. Milk."
□ 3. Orange juice."
□ 4. Coca Cola™."

15. AF A client is at 24 weeks' gestation. The nurse is reviewing the report of laboratory tests as noted below.

LABORATORY RESULTS

Test	Result
Blood type	A-positive
Blood glucose	90 mg/dL
VDRL	Positive
Rubella titer	1:16

The nurse should report which of these results to the health care provider?

□ 1. Blood type.
□ 2. VDRL.
□ 3. Blood sugar.
□ 4. Rubella titer.

16. AF The nurse is reviewing a pregnant client's immunization record. Which of the following immunizations are contraindicated during pregnancy and are not updated at this time? Select all that apply.

□ 1. Tetanus.
□ 2. Rubella.
□ 3. Mumps.
□ 4. Chickenpox.
□ 5. Live attenuated influenza vaccine (LAIV).
□ 6. Hepatitis B.

17. The nurse is teaching a class for pregnant women. The nurse should instruct which of the following clients that limitations on exercise are needed to prevent complications?

□ 1. Client who is 16 years of age and a member of the swim team.
□ 2. Client who is 26 years of age with mitral valve prolapse.
□ 3. Client who is 30 years of age and a physical education teacher.
□ 4. Client who is 39 years of age with gestational diabetes.

18. The nurse is teaching a class about breastfeeding to pregnant women who wish to breast-feed their newborns. Which of the following client statements indicate successful teaching has been accomplished?

- □ 1. "I need to avoid using soap on the nipples."
- □ 2. "I need to wear a bra with elastic straps."
- □ 3. "I will increase my caloric intake 1,000 calories a day."
- □ 4. "I will use nipple rolling to toughen my nipples."

19. AF A woman in the third trimester of pregnancy asks the nurse why she is having an ultrasound at this time. The nurse informs the client that an ultrasound is a means of obtaining more information about which of the following? Select all that apply.

- □ 1. The cause of preterm labor.
- □ 2. The position of the placenta.
- □ 3. The size of the fetus.
- □ 4. The position of the fetus.
- □ 5. The maturity of the fetal lungs.
- □ 6. The amount of amniotic fluid.
- □ 7. The ability of the fetus to undergo the stress of an induction.

20. A woman who is 3 months pregnant has pneumonia. The HCP has prescribed amoxicillin (Amoxil). The nurse should:

- □ 1. Question the order.
- □ 2. Instruct the woman to stop taking the medication.
- □ 3. Advise the woman to take the medication with her usual diet.
- □ 4. Inform the woman that this drug has been known to demonstrate adverse fetal effects.

Answers and Rationales

1. 2 This woman has been pregnant 4 times, including the current pregnancy (Gravida 4). She carried two pregnancies to term or beyond 37 weeks' gestation. Even though a pregnancy ended with twins, it counts as one pregnancy (Term 2). Her third pregnancy ended with a premature birth at 7 months. Although the child did not survive, it counts as a premature birth (Premature 1). She has had no terminations of a pregnancy, elective or spontaneous, before viability or 20 weeks (Abortion 0). She has three living children, the twins and the little girl (Living Children 3). (A)

2. 3 The first voided specimen in the morning is the most concentrated and contains levels of hCG approximately the same as those in the blood serum. Random urine samples usually have lower levels. Drinking excessive fluids may dilute the specimen and give a false-negative reading. Urine tests are sensitive at about 26 days after conception. Levels of hCG increase until they peak at about 60 to 70 days of gestation, then decline until about 140 days of gestation. The hCG level remains stable until about 30 weeks, and then gradually declines until term. (H)

3. 4 According to Nagele's rule, after determining the first day of the last menstrual period, subtract 3 months and add 7 days. Adjust the year if necessary. (A)

4. 2 Screening tests performed during a prenatal visit help the nurse identify potential complications and health problems so that an appropriate plan of care can be initiated. Lack of uterine growth and inappropriate weight gain or loss may alert the nurse to potential problems but do not explain why all of the screening measures are done. Telling a client that a test is "routine" is not a satisfactory explanation. (R)

5. 3 Data related to a woman's menstrual history are used to determine expected date of delivery (EDC or EDD). Other information from the woman's health history and her family's health history helps to provide information about the potential for early delivery and a twin pregnancy, but are not directly related to the woman's menstrual history. Information about the use of contraception may help determine if the pregnancy was planned. (M)

6. 2 Gestational age refers to the age of the fetus, usually expressed in weeks. (A)

7. 3 At 20 to 22 weeks' gestation the level of the fundus of the uterus should be at the umbilicus. Fundal height should correlate with other measurements of the length of the pregnancy, such as information about the first day of the woman's last menstrual period and ultrasound measurements done earlier in the pregnancy. If the fundal height is lower than expected, intrauterine growth retardation is suspected. If it is higher, other problems may be present such as polyhydramnios or a twin pregnancy. (M)

8. 1 Morning sickness occurs in 50% to 70% of pregnant women. Avoiding an overloaded or empty stomach may help. Eating dry carbohydrates upon awaking has been found to be helpful. Morning sickness usually subsides within the first trimester as hormone levels stabilize; for most women, it does not last throughout the pregnancy. Although there is some evidence that morning sickness may have an emotional component as the woman adjusts to being pregnant, there is no evidence that anxiety directly affects the fetus unless it results in poor health habits in the pregnant woman. (H)

9. 3 GI tract mobility slows because of the affect of progesterone on smooth muscle, resulting in increased absorption of water and dry, hard stools. Compression from the enlarging uterus and the iron in prenatal vitamins add to the problem. Increasing fluid intake, exercising, and eating foods high in fiber will help. Mineral oil blocks the absorption of fat soluble vitamins in the GI tract. Laxatives are not recommended without consulting a HCP because they may trigger premature labor, especially in the third trimester. Vitamins with iron are needed for the production of RBCs in the mother, and assure a source of iron for the fetus. Foods high in protein are also essential for tissue growth and RBC production in the mother and the fetus, and usually do not increase constipation. (H)

10. 1 Leg cramps result from muscle spasms caused by a variety of changes in the body during pregnancy. Extending the knee and dorsiflexing the toe can help relax the leg muscles and relieve the spasm. Homans sign is assessed to rule out a blood clot when a woman complains of leg cramps. However, even with a negative Homans sign, rubbing the leg is avoided in case a clot is present. Iron and vitamin C are not related to muscle spasms. Warmth rather than cold is used to relieve sore, cramping muscles when the possibility of clots has been ruled out. (H)

11. 4 Vaginal bleeding in the first trimester may indicate a threatened or actual abortion and needs to be assessed by a HCP. There are also benign situations when bleeding occurs in the first trimester, but more serious problems need to be ruled out. Fetal movement is not felt in the first trimester. Nausea and urinary frequency are expected during this time. (R)

12. 2 Positive indications of pregnancy are directly attributed to the fetus and include the presence of a fetal heart beat distinct from that of the mother, fetal movement felt by someone other than the mother, and visualization of the fetus by ultrasound or other methods. A positive home pregnancy test and Braxton Hicks contractions are probable indicators, but can have other explanations. A missed period strongly suggests pregnancy in a woman having unprotected sexual activity, but also can have other causes. (C)

13. 2 The nurse instructs the client that lying on her back during the end of pregnancy causes the enlarged uterus to compress the descending aorta and the vena cava and reduce circulation to the kidneys and uterus. The nurse tells the client to lie on her side to relieve pressure on those organs. The woman's position when lying down does not affect nocturia, backache, or the potential for increased uterine activity and premature labor. (H)

14. 3 Iron absorption is facilitated by acid (empty stomach or juice containing ascorbic acid). Iron absorption is hampered by calcium (milk) and caffeine (tea and cola drinks). (D)

15. 2 The nurse reports the results of the VDRL to the HCP. The pregnant client must be treated for syphilis to prevent perinatal transmission of the disease. The rubella titer and blood sugar values are within normal range. The blood type is not a significant factor in this situation. (A)

16. 2, 3, 4, 5 During pregnancy, live virus immunizations are not administered because of potential teratogenicity. These immunizations include chickenpox, rubella, mumps, small pox, and live attenuated influenza vaccine. Vaccines containing killed viruses (tetanus, diphtheria, hepatitis B) may be administered, and in fact are recommended by the CDC if the immunizations are not up to date. (H)

17. 2 Pregnant clients experiencing mitral insufficiency or mitral valve prolapse have difficulty with the left ventricle moving the volume of blood forward that has been received from the left atrium. The normal physiologic tachycardia of pregnancy shortens diastole (artrial contraction) and decreases the time available for blood to flow across the valve. Physical exercise resulting in extreme exertion will place both the mother and fetus at risk. The client who is 16 years of age can obtain exercise as tolerated because of her age and state of physical fitness. The client who is 30 years of age can also exercise and does not need to unnecessarily limit her activity related to her job. The client who is 39 years of age is instructed to incorporate exercise gradually into a daily routine if she did not exercise prior to the pregnancy; additionally, exercise is important because of her gestational diabetes. (H)

18. 1 Clients are instructed to use only warm water to cleanse the nipples after breast-feeding. Soap is harsh and dries out the skin tissue, leading to cracked and sore nipples. The client is advised to select a bra with wide shoulder straps for good support. The caloric intake for a breast-feeding mother is 2,500 calories per day. Toughening the nipple is no longer advocated, and the nipple rolling method is no longer encouraged. (H)

19. 2, 3, 4, 6 An ultrasound provides information about the position of the fetus, position of the placenta, the size of the fetus, and the amount of amniotic fluid present. An ultrasound does not provide information directly about the cause of preterm labor, the maturity of the fetus's lungs, or the ability of the fetus to undergo the stress of labor. (R)

20. 3 Amoxicillin (Amoxil) is categorized by the FDA as a Category B drug, in which controlled studies in animals have not shown a fetal risk and fetal risk has not been reproduced in human studies. The drug is considered safe, and therefore the nurse does not question the order. The client is instructed to continue to take the full dose of the medication as prescribed. Category X drugs such as warfarin (Coumadin) have demonstrated fetal risk, and the risk to the fetus outweighs the benefits; therefore, the drugs are contraindicated during pregnancy. (D)

chapter

5 Complications of Pregnancy

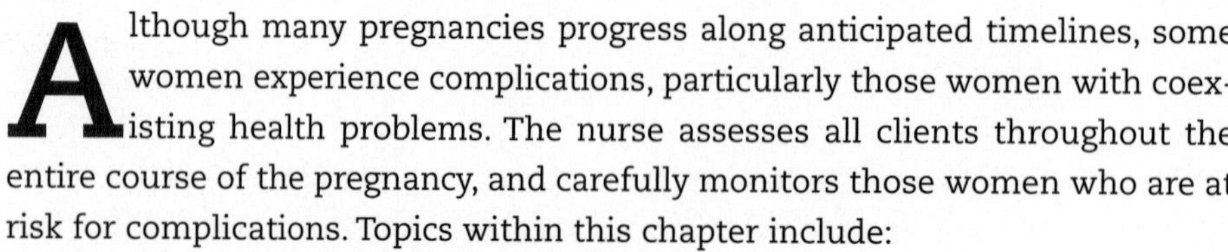

Although many pregnancies progress along anticipated timelines, some women experience complications, particularly those women with coexisting health problems. The nurse assesses all clients throughout the entire course of the pregnancy, and carefully monitors those women who are at risk for complications. Topics within this chapter include:

- Bleeding Disorders of Pregnancy: Abortion
- Cardiac Disease
- Abruptio Placenta
- Placenta Previa
- Type 1 and Gestational Diabetes
- Ectopic Pregnancy
- Gestational Trophoblastic Disease (Hydatid Mole)
- Hyperemesis of Pregnancy
- Infections
- Hypertensive Disorders of Pregnancy

Bleeding Disorders of Pregnancy: Abortion

I. Definition: Abortion, a bleeding disorder of pregnancy, is the spontaneous or elective termination of a pregnancy. Elective abortion occurs prior to the age of fetal viability, which varies by state law. This section discusses spontaneous abortion, the lay term for which is *miscarriage*.
  A. Types of spontaneous abortion
    1. Threatened: Unexplained bleeding, cramping with closed cervix that continues until the pregnancy is lost
    2. Missed: Fetus dies in utero but is not expelled
    3. Inevitable, or complete: All products of conception are expelled
    4. Incomplete: Fetus usually expelled, with placenta remaining in utero
    5. Septic: Infection present
    6. Recurrent: Three or more losses at 20 weeks' gestation or less
  B. Possible causes
    1. Genetic defects
    2. Maternal illness
    3. Exposure to chemicals
    4. No known etiology (occurs 50% of the time)
  C. Indications
    1. Vaginal bleeding
    2. Cramping

II. Nursing process
  A. Assessment
    1. Assess for risk factors prior to and during pregnancy.
      a. Prior losses
      b. Maternal disease (e.g., thyroid, genetic abnormalities, abnormalities of genitourinary track, environmental exposure, trauma, etc.)
    2. Perform a detailed maternal medical and pregnancy history, and history of allergies.
    3. Assess vital signs and fetal heart tones (FHTs) if more than 10 weeks' gestation.
    4. Assess count and weigh pads.
    5. Assess for presence of shock.
    6. Obtain diagnostic tests.
      a. Human chorionic gonadotrophin (hCG) levels
      b. Ultrasound
  B. Analysis
    1. Anticipatory Grieving related to risk of loss of pregnancy
    2. Acute Pain related to uterine cramping
    3. Fear related to potential for losing pregnancy
  C. Planning
    1. Maintain pregnancy by bed rest, decreased activity, and pelvic rest.
    2. Intervene during loss of pregnancy if medically indicated (maternal hemorrhage) to ensure safe maternal outcome.
    3. Provide support to parents during grieving process.
  D. Implementation
    1. Provide client teaching about the following:
      a. Possible outcomes of pregnancy given current bleeding, cramping, or cervical status
      b. Physical process of loss of pregnancy if at home or hospitalized
      c. Indications of blood loss, and the need to seek medical intervention
      d. Follow-up care, diet, activity, birth control after abortion is complete or current problem resolves
    2. Assess vital signs, bleeding, and cramping.
    3. Determine blood type and Rh status.
    4. If dilation and curettage (D&C), induction of labor, or dilation and suction if all products of conception not expelled (missed abortion):
      a. Perform assessments as previously mentioned.
      b. Insert IV line with large catheter for blood if needed.
      c. Obtain consents.
    5. Provide spiritual care if desired.
    6. Maintain bed rest through recovery.
    7. Administer Rh immune globulin postoperatively if Rh negative.

CN

III. Client needs
  A. Physiologic adaptation
    1. Inevitable, complete abortion
      a. Vaginal bleeding, cervix opens
      b. Body unable to maintain live fetus in utero, resulting in pregnancy loss and passing of all contents
    2. Missed abortion
      a. Fetal death without expulsion of fetus or placenta
      b. Induction of labor, D&C, or use of medication, depending on fetal size and age
    3. Threatened abortion
      a. Vaginal bleeding, cervix remains closed
      b. Threat to pregnancy declines, bleeding and cramping stop, pregnancy maintained
      c. Bed rest until bleeding decreases or ceases
  B. Management of care: Care of the client with a bleeding disorder of pregnancy requires critical

thinking skills and knowledge of assessment, and teaching and evaluation methods unique to the RN role. These skills cannot be delegated to an LPN or UAP.

1. Consult with an HCP about the probability of pregnancy outcome.
2. Review diagnostic tests (hCG level, ultrasound, Rh status, and hematocrit and hemoglobin if surgery is indicated).
3. Instruct client on discharge about the need to return to the health care setting if bleeding and cramping persist. Client discharged to pass products of conception if early, uncomplicated pregnancy with minimal bleeding and cramping.
4. If D&C or induction indicated:
   a. Preoperative care
      (1) Obtain consent, vital signs, IV, ultrasound.
      (2) Communicate with anesthesiologist.
      (3) Determine Rh status.
   b. Postprocedure care
      (1) Assess vital signs, fundal height, and lochia for bleeding every 15 min for the first hour.
      (2) Assess level of consciousness every 15 min for the first hour.
      (3) Advise activity as tolerated.
      (4) Instruct client to refrain from intercourse until bleeding stops.
      (5) Advise diet as tolerated.

C. Safety and infection control
   1. Instruct client to abstain from intercourse until bleeding stops.
   2. Initiate birth control if another pregnancy is not desired at this time.
   3. Instruct client to return to HCP if experiencing bleeding heavier than period or a foul odor, fever, or continued cramping or backache.

D. Health promotion and maintenance: Genetic counseling may be indicated if there is recurrent abortion.

E. Psychologic integrity
   1. Support need to grieve.
   2. Provide chaplain as needed.
   3. Refer to support groups.

F. Basic care and comfort
   1. Provide comfort measures as needed (e.g., analgesics, and rest and sleep opportunities).
   2. Provide emotional support by answering questions, encouraging client ventilation of emotions and fears, and providing grief counseling as needed.
   3. Determine and report changes in physical status (increased bleeding, signs of infection).
   4. Offer medication for cramping.

G. Reduction of risk potential
   1. Keep client on bed rest until bleeding stops if pregnancy is able to be maintained.
   2. Instruct "pelvic rest": No intercourse, with gradual return of physical activity.

H. Pharmacologic and parenteral therapies: Client will state the purpose for and associated side effects of all medications.
   1. Induction of labor by intravaginal prostaglandin E_2 or intravaginal misoprostol (Cytotec) if pregnancy is greater than 12 weeks
   2. Conscious sedation for D&C
   3. Ibuprofen, 800 mg po, for cramping postoperatively
   4. RhoGAM if Rh-negative

Cardiac Disease

I. Definition: A variety of cardiac problems could preexist or be caused by pregnancy and could impact maternal and fetal health during the pregnancy. Women with a history of cardiac disease are currently being treated earlier in life during their childbearing years and are choosing to have children. Older women with cardiovascular disease related to aging are bearing children later in life and may experience the pregnancy along with cardiac disease. One percent of all pregnancies are complicated by cardiac disease.

A. Heart disease in pregnancy is classified by the degree of client limitation. The New York Heart Association Cardiac Disease Classification is as follows:
   1. Class 1—disease with no limitation of physical activity; no pain or insufficiency
   2. Class 2—disease with slight limitation of activity; fatigue, dyspnea, palpitations result
   3. Class 3—disease with marked limitation of activity; minor activity causes excessive fatigue, palpations, and dyspnea
   4. Class 4—disease with inability to perform any activity without discomfort; cardiac insufficiency, angina may result at rest

B. Types of cardiac disease
   1. Congenital, may be caused by congenital anomalies
   2. Acquired, such as rheumatic heart disease and mitral valve disease
   3. Ischemic, such as ischemic heart disease

II. Nursing process

A. Assessment
   1. Obtain a detailed health history including cardiac history, prior pregnancies, medications (prenatal vitamins, ferrous sulfate, cardiac medications), and surgeries.

2. Perform a comprehensive physical assessment, including indications of cardiac changes during pregnancy (see also management of care).
   a. Increased heart rate
   b. 40% to 50% increase in blood volume
   c. Increased cardiac output and stroke volume
3. Perform fetal assessment.
   a. Ultrasound
   b. Nonstress testing (NST), fetal monitoring for late decelerations
   c. Biophysical profile to determine whether rate of fetal growth is currently adequate (intrauterine growth restriction indicates poor perfusion and poor growth) or if fetal demise
4. Assess nutritional status (see implementation).
5. Obtain diagnostic tests.
   a. ECG
   b. Chest x-ray
   c. Echocardiogram
   d. CBC for anemia

B. Analysis
1. Activity Intolerance related to decreased cardiac output
2. Risk for Fetal Injury related to effect of cardiac disease on pregnancy
3. Health-Seeking Behaviors related to impact of pregnancy on heart disease
4. Knowledge Deficit related to effect of cardiac disease on pregnancy
5. Anxiety related to unknown pregnancy and fetal outcome
6. Interrupted Family Process related to inability to continue normal family activities
7. Risk for Impaired Parenting related to inability to care for other children if the mother has other children
8. Risk for Imbalanced Fluid Volume related to changes resulting from movement of fluid from extracellular to intravascular spaces

C. Planning
1. Provide client and family teaching.
2. Relieve pain.
3. Manage weight and nutrition status.

D. Implementation
1. Assess nutrition and provide client teaching about diet.
   a. 2,400 calorie pregnancy diet—sufficient calories for fetal growth but not maternal adipose tissue deposition.
   b. Sodium restriction depends on type of cardiac problem.
2. Monitor patterns of weight gain.
3. Monitor baseline vital signs; assess changes over time.
4. Elevate client's legs at frequent intervals.
5. Apply elastic stockings as needed.
6. Administer medications (see pharmacologic and parenteral therapies).
7. Provide continuous assessment of client health status, health promotion activities, and educational needs.
8. Provide client teaching regarding danger signs indicating need to contact HCP.
9. Administer epidural for labor analgesia or anesthesia, if desired (less taxing on cardiac system).
10. Provide assistance with open glottis pushing, if indicated (laboring down, forceps, vacuum).

E. Evaluation
1. Client identifies signs and symptoms indicating worsening cardiac disease.
2. Client's cardiac status remains stable during pregnancy, labor, and delivery.
3. Infant is free from complications as result of maternal cardiac disease.

CN

III. Client needs

A. Physiologic adaptation
1. Heart murmurs occur in many well pregnant women and disappear after pregnancy.
2. By 28 weeks' gestation, a 40% to 50% blood volume increase has occurred. If the heart has been compromised, cardiac output may be compromised and maternal tissues and the fetus may not be perfused adequately.
3. Heart rate increases 10 to 15 beats per minute.
4. Cardiac output increases 30% to 50% by end of second trimester, and decreases as term nears.
5. Progesterone causes vasodilation.

B. Management of care: Care of the client with cardiac disease requires critical thinking skills and knowledge of assessment, and teaching and evaluation methods unique to the RN role. These skills cannot be delegated to an LPN or UAP.
1. Delegate responsibly those activities that can be delegated, including monitoring of intake and output, and baseline vital signs for the stable client. All monitoring information is reported to the RN.
2. Provide prenatal management of care.
   a. Refer client to preconception counseling with cardiologist to determine ability of client with cardiac disease to

carry pregnancy (e.g., Class I and Class II are usually able to carry pregnancy to term).
   b. Establish collaborative health care environment with OB, nursing staff, and internist/cardiologist.
   c. Assess cardiac status for symptoms of cardiac decompensation, congestive heart failure, or pulmonary edema (e.g., chest pain with activity, dyspnea, fainting with exertion, orthopnea). Assess client for activity level causing shortness of breath, dyspnea, cough, edema, jugular vein distention, as well as capillary refill and lung sounds. Obtain record of:
      (1) Category, how acquired.
      (2) Prior pregnancies, medications (prenatal vitamins, ferrous sulfate, cardiac medications), and surgeries.
3. Provide management of care during labor and delivery.
   a. Continue antepartal assessment.
   b. Use fetal monitoring for late decelerations and hypoxia.
   c. Maintain maternal oxygenation saturation status.
   d. Prepare client for potential forceps, vacuum delivery, or "laboring down" to decrease need to push.
   e. Prepare client for possible cesarean section if there is presence of significant cardiac decompensation and an inability to tolerate stress of labor.
   f. Monitor hemodynamic status as needed.
   g. Reduce stress and pain levels to maintain normal heart rate and BP.
4. Provide management of care during postpartum period.
   a. Continue antepartal assessments, looking specifically for problems associated with fluid shifts (increase in respiratory rate or distress, tachycardia).
   b. Assure adequate rest.
   c. Ambulate client to prevent thrombophlebitis.

C. Safety and infection control: Assess client for risk of thrombophlebitis during postpartum period; this is a critical time of readjustment because of excessive fluid volume re-entering the vascular system.

D. Health promotion and maintenance: Provide client and family teaching concerning the need for rest, activity changes, and potential limitations; continued care by cardiologist; and a support system.

E. Psychologic integrity
   1. Assist client to understand limitations caused by pregnancy.
   2. Assist client to plan for diversional activities.
   3. Encourage client to work with support system.

F. Basic care and comfort
   1. Provide comfort measures as needed (e.g., rest and sleep opportunities).
   2. Provide emotional support by answering questions, and encouraging client ventilation of emotions and fears concerning pregnancy and pregnancy outcome based on current knowledge of cardiac disease related to pregnancy.
   3. Support learning needs by educating client concerning cardiac disease in pregnancy, referring to support and resources as needed.
   4. Determine and report changes in physical status (e.g., shortness of breath, excessive edema, difficulty breathing with or without activity, chest pain).

G. Reduction of risk potential: Assess client for risk of heart failure and thrombophlebitis.

H. Pharmacologic and parenteral therapies: Client will state the purpose for and associated side effects of all medications used to treat cardiac disease during pregnancy.
   1. Antibiotics if taken prior to pregnancy (penicillin is not teratogenetic during pregnancy)
   2. Antibiotics given for any surgical procedures, labor, or dental work
   3. Docusate sodium—100 mg po twice a day as stool softener to prevent straining
   4. Heparin therapy—replaces warfarin (Coumadin) therapy during pregnancy as heparin does not cross the placenta
   5. Oxytocin—Pitocin 20 units/1,000 ml times 2 postpartum to control bleeding; used with caution related to blood volume increase and constrictive nature of Pitocin
   6. Prenatal vitamins once daily
   7. Ferrous sulfate—325 mg twice daily po to prevent anemia
   8. Other medications include:
      a. Furosemide (Lasix)
      b. Digitalis
      c. Beta-blockers (Inderal)

Abruptio Placenta

I. Definition: Abruptio placenta is an episode of premature separation of a normally implanted placenta after 20 weeks' gestation. Separation may be complete or partial, and may result in external or concealed bleeding. Areas that are separated may be small, or large enough to detach either part of or the entire placenta. Perfusion of the infant varies with the degree of detachment, ranging from no fetal distress to fetal demise. If delivery does not occur with the acute episode, the pregnancy may continue.

II. Nursing process

A. Assessment

1. Perform a comprehensive physical assessment at initiation of prenatal care, including signs and symptoms of placental abruption.
   a. Rigid, boardlike uterine tone, painful uterus with sustained tetanic uterine contractions
   b. Dull backache and/or abdominal pain
   c. Uterine contractions mild to firm or frequent with increased tone
2. Obtain a detailed health history, including past medical and surgical history, psychosocial history, and history of prior pregnancies (see risk factors).
3. Assess risk factors for abruption.
   a. Maternal hypertension
   b. Cigarette smoking
   c. Multiparity
   d. Prior abortions
   e. Cocaine and methamphetamine use
   f. Abdominal trauma
   g. Short umbilical cord
4. Assess vital signs, FHTs, fundal height, vaginal discharge, fetal movement, and any changes each prenatal visit.
   a. Fetal heart rate pattern may remain reassuring or become nonreassuring with decreased variability, late decelerations, decreased baseline and then absence of FHTs.
   b. Shock may occur with significant blood loss (vaginal or concealed), confusion as bleeding and shock progresses.
5. Obtain diagnostic tests.
   a. Ultrasound for diagnosis, placental location, clot visualization
   b. Clotting studies
      (1) PT, PTT
      (2) Platelet count
      (3) D-dimer
      (4) Fibrinogen, fibrin split products
      (5) Hematocrit (Hct) and hemoglobin (Hgb)

B. Analysis

1. Impaired Gas Exchange with Fetal Distress related to decreased placental blood flow
2. Acute Pain related to tissue ischemia
3. Anxiety related to unknown maternal and fetal outcome
4. Ineffective Tissue Perfusion: Fetal, related to lack of blood and oxygen to support life
5. Risk for Dysfunctional Grieving related to loss of child

C. Planning

1. Maintain adequate tissue perfusion for mother and infant.
2. Provide pain relief.
3. Manage fetal distress and maternal blood loss.
4. Provide client teaching regarding risk factors.
5. Observe and document current labor progress.
6. Monitor for worsening condition of mother and infant.
7. Explain status of problem and plan of care.
8. Reassure client.

D. Implementation (see management of care)

E. Evaluation

1. Infant remains in utero until term with no complications from abruption.
2. Infant is delivered without complications or long-term sequelae.
3. Client's condition remains stable throughout the perinatal period.

CN

III. Client needs

A. Physiologic adaptation

1. Uterus responds to stimuli (hypertension, trauma, cocaine, etc.) by contracting swiftly, resulting in placenta being pulled away from inside of uterus either partially or completely. Bleeding inside the uterus causes uterine irritability and sustained, painful uterine contractions (tetany). Uterine contractions:
   a. Decrease fetal and uterine blood supply, potentially causing hypoxia to infant and uterus as well as pain to mother.
   b. Eliminate oxygen to infant, causing fetal distress; poor oxygenation, if severe enough, can lead to fetal death.
2. Uterus remains contracted and painful until the source has been eliminated: Amount of vaginal or concealed bleeding depends on location and amount of placental detachment and ability of body to clot; large amount of bleeding into uterus can lead to maternal shock.
3. During a major abruption, maternal clotting factors are consumed; if all clotting factors are used, the mother has no

resources to carry out normal clotting in the remainder of body and can lead to disseminated intravascular coagulation.

4. When small abruptions occur, the remainder of the placental tissue can support fetal oxygenation. The fetus may be adequately perfused and have no distress, thus facilitating continuation of the pregnancy.

B. Management of care: Care of the client with abruptio placenta requires critical thinking skills and knowledge of assessment, and teaching and evaluation methods unique to the RN role. These skills cannot be delegated to an LPN or UAP.
   1. Assess risk factors; past medical and drug history; prior pregnancies; events of current pregnancy; signs and symptoms of abruption; trauma to abdomen; maternal and fetal vital signs, and contraction pattern.
   2. Provide client and family teaching about abruptio placenta and plan of care as time permits during acute stage.
   3. If delivery is necessary (acute phase, involving large abruption):
      a. Request clotting studies (see diagnostic studies in assessment section), and Hct, Hgb, platelets.
      b. Type and screen/crossmatch for blood replacement.
      c. Establish an IV line with large-bore intracatheter and administer fluids to replace volume.
      d. Replace blood, plasma, and platelets as needed.
      e. Monitor intake and output with precise blood loss.
      f. Assure that no vaginal examinations are performed.
      g. Prepare for cesarean section if blood loss cannot be stopped or if fetal distress exists or continues.
      h. Mobilize nursing and medical resources (anesthesiologists, surgery teams, neonatologists).
      i. Use continuous fetal monitoring particularly cognizant of signs of fetal distress (late decelerations, loss of variability and accelerations, sinusoidal patterns, terminal bradycardia).
      j. Assess maternal vital signs, and perform labor assessments every half hour.
      k. Administer oxygen at 10 to 12 L/min via mask.
      l. Place client in lateral position for best fetal perfusion.
   4. If delivery is not necessary immediately (expectant management for small abruption):
      a. Assess fetal and contraction monitoring.
      b. Monitor maternal vital signs.
      c. Monitor vaginal bleeding.
      d. Obtain a biophysical profile as needed.
      e. Obtain ultrasound as needed.
      f. Administer betamethasone (Celestone), 12 mg IM every 24 hr times 2, to mature fetal lungs if needed.
      g. Instruct client prior to discharge concerning need to return to hospital with abdominal pain, vaginal bleeding, or contractions.
      h. Facilitate follow-up care in office or home setting.

C. Safety and infection control
   1. Anticipate potential for postpartum hemorrhage (depletion of clotting factors).
   2. Anticipate potential for disseminated intravascular coagulation if abruption is unresolved.

D. Health promotion and maintenance: Provide client and family teaching concerning risk factors for abruption and ways to identify behaviors to minimize risk factors (see reduction of risk potential).

E. Psychologic integrity
   1. Explain medical problem and plan of care to allay fear for client and infant.
   2. Assist client and family in coping with changes.
   3. Identify stress factors and anxiety that may interfere with recovery.
   4. Refer to counseling and support groups to assist the client with meeting outcomes.
   5. Assess client's ability to manage independently, including social support and home health care needs.

F. Basic care and comfort
   1. Provide adequate pain management.
   2. Ensure maternal and fetal physical safety.
   3. Identify and notify HCP of changes that identify condition is worsening (signs of infection, increased bleeding, change in maternal and fetal vital signs, contraction pattern).
   4. Support client's emotional needs by providing opportunities to ask questions and ventilate fears or concerns.

G. Reduction of risk potential
   1. Provide client and family teaching regarding health behaviors that promote a healthy pregnancy and specifically decrease the risk of abruption.
      a. Eliminate all forms of tobacco.
      b. Eliminate or control hypertension.
      c. Refrain from recreational drug use.
      d. Avoid trauma and abusive situations.

2. Notify HCP immediately of vaginal bleeding and abdominal pain.

H. Pharmacologic and parenteral therapies: Client will state the purpose for and associated side effects of all medications used to treat abruptio placenta.
   1. Betamethasone (Celestone), 12 mg IM every 24 hr times 2, to facilitate fetal lung maturity
   2. IV line to maintain access and infuse fluids
   3. Platelets, blood volume expanders, PRBCs, depending on current status to replace clotting factors and platelets in maternal system

Placenta Previa

I. Definition: Placenta previa is the attachment of the placenta in the lower uterine segment, near or covering the internal cervical os; the condition is first identified in the second trimester with a self-limiting bleeding incident followed by more prolonged bleeding episodes as pregnancy continues. Bleeding recurs at any time during the remainder of pregnancy, particularly as cervix softens and dilates. Maternal blood loss can occur very rapidly with fetal oxygenation responding proportionately to maternal BP and cardiac output changes. Bleeding ends as a clot forms in cervical opening. Fetus may lie in an abnormal position (other than cephalic) as placenta occupies the portion of pelvis where the fetal head usually lies. Placenta previa occurs approximately in 1 in 200 pregnancies and the occurrence rate doubles in women who have had more than five children. Placenta previas are classified as:
   A. Complete/total—placenta covers the entire cervical os.
   B. Partial/incomplete—placenta covers a portion of the internal cervical os.
   C. Low-lying/marginal—placenta is located in the lower uterine segment but does not cover the os.

II. Nursing process
   A. Assessment
      1. Perform a comprehensive physical assessment at initiation of prenatal care, including assessment for signs and symptoms of placenta previa.
         a. Painless bright red vaginal bleeding (a classic sign) after 24 weeks' gestation
         b. FHTs remain within normal limits unless there is excessive blood loss
         c. Soft, nontender uterus with normal tone
         d. Bleeding episodes increase in frequency and duration
      2. Obtain a detailed health history, including past medical and surgical history, and obstetric history.
      3. Assess risk factors for placenta previa.
         a. Multipara
         b. Prior placenta previa
         c. Prior caesarean section or uterine surgery creating scars
         d. Smoking
         e. Elderly gravida
         f. Large placenta
      4. Assess vital signs, FHTs, fundal height, vaginal discharge, fetal movement, and variations and changes at each prenatal visit.
      5. Assess for presence or absence of clots with bleeding (indicates normal clotting ability).
      6. Obtain diagnostic tests.
         a. Ultrasound for placental location
         b. Clotting studies
            (1) PT, PTT
            (2) Platelet count
            (3) D-dimer
            (4) Fibrinogen, fibrin split products
         c. Hct, Hgb
   B. Analysis
      1. Ineffective Tissue Perfusion: Cardiovascular, related to decreased arterial blood flow
      2. Risk for Decreased Cardiac Output related to decreased arterial blood flow
      3. Anxiety (maternal) related to unknown outcome for client and infant
      4. Risk for Injury related to emergency delivery
      5. Risk for Infection related to blood loss and open vessels near cervix
   C. Planning
      1. Provide continual fetal monitoring.
      2. Prevent injury.
      3. Maintain tissue perfusion within normal limits.
      4. Monitor vital signs.
      5. Prevent anxiety.
   D. Implementation
      1. Discuss with HCP if infant is mature enough to deliver during particular bleeding episode.
      2. Determine maternal and fetal risks and benefits concerning continuing pregnancy or delivery with each bleeding episode.
      3. Avoid vaginal examinations as they may tear placenta adhering to cervix.
      4. Provide continual fetal monitoring during bleeding episode.
      5. Monitor maternal vital signs, vaginal bleeding.
      6. Document input and output including peripads and protective bed pads.
      7. Monitor for safety of client with ambulation after bleeding episode.
   E. Evaluation
      1. Client's vital signs remain stable.

2. Fetal heart rate remains stable, with moderate variability, range of 110 to 160 beats per minute with accelerations and no deceleration patterns.
3. Client's blood loss remains minimal.
4. Client displays no tension or anxiety.
5. Client's tissue perfusion is within normal limits as evidence by O_2 saturations, stable vital signs, and minimal blood loss.
6. Client delivers mature infant by cesarean or vaginal delivery without maternal morbidity.

CN

III. Client needs

A. Physiologic adaptation
1. As cervix softens and begins to change during pregnancy, bleeding episodes begin and repeat as more of the placental area is exposed.
2. The amount of blood lost during each bleeding episode increases as the pregnancy continues.

B. Management of care: Care of the client with placenta previa during bleeding episodes with no anticipated delivery requires critical thinking skills and knowledge of assessment, and teaching and evaluation methods unique to the RN role. These skills cannot be delegated to an LPN or UAP.
1. Document comprehensive physical assessment at initiation of prenatal care (see assessment); assess maternal and fetal vital signs, FHTs, fundal height, vaginal discharge, fetal movement.
2. Participate in assessing, preparing for, collecting samples, interpreting diagnostic studies (see diagnostic studies).
3. Validate that bleeding is from placenta previa.
   a. Painless, bright red vaginal bleeding (classic sign), sudden onset after 24 weeks' gestation
   b. FHTs remain within normal limits unless excessive blood loss
   c. Soft, nontender uterus with normal tone
4. Administer blood, plasma, platelets if blood loss is excessive, or if fetal or maternal hypoxia exists.
5. Maintain an IV infusion with large-bore intracatheter and regulate fluids to replace volume.
6. Type and screen/crossmatch/administer blood, plasma, platelets replacement as needed.
7. Monitor intake and output with precise blood loss.
8. Assure there are no vaginal examinations.
9. Prepare for cesarean section if blood loss does not decrease and stop or if fetal distress exists or continues.
10. Mobilize nursing and medical resources (anesthesiologists, surgery teams, neonatologists).
11. Provide continuous fetal monitoring particularly cognizant of late decelerations, loss of variability, no accelerations, sinusoidal patterns, and terminal bradycardia.
12. Monitor maternal vital signs.
13. Administer oxygen at 10-12 L/min via mask as needed.
14. Position client in left lateral position with wedge for best perfusion.
15. Administer betamethasone (Celestone), 12 mg IM every 24 hr times 2, to facilitate fetal lung maturity if delivery can be delayed 48 hr, and infant is preterm.
16. Prepare client for discharge to home when bleeding stops for 72 hr, no preterm labor and fetal well-being exists. Provide client and family education.
   a. Instruct client about home care needs and refocus on antepartum home care (see reduction of risk potential).
   b. Instruct client that delivery will be by cesarean section when infant completes 37 weeks, lungs are mature, or when an episode of bleeding threatens life of mother or infant.
      (1) Discuss alternate courses of action such as vaginal delivery if placenta previa is marginal or low lying.
      (2) Develop plan of care based on client preferences.
17. Perform ongoing assessments.
   a. Obtain biophysical profile as needed.
   b. Monitor vital signs, contractions, and infant for preterm labor.
   c. Initiate home fetal monitoring if indicated.
   d. Initiate HCP or home visits weekly.
   e. Monitor maternal activity level.
   f. Monitor uterine activity level.
   g. Assure client adherence to health care plan.
   h. Perform ultrasound as needed to evaluate position change of placenta (as growth occurs during pregnancy, placenta may be drawn into lower uterine segment).
18. Evaluate client understanding of current plan of care and ways the client can assist in her own care and recovery.
19. Review plan of care and standards of care to develop alternative strategies useful in caring for this type of client.

C. Safety and infection control: Prevent falls for mother and monitor infant for orthostatic hypotension and hypoxia as a result of blood loss, hypotension, and anemia from blood loss.

D. Health promotion and maintenance: Provide client and family teaching.
   1. Continue pregnancy diet at home with increased iron intake.
   2. Practice healthy behaviors to promote a healthy pregnancy and prevent injury.

E. Psychologic integrity: Discuss support network for client, work situation, care of other children, and provide referrals as needed.

F. Basic care and comfort
   1. Provide comfort measures as needed (e.g., rest and sleep opportunities).
   2. Provide emotional support by answering questions, encouraging client ventilation of emotions and fears, and providing grief counseling as needed.
   3. Determine and report changes in physical status such as increased bleeding, signs of infection, or fetal distress.

G. Reduction of risk potential: Provide client and family teaching regarding home care needs and refocus on antepartum home care.
   1. Discuss need for quick return to hospital with vaginal bleeding, lack of fetal movement, or beginning of contractions.
   2. Advise limited activity level during remainder of pregnancy to relieve pressure on cervix (may include bed rest); encourage left lateral position when resting.
   3. Advise pelvic rest (no intercourse, douching, or placing anything in vagina); discuss other methods of mutual pleasuring if needed.

H. Pharmacologic and parenteral therapies: Client will state purpose for and associated side effects of medications used to treat placenta previa.
   1. Ferrous sulfate, 325 mg po twice a day to treat anemia created by bleeding of placenta previa
   2. IV lactated Ringer to replace blood fluid volume during bleeding episode
   3. Platelets, blood volume expanders, packed red blood cells (PRBCs) depending on current status to replace clotting factors, and platelets in maternal system

Type 1 and Gestational Diabetes

I. Definition: Type 1 diabetes is a chronic autoimmune disorder of carbohydrate metabolism resulting in altered glucose production or resistance of the cells to the insulin being secreted. Proteins, fats, and carbohydrates are inadequately metabolized. The resulting hyperglycemia affects multiple organ systems including the eyes, nervous system, cardiovascular, renal, and hepatic systems. (See Chapter 27 for further information about diabetes mellitus.) Diabetes in pregnancy is classified according to the White classification, beginning with gestational diabetes and ending with diabetes with severe complications.

A. Insulin resistance increases as a result of human placental lactogen (HPL), estrogen, progesterone, adrenal cortisol, placing additional stress on the pregnancy and creating a temporary diabetic state that typically ends with the delivery of the placenta.

B. Insulin needs are low in the first trimester and become elevated in the second and third trimesters.

C. Risk to fetus/neonate occurs because of unstable, elevated blood glucose levels. Risks include macrosomia, hypoglycemia, hyperbilirubinemia, respiratory distress syndrome, congenital anomalies, and hypocalcemia.

II. Nursing process

A. Assessment
   1. Obtain a detailed health history including allergies, prior hospitalizations with pregnancy and diabetes, psychosocial history, and family medical history.
   2. Perform a comprehensive physical assessment at first prenatal visit.
   3. Assess risk factors to pregnancy as a result of diabetes.
      a. Maternal—obesity, hypertension, hydramnios, pre-eclampsia/eclampsia, ketoacidosis, and dystocia.
      b. Infant—congenital anomalies (heart, CNS, skeletal system), macrosomia, respiratory distress syndrome, hyperbilirubinemia, and intrauterine growth retardation.
   4. Assess risk factors for gestational diabetes.
      a. Maternal—prior large for gestational age (LGA) birth, client older than 40 years of age, first-degree relative with diabetes, prior stillborn, and cultural susceptibility (Hispanic, African American, Southeast Asian background)
      b. Infant—macrosomia, malformation, or congenital anomalies
   5. Perform diabetes-related assessments.
      a. Polyuria, polydipsia, polyphagia
      b. Ketonuria, glycosuria, recurrent infections
   6. Perform pregnancy-related assessments.
      a. Fundal height, weight gain
      b. FHTs, fetal movement
      c. Vital signs

7. Obtain diagnostic tests.
   a. Ultrasound
   b. Biophysical profile
   c. Kick count
   d. NST
   e. Oxytocin challenge test
   f. Blood glucose levels
      (1) Fasting blood glucose: Any time during pregnancy
      (2) Hemoglobin A1c: Any time during pregnancy
      (3) Blood glucose level: Every 1 hr during labor

B. Analysis
1. Risk for Injury: Maternal, related to possible complications of hypoglycemia and hyperglycemia
2. Risk for Injury: Fetal, related to possible complications of hypoglycemia and hyperglycemia
3. Health-Seeking Behaviors related to desire for healthy outcome of pregnancy complicated by diabetes
4. Knowledge Deficit related to management of diabetes
5. Risk for Anxiety related to management of diabetes
6. Risk for Imbalanced Nutrition: More than Body Requirements, related to diabetes

C. Planning
1. Maintain blood glucose between 70 and 110 mg/dl.
2. Provide client teaching about appropriate health behaviors.
3. Identify and manage possible complications of mother and fetus associated with diabetes in pregnancy.
4. Involve a multidisciplinary health care team including obstetrician, endocrinologist, nursing staff, and dietitian.
5. Provide client teaching on all aspects of balancing diabetes and pregnancy for healthy maternal and fetal outcomes.

D. Implementation
1. Provide interventions during antepartum period: Type 1 diabetes.
   a. Provide client teaching regarding the following:
      (1) Pregnancy and its impact on diabetes
      (2) Preventing complications by maintaining normal blood glucose levels through diet, exercise, insulin, and glucose monitoring
      (3) Signs and symptoms and interventions for hypo- and hyperglycemia
      (4) Perceived change in fetal activity
      (5) Plan of care through pregnancy
   b. Review normal glucose and insulin changes and needs during pregnancy.
   c. Discuss importance of normal maternal glucose levels on infant well-being.
   d. Review anticipatory guidance, need for additional obstetric care because of diabetes.
   e. Refer to dietitian to ensure appropriate dietary intake.
   f. Refer supplemental food program assistance for mother, infant, and other children, if needed.
   g. Administer medications such as insulin, prenatal vitamins, ferrous sulfate as ordered (see pharmacologic and parenteral therapies).
2. Provide interventions during antepartum period: Gestational diabetes.
   a. Emphasize importance of continued, frequent antenatal care.
   b. Emphasize identification of learning needs by client with a new disease process.
   c. Provide client teaching regarding the following:
      (1) Gestational diabetes
      (2) Preventing complications by maintaining normal blood glucose levels through diet, exercise, insulin use, and glucose monitoring
      (3) Signs and symptoms and interventions for hypo- and hyperglycemia
      (4) Perceived change in fetal activity
      (5) Plan of care through pregnancy
   d. Review normal glucose changes and needs during pregnancy.
   e. Assess normal maternal and infant development to determine deviations and prevent complications (kick count, NST, biophysical profile, amniocentesis).
   f. Review anticipatory guidance and need for additional obstetric care resulting from diabetes.
      (1) Refer to dietitian to ensure appropriate dietary knowledge.
      (2) Refer to social work if resources are not available for dietary intake.
      (3) Refer supplemental food program assistance for mother, infant, and other children, if needed.
      (4) Administer medications that may be used in treatment of gestational diabetes: Insulin, prenatal vitamins, ferrous sulfate (see pharmacologic and parenteral therapies).

3. Provide interventions during intrapartum period: Type 1 and gestational diabetes.
    a. Assess blood glucose levels hourly.
    b. Maintain adequate hydration with IV fluids and clear liquids.
    c. Provide continuous fetal monitoring.
    d. Prepare for fetal distress or difficult delivery even with no anticipated problems.
4. Provide interventions during postpartum period: Type 1 and gestational diabetes.
    a. Monitor blood glucose levels, which should quickly return to prepregnancy levels after delivery of placenta (breastfeeding further lowers blood glucose levels as metabolism increases to produce milk).
    b. Monitor maternal insulin requirements, which will return to prepregnancy levels for clients with type 1 diabetes.

E. Evaluation
1. Client delivers healthy, full-term infant.
2. Client maintains stable vital signs and blood glucose levels through delivery.
3. Client adheres to nutrition, exercise, and insulin requirements of diabetes and pregnancy.
4. Client adheres to nutritional requirements of gestational diabetes.

CN

III. Client needs

A. Physiologic adaptation
1. Insulin needs are low in first trimester because of nausea and vomiting associated with pregnancy, and low requirements of growing fetus.
2. Insulin antagonists produced by body as HPL decrease tissue sensitivity or ability to use maternal insulin.
3. Maternal glucose crosses the placenta; insulin does not.
4. High maternal glucose levels cross placenta and cause fetus to produce greater amounts of insulin to process glucose, causing the LGA infant.
5. Excessive insulin production in the fetus causes a decrease in surfactant production and increases the risk of respiratory distress syndrome.
6. Delivery of placenta is the point where insulin requirements return to prepregnancy levels.
7. Elevated glucose levels place client at increased risk for infection (UTIs, pyelonephritis, candidiasis).
8. Gestational diabetes diagnosed in the second trimester as HPL and insulin resistance increase, and physiologic needs of pregnancy increase.

B. Management of care: Care of the pregnant client with diabetes requires critical thinking skills and knowledge of assessment, and teaching and evaluation methods unique to the RN role. These skills cannot be delegated to an LPN or UAP.
1. Delegate responsibly those activities that can be delegated, including basic care needs and vital sign checks for the stable client. All monitoring information is reported to the RN.
2. Perform comprehensive physical assessments at beginning of pregnancy, during labor, and postpartum, and as needed during pregnancy.
3. Provide information on changes in client status to all HCPs on interdisciplinary team.
4. Facilitate collaborative care among endocrinologist, obstetrician, nutritionist, and nursing staff.
5. Provide interventions for type 1 diabetes.
    a. Prior to conception, assess client with type 1 diabetes for:
        (1) Type and etiology of diabetes, glucose control (Hgb A_{1c}).
        (2) Present complications of diabetes.
        (3) Diet and insulin regimen.
        (4) Knowledge of diabetes and its control.
        (5) Client commitment to diabetes control.
    b. Antenatal
        (1) Initiate tests per order of HCP and review results.
            (a) NST
            (b) Ultrasound for dating, size
            (c) Biophysical profile
            (d) Contraction stress tests
        (2) Reinforce self-care behaviors.
            (a) Glucose monitoring 4 times a day
            (b) Insulin administration
            (c) Balanced diet at approximately 2,500 calories per day and/or refer to dietitian
            (d) Exercise daily
            (e) Fetal kick counts
            (f) Monitoring for hypo-/hyperglycemia
        (3) Reinforce diet, exercise, and insulin as treatment for diabetes during the second and third trimesters as HPL and insulin resistance increase, and physiologic needs of pregnancy increase.

(4) Assess fetal status of the nondiabetic pregnant client at minimum in first trimester and with increased frequency during third trimester, or at any indication of declining fetal condition.

c. Labor and delivery
(1) Provide client and family teaching.
(2) Perform maternal physical assessment and monitoring.
(3) Perform fetal and contraction monitoring.
(4) Administer IV fluids without glucose.
(5) Administer insulin drip as needed.
(6) Check blood glucose levels hourly.
(7) Assess urine for protein and glucose.
(8) Prepare for fetal distress, dystocia, macrosomia, respiratory distress, and hypoglycemia even with fetal well-being.

d. Postpartum
(1) Provide client and family teaching.
(2) Perform normal postpartal maternal and infant care.
(3) Assess for infection.
(4) Provide continued blood glucose monitoring.
(5) Anticipate lowering of blood glucose levels and return of insulin needs to prepregnancy levels.
(6) Monitor infant diligently for hypoglycemia.

5. Provide interventions for gestational diabetes.
a. Antenatal
(1) Screen for gestational diabetes. (All pregnancies screened for gestational diabetes at 24 to 28 weeks' gestation.)
(2) On diagnosis, provide client teaching about the following:
(a) Glucose monitoring 4 times a day
(b) Insulin administration, if needed
(c) Balanced diet at approximately 2,500 calories per day and/or refer to dietitian
(d) Daily exercise
(e) Fetal kick counts (three to four kicks per hour)
(f) Monitoring for hypo-/hyperglycemia

b. Labor and delivery (see interventions for type 1 diabetes).

c. Postpartum (see interventions for type 1 diabetes).

C. Safety and infection control
1. Assess client for infection (pyelonephritis, vaginal infections) and Pre-eclampsia at each antenatal visit. These occur more frequently in diabetes.
2. Assess client support systems to prevent injury (hypo- and hyperglycemia) while in home setting.
3. Assess for neonatal effects as a result of diabetes.
a. Congenital anomalies (cardiac, skeletal, and neurologic as a result of maternal hyperglycemia)
b. Respiratory distress syndrome as a result of hyperinsulinemia in fetus with resultant decrease in surfactant production
c. Birth injury (fractured clavicles, shoulder dystocia, hyperbilirubinemia, hypocalcemia)
d. Fetal demise (greatest risk at period over 36 weeks)
e. Intrauterine growth restriction: Perfusion of mother and infant decreases as client's diabetes classification worsens; the fetus is also compromised and may be growth-retarded as the result of lack of oxygen and nutrients in system.

D. Health promotion and maintenance
1. Type 1 diabetes
a. Prepregnancy
(1) Provide anticipatory guidance to maintain glucose levels and prevent hypoglycemia or ketoacidosis.
(2) Provide client teaching—normal glucose levels are key to birthing infant without congenital anomalies, hypoglycemia, and hyperbilirubinemia.

b. Antenatal
(1) Provide client teaching about:
(a) Effect of diabetes on pregnancy.
(b) Preventing complications by maintaining normal blood glucose levels through diet, exercise, insulin use, and glucose monitoring.
(c) Signs and symptoms and interventions for hypo-and hyperglycemia.
(d) Perceived change in fetal activity.
(e) Plan of care.
(2) Assess normal maternal and infant development to determine

deviations and prevent complications (kick count, NST, biophysical profile, amniocentesis).

2. Gestational diabetes
   a. Antenatal
      (1) Assess lifestyle behaviors and cultural backgrounds placing client at risk (African Americans, Hispanics, American Indians, and Southeast Asians; obesity; family history of type 2 diabetes).
      (2) Provide client teaching about:
      (a) Gestational diabetes.
      (b) Preventing complications by maintaining normal blood glucose levels through diet, exercise, insulin use, and glucose monitoring.
      (c) Signs and symptoms and interventions for hypo-and hyperglycemia.
      (d) Perceived change in fetal activity.
      (e) Plan of care.
      (f) How to monitor blood glucose levels, signs and symptoms of hypo-/hyperglycemia, and fetal movement.
      (g) Need to maintain normal blood glucose to optimize potential for healthy infant and to prevent complications.
      (h) Dietary management—three meals, three snacks per day, totaling at 2,500 calories per day.

E. Psychologic integrity
   1. Assist client and family in coping with lifestyle, dietary and insulin needs, and changes in each of these areas that may be needed during pregnancy.
   2. Evaluate family as support system for client.

F. Basic care and comfort
   1. Provide comfort measures as needed (e.g., rest and sleep opportunities).
   2. Provide emotional support by answering questions and encouraging ventilation of emotions and fears.
   3. Support learning needs by educating concerning disease and pregnancy, referring to support, and providing resources as needed.
   4. Determine and report changes in physical status (hypo-/hyperglycemia, decreased or lack of fetal movement).

G. Reduction of risk potential
   1. Administer 50 g of glucola at 24 to 28 weeks' gestation for all pregnant women for diagnosis.
   2. Evaluate infant and maternal status throughout pregnancy.
   3. Conduct blood glucose testing a minimum of 4 times daily.
   4. Maintain blood glucose level within normal limits.
   5. Use NST, fetal kick counts beginning at approximately 32 weeks to provide early detection of fetal problems.
   6. Encourage prenatal visits more frequently (weekly).
   7. Advise a balanced pregnancy diet with snacks.
   8. Ensure exercise daily.
   9. Provide client teaching about:
      a. Hypo-/hyperglycemia signs and symptoms and treatment.
      b. Decreased or lack of fetal movement.
      c. Need for more frequent antenatal care.

H. Pharmacologic and parenteral therapies: Client will state the purpose for and associated side effects of all medications used to treat diabetes.
   1. Antenatal
      a. Prenatal vitamins, one daily
      b. Ferrous sulfate, 325 mg po twice daily if anemic
      c. Insulin therapy on sliding scale based on pregnancy and prepregnancy needs to maintain blood glucose of 70 to 110 mg/dl
   2. Labor and delivery
      a. IV fluids without glucose at 125 ml/hr
      b. Insulin drip on sliding scale if unable to maintain blood glucose during labor
         (1) Maintains blood glucose level between 70 and 110 mg/dl
         (2) Side effects such as hypoglycemia; ketoacidosis can occur if the client does not receive enough insulin
         (3) Insulin antagonists decrease tissue sensitivity or ability to use maternal insulin
   3. Postpartum
      a. Resume prenatal vitamins, if breastfeeding
      b. Ferrous sulfate, 325 mg po twice daily
      c. Insulin needs return to prepregnancy level if bottle feeding
      d. Insulin needs may be slightly lower than prepregnancy levels if breastfeeding (increase basal metabolic rate to produce breast milk).

Ectopic Pregnancy

I. Definition: An ectopic pregnancy occurs when a fertilized egg becomes implanted outside the uterus, usually in the fallopian tube. Implantation can also occur in the abdomen. Signs, symptoms, and nursing care depend on the location of the implantation and the gestational age of the pregnancy. The earlier the ectopic pregnancy is diagnosed, the greater the opportunity for medication as intervention rather than surgery.

II. Nursing process
- A. Assessment
  1. Obtain a complete health history including history of:
     - a. Pelvic inflammatory disease.
     - b. Sexually transmitted infections (STIs).
     - c. Tubal ligations.
  2. Assess for missed periods, and tenderness or pain on lower right or left side of abdomen.
  3. Assess for dark brown or red bleeding.
  4. Obtain date of last normal period.
  5. Obtain diagnostic tests.
     - a. Ultrasound
     - b. Beta hCG levels
     - c. Serum progesterone levels
- B. Analysis
  1. Risk for Maternal Injury related to rupture of fallopian tube.
  2. Acute Pain related to swelling and/or rupture of fallopian tube.
  3. Ineffective Tissue Perfusion: Cardiovascular, related to blood loss secondary to rupture of ectopic pregnancy.
  4. Risk for Anemia related to blood loss secondary to rupture of fallopian tube.
  5. Anticipatory Grieving related to pregnancy loss.
  6. Powerlessness related to loss of pregnancy secondary to ectopic pregnancy.
- C. Planning
  1. Provide interventions to prevent rupture of fallopian tube.
  2. Discuss possibility of surgery if the tube is in danger of rupturing or if it ruptures.
  3. Provide support for grieving process.
  4. Minimize client pain and blood loss.
- D. Implementation
  1. Treat ectopic pregnancy with either medication or surgery depending on stage of pregnancy and condition of mother.
  2. Provide client teaching concerning current and future pregnancy.
- E. Evaluation
  1. Client's ectopic pregnancy is identified and treated before tubal rupture occurs.
  2. Client has no signs or symptoms of infection or hemorrhage as a result of pregnancy or surgery.
  3. Client works through the grieving process after the loss of pregnancy.
  4. Client is aware of factors placing her at risk for future ectopic pregnancies.
  5. Client identifies and uses support systems.

CN

III. Client needs
- A. Physiologic adaptation
  1. Early pregnancy signs and symptoms present as with a normal pregnancy.
  2. Pain on the right or left side begins as distention of fallopian tube occurs and continues until intervention or rupture take place.
  3. Bleeding and potentially shock begin when rupture occurs.
- B. Management of care: Care of the client with ectopic pregnancy requires critical thinking skills and knowledge of assessment, and teaching and evaluation methods unique to the RN role. These skills cannot be delegated to an LPN or UAP.
  1. Surgical intervention:
     - a. Provide preoperative and postoperative care.
     - b. Assess maternal vital signs and blood loss.
     - c. Obtain diagnostic tests.
       - (1) CBC, Hct, Hgb, type and cross-match for blood prior to surgery
       - (2) Blood type, Rh status
       - (3) Ultrasound
     - d. Administer IV for fluid volume replacement and medication administration.
  2. Chemical intervention: Ectopic pregnancy is unruptured, less than 4 cm in diameter by ultrasound.
     - a. Methotrexate IM X 1
     - b. Weekly hCG levels after therapy, anticipating downward trends
- C. Safety and infection control
  1. Identify risk factors for any pregnant woman.
  2. Provide client teaching to prevent STIs and preserve fallopian tube function.
  3. Encourage seeking health care early in pregnancy to prevent need for surgery.
  4. Limit number of vaginal examinations as these may rupture tube, causing further bleeding.
  5. Recognize that vaginal blood loss is not an accurate indication of true blood loss.
  6. If vaginal bleeding is present, assess for signs of shock: tachycardia, hypotension, shoulder pain, vertigo.

D. Health promotion and maintenance: Instruct client to avoid becoming pregnant for 3 months after surgical or medication intervention.
E. Psychologic integrity
   1. Monitor client during grieving process.
   2. Evaluate support systems of client.
F. Basic care and comfort
   1. Provide comfort measures as needed (e.g., analgesics, rest and sleep opportunities).
   2. Provide emotional support by answering questions, encouraging ventilation of emotions and fears, and providing grief counseling as needed.
   3. Determine and report changes in physical status, including:
      a. Increased bleeding, signs of infection.
      b. Increased pain levels.
G. Reduction of risk potential
   1. Provide client teaching concerning risk factors for ectopic pregnancy.
   2. Inform client of risk of future ectopic pregnancy and future fertility.
   3. Provide client teaching concerning side effects of methotrexate, if used.
   4. Advise client to obtain pelvic rest (avoiding intercourse, use of tampons for 6 weeks postinterventions).
   5. Eliminate risk of ectopic pregnancy by preventing STIs with use of condoms.
H. Pharmacologic and parenteral therapies: Client will state the purpose for and associated side effects of all medications used to treat ectopic pregnancy.
   1. Methotrexate IM X 1
   2. Avoidance of sun during treatment
   3. IV for fluid volume replacement if needed
   4. Blood products for RBC replacement

Gestational Trophoblastic Disease (Hydatidiform Mole)

I. Definition: Gestational trophoblastic disease refers to a pregnancy that results in proliferation and degeneration of the trophoblastic villi and never contains a viable pregnancy. During degeneration, the cells fill with clear fluid and appear as clear, fluid-filled vesicles that develop as grapelike clusters. Disease may be classified as complete mole, with incomplete chromosomal material, or partial mole, with portions of the villi developing normally while other layers contain triple chromosomes.

II. Nursing process
A. Assessment
   1. Assess for indications including:
      a. Fundal height greater than gestational age as determined by last menstrual period.
      b. Presence of excessive nausea and vomiting.
      c. Symptoms of pre-eclampsia (hypertension).
      d. By 16 weeks' gestation, dark brown or red vaginal bleeding; as bleeding becomes more perfuse, the clear fluid-filled vesicles are also expelled.
      e. Vital signs with potentially elevated BP.
      f. Absence of FHTs.
   2. Obtain diagnostic tests.
      a. Ultrasound
      b. CBC, platelets prior to surgery
      c. hCG levels
B. Analysis
   1. Disturbed Thought Process related to anger from loss of "normal" pregnancy
   2. Anxiety related to surgical removal of molar pregnancy
   3. Fear related to surgical removal of molar pregnancy
   4. Risk for Ineffective Coping related to feelings of loss related to removal of pregnancy thought to be normal
   5. Deficient Fluid Volume related to removal of uterine vesicles
   6. Anxiety related to risk of carcinoma
C. Planning
   1. Minimize pain associated with surgery.
   2. Provide client teaching concerning disease, interventions (surgery), recovery, and future pregnancy.
   3. Engage support system to assist client.
   4. Refer to support groups after surgery.
D. Implementation
   1. Perform comprehensive physical and psychosocial assessments while providing care.
   2. Provide information on changes in client status to the HCP and appropriate members of the health care team.
   3. Establish IV for fluid volume replacement prior to surgery.
   4. Provide client teaching concerning anesthesia, surgical, and recovery procedures.
   5. Monitor vital signs, especially BP.
   6. Maintain accurate intake and output.
   7. Evaluate vaginal bleeding pre- and post-surgery.
   8. Provide preoperative and surgical recovery care per protocol with vital signs, orientation, vaginal bleeding, mobility, O_2 saturation, and grief response.
   9. Monitor client for potential problems such as increased vaginal bleeding, increased BP, tachycardia, and pallor.
E. Evaluation
   1. Client experiences minimal pain.
   2. Client tolerates surgery without side effects.

3. Client progresses through grieving process without difficulty or guilt.
4. Client does not become pregnant and remains without hCG for 1 year.
5. Client remains free of choriocarcinoma.

CN

III. Client needs
 A. Physiologic adaptation
  1. Trophoblastic tissues proliferate and become edematous without sufficient blood supply from fetus; develop into grapelike cluster.
  2. Excessive levels of hCG are produced by overgrown trophoblastic cells; with increased hCG levels, nausea and vomiting are increased and continue past first trimester.
  4. Vesicles cause uterine distention greater than normal uterine size for gestational age; uterine size greater than expected for weeks of pregnancy.
  5. Anticipate BP to be elevated as part of disease process.
 B. Management of care: Care of the pregnant client with gestational trophoblastic disease requires critical thinking skills and knowledge of assessment, and teaching and evaluation methods unique to the RN role. These skills cannot be delegated to an LPN or UAP.
  1. Delegate responsibly those activities that can be delegated, including basic care needs and vital sign checks for the stable client. All monitoring information is reported to the RN.
  2. Establish IV for fluid volume replacement prior to surgery.
  3. Review laboratory studies, particularly CBC and platelets.
  4. Type and screen for blood products, if needed, prior to dilation and suction.
  5. Provide client and family teaching regarding anesthesia, surgical, and recovery procedures (see also safety and infection control and reduction of risk potential).
  6. Monitor vital signs, especially BP, elevated related to disease process.
  7. Document intake and output.
  8. Evaluate vaginal bleeding pre- and post-surgery.
  9. Provide preoperative and surgical recovery care per agency policy with attention to monitoring vital signs, keeping the client orientated, documenting vaginal bleeding, assuring mobility, monitoring O_2 saturation, and assessing grief response.
  10. Recognize potential complications, including:
   a. Increased vaginal bleeding.
   b. Increased BP.
   c. Tachycardia.
   d. Pallor.
  11. Communicate information on changes in client status to HCP and appropriate members of health care team.
 C. Safety and infection control: Provide client and family teaching.
  1. Report any of the following to the HCP after surgery: foul vaginal odor, abnormal bleeding, and/or fever.
  2. Use methotrexate as follow-up chemotherapy after hydatidiform mole evacuation, if prescribed.
  3. Follow-up with 1 month checks of hCG levels for 1 year.
 D. Health promotion and maintenance
  1. Instruct client to obtain diet high in iron to replace lost RBCs.
  2. Discuss use of contraception for 1 year after molar evacuation.
 E. Psychologic integrity
  1. Monitor client for anxiety and fear related to surgical procedure.
  2. Refer client to support groups for grief counseling related to loss of "normal" pregnancy.
 F. Basic care and comfort
  1. Provide comfort measures as needed (e.g., nutritious diet, and rest and sleep opportunities).
  2. Support learning needs by educating client concerning disease and needs for follow-up care.
  3. Determine and report changes in physical status to include recurrent nausea and vomiting, and vaginal bleeding.
 G. Reduction of risk potential: Provide client and family teaching.
  1. Seek medical care for pain and bleeding when it occurs.
  2. Notify HCP in subsequent pregnancies for ultrasound verification of normal pregnancy as there is four- to fivefold increased risk for second molar pregnancy.
  3. Obtain and use birth control for 1 year after molar pregnancy.
  4. Have hCG levels drawn every month for 1 year to validate absence of pregnancy and that all of molar pregnancy is removed.
 H. Pharmacologic and parenteral therapies: Client will state the purpose for and associated side effects of all medications used to manage gestational trophoblastic disease, including methotrexate course of chemotherapy.
  1. Teach client to avoid sun exposure and alcohol intake.
  2. Ensure cautious use for client with infection.

Hyperemesis of Pregnancy

I. Definition: Hyperemesis of pregnancy refers to nausea and vomiting of pregnancy severe enough in the first trimester to lead to dehydration, electrolyte imbalance, and significant weight loss. Hyperemesis may also continue into the second trimester. The condition occurs in one in 200 to 300 women. Nausea and vomiting do not allow the client to maintain normal nutrition. The etiology is unknown.

II. Nursing process

A. Assessment

1. Obtain a detailed health history, psychosocial history, and history of nausea and vomiting (daily, and in prior pregnancies), and eating patterns, including daily food intake.
2. Assess fluid status: intake and output, and skin tenting.
3. Assess weight on day-to-day basis; weight trend prior to and during pregnancy.
4. Obtain diagnostic tests.
   a. Hct hemoconcentration due to dehydration associated with vomiting and fluid losses
   b. Urine testing for ketones, pH level

B. Analysis

1. Deficient Fluid Volume related to nausea and vomiting of pregnancy
2. Ineffective Coping related to stress of pregnancy

C. Planning

1. Promote hospitalization and NPO status for 24 hr; advance diet as tolerated.
2. Administer IV fluids to rehydrate and maintain electrolyte balance.
3. Provide slow introduction of food and fluid after being NPO.
4. Initiate home health follow-up to assess wellness.
5. Maintain TPN if hospitalization and NPO status do not reduce or solve nausea and vomiting.

D. Implementation (see management of care)

E. Evaluation

1. Client remains free of nausea and vomiting during remainder of pregnancy.
2. Client maintains 2,500 calorie diet for a healthy maternal and infant outcome.

CN

III. Client needs

A. Physiologic adaptation

1. Nausea and vomiting is attributed to hCG and progesterone levels.
2. Increased functioning of the thyroid as a result of hCG may cause nausea and vomiting in pregnancy.

B. Management of care: Care of the pregnant client with hyperemesis requires critical thinking skills and knowledge of assessment, and teaching and evaluation methods unique to the RN role. These skills cannot be delegated to an LPN or UAP.

1. Delegate responsibly those activities that can be delegated, including basic care needs, vital sign checks, and assessments and detailed documentation of past and current nausea and vomiting (all monitoring information is reported to the RN).
   a. How late in day nausea and vomiting continues
   b. Number of times a day client vomits
   c. Amount of emesis each time client vomits
   d. Client's feelings related to pregnancy
2. Maintain client NPO status for first 24 hr.
3. Initiate IV infusion to eliminate dehydration and maintain hydration.
4. Administer medications.
5. Monitor input and output, and daily weights.
6. Assess vital signs per agency protocol.
7. After 24 hr, introduce clear liquids slowly, then crackers, and slowly advance to regular diet if tolerated without nausea and vomiting.
8. Monitor all episodes of nausea and vomiting.
9. Provide quiet, nonstimulating environment conducive to rest.
10. Monitor for signs and symptoms of dehydration: skin tenting, urine testing for color, pH, ketones.
11. Assess FHTs according to age of fetus.
12. Communicate information on change in client status to the HCP and members of health care team.
13. Provide consultations with dietitian.

C. Safety and infection control: Prevent risk to health of client and fetus (see health promotion and maintenance).

D. Health promotion and maintenance: Provide client and family teaching.

1. Avoid consuming spicy foods and strong-smelling foods.
2. Ask for medication when nausea and vomiting begin rather than waiting until vomiting is inevitable.

E. Psychologic integrity

1. Encourage family support systems.
2. Evaluate client's acceptance of pregnancy.

F. Basic care and comfort

1. Provide comfort measures as needed (e.g., rest and sleep opportunities).

2. Provide emotional support by answering questions and encouraging ventilation of emotions and fears concerning pregnancy.
3. Support learning needs by educating concerning hyperemesis in pregnancy, referring to support resources as needed.
4. Determine and report changes in physical status—dehydration, ketones, urine, and excessive weight loss.

G. Reduction of risk potential: Ensure small, frequent meals and no strong odors to foods; separate foods from liquids; provide attractive food presentation; assure hot foods are hot and cold foods are cold.

H. Pharmacologic and parenteral therapies: Client will state the purpose for and associated side effects of all medications used to treat hyperemesis of pregnancy.
1. Ondansetron (Zofran)
2. Promethazine (Phenergan)
3. Hydroxyzine (Vistaril)

Infections

I. Definition: Infections in pregnancy describe an inflammation of tissue with many potential etiologies: (a) viral—may have no cure, such as AIDS, herpes; (b) bacterial—treated with antibiotics; (c) fungal; and (d) protozoan and parasitic. During pregnancy both the mother and fetus may be threatened by the infection and both need to be considered in treatment plans. Treatment options depend on etiology of the infection, normal course, outcomes of the infective process, age of the pregnancy, and effects of the medications on the mother and the fetus. (See Table 5-1 for detailed information on each infection.)

II. Nursing process

A. Assessment
1. Perform a comprehensive physical assessment, including assessment for signs and symptoms.
2. Obtain a detailed health history, including history of sexual activity and lifestyle behaviors (IV drug abuse, alcohol use, nutrition, levels of stress, and fatigue).
3. Assess characteristics of body systems and areas affected by infection.
4. Obtain diagnostic tests.
   a. Blood draw, swab of area
   b. Culture and sensitivity
   c. Microscopic analysis

B. Analysis
1. Anxiety related to effects of infection on pregnancy
2. Disturbed Body Image related to infection
3. Deficient Knowledge related to infection
4. Acute Pain related to effects of infection
5. Ineffective Coping related to infection status
6. Sexual Dysfunction related to active disease process
7. Social Isolation related to effect of disease process on relationships
8. Risk for Maternal Injury related to infection
9. Risk for Fetal Injury related to infection

C. Planning
1. Provide client and family teaching (see health promotion and maintenance).
3. Administer treatment specific for infection.
4. Test for cure of infection if indicated.
5. Refer to support groups as needed.
6. Use barrier precautions, and hand hygiene appropriate for type of infection.

D. Implementation (see management of care)

E. Evaluation
1. Client has no recurrence of infection or disease.
2. Client participates in measures to prevent recurrence or prevent transmission of an infection or a disease to partner.
3. Client's infection is cured by selected treatment without injury to the fetus.
4. Client correctly identifies precautions in sexual practices to prevent transmission to others.

CN

III. Client needs

A. Physiologic adaptation: Depending on type, infection may be transmitted to infant transplacentally, during birth process, breast-feeding, or by after birth exposure from parent. Infections acquired during first 3 months of pregnancy (when fetal development is occurring) are most teratogenic.
1. For infection without cure, goal is to minimize symptoms and exposure of others to disease.
2. Exposure to medications used to treat infections may be teratogenetic to fetus. Treatment may be delayed until first trimester is completed and risk of teratogenetic effects are decreased (metronidazole [Flagyl]).
3. Fetal risk of contracting noncurable infections is often improved with initiation of treatment as soon as the pregnancy is diagnosed (AIDS).

B. Management of care: Care of the pregnant client with infection requires critical thinking skills and knowledge of assessment, and teaching and evaluation methods unique to the RN role. These skills cannot be delegated to an LPN or UAP.
1. Assess for signs and symptoms of infection.
2. Perform culture or draw blood specific to type of infection.

Table 5-1 Infections During Pregnancy

Condition, Etiology	Transmission, Maternal Signs and Symptoms (S&S)	Fetal/Neonatal Effects, S&S, Implications for Pregnancy
TOXOPLASMOSIS Parasite: *Toxoplasma gondii* Transplacental transmission	• Transmission: Acquired by consuming raw/undercooked meat, handling infected cat litter • Labs: Levels of IgG (long-term prior infection) and IgM (acute infection) • S&S: Rash, flulike symptoms • Rx: Pyrimethamine, sulfadiazine	• Dx: Fetal blood samples for IgM (best testing); may be infected at birth or may be congenital • S&S: Asymptomatic chorioretinitis, hydro- or microcephaly • Rx: Sulfa
HEPATITIS A (Infectious hepatitis)	• Transmission: Spread by droplets, hands, poor hand hygiene, especially after bowel movement • S&S: Flulike symptoms; may cause spontaneous abortion, premature labor, in utero fetal demise • Treatment: Gamma globulin	• Fetal anomalies if exposed in first trimester; may cause spontaneous abortion, PTL, in utero fetal demise • Treatment: Gamma globulin given to exposed infants
HEPATITIS B	• Transmission: Spread like HIV (needles, syringes, blood, sex, body fluid exchange), and transplacentally • Dx: Positive for hepatitis B surface antigen • S&S: Fever, rash, anorexia, malaise, jaundice RUQ pain • Treatment: All mothers screened at first prenatal visit; inoculation during pregnancy is OK	• S&S: PTL and birth involves infection during birth process • Treatment: Hepatitis B immune globulin; hepatitis B vaccine
RUBELLA 3-day or German measles	• Transmission: Droplet • S&S: Fever, rash, mild lymphedema • Potential outcome is miscarriage • Dx: Maternal titer more than 1:16, immune; titers between 1:16 and 1:8, indeterminate; less than 1:8, nonimmune • Treatment: No rubella vaccination during pregnancy related to risk of anomalies; rubella vaccine given postpartum, no pregnancy for 3 months after vaccine	• Risk of congenital anomaly highest if exposed in first trimester, more subtle after fourth month • S&S: Hearing loss, cataracts, cardiac defects, IUGR • Rx: Isolate infant until non infective
CYTOMEGALOVIRUS (CMV) Incubation 28-60 days	• Transmission: Respiratory (droplet) or sexually transmitted; at-risk women are those working in day care, nurses in pediatric setting • Transmission to fetus: transplacental, birth canal, breast-feeding • Dx: IgG and IgM antibody testing • S&S: Asymptomatic illness or flulike symptoms • RX: None, symptom management; antiviral therapy may be used	• S&S: Asymptomatic or mental retardation, deafness, blind, seizures • Implications: CMV develops in infants born to mothers who had primary infection in pregnancy • Implications: Children in day care settings usually test positive

HERPES SIMPLEX VIRUS I AND II
Transmitted by person actively shedding virus
Incubation 2-10 days
Shedding for 3 mo after primary infection
1-2 days after recurrent infection
	• Transmission:
	  • Labor: Ascending infection after rupture of membrane (ROM)
	  • Transplacentally if primary infection is during pregnancy
	• Transmission prevention: Cesarean section if ROM less than 4-6 hr. After 6 hr ROM, infants usually infected and can deliver vaginally
	• Dx: Cell culture
		• Transmission:
		  • Transplacental
		  • Ascending during labor
		  • Infected birth canal
		  • Directly by family
		• S&S: First and second week of life with vesicles or encephalitis, or all system involvement
		• RX: Acyclovir used in mothers and infants

(Continued)

Table 5-1 Infections During Pregnancy (*Continued*)

Condition, Etiology	Transmission, Maternal Signs and Symptoms (S&S)	Fetal/Neonatal Effects, S&S, Implications for Pregnancy
HERPES SIMPLEX VIRUS I AND II (continued)	• S&S: • Vesicles on mucous membranes, external genitalia; women more severely infected than men • Primary lesions most virulent, painful • Stress reactivates virus	
AIDS Spread by exchange of body fluids, breast-feeding, transplacentally	• At-risk groups: Women with partners from geographic area where prevalent; IVDA, persistent, recurrent STDs, history of multiple partners; persons with blood transfusions between 1978 and 1985 • S&S: See cough, pneumonia, diarrhea, oral lesions, weight loss. See also Chapter 29 • Dx: EIA, Western blot test • Pregnancy not encouraged • Prenatal period: Symptomatic HIV women have PTL, infections, IUGR, stillbirths treated with antivirals. Educate and treat for alcohol, drug use, sex practices • Intrapartum period: External fetal monitoring, cesarean section, treat with AZT during labor • Postpartum period: Continue antiviral treatment. HIV virus can be transmitted via breast-feeding; the risk of transmission is reduced if the mother is being treated.	• Implications: Newborns will have + antibodies for HIV, at birth will be asymptomatic, 20%-30% will remain positive by 15-18 months and will develop AIDS • Transmission to newborn in three ways: • Maternal circulation (horizontal transmit) • Labor and delivery: Inoculation or ingestion of maternal blood and other infected fluids, EFM (vertical transmit) • Breast milk • Treatment: Zidovudine for 6 weeks (counseling, immunizations); bathe infant as soon as possible before injections • If no treatment, the risk of transmission to infant is 20%-30% • If treated, the risk for transmission to infant is less than 2%
GONORRHEA *Neisseria gonorrhoeae* Spread by direct contact with infected lesions Vertical transmission to infant Incubation 2-5 days	• Risk factors: Age less than 20 years, early onset of sex, multiple partners, coexists with chlamydia • S&S: Asymptomatic, dysuria, green-yellow discharge, PID, chronic pain • Treatment: Rocephin, cefixime; all recent partners treated • In pregnancy: PTL, premature rupture of membranes. Postpartum endometritis: at risk (prior to pregnancy) and in pregnancy.	• S&S: Ophthalmia neonatorum, sepsis • Rx: Erythromycin both eyes at birth, ceftriaxone
SYPHILIS Treponema pallidum, spirochete Incubation 10-90 days	• Transmission: Skin, mucous membranes by direct lesion contact, placental • Dx: RPR, VDRL; three stages: • Primary chancre: painless ulcer at entry point (most infectious) • Secondary: red macules on soles, palms, lymphadenopathy • Tertiary: Internal organs, CV, CNS • Rx: • Penicillin G 2.4 million units IM for primary and secondary • 7.2 million units for tertiary • Tetracycline or doxycycline; tetracycline contraindicated in pregnancy • Test client at first prenatal visit and at 36 weeks' gestation • Treat partner concurrently	• S&S: Depends on number of weeks' gestation • Abortion, PTL • Transferred to infant in utero begin at 16 weeks' gestation • 50% of infected neonates die

Condition, Etiology	Transmission, Maternal Signs and Symptoms (S&S)	Fetal/Neonatal Effects, S&S, Implications for Pregnancy

CHLAMYDIA
Chlamydia trachomatis
	• Risk factors: Female less than 20 years of age; low economic status; multiple sex partners
	• S&S: Asymptomatic, or mucopurulent discharge, bleeding, dysuria; may have GC also
	• Dx: Lab culture (takes 4–7 days); cultures at first prenatal visit
	• Rx: Doxycycline, azithromycin (may lead to PID, infertility, sterility); treat partner concurrently
		• Implications: Stillbirth, PTL, conjunctivitis, pneumonia
		• Rx :
		  • All newborns' eyes are treated with erythromycin regardless of exposure
		  • Oral erythromycin for 2 weeks for systemic chlamydia

TUBERCULOSIS (TB) *Mycobacterium tuberculosis*	• S&S: Positive PPD (TB skin test) and chest x-ray (skin testing is safe in pregnancy, chest x-rays after 20 weeks are safe with shield). S&S include cough, fever, chills, night sweats • Treatment: Isoniazid (INH) with vitamin B_6 to prevent neurotoxicity in infant	• Transmission: Occurs by aspirating infected amniotic fluid, airborne; isolate infant from mother if infant is negative, mother has positive sputum culture • S&S: Fever, lethargy, failure to thrive • Dx and Rx: Skin test infant at birth; if positive, placed on isoniazid and retested in 3-4 months

HUMAN PAPILLOMAVIRUS
Genital warts called condylomata acuminate, incubation 3-6 months
Most common viral STI
Causes cervical cancer
	• Risk: Multiple partners, genital contact with infected person
	• Dx: Colposcopy, direct visualization, biopsy, pap smear
	• S&S: Highly contagious warts on labia, vulva, anus, rectum, etc. (occurs at entry site, direct skin to skin contact); worsens during pregnancy
	• Rx:
	  • No Rx eradicates all of virus. Iodine compounds, laser, cryotherapy, electrocautery. Recurrence 70%; not for use during pregnancy
	  • Pregnancy causes overgrowth, increases friability of lesions
	  • Condom use
		• S&S: Hoarseness, abnormal cough, cry, respiratory or laryngeal papillomatosis

VARICELLA
Primary infection is chicken pox, secondary is shingles
Incubation: 2-3 weeks
	• Transmission: Transplacental
	  • 90% of women are immune based on prior immunization or having had disease
	  • Greatest risk to infant when maternal infection less than 5 days before delivery to 2 days after delivery
	• Treatment: VZIG (varicella zoster immune globulin); must be given within 72 hr of exposure to be effective. (↓effects on fetus)
		• Rx: VZIG at birth; acyclovir

GROUP B STREPTOCOCCUS (GBS, GBBS) (Leading cause of life-threatening perinatal infections in United States)	• 10%-30% of pregnant women carry micro-organisms as normal vaginal flora in GI, GU track • Effects: miscarriage, stillbirth, preterm birth, fever septicemia, puerperal infection • Risk factors: African American women; less than 20 years of age; history of prior birth with GBS; multiple gestation; heavy colonization of bacteria; planned cesarean section not treated	• Leading cause of neonatal sepsis and meningitis. Other effects: blindness, deafness, MR, learning disabilities, death. • <u>Early onset:</u> S&S of sepsis usually present within 72 hr after birth • <u>Late onset:</u> 8 days to 3 months. • Meningitis • Treatment: Antibiotics

(Continued)

Table 5-1 Infections During Pregnancy (*Continued*)

Condition, Etiology	Transmission, Maternal Signs and Symptoms (S&S)	Fetal/Neonatal Effects, S&S, Implications for Pregnancy
GROUP B STREPTOCOCCUS (continued)	• Dx: All women cultured at 35-37 weeks' gestation; if positive, Rx in labor • Rx: Penicillin, 5 million units loading dose, IVSS, then 2.5 million units every 4 hr during labor. Want 4-6 hr from first dose to delivery	
BACTERIAL VAGINOSIS *Gardnerella*	• S&S: Fishy vaginal odor, discharge profuse, thin, gray white, "clue cells" present • Rx: Metronidazole (Flagyl) 250 mg three times a day for 7 days; no alcohol during Rx; no Rx in first trimester; associated with PTL, chorioamnionitis, UTIs	• Implications: May cause PTL and birth
CANDIDIASIS *Candida albicans*	• Risk factors: Antibiotic therapy, diabetes, pregnancy, obesity, diets high in refined sugars • S&S: Vaginal, vulvar itching, swelling and redness, discharge is thick, white, cottage cheesy in patches attached to vaginal walls, wet smear shows yeast • Rx: Miconazole (Monistat), clotrimazole (Gyne-Lotrimin)	• Implications: Infant may contract during delivery; may be transferred to maternal nipples with breast-feeding
TRICHOMONAS	• S&S: Asymptomatic or yellow/green/ frothy malodorous discharge, inflamed vulva, cervix, itchy • Dx: Can see protozoa swimming on smear • Rx: Metronidazole 2 g po; treat partner concurrently	• Transmission: Infant contacts through contact in birth canal
URINARY TRACT INFECTION Usually *Escherichia coli*	• Risk factors: History of UTI, sickle cell trait, diabetes, pregnancy, poor hygiene. If not treated, may lead to pyelonephritis • Dx: Urinalysis with more than 100,000 in colony count. Protein, WBCs, bacteria in urine • Rx: Increase oral fluid intake; monitor intake and output, and S&S of pyelonephritis; antibiotics; education regarding hygiene	• No implications

3. Notify appropriate health care agencies (state board of health) of particular infections and diagnoses.
4. Facilitate follow-up outpatient testing as needed.
5. Assess for home health care needs.
6. Provide client and family teaching about infection, including:
   a. Medications, effects, and side effects of medication.
   b. Self-assessment for recurrence of infection.
   c. Risk of transmission of infections to sexual partners and methods to prevent transmission.
   d. Role of infection in future childbearing.

C. Safety and infection control
   1. Facilitate health behavior teaching to prevent infection or disease for all sexually active and presexually active individuals:
      a. Safest sex is abstinence.
      b. Use condoms for prevention of STIs and birth control.
   2. Advise partners of clients with STIs to be treated concurrently.

D. Health promotion and maintenance: Provide client and family teaching.
   1. Practice self-care behaviors to prevent recurrences and exposure of others.
   2. Practice health behaviors that promote a healthy lifestyle.

E. Psychologic integrity
   1. Assist client and family in coping with sexual practice and lifestyle changes.
   2. Identify stress factors and anxiety that may interfere with recovery.
   3. Refer to support groups and counseling appropriate for infection or disease process.

F. Basic care and comfort: Discuss methods to provide physical comfort based on type of infection.

G. Reduction of risk potential: Identify pharmacotherapy for consideration to prevent recurrence and decrease effects of infection or disease.

H. Pharmacologic and parenteral therapies: Client will state purpose, dosage, timing, and side effects of medications to treat infection or disease. These therapies may include:
   1. Antiviral medications
   2. Antibiotics
   3. Antiparasitic agents
   4. Immunizations

Hypertensive Disorders of Pregnancy

I. Definition: Hypertensive disorders of pregnancy may be pre-existing or may occur during pregnancy. (See also Chapter 20 for discussion of management of clients with hypertension.) Hypertensive disorders complicate 12% to 20% of pregnancies, with certain populations being at highest risk (Native Americans, African Americans, Hispanics). Hypertension is the most common medical complication in pregnancy and a leading cause of maternal morbidity and mortality in the world. Treatment is aimed at containing the hypertension, preventing seizures, and preventing fetal and maternal mortality.

A. Types of disorders
   1. Chronic hypertension: Hypertension existing before 20 weeks' gestation and sustained after 12 weeks postpartum; often occurs prior to pre-eclampsia
   2. Pre-eclampsia (gestational hypertension): An elevation of blood pressure after 20 weeks' gestation accompanied by proteinuria. Pre-eclampsia, gestational hypertension, or pregnancy-induced hypertension describes the same pregnancy-related condition, which is classified as mild or severe:
      a. Mild pre-eclampsia includes hypertension greater than 140/90, but less than 160/110, 4 to 6 hr apart within 7 days, and proteinuria 300 mg or greater in 24 hr. This disorder can be managed from home.
      b. Severe pre-eclampsia requires hospitalization and aggressive medical treatment. The disorder involves more than one of the following: BP elevations of 160/110 or greater, proteinuria of more than 2 g in 24-hr urine sample, oliguria of greater than 30 ml/hr, headaches, dizziness, epigastric pain, blurred vision, pulmonary edema, epigastric pain, thrombocytopenia, liver dysfunction or development of HELLP syndrome (see following description) or eclampsia.
   3. Eclampsia: Pre-eclampsia complicated by a seizure or coma hospitalization and aggressive medical treatment is required.
   4. HELLP syndrome: Liver dysfunction indicating worsening pre-eclampsia. Usually develops before 36 weeks' gestation. Clients with this syndrome require hospitalization and need to deliver regardless of gestational age because of the risks to the mother. Morbidity and mortality rates for mothers and infants are very high. The acronym identifies the changes that occur:
      a. Hemolysis—destruction of RBCs
      b. EL—indicating elevated liver enzymes (LDH more than 600 International Units per liter, AST more than 70 International Units per liter), and
      c. LP—low platelets at a level of less than 150,000 mm^3.

B. Etiology: The precise etiology of pre-eclampsia is unknown. The only cure is delivery of the infant and placenta as pre-eclampsia is based on the presence of trophoblastic tissue. Pathophysiology of pre-eclampsia centers around the inability of spiral arteries to dilate, an inflammatory response that is exaggerated, and a dysfunctional endothelial cell response. The client exhibits decreased perfusion, decreased plasma volume, and changes in the clotting cascade and the endothelium.

C. Indications: Classic signs and symptoms include hypertension and proteinuria. Edema is more severe than swelling of the lower extremities normally associated with normal pregnancy and involves sudden weight gain and edema of hands and face.

D. Complications: Pre-eclampsia places a woman at risk for abruptio placenta, congestive heart failure, cerebral edema, hemorrhage, stroke, DIC, renal failure, and hepatic failure. Fetal risks include hypoxia and intrauterine growth retardation as a result.

II. Nursing process

A. Assessment

1. Obtain a detailed health history, including history of allergies, prior hospitalizations with pregnancy, psychosocial history, and family medical history.
2. Perform a comprehensive physical assessment including vital signs and SpO_2.
3. Assess for risk factors prior to pregnancy.
   a. Primigravida
   b. Multiparity with a different father for current fetus
   c. Client age over 35 years or under 17 years
   d. Diabetes
   e. Pre-eclampsia in prior pregnancy
   f. Family history of pre-eclampsia
   g. Obesity
   h. Pre-existing renal, vascular, or hypertensive disease
4. Assess for risk factors for developing pre-eclampsia during pregnancy.
   a. Multiple gestation
   b. Hydatiform mole
   c. First pregnancy
5. Assess outcome of results of maternal risk factors.
   a. Seizure activity, clonus, exaggerated reflexes, headache, cerebral edema
   b. Thrombocytopenia, pulmonary edema, increased ocular pressure
   c. Hepatomegaly leading to epigastric pain
6. Assess outcome of risk to fetus.
   a. Intrauterine growth retardation
   b. Hypoxia during labor and delivery
7. Obtain diagnostic tests.
   a. Ultrasound
   b. Biophysical profile
   c. Kick count
   d. CBC
   e. LDH, AST, PT, PTT, fibrinogen

B. Analysis

1. Risk for Maternal Injury related to pre-eclampsia
2. Risk for Fetal Injury related to pre-eclampsia
3. Health-Seeking Behaviors related to desire for healthy outcome of pregnancy complicated by diabetes
4. Knowledge Deficit related to altered management of pregnancy by diagnosis of pre-eclampsia
5. Risk for Anxiety related to outcome of health problem
6. Compromised Family Coping related to maternal separation from family
7. Ineffective Tissue Perfusion: Cardiovascular, related to effects of pre-eclampsia
8. Impaired Gas Exchange to mother and fetus related to maternal vasospasms and hypovolemia
9. Ineffective Tissue Perfusion related to pulmonary edema
10. Risk for Hepatic Injury related to hypertension

C. Planning

1. Reduce BP to normal limits.
2. Prevent seizures, cerebral edema, and stroke.
3. Prevent renal disease and hepatic complications.
4. Deliver healthy infant at full term without complications through vaginal delivery with oxytocin (Pitocin) induction if indicated.

D. Implementation (see management of care)

E. Evaluation

1. Client and caregivers detect signs of worsening pre-eclampsia in the home setting.
2. Client explains pre-eclampsia, its treatment, and possible complications.
3. Client maintains stable vital signs and experiences no seizures.
4. Client delivers a healthy, full-term infant with no complications.

CN

III. Client needs

A. Physiologic adaptation: Decreased levels of perfusion occur as result of hypertension. Vasospasms result in fluid shifts from intravascular to intracellular spaces, intravascular coagulation, and sensitivity to angiotensin II. This results in:

1. Edema (generalized, pulmonary) leading to facial, hand, and abdominal edema
2. Hemolysis of RBCs leading to decreased Hgb and Hct
3. Cerebral spasms leading to blurred vision, seizures

4. Microemboli leading to elevated liver enzymes, nausea and vomiting, right upper quadrant pain, liver rupture
5. Clumping of platelets and fibrin deposits leading to thrombocytopenia

B. Management of care: Care of the pregnant client with hypertensive disorders of pregnancy requires critical thinking skills and knowledge of assessment, and teaching and evaluation methods unique to the RN role. These skills cannot be delegated to an LPN or UAP.
1. Facilitate collaborative care among endocrinologist, obstetrician, nutritionist, and nursing staff.
2. Document physical assessments and care to the client with pre-eclampsia antenatally, during labor and delivery, and postpartally.
3. Provide information on changes in client status to all HCPs on interdisciplinary team.
4. Plan home care for client with mild pre-eclampsia and follow through with home or office visit to assess change in maternal/fetal status. Provide client and family teaching for care in the home environment:
   a. Self-monitoring for worsening condition
      (1) Edema of face and hands
      (2) Worsening headaches
      (3) Visual changes, epigastric pain
      (4) Nausea/vomiting
   b. Self-monitoring for worsening fetal status
      (1) Kick count
      (2) Perceived change in fetal activity
   c. Need for frequent prenatal assessments with
      (1) NST
      (2) Biophysical profile
      (3) Ultrasound to monitor growth
   d. Resting on left side
   e. Daily weights
   f. Urine testing for protein, glucose
5. Plan hospital care for client with severe pre-eclampsia.
   a. Establish an IV infusion and maintain at "keep open" rate.
   b. Begin magnesium sulfate therapy to prevent seizures.
      (1) Loading dose 4 to 6 g over 15 to 30 min followed by maintenance dose of 1 to 3 g/hr
      (2) Calcium gluconate (1 g IV or 10 ml of 10% solution) available as anecdote for magnesium toxicity
   c. Use continuous maternal, fetal, and contraction monitoring if antenatal.
   d. Assess:
      (1) Input and output.
      (2) Reflexes 3+ to 4+.
      (3) Pulmonary edema: Breath sounds and oxygen saturation.
      (4) Urine testing for protein (3+, 4+), specific gravity.
      (5) 24-hr urine for protein (greater than 5 g equals severe pre-eclampsia).
      (6) Headache, dizziness, blurred vision, epigastric pain, visual disturbances, level of consciousness, and oliguria.
      (7) Clonus one or more beats.
      (8) Diagnostic studies, including:
         (a) CBC: Decreased Hct.
         (b) LDH: Greater than 600 International Units per liter.
         (c) AST: Greater than 70 International Units per liter.
         (d) PT: Unchanged.
         (e) PTT: Unchanged.
         (f) Fibrinogen: Unchanged.
      (9) Presence of magnesium toxicity:
         (a) Respiratory rate less than 12.
         (b) Decreased or absent reflexes.
         (c) Disorientation.
      (10) Vital signs, particularly BP and respiratory rate.
   e. Administer oxygen as ordered (2 to 4 liters per mask or canula) as needed to maintain adequate perfusion.
   f. Limit fluid intake to 125 ml/hr to prevent pulmonary edema.
   g. Administer antihypertensive medications.
   h. Conduct neurologic assessment for headaches, level of consciousness, visual disturbances, and nausea and vomiting.
6. Plan hospital care for client with eclampsia: Care for severe pre-eclamptic and with onset of seizure.
   a. Maintain patent airway.
   b. Administer oxygen as ordered.
   c. Protect from injury.
   d. Provide continuous fetal and contraction monitoring if pregnant.
   e. Administer medication for seizures.
      (1) Magnesium sulfate
      (2) Diazepam (Valium) 5 to 10 mg IV to halt seizures

7. Plan hospital care for client with HELLP syndrome.
    a. Transfer to tertiary care center.
    b. Use invasive hemodynamic monitoring.
    c. Document assessments/interventions for severe pre-eclampsia.
    d. Monitor labor leading to vaginal delivery over cesarean section.

C. Safety and infection control
1. Use padded side rails and dim lights for nonstimulating environment to minimize overstimulation of CNS.
2. Prepare and have medications, oxygen, and suction available in case of seizures.

D. Health promotion and maintenance: Provide client and family teaching about preventing more severe pre-eclampsia by maintaining bed rest in left lateral position even though the client feels well.

E. Psychologic integrity
1. Assist client and family in coping with lifestyle changes.
2. Stress importance of supportive family members and environment.

F. Basic care and comfort
1. Provide physical comfort measures as needed (e.g., rest and sleep opportunities, and pain medication).
2. Determine and report changes in physical status.
    a. Presence or increase in clonus and/or seizure activity.
    b. Decrease in urinary output.
    c. Complaints of epigastric pain, headache, and/or visual disturbances.

G. Reduction of risk potential
1. Remind client to follow recommendations of HCP.
2. Conduct NST and fetal kick counts beginning at approximately 32 weeks' gestation.
3. Instruct client to have weekly prenatal visits.
4. Ensure a balanced pregnancy diet.

H. Pharmacologic and parenteral therapies: Client will state purpose for and associated side effects of all medications used to treat hypertensive disorders of pregnancy.
1. Medications used to manage hypertension (see discussion of hypertension in Chapter 20)
2. Magnesium sulfate therapy to prevent seizures: Loading dose 4 to 6 g over 15 to 30 min followed by maintenance dose of 1 to 3 g/hr
4. Calcium gluconate (1 g IV or 10 ml of 10% solution) available as anecdote for magnesium toxicity
5. Hydralazine 5 to 10 mg IV for acute hypertension
6. Methyldopa (Aldomet) during pregnancy on a long-term basis because of its safety in pregnancy
7. Labetalol hydrochloride (Normodyne)—IV bolus/infusion

Bibliography

Klossner, N. J., & Hatfield, N. (2005). *Introduction to maternity and pediatric nursing*. Philadelphia: Lippincott Williams & Wilkins.

Pillitteri, A. (2006). *Maternal & child health nursing: Care of the childbearing and childrearing family* (5th ed.). Philadelphia: Lippincott Williams & Wilkins.

Simpson, K. R., & Creehan, P. A. (2007). *AWHONN's perinatal nursing* (3rd ed.). Philadelphia: Lippincott Williams & Wilkins.

Witt, C. (2007). *Advances in neonatal care*. Philadelphia: Lippincott Williams & Wilkins.

CHAPTER 5

Practice Test

Bleeding Disorders of Pregnancy: Abortion

1. A woman has an incomplete abortion (miscarriage) at 12 weeks' gestation. After a D&C, she returns to the women's unit. After assessing the vital signs and amount of bleeding, the nurse should next:

□ 1. Assess level and consistency of the fundus.
□ 2. Confirm client's blood type and Coombs' status.
□ 3. Read postoperative orders written by the HCP.
□ 4. Request that the grief counselor visit the client in the morning.

2. AF The nurse is providing discharge instructions to a woman who has had a D&C following an incomplete abortion (miscarriage). Which of the following instructions does the nurse include in the discharge plan? Select all that apply.

□ 1. Abstain from sexual relations for 6 weeks.
□ 2. Report temperature over 101°F to HCP.
□ 3. Remain on bed rest for 3 days following the surgery.
□ 4. Take analgesics as prescribed for 2 to 3 days.
□ 5. Avoid heavy lifting until the bleeding stops.

Cardiac Disease

3. A client is 10 weeks' pregnant, has class III cardiac disease, and is taking Digoxin. The nurse teaches the client to take which of the following measures?

□ 1. Increase fluid intake.
□ 2. Rest in bed a large part of the day.
□ 3. Have a nonstress test (NST) in the third trimester.
□ 4. Be placed on anticoagulation therapy.

4. During labor a client with a history of class III heart disease will:

□ 1. Be unable to receive epidural anesthesia.
□ 2. Be kept on her side with her head elevated.
□ 3. Not have an IV infusion to avoid fluid overload.
□ 4. Be encouraged to push to avoid the need for forceps.

Abruptio Placenta

5. AF The nurse is assessing a woman who is at 24 weeks' gestation. Which of the following place this woman at risk for abruptio placenta? Select all that apply.

□ 1. Client smokes 10 cigarettes per day.
□ 2. Client has delivered five other children.
□ 3. Client is 26 years of age.
□ 4. Client walks 2 miles five times a week.
□ 5. Client tripped and fell on her abdomen 4 weeks ago.

Placenta Previa

6. A multipara is admitted to the hospital at 36 weeks' gestation. The client indicates that she has experienced a gush of painless bright red blood from her vagina. The client is most likely experiencing which of the following?

□ 1. Placenta previa.
□ 2. Abruptio placenta.
□ 3. Ectopic pregnancy.
□ 4. Trophoblastic disease.

Type 1 and Gestational Diabetes

7. At 28 weeks' gestation, a pregnant client is tested for gestational diabetes. The client asks, "Why am I being tested? There is no history of diabetes in my family." The nurse should explain that she is being tested because pregnancy causes:

□ 1. Changes in protein metabolism.
□ 2. Changes in carbohydrate metabolism.
□ 3. Decreased insulin resistance.
□ 4. Decreased insulin secretion.

8. The nurse is reviewing the chart of a client in a prenatal clinic who is G3P2. Which of the following situations alerts the nurse to the possible presence of gestational diabetes in this woman?

□ 1. Client was diagnosed with an eating disorder as an adolescent.
□ 2. Fetus has been determined to be small for gestational age (SGA).
□ 3. Client has had recurrent monilial vaginitis that does not respond to treatment.
□ 4. Client has been diagnosed with oligohydramnios.

9. In discussing management of insulin and diet with a G4P3 pregnant, type 1 diabetic woman, the nurse should:

- □ 1. Emphasize the fact that her prescribed prepregnant diet will still be suitable.
- □ 2. Explain that high parity contributes to depletion of maternal nutrient stores.
- □ 3. Explain that diet and insulin needs may vary at different times during pregnancy.
- □ 4. Instruct her to regulate her diet and insulin on the basis of urine tests for sugar.

10. Which of the following is the reason for conducting an NST after 35 weeks' gestation in a woman whose pregnancy is complicated by diabetes?

- □ 1. Fetus may be less active in a diabetic woman.
- □ 2. Placenta may be less able to carry oxygen because of vascular changes from the diabetes.
- □ 3. Diabetic mother is more likely to develop an infection, so needs to be delivered early.
- □ 4. Diabetic mother may have a very large infant, causing continuous peritoneal dialysis.

Ectopic Pregnancy

11. AF A client is hospitalized with a ruptured tubal pregnancy (ectopic pregnancy). The nurse should do which of the following? Select all that apply.

- □ 1. Increase oral fluids.
- □ 2. Place the woman on bed rest.
- □ 3. Prepare the woman for a cesarean delivery.
- □ 4. Start an IV.
- □ 5. Wait for the fetus to be expelled.
- □ 6. Monitor the woman for shock.

Gestational Trophoblastic Disease (Hydatidiform Mole)

12. A woman in her twelfth week of pregnancy presents with these signs: persistent headache, hypertension, some visual disturbances, intermittent reddish brown or dark brown discharge, and a fundal measurement larger than expected for her estimated date of confinement (EDC). These symptoms indicate which of the following?

- □ 1. Threatened abortion
- □ 2. Ectopic pregnancy
- □ 3. Hydatidiform mole
- □ 4. Pregnancy-induced hypertension

Hyperemesis of Pregnancy

13. AF A client has hyperemesis gravidarum. The nurse is assessing the client for potential risks to her health and that of her fetus. The nurse reviews the integrated history and physical database as noted below.

Name *Chistine Smith, RN* Date *3/12/09*

GASTROINTESTINAL

Stool: ✓ Formed; ___ Loose; ___ Liquid; ___ Mucus; ___ Ostomy; ___ Incontinent
Color: ✓ Brown; ___ Black; ___ Red tinged; ___ Bloody
Diarrhea: ___
Constipation: ___
Abdomen: ✓ Soft; ___ Rigid; ___ Nontender; ___ (Location)
Bowel sounds: ✓ Present; ___ Absent; ___ Hypoactive; ___ Hyperactive

Obese ___; Thin ___; Emaciated ✓; Nourished ___
*NUTRITION:
___ Special diet
___ Tube feeding
___ Chewing problem
___ Swallowing problems
✓ Nausea/vomiting
___ Poor appetite
✓ Wt (loss)/gain *5* lb
*Refer to dietitian if any

GENITOURINARY/REPRODUCTIVE

Color of urine: ___ Yellow; ✓ Amber; ___ Pink/Red tinged; ___ Brown; ___ Orange; ___ Clear; ___ Cloudy

___ Ileo-conduit
___ Incontinent ___ Catheter in place
___ Frequency ___ Urgency
___ Difficulty in initiating stream
___ Pain ___ Burning
___ Oliguria ___ Anuria
___ Dialysis

Access site: ___ Date of last dialysis: ___
Comments: ___
Date of LMP ___ Date of last PAP ___
Breast self-exam ___ ___ Yes ___ No
Use of contraceptives: ___ Yes (type ___) ___ No ___ N/A
Vaginal discharge: ___ Yes (describe ___) ___ No
Bleeding: ___ Yes (amount ___) ___ No
Pregnancies:
Pregnant ✓ Yes ___ Weeks ___ Gravida ___ Para ___ No
Date of last prostate exam ___
Testicular self-exam ___ Yes ___ No
Comments: *Skin dry with poor turgor, Hemoglobin 14 gm/dL, Hematocrit 40%, Potassium is 3.0 mEq/L, Sodium is 140 mEq/L*

The nurse bases the care plan on data that indicate the client has signs of:

- □ 1. Dehydration.
- □ 2. Hyperkalemia.
- □ 3. Anemia.
- □ 4. Active bowel sounds.

Infections

14. Care for the pregnant woman who is HIV-positive includes:

- □ 1. Retesting for HIV antibodies every trimester.
- □ 2. Decreasing exposure to infection.
- □ 3. Wearing gloves whenever any care is given.
- □ 4. Counseling about the need to abstain from all sexual activity during pregnancy.

Hypertensive Disorders of Pregnancy

15. A multipara is scheduled for admission to the hospital for severe gestational hypertension. The nurse should take which of the following measures?

- □ 1. Monitor BP every shift.
- □ 2. Assess level of consciousness once every 4 hr.

□ 3. Check for Homans sign every 4 hr.
□ 4. Insert a Foley catheter for accurate hourly measurement of urine output.

16. AF The nurse is assessing a woman who is 20 weeks' pregnant. Which information on the client's prenatal record indicates that she is at increased risk for pre-eclampsia? Select all that apply.
□ 1. Anemic before pregnancy.
□ 2. 16 years of age.
□ 3. Chronic renal disease.
□ 4. A single fetus.
□ 5. Obesity.
□ 6. Bleeding in the first trimester.
□ 7. Fatigue in the second or third trimester.
□ 8. A family history of pre-eclampsia.

17. The nurse is caring for a woman who is 8 months' pregnant and admitted to the hospital with eclampsia. The client is receiving magnesium sulfate. The nurse monitors the effectiveness of the drug by noting which of the following?
□ 1. Decreased BP
□ 2. Pain relief
□ 3. Less anxiety
□ 4. Prevention of labor contractions

18. A client who is 8 months' pregnant is admitted to the hospital because of hypertension. The client is receiving a magnesium sulfate infusion. The nurse monitors the client for side effects of the drug. Which one of the following side effects is expected?
□ 1. Chills and shaking.
□ 2. Flushing.
□ 3. Epigastric pain.
□ 4. Irritability.

19. The nurse in a prenatal clinic is reviewing charts of pregnant women seen that day. Which of the following information indicates that the nurse should call the client and have her return to the clinic the next day for follow-up to assess her for potential worsening of pre-eclampsia?
□ 1. "Two months pregnant—abdominal discomfort at times accompanied by small amounts of vaginal spotting, BP 146/100."
□ 2. "Seven months pregnant—BP 150/110, proteinuria, gained 10 lb in last 2 weeks."
□ 3. "Three months pregnant—BP 90/64, occasional headache after using eyes for fine work."
□ 4. "Six months pregnant—epigastric discomfort after meals, headaches after exercise, BP 128/80, gained 8 lb since last visit."

20. AF Which of the following risk factors are associated with the development of pre-eclampsia? Select all that apply.
□ 1. ABO incompatibility.
□ 2. Family history.
□ 3. Chronic hypertension.
□ 4. Chronic renal disease.
□ 5. Maternal age 20 to 40 years.
□ 6. Multiparity.
□ 7. Obesity.

Answers and Rationales

1. 2 After an abortion (miscarriage) a client's Rh and Coombs status is evaluated to find if the client should receive immune globulin D (RhoGAM). After an abortion at 12 weeks' gestation, the fundus is not palpable. While reading the orders and requesting a grief counselor are important, they are not the first priority. (R)

2. 2, 4, 5 The nurse instructs a client that after a D&C she should monitor herself for signs of infection and report signs such as an elevated temperature to the HCP. The client may experience cramping and lower back or pelvic pain; the nurse instructs the woman to take analgesics as prescribed. The nurse also advises the woman to avoid strenuous activity and lifting until the bleeding has stopped, and to abstain from sexual relations for 2 weeks. The client remains on bed rest for the day of surgery, but can resume normal activities as tolerated on the next day. (H)

3. 2 Because women with class III heart disease are symptomatic with ordinary activity, bed rest for a large part of the day is recommended. Increasing fluid intake is not recommended. The use of anticoagulation drugs is only recommended for the client at increased risk for clot formation during pregnancy. Some cardiac conditions do put women at increased risk, but it is not a general recommendation. Third trimester NSTs are more commonly recommended for women who are diabetic. (R)

4. 2 During labor, cardiac function is supported by keeping the woman's head and shoulders elevated and body parts resting on pillows. The side-lying position facilitates hemodynamics in the mother and better placental profusion. Discomfort causes stress for the mother. Epidural analgesia provides safe relief of pain without some of the complications associated with narcotics; hypotension is avoided. If there are no obstetric problems, a vaginal delivery is recommended. Forceps or vacuum extraction is used if needed to shorten the second stage of labor and lessen the workload on the heart from prolonged pushing. Fluid load is carefully monitored. An IV infusion through a pump facilitates meeting fluid need without the danger of overload. (M)

5. 1, 2, 5 The risk factors for abruption placenta include smoking, multiparity, advanced maternal age, and history of falling. This client has three risk factors. Exercising and her young age are not risks for this client. (R)

6. 1 Painless bright red bleeding is usually indicative of a placenta previa. An ultrasound validates diagnosis. Bleeding from an abruption is usually darker and painful. An ectopic pregnancy or trophoblastic disease (hydatidiform mole) is not seen in the third trimester. (R)

7. 2 During pregnancy, placental hormones cortisol and insulinase increase insulin resistance, causing changes in carbohydrate metabolism. Protein metabolism is not altered, although protein needs increase by about 10 g per day to meet needs of maternal and fetal tissue development. Insulin secretion is not altered by pregnancy. (A)

8. 3 Recurrent infections, especially monilial vaginitis that is difficult to treat, are seen in women with high concentrations of glucose in their urine. A diabetic woman is likely to have more than normal amniotic fluid (polyhydramnios) and an LGA fetus. An eating disorder is unrelated to diabetes. (R)

9. 3 For insulin-dependent diabetics, diet and insulin requirements vary during pregnancy. Insulin needs may decrease during the first trimester especially if the mother is unable to eat because of nausea. Glucose is also used by the growing fetus. In the second trimester, a hormone called insulinase produced by the mother protects the fetus from hypoglycemia and acts as an insulin antagonist in the mother decreasing insulin's effectiveness and making it necessary for the woman to increase her daily dose. By the third trimester insulin needs may double or more, but usually level off by 36 weeks. Insulin doses are titrated based on frequent testing of blood glucose levels. Blood glucose tests are far more accurate than urine tests used for screening. Diet modifications are also necessary depending on the mother's symptoms (nausea and vomiting), her activity level, and blood glucose levels. High parity is unrelated to insulin needs. (H)

10. 2 Because of changes in the blood vessels in the placenta of a diabetic woman, as she approaches the end of her pregnancy the functioning of the placenta is assessed at frequent intervals. If the placenta is not able to provide adequate oxygen to the fetus because of circulatory problems from damage to blood vessels, the fetus is delivered early in order to prevent damage to the fetus and even death. An NST assesses whether the fetus can respond to the need for more oxygen with movement or contractions by increasing the heart rate; if so, delivery can be postponed. The test is repeated every 3 to 4 days. Infection and an LGA infant may complicate a diabetic woman's pregnancy, but other assessments are needed to monitor for these conditions. The fetus is not likely to be less active unless other problems exist. (R)

11. 2, 4, 6 If the fallopian tube is ruptured, surgery may be indicated to repair or remove the tube. The client is prepared for surgery and assessed for active bleeding (either external or internal) as well as signs of shock. Findings might include hypotension, tachycardia, and vertigo. Blood loss can be significant. The woman is kept NPO and an IV infusion is started. Because there is no fetus in the uterus, no fetus will be spontaneously passed; it is much too early for a cesarean delivery. (M)

12. 3 Persistent headache, hypertension, some visual disturbances, intermittent reddish brown or dark brown discharge, and a fundal height measurement larger than expected for estimated date of confinement are all signs of a hydatidiform mole. A threatened abortion presents with bright red bleeding and normal or low BP. A woman experiencing an ectopic pregnancy complains of pain on one side of her abdomen and has a normal to lower BP. There will be no vaginal discharge or larger than expected fundal height with pregnancy-induced hypertension. (R)

13. 1 Because of severe vomiting, the client with hyperemesis gravidarum can become easily dehydrated as noted by decreased urine output and poor skin turgor; the nursing care plan is designed to manage the dehydration, likely through IV fluid replacement. Electrolyte imbalance may also occur with hyperemesis gravidarum, and typically the potassium is low (hypokalemia) rather than high (hyperkalemia); the sodium is within normal limits. The client's hemoglobin and hematocrit are within normal limits and anemia is not present as a result of the vomiting. Bowel sounds are normal for this client. (R)

14. 2 Because of the woman's compromised immune system, she is counseled to avoid exposure to infection. Retesting for HIV antibodies is not necessary once the presence of the disease is confirmed. Wearing gloves is recommended only when it is likely that the nurse will be exposed to body fluids when giving care. Sexual activity can continue as long as there are no contraindications because of pregnancy complications and the couple uses appropriate protection such as a condom. (M)

15. 4 Because of the potential for worsening of the woman's condition, careful monitoring of this client is essential. Accurate measurement of urine output hourly is very important because an output below 30 ml/hr needs to be reported and treated. BP is measured every 2 hr or more frequently if a rise is found. Level of consciousness is monitored continually. Homans sign is performed less frequently unless there is reason to suspect a blood clot in the lower extremities. (M)

16. 2, 3, 5, 8 Maternal age (client age younger than 19 years or over 40 years), chronic renal disease, diabetes, obesity, a multifetal gestation, a primigravida, a family history of pre-eclampsia, or a pregnancy with a new partner are some factors that put a woman at increased risk for pre-eclampsia. Anemia and bleeding early in the pregnancy put a woman at risk for other pregnancy complications. A single fetus and fatigue in the later half of pregnancy are not related to pre-eclampsia. (R)

17. 3 Magnesium sulfate prevents progression of the hypertension of eclampsia by lowering the BP. The drug does not cause pain relief, decreased anxiety, or prevention of contractions. (D)

18. 2 Magnesium sulfate causes vasodilation, which results in increased warmth and flushing. Chills and shaking are common after birth. Epigastric pain is a sign of progressing pre-eclampsia. Magnesium sulfate is a CNS depressant and would not cause increased irritability. (D)

19. 2 This client may have pre-eclampsia, which is a syndrome during pregnancy that usually occurs after 20 weeks' gestation. Pre-eclampsia is characterized by an elevation in BP of 30 points systolic and 15 points diastolic above the prepregnant BP, as well as proteinuria. A weight gain of 10 lb or more in 2 weeks may indicate edema, including cerebral edema, beyond what is expected during pregnancy. If a woman exhibits elevated BP in the first trimester, it is labeled *chronic hypertension* and may have been present before the pregnancy. The woman with this diagnosis is carefully monitored for the development of pre-eclampsia after 20 weeks' gestation and is taught what symptoms to report to her HCP. Epigastric pain with a normal BP may be a symptom of acid reflux or heartburn. (M)

20. 2, 3, 4, 7 Risk factors for pre-eclampsia include Rh incompatibility, family history, chronic hypertension, maternal age less than 19 years and older than 40 years, primigravidity or first pregnancy with a new partner, obesity, and multiple gestation. ABO incompatibility, maternal age 20 to 40 years, and multiparity are not considered risk factors. (M)

chapter

6

The Birth Experience

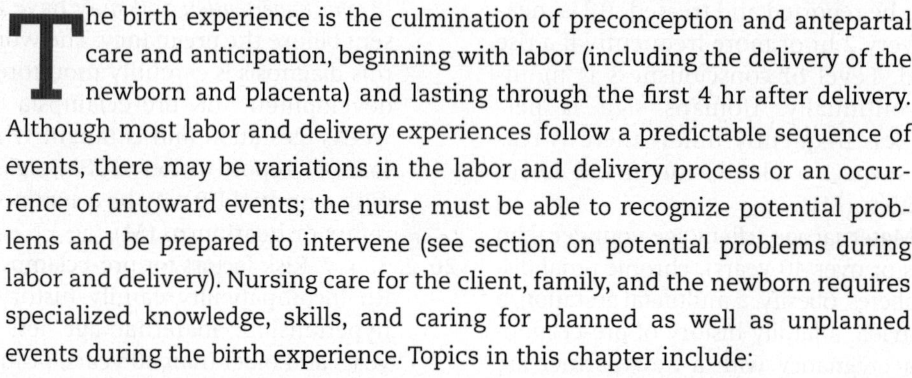

The birth experience is the culmination of preconception and antepartal care and anticipation, beginning with labor (including the delivery of the newborn and placenta) and lasting through the first 4 hr after delivery. Although most labor and delivery experiences follow a predictable sequence of events, there may be variations in the labor and delivery process or an occurrence of untoward events; the nurse must be able to recognize potential problems and be prepared to intervene (see section on potential problems during labor and delivery). Nursing care for the client, family, and the newborn requires specialized knowledge, skills, and caring for planned as well as unplanned events during the birth experience. Topics in this chapter include:

- Normal Labor and Delivery
- Potential Problems During Labor and Delivery
- Procedures Used During Labor and Delivery
- Preterm Labor
- Dystocia
- Disseminated Intravascular Coagulation
- Cesarean Section
- Vaginal Birth After Cesarean Section

Normal Labor and Delivery

I. Definition: The sequence of events occurring between 38 and 42 weeks' gestation, beginning with initiation of labor, birth of the infant, delivery of placenta, through first 2 to 4 hr postpartum.

A. Stages of labor

1. Stage 1: Initiation of labor through 10-cm cervical dilation; is longest stage, with three phases (early or latent, active, and transition). Physiologically, the uterus contracts and relaxes at frequent intervals as a response to maternal hormones.
   a. Estrogens stimulate uterine contractions; prostaglandins soften the cervix and play a role in the rising level of estrogen.
   b. Decreasing progesterone levels allow the body to initiate and continue contractions, and efface (thin, 0% to 100%) and dilate (open, 0 to 10 cm) the cervix.
2. Stage 2: 10-cm dilation through birth of infant. Once fully dilated, involuntary contractions (primary force of labor) and maternal pushing (secondary force of labor) augment the expulsive effort culminating in birth. The fetus changes position during the birth process (cardinal movements of labor) to accommodate the maternal pelvis; positions include:
   a. Descent
   b. Flexion
   c. Internal rotation
   d. Extension
   e. Restitution
   f. External rotation
   g. Expulsion
3. Stage 3: Delivery of the placenta; contractions continue, resulting in expulsion of the placenta.
4. Stage 4: Delivery of the placenta through the first 2 to 4 hr postpartum. Physiologically, the first 2 to 4 hr after delivery begins the physical and emotional readjustment to the nonpregnant state with a rapid change in hormones after placental delivery.

B. True labor is differentiated from false labor by effacement and dilation of the cervix.

C. Influences on labor: Four critical factors (the four Ps of childbearing): Powers, Passenger, Passageway, and Psyche

1. **Powers** (contractions): Involuntary contraction of uterus during the first three stages of labor cause the cervix to:
   a. Efface: Shortening and thinning expressed as a percentage from 0 to 100.
   b. Dilate: Opening of cervix from 0 to 10 cm.
2. **Passenger** (fetus): Size and position of fetus influences its ability to maneuver through the maternal birth canal.
3. **Passageway** (birth canal): Soft tissues of vagina, the cervix along with the maternal bony pelvis surrounding the infant during the delivery, impact the ability to descend through the pelvis. There are situations in which a normal pelvis is not large enough for an infant to deliver; conversely, there are situations in which a small pelvis is adequate for a small infant.
4. **Psyche** (mind): The mental experience of labor and delivery is influenced by the length of time required, perception of pain, desire for child, and support offered.

D. Terms associated with birthing:

1. Presentation: Portion of infant entering pelvis first (head, feet, buttocks, hand, etc.)
   a. Breech: Buttocks or feet as presenting part, usually resulting in cesarean delivery for a first-time mother
      (1) Complete: Knees and hips flexed, thighs on abdomen
      (2) Frank: Hips flexed, knees extended
      (3) Footling: One or both feet as presenting part
   b. Cephalic/vertex: Head as presenting part in 95% of deliveries; the occiput is usually seen first
2. Lie: Relationship of long axis of mother to long axis of infant, either transverse or longitudinal. Transverse lie requires cesarean section if fetal rotation does not occur. Vertical lie results in head or buttocks/feet as the presenting part.
3. Station: Measurement in centimeters of decent of biparietal diameter of fetal head in relation to maternal ischial spines. Ranges from −5 (5 cm above level of spines) to +5 (5 cm below level of spines and fetal head is on the perineum). Fetus is at 0 station (engagement) when biparietal diameter is level of ischial spines.
4. Position: Fetal position (landmark on presenting part) in relation to maternal pelvis; indicated by letters:
   a. Relationship of left or right **(L or R)** side of the mother to presenting part of infant (occiput **[O]** vertex presentation, mentum **[M]** in a face presentation, sacrum **[S]** in breech presentation, and acromion process of the scapula **[Sc]** in a shoulder presentation) and anterior or posterior **(A or P)** of maternal pelvis.

b. When put together, these characteristics determine fetal position as fetus exits the mother. Examples include **ROA** (right occiput anterior) and **LOA** (left occiput anterior), which are the most common positions. Many variations exist (e.g., **LOP**, **ROP**, and **LSA**).

5. Mechanisms of labor/cardinal movements: Movements the fetus completes as birth occurs.
   a. Engagement: Biparietal diameter of fetal head reaches level of ischial spines
   b. Descent: Downward movement of fetus through maternal pelvis
   c. Flexion: The fetal chin tucks onto chest
   d. Internal rotation: Movement of fetal head from transverse to anterior posterior position as it accommodates the pelvic inlet and midpelvis
   e. Extension: Movement of fetal head as it emerges onto the perineum as the face and head become visible
   f. Restitution: Turning of infant head to face the right or left leg of mother, bringing the head in the correct relationship to the fetal back
   g. External rotation: The fetal shoulders rotate internally to an anterior posterior position, further turning the fetal head to one side or the other
   h. Expulsion: The upper shoulder rotates under the maternal symphysis and is born, followed by the posterior shoulder and the remainder of the infant
6. Attitude: Relationship of fetal body parts to one another. Normal attitude is flexion, where fetus is curled on itself with chin on chest, arms and legs folded: "fetal position."
7. Premonitory signs of labor: Physical changes indicating that time of labor is nearing. These include:
   a. Lightening or dropping: Fetus moves deeply into maternal pelvis 2 weeks before delivery in primipara and at time of labor and delivery for multiparas. "Lightens" maternal perception of fetal burden as mother can breathe more easily.
   b. Loss of mucous plug: As cervix softens and begins to open, the protective plug of mucus in the cervix is lost, often with small amount of blood.
   c. Burst of energy: Client uses her energy to prepare for childbearing and the new infant, and can enter labor tired.
   d. Increase in Braxton Hicks contractions.
   e. Increase in vaginal discharge.
8. Engagement: Largest diameter (biparietal) of presenting part reaches or passes maternal pelvic inlet.
9. Leopold maneuvers: Four maneuvers by HCP to determine fetal engagement and positioning:
   a. First: Palpate maternal fundus to determine fetal part that is present. Place hands on fundus and palpate for firmness, round (head), or softness, irregularity (buttocks).
   b. Second: Place hands on either side of abdomen, applying firm, gentle pressure on one side and then the other. Side with fetal back will palpate long and firm and the side with arms and legs will be irregular and lumpy.
   c. Third: Fetal position is determined by placing thumb and forefinger of one hand in C shape immediately above the symphysis, palpating the portion of fetus that is located there. It will feel firm (head) or soft (buttocks).
   d. Fourth: Fetal descent is determined by placing one hand on each side of maternal abdomen and sliding hands down to symphysis, palpating for head or buttocks of infant.
10. Episiotomy: Incision into perineal body to facilitate birth of infant. Two types: Midline (incision toward the rectum) and mediolateral (incision from posterior vagina at a 45-degree angle into muscle).
11. Lacerations: Tears in perineal tissue as a result of distention by fetal head. Four degrees:
    a. First degree: Through skin, mucous membrane
    b. Second degree: Tears through skin, mucous membrane, and muscle of perineal body
    c. Third degree: Through skin, mucous membrane, muscles, and rectal sphincter
    d. Fourth degree: Through skin, mucous membrane, muscle, rectal sphincter, and rectal wall
12. Amniotomy: Artificial rupture of membranes. Augments labor contractions.
13. Premature rupture of membranes: Rupture of membranes before the onset of labor.

II. Nursing process

A. Assessment

1. Assess client in stage 1 labor (beginning of labor to 10 cm dilation).
   a. Phase 1: Early or latent phase, 0 to 3 cm dilation:
      (1) Pain level: Contractions tolerated with concentration.

(2) Contractions: Irregular; every 5 to 10 min with mild intensity (25 to 45 mmHg); lasting half a minute to one full minute.
(3) Emotional status: Client is lighthearted, excited, talkative, and happy that labor is beginning.

b. Phase 2: Active phase, 4 to 7 cm dilation:
(1) Pain level: Pain is more intense, often with need for medication.
(2) Contractions: Every 2 to 5 min with moderate to strong palpation (45 to 75mmHg).
(3) Emotional status: Client is more serious, quieter, absorbed in work of labor, and less self-confident.

c. Phase 3: Transition phase, 8 to 10 cm dilation:
(1) Physical changes: Indicate transition; include increase in bloody show, urge to push, backache, nausea, vomiting, and trembling.
(2) Contractions: Every 2 to 3 min, strong in intensity, lasting 1 to 2 min.
(3) Emotional status: Client is irritable, discouraged, tired; exhibits decreased ability to cope and relax if unmedicated.

2. Assess client in stage 2 labor (10 cm through birth of infant).
   a. Fetal descent usually from 0 station to +5 cm to birth.
   b. Emotional status: Client is intent, cooperative, dozing between contractions.
3. Assess client in stage 3 labor (birth of infant through delivery of placenta): Client exhibits emotional status that is excited and focused on infant rather than self, unless in severe pain.
4. Assess client in stage 4 labor (delivery of placenta through 4 hr postpartum): Client is tired, but unable to sleep; exhibits symptoms of hunger and thirst; is excited, and relives and reviews birth experience; demonstrates bonding with infant and significant other. Assessment also involves:
   a. Recovery room maternal assessment.
   b. Newborn assessment, stabilization, and Apgar score.

B. Analysis
1. Acute Pain related to uterine contractions and cervical dilation
2. Powerlessness related to duration and inability to control labor
3. Anxiety related to unknown maternal and fetal outcome
4. Ineffective Coping related to unpredictability of labor
5. Deficient Knowledge related to first childbearing experience, inability to participate in childbirth classes
6. Risk for Social Isolation related to unfamiliar environment, lack of support persons
7. Risk for Deficient Fluid Volume related to decreased intake during labor
8. Fatigue related to long labor process
9. Risk for Infection related to rupture of membranes (ROM), episiotomy

C. Planning
1. Promote normal labor and delivery process.
2. Prevent injury or complications to mother and infant.
3. Monitor vital signs.

D. Implementation
1. Provide continuous fetal and maternal assessment.
2. Coordinate activities depending on current stage and phase of labor.
3. Have delivery table and equipment available at appropriate time.
4. Assist with pharmacologic and nonpharmacologic comfort and coping techniques.
5. Check all equipment to assure proper working condition (oxygen, suction, resuscitation equipment).
6. Notify HCP in adequate time to be present for delivery.

E. Evaluation
1. Client affirms satisfaction with labor and delivery process.
2. Client delivers in normal time frame without injury or complications with vital signs within normal limits.
3. Infant is delivered without injury with Apgar score of more than 7 at 1 and 5 min with no anomalies or complications.

CN

III. Client needs

A. Physiologic adaptation
1. Normal physical changes occurring during the labor process include:
   a. WBCs increase up to 25,000 mm^3 (increase in neutrophils in response to stress and tissue trauma).
   b. Dehydration occurs as a result of NPO status or clear liquid status; profuse perspiration; insensible water loss from increased respirations.
   c. Cardiac output increases.
   d. Respiratory rate increases, altering acid base balance.

e. Gastric motility decreases, often resulting in nausea and vomiting during transition with risk of aspiration.
f. Pain present as a result of hypoxia of uterine muscle cells during contractions, stretching of lower uterine segment, dilation of cervix, and distention of perineum and vagina.

2. Maternal positioning may cause vena cava or hypotensive syndrome from pressure on vena cava; the nurse positions client on left side to facilitate venous return to the heart.
3. Fetal heart rate (FHR) to remain between 110 and 160 beats per minute, moderate variability, accelerations with fetal movement, and no decelerations.

B. Management of care: Care of the client during labor and delivery requires critical thinking skills and knowledge of assessment, and teaching and evaluation methods unique to the RN role. These skills cannot be delegated to an LPN or UAP.

1. Delegate responsibly those activities that can be delegated, including basic care needs and vital sign checks. All monitoring information is reported to the RN.
2. Manage all aspects of care during labor; consult with HCP when problems arise and at time of delivery.
3. Provide nursing interventions during stage 1 labor—phase 1 (on admission/early phase).
   a. Conduct physical and obstetric assessment (bloody show, ROM for color, odor, amount), review of laboratory data, last food intake (in case of need for surgery).
   b. Determine client's birth plan, support system, prior child-birthing experiences, medical conditions, and coping skills to develop plan of care; consider analgesia or anesthesia needs, fears and concerns.
   c. Conduct vaginal examination for effacement, dilation, presenting part, station, position on admission, and as needed.
   d. Notify HCP of admission, condition of mother (emotional status, cervical effacement and dilation, station), and fetus (fetal heart baseline, accelerations, variability, deceleration patterns).
   e. Obtain laboratory studies obtained per HCP protocol as needed, urine analyzed for protein, glucose, check blood glucose level (Accu-Chek) every 4 hr for gestational diabetic and insulin-dependent diabetes mellitus.
   f. Provide information on changes in client status to the HCP and appropriate members of the multidisciplinary team (pediatricians, special care nursery staff).
   g. Monitor client for indications that labor is not progressing normally: fetal distress (decreased variability, lack of accelerations, late decelerations, severe or prolonged variable decelerations), change in maternal vital signs, increase in temperature, increase or decrease in blood pressure, vaginal bleeding, hypo- or hypertonic labor, excessive fear or pain (age, gravida, parity, etc.).
   h. Evaluate risk factors that may impact labor.
   i. Assess frequency, intensity, and duration of contractions (normal is every 2 to 3 min, moderate intensity, lasting 60 to 90 s and causing effacement and dilation of cervix).
   j. Evaluate impact of interventions on labor progress.
   k. Establish infusion of IV fluids or saline lock in place for access if needed and to maintain hydration.
   l. Review laboratory analysis of hematocrit, hemoglobin, glucose screen, maternal serum alpha-fetoprotein screen (MSAFP), hepatitis B surface antigen (HbsAg), blood type, Rh, sickle cell screen, rubella titer, urinalysis, gonorrhea, chlamydia, syphilis screen, pap smear, and determine impact of each abnormal result on labor process.
   m. Assess laboring client (vital signs, contraction pattern, pain and coping level) every half hour.
   n. Offer clear fluids, ice chips, or NPO status.
   o. Instruct client and family about:
      (1) Medications available during labor process (analgesics, regional anesthesia, etc.).
      (2) The labor process, physical and emotional changes as labor progresses.
      (3) Comfort strategies for nurse and other support persons/coaches to use to assist labor client (back rubs, use of warm and cool compresses, breathing and relaxation techniques, aroma therapy, acupuncture, and environmental changes).

(4) Self-care behaviors available to mother (hydrotherapy pool, shower, labor ball, doula).

4. Provide nursing interventions during stage 1 labor—phase 2 (active phase).
   a. Assist client with breathing, relaxation, comfort measures as needed.
   b. Anticipate need for regional anesthesia.
   c. Support breathing and relaxation, self-care measures if unmedicated.
   d. Document vital signs, fetal monitoring every half hour.
   e. Have client empty bladder every 2 to 4 hr as needed (allows fetus to descend).
   f. Document intake and output.
   g. Participate in amniotomy as needed:
      (1) Monitor FHR immediately after artificial rupture of membranes (AROM).
      (2) Document color, odor, amount of amniotic fluid and changes occurring during labor.
   h. Offer clear liquid diet, ice chips.
   i. Conduct vaginal examinations only as needed.
5. Provide nursing interventions during stage 1 labor—phase 3 (transition phase).
   a. Document vital signs every half hour.
   b. Note fetal and contraction monitoring continuously, observing for early decelerations.
   c. Document intake and output.
   d. Offer support and reassurance.
   e. Assist client to void every 2 to 4 hr as needed.
   f. Assist client with breathing, relaxation, comfort measures as needed.
   g. Monitor for analgesia needs.
   h. Provide client and family teaching as needed regarding process of labor and delivery.
   i. Perform vaginal examinations only as needed.
6. Provide nursing interventions during stage 2 labor.
   a. Provide client and family teaching regarding process of laboring down or pushing.
   b. Monitor FHR during and after contractions.
   c. Monitor changes in station of fetus from 0 to +5 and fetal response with each contraction (reassuring FHT with no decelerations, moderate variability, accelerations present).
   d. Observe maternal response to pushing (fatigue, dehydration, resting between contractions).
   e. Prepare for delivery (delivery table and warmer set up and suction and oxygen checked, preheat warmer).
   d. "Iron" (smooth out) perineum to decrease need for episiotomy.
   g. Notify HCP and pediatrician of client's progress.
7. Provide nursing interventions during stage 3 labor.
   a. Note time, fetal position, type of delivery; assign Apgar score and stabilize infant.
   b. Anticipate maternal and fetal responses and needs.
   c. Note and document length of time from delivery of infant to delivery of placenta.
   d. Begin infusion of 20 units of oxytocin (Pitocin) in 10,000 ml of lactated Ringer or 20 units Pitocin IM if no IV line is available.
   e. Monitor type of episiotomy, lacerations, and repairs and implement strategies for healing.
      (1) Apply ice to perineum after repair.
      (2) Instruct client on care of episiotomy/lacerations, topical products to decrease swelling and eliminate pain.
      (3) Instruct client on use of medication and positioning to decrease pain.
8. Provide nursing interventions during stage 4 labor.
   a. Plan for recovery assessment every 15 min for 4 times, every 1 hr for 2 times, then every 8 hr. Includes fundus, lochia, bladder, mobility, orientation, vital signs, pain.
   b. Assist mother with breast or bottle feeding.
   c. Conduct physical assessment of infant; administer medications.
   d. Provide time for bonding within family.

C. Safety and infection control
1. Conduct vaginal examinations only when indicated throughout labor.
2. Observe clear, odorless amniotic fluid is normal with ROM. Meconium-stained fluid indicates fetal distress has occurred and need to plan vigilant fetal monitoring with neonatal resuscitation-certified staff at delivery. Meconium-stained fluid is common with breech deliveries.
3. Interpret fetal heart monitoring and contraction monitoring approximately every half hour.
   a. Baseline: Average FHR without contractions is between 110 and 160 BPM.

b. Tachycardia: Increase in FHR above 160 BPM lasting 10 min or longer.
 (1) Etiology: Anemia, maternal fever, dehydration, medications such as atropine, ritodrine (Yutopar), and terbutaline (Brethine).
 (2) Interventions: Assess maternal Hct, Hgb; medications administered; maternal temperature, hydration status; and length of ROM for potential etiology. Analyze trends over time in labor; report abnormal results of analysis to HCP.

c. Bradycardia: Decrease in heart rate below 110 BPM lasting 10 min or longer.
 (1) Etiology: Hypoxia, maternal hypotension, cord compression, medications such as analgesics.
 (2) Interventions: Analyze situation at hand for potential etiology. Turn mother to left side (increase perfusion), begin oxygen by mask at 8 to 10 L/min, increase plain IV fluid rate, notify HCP.

d. Accelerations: Transient increase in FHR as response to fetal movement. To be considered acceleration, the heart rate must increase by 15 beats and last for 15 s; this is a sign of fetal well-being and is reassuring.

e. Variability: Beat-to-beat irregularity in FHR. Two to six cycles expected in 1 min and is a response ofthe sympathetic and parasympathetic systems; may be charted as:
 (1) Absent: No beats of variability
 (2) Minimal: One to five beats of variability
 (3) Moderate: Six to 25 beats of variability (sign of fetal well-being)
 (4) Marked: More than 25 beats of variability

f. Early decelerations: Drop in FHR that inversely mirrors the pattern of the contraction.
 (1) Etiology: Indicates fetal head compression and is normally seen during transition and pushing phases of labor.
 (2) Interventions: If client is pushing—no interventions; document as normal for this part of labor. If occurs earlier in labor, consider risk for cephalopelvic disproportion.

g. Variable decelerations: Rapid decrease in FHR during a contraction with a rapid return to the baseline by the end of the contraction. Decelerations are variable and can be V, U, or W in shape.
 (1) Etiology: Indicates cord compression.
 (2) Interventions: Turn client to side to relieve cord compression; if unrelieved, turn to opposite side.

h. Late decelerations: Subtle or obvious decreases in FHR that is late in returning to the baseline (e.g., returns to the baseline after the contraction is over; nonreassuring fetal heart pattern). This is the only deceleration pattern that returns to the baseline after the contraction is over.
 (1) Etiology: Uteroplacental insufficiency resulting in lack of oxygen to fetus. Any condition associated with pregnancy that can decrease/limit oxygenation to the fetus may cause late decelerations, including: diabetes, pre-eclampsia, postterm pregnancy, tetanic contractions, and other maternal disease processes.
 (2) Interventions (prioritized):
  (a) Discontinue Pitocin if infusing—prevents further artificial contraction of uterine muscle, increasing ability of oxygen to move to fetus.
  (b) Turn client to side—improves venous return to heart, etc.
  (c) Administer oxygen by facial mask at 8 to 10 L/min—increases oxygen available to maternal system.
  (d) Increase mainline plain IV fluid rate—increases volume of fluid, transports oxygen moving through system.
  (e) Notify HCP—communicates awareness of problem and interventions instituted.

4. Analyze contraction patterns.
 a. Frequency: Beginning of one contraction to the beginning of the next. Must have minimum of three contractions to evaluate the pattern.
 b. Intensity: How firm the contraction is in the fundus: documented as mild, moderate, and firm if palpated; if measured internally, millimeters of mercury represents actual intensity.
 c. Duration: The length of the contractions, averaging 60 to 90 s during active labor.

D. Health promotion and maintenance
   1. Offer clear fluids, ice chips, NPO during labor. Fluids, food as tolerated after delivery.
   2. Provide rest as much as possible during labor for conservation of energy.

E. Psychologic integrity
   1. Reinforce prenatal education, listen to client needs, provide support, reduce stress and anxiety as needed.
   2. Evaluate support person(s) at bedside and how well person is working with client; offer suggestions as needed.
   3. Provide emotional support (answer questions, encourage ventilation of emotions and fears concerning labor and delivery).

F. Basic care and comfort: Provide comfort measures, including rest and sleep opportunities, and medication as needed.

G. Reduction of risk potential
   1. Assure bed rest after ROM or if dilated more than 5 cm.
   2. Monitor for foul odor in amniotic fluid, rising maternal temperature or FHR.
   3. Analyze fetal and contraction monitoring.
   4. Administer penicillin for positive group B streptococcal infection and positive group B streptoccocal status on admission and every 4 hr.

H. Pharmacologic and parenteral therapies: Client will state the purpose for and associated side effects of all medications used during labor and delivery.
   1. Nonpharmacologic methods of pain control include:
      a. Therapeutic touch, acupressure, massage, counter pressure, hot and cold compresses.
      b. Position changes, ambulation, birthing ball, Jacuzzi, showers, breathing techniques, visualization, biofeedback.
   2. Early labor medications include:
      a. Barbiturates: Secobarbital (Seconal) 100 mg PO to provide therapeutic rest, light sleep, or alter dysfunctional labor pattern sedation in early labor when delivery is not anticipated for 8 to 12 hr. Caution: No anecdote available. If crosses placenta, can cause newborn CNS depression.
      b. Tranquilizers: Hydroxyzine (Vistaril), promethazine (Phenergan) 25 mg IM, or slow IV push as antianxiety, muscle relaxants, antiemetics, and to potentiate narcotics.
      c. Narcotics: Meperidine (Demerol), butorphanol (Stadol), nalbuphine (Nubain), fentanyl (Sublimaze) IM or slow IV push to alter sensation of pain; inability to cope may decrease uterine activity. Caution: Have narcotic antagonist naloxone (Narcan) on hand if medication is in maternal system less than 2 hr before birth.
   3. Active labor medications include:
      a. Epidural: Various medications used to relieve pain in pelvis and lower extremities: bupivacaine, ropivacaine, morphine (Duramorph). Want epidural to partially wear off to facilitate pushing; re-dose for delivery and repair. Maternal hypotension can occur shortly after administration and may lead to fetal distress; when using an epidural, the nurse provides the following measures:
         (1) Take maternal vital signs every 2 to 5 min for 15 min after epidural.
         (2) Preload mother with 500 ml IV fluid bolus immediately before epidural placement to prevent hypotension.
      b. Ephedrine: Anecdote for hypotension associated with epidural.
      c. Intrathecal narcotic: Narcotic in subarachnoid space with pain relief and ability to maintain mobility. Maternal side effects include urinary retention, respiratory depression, pruritus, and nausea and vomiting.
      d. Paracervical block: Lidocaine (Xylocaine) injected at the level of the uterine and pelvic plexuses to provide analgesia during first stage of labor. Fetal bradycardia can occur in up to 50% of clients, and the nurse should monitor FHR.
   4. Medications used during delivery include:
      a. General anesthesia for emergency cesarean delivery. Nurse assures an IV line is present, client is NPO, consents are signed, and oral antacid (sodium citrate [Bicitra]) has been administered to decrease gastric acid production.
         (1) Maternal side effect: Aspiration.
         (2) Newborn side effect: If anesthesia transferred to infant prior to delivery, may result in respiratory depression, hypotonic infant. Infant needs to be delivered within 5 min of mother being put to sleep to prevent "sleepy" infant.

b. Continuation of epidural for vaginal or cesarean birth.
c. Pudendal block: Local anesthetic (lidocaine, Xylocaine, etc.) injected intravaginally at level of pudendal nerves prior to delivery. Perineal area numb for repair and 1 to 2 hr postpartum. No maternal or infant side effects.
d. Local anesthetic (Xylocaine or lidocaine) for repair of lacerations/episiotomy.
e. Natural pressure anesthesia: Created as the head distends the perineum. While the head remains on the perineum, the anesthesia remains and an episiotomy can be made without pain. Local anesthesia will be needed for episiotomy repair because the pressure of the head has been removed.

5. Penicillin: 5 million units IV followed by 2.5 million units every 4 hr for positive group B streptoccocal status.
6. Oxytocin (Pitocin): 20 units in 1 L IV fluid twice postpartum for prevention of hemorrhage.

Potential Problems During Labor and Delivery

I. Definition: Variations in the labor and delivery process, or an occurrence of untoward events requires that the nurse recognize potential problems and be prepared to intervene. Some potential problems include cord prolapse, precipitous labor and delivery, amniotic fluid embolism, and postterm labor.

Cord Prolapse

I. Definition: Cord prolapse involves a loop of the umbilical cord slipping past the presenting portion of the fetal head; the cord may slip entirely past the fetal head with ROM. As the fetal head moves down in the pelvis, the cord is compressed, creating fetal distress, decelerations, and hypoxia. Delivery is the only intervention to relieve the cord compression. Cord prolapse is a medical and nursing emergency.

II. Management of care

A. Assess client to determine risk factors.
1. ROM
2. Fetus at a negative station
3. Premature ROM
4. Fetus with abnormal presentation
5. Multiple gestations
6. Polyhydramnios

B. Observe continuously fetal monitor strip in client at risk.
C. After ROM (artificial or spontaneous), monitor fetal heart for 10 min for decelerations indicating cord compression or prolapse.
D. If decelerations are observed, activate emergency call system while reassuring client.
E. Place gloved hand with upward gentle pressure on presenting part to relieve cord compression.
F. Direct medical support personnel to place client into Trendelenburg position.
G. Notify HCP.
H. Continue to maintain gentle support of fetal head while support staff prepares client for surgery; gentle support is continued until fetus is delivered by cesarean section.
I. Prepare for immediate vaginal delivery if cervix is 10 cm dilated and completely effaced.
J. Reassure client; talk client through procedures occurring for rapid cesarean section.

Precipitous Labor and Delivery

I. Definition: Precipitous labor and delivery refers to extremely rapid labor and delivery (completed in 3 hr or less). Risk factors include the following:
A. Prior rapid delivery
B. Multiparity
C. Induction or amniotomy

II. Management of care: Have terbutaline (Brethine) on hand to decrease strength and frequency of contractions.

Amniotic Fluid Embolism

I. Definition: Amniotic fluid embolism occurs when amniotic fluid enters maternal circulatory system through an open uterine blood sinus and is then carried to lungs as embolus. Amniotic fluid embolism can occur during labor, delivery, or postpartum period, and is a medical and nursing emergency. This complication occurs in one in 8,000 deliveries.

II. Management of care

A. Monitor client for indications.
1. Respiratory distress
2. Cough that is bloody or frothy
3. Hypotension
4. Shock
5. Cardiac arrest
6. Hemorrhage related to coagulation defects
7. Uterine atony

B. Provide or assist with interventions as needed.
1. Oxygen by mask at 8 to 10 L/min
2. Intubation with mechanical ventilation
3. Cardiopulmonary resuscitation
4. IV fluids

5. Packed red blood cells (PRBCs), platelets for coagulation defects
6. Foley catheter with hourly intake and output

C. Prepare for emergency delivery after maternal stabilization.
D. Inform family of emergency situation and provide support as needed.

Postterm Labor

I. Definition: Postterm labor refers to labor occurring after completion of 42 weeks' gestation. The volume of amniotic fluid decreases as fetus becomes postterm. Placental function decreases as pregnancy becomes postmature.

II. Management of care
   A. Validate client is postterm based on quickening, ultrasound in first trimester, initial fetal heart tones.
   B. Review results of diagnostic testing.
      1. Ultrasound validates postterm status
      2. Biophysical profile assesses fetal status
      3. Nonstress test assesses fetal status
      4. Fetal kick counts
      5. Fundal height correlation with estimated date of confinement
   C. Provide client and family teaching.
      1. Instruct client to report decrease or change in fetal movement.
      2. Discuss rationale for induction process (decrease in placental function).
   D. Plan care for client during labor.
      1. Implement continuous fetal and contraction monitoring.
      2. Prepare for potential cervical ripening and induction.
      3. Assess risk status of fetus related to potential uteroplacental insufficiency.
      4. Prepare for fetal distress cord compression resulting from decreased amniotic fluid.
      5. Prepare for potential meconium aspiration and asphyxia.
      6. Prepare for amnioinfusion to cushion cord.

Procedures Used During Labor and Delivery

I. Definition: Procedures used during labor and delivery may include induction of labor, cervical ripening, external version, forceps delivery, or vacuum extraction.

Induction of Labor

I. Definition: Artificial stimulation of uterine contractions prior to initiation of spontaneous uterine contractions for the purpose of achieving a vaginal birth; may be mechanical or pharmacologic interventions.
   A. Assess client for indications for induction.
      1. Maternal health problems: hypertension, diabetes mellitus, pre-eclampsia
      2. Fetal health problems: diabetes mellitus, postterm pregnancy, isoimmunization
      3. Fetal death
   B. Monitor client during each phase.
      1. Preinduction cervical ripening (see also section on cervical ripening):
         a. Form of prostaglandin swallowed or placed in, near, or around cervix to soften and efface cervix and to initiate contractions.
         b. A laminaria of seaweed may be placed in cervix to create the same effects.
      2. Labor induction with Pitocin: use of oxytocin (Pitocin) to stimulate contractions after cervical ripening.

II. Management of care
   A. Obtain a reactive nonstress test as ordered.
   B. Perform a vaginal examination for evidence of cervical ripening.
   C. Use fetal monitor strip prior to initiation of oxytocin (Pitocin) per hospital protocol.
   D. Observe fetal and contraction monitoring.
   E. Maintain an IV infusion with oxytocin (Pitocin) infused via pump as secondary line.
   F. Administer oxytocin (Pitocin) per agency protocol.
   G. Prepare for hyperstimulation and potential fetal distress.
      1. Discontinue oxytocin (Pitocin).
      2. Position client on left side.
      3. Administer oxygen at 8 to 12 L/min via mask.
      4. Maintain IV infusion and increase rate of infusion as needed.
      5. Notify HCP.
      6. Prepare for cesarean section.
   H. Implement protocol for hyperstimulation if needed.
   I. Administer medications as ordered.
      1. Prostaglandin E_2: Prostaglandin gel (Prepidil), 0.5 mg, or insert dinoprostone (Cervidil), 10 mg
      2. Prostaglandin E_1: Misoprostol (Cytotec; synthetic prostaglandin E; placed in cervix or swallowed)
      3. Pitocin: Oxytocin for labor induction

Cervical Ripening

I. Definition: Process of causing the cervix to soften and dilate prior to labor and delivery.

II. Management of care
  A. Explain procedure to client and family.
  B. Obtain admission physical, psychosocial, history of subsequent pregnancies, and assessment.
  C. Review Bishop score completed by HCP.
  D. Review indications for induction.
  E. Obtain maternal vital signs per protocol.
  F. Use fetal monitoring with reassuring monitor strip prior to initiation of cervical ripening per hospital protocol.
  G. Note fetal and contraction monitoring for hyperstimulation and responses to medication per protocol.
  H. Promote safety and infection control.
    1 Keep client in supine position with wedge for 1 to 2 hr with initial and subsequent doses of intravaginal medication.
    2. Maintain a saline lock or IV line for parenteral access.

External Version

I. Definition: External version involves external manipulation of fetus in utero from abnormal position to vertex presentation after 34 weeks' gestation.
II. Management of care
  A. Use fetal and contraction monitoring for half hour prior to procedure.
  B. Explain to client the procedure, and sensations to expect; obtain consent as needed.
  C. Document fetal position, placental location.
  D. Validate that Rh-negative mothers have received RhoGAM at 28 weeks' gestation.
  E. Maintain IV infusion and maintain fluid balance.
  F. Administer terbutaline (Brethine) for uterine relaxation.
  G. Support client during version procedure.
  H. Monitor maternal pain level during procedure.
  I. Use fetal and contraction monitoring after the procedure until contractions cease, FHR at baseline with moderate variability, and no decelerations and accelerations are present.
  J. Provide client teaching before discharge regarding what to report to HCP:
    1. ROM
    2. No fetal movement
    3. Initiation of labor
    4. Vaginal bleeding
  K. Have Terbutaline at bedside to relax uterus after the procedure if needed.

Forceps Delivery

I. Definition: Forceps delivery involves delivery of fetal head with assistance of interlocking blades placed around head during delivery.
II. Management of care
  A. Explain to client the procedure, and sensations to expect; obtain consent as needed.
  B. Use fetal and contraction monitoring continuously.
  C. Assist client to empty bladder.
  D. Monitor maternal pain level during procedure.
  E. Assess neonate postdelivery for:
    1. Lacerations, bruising, palsy, asymmetry of face.
    2. Ability of infant to suck and swallow.
  F. Apply ice to maternal perineum postperineal repair as needed.
  G. Offer medication for perineal pain (e.g., topical anesthetics).
  H. Instruct client about care to perineum (wipe front to back, use of spray bottle/peribottle).

Vacuum Extraction

I. Definition: Vacuum extraction involves delivery of fetal head with assistance of a suction device attached to fetal scalp during delivery.
II. Management of care
  A. Explain to client the procedure, and sensations to expect; obtain consent as needed.
  B. Use fetal and contraction monitoring continuously.
  C. Assist client to empty bladder.
  D. Encourage maternal pushing with contractions.
  E. Assess neonate postdelivery for:
    1. Lacerations, bruising, caput succedaneum
    2. Cephalohematoma
    3. Cerebral trauma
  F. Use ice, topical anesthetics to perineum postperineal repair as needed.
  G. Offer medication for maternal perineal pain.
  H. Provide comfort measures (tucks, side-lying position).
  I. Instruct client about care to perineum (wipe front to back, use of spray bottle/peribottle).

Preterm Labor

I. Definition: Preterm labor (PTL) is labor resulting in cervical effacement and dilation occurring between 20 to 37 weeks' gestation. One in eight infants is born prematurely, with PTL as the most common obstetric complication accounting for more than 80% of neonatal deaths. Precise etiology of PTL is unknown although an infection is commonly seen.
  A. Indications
    1. Contractions increasing in frequency, intensity, and duration
    2. Lower abdominal pressure or backache
    3. Changes in vaginal discharge or initiation of bloody show
    4. Intestinal cramping

B. Risk factors: PTL is a risk for any pregnant client; additional risk factors include:
   1. Preterm labor in prior pregnancies.
   2. Prior episodes of PTL in current pregnancy.
   3. Any situation that over distends uterus (polyhydramnios, multiple gestation).
   4. Domestic violence.
   5. Inadequate nutrition.
   6. Use of drugs, alcohol.
   7. Smoking.

II. Management of care
A. Assessment
   1. Perform a comprehensive physical assessment including assessment of weeks' gestation, viability of fetus, ROM.
   2. Assess client for risk factors as noted here.
   3. Assess client knowledge of benefit of prolonging pregnancy.
   4. Assess client's desire to continue pregnancy to term.
   5. Obtain diagnostic tests.
      a. Fetal fibronectin
      b. Ultrasound for cervical length
      c. Home uterine contraction monitoring
      d. Vaginal cultures for any sexually transmitted infection, such as gonorrhea, chlamydia, bacterial vaginosis
      e. Urinalysis, culture, and sensitivity if urinary tract infection (UTI)

B. Analysis
   1. Anxiety related to unknown fetal outcome
   2. Situational Low Self-Esteem related to inability to carry infant to term
   3. Activity Intolerance related to boredom and activity restrictions at home or during hospitalization
   4. Compromised Family Coping related to loss of income of client, need for child care

C. Planning
   1. Provide client teaching about risk factors to prevent PTL.
   2. Monitor status of PTL.
   3. Complete interventions on decision to intervene or deliver.
   4. Provide emotional support.
   5. Prepare for possible loss of infant.
   6. Refer to community support systems.

D. Implementation (see management of care)

E. Evaluation
   1. Client delivers a full-term healthy infant.
   2. Client's PTL abates with treatment by client and/or HCPs.

III. Client needs
A. Physiologic adaptation
   1. Fetal fibronectin present during weeks 22 to 34 indicates an increased risk of PTL, the absence of fetal fibronectin is a better indicator that the pregnancy will continue for more than 2 weeks.
   2. Maternal muscle wasting can occur with prolonged bed rest.
   3. Prolonged bed rest may place client at risk for thrombophlebitis.
   4. Shortening of cervical length or a short cervix may indicate a risk for PTL.

B. Management of care: Care of the client during PTL requires critical thinking skills and knowledge of assessment, and teaching and evaluation methods unique to the RN role. These skills cannot be delegated to an LPN or UAP.
   1. Monitor client for indications of PTL at each prenatal visit:
      a. Feelings of pelvic pressure
      b. Presence of menstrual-like cramps, dull backache, intestinal cramping, heaviness or aching in thighs, bloody show
      c. Contractions less than 10 min apart
      d. Increase or change in vaginal discharge
   2. Refer client to home health services to implement home uterine monitoring, etc.
   3. Provide client teaching about, and implement care for, client undergoing PTL diagnostic testing:
      a. Fetal fibronectin: Presence indicates possibility of PTL in 7 to 14 days.
      b. Transvaginal ultrasound: Cervical length less than 2.5 cm has greater risk of PTL before 35 weeks' gestation.
      c. Home uterine monitoring: Provides data to HCP supporting interventions if more than eight contractions per hour and cervical effacement and dilation.
   4. With hospitalization for treatment of PTL, the nurse will:
      a. Assess fetal and contraction monitoring to assess fetus and frequency, intensity, and duration of contractions every half hour.
      b. Monitor vital signs per labor protocol (every half hour).
      c. Maintain IV fluids to hydrate, provide access for medications.
      d. Administer medication per HCP orders to decrease, or eliminate contractions.
         (1) Magnesium sulfate: 4 to 6 g over half hour as loading dose and 1 to 3 g/hr until contractions cease for 24 hr
         (2) Magnesium levels to determine if dosages are in therapeutic range
         (3) Betamethasone (Celestone): 12 mg IM every 24 hr times 2 to initiate fetal lung maturity

e. Test for infection as needed (urinalysis, cultures for chlamydia, gonorrhea).
f. Keep client NPO or clear liquid diet until contractions cease.
g. Monitor laboratory results as needed (CBC, platelets).
h. Alert perinatologist, NICU staff.
i. Facilitate conference between perinatology and parents of infant to discuss and make decisions concerning resuscitation efforts to be made when infant is born, if viability is uncertain.
j. Prepare for preterm birth.

C. Safety and infection control
1. With use of tocolytic drugs, monitor for hyperglycemia, pulmonary edema, tachycardia of mother and/or infant.
2. With use of magnesium sulfate, monitor for magnesium toxicity (respiratory rate 12 or higher), absent reflexes, and disorientation every half hour.
3. After treatment for PTL and in preparation for returning to home undelivered, provide client teaching about:
a. Adequate hydration, diet.
b. Refraining from activities stimulating contractions (sexual intercourse, nipple stimulation, prolonged standing, strenuous activity).
c. Need for more frequent prenatal care appointments.
d. Activities to occupy time if on bed rest.
e. Support systems, personal empowerment, emotional support.
f. Reactivate home health services.

D. Health promotion and maintenance: Antenatally, the RN performs the following interventions:
1. Instruct all childbearing clients concerning need for prenatal care.
2. Provide written guidelines to prevent PTL to all prenatal clients.
3. Emphasize strategies to implement if PTL occurs:
a. Stop activity and rest on side.
b. Empty bladder.
c. Drink two to three glasses of water.
d. Palpate contractions and monitor for 1 hr.
e. Call HCP if contractions continue.

E. Psychologic integrity
1. Evaluate support systems of client.
2. Provide diversional materials of client's choice (reading, games, crossword puzzles, sudoku) while hospitalized.

F. Basic care and comfort
1. Implement comfort measures for client, including pain medication, sleep, and rest.
2. Provide emotional support (answer questions, encourage ventilation of emotions and fears concerning PTL).
3. Support learning needs by educating concerning PTL (signs and symptoms of PTL, times to call HCP, interventions to prevent PTL).
4. Refer to resources enabling client to carry pregnancy to term.

G. Reduction of risk potential: At each prenatal visit, the nurse provides the following interventions:
1. Re-educate client regarding signs and symptoms of PTL.
2. Assess client for PTL signs and symptoms.
3. Assess client for infection.

H. Pharmacologic and parenteral therapies: Client will state the purpose for and associated side effects of all medications used for PTL.
1. Medications administered in hospital setting:
a. Corticosteroids administered to facilitate fetal lung maturity at least 2 days prior to delivery; includes betamethasone (Celestone)
b. Tocolytic therapy
(1) Magnesium sulfate, IV
(2) Ritodrine (Yutopar), IV
(3) Terbutaline sulfate (Brethine), IV, SC, PO, pump
(4) Indomethacin (Indocin), PO
(5) Nifedipine (Procardia), PO
2. Medications self-administered by client in home setting: Tocolytic therapy:
a. Terbutaline sulfate (Brethine), PO, pump, or SC
b. Indomethacin (Indocin), PO
c. Nifedipine (Procardia), PO

Dystocia

I. Definition: Dystocia is difficult or abnormal labor. The normal labor pattern can be disrupted by the following:
A. Change in the uterine contractions (hypo-/hypertonic contractions)
1. Hypotonic contractions: Contractions that occur less than three times in 10 min and continue to decrease in frequency, intensity, and duration. These clients often have a normal latent phase of the first stage of labor and hypotonic contractions occur in the active phase. Interventions include oxytocin (Pitocin) augmentation and/or amniotomy.
2. Hypertonic contractions: Contractions that occur during the latent phase, are painful, frequent, and have an elevated contraction

baseline. This pattern causes hypoxia to the uterine muscle and pain as a result. These clients are often very tired and treatment is a 4- to 6-hr rest period with client usually waking in active labor.

B. Alterations in the pelvis (contracted, cephalopelvic disproportion): A contracted pelvis is not large enough for a normal-sized infant to navigate through. On the other hand, the pelvis may be adequate in size but the fetal head is enlarged. Both result in dystocia.

C. Position, size, or number of fetuses (multifetal pregnancy):
  1. Abnormal position: An infant in a position other than vertex can create dystocia. In many instances, the abnormal positioning (shoulder presentation, breech) will result in a cesarean section for the client or a prolonged labor (occiput posterior position).
  2. Carrying more than one fetus may cause dystocia as the uterine muscle is often unable to coordinate the work of the uterine musculature. If the infants are in positions other than vertex, a cesarean section is anticipated.

II. Nursing process

A. Assessment
  1. Assess client for risk factors (marginal size of pelvis, forceps or vacuum extraction in prior births, oxytocin [Pitocin] augmentation in prior labors, or dystocia in prior pregnancies).
  2. Obtain diagnostic tests.
     a. Ultrasound for fetal positioning
     b. X-rays to determine diameters of fetal head and maternal pelvis
     c. Fetal monitoring for fetal well-being and maternal contraction patterns
  3. Assess presence of pain and labor coping.

B. Analysis
  1. Risk for Injury related to complicated delivery
  2. Anxiety related to unknown fetal outcome
  3. Deficient Knowledge related to no prior experience with abnormal labor process

C. Planning
  1. Anticipate delivery of healthy infant.
  2. Instruct client concerning testing, procedures, and plan of care.
  3. Anticipate the mother and fetus to progress through labor without complications.
  4. Anticipate resolution of the situation causing dystocia without maternal or fetal injury.

D. Implementation
  1. Assess client, contraction, and fetal heart patterns.
  2. Provide emotional support.
  3. Assess infant for signs of well-being after delivery.
  4. Provide interventions for dystocia.
     a. Hypotonic contractions: Oxytocin (Pitocin), amniotomy
     b. Hypertonic contractions: Medication to provide therapeutic rest for client (meperidine [Demerol], morphine sulfate, nalbuphine [Nubain])
     c. Abnormal positioning: Notify HCP, who will determine plan of care; interventions may include:
        (1) External version
        (2) Cesarean section

E. Evaluation
  1. Client evaluates pain and anxiety as resolved.
  2. Infant is delivered without health complications, and with an Apgar score of 9 or 10.
  3. Client states she is knowledgeable about plan of care.
  4. Client progresses without complications through labor with medical and nursing interventions to remediate dystocia.

III. Client needs

A. Physiologic adaptation
  1. Normal labor
     a. Size of maternal pelvis and fetal head should allow descent at 1 cm/hr.
     b. Maternal contractions should average three in 10 min, last approximately 1 min, and are of moderate intensity.
  2. Dystocia
     a. With abnormal positioning, the fetus is unable to move through pelvis at normal rate.
     b. Contractions in dystocia originate miduterus rather than the fundus, as occurs in normal labor.

B. Management of care: Care of the client experiencing dystocia requires critical thinking skills and knowledge of assessment, and teaching and evaluation methods unique to the RN role. These skills cannot be delegated to an LPN or UAP.
  1. Assess client contraction and fetal heart patterns.
  2. Provide emotional support.
  3. Assess neonate for signs of well-being after delivery.
  4. Provide interventions for dystocia.
     a. Hypotonic contractions: Oxytocin (Pitocin), amniotomy
     b. Hypertonic contractions: Medication to provide therapeutic rest for client

(meperidine [Demerol], morphine sulfate, nalbuphine [Nubain])

c. Abnormal positioning
(1) Notify HCP, who will determine plan of care.
(2) Interventions may include:
(a) External version.
(b) Cesarean section.

C. Safety and infection control
1. Assess mother for dehydration and fatigue.
2. Assess fetus for hypoxia and acidosis based on monitoring.

D. Health promotion and maintenance
1. Instruct client and family concerning anticipated plan of care.
2. Encourage support system to provide comfort measures (e.g., back rubs, warm and cool compresses).

E. Psychologic integrity: Incorporate support system into client care to support client and labor process.

F. Basic care and comfort
1. Provide comfort measures as client experiences dystocia, including sleep and rest opportunities, and pain medication as needed.
2. Provide emotional support (answer questions, encourage ventilation of emotions and fears concerning dystocia and its impact on labor and delivery).
3. Support learning needs by educating client and family about dystocia.

G. Reduction of risk potential
1. Identify potential problems as early in pregnancy or labor as possible.
2. Provide continuous monitoring during labor process.

H. Pharmacologic and parenteral therapies: Client will state the purpose for and associated side effects of all medications used for dystocia.
1. Oxytocin (Pitocin) per induction protocol
2. Nalbuphine (Nubain), promethazine (Phenergan), meperidine (Demerol), morphine sulfate

Disseminated Intravascular Coagulation

I. Definition: Disseminated intravascular coagulation (DIC) is a clotting/coagulation disorder appearing after a complication of pregnancy consumes the body's clotting factors causing external and internal bleeding throughout the body. Concurrently, microemboli occlude small vessels, leading to tissue and organ hypoxia. The woman is clotting and bleeding simultaneously. DIC can occur prior to, during, or after delivery, and is a medical and nursing emergency.

II. Nursing process

A. Assessment
1. Perform a comprehensive physical assessment at initiation of prenatal care: Vital signs, fetal heart tones, fundal height, vaginal discharge, fetal movement, any changes each prenatal visit.
2. Assess for risk factors for DIC, serious obstetric complications, and precipitating events such as:
a. Abruptio placenta
b. Abortion
c. Fetal demise
d. Cardiac arrest
e. Sepsis
f. Amniotic fluid embolism
g. Hydatidiform mole
3. Obtain a detailed health history including past medical and surgical history, psychosocial history, and history of prior pregnancies.
4. Assess for signs and symptoms of DIC.
a. Bleeding from recently abraded sites: gums, IV puncture sites, incision sites, uterus, episiotomy
b. Bleeding is without evidence of clot formation
c. Petechiae formation on skin
d. Signs and symptoms of shock with significant blood loss
e. Fetal distress as evidenced by decreased variability, absence of accelerations, late decelerations
6. Obtain diagnostic tests.
a. Clotting studies
(1) Prothrombin time (PT), and partial thromboplastin time (PTT) (prolonged)
(2) Platelet count less than 50,000/mm^3 (normal = 140,000 to 400,000/mm^3)
(3) D-dimer-positive (diagnostic of DIC)
(4) Fibrin split products (present, elevated, or both)
(5) Fibrinogen level less than 100 mg/dl (normal is 300 to 600 mg/dl during pregnancy)
b. Hct and Hgb (decreased)

B. Analysis
1. Impaired Gas Exchange and fetal distress related to decreased placental blood flow
2. Acute Pain related to tissue ischemia
3. Anxiety related to unknown outcome
4. Ineffective Tissue Perfusion: Cardiopulmonary, related to hypoxia

5. Ineffective Coping related to fear or confusion as bleeding/shock progresses

C. Planning
1. Assist with elimination of causative agent.
2. Oxygenate client and fetus.
3. Relieve pain.
4. Manage fetal distress.
5. Type and crossmatch for blood, replace maternal blood loss through blood, packed cells, and volume-expanding products.
6. Promote delivery of fetus to preserve life.
7. Monitor for worsening condition of mother and fetus.
8. Observe and document current labor progress.
9. Provide client teaching about risk factors.
10. Explain status of problem and plan of care to family.

D. Implementation (see management of care)

E. Evaluation
1. Client's underlying etiology is identified and treated quickly.
2. Client's vital signs remain stable.
3. Client's laboratory studies return to normal.
4. Infant is delivered or remains stable in utero.

CN

III. Client needs

A. Physiologic adaptation: DIC can occur prior to, during, or after delivery.
1. A serious complication occurs in the pregnancy or the labor and delivery process causing clotting factors and platelets to be depleted. Simultaneously, fibrin clots begin to form and clot lysis occurs.
2. Hemorrhage occurs from the lack of clotting factors and microemboli cause small vessels to obstruct, causing tissue hypoxia.

B. Management of care: Care of the client with DIC requires critical thinking skills and knowledge of assessment, and teaching and evaluation methods unique to the RN role. These skills cannot be delegated to an LPN or UAP.
1. Check maternal vital signs and perform labor assessments every half hour or as indicated by maternal condition.
2. Perform continuous fetal monitoring, particularly cognizant of late decelerations, loss of variability and accelerations, sinusoidal patterns, terminal bradycardia.
3. Initiate IV infusion with large-bore intracatheter and fluids to replace volume.
4. Verify that order for laboratory clotting studies, CBC, platelets, type and crossmatch for blood has been submitted review results for nursing implications.
5. Assist client into left lateral position for best perfusion.
6. Mobilize nursing and medical resources (anesthesia, surgery teams, neonatologists).
7. Monitor intake and output precisely.
8. Prepare for cesarean section if blood loss cannot be stopped or if fetal distress exists or continues.
9. Administer blood, plasma, platelets replacement as ordered.
10. Administer oxygen at 10 to 12 L/min via mask.

C. Safety and infection control
1. Anticipate possibility of DIC with history of risk factors.
2. Anticipate possibility of DIC when problems in pregnancy are identified.

D. Health promotion and maintenance: Emphasize health promotion behaviors during pregnancy, including adequate prenatal care, and excellent self-care, including rest, eating well, exercise, and positive outlook.

E. Psychologic integrity
1. Assist client and family in coping with changes.
2. Identify stress factors and anxiety that may interfere with recovery.
3. Refer client to counseling and/or support group.

F. Basic care and comfort: Provide adequate pain management and maternal and fetal safety.

G. Reduction of risk potential
1. Identify risk factors for DIC during antenatal care.
2. Provide client and family teaching about signs or symptoms of an abnormality during pregnancy, and the need to seek care.

H. Pharmacologic and parenteral therapies: Client will state the purpose for and associated side effects of all medications used to manage DIC.
1. IV infusion of lactated Ringer
2. Platelets, blood volume expanders, PRBCs to replace depleted clotting factors and blood volume

Cesarean Section

I. Definition: Cesarean section (C-section) is the delivery of the fetus through incision in abdomen and uterus. Cesarean sections are either planned or emergent and are determined to be necessary by the HCP based on health of mother, fetus, or both. The current cesarean section rate in the United States is approximately 29%. Mortality rates are approximately 6 in 100,000 women.

A. Indications for elective cesarean section
   1. Cephalopelvic disproportion
   2. Active herpes, type II
   3. Breech presentation
   4. HIV
   5. Placenta previa
   6. Maternal neoplasm, tumors
B. Indications for emergency cesarean section
   1. Fetal distress
   2. Prolapsed cord
   3. Abruptio placenta
   4. Failure to progress in labor
   5. Severe pre-eclampsia
   6. Cephalopelvic disproportion
C. Types of incisions
   1. Classic: Vertical incision into abdomen and uterus. Used for emergency cesareans and in repeat cesareans with prior classic incision; may result in greater blood loss.
   2. Low segment: Horizontal incision into abdomen with either vertical or horizontal incision into uterus. Horizontal incision into uterus results in:
      a. Less blood loss.
      b. Cosmetically pleasing.
      c. Less likelihood of uterine rupture in future pregnancies.

II. Nursing process

A. Assessment
   1. Assess L/S (lecithin to sphingomyelin) ratio of 2:1 indicating mature fetal lungs.
   2. Assess for risk factors prior to and during pregnancy.
      a. Prior cesarean sections
      b. Type of incision into uterus
      c. Rationale for prior cesarean section (s)
B. Analysis
   1. Anticipatory Grieving related to risk of loss of vaginal delivery
   2. Acute Pain related to incisions
   3. Fear related to unknown outcomes of surgery
   4. Risk for Infection related to altered skin integrity
   5. Risk for Hemorrhage related to surgical procedure
C. Planning
   1. Provide client and family teaching about the procedure.
   2. Maintain mother's blood loss at less than 1,000 ml.
   3. Prevent pain during procedure.
D. Implementation
   1. Planned cesarean section
      a. Obtain presurgical laboratory studies as outpatient (CBC, platelets).
      b. Admit client at term.
      c. Keep client NPO for 6 to 8 hr prior to procedure.
      d. Obtain admission histories, physical assessments, consents, anesthesia consult, education concerning procedure, IV, Foley catheter, fetal monitoring.
      e. Prepare for surgery with appropriate "time outs" per agency safety standards.
      f. Admit mother and infant to postpartum unit in stable condition.
   2. Emergency cesarean section
      a. Instruct client about procedure as time permits.
      b. Activate emergency protocols for unit as needed.
      c. Coordinate team assisting with consents, teaching, IV, Foley catheter, fetal monitoring, anesthesia, and the surgical procedure.
E. Evaluation
   1. Client is knowledgeable concerning procedure.
   2. Client's blood loss remains less than 1,000 ml.
   3. Client remains afebrile without pain during procedure.
   4. Client has sufficient support systems during cesarean section.
   5. Infant has Apgar score of 9 or 10 with no anomalies.

III. Client needs

A. Physiologic adaptation
   1. Fetus physically unable to fit through pelvis
   2. Fetus unable to tolerate process of labor
B. Management of care: Care of the client undergoing a cesarean section requires critical thinking skills and knowledge of assessment, and teaching and evaluation methods unique to the RN role. These skills cannot be delegated to an LPN or UAP.
   1. Assess the following:
      a. Fetal monitoring
      b. Maternal vital signs
      c. Status of membranes (color, odor, amount), bleeding
      d. Maternal emotional status
   2. Administer antacid prior to surgery.
   3. Place a Foley catheter.
   4. Remove dentures, contacts lenses.
C. Safety and infection control
   1. Maintain aseptic technique throughout procedures.
   2. Provide time outs as indicated in standard of care.
   3. Administer prophylactic antibiotics after delivery of placenta.

D. Health promotion and maintenance
   1. Encourage client participation in childbirth education discussions of cesarean section deliveries.
   2. Provide client teaching about symptoms, and instruct to report symptoms immediately.
E. Psychologic integrity
   1. Provide constant emotional support to client and partner.
   2 Encourage support network to assist family on return home.
F. Basic care and comfort
   1. Provide comfort measures as needed, including rest and sleep opportunities during hospitalization.
   2. Provide emotional support (e.g., answer questions, encourage ventilation of emotions and fears concerning surgical procedure and pregnancy outcome).
   3. Support learning needs by educating concerning the surgical procedure and care before and after surgery.
   4. Refer to support groups and resources as needed.
G. Reduction of risk potential: Alert neonatal staff and assure presence for delivery if indicated.
H. Pharmacologic and parenteral therapies: Client will state the purpose for and associated side effects of all medication used for cesarean section.
   1. Analgesia and anesthesia for surgical procedure (general if emergency; spinal, epidural, combination of epidural/spinal for nonemergent procedure)
   2. Analgesia available after surgery (narcotic and nonnarcotic analgesics, NSAIDs)

Vaginal Birth After Cesarean Section

I. Definition: Vaginal birth after cesarean (VBAC) describes a woman who gives birth vaginally after having at least one cesarean section with a prior delivery.

II. Management of care
A. Assessment
   1. Assess for low transverse uterine incision in prior cesarean.
   2. Assess reason for prior cesarean not present in this pregnancy (breech, fetal distress, etc.).
   3. Assess cervix soft, anterior.
B. Analysis
   1. Fear related to possible need for repeat cesarean section
   2. Risk for Impaired Skin Integrity related to uterine rupture
C. Planning
   1. Provide client and family teaching regarding labor process and procedures.
   2. Prevent fetal distress or uterine rupture.
D. Implementation
   1. Obtain admission history, physical assessments, consents, anesthesia consult, education concerning procedure, IV as for any vaginal delivery.
   2. Assess for pre-existing reason indicating need for repeat cesarean section.
   3. Monitor labor process with continuous fetal monitoring.
   4. Monitor labor progress against normal labor continuum.
E. Evaluation
   1. Client is knowledgeable concerning labor process and procedures necessary if repeat cesarean section is indicated.
   2. Client progresses through labor in normal time frames without fetal distress or uterine rupture.
   3. Infant is born with Apgar score between 9 and 10 with no anomalies.

CN

III. Client needs
A. Physiologic adaptation
   1. Fetus at term, physically able to fit through pelvis.
   2. Fetus appears able to tolerate process of labor.
   3. Prior uterine incision is low transverse.
B. Management of care: Care of the VBAC client requires critical thinking skills and knowledge of assessment, and teaching and evaluation methods unique to the RN role. These skills cannot be delegated to an LPN or UAP.
   1. Implement all actions and assessments identified in normal labor.
   2. Maintain continuous fetal monitoring.
   3. Maintain continuous contraction monitoring.
   4. Observe labor process for possibility of uterine rupture.
C. Safety and infection control
   1. Use aseptic technique throughout labor and delivery.
   2. Monitor for labor complications, dystocia.
D. Health promotion and maintenance
   1. Provide client teaching concerning VBAC process and possibility of repeat cesarean section.
   2. Identify signs of dysfunctional labor and fetal distress as they appear.
   3. Treat emerging complications as they develop.

E. Psychologic integrity
 1. Provide emotional support to client and partner during labor.
 2 Inform client concerning progress of this labor.
 3. Assist client with coping should cesarean section become necessary.

F. Basic care and comfort: Provide comfort measures as needed for normal labor.

G. Reduction of risk potential
 1. Assure client meets criteria for VBAC.
 2. Alert neonatal staff for delivery if indicated.

H. Pharmacologic and parenteral therapies: Client will state the purpose for and associated side effects of all medications used for VBAC.
 1. Analgesia and anesthesia as indicated for normal labor
 2. Analgesia and anesthesia as indicated if cesarean section

Bibliography

Klossner, N. J., & Hatfield, N. (2005). *Introduction to maternity and pediatric nursing*. Philadelphia: Lippincott Williams & Wilkins.

Pillitteri, A. (2006). *Maternal & child health nursing: Care of the childbearing and childrearing family* (5th ed.). Philadelphia: Lippincott Williams & Wilkins.

Simpson, K. R., & Creehan, P. A. (2007). *AWHONN's perinatal nursing* (3rd ed.). Philadelphia: Lippincott Williams & Wilkins.

Witt, C. (2007). *Advances in neontal care*. Philadelphia: Lipincott Williams & Wilkins.

CHAPTER 6

Practice Test

Normal Labor and Delivery

1. The nurse is performing a vaginal examination on a client in labor. The nurse finds the fetal presenting part 1 cm above the ischial spines. The nurse should chart the station as:
- ☐ 1. −1 Station.
- ☐ 2. +1 Station.
- ☐ 3. Engaged.
- ☐ 4. Floating.

2. The nurse is managing a pregnant client's second stage of labor. The nurse should intervene when observing which of the following? The woman is using:
- ☐ 1. Closed glottis pushing.
- ☐ 2. Open glottis pushing.
- ☐ 3. "Rest and descent."
- ☐ 4. Squatting while pushing.

3. A client in labor received an epidural for pain management. Before receiving the epidural, the client's BP was 124/76. Ten minutes after receiving the epidural, the client's BP is 98/56 and the mother is vomiting. Before calling the HCP, the nurse should:
- ☐ 1. Decrease the IV fluid rate.
- ☐ 2. Turn the client to her side.
- ☐ 3. Catheterize the client.
- ☐ 4. Perform a vaginal examination.

4. A pregnant client at 38 weeks' gestation comes to the labor room because "my bag of waters broke." The HCP asks the nurse to verify spontaneous ROM using Nitrazine paper. The nurse observes that the Nitrazine paper turns bright blue. The nurse's NEXT action should be to:
- ☐ 1. Notify the HCP that the membranes are ruptured.
- ☐ 2. Perform a sterile vaginal examination to assess the cervix.
- ☐ 3. Document the findings of the Nitrazine test.
- ☐ 4. Offer the client a sterile sanitary pad after performing perineal care.

5. The HCP performs a vaginal examination on a woman in active labor and tells the nurse the client is 5 cm, 50%, −1, and right occiput posterior (ROP). The nurse should assess the maternal vital signs, FHR, and uterine activity at least every:
- ☐ 1. 60 minutes.
- ☐ 2. 30 minutes.
- ☐ 3. 10 minutes.
- ☐ 4. 5 minutes.

6. A client in the second stage of labor who planned an unmedicated birth is in severe pain because the fetus is in the ROP position. The nurse should position the client in which of the following positions for pain relief?
- ☐ 1. Lithotomy.
- ☐ 2. Right lateral position.
- ☐ 3. Hands and knees.
- ☐ 4. Tailor sitting.

7. AF The nurse performs Leopold maneuvers on a client who is 36 weeks pregnant to assess the best place to locate the fetal heart tones (FHTs). The nurse feels a soft part in the fundus, smooth surface on the right maternal abdomen, and an irregular surface on the left maternal abdomen. Based on these findings, place an "X" on the following image where the nurse will find the FHTs with a Doppler.

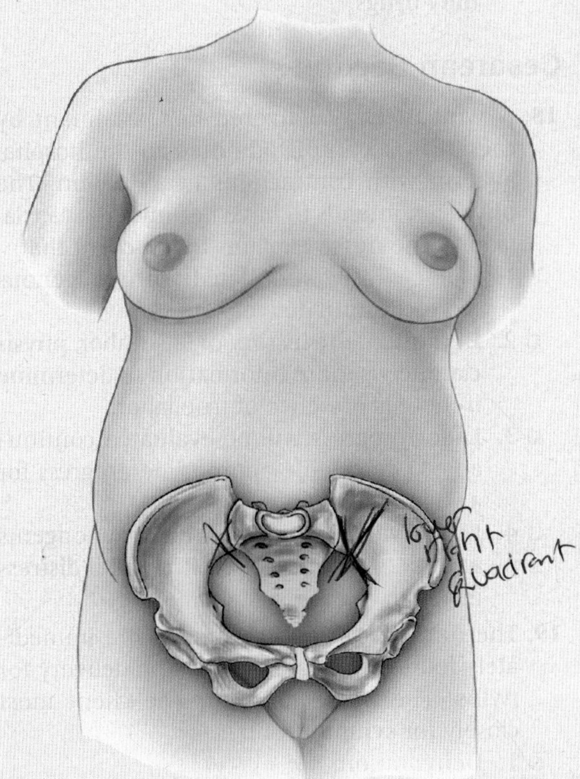

8. A laboring woman's cervix is dilated 6 cm and the presenting part is at a −2 station. Her membranes have just ruptured. Which nursing action takes priority?
- □ 1. Timing of contractions.
- □ 2. Assessing BP.
- □ 3. Determining the station of the presenting part.
- □ 4. Assessing the FHR.

Potential Problems During Labor and Delivery

9. During delivery the nurse notes a prolapsed cord. The nurse should first:
- □ 1. Prepare the parents for the potential loss of the infant.
- □ 2. Relieve pressure on the cord and prepare the woman for an emergency cesarean section.
- □ 3. Clamp the part of the cord that protrudes from the vagina.
- □ 4. Initiate an oxytocin (Pitocin) drip to affect delivery as soon as possible.

10. AF Which of the following indicate amniotic fluid emboli in a woman in the second stage of labor? Select all that apply.
- □ 1. Dyspnea.
- □ 2. Hypotension.
- □ 3. Tachycardia.
- □ 4. Elevated fever.
- □ 5. Bleeding from IV puncture site.
- □ 6. Cloudy, foul-smelling amniotic fluid.
- □ 7. Cardiac arrest.

Procedures Used During Labor and Delivery

11. AF The nurse is caring for a labor patient at 41 weeks' gestation who is being induced with oxytocin (Pitocin). The nurse observes the following pattern on the electronic fetal monitor tracing.

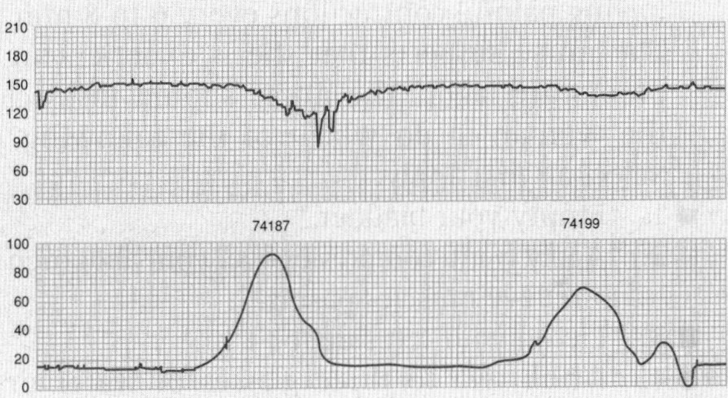

The nurse should do which of the following? Select all that apply.
- □ 1. Continue routine labor care.
- □ 2. Discontinue the oxytocin infusion.
- □ 3. Administer oxygen by mask at 8 to 10 L/min.
- □ 4. Turn the woman to her side.
- □ 5. Lift the presenting part off the umbilical cord.
- □ 6. Increase the rate of the maintenance IV.
- □ 7. Notify the HCP.

12. The nurse is monitoring a laboring client who is receiving oxytocin (Pitocin) for labor stimulation. The contractions are 2 min apart and lasting 90 s. The fetal heart baseline is in the 140s. Three contractions occur in rapid succession and the FHR decreases to 110. The nurse should next:
- □ 1. Start oxygen per mask.
- □ 2. Turn the mother to her side.
- □ 3. Evaluate the maternal pain level.
- □ 4. Stop the oxytocin (Pitocin).

13. A client in labor is receiving oxytocin (Pitocin). During labor the nurse observes decelerations in the FHR that are not associated with contractions. The nurse should:
- ☐ 1. Change the client's position.
- ☐ 2. Start oxygen per tight face mask.
- ☐ 3. Increase the IV fluid rate.
- ☐ 4. Discontinue oxytocin (Pitocin).

14. The nurse is caring for a primigravida at term with ruptured membranes. She had contractions every 5 min lasting 60 s on admission. After 2 hr, the contractions are now every 10 min and last 30 s. If there is no evidence of cephalopelvic disproportion, the nurse should prepare the client to receive which of the following?
- ☐ 1. Oxytocin (Pitocin).
- ☐ 2. An epidural anesthesia.
- ☐ 3. Terbutaline.
- ☐ 4. Morphine.

Preterm Labor

15. AF A woman who is 31 weeks' pregnant is having painful contractions every 6 to 8 min. The nurse suspects that she is experiencing premature labor. The nurse should instruct the woman to do which of the following? Select all that apply.
- ☐ 1. "Empty your bladder."
- ☐ 2. "Apply warm compresses over your abdomen to relieve muscle spasms."
- ☐ 3. "Lie on your left side for 1 hr."
- ☐ 4. "Drink two to three glasses of water or juice."
- ☐ 5. "Try to relax by reading a book or watching TV."
- ☐ 6. "Avoid touching your abdomen."
- ☐ 7. "Go to the clinic if the contractions do not abate in 1 hr."
- ☐ 8. "Report any bleeding or leakage of fluid from the vagina."

Dystocia

16. After delivery of the head, the client develops shoulder dystocia. The nurse can assist the HCP by performing which of the following interventions?
- ☐ 1. Apply suprapubic pressure to push the shoulder under the pubic bone.
- ☐ 2. Apply fundal pressure as the physician pulls from below.
- ☐ 3. Assist with the application of special forceps.
- ☐ 4. Increase oxytocin (Pitocin) in small increments as long as the infant's heartbeat remains above 110.

Disseminated Intravascular Coagulation

17. Which of the following women who are in labor is at greatest risk for DIC?
- ☐ 1. Client who is 24 years of age delivering twins.
- ☐ 2. Client who is 30 years of age with an amniotic fluid embolus.
- ☐ 3. Client who is 15 years of age and a primipara.
- ☐ 4. Client who is 40 years of age who took fertility drugs.

Cesarean Section

18. A woman who delivered her last infant by caesarean section is admitted to the hospital at term with contractions every 5 min. The physician intends to have her undergo "a trial labor." The nurse explains to the client that:
- ☐ 1. Labor will be stimulated with exogenous oxytocin until delivery.
- ☐ 2. Because of the history of false labor, physician needs more information to determine if there is presence of true labor.
- ☐ 3. Labor progress will be evaluated continually to determine appropriate progress for a vaginal delivery.
- ☐ 4. Labor will be arrested with tocolytic agents after a 2-hr period even if no fetal distress is noted.

19. The nurse is caring for a multipara immediately following a cesarean section delivery for twins. The nurse monitors the client most closely for symptoms of:
- ☐ 1. Dehydration.
- ☐ 2. Hypertension.
- ☐ 3. Immobility.
- ☐ 4. Hemorrhage.

Vaginal Birth After Cesarean

20. Which of the following women is the best candidate for VBAC?
- ☐ 1. Client who had an emergency cesarean section because of fetal distress during her last delivery and has a classic incision.
- ☐ 2. Client who had a breech presentation in her last pregnancy; this pregnancy is a vertex presentation.
- ☐ 3. Client who dilated to 6 cm in her last delivery and failed to progress beyond this point despite 5 more hours of labor.
- ☐ 4. Diabetic client whose last infant was over 10 lb; this infant is larger, as seen on ultrasound.

Answers and Rationales

1. 3 If the presenting part is above the ischial spines 1 cm, the station is −1. If the presenting part is 1 cm below the ischial spines, the station is +1. Engaged and floating are not descriptive of station. (A)

2. 1 Closed glottis pushing is associated with fetal hypoxia and subsequent acidosis. Open glottis pushing, "rest and descent," and squatting have positive influences on second-stage of labor and birth. (A)

3. 2 The nurse turns the client to the side to reduce pressure on the abdominal aorta. The IV fluid rate would be increased, not decreased. There is no information indicating the client has a full bladder or requires a vaginal examination. (D)

4. 1 Nitrazine paper responds to alkaline fluids by changing blue; amniotic fluid is alkaline so the color verifies that the membranes are ruptured. The nurse notifies the HCP that membranes are ruptured so that a plan of action can be developed. Rupture of membranes in the absence of labor increases the risk of infection. Vaginal examinations are limited until labor is initiated. Wearing a sanitary pad increases the potential for infection. Documentation of the Nitrazine test is completed after notifying the HCP. (M)

5. 2 Standards of care require that the client in active labor (4 to 7 cm) has vital signs, FHR, and uterine activity assessed every 15 to 30 min. Vital signs, FHR, and contractions are assessed every 30 to 60 min during latent labor (0 to 3 cm). During transition (8 to 10 cm) the vital signs are assessed every 15 to 30 min. (R)

6. 3 Placing the client in the hands and knees position pulls the fetal head away from the sacral promontory (relieving pain) and facilitates rotation of the fetus to the anterior position. Lithotomy is the position preferred by some HCPs for delivery but does not facilitate rotation. The right lateral position will perpetuate the ROP position. Tailor sitting facilitates descent in OA positions. (M)

7. Correct answer: "X" is in the right lower quadrant. Leopold maneuvers indicate that the FHTs will be located in the right lower quadrant. The smooth surface on the maternal right abdomen is the fetal back; the irregular surface on the left reflects fetal arms and legs. The soft part in the uterine fundus is the fetal buttocks. The heart is best heard through the fetal back or shoulder. (M)

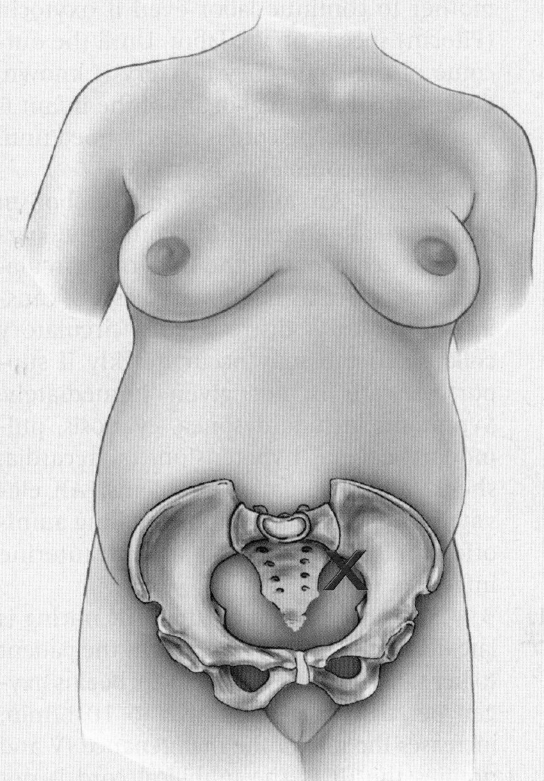

8. 4 When membranes rupture, the first nursing action is to assess the FHR. With the gush of fluid accompanying rupture of the membranes, there is the possibility that the umbilical cord has come down between the fetal head and the mother's pelvis, compromising circulation in the cord and oxygenation to the fetus. This is especially likely to happen if the presenting part is at a minus station. Although the other assessments need to continue during labor, they do not take priority over assessing fetal well-being when membranes rupture. (R)

9. 2 The most important step for the nurse to take when there is a cord prolapse is to relieve pressure on the cord so that the infant continues to get oxygen through the cord. This is accomplished by placing the hand in the vagina and pushing the head up in the pelvis, making more room between the infant's head and the mother's bony pelvis. The infant is delivered as soon as possible by cesarean section. The relief of pressure on the cord must be continuous until delivery; therefore, the nurse calls for help because others will need to assist in preparing the woman for surgery. There is not time in this emergency to allow the mother to continue labor even if oxytocin (Pitocin) speeds up the labor. Until the outcome of the emergency delivery is known, discussion of potential death of the infant is inappropriate. The cord is not clamped until the infant is completely born. (M)

10. 1, 2, 3, 5, 7 An amniotic fluid embolism occurs when amniotic fluid containing particles of debris enters the maternal circulation and obstructs pulmonary vessels, causing respiratory distress and circulatory collapse. Death may occur quickly if supportive care is not given immediately. Symptoms include dyspnea, cyanosis, pulmonary edema, hypotension, tachycardia, shock, and coagulation problems. An elevated fever and cloudy, foul-smelling amniotic fluid are related to an intrauterine infection. (R)

11. 2, 3, 4, 6, 7 The pattern on the FHR tracing is late decelerations. The nurse turns the patient to her side, discontinues oxytocin, begins oxygen per tight face mask at 8 to 10 L/min, increases the rate of the maintenance IV and notifies the HCP. The umbilical cord is not prolapsed at this point. Amnioinfusion may be performed if the tracing shows variable decelerations. (M)

12. 4 The client is experiencing hyperstimulation from the oxytocin (Pitocin). The priority action is to discontinue the oxytocin. Oxygen may improve the fetal oxygenation, but the fetus is responding to the hyperstimulation pattern. Turning the mother to her side may improve perfusion of the placenta, but only after hyperstimulation is corrected. The maternal pain level does not immediately influence the FHR. (S)

13. 1 Variable decelerations have no relationship to contractions and are related to intermittent compression of the umbilical cord. The appropriate nursing action is to reposition the client, which may reduce compression on the umbilical cord. It is not necessary to start oxygen at this time as repositioning the client may reduce the cord compression. Increasing the IV fluid rate or discontinuing oxytocin (Pitocin) will not relieve the cord compression. (M)

14. 1 Oxytocin (Pitocin) is used to stimulate labor, making the contractions stronger and closer together. An epidural may help the woman relax by relieving pain, but may also slow labor even more. Terbutaline is used to stop contractions, especially with premature labor. Morphine is a narcotic that is usually not used in labor because of the respiratory suppression affect of the drug on the infant after birth. (D)

15. 1, 3, 4, 7, 8 The nurse advises the woman to first empty her bladder because a full bladder can cause uterine contractions. The client is advised to lie on her left side because rest may lessen the contractions and that position is best for placental profusion, and to hydrate with oral fluids because dehydration can cause contractions. If the contractions do not abate in an hour or the woman experiences ROM or bleeding, she is advised to come into the clinic or emergency department to be assessed for premature labor. The nurse also instructs the client how to palpate contractions. Warm compresses and touching the abdomen do not affect premature labor. Telling a woman to relax and ignore her symptoms is not appropriate. (M)

16. 1 When a shoulder dystocia is diagnosed, the nurse applies pressure over the pubic bone while the HCP applies traction to the head. This maneuver helps move the shoulder under the pubic arch. Applying fundal pressure is contraindicated because it pushes the shoulder tighter against the pelvic bone and can cause a ruptured uterus. Forceps are not used because the head is already delivered. Oxytocin (Pitocin) is dangerous and ineffective in relieving the problem in this emergency situation. (M)

17. 2 Clients with amniotic fluid emboli are at risk for DIC; the nurse monitors this client for bleeding, signs of shock, and fetal distress. Having twins, being a primipara, or taking fertility drugs are not precipitating factors for DIC. Maternal age is not correlated with DIC. (A)

18. 3 A trial of labor in this context means that the woman is allowed to go into labor and her progress is assessed by cervical dilatation and effacement as well as fetal descent evaluated to determine whether to allow the labor to progress to delivery. If there are indications that labor is not progressing, other means of delivery are considered. Labor stimulation is used cautiously and may not be safe. A history of false labor is not relevant. If fetal distress is noted and an emergency cesarean section cannot be done immediately, tocolytic agents may be considered to stop contractions. (A)

19. 4 Because this woman has had other pregnancies and her uterus was overstretched with twins, her uterus may have difficulty contracting to control bleeding. She is at greatest risk for hemorrhage. The client may become dehydrated from diaphoresis and lack of fluid intake; the nurse monitors intake and output carefully, but that is not the priority at this time. Increased BP is not common following cesarean section. The woman is not immobile and can be encouraged to move all extremities. (M)

20. 2 The best candidate for a VBAC is a woman who had a cesarean section in her last delivery because of a problem related to the infant that is not repeated in this pregnancy. The woman with the breech presentation in her last delivery and a vertex presentation in this pregnancy would be the best candidate, especially if she has had other vaginal deliveries. The woman who was unable to dilate beyond 6 cm (failure to progress) is likely to experience the same problem with this delivery. The woman with the very large infant is likely to experience cephalopelvic disproportion with this delivery if she experienced cephalopelvic disproportion with her last infant who was large. A classic cesarean section scar is a contraindication for a VBAC because that type of scar may not be strong enough to withstand the stress of hours of uterine contractions and may result in a uterine rupture. (A)

chapter 7

Postpartum Care

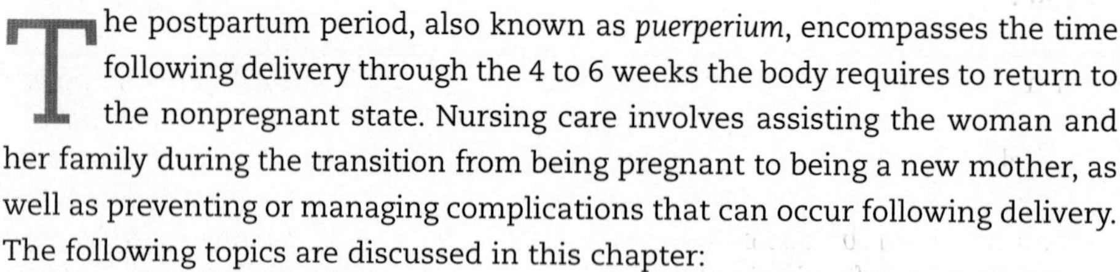

The postpartum period, also known as *puerperium*, encompasses the time following delivery through the 4 to 6 weeks the body requires to return to the nonpregnant state. Nursing care involves assisting the woman and her family during the transition from being pregnant to being a new mother, as well as preventing or managing complications that can occur following delivery. The following topics are discussed in this chapter:

- Postpartum Care Following Vaginal or Cesarean Delivery
- Postpartum Infections
- Postpartum Bleeding Disorders: Postpartum Hemorrhage
- Thromboembolic Disease
- Psychiatric Disorders

Postpartum Care Following Vaginal or Cesarean Delivery

I. Definition: Care for the postpartum client begins immediately after delivery.

Approximately 75% of all deliveries are vaginal and the remaining 25% are cesarean. The client who has had a cesarean section is also recovering from surgery and needs postpartum as well as postsurgical care.

II. Nursing process

A. Assessment

1. In addition to vital signs and pain level, the eight areas pertinent to assessment of a postpartum client can be remembered by the acronym **BUBBLE HEN**: **B**reasts, **u**terus, **b**owels, **b**ladder, **l**ochia, **e**pisiotomy, **H**omans sign, **e**motions, and **n**utrition.
2. Additional postpartum assessments include:
   a. Maternal and infant bonding and attachment.
   b. Psychosocial stage: Taking in, taking hold, or letting go.
   c. Education and support system needs.
   d. Immunization needs prior to discharge (Rh immune globulin [RhoGAM], rubella vaccine).
   e. Contraceptive needs and preferences.
   f. Cultural and religious beliefs, needs, and practices affecting maternal and infant care.
   g. Breast and/or bottle feeding practice (breast and nipple assessment for bruising, cracking, and soreness).
3. Additional assessments following cesarean section include:
   a. Incision site; remember the acronym REEDA (redness, edema, ecchymosis, discharge, and approximation).
   b. Bowel sounds, assess all four quadrants; flatus.
   c. Lung fields (all aspects).
   d. Foley catheter.
   e. Return of sensation, level of consciousness, and orientation after recovery.
   f. Use of patient-controlled analgesia (PCA), pain medications after surgery.
   g. Ambulation.
   h. Diagnostic tests, including CBC, platelets postpartum as needed.

B. Analysis

1. Urinary Retention related to trauma to perineum
2. Constipation related to slowed peristalsis
3. Acute Pain related to perineal trauma, hemorrhoids, incision (episiotomy, lacerations, cesarean section), and uterine cramping
4. Impaired Skin Integrity related to lacerations, episiotomy, cesarean section incision, nipple trauma
5. Impaired Parenting related to inability to assume parenting role
6. Risk for Impaired Parent/Infant/Child Attachment related to maternal age, unwanted pregnancy
7. Imbalanced Nutrition: Less than Body Requirements related to lifestyle, lack of knowledge
8. Disturbed Sleep Pattern related to care of newborn, hospital routine
9. Deficient Knowledge related to first-time parenting
10. Risk for Injury related to effects of anesthesia
11. Risk for Deficient Fluid Volume related to postpartum hemorrhage, uterine atony
12. Risk for Infection related to altered tissue integrity
13. Impaired Physical Mobility related to surgical procedure

C. Planning

1. Facilitate voiding when bladder is full or after Foley removal.
2. Encourage spontaneous bowel movements by 3 days postpartum.
3. Manage pain by comfort measures and medication.
4. Provide client and family teaching per hospital protocol regarding:
   a. Parenting activities (e.g., feeding, comfort, diaper changes begin shortly after birth, or with ambulation for cesarean section client).
   b. Maternal health care needs:
      (1) Adequate nutrition to repair tissues, prevent anemia, meet infant breast-feeding needs.
      (2) Personal physical care for self, incision, or episiotomy.
5. Support opportunities for bonding and attachment.
6. Initiate breast or bottle-feeding per client's preference.
7. Encourage ambulation when client is physically stable.
8. Immunize client as needed before discharge.

D. Implementation

1. Offer bedpan, as needed, or assist client to toilet every 4 hr if uterus is deviated to side, or elevated in abdomen above position it was in the previous check. Catheterize if necessary. Measure urine until output is at least 300 ml and bladder is empty.

2. Encourage bowel function by increased ambulation, fluids, and fiber.
3. Offer pain medication before breast-feeding if client has severe after-pains, and for other discomfort. Investigate unexpected or severe pain.
4. Facilitate rooming-in as much as possible—teach parents how to identify and respond to cues of the infant.
5. Follow breast-feeding protocols of hospital (e.g., feeding on demand, but waking infant every 4 hr during the first 3 days to feed; if under 6 lb, every 3 hr).
6. Assist with ambulation the first time (within 4 hours of vaginal delivery and when legs have sensation if the client had a cesarean section).
7. Administer RhoGAM within 72 hr following delivery, rubella vaccine if titer is negative prior to discharge.

E. Evaluation
1. Client initiates bonding, attachment, and parenting roles.
2. Client copes with mood changes ("postpartum blues").
3. Client's voiding and stooling return to normal pattern.
4. Client's uterus and lochia follow expected postpartum patterns.
5. Client resumes nutritious diet.
6. Client's pain is managed adequately.
7. Client remains free of infection; cesarean delivery incision/episiotomy heals without complications.
8. Client verbalizes adequate knowledge to care for self and infant.
9. Client is released to home having received appropriate immunizations.
10. Client makes appointment for follow-up care for self and infant.
11. Client's follow-up care is initiated.
12. Client's decision for birth control is discussed.

CN

III. Client needs

A. Physiologic adaptation
1. Physiologic and emotional return to non-pregnant state takes 4 to 6 weeks. Placental site heals in 6 weeks, while endometrial area heals in 2 to 3 weeks. Cesarean section skin incision heals in 1 to 2 weeks, and uterine incision heals in 4 to 6 weeks.
2. Typical progression of return to prepregnancy state:
   a. Fundus is firm at umbilicus or lower when checked in supine position; bleeding will saturate less than one pad per hour and continues to decrease daily.
   b. Fundal height decreases at umbilicus immediately after delivery, rises to one fingerbreadth above the umbilicus at 12 hr after delivery then decreases 1 cm per day.
   c. Lochia changes include:
      (1) Rubra (red) 1 to 2 days postpartum
      (2) Serosa (pink, serosanguinous) 3 to 10 days postpartum
      (3) Alba (off-white) 11 days to 6 weeks postpartum
   d. Postpartum blues may occur 3 to 5 days postpartum as the result of fluctuating hormones, fatigue, and added responsibilities.
3. After pains more severe in multigravida, breast-feeding client, or client with twins, polyhydramnios, LGA infant, as uterus contracts, relaxes, and contracts again.
4. Postpartum diuresis occurs in first 5 days postpartum, accounts for approximately 5 lb loss of pregnancy induced fluid now returning to intravascular spaces.
5. Vital signs: Pulse rate post delivery is 50 to 70 beats per minute (BPM), temperature less than 100.4°F in first 24 hr postpartum as result of dehydration, BP orthostatic hypotension for 48 hr postpartum as the result of splanchnic engorgement.
6. Peristalsis returns slowly after manipulation of bowel during cesarean section.
7. Adjustment to change in family structure and responsibilities begins immediately.
8. Laboratory studies:
   a. WBC count: Neutrophils less than 25,000/mm^3 considered normal for 10 to 12 days postpartum
   b. Clotting factors: Remain elevated during puerperium-increased risk for thrombophlebitis
   c. Hematocrit may be elevated as the result of dehydration

B. Management of care: Care of the postpartum client requires critical thinking skills and knowledge of assessment, and teaching and evaluation methods unique to the RN role. These skills cannot be delegated to an LPN or UAP.
1. Delegate responsibly those activities that can be delegated, including basic care needs and vital signs for stable clients. All monitoring information is reported to the RN.
2. Perform comprehensive assessments for client with a vaginal delivery and cesarean section.

a. Assess breast, uterus, bowel, bladder, lochia, emotions, Homans sign, nutrition, episiotomy, and vital signs every 8 hr.
b. Initiate focused assessment in areas of other health care problems as needed.
c. Monitor IV fluids:
(1) 20 units of oxytocin (Pitocin) in first 2 L of fluids postpartum
(2) Discontinue IV infusion when bleeding is scant, fundus remains firm at umbilicus and at midline
d. Assess sensation in extremities; maintain bed rest until sensation returns.
e. Assess bonding and attachment, and psychosocial stage progression.
f. Assess need for and give RhoGAM, rubella vaccine prior to discharge if appropriate candidate.
g. Evaluate client against norm for change in fundal height and lochia.

3. Provide client care and teaching for breast-feeding:
a. Perform nipple assessment: Obtain history of breast surgeries (e.g., augmentation, reduction, biopsies, or trauma).
b. Initiate breast-feeding within 1 hr of delivery. If infant is unable to be put to breast, use hospital-grade breast pump within 4 to 6 hr of delivery.
c. Position client for comfort during breast-feeding. For infant: Cross-cradle, side-lying, cradle; for mother: Sitting with back support, use of pillows to support infant.
d. Ensure proper alignment of infant: Ear, shoulder, and hips in straight alignment.
e. Promote infant's latching on to breast:
(1) Ensure infant's mouth is open wide, with tongue down.
(2) Bring infant into breast covering ¾ to 1 in. of breast tissue into infant's mouth.
(3) Position chin to touch breast tissue.
(4) Use infant's lips as flanges.
(5) Listen for sucking and swallowing; watch for swallowing (chin drop and ear wiggle for transfer of breast milk).
f. Direct breast-feed on one breast, and then on second breast, if needed. Instruct client to begin next feed on side fed on the least during previous feed.
g. Inform client of no time limits at breast: 8 to 12 times at breast in 24 hr; avoid pacifiers and artificial nipples with formula for at least first 10 days.
h. Inform client that uterine cramping is due to release of oxytocin and prostaglandins during breast-feeding; use ibuprofen for relief control.
i. Inform client that breast engorgement can present after 3 days postpartum: Breast-feeding frequently (8 to 12 times in 24 hr) is best prevention; relieve discomfort through warm shower, cool compress to breast, and anti-inflammatory medication.
j. Inform mother about medications that could cause a decrease milk supply:
(1) Estrogen-/progestin-based contraceptives may decrease milk supply when used prior to 6 weeks postpartum when milk supply is well established.
(2) Use barrier contraception prior to 6 weeks.
k. Inform client about contraindications to breast-feeding:
(1) Ingestion of medications that may enter milk supply in large quantities (lithium, street or chemotherapy drugs)
(2) Presence of AIDS, HIV-positive, or TB
(3) Use of antibiotics and cold remedies acceptable in breast-feeding, but pseudoephedrine, diphenhydramine may decrease milk supply
l. Discuss prevention of sore nipples (soreness indicates poor and/or incorrect latch) such as coating nipple with colostrum, mother's milk, or lanolin. Additional steps include:
(1) Ensure adequate latch: Infant mouth covers areola.
(2) Break suction before removing infant from breast by inserting finger into infant's mouth.
(3) Practice good breast care: Expose nipples to air; keep nipples dry between feedings; change nursing pads frequently; avoid soap on nipples.

4. Provide client care and teaching for bottle feeding.
a. Wear support or sports bra for first week postpartum.
b. Avoid stimulation to nipples.
c. Treat engorgement with continual use of supportive bra, cool packs to breasts, anti-inflammatory medications for pain.

5. Assess pain every 2 hr.
   a. For uterine cramping, promote voiding, ambulation, and medications including:
      (1) Prostaglandin inhibitors (ibuprofen [Motrin], naproxen [Anaprox, Aleve]).
      (2) Narcotics, if unrelieved (hydrocodone [Vicodin], oxycodone [Percocet]).
   b. For perineal pain related to episiotomy, hemorrhoids, provide pain medication in addition to increasing comfort measures (e.g., position changes, topical anesthetic medication, sitz baths).
6. Provide interventions for inability to void.
   a. Apply ice to perineum after delivery.
   b. Use "in and out" catheter if unable to void every 6 to 8 hr or when fundus is above umbilicus, off to right or left, or bleeding is increased.
   c. Encourage fluids.
   d. Monitor intake and output for evidence of dehydration.
   e. Measure first two spontaneous voids for minimum of 200 to 300 ml each void.
7. Provide interventions for constipation.
   a. Advise 8 to 10 glasses of fluid per day.
   b. Initiate diet with adequate fiber.
   c. Administer stool softeners: Docusate sodium 100 mg PO twice a day.
8. Initiate diagnostic studies postpartum including CBC and platelets first day postpartum if hemorrhage or anemia has occurred, or client has abnormal clotting history; culture and sensitivity if infection is suspected.
9. Provide additional interventions for cesarean client.
   a. Assess incision, lung fields, every 4 hr.
   b. Administer IV fluids: Maintain IV fluids 12 to 24 hr postpartum; change to intermittent infusion catheter lock when retaining clear liquid diet and bowel sounds are present without nausea or vomiting.
   c. Keep Foley catheter to gravity drainage for approximate 12 hr postpartum.
      (1) Assess for color odor and volume (more than 30 ml/hr)
      (2) Accurate intake and output until IV infusion is discontinued and client has voided two times with complete emptying of the bladder
   d. Assist client to turn cough, deep breathe every 2 hr or use incentive spirometry every 2 hr.
   e. Assist client to perform leg exercises every 2 hr or use pneumatic leg cuffs until ambulatory.
   f. Assess bowel sounds every 4 hr until client is passing flatus.
   g. Assess pain every 2 hr.
      (1) Use nonpharmacologic pain control, client relaxation, focused breathing, relaxation
      (2) PCA for pain control with morphine or meperidine (Demerol) for 12 to 24 hr postpartum
      (3) Change to medications by mouth following PCA (hydrocodone [Vicodin], oxycodone [Percocet])
10. Provide information on changes in client status to health care providers (HCPs) of the multidisciplinary team.
11. Instruct client about care for self and infant (see also Chapter 8).

C. Safety and infection control
1. Instruct client to make 4- to 6-week follow-up appointment with HCP.
2. Instruct client to inform HCP after hospital discharge of:
   a. Temperature greater than 100.4°F.
   b. Saturation of more than one pad in 1 hr.
   c. Clots size of fist.
   d. Bleeding that has foul odor or returns to red after being pink, dark brown, or off-white.
   e. Headaches with visual disturbances, epigastric pain.
   f. Feelings or thoughts of wanting to not care for or hurt self or infant.
   g. Pain in calves, breasts, or bladder area.
   h. Inability to void and burning or pain with voiding.
   i. Complications related to incision (if client had a cesarean section); inspection should occur daily for any further redness, bleeding, separation, or discharge.
3. Assist client out of bed first time.
4. Instruct client on care of perineum to prevent infection, including wiping front to back one time only with tissue; use of spray; bottle or peribottle to clean perineum until perineal pain is no longer experienced.
5. Review plan of care to determine if care is consistent with best practices of the profession and has provided the best outcomes for this client based on the situation.

D. Health promotion and maintenance
1. Provide environment supportive of bonding and attachment process. Encourage

contact by providing space for parents and family. Provide teaching as needed.

2. Assist client to evaluate support systems, and determine need for assistance.
3. Instruct client about basic care following discharge from hospital, including managing common discomforts after delivery.
   a. Rest when infant sleeps; nap during daytime; have support system to help cook, clean, care for other children.
   b. Lift nothing heavier than infant for 2 weeks.
   c. Perform perineal care until perineum is no longer sensitive; treat perineal discomfort.
      (1) Squeeze buttocks together before sitting in chair, then relax muscles.
      (2) Avoid standing for long periods of time to reduce pressure on perineal area.
      (3) Use sitz bath four times a day after first 24 hr postpartum.
   d. Obtain adequate nutrition.
      (1) Eat balanced diet with adequate nutritional content; drink to thirst.
      (2) Consume iron-rich foods if anemic.
      (3) Refrain from weight loss program until discussed with HCP at 6 weeks.
      (4) Consume an additional 300 to 500 calories per day if breast-feeding.
   e. Perform breast care (for breast-feeding and bottle-feeding client).
      (1) For breast-feeding client:
         (a) Wear supportive bra 24 hr per day.
         (b) Drink a glass of fluid each time infant nurses.
         (c) Increase diet by 300 to 500 calories of healthy food per day.
      (2) For bottle-feeding client:
         (a) Wear supportive bra, sports bra, or binder for 24 hr per day.
         (b) Avoid stimulation to breast: have shower water run on shoulders rather than breasts; refrain from using breast pump or removing colostrum.
         (c) Treat engorgement by supportive bra, cold packs to breasts, and anti-inflammatory medications.
   f. Resume intercourse when no active bleeding, perineum healed, or have 4 to 6 week postpartum check; also avoid douching, or tampons until follow-up visit with HCP.
   g. Shower, shampoo as needed.
   h. Wait 2 weeks to drive after vaginal delivery, and wait 4 weeks to drive after cesarean section.

E. Psychologic integrity
1. Assess client stages of postpartum psychosocial adjustment.
   a. Taking in: First 2 days postpartum as evidenced by focus on own well-being and needs, reviewing labor and delivery process
   b. Taking hold: Days 3 through 10 postpartum as evidenced by shifting focus to care of infant and learning tasks involved
   c. Letting go: Day 11 through 6 weeks postpartum as evidenced by preparing to return to work, allowing others to care for infant
2. Provide interventions for altered parenting, and to facilitate bonding and attachment.
   a. Encourage participation in infant care; provide teaching regarding care needs of infant and role model care.
   b. Create a supportive environment for questions and answers, bonding, and attachment.
   c. Provide bonding time as soon after birth as possible.
   d. Provide positive reinforcement.

F. Basic care and comfort
1. Encourage care of infant and self.
2. Provide comfort measures as needed, including rest and sleep opportunities, and pain relief as needed.
3. Provide emotional support (e.g., answer questions, encourage ventilation of emotions and fears while in hospital environment).
4. Support learning needs by educating concerning postpartum care of mother and infant.
5. Refer to support groups, resources as needed or desired by client.

G. Reduction of risk potential
1. Provide information regarding birth control options including methods of birth control available and appropriate for infant feeding situation; suggest use of foam and condoms prior to check-up with HCP.
2. Provide community resources for identified problems and/or as support such as La Leche League, breast-feeding support groups, new mothers groups, hospital warm lines.

H. Pharmacologic and parenteral therapies: Client will state the purpose, dosage, timing, effects,

and side effects of specific medications used during postpartum.
1. Medications used at home:
   a. Docusate sodium, 100 mg PO twice a day for constipation
   b. Ibuprofen, 800 mg PO every 6 to 8 hr as needed for pain
   c. Prenatal vitamins, 1 PO every day
   d. Ferrous sulfate, 325 mg PO bid
   e. Naproxen sodium (Anaprox, Aleve, Naprosyn) for pain and inflammation
   f. Hydrocodone/acetaminophen (Vicodin), one to two tablets every 4 to 6 hr as needed for pain with limit of eight in 24-hr period
   g. Acetaminophen, codeine phosphate (Tylenol with codeine), one to two tablets PO every 4 to 6 hr as needed for pain
   h. Simethicone 80 mg PO four times a day, as needed for gas
2. Medications used in hospital setting:
   a. Ketoralac (Toradol) 30 mg every 6 hr as needed for pain after cesarean section
   b. Meperidine (Demerol) per PCA
   c. Morphine per PCA

Postpartum Infections

I. Definition: Postpartum infection is characterized by a temperature of 100.4°F or higher, for more than 24 hr after delivery on 2 consecutive days within the first 10 days postpartum. Infection occurs in approximately 6% of all births in the United States. Other occasions that may cause temperature elevation include a cesarean section, dehydration in the first 24 hr after birth, and breast engorgement.

A. Possible sites for infection
1. Urinary tract
2. Cervix, vagina, endometrium (endometritis)
3. Uterus (metritis), connective tissue of uterus (parametritis), or pelvic organs outside the uterus such as the fallopian tubes (salpingitis)
4. Breast(s) (mastitis)
   a. Infection occurs in 2% to 5% of lactating women within 2 to 4 weeks after delivery
   b. Risk factors include nipple trauma, milk stasis, poor hand hygiene, failure to empty breasts, and obstruction of milk ducts
5. Ovaries (oophoritis)
6. Incision/wound site

B. Causative organisms
1. Group B streptococcus
2. *Staphylococcus aureus*
3. *Chlamydia trachomatis, Clostridium*
4. *Escherichia coli*

II. Nursing process

A. Assessment
1. Assess factors placing client at risk for infection.
   a. Anemia
   b. Multiple vaginal examinations and/or catheterizations during labor
   c. Poor personal hygiene (including poor hand hygiene)
   d. Poor nutritional habits
   e. Diabetes
   f. Prolonged rupture of membranes
   g. Hemorrhage
   h. Trauma at delivery
2. Assess for general indications of infection.
   a. Presence of temperature greater than 100.4°F after first 24 hr after delivery within first 10 days postpartum
   b. Redness, edema, approximation, ecchymosis, or discharge at incision site
   c. Presence of headache, vertigo, malaise, anorexia, chills, backache
   d. Pain at infection site
   e. Pain and/or burning on urination, costovertebral angle
   f. Costovertebral angle or flank pain
3. Assess for infection by site involved.
   a. Urinary tract
      (1) Dysuria
      (2) Urge to void with small volume actually being emptied
      (3) Hematuria
      (4) Distended bladder
      (5) Nausea, vomiting
      (6) Increased vaginal bleeding related to distended bladder
      (7) History of catheterization(s) during labor
      (8) Low-grade fever with cystitis, high fever with pyelonephritis
      (9) Pain in flank or costovertebral angle in pyelonephritis
   b. Breast(s) (mastitis)
      (1) Painful, reddened, or tender area of breast(s)
      (2) Flulike symptoms of fever, chills, lethargy
      (3) Traumatized, cracked, or bleeding nipples from breast-feeding
      (4) Elevated temperature, pulse rate
      (5) History of missed, short, inconsistent feedings, engorgement

c. Cervix, vagina, endometrium (endometritis); uterus (metritis); pelvic organs outside the uterus (salpingitis); connective tissue of uterus (parametritis); and ovaries (oophoritis)
   (1) Pulse greater than 100
   (2) Abdominal and/or uterine pain or tenderness
   (3) Flulike symptoms: temperature, aches, lethargy
   (4) Backache
   (5) Lochia with foul odor, abnormal in amount
   (6) Rubra lochia for prolonged period of time
   (7) Uterus does not decrease in size at expected rate (remains palpable after 9 days postpartum)
d. Assess incision/wound site for the following:
   (1) Redness, edema, and/or purulent discharge from incision site
   (2) Cellulitis surrounding incision
   (3) Separation of incision site

4. Obtain diagnostic tests.
   a. WBC for rapid increase in number of WBC above labor values
   b. Increase in sedimentation rate

B. Analysis
1. Acute Pain related to infection
2. Interrupted Family Processes related to postpartum infection
3. Ineffective Thermoregulation related to infective process
4. Impaired Parenting related to difficulty bonding and fear of giving infant infection
5. Deficient Knowledge related to no prior experience with postpartal infections
6. Impaired Tissue Integrity related to labor and delivery process

C. Planning
1. Diagnose and initiate treatment of infection in early stages.
2. Maintain ability of client to care for infant.
3. Use support systems to provide assistance if needed.
4. Instruct client's support system to care for infant, allowing rest for client.
5. Provide client teaching concerning medications effects, side effects, and actions.

D. Implementation
1. Evaluate client response to interventions.
2. Provide client teaching regarding current condition, assessments, and interventions.
3. Encourage 2,400 calorie diet to repair and heal tissue.
4. Obtain culture and sensitivity of infected area or lochia prior to initiating antibiotic therapy.
5. Administer antibiotics.
6. Plan comfort measures, including linen and gown changes, back rub, cool cloths, showers, and frequent rest periods.
7. Increase oral fluids to 3,000 ml per day.
8. Administer analgesics as needed.
9. Administer medications to lower temperature (aspirin, acetaminophen [Tylenol]).
10. Observe universal precautions.
11. Perform frequent hand hygiene.

E. Evaluation
1. Client is pain free, afebrile within 24 hr, and resting adequately.
2. Client's infection causes no further complications.
3. Client and infant parenting and bonding does not experience delay.
4. Client successfully breast-feeds.
5. Client allows support persons to care for infant in hospital and at home.
6. Client completes medication regimen.

CN

III. Client needs

A. Physiologic adaptation
1. Inflamed or infected tissue heals more slowly or may not heal at all.
2. Anemia slows healing process.

B. Management of care: Care of the client with a postpartum infection requires critical thinking skills and knowledge of assessment, and teaching and evaluation methods unique to the RN role. These skills cannot be delegated to an LPN or UAP.
1. Delegate responsibly those activities that can be delegated, including basic care needs for the stable client and the assessments for the following (all monitoring information is reported to the RN):
   a. Vital signs every 4 hr and before and after antipyretic agents
   b. Infection site for edema, redness, discharge, approximation if applicable, pain, purulent drainage, odor lochia
   c. Infection site for pain
   d. Presence of headache, vertigo, malaise, anorexia, chills, backache
2. Perform comprehensive assessments for indications of infection specific to infection site (see section on assessment).
3. Provide care specific to site and type of infection.
   a. Urinary tract infections:
      (1) Assist client to empty bladder completely and frequently.

(2) Instruct client to wipe from front to back after urination, wear cotton underwear, and loose-fitting clothes.
(3) Maintain intake and output.

b. Mastitis:
(1) Feed infant every 2 hr to empty breasts.
(2) Wear supportive bra 24 hr per day.
(3) Latch infant on to cover entire areola (eliminate nipple cracking).
(4) Rotate feeding positions.

c. Incision/wound infection: With open wound, provide wet-to-dry dressing changes; medicate client prior to dressing changes.

d. Infection of cervix, vagina, endometrium, pelvic organs, outside the uterus, ovaries, connective tissue: Assess changes in color, odor, amount of vaginal discharge during antibiotic therapy.

C. Safety and infection control
1. Observe universal precautions for all clients.
2. Initiate isolation if indicated.
3. Maintain client in Semi-Fowler position to facilitate drainage if appropriate.

D. Health promotion and maintenance: Provide perineal care.

E. Psychologic integrity
1. Inform client and family of status and progress.
2. Encourage visitors if client is stable, hospitalization prolonged, and client is interested.

F. Basic care and comfort
1. Provide comfort measures as needed, including rest and sleep opportunities, and relief of pain through nursing measures or medication.
2. Provide emotional support (answer questions, encourage ventilation of emotions and fears while in health care environment).
3. Support learning needs by providing client teaching specific to infection process.
4. Determine and report changes in emotional or physical status.
5. Refer to resources as needed.

G. Reduction of risk potential: Provide client and family teaching about the need for rest, a nutritious diet, and the need to complete medication regimen.

H. Pharmacologic and parenteral therapies: Client will state the purpose for and associated side effects of antipyretics and antibiotic therapy used to treat postpartum infection. Medication used depends on site, culture, and sensitivity results.

Postpartum Bleeding Disorders: Postpartum Hemorrhage

I. Definition: Postpartum hemorrhage is defined by amount of blood loss and the time frame in relation to the delivery. For a vaginal delivery, hemorrhage is loss of more than 500 ml; for a cesarean section, hemorrhage is defined as a loss of more than 1,000 ml in a 24-hr period. Postpartum hemorrhage can occur within the first 24 hr after delivery (early hemorrhage) and after 24 hr postpartum through 6 weeks postpartum (late hemorrhage). Causes for postpartum hemorrhage are as follows:

A. Uterine atony: Lack of contraction by the postpartum uterus. Complicates 5% of births. Uterine atony is associated with polyhydramnios, macrosomia, multiparity, multifetal gestation, chorioamnionitis, use of magnesium sulfate, and rapid or prolonged labor and delivery. Indicated by:
a. Flaccid, "boggy" uterus after delivery of placenta
b. Increasing fundal height as blood collects in uterus. Bleeding occurs within the uterus if the muscles do not contract around blood vessels. As bleeding continues and uterus enlarges, it becomes less able to contract. Blood may be retained in the uterus without evidence of a large amount of external vaginal bleeding.

B. Lacerations of the genital tract: Includes tears in the cervix, vagina, and perineum and results in a continuous trickle of bright blood while the uterus remains contracted.

C. Hematomas: Collection of blood encapsulated beneath skin surface of perineum, vagina, or in the retroperitoneal area. Associated with forceps or rapid delivery. Indicators include pain, blue discoloration to genital area, pressure in rectal or vaginal area.

D. Retained placenta: Placenta adheres to inside of uterus for more than 30 min after delivery. Areas within uterus with membranes or placenta attached cannot contract around blood vessels causing hemorrhage. Indicated by excessive bleeding postpartum.

E. Inversion of uterus (medical emergency): The fundus prolapses through the cervix into the vagina or onto the perineum. Inversions are designated as partial or complete. Indicated by palpation of soft, round mass in vagina or visualization of mass in the vagina or protruding onto perineum after delivery.

F. Subinvolution: Failure of uterus to return to prepregnant state as result of infection or retained placental fragments. Usually recognized at postpartum check when uterus is boggy and larger than normal and/or lochia has continued; excessive for the postpartum time frame and may have a foul odor.

II. Nursing process

A. Assessment

1. Perform a comprehensive physical assessment; assess for indications related to cause of postpartum hemorrhage (see indications in definition section).
2. Perform general assessments related to postpartum hemorrhage.
   a. Monitor vital signs and trends over time (vital signs may be unreliable as indicator of shock as body has a 40% to 50% increase in blood volume during pregnancy).
   b. Note location and firmness of fundus.
   c. Palpate bladder for distention and filling.
   d. Assess bleeding in relationship to firmness of uterus.
   e. Examine entire placenta after delivery or review documentation of visualization of all parts of placenta after delivery.
   f. Assess lochia for color, odor, and amount.
   g. Assess for risk factors.
   h. Visualize perineum for blue discoloration and presence of swelling or edema.
3. Obtain diagnostic tests (depending on etiology of bleeding).
   a. CBC with platelets
   b. Blood type, antibody screen if potential need to transfuse

B. Analysis

1. Deficient Fluid Volume related to blood loss secondary to hemorrhage
2. Ineffective Tissue Perfusion: Cardiopulmonary related to decreased blood volume
3. Risk for infection related to invasion of tissue by microorganisms
4. Fatigue related to low hematocrit and hemoglobin secondary to hemorrhage
5. Risk for Interrupted Family Processes related to inability to care for self or infant

C. Planning

1. Identify client at risk for hemorrhage.
2. Assess frequently to determine hemorrhage in initial stages before complications result.
3. Intervene at earliest signs of hemorrhage.

D. Implementation

1. Perform comprehensive assessments as previously listed.
2. Massage uterus until firm, express clots; teach client light uterine massage.
3. Ask client to void every 2 hr.
4. Continue IV fluids.
5. Monitor vital signs per protocol and assessing for trends.
6. Catheterize if needed.
7. Administer medications specific to etiology to decrease bleeding (see pharmacologic and parenteral therapies).
8. Monitor intake and output, including vaginal bleeding.

E. Evaluation

1. Client continues bonding with infant.
2. Client's bleeding transitions from rubra to serosa to alba within 2 weeks.
3. Client's vital signs remain within normal values.
4. Client loses less than 500 ml (vaginal delivery) or less than 1,000 ml (cesarean section) in 24 hr.

CN

III. Client needs

A. Physiologic adaptation: Vital signs postpartum may not indicate shock initially as the woman has had a 40% to 50% volume increase during pregnancy.

B. Management of care: Care of the client with a postpartum hemorrhage requires critical thinking skills and knowledge of assessment, and teaching and evaluation methods unique to the RN role. These skills cannot be delegated to an LPN or UAP.

1. Uterine atony
   a. Perform initial assessments and interventions as noted in implementation.
   b. Administer medications to contract uterus; if medication not effective, use bimanual compression of uterus.
   c. If compression is not effective, promote exploration of interior of uterus by HCP for retained fragments.
   d. If exploration of the uterus is not effective, uteroovarian, uterine, and hypogastric vessel ligation may be needed.
   e. Promote hysterectomy as last resort to stop bleeding.
2. Lacerations of the genital tract
   a. Provide initial assessments and interventions as noted in implementation; bleeding does not stop with firm uterus.

   b. Promote visualization of vagina, cervix, and rectum for bleeding.
   c. Promote ligation, coagulation of bleeding areas.
3. Hematomas
   a. Provide initial assessments and interventions as noted in implementation.
   b. Promote continued assessment for further bleeding and increase in size and discoloration in perineal area.
   c. Assess for perineal pressure; need to have bowel movement; increasing pain where the cause cannot be identified.
   d. Apply cold/ice packs to area if external.
   e. Promote ligation of vessels, evacuation of hematoma.
4. Retained placental fragments
   a. Provide initial assessments and interventions as noted in implementation.
   b. Promote uterine exploration with continued bleeding.
   c. Administer medications to decrease bleeding.
   d. Promote D&C to remove retained fragments.
5. Inversion of uterus (medical emergency)
   a. Provide initial assessments and interventions as noted in implementation.
   b. Provide continuous assessment and treatment for shock per HCP orders.
   c. Promote uterine relaxation with anesthesia or tocolytics.
   d. Re-invert uterus.
   e. After uterus is restored to normal position, administer oxytocin (Pitocin) and potentially other medications to contract uterus per HCP's orders.
   f. Administer antibiotics, recovery procedures.
6. Subinvolution
   a. Provide initial assessments and interventions as noted in implementation.
   b. Promote diagnosis by HCP with treatment specific to etiology.
   c. Promote initiation of antibiotic therapy, if infected.
   d. Promote removal of retained fragments by D&S or D&C.
   e. Administer medication to contract uterus after surgery.

C. Safety and infection control: Provide client and family teaching.
   1. Report any vaginal bleeding heavier than a period.
   2. Empty bladder every 2 to 3 hr regardless of urgency.
   3. Report any signs and symptoms that seem unusual.

D. Health promotion and maintenance: Encourage client to inform HCP of abnormal changes in bleeding postpartum.

E. Psychologic integrity
   1. Assist client and family in coping with complications of childbirth; suggest coping strategies and encourage client to choose those fitting the situation.
   2. Assist client to identify stress factors and anxiety that may interfere with recovery.

F. Basic care and comfort
   1. Provide comfort measures as needed, including rest and sleep opportunities, and relief of pain through nursing measures or medication.
   2. Provide emotional support (e.g., answer questions, encourage ventilation of emotions and fears while in health care environment).
   3. Support learning needs by providing teaching specific to bleeding disorders postpartum.
   4. Determine and report changes in emotional or physical status (passage of blood clots, bright red bleeding, saturating a pad an hour).
   5. Refer to resources as needed.

G. Reduction of risk potential (care for any postpartal client)
   1. Identify factors placing client at risk for bleeding disorders.
   2. Validate client's most recent hematocrit and hemoglobin levels.
   3. Evaluate client for orthostatic hypotension until client is consistently stable.
   4. Promote slow ambulation, with assistance until client is stable.

H. Pharmacologic and parenteral therapies: Client will state the purpose for and associated side effects of medications used to treat postpartum bleeding disorders. Medications are specific to etiology to decrease bleeding:
   1. Continue infusion of 10 to 40 units of oxytocin (Pitocin) per liter of IV fluids as ordered
   2. Methylergonovine (Methergine), 0.2 mg IM
   3. Prostaglandin E_2 (Prostin, Hemabate), 0.25 mg IM into uterine muscle during cesarean section as needed for continuous uterine contraction
   4. Misoprostol (Cytotec), 400 to 800 mcg vaginally or rectally

Thromboembolic Disease

I. Definition: Inflammation of blood vessels with potential formation of a blood clot inside the vessel. Women are at a high risk during pregnancy and postpartum as a result of venous stasis and high levels of coagulation factors. Clotting disorders often develop after returning home rather than during hospitalization, indicating an education need for clients at risk. Types of clotting disorders include the following:
   A. Superficial vein thrombosis: Involves the superficial saphenous vein with little risk of pulmonary embolism. Superficial leg vein disease is characterized by pain and tenderness with a positive Homans sign.
   B. Deep vein thrombosis: Involves the deep veins anywhere from the foot to the iliofemoral region. Pain will occur at the point that is affected.
   C. Pulmonary embolism: Occurs when a clot dislodges from a deep vein and is carried to the lung system, where it obstructs pulmonary blood flow. Signs and symptoms include difficulty breathing, a productive cough and hemoptysis, and tachycardia.

II. Nursing process
   A. Assessment
      1. Assess for risk factors putting client at risk for blood clots, including cesarean section, smoking, client older than 35 years of age, prior blood clots, obesity, trauma to extremities during delivery, and diabetes.
      2. Assess vital signs every 4 hr.
      3. Assess for signs and symptoms.
         a. Edema, swelling, and warmth of leg
         b. Tenderness in vein
         c. Low-grade fever
         d. Positive Homans sign
      4. Obtain diagnostic tests.
         a. Venogram
         b. Doppler ultrasound
   B. Analysis
      1. Acute Pain related to inflammation, tissue hypoxia, and clot formation
      2. Impaired Parenting related to limited ambulation as result of clotting disorder
      3. Ineffective Tissue Perfusion: Cardiopulmonary, related to poor venous circulation
      4. Interrupted Family Processes related to limited ambulation
      5. Risk for Impaired Parenting related to limited ambulation
   C. Planning
      1. Diagnose and initiate treatment in early stages.
      2. Maintain ability of client to care for infant.
      3. Use support systems to provide assistance if needed.
      4. Instruct client's support system to care for infant, allowing rest for client.
   D. Implementation (see management of care)
   E. Evaluation
      1. Client's disease (inflammation) is treated without complications (e.g., embolus, immobility).
      2. Client verbalizes medication, effects, and side effects to report, and dosage at time of discharge.
      3. Client and infant bonding does not experience delay.
      4. Client verbalizes self-care measures and medical regimen for postpartum.
      5. Client is pain-free, afebrile within 24 hr, and resting adequately.
      6. Client's support persons assume management of home situation.

CN

III. Client needs
   A. Physiologic adaptation
      1. Inflamed or infected tissue heals more slowly.
      2. Fibrinogen levels remain elevated after delivery.
      3. Positioning during delivery may cause pooling of blood in lower extremities.
      4. Cesarean section may traumatize vessels in lower abdominal area and increase risk for inflammation.
   B. Management of care: Care of the client with thromboembolic disease requires critical thinking skills and knowledge of assessment, and teaching and evaluation methods unique to the RN role. These skills cannot be delegated to an LPN or UAP.
      1. Delegate responsibly those activities that can be delegated, including basic care needs and vital signs for the stable client. All monitoring information is reported to the RN.
      2. Perform comprehensive physical assessments and provide care for clients with postpartal inflammation.
         a. Assess vital signs every 4 hr, looking for slight elevation of temperature.
         b. Assess site of inflammation for edema, redness, paleness, and pulses.
      3. Provide client teaching regarding current condition, assessments, interventions, and plan of care while being hospitalized and when returning home.
      4. Provide interventions as follows:
         a. Superficial vein disease
            (1) Complete assessment strategies.
            (2) Keep leg elevated.

(3) Administer analgesics, if needed.
(4) Apply warm heat.
(5) Promote early ambulation.
(6) Prevent client standing for long periods of time (avoid venous stasis).
(7) Apply support stockings (reduce venous congestion).
(8) Administer heparin therapy as ordered.
(9) Promote coagulation studies as indicated by HCP.
(10) Monitor vaginal bleeding changes related to heparin therapy.

b. Deep vein thrombosis
(1) Complete assessment strategies.
(2) Promote bed rest with leg elevated.
(3) Administer analgesics as needed.
(4) Apply warm heat.
(5) Promote IV heparin therapy followed by oral therapy for 3 months.
(6) Implement warfarin (Coumadin) therapy if not breast-feeding.
(7) Promote coagulation studies as indicated by HCP.
(8) Monitor vaginal bleeding changes related to coagulation therapy.

c. Pulmonary embolism
(1) Promote immediate problem identification based on signs and symptoms of dyspnea, shortness of breath, tachypnea, sudden cough with blood-tinged sputum, chest pain, cyanosis, loss of consciousness.
(2) Promote immediate treatment including CPR if indicated, IV O_2 at 8 L/min, support and maintenance of circulation if indicated.
(3) Promote coagulation therapy for 6 months per HCP: warfarin (Coumadin), heparin.

C. Safety and infection control
1. Avoid prolonged placement in stirrups.
2. Maintain hydration during labor and delivery.

D. Health promotion and maintenance
1. Instruct client to avoid use of aspirin, ibuprofen and other NSAIDs while on anticoagulant therapy.
2. Instruct client about use of herbals that interact with anticoagulant therapy (garlic, ginger, ginkgo).
3. Observe warning signs of hemorrhage from anticoagulant therapy such as:
(1) Bleeding gums, bleeding in stools or urine, nose bleeds.
(2) Petechia, increased vaginal bleeding, bruising.
4. Obtain laboratory studies that monitor clotting time (international normalized ratio less than 5; activated partial thromboplastin time, 30 to 45 s).
5. In preparation for discharge, involve significant other or family in discharge teaching as support for client.

E. Psychologic integrity
1. Inform client and family of status and progress of specific clotting disorder.
2. Encourage visitors and interaction with and care of infant if client is stable or hospitalization is prolonged.

F. Reduction of risk potential: Provide client and family teaching.
1. Obtain rest and nutritious diet.
2. Complete medication regimen.
3. Perform self-care measures.
a. Avoid crossing legs.
b. Take frequent rest breaks when riding in the car.
c. Identify history in subsequent pregnancies.

G. Pharmacologic and parenteral therapies: Client and family will state the purpose for and associated side effects of all medications used to treat thromboembolic disease.
1. Heparin therapy
2. Warfarin (Coumadin)
3. Protamine sulfate as anecdote
4. Aspirin may be implemented as anticoagulant therapy and not for pain control.

Psychiatric Disorders

I. Definition: Postpartum-onset psychiatric disorders are classified as one syndrome with three subgroups: Postpartum adjustment reaction with mood depression, postpartum psychosis, and postpartum depression.

A. Postpartum adjustment reaction with mood depression, also known as *baby blues,* is thought to take place because of the change in hormonal levels the mother is undergoing, as well as psychologic adaptation.
1. Symptoms, which can occur 3 to 5 days after delivery include client feeling overwhelmed, tired, irritable, and unable to cope; tears may occur at any time.
2. Affects at least 50% of all new mothers. Unlike postpartum depression or postpartum psychosis, the syndrome is usually self-limiting.

3. Treatment typically involves support from family, obtaining sufficient rest, and if symptoms do not resolve, the client may need counseling, referral to a mental health professional, and use of medication. The nurse should refer all clients who express thoughts of suicide or harm to newborn to a mental health professional.

B. Postpartum psychosis is a severe mental illness, often viewed as pre-existing depression with childbearing as a precipitating crisis.
   1. Symptoms include client's experiences of delusions or hallucinations with potential intent to harm herself or the infant resulting from loss of touch with reality.
   2. Postpartum psychosis is rare, occurring in 1 to 2 in 1,000 births. Symptoms occur within 6 weeks to 3 months of delivery. If not treated, there is a risk of suicide and infanticide in about 5% of women.
   3. Treatment involves intervention of mental HCPs who administer antipsychotic medication and provide counseling.

C. Postpartum depression, also called *perinatal depression,* is depression that occurs up to 1 year after delivery. The depression affects the well-being of the woman and requires treatment by an HCP.
   1. Symptoms include sadness as well as feelings of anxiousness expressing feelings of loss.
   2. Affects 10% to 20% of women. Usually begins during the fourth postpartum week and often lasts up to 1 year.
   3. Treatment typically involves counseling and medication.

II. Nursing process

A. Assessment
   1. Assess factors putting client at risk for depression, blues, or psychosis.
      a. Prior depression or history of psychosis, with or without pregnancy
      b. Unplanned or unwanted pregnancy
      c. Single parenting (lack of support and/or poor relationship with parents or father of the infant)
      d. Low self-esteem and stress
   2. Perform client and family interview assessing feelings of loss of control, overwhelming responsibility, feelings of sadness without precipitating etiology, hallucinations or delusions, threats to harm self or infant.
   3. Assess for presence of hallucinations or delusions, and threats to harm self or infant.
   4. Assess for degree of sadness, perceived stress level of client, and general signs and symptoms including irritability, lack of interest in activities, crying, insomnia, inability to concentrate, and disturbed body image.
   5. Complete postpartum depression scales, with sensitivity to potential for altered perception of discussions by client.

B. Analysis
   1. Ineffective Coping related to postpartum depression
   2. Impaired Parenting related to postpartum depression
   3. Compromised Family Coping related to new parenting situation
   4. Ineffective Coping related to alteration in lifestyle, responsibilities within family

C. Planning
   1. Provide client teaching postpartum concerning postpartum emotional reactions.
   2. Diagnose and initiate treatment in early stages with antidepressants, behavior therapy per HCP.
   3. Maintain ability of client to care for infant.
   4. Use support systems to provide assistance if needed.
   5. Instruct client's support system concerning signs and symptoms to contact HCP, while facilitating rest for client.

D. Implementation
   1. Perform assessments as previously mentioned.
   2. Identify potential or actual problem.
   3. Refer client to appropriate obstetric or psychiatric service.
   4. Refer for follow-up home visit.

E. Evaluation
   1. Client verbalizes understanding of emotional reactions and illness that can occur postpartum.
   2. Client's disease is treated without threats or injury to mother, infant, or family.
   3. Client verbalizes names of mood-stabilizing and antipsychotic medication, dosages, effects, and side effects to report at time of discharge.
   4. Client and infant parenting and bonding develop at normal rate.
   5. Client verbalizes self-care measures and medical regimen for postpartum time.
   6. Client and support persons are able to assist with management of home situation, if needed.
   7. Client and infant are safe.
   8. Client uses appropriate coping strategies.

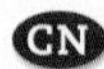

III. Client needs
  A. Physiologic adaptation: Contributing factors for postpartum-onset psychiatric disorders include:
    1. Rapid shift in estrogen, progesterone, and corticotrophin-releasing hormone alter client perceptions of situation at hand.
    2. Fatigue, loss of sleep heighten physical changes occurring as result of labor and delivery.
  B. Management of care: Care of the client with a psychiatric disorder requires critical thinking skills and knowledge of assessment, and teaching and evaluation methods unique to the RN role. These skills cannot be delegated to an LPN or UAP.
    1. Delegate responsibly those activities that can be delegated, including basic care needs and vital signs for the stable client.
    2. Assess client and family (see assessment section).
    3. Provide client and family teaching regarding current obstetric condition, assessments, interventions, and plan of care while being hospitalized and when returning home.
    4. Refer client to mental HCP.
  C. Safety and infection control: Provide client and family teaching.
    1. Continue appointments with mental HCPs.
    2. Contact mental HCP on feelings of suicide, presence of delusions or hallucinations, or feelings of inadequacies in caring for self or infant.
    3. Use strategies to cope with mental health problems at home as indicated by mental HCPs.
  D. Health promotion and maintenance: Provide client and family teaching concerning potential for depression and psychosis.
  E. Psychologic integrity
    1. Encourage participation in individual or group therapy as ordered.
    2. Inform client and family of status and progress.
    3. Encourage visitors if client is stable, hospitalization is prolonged, and client is interested.
  F. Basic care and comfort
    1. Provide comfort measures as needed, including rest and sleep opportunities.
    2. Provide emotional support (e.g., answer questions, encourage ventilation of emotions and fears while in safe environment).
    3. Support learning needs by educating concerning postpartum depression referring to support, resources as needed.
    4. Determine and report changes in emotional or physical status.
  G. Reduction of risk potential
    1. Provide client teaching.
      a. Inform HCPs about prior depression or psychosis if client becomes pregnant in the future (high rate of recurrence in subsequent pregnancies).
      b. Obtain rest, eat nutritious diet, and practice self-care.
      c. Use support systems.
      d. Complete medication regimen; continue with follow-up care with mental HCPs.
    2. Discuss risks of medications in breast milk if breast-feeding.
  H. Pharmacologic and parenteral therapies: Client and family will state the purpose for and associated side effects of all medications used to treat psychiatric disorders.
    1. Antidepressants: Used with caution in breast-feeding client. Selective serotonin reuptake inhibitors include fluoxetine (Prozac), paroxetine (Paxil), and sertraline (Zoloft).
    2. Antipsychotic drugs: Used with caution in breast-feeding client.

Bibliography

Klossner, N. J., & Hatfield, N. (2005). *Introduction to maternity and pediatric nursing*. Philadelphia: Lippincott Williams & Wilkins.

Pillitteri, A. (2006). *Maternal & child health nursing: Care of the childbearing and childrearing family* (5th ed.). Philadelphia: Lippincott Williams & Wilkins.

Simpson, K. R., & Creehan, P. A. (2007). *AWHONN's perinatal nursing* (3rd ed.). Philadelphia: Lippincott Williams & Wilkins.

Witt, C. (2007). *Advances in neonatal care*. Philadelphia: Lippincott Williams & Wilkins.

CHAPTER 7

Practice Test

Postpartum Care Following Vaginal or Cesarean Delivery

1. The nurse is assessing a client who experienced a spontaneous vaginal delivery. On the second postpartal day, the nurse assesses the client's lochia. Which of the following is expected? The lochia is:
- □ 1. Light pink to brown in color and scant in amount.
- □ 2. Bright red in color and light to moderate in amount.
- □ 3. Bright red in color with clots and heavy in amount.
- □ 4. Light pink in color and heavy in amount.

2. AF The nurse is providing care for a client following delivery; the client has a fourth-degree episiotomy and is complaining of constipation. The nurse can suggest the woman try using which of the following? Select all that apply.
- □ 1. Stool softeners.
- □ 2. High-roughage diet.
- □ 3. Sitz baths.
- □ 4. Suppository.
- □ 5. Increased fluids.

3. The nurse making rounds enters the postpartum client's room and overhears her talking to a friend on the telephone: "I used the breathing and it worked. I pushed about four times and the baby just slipped out." The nurse recognizes this as a sign that the mother is in which of the following stages?
- □ 1. Dependent: Taking-in phase of maternal postpartum adjustment.
- □ 2. Dependent-independent: Taking-hold phase of maternal postpartum adjustment.
- □ 3. Dependent-interdependent: Taking-on phase of maternal postpartum adjustment.
- □ 4. Interdependent: Letting-go phase of maternal postpartum adjustment.

4. AF The nurse is making a postpartum visit at the home of a client who delivered 14 days earlier. After assessing the vital signs (temperature, 99°F; pulse, 88 BPM; respiration rate, 20 breaths per minute; and BP 112/60), the nurse records other findings as follows:

Breasts	Heart	Lungs	Abdomen
Soft ✓ Firm Ø Nipples intact ✓ Cracks Ø Blisters Ø	Regular rate, 88	Clear ✓	Soft ✓ Distended Ø Bowel sounds ✓ Fundus firm ✓ Midline ✓ 4 FB ⇓ U Nontender ✓ Bladder empty ✓

Perineum	Lochia	Extremities
Midline episiotomy redness Ø Ecchymosis Ø Edema Ø Discharge Ø Approximated ✓ Hemorrhoids Ø	Serosa	Legs: 1+ ankle edema Redness Ø Tenderness Ø Homans Ø

Which finding indicates delayed involution?
- □ 1. Vital signs.
- □ 2. Fundus.
- □ 3. Lochia.
- □ 4. Edema of the ankles.

5. The nurse is teaching the client about breastfeeding. Which of the following observations indicates the need for additional teaching?
- □ 1. Client brings infant's mouth to the nipple to latch on.
- □ 2. Client holds the infant in the cradle hold.
- □ 3. Client pulls the infant from the breast after 5 min of nursing.
- □ 4. Client places the infant at the breast when cues to hunger are present.

6. The nurse is providing care to a client who is Rh-negative and just delivered her first infant. The HCP has written an order to administer Rh immune globulin (RhoGAM) if indicated. The nurse administers the RhoGAM if the infant is:
- □ 1. Rh-positive and the Coombs test is negative.
- □ 2. Rh-positive and the Coombs test is positive.
- □ 3. Rh-negative and the Coombs test is negative.
- □ 4. Rh-negative and the Coombs test is positive.

7. The nurse is providing care to a client following delivery. The client is bottle-feeding her infant, and her breasts are engorged. The nurse should suggest the woman do which of the following to relieve the engorgement?
- □ 1. Run warm water over the breasts in the shower.
- □ 2. Use a breast pump to remove milk from the breasts.
- □ 3. Wear a snug support bra with Ace binder.
- □ 4. Apply cool cabbage leaves to the breast under the bra.

8. When palpating the abdomen of a woman with a vaginal delivery 2 hr ago, the nurse has difficulty locating the fundus because it is "boggy." The nurse's first action is to:
- □ 1. Notify the HCP.
- □ 2. Start an IV with oxytocin (Pitocin).
- □ 3. Massage the fundus.
- □ 4. Catheterize the client.

9. On the second postpartum day the client has lochia rubra. The nurse should:
- □ 1. Record the finding on the client's chart.
- □ 2. Place the woman on bed rest.
- □ 3. Report the finding to the HCP.
- □ 4. Start an IV infusion of normal saline.

10. The nurse is caring for a mother who delivered her second child 24 hr ago. While she is nursing her new daughter, she complains about experiencing menstrual-like cramps. She states "This did not happen when I had my first baby." The nurse should tell the client:
- □ 1. "I will notify your doctor; there is a possibility that you have retained some placental fragments."
- □ 2. "You are probably experiencing these cramps because you had such a long labor."
- □ 3. "You received oxytocin (Pitocin) after delivery. It will wear off in the next 48 hours."
- □ 4. "Your infant's suckling stimulates contraction of both your uterus and your milk cells; women especially feel this with their second or third infant."

11. When a client ambulates to the bathroom after sleeping 5 hr on the first postpartum day, she calls the nurse because of a gush of bright red blood. The nurse should explain to the client that likely the gush of blood is:
- □ 1. Abnormal bleeding and a sign that a postpartum hemorrhage is likely.
- □ 2. Blood pooling in the vaginal vault that was discharged when the mother stood up.
- □ 3. Bladder spasms from a full bladder.
- □ 4. Segments of the placenta are still in the uterus.

12. The nurse examines the breast of a primipara 12 hr after delivery. Which of the following is expected at this time?
- □ 1. Soft, no change from delivery.
- □ 2. Harder than before delivery.
- □ 3. Tender to touch.
- □ 4. Smaller than before delivery with a small amount of bloody discharge.

Postpartum Infections

13. AF The nurse should instruct a breast-feeding mother that the best way to prevent mastitis is to do which of the following? Select all that apply.
- □ 1. Bottle-feed until the milk comes in.
- □ 2. Take antibiotics during labor.
- □ 3. Prevent nipple fissures by carefully positioning the infant during feedings.
- □ 4. Drink plenty of fluids.
- □ 5. Use a nipple shield.
- □ 6. Remove the infant from the breast by inserting a finger in his mouth to break the suction.

14. The nurse is assessing a client 24 hr following a vaginal delivery. Which of the following indicates puerperal sepsis (endometritis) and should be reported to the HCP?
- □ 1. Malaise and foul-smelling, profuse lochia.
- □ 2. Edema and hypertension.
- □ 3. Lower abdominal cramping and cloudy urine.
- □ 4. Dizziness and hypotension.

Postpartum Bleeding Disorders: Postpartum Hemorrhage

15. The nurse is providing care for of a group of clients following delivery. Which of the following clients is at low risk for postpartum hemorrhage and can be cared for last?
- □ 1. Primigravida who was induced for 24 hr prior to delivery.
- □ 2. Multigravida who delivered her sixth child.
- □ 3. Multigravida who had a cesarean section for triplets.
- □ 4. Primigravida who pushed for 2 hr.

16. A client who delivered a healthy newborn 4 hr ago reports to the nurse that she has noticed a marked increase of bright red bleeding on her perineal pad in the last hour. The nurse assesses the client's uterine fundus and notes that it is firm and in the midline. The client has voided 600 ml of urine in the last hour. The nurse should first:

□ 1. Administer heparin (Lovenox).
□ 2. Assist the client to change her perineal pad.
□ 3. Administer oxytocin (Pitocin).
□ 4. Notify the HCP.

Thromboembolic Disease

17. On the second day following a vaginal delivery, a primipara is diagnosed with thrombophlebitis. The HCP orders heparin (Lovenox) IV, which is expected to:
□ 1. Relax the smooth muscles.
□ 2. Prevent deep vein thrombosis.
□ 3. Increase uterine contractions.
□ 4. Manage infection.

18. AF The nurse is assessing a woman who had a vaginal delivery 28 hr ago. The client is complaining of pain and tenderness in her right leg. Where should the nurse palpate to obtain further information about the pain? Identify the location by placing an "X" on the following image:

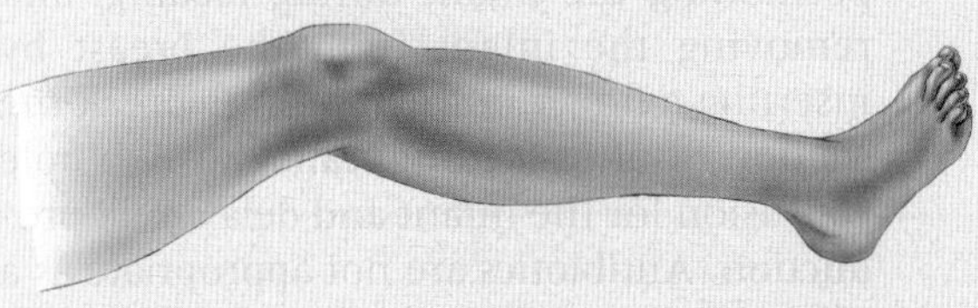

Psychiatric Disorders

19. AF After delivery of twins, the nurse is assessing a client for postpartum depression. Which of the following increases the risk of postpartum depression (peripartal mood disorder)? Select all that apply.
□ 1. Adolescence.
□ 2. Race (African American).
□ 3. Child care stress.
□ 4. Less than high school education.
□ 5. Support from husband.
□ 6. History of depressive mood disorder.
□ 7. Unplanned/unwanted pregnancy.

20. A husband tells the nurse that his wife, who delivered 6 weeks ago, is sad all the time and overwhelmed by the responsibility of caring for her infant. He states that when he came home from work, the infant's clothing had formula stains and the diaper was very dirty. The mother could not remember when she had last fed the infant. The nurse should:
□ 1. Assess how much help the mother has in caring for her infant.
□ 2. Explain that for some new mother's "baby blues" take longer to resolve.
□ 3. Advise the husband to bring his wife to an HCP today.
□ 4. Ask the father if the mother has a good relationship with her mother.

Answers and Rationales

1. 2 For the first 3 to 5 days after delivery, the lochia is bright red and moderate in amount. Bright red lochia with clots and heavy flow is not expected. Scant light pink to brown lochia is serosa and is not expected on the second postpartum day. (A)

2. 1, 2, 3, 5 The nurse suggests that the woman eat a high-roughage diet and increase her fluid intake. The nurse also suggests the woman use mild stool softeners if needed. A sitz bath may relieve pain and swelling in the area and make having a stool less painful. Suppositories and enemas are contraindicated in the presence of a fourth-degree episiotomy as they will distend the rectum and potentially stretch or tear the episiotomy. (S)

3. 1 The client's conversation reviews the birth experience, evidence of the dependent: taking-in phase. During the dependent-independent: taking-hold phase, the mother exhibits eagerness to learn and practice care of the infant and self. Focus on the family as a unit with interacting members is evidence of the interdependent: letting-go phase. The dependent-interdependent is not a phase of maternal postpartum adjustment. (P)

4. 2 The fundus descends at the rate of one to two fingerbreadths per day and by 2 weeks is no longer a pelvic organ. The vital signs, breasts, heart, lungs, abdomen (with exception of fundus), lochia, perineum, and extremities are within normal limits. (M)

5. 3 Pulling the infant from the breast can result in injury to the nipple. The correct way to unlatch is to place a finger next to the nipple and gently breaking the suction. The infant is always brought to the nipple rather than pulling the nipple and breast toward the infant. The cradle hold is a common breast-feeding position. To establish adequate milk supply, place the infant at breast whenever cues to hunger (mouthing, sucking) are present. (M)

6. 1 The mother receives RhoGAM if the infant is Rh-positive and the Coombs test is negative, indicating that there are no circulating antibodies to Rh-positive blood in the maternal system. (D)

7. 4 Cabbage leaves tucked into the bra relieve engorgement. Allowing warm water to run over the breasts may result in milk ejection and the breast will be stimulated to make more milk. Using a breast pump will also stimulate the breasts to produce milk. Wearing a snug bra and an Ace binder will not relieve engorgement, but may prevent further filling. (M)

8. 3 The most frequent cause of excessive bleeding after childbirth is uterine atony or failure of the uterine muscle to contract firmly. An appropriate first action to restore good tone is stimulation by gently massaging the uterine fundus until it is firm. If this intervention is not successful in restoring muscle tone, the woman is encouraged to empty her bladder. If she is unable to completely empty the bladder, catheterization may be necessary. If bleeding is excessive and muscle tone does not improve, it is necessary to notify the HCP. After a careful assessment for the cause of the problem, IV oxytocin (Pitocin) may be used to restore uterine muscle tone. (M)

9. 1 Initially, lochia is bright red. It consists mainly of blood and decidual debris from the shedding of the uterine lining. It is labeled *lochia rubra*; the nurse records the finding on the client's chart. After 3 to 4 days the discharge becomes pale pink or brown and is called *lochia serosa*. In about 10 days to 2 weeks, the discharge becomes yellow or white. The discharge may last up to 6 weeks. If the lochia becomes bright red after it has changed to pink, brown, or yellow, the woman is advised to get off her feet and rest. If the bright red bleeding continues, she is advised to contact her HCP. It is not necessary to start an IV infusion as the finding is normal. (M)

10. 4 "Afterpains" are uncomfortable cramping-like pains caused by periodic relaxation and vigorous contraction of the uterus. They are stronger and more painful after second and subsequent pregnancies. Breast-feeding and exogenous oxytocic medication usually cause these afterpains to intensify because both stimulate uterine contractions. Oxytocin (Pitocin) given during labor is out of the mother's system after 24 hr. A long labor and retained placental fragments would more likely cause the uterus to relax, not contract. (C)

11. 2 Blood pools in the vagina when a woman is lying on her back. It will leak out when she stands up. If the discharge lessens after this initial gush, no further intervention is needed. If heavy bleeding continues, the uterine fundus is palpated to be sure it is firm and in the midline, and the woman is asked to empty her bladder. If the bleeding continues after attempts to control it fail, retained placental tissue may be suspected. (M)

12. 1 The breasts are soft for the first few days after delivery before the milk supply comes in. The nurse encourages the mother to place the infant on the breast during this period because sucking stimulates milk production and the infant will get colostrum, a clear, yellowish fluid higher in protein and minerals than mature milk and rich in immunoglobulins. (C)

13. 3, 6 Irritation of the nipple with the development of fissures and a route for infection to enter the breast is best prevented by careful positioning the infant during feeding, and removing the infant from the breast by inserting a finger in the mouth to break the suction. Bottle-feeding can cause nipple confusion for the infant and delay milk production. Antibiotics are not appropriate as a preventive strategy for mastitis. Nipple shields are used for inverted nipples. Plenty of fluids and a healthy diet are very important for successful breast-feeding but do not prevent mastitis. (H)

14. 1 Foul-smelling, profuse lochia, and chills, fever, and malaise are symptoms of endometritis. Edema and hypertension are signs of pre-eclampsia, eclampsia, or the HELLP syndrome (hemolysis, elevated liver enzymes, and low platelets). Lower abdominal cramping and cloudy urine are signs of a urinary tract infection. Dizziness and hypotension may be signs of significant blood loss. (S)

15. 3 Increased risk for postpartum hemorrhage is associated with grand multiparity, multiple gestation, macrosomia, hydramnios, rapid or prolonged labor, and use of oxytocin for labor induction or augmentation. The woman who had a cesarean section is at least risk because of the controlled delivery. (M)

16. 4 Because the uterine fundus is firm and in the midline, and the woman has emptied her bladder, the nurse suspects that the source of the bleeding is not a boggy uterus but from another cause and notifies the HCP. The most likely source of the bleeding 2 to 4 hr after delivery is a vaginal or cervical tear or bleeding from the site of the episiotomy. The client is not experiencing clotting disorders and heparin (Lovenox) is contraindicated at this time. After notifying the HCP, the nurse assists the client to change the perineal pad and obtains accurate measurement of the amount of bleeding. Because the source of the bleeding is not the uterus, oxytocin (Pitocin), a drug used to increase contraction of uterine muscles, will not be helpful. (S)

17. 2 Heparin (Lovenox) is used to treat thrombophlebitis and prevent deep vein thrombosis. Terbutaline is a smooth muscle relaxant and is used to treat premature labor; oxytocin (Pitocin) is used to increase smooth muscle contraction in the uterus; antibiotics are used to manage infections; none of these are outcomes of the use of heparin (Lovenox). (D)

18 The nurse asks the client to dorsiflex the foot of the right leg, while palpating the calf. Pain on dorsiflexion indicates the presence of deep vein thrombosis (Homans sign). The involved area will be warm to touch. (A)

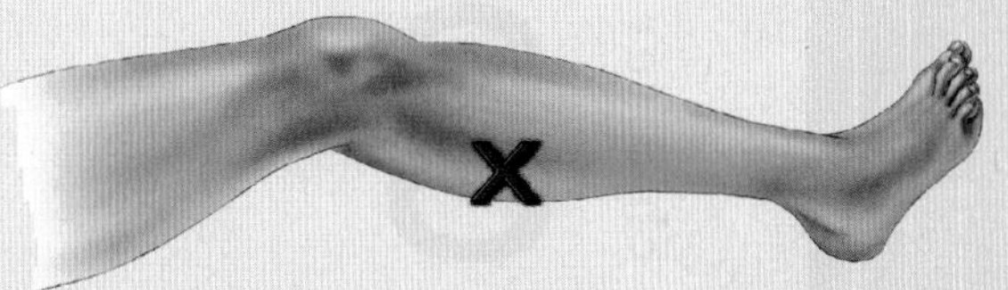

19. 1 2, 3, 4, 7 Risk factors for postpartum depression include prenatal depression, previous depressive disorder, life stress, lack of social support, prenatal anxiety, marital dissatisfaction, child care stress, maternity blues, African American race, being an adolescent mother, less than high school education, and unplanned/unwanted pregnancy. (P)

20. 3 This client is evaluated for postpartum depression as soon as possible, preferably that day. The nurse advises the client's husband to avoid leaving her alone with the infant until she has been seen by an HCP and depression is ruled out. Six weeks postpartum is beyond the time when baby blues is an appropriate explanation for sadness and inability to safely care for the infant. Although it is harder for some mothers to adjust to the responsibility for infant care, especially if she has a poor support system and no help, she must be evaluated for more serious depression before she is allowed to continue to care for the infant alone. (P)

chapter 8

The Neonatal Client

Most pregnancies, particularly those in which there has been adequate prenatal care, result in the birth of a healthy neonate. During delivery and postpartum, the nurse assesses the neonate, promotes family bonding, and instructs the family about care of their neonate. Occasionally, the neonate may be born before the expected due date (preterm) or after the due date (postterm), or be small or large for gestational age, and the nurse plans care accordingly. The nurse must be alert to the potential for health problems of the neonate and collaborate with the health care team to manage care. Topics and neonatal health problems discussed in this chapter include:

- Healthy Neonate
- Preterm Neonate
- Postterm Neonate
- Neonate Small for Gestational Age
- Neonate Large for Gestational Age
- Hypoglycemia
- Infant of Diabetic Mother
- Hyperbilirubinemia
- Respiratory Distress
- Infection and Sepsis
- HIV and AIDS
- Drug-Exposed Neonate
- Fetal Alcohol Spectrum Disorder

Healthy Neonate

I. Definition: A term neonate is born between 38 and 42 weeks' gestation. The healthy neonate is free of complications from labor and delivery as well as health problems that can result from genetic or maternal health problems.

II. Nursing process
 A. Assessment
  1. Obtain a detailed health history.
   a. Maternal history: Blood type, age, presence of chronic disease, infections, TORCH, group B beta streptococcus, drug use, maternal infections (if mother is positive for infection, neonate is assessed and observed for signs and symptoms of sepsis)
   b. Prenatal history: Estimated date of confinement, complications with pregnancy, labor and delivery history, use of analgesia or anesthesia
   c. Timing of assessment: Apgar cores, hours of age
   d. Neonate and parent interaction: Attachment and bonding
   e. Infant at risk: Birth weight, gestational age, type and length of newborn illness, environmental factors, maternal factors, maternal-infant separation
  2. Perform a comprehensive physical assessment.
   a. General appearance
    (1) Awake and sleep states:
     (a) Alert states—drowsy, wide awake, active awake, crying
     (b) Sleep states—deep or quiet sleep, active REM
    (2) Color: Pink with pink mucous membranes and nail beds, appropriate for race and ethnic heritage; assess for jaundice by blanching over boney prominence such as the forehead or chin, acrocyanosis is normal in the first 24 to 48 hr
    (3) Posture: Flexed position with extremities brought to midline
    (4) Respiratory: Nonlabored, rate 30 to 60 breaths per minute, clear and equal breath sounds, symmetrical chest excursion
    (5) Symmetry of body parts and movement
   b. Body measurements
    (1) Weight: Normal range, 2,500 to 4,000 g (5 lb 8 oz to 8 lb 13 oz); total weight loss should not be greater than 10% for term neonates and 15% for preterm neonates. Weight regained by 2 weeks if nutrition is adequate. Weighing at approximately the same time each day helps with accurate comparisons.
    (2) Length: Normal range, 48 to 52 cm (18 to 22 in.).
    (3) Head circumference: Normal range, 32 to 37 cm (12.5 to 14.5 in.); measured over the most prominent part of the occiput and just above the eyebrows—occipital frontal circumference (OFC).
    (4) Chest circumference: Normal range, 30 to 35 cm (12 to 14 in.); measured at the lower edge of scapulas and over nipple line. Generally 2 cm less than head circumference.
    (5) Abdominal circumference: Measured at the level of the umbilicus with the bottom edge of the measuring tape at the top of the umbilicus. Generally smaller than or equal to chest circumference.
   c. Vital signs
    (1) Heart rate: 120 to 160 beats per minute (apical) but may be as low as 80 while sleeping and as high as 180 when crying); assess for full minute to document rate, rhythm, position of the apical impulse, and intensity and presence of murmurs. Transient murmurs are considered normal because of incomplete closure of the ductus arteriosus or foramen ovale.
    (2) Peripheral pulses: Examine in all extremities, assessing for lags, strength, discrepancies, and rate variations.
    (3) Respirations: 30 to 60 breaths per minute; predominantly diaphragmatic; periods of apnea up to 20 s without changes in color or heart rate is considered normal. Count respirations for a full minute to achieve an accurate assessment because of episodic breathing. Breath sounds are clear and equal.
    (4) BP: 80/45 to 60/40 at birth. Assess perfusion, presence and quality of pulses, capillary refill (less than

2 to 3 s when skin is blanched; upper and lower extremities are equal).
(5) Temperature: 36.0°C to 37.0°C (96.8°F to 98.6°F) is most commonly assessed by axillary, continuous skin method with placement of servo control; rectal and tympanic temperatures can also be used.

d. Skin characteristics
(1) Color: Pink, general body color including mucous membranes; unhealthy skin colors include:
(a) Ruddy—indicates increased hematocrit
(b) Pale—indicates decreased hematocrit
(c) Cyanosis—(bluish color to skin and mucous membranes) indicates decreased oxygenation to the blood
(d) Jaundice—(yellowish discoloration of the skin, progresses in a cephalocaudal manner, is assessed by blanching skin over boney prominence, may be seen in the sclera or on the gum line) indicates increasing bilirubin
(2) Turgor: Indicates hydration, elasticity; returns to normal shape rapidly when tented
(3) Common variations of skin color that require no intervention:
(a) Acrocyanosis—peripheral cyanosis, bluish discoloration of hands and feet; normal first few hours after birth; caused by poor peripheral circulation resulting in vasomotor instability
(b) Mottling—lacy pattern of dilated blood vessels under the skin, due to general circulation fluctuations
(c) Harlequin sign—division of body with a line from head to toe causing half of the body to be pink and the other half of the body to be pale in color; caused by a vasomotor disturbance in the blood vessels where one side dilates and the other side contracts
(d) Erythema toxicum—*newborn rash,* perifollicular eruption of lesions that are firm, small (1 to 3 mm), white or pale yellow papule or pustule with an erythematous base (unknown cause)
(e) Vernix caseosa—protective white cheeselike substance that covers the skin; appears at approximately 20 to 24 weeks' gestation and decreases as the neonate approaches term, when it is only seen in the creases of the legs, arms, and genitals
(f) Milia—sebaceous glands that appear as raised white spots on the face, especially across the nose and chin
(g) Telangiectatic nevi/stork bites—pink to reddish patches on the nape of the neck, eyelids, nose, and lower occipital bone; usually fade by 2 years of age
(h) Mongolian spots—bluish-black macular areas usually on the dorsal area of the buttocks. Found in dark skinned races, Asians, and Pacific Islanders. Careful documentation is important so not to confuse with child abuse. Usually fade by 2 years of age
(i) Nevus flammeus—also called *port wine stain,* is an elevated, sharply demarcated, red to purple area of capillary angioma below the skin. Does not fade; may be associated with Sturge-Weber syndrome
(j) Nevus vasculosus—also called *strawberry mark* or *strawberry hemangioma*; enlarged capillaries in the dermal and subdermal layers, with raised, clear delineation and rough surface; these increase in size until about 8 months and then begin to recess

e. Head
(1) Large for body size: Approximately one fourth of body size
(2) Sutures: Overriding, approximated, separated, fused (fusion in the neonate is an abnormal finding)
(3) Molding: Asymmetry caused by cranial bone movement during labor and delivery

(4) Fontanelles
(a) Anterior—diamond-shaped, 3 to 4 cm long and 2 to 3 cm wide; closes by 18 to 24 months of age
(b) Posterior—triangular-shaped, formed by the parietal and occipital bone, 0.5 by 1 cm; closed by 8 to 12 weeks of age
(5) Birth injuries
(a) Ecchymosis and petechiae seen on face with rapid second-stage or shoulder dystocia
(b) Forceps or vacuum extractor marks
(c) Cephalhematoma—caused by a collection of blood between the periosteum and a cranial bone; does not cross suture lines; resolves over a few weeks or months without treatment
(d) Caput succedaneum—soft tissue swelling of scalp; crosses suture line; fluid is usually reabsorbed within 12 hr to first few days of life
(e) Subgaleal hemorrhage—blood collected between the connective tissues of the occipital and frontal muscles; swelling that crosses suture lines; fluctuates when palpated; fullness may be noted in the neck, may be fatal

f. Eyes
(1) Color: Usually blue-gray or brown, sclera white, clear lens and iris
(2) Movement: Eyelid with blink reflex, symmetrical movement of eyes; may be cross-eyed and exhibit strabismus
(3) Eyelids: Without redness or swelling, may have edema related to eye prophylaxis
(4) Conjunctivitis: Pink without drainage
(5) Subconjunctival hemorrhage: May be present
(6) Red reflex: Present

g. Ears
(1) Placement: Top of ear above an imaginary line drawn from the inner canthus to the outer canthus of the eye to the ear
(2) Shape: Incurving of top two thirds of pinna in term neonate; preterm neonates have less cartilage in pinna
(3) Preauricular skin tags: Neonates are evaluated for hearing loss

h. Nose
(1) Patency: Neonates are obligate nose breathers; nose is clear and free from mucus. If respiratory distress is noted, patency is evaluated.
(2) Choanal atresia: Congenital blockage of the passageway between nose and pharynx

i. Mouth
(1) Lips and mucous membranes: Pink, symmetrical movement
(2) Cleft lip/palate: Assess for intactness of lips, hard and soft palate
(a) Precocious teeth—usually central incisor, and are usually removed if loose to prevent aspiration
(b) Epstein's pearls—cysts on hard palate
(c) *Candida albicans*—commonly know as *thrush;* white patches adhering to mucous membranes
(d) Tongue-tied—frenulum tissue extending to tip of tongue

j. Neck
(1) Muscle tone: Term neonates able to hold head up for a few seconds while in a prone position
(2) Masses: No masses present
(3) Clavicles: Inspected for intactness; careful assessment is needed for LGA neonates, shoulder dystocia, or difficult deliveries

k. Chest
(1) Chest movement: Symmetrical; assess for retractions
(2) Heart: Normal rate and rhythm, range 120 to 160 beats per minute; measure over full minute for adequate rate assessment; transient murmurs may be heard
(3) Pulses: Bilateral and equal; assess brachial, radial, femoral, and pedal
(4) Lungs: Breath sounds clear and equal; assess rate for full minute because of periodic breathing to obtain accurate assessment (breath sounds could be course at birth and clear as respirations are established)
(5) Breast development depends on gestational age

l. Abdomen
(1) Umbilical cord: Three vessels, two arteries, one vein; dries and sloughs off in 7 to 10 days. Observe for redness, drainage, and/or bleeding.

(2) Bowel sounds: May be present at or shortly after birth in all four quadrants
(3) Shape: Flat, slightly rounded, no distention or firmness

m. Genitals
(1) Female/male: Easily differentiated; assess for voiding
(a) Female
- Pseudomenstruation—small amount of vaginal bleeding related to maternal hormonal influences
- Vaginal skin tags may be present

(b) Male
- Hypospadias—opening of urinary meatus on the underside of the glans
- Epispadias—opening of urinary meatus on the upper side of the glans
- Phimosis—prolonged erection
- Scrotum—assessment for descent of testicles
- Hydrocele

(2) Anus: Assess for patency

n. Extremities
(1) Arms: Equal and symmetrical movement
(a) Brachial palsy—birth injury related to edema and hemorrhage of the nerve sheath at the level of C5 to T1
(b) Erb-Duchenne paralysis—birth injury related to edema and hemorrhage of the nerve sheath at the level of C5 to C7

(2) Hands/feet: Five digits on each
(a) Polydactyly—increased number of fingers or toes
(b) Syndactyly—webbing between fingers or toes
(c) Simian crease—palmer crease transversing the hand; indicator of possible chromosomal abnormality

(3) Legs: Equal and symmetrical movement
(a) Ortolani and Barlow maneuvers—assessment of hip stability, dislocated or dislocatability
(b) Symmetrical gluteal fold—assessment for congenitally dislocated hips

(4) Feet: Talipes equinovarus versus positional clubfoot
(5) Back: Intact and smooth; assess for sacral dimple, and absence of tuffs of hair

3. Perform neurologic assessment—includes state of alertness, resting posture, cry, quality of muscle tone, and motor activity.
a. Tonic neck reflex
b. Grasping reflex
c. Moro reflex
d. Rooting reflex
e. Sucking reflex
f. Babinski reflex
g. Trunk incurvation

4. Assess gestational age—gestational age is a clinical picture of the neonate; one or two characteristics do not indicate gestational age.
a. Perform within first 4 hr of life to enable HCP to address age-related issues or problems.
b. Use the Ballard assessment tool (modified from the Dubowitz score to increase simplicity and decrease stress on the neonate)—total scores range from −10 to 50; assists in determining gestational age between 20 and 44 weeks' gestation. Two components of the Ballard assessment tool:
(1) Neuromuscular maturity
(a) Posture: Score 0 to 4
(b) Square window (wrist): Score −1 to 4
(c) Arm recoil: Score 0 to 4
(d) Popliteal angle: Score −1 to 5
(e) Scarf sign: Score −1 to 4
(f) Heel to ear: Score −1 to 4

(2) Physical maturity
(a) Skin: Score −1 to 5
(b) Lanugo: Score −1 to 4
(c) Plantar surface: Score −1 to 4
(d) Breast: Score −1 to 4
(e) Eye/ear: Score −1 to 4
(f) Genitals, male/female: Score −1 to 4

5. Obtain diagnostic tests—Based on the condition of the neonate.
a. Hemoglobin/hematocrit
b. Blood type ABO Rh
c. Coombs
d. Bilirubin
e. Newborn screen—test varies by state. Common screens are for cystic fibrosis, galactosemia, congenital adrenal hyperplasia, hypothyroidism, biotinidase deficiency, phenylketonuria, maple syrup urine disease, and hemoglobinopathies.
f. Glucose

g. CBC differential
h. Blood culture
i. Blood gas
j. Hearing test

B. Analysis
1. Risk for Ineffective Breathing Pattern related to retained lung fluid and mucus
2. Ineffective Peripheral Tissue Perfusion related to ineffective thermoregulation
3. Imbalanced Nutrition: Less Than Body Requirements related to inadequate intake
4. Impaired Urinary Elimination related to inadequate fluid intake or meatal edema secondary to circumcision
5. Risk for Infection related to immature immune system, birth trauma, invasive procedures such as heel sticks or venipunctures, circumcision site, cord healing, maternal history of infection at the time of delivery
6. Deficient Knowledge related to lack of experience or information about infant care and feeding
7. Risk for Injury related to knowledge deficit about car seat safety and sleep positions
8. Impaired Family Processes related to addition of new family member, role change, and demands on care givers
9. Risk for Imbalanced Body Temperature related to evaporation, radiant, conductive, and convective heat losses
10. Ineffective Airway Clearance related to increased mucus

C. Planning
1. Support transition to extrauterine life by decreasing pulmonary vascular resistance, and increasing systemic vascular resistance.
2. Maintain temperature in neutral thermal environment.
3. Prevent infection.
4. Provide adequate nutrition for growth and development.
5. Promote maternal-infant bonding and interaction.
6. Prevent cold stress.
7. Instruct caregiver on adequate voiding and stooling behavior.
8. Instruct caregiver on sleep/wake cycles.
9. Instruct caregiver regarding: safety/car seats, safe sleep positions (AAP recommends supine sleeping).

D. Implementation: Initial care by the nurse involves monitoring vital signs and protecting the airway by removing secretions from the mouth and then nose. (See also management of care.)

E. Evaluation
1. Infant's vital signs are stable, respiratory efforts are nonlabored, and temperature is in normal range.
2. Infant is voiding six to eight times in a 24-hr timeframe.
3. Infant is stooling at least one time in 24 hr and may stool each feeding; there is no water ring around stool.
4. Infant's cord is clean, dry, and without redness.
5. Infant is eating every 2 to 4 hr, maintaining blood glucose 50 to 110 mg/dl.
6. Infant is sleeping in safe supine position.
7. Infant is sleeping 20 of 24 hr, with variation in alert and sleep states.
8. Infant's caregiver is able to feed, bathe, diaper, and handle neonate with ease.

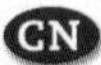

III. Client needs

A. Physiologic adaptation
1. Respiratory: At 20 to 24 weeks' gestation, the alveolar duct begins to differentiate into type I and type II cells. Type II cells are responsible for the production of surfactant; these cells continue to increase in number as the neonate approaches term.
   a. Initiation of breathing requires two major changes:
      (1) Lung expansion must take place with pulmonary ventilation being established
      (2) Pulmonary circulation must be increased
   b. In order for breathing to happen successfully, four events must occur:
      (1) Mechanical stimuli—removal of lung fluid as fetus passes through the birth canal, then chest recoil creating negative intrathoracic pressure causing passive inspiration
      (2) Chemical stimuli—an inspiratory gasp triggered by the elevation in PCO_2 and decrease in pH and PO_2; this triggers the aortic and carotid chemoreceptors, initiating impulses that stimulate the respiratory center in the medulla
      (3) Thermal stimuli—cold stimulates nerve endings in the skin and the response by the neonate is rhythmic respirations (at birth the ambient temperature drops from 37°C to 23.9°C [98.6°F to 75°F]); use caution to prevent cold stress
      (4) Sensory stimuli—these include tactile, auditory, and visual stimulation during and after birth, such as

drying the neonate and placing skin to skin with the mother

c. Factors that may work against the first breath:
   (1) Alveolar surface tension
   (2) Viscosity of lung fluid
   (3) Degree of lung compliance

2. Cardiac: With the first breath, the pressure in the left atrium increases as blood returns from the pulmonary veins, pressure drops in the right atrium, and systemic vascular resistance increases.
   a. Five major adaptations that occur:
      (1) Increased aortic pressure and decreased venous pressure
      (2) Increased systemic pressure and decreased pulmonary artery pressure
      (3) Closure of the foramen ovale
      (4) Functional closure of the ductus arteriosus
      (5) Functional closure of the ductus venosus
   b. Evaluate with a cardiac echo unresolved murmurs that occur with cyanosis.
3. Thermoregulation: Closely related to metabolism and oxygen consumption. It is important to maintain a neutral thermal environment (NTE) where oxygen usage and metabolism is minimal; the amount of subcutaneous fat, thickness of epidermis, and closeness of blood vessels to skin have influence on the NTE. Flexed position of term neonate reduces heat loss, and preterm neonates have limited flexion ability.
4. Thermogenesis: Increased basal metabolic rate, muscular activity, and nonshivering thermogenesis is triggered by a release of norepinephrine by the adrenal gland and in brown fat (first appears 26 to 30 weeks' gestation, located on midscapula, axillas, around neck, kidney, and adrenal glands); this causes brown fat triglycerides to metabolize into glycerol and fatty acids, which are used for energy and result in acidosis.
5. Hepatic: Liver palpated 2 to 3 cm below the right costal margin. Liver stores iron; functions in carbohydrate metabolism and in the conjugation of bilirubin; absence of intestinal flora, which is necessary for the production of vitamin K, phytonadione (AquaMEPHYTON) is given to prevent hemorrhagic disease of the newborn.
6. GI: By 36 to 38 weeks' gestation, the neonate has the ability to transport nutrients with the presence of adequate enzymes and digest most simple carbohydrates, fats, and proteins. Bowel sounds are present within the first 30 to 60 min of life and the neonate can be fed during this time frame if showing no signs of distress.
7. Urinary: Neonatal kidney by 34 to 36 weeks' gestation has a full complement of functioning nephrons and a decreased glomerular filtration rate; therefore, unable to dispose of water quickly when necessary, and the juxtamedullary portion of the nephron has limited capacity to reabsorb HCO_3 and H+ and concentrate urine. The ability to concentrate urine fully is achieved by 3 months of age.
8. Immunologic: A neonate's inflammatory response has a limited ability to recognize, localize, and destroy invasive bacteria. Signs and symptoms of infection are often vague and subtle.

B. Management of care: Care of the neonate requires critical thinking skills and knowledge of assessment, and teaching and evaluation methods unique to the RN role. The following skills cannot be delegated to an LPN or UAP.
1. Provide initial care.
   a. Monitor vital signs.
   b. Protect airway by removing secretions from the mouth and then nose.
   c. Perform complete physical assessments with evaluation for risk factors (completed within 2 hr of life).
   d. Provide cord care after clamped for first 24 hr; remove clamp, keep dry, and clean with sterile water if soiled (sloughs off in 7 to 10 days).
   e. Administer medications to protect from hemorrhagic disease of the newborn, eye pathogens, and hepatitis B.
2. Delegate responsibly those activities that can be delegated. All monitoring information is reported to the RN. Tasks include:
   a. Deliver care to protect temperature stability; keep neonate away from drafts, away from windows, hat on head for first 24 hr, and lightly covered.
   b. Bathe infant to remove blood-borne pathogens, taking care not to cause cold stress.
   c. Implement feeding.
      (1) Breast—on demand, at least every 2 to 4 hr; observe for proper positioning and latching, rhythmic suck, swallow, breathing, and burping
      (2) Bottle-feeding—on demand at least every 3 to 4 hr; observe for proper

positioning, rhythmic suck, swallow, breathing, and burping
   d. Provide care of the circumcised and noncircumcised penis.
   e. Provide SIDS prevention: Position supine, with feet to foot of bed, covered with light blanket to nipple line.
3. Instruct client to adhere to follow-up appointments with HCP.
4. Discuss with client the importance of frequent follow-up care in first year of life to assess proper growth and development, and promote meeting of developmental milestones.
5. Explore support groups available in area for new parents; these may focus on new mothers and activities such as breast-feeding or infant play groups.

C. Safety and infection control
1. Perform proper identification confirmation: Identification bracelets for mothers, significant other, and neonates; foot printing in the delivery room before mother and infant are separated. Many institutions have infant abductions security systems in place.
2. Perform frequent hand hygiene and instruct parents on the benefits and infection reduction associated with good hand hygiene.
3. Instruct parents on care for umbilical cord—call HCP if redness, foul odor, bright red bleeding, or greenish yellow drainage is noted.
4. Promote immunizations: Follow current CDC guidelines. The AAP recommends routine vaccination of neonates with hepatitis B before initial discharge from hospital.

D. Health promotion and maintenance
1. Instruct parents on signs of distress such as color change, breathing, or behavior.
2. Maintain NTE-oxygen consumption and metabolism increases as temperature is above or below normal range.
3. Monitor temperature every 30 min until client stable for 2 hr (temperature should stabilize in 8 to 12 hr); then monitor at least every 8 hr or according to agency policy.
4. Avoid cold stress to decrease oxygen consumption, depletion of glycogen stores, and metabolism of brown fat.
5. Instruct parents on heat loss by convection, radiation, evaporation, and conduction.
6. Place neonate under radiant warmer with servo control or incubator, as necessary.
7. Place hat on neonate's head for first 24 hr.

E. Psychologic integrity
1. Facilitate parent-newborn attachment by encouraging eye-to-eye contact, parents bathing infant, and calling infant by given name, and explaining neonatal behaviors to parents.
2. Instruct parents regarding periods of reactivity.
   a. First period of reactivity—lasts approximately 30 min after birth; neonate is awake, alert, and has a strong suck. This a good opportunity to initiate breast-feeding: heart rate and respiratory rate may be increased.
   b. Period of inactivity to sleep phase—neonate goes into a deep sleep from 2 to 4 hr, is difficult to wake, and usually not interested in suckling; respirations and heart rate usually return to baseline.
   c. Second period of reactivity—neonate is again alert and awake for approximately 4 to 6 hr; an increase in respiratory rate and gastric mucus may be seen. Neonate responds by gagging, choking, and regurgitation, and may be interested in suckling. GI tract becomes more active.
3. Instruct parents regarding characteristics of behavioral (sleep and alert) states (see assessment).

F. Basic care and comfort
1. Offer anticipatory guidance.
2. Instruct parents on immature cardiac sphincter and regurgitation: normal during the neonatal period; avoiding overfeeding; frequent burping helps to decrease amount of regurgitation.
3. Ensure adequate growth. Weight gain should be 15 to 30 g per day and increase 1.0 cm to body length per week.
   a. Provide 95 to 130 kcal/kg per day (breast milk contains more medium chain triglycerides and lipase than cow's milk and is more readily absorbed).
   b. Encourage healthy neonates to feed (breast or bottle) during the first period of reactivity; signs of readiness include rooting and sucking behaviors when lips or cheek are stimulated, active bowel sounds, and lack of abdominal distention.
4. Monitor stool.
   a. Meconium—usually passed within 8 to 24 hr after birth; consists of amniotic fluid, intestinal secretions, and shed

mucosal cell (dark green or black, thick, and tarry in appearance)
   b. Transitional stools—part meconium and part fecal material (thinner brown to green)
   c. Stool appearance—depends on method of feeding; ranges between formed soft brown stool (in bottle-fed neonate) to mushy yellow (in breast-fed neonate)
   d. Stool patterns—stool at least one time per day; breast-feed neonate may stool more frequently
5. Monitor voiding patterns. Neonate may void at birth; normal voiding is between 24 and 48 hr. Inform parents that 6 to 10 wet diapers in a 24-hr period is an indicator of adequate fluid intake. Instruct parents to:
   a. Report if neonate does not void between 24 and 48 hr after birth: should be assessed for adequate intake, bladder distention, restlessness, and symptoms of pain.
   b. Report any blood in urine; pseudomenstruation is normal in females and some bleeding is normal in circumcised males. Urates or brick dust is a normal finding in both males and females.
6. Bathe neonate: First bath is performed once neonate is determined to have stable vital signs and has made the appropriate cardiopulmonary transition. Protect temperature while bathing (rewarm as necessary) and assess temperature after bath to ensure thermoregulation.
7. Provide skin care to prevent breakdown; use mild soap or clear water; keep perianal and buttocks clean and dry to prevent diaper dermatitis.
8. Provide current information to parents regarding circumcision so an informed decision can be made: circumcision based on cultural, social, and family tradition; AAP policy does not recommend routine circumcision and acknowledges there are medical indications. Also provide client teaching about the following:
   a. For circumcised male neonate:
      (1) Risks and outcomes, such as hemorrhage, infection, difficulty in voiding, pain, progressive stenosis of urethral meatus
      (2) Performed when neonate is well stabilized and free from infection; may be done in the hospital or as part of a religious ceremony
      (3) Pain-management techniques include oral glucose, nonnutritive sucking, and swaddling
   b. For uncircumcised male neonate, use good hygiene practices. Occasionally during the daily bath, gently retract and wash glans with soap and water; if retraction does not happen, do not force.

G. Reduction of risk potential
1. Assure safe sleep positioning: supine (back) for sleeping. The AAP guidelines for safe sleep and SIDS prevention include placing feet to foot of crib, covering with light blanket to nipple line, and taking care not to overheat the neonate.
2. Give "tummy time" during wakeful play periods but care-provider must observe the neonate.
3. Prevent shaken baby syndrome: Provide parental teaching regarding safe handling of infant; it is NEVER okay to shake an infant or small child.
4. Avoid smoking around the neonate; smoking leads to increased respiratory and ear infection as well as increased incidence of SIDS.
5. Maintain car seat safety. Instruct parents that an approved car seat is needed to go home from hospital; the safest spot is the middle back seat, in rear-facing position for children under 20 lb. It is very important that parents read and follow manufacturer's instruction.

H. Pharmacologic and parenteral therapies: Client family will state the purpose for and associated side effects of all medications.
1. Vitamin K1 phytonadione (AquaMEPHYTON): Single dose of 0.5 to 1.0 mg parenterally within 1 hr of birth; given in the middle third of the vastus lateralis muscle in the lateral aspect of the thigh to prevent complications of hemorrhagic disease of the newborn.
2. 0.5% erythromycin (Ilotycin Ophthalmic) for the prevention of *Neisseria gonorrhoeae* and *Chlamydia*; instilled into lower conjunctival sac, may be delayed up to 1 hr to promote maternal infant interaction. Other agents that may be used include tetracycline; some may cause a chemical conjunctivitis.
3. Hepatitis B vaccine (Engerix-B, Recombivax HB): 0.5 ml (10 mcg) IM in the middle third of the vastus lateralis muscle of the lateral aspect of the thigh; given at birth to 2 months of age. Second dose is given at least 1 month after the first; third dose at

least 2 months after second dose, but not before 6 months of age. If mother is positive for HBsAg the vaccine is given in the first 12 hr of life. Side effects from vaccine include erythema, swelling, warmth, irritability, or low-grade fever.

Preterm Neonate

I. Definition: A preterm neonate is one who is born less than 37 weeks' gestation.
   A. Incidence is approximately 8% of births in United States
   B. Risk factors
      1. Maternal-inadequate prenatal care
      2. Lower socioeconomic status
      3. Substance abuse
      4. Chronic medical conditions
      5. Urinary tract infections
      6. Incompetent cervix
      7. Premature rupture of membranes
      8. Multiple gestations

II. Nursing process
   A. Assessment
      1. Physical appearance:
         a. Skin—usually pink or ruddy, may be thin or translucent with blood vessels visible
         b. Decreased subcutaneous fat
         c. Large head for body size
         d. Presence of lanugo
         e. Minimal ear cartilage
         f. Short nails
         g. Flaccid tone
         h. Diminished reflexes
      2. Respiratory status: Skin for blue coloring; increased respiratory rate; grunting, nasal flaring, retractions (substernal, intercostal, subcostal, and suprasternal), increased effort, increased work of breathing; decreased lung compliance; decreased breath sounds; irregular breathing patterns; apnea and bradycardia
      3. Cardiac status: Patent ductus arteriosus as evidenced by murmur; increased respiratory effort, decreased gas exchange, bounding pulses
      4. Thermoregulation: Body temperature, environmental temperature, amount of subcutaneous fat, glucose levels, and oxygen requirement
      5. GI system: Feeding tolerance each feeding, residuals, vomiting, abdominal distention, increasing abdominal girth, bowel sounds, bowel loops, stool pattern and consistency, presence of gag reflex
      6. Presence of intraventricular hemorrhage: Vulnerability; neonates less than 1,500 g and less than 34 weeks' gestation, decreased BP, decreased oxygenation saturation, increased irritability, decreasing hematocrit, full or bulging anterior fontanel
      7. Sepsis: Hypotension, behavior or feeding change, temperature instability, changes in respiratory status
      8. Family interaction with neonate (interaction may be limited)
   B. Analysis
      1. Impaired Gas Exchange related to immature pulmonary system and decrease surfactant production
      2. Ineffective Breathing Pattern related to immature CNS
      3. Decreased Cardiac Output related to hypotension and decreased tissue perfusion secondary to patent ductus arteriosis
      4. Ineffective Thermoregulation related to decreased subcutaneous fat, decreased glycogen stores, and decreased brown fat
      5. Imbalanced Nutrition: Less Than Body Requirements related to decreased suck, swallow-breathing coordination, and decreased ability to absorb nutrients
      6. Risk for Imbalanced Fluid Volume due to potential for Intraventricular Hemorrhage related to fragile capillary network of the germinal matrix
      7. Risk for Infection related to immature immune system, immature skin, and invasive procedures
      8. Ineffective Coping related to unexpected delivery and unrealistic expectations
   C. Planning
      1. Support respiratory effort.
      2. Support immature body systems (CNS, GI, and renal).
      3. Prevent infection.
      4. Maintain temperature in neutral thermal environment.
      5. Provide adequate nutrition for growth and development.
      6. Promote maternal and infant bonding and interaction.
   D. Implementation
      1. Assess breath sounds, respiratory effort, and oxygen saturation.
      2. Support oxygen requirements as needed to maintain PaO_2 mmHg.
      3. Use oxygen mask, nasal cannula, head hood, CPAP, or mechanical ventilation; use heat and humidity as soon a possible.
      4. If apneic, gently stimulate to encourage breathing; respiratory support may be

necessary; methylxanthine drugs may be used.

5. Assess cardiac status by auscultation of rate and rhythm.
6. Assess pulses, attention to bounding femoral pulses.
7. Maintain a neutral thermal zone; use support of radiant warmer or incubator.
8. Provide positioning for patent airway; avoid hyperextending the neck.
9. Position for flexed posture to decrease surface area and conserve heat.
10. Provide 95 to 130 kcal/kg per day for adequate growth.
11. Increase feedings as tolerated; may need to be fortified to increase calorie content, breast milk, or formulas.
12. Administer enteral (oral) feedings; may be by mouth or via oral/nasal gastric tube.
13. Administer total parenteral nutrition as needed if neonate is unable to tolerate enteral feedings.
14. Provide calories to enable a consistent weight gain of 20 to 30 g per day.
15. Provide increased calcium, phosphorus, and vitamin D; provide nutrition with higher concentration of whey protein than casein.
16. Include parents in care of neonate, including temperature taking, diaper changing, and feeding as condition allows.
17. Prevent infection by meticulous hand hygiene.

E. Evaluation

1. Infant gains 20 to 30 g per day, increases in OFC and length of 1 cm per week.
2. Infant demonstrates stable respiratory status.
3. Infant maintains temperature stability.
4. Infant remains free from infection.
5. Infant demonstrates growth and development appropriate for gestational age.
6. Infant expresses optimum neuromuscular development.
7. Parents verbalize comfort in providing care in home setting.

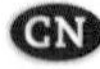

III. Client needs

A. Physiologic adaptation

1. Respiratory—decreased surfactant production due to lung immaturity, alveolar collapse, and decreased oxygenation and ventilation; decreased amounts of surfactant with decreased lung compliance.
2. Lower pulmonary vascular resistance leads to increased left-right shunting. Blood takes path of least resistance (through the ductus arteriosus), increasing blood flow back into the lungs and decreasing gas exchange and oxygenation.
3. Cardiac—ductus arteriosus responds to oxygen; preterm neonates are at high risk for becoming hypoxic, thus causing the ductus to remain open. This allows blood to bypass the lungs, sending decreased oxygenated blood to the body and oxygenated blood back to the lungs.
4. Thermoregulation—neonates have limited ability to produce heat because of large surface area in relation to body mass and because of the neonate's inability or limited ability to flex keeps surface area large, thus decreasing the ability to conserve heat. The neonate also has decreased brown fat available for metabolism, decreased glycogen stores in the liver, limited subcutaneous fat, and decreased ability for muscle activity. The skin is thin, which allows for increased insensible water loss due to increased skin permeability, decreased ability for vasoconstriction of superficial blood vessels, and heat conservation.
5. GI—decreased stomach size, immature esophageal cardiac sphincter, poor suck-swallow-breath coordination, high caloric demand for growth and increased oxygen requirements, limited ability to convert some essential amino acid to nonessential amino acids, difficulty absorbing saturated fats, deficiency of calcium and phosphorus as a result of two thirds of minerals deposited in last trimester.
6. Apnea of prematurity—breathing cessation of 20 s or longer, or breathing cessation for less than 20 s with color change and bradycardia due to neurologic immaturity; presents usually between 2 and 7 days of life.
7. Renal—glomerular filtration rate is lower because of prematurity, decreased renal perfusion, limited ability to concentrate urine, or to excrete excess amounts of fluid, limited ability to excrete drugs, reduced buffering capacity predisposing neonate to metabolic acidosis.
8. Hepatic and hematologic—iron is stored in the liver, especially in the last trimester. Neonates born before this have low stores of iron; anemia can become a problem because of frequent blood sampling.
9. Greater risk for infection because of immature immunity—most passive immunity acquired in the last trimester, leaving neonate with few antibodies at birth; skin is thin and easily excoriated, making easy access for infections.

B. Management of care: Care of the neonate requires critical thinking skills and knowledge of assessment, and teaching and evaluation methods unique to the RN role. The following skills cannot be delegated to an LPN or UAP.

1. Monitor PaO_2. Critical to prevent retinopathy of prematurity, which is multifactorial in origin; causes injury to developing vascular system of the retina, leading to ischemia and hemorrhage, scarring and retinal detachment.
2. Manage fluid infusion rates and osmolality to prevent intraventricular hemorrhage, which occurs because of the immature germinal matrix.
3. Provide respiratory care. Support with minimal supplemental oxygen. Pulse oximetry is necessary to monitor oxygen saturation; nasal cannula, oxygen mask, CPAP, or ventilator support might be necessary.

C. Safety and infection control
1. Practice strict hand hygiene.
2. Separate equipment for each neonate.
3. Isolate each infant according to standard precautions.
4. Use strict aseptic technique with IV tubing changes; provide changes in IV fluids every 24 to 48 hr according to hospital policy.

D. Health promotion and maintenance
1. Provide thermoregulation—use warmed humidified oxygen, use incubator or heat shield, avoid placing neonate in contact with cold surfaces, keep skin dry, use radiant warmers and incubators with servo control; keep cribs, warmers, and incubators away from drafts and direct sources of sunlight.
2. Ensure adequate growth—provide 95 to 130 kcal/kg per day; OFC and length should increase at 1 cm per week as an indicator of adequate growth.

E. Psychologic integrity
1. Provide family with photographs.
2. Encourage journaling by family to note neonate's journey and progress.
3. Provide family with phone number to NICU and encourage phone calls from family for updates on condition.
4. Call neonate given name as soon as it is known; use name cards at bedside.
5. Promote positive parent-infant attachment; offer photographs, call neonate by correct gender and given name, encourage eye contact between neonate and parent, and encourage skin-to-skin holding.

F. Basic care and comfort
1. Skin care: Keep skin clean and dry; assure minimal use of products on skin; remove potential skin irritants such as skin preparation and materials used for monitoring or diagnostic procedures.
2. Developmental care: Flexion with positioning, nesting or swaddling, gentle touch; self-consoling activities such as hand-to-mouth activities, nonnutritive sucking.
3. Pain reduction: Use nonpharmacologic pain-reduction methods such as swaddling and nonnutritive sucking; analgesic and sedatives may be necessary.
4. Feedings: Neonate requires 95 to 130 kcal/kg per day for growth and development; requires more protein than term neonate. Formula or breast milk may need fortification from 20 kcal/oz to 22, 24, 27, or 30 cal/oz. Weight gain should be 20 to 30 g per day.
   a. Types of feeding include bottle, breastfeeding, gavage, and total parenteral nutrition.
   b. Provide client teaching about feeding related issues, including reading behavioral cues, feeding technique and patterns, voiding and stool patterns, normal growth patterns, and signs and symptoms of feeding difficulties or intolerance.

G. Reduction of risk potential
1. Evaluate ability of neonate to ride in car seat for the time it requires to reach home or 1 hr, whichever is greater, without oxygen desaturation.
2. During sleep, position neonate on back with feet to foot of bed with light blanket to axilla.
3. Prevent shaken baby syndrome (100% preventable)—encourage positive parent-infant attachment, instruct parents on danger of shaking a neonate.
4. Prevent infection in home environment—require visitor to perform hand hygiene before handling neonate, limit number of visitors in the first 8 weeks of life, limit visitors to individuals who are healthy (no rashes, coughs, runny noses, or fevers).
5. Screen and protect against respiratory syncytial virus.

H. Pharmacologic and parenteral therapies: Client family will state the purpose for and associated side effects of all medications.
1. Fluids—start at 80 to 100 mL/kg per day and increase about 20 mL/kg per day up to 160 to 200 mL/kg per day based on neonate's diagnosis and gestational age

2. Caffeine—maintenance dose 5 to 8 mg/kg; can be given PO or IV. Treats neonatal apnea; side effects include restlessness, vomiting, and tachycardia

Postterm Neonate

I. Definition: A postterm neonate is one who is born after 42 weeks' gestation.
  A. Incidence is approximately 4% to 18% of births in United States
  B. Risk factors
    1. Primiparity
    2. High multiparity
    3. Inaccurate estimation date of birth
    4. Past history of prolonged pregnancy
II. Nursing process
  A. Assessment
    1. Physical appearance—may be of normal size and health, may be thin and long-bodied. Look for dry and cracked skin, long nails beyond the fingertips, no vernix present; alert, wide-eyed appearance; creases covering the soles of the feet; abundant scalp hair; weight may be over 4,000 g.
    2. Birth injury related to large size: Erb palsy, fractures of clavicle or skull.
    3. Postmaturity syndrome: Postmature newborns are those born after 42 weeks in the uterus. Only 5% of postterm neonates experience postmaturity syndrome. Mortality rate in postmaturity syndrome is 2 to 3 times higher than postterm deaths because of inadequate fetal and placental reserves. Risks for postmaturity include:
      a. Hypoglycemia
      b. Utero hypoxia resulting in meconium staining or meconium aspiration
      c. Increased RBC production resulting from hypoxic state in utero
      d. Hypoxic state resulting in possible seizures
      e. Thermoregulation—instability due to wasting of subcutaneous fat
    4. Presence of pain along with each vital sign assessment.
  B. Analysis
    1. Risk for Injury related to increased size at birth
    2. Hypothermia related to decreased subcutaneous fat
    3. Imbalanced Nutrition: Less Than Body Requirements related to increased glucose utilization in utero and decreased placental perfusion
    4. Impaired Gas Exchange in lungs and cellular level related to airway obstruction from meconium aspiration
    5. Risk for Ineffective Tissue Perfusion related to increase RBC production
    6. Risk for Seizures related to hypoxia and/or hypoglycemia
  C. Planning
    1. Provide comfort measures if birth injury has occurred.
    2. Support temperature to prevent cold stress so calories are used for brain and tissue growth.
    3. Provide nutrition to support brain and tissue development.
    4. Provide respiratory support to compromised neonate.
  D. Implementation
    1. Monitor vital signs for adequate oxygen consumption.
    2. Maintain thermoregulation.
    3. Assess for birth injury, assessing for symmetrical movement of face and arms, and absence of trauma to scalp and head (if forceps or vacuum extractor was used).
    4. Assess for decreased neurologic response or seizure activity related to hypoxia.
    5. Monitor glucose carefully because of increased utilization, thus decreased stores.
    6. Provide glucose (breast- or bottle-feeding preferred if neonate's status allows at 1 to 2 hr of age) to protect the CNS.
    7. Assess respiratory status for signs of respiratory distress due to meconium aspiration.
    8. Monitor hematocrit to determine the presence or extent of polycythemia.
  E. Evaluation
    1. Infant has effective respirations for adequate gas exchange.
    2. Infant has normal glucose levels for growth, development, and CNS protection.
    3. Infant has stable temperature to minimize metabolic demands.
    4. Infant has adequate pain management.

CN

II. Client needs
  A. Physiologic adaptation
    1. Macrosomia—assess for birth injury related to increase body size.
    2. Respiratory distress—possible decreased surfactant production due to chronic hypoxemia; possible pulmonary hypertension and possible meconium aspiration.
  B. Management of care: Care of the postterm neonate requires critical thinking skills and knowledge of assessment, and teaching and evaluation methods unique to the RN role.

The following skills cannot be delegated to an LPN or UAP.

1. Assess for brain injury, fractures of clavicle or skull, nerve damage to face, arm, or diaphragm.
2. Assess for seizures related to possible hypoxic insults.

C. Safety and infection control: Provide skin care; observe for breakdown due to dryness of skin.

D. Health promotion and maintenance: Provide thermoregulation. Use warmed humidified oxygen; avoid placing neonate in contact with cold surfaces; keep skin dry; use radiant warmers and incubators with servo control; keep cribs and warmers away from drafts and direct sources of sunlight.

E. Psychologic integrity: Provide parental teaching about appropriate developmental levels.

F. Basic care and comfort
1. Provide nutrition for growth and development, usually 120 kcal/kg per day.
2. Manage glucose levels; assess for decreased glucose stores as high rate of glucose use may have occurred in utero.

G. Reduction of risk potential: Assess for potential risks (see analysis section).

H. Pharmacologic and parenteral therapies: Administer oxygen and parentereal fluids as previously noted.

Neonate Small for Gestational Age

I. Definition: Small for gestational age (SGA) neonates at birth are below the tenth percentile on the intrauterine growth curve. SGA neonates may be preterm, term, or postterm.

A. SGA neonates are at risk for perinatal asphyxia, polycythemia, hypothermia, hypoglycemia, intrauterine infections, hypocalcemia, congenital malformations, and cognitive disabilities.

B. SGA and intrauterine growth restriction (IUGR) are not necessarily interchangeable. The IUGR pregnancies are pregnancies of advanced gestational age and limited fetal growth. IUGR can be symmetric (proportional) or asymmetric (disproportional). Causes of IUGR include:
1. Maternal cause—multiple gestations, lack of prenatal care, primiparity, grand multiparity, inadequate nutritional intake, age (under 16 or over 40 years), chronic disease, substance abuse, tobacco use, diminished blood flow to the uterus
2. Fetal factors—congenital infections, congenital malformations, chromosomal syndrome, and inborn errors of metabolism

II. Nursing process

A. Assessment: Assess physical appearance of a neonate who is SGA.
1. Large head in relation to chest and abdomen
2. Small or decreased subcutaneous fat
3. Loose skin
4. Long and thin in appearance
5. Small amounts of scalp hair
6. Sunken abdomen

B. Analysis
1. Imbalanced Nutrition: Less Than Body Requirements related to increased metabolic needs
2. Impaired Gas Exchange related to retained lung fluid
3. Hypothermia related to decreased subcutaneous fat
4. Risk for Impaired Tissue Perfusion related to polycythemia
5. Risk for Impaired Parenting related to unrealistic expectations

C. Planning
1. Provide adequate nutrition to allow brain and tissue growth.
2. Provide respiratory support to compromised neonate.
3. Support temperature to allow use of calories for growth.
4. Encourage maternal-infant bonding and interaction.
5. Assess for prenatal infection such as those found in a TORCH screen.

D. Implementation
1. Provide adequate nutrition for growth and development.
2. Assess and plot growth on neonatal growth charts.
3. Assess for respiratory alterations and support with oxygen if necessary.
4. Maintain neutral thermal environment.
5. Treat prenatal infections as identified by TORCH screen or other diagnostics such as cultures.

E. Evaluation
1. Infant has normal respiratory effort and rate with adequate gas exchange.
2. Infant experiences temperature and glucose stability.
3. Infant experiences 15- to 30-g weight gain in 24 hr.
4. Parents have a clear understanding of the needs for positive outcomes.
5. Infant is free from infection.

CN

III. Client needs

A. Physiologic adaptation

1. Instruct parents about the risk of hypoglycemia and the importance of frequent feeding to maintain glucose levels.
2. Monitor for hyperviscosity related to increase RBC production as a result of chronic perinatal asphyxia.

B. Management of care: Care of the neonate who is SGA requires critical thinking skills and knowledge of assessment, and teaching and evaluation methods unique to the RN role. The following skills cannot be delegated to an LPN or UAP.
   1. Provide respiratory support if necessary.
   2. Provide continued evaluation of congenital malformation.
   3. Monitor for seizure activity related to asphyxia.
   4. If neonate has positive findings on TORCH screen, consider not allowing a pregnant HCP to administer care.

C. Safety and infection control: Screen and monitor for TORCH infections.

D. Health promotion and maintenance
   1. Monitor for cold stress from decreased subcutaneous fat.
   2. Instruct parents on proper thermoregulation, such as keeping neonate out of drafts.

E. Psychologic integrity: Assist parents to adapt to needs of their newborn.

F. Basic care and comfort
   1. Provide 95 to 130 kcal/kg per day for adequate growth and development.
   2. Monitor glucose for hypoglycemia related to increased utilization.

G. Reduction of risk potential: Assess for potential risks (see analysis section).

H. Pharmacologic and parenteral therapies: Use oxygen as needed; maintain adequate fluid and nutritional intake with parentereal fluids as ordered.

Neonate Large for Gestational Age

I. Definition: A large for gestational age (LGA) is a neonate whose birth weight is at or above the ninetieth percentile according to the intrauterine growth curve.
   A. Etiology may involve miscalculation of date of conception, maternal diabetes, genetic predisposition, multiparity, male infants, or transposition of the great vessels.
   B. LGA neonates are at risk for inadequate nutrition, respiratory distress, and birth injuries.

II. Nursing process
   A. Assessment
      1. Physical appearance—generally proportional body size and presence of macrosomia
      2. Motor skills (may be poor)
      3. Ability of neonate to take feedings (may have difficulty)
      4. Presence of birth injuries because of large size—includes bruising, shoulder dystocia, brachial plexus palsy, facial paralysis, phrenic nerve palsy, skull fracture, cephalhematoma, intercranial hemorrhage, asphyxia, and fractured clavicle
      5. Respiratory status due to potential for retained lung fluid—seen more frequently with cesarean section delivery, which occurs at a greater rate because of increased neonatal size
      6. Presence of hypoglycemia, polycythemia, and/or hyperviscosity
      7. Presence of pain along with assessment of vital signs
   B. Analysis
      1. Impaired Gas Exchange related to retained lung fluid associated with cesarean section birth
      2. Imbalanced Nutrition: Less Than Body Requirements related to increased glucose utilization
      3. Risk for neurovascular dysfunction related to hypoxia or birth injury
      4. Risk for Injury related to birth process and macrosomia
      5. Risk for Impaired Parent/Infant/Child Attachment related to maternal fear of further injuring neonate
      6. Acute Pain related to birth injury
   C. Planning
      1. Support respiratory effort.
      2. Provide nutrition for brain and tissue growth.
      3. Provide glucose to prevent hypoglycemia.
      4. Provide thermoregulation.
      5. Provide comfort measures if birth injury is present.
   D. Implementation (see management of care)
   E. Evaluation
      1. Infant has normal respiratory effort and rate with adequate gas exchange.
      2. Infant maintains glucose above 50 mg/dl.
      3. Infant has adequate nutrition to support normal brain and tissue growth.
      4. Infant experiences temperature stability.
      5. Infant is free from injury.

CN

III. Client needs
   A. Physiologic adaptation: If birth injury has occurred due to macrosomia, instruct parents on proper handling of neonate.
   B. Management of care: Care of the LGA neonate requires critical thinking skills and knowledge

of assessment, and teaching and evaluation methods unique to the RN role. The following skills cannot be delegated to an LPN or UAP.
1. Monitor respiratory effort and support as necessary.
2. Assist parent in understanding feeding readiness cues.
3. Monitor for hypoglycemia at 1 hr of age and until glucose levels are stable above 50 mg/dl.
4. Provide feeding as soon after birth as possible; IV glucose may be necessary.
5. Assist parents to understand how to arouse and console neonate.
6. Provide parental teaching regarding any birth injuries.
7. Provide for pain management if birth injury has occurred.

C. Safety and infection control: Prevent further injury and infection.
D. Health promotion and maintenance: Provide parental teaching regarding care for infant.
E. Psychologic integrity: Instruct parents on proper growth and development and behavioral expectations.
F. Basic care and comfort: Assess pain levels of neonates with birth injury and treat as necessary with nonpharmacologic interventions such as swaddling, positioning, and nonnutritive sucking. Use pharmacologic methods if necessary (e.g., Sweet-Ease, acetaminophen [Tylenol], or morphine).
G. Reduction of risk potential: Assess for potential risks (see analysis section).
H. Pharmacologic and parenteral therapies: Client will state the purpose for and associated side effects of all medications.
1. Acetaminophen (Tylenol)—maintenance dose 12 mg/kg PO; used for treatment of mild-to-moderate pain. Monitor for liver toxicity, rashes, fever, thrombocytopenia, leukopenia, and neutropenia.
2. Morphine—dose 0.05 to 0.2 mg/kg IV over 5 min; usually repeated every 3 to 4 hr; used for analgesia, sedation, and treatment of opioid withdrawal. Monitor for decreased respiratory effort and decreased bowel function. Assess bladder for urinary retention if output is decreased.
3. Lorazepam—dose 0.05 to 0.1 mg/kg IV slow push; used as an anticonvulsant. Monitor for respiratory depression and CNS depression.
4. Phenobarbital—maintenance dose 3 to 4 mg/kg per day; used as an anticonvulsant. May be given PO or IV; if IV, monitor for extravasation and phlebitis and respiratory depression.

Hypoglycemia

I. Definition: Hypoglycemia in a neonate is defined as a blood sugar of less than 40 to 50 mg/dl (normal blood sugar is 50 to 110 mg/dl).

II. Nursing process

A. Assessment
1. Risk for hypoglycemia—includes infants of diabetic mothers; infants who are preterm, SGA, LGA, postterm, septic, or stressed; and neonates with shock, respiratory distress, or cardiac disease.
2. Signs and symptoms
   a. Presence of jitteriness, twitching, tremors, irritability, high-pitched or weak cry (untreated hypoglycemia can lead to hypoglycemic seizures)
   b. Increased respiratory rate, increased work of breathing, apnea, cyanosis
   c. Temperature instability
   d. Lethargy
   e. Inadequate suck-swallow coordination; poor feeding
   f. Shrill cry

B. Analysis
1. Imbalanced Nutrition: Less Than Body Requirements related to increased glucose use secondary to physiologic stress
2. Ineffective Breathing Pattern related to tachypnea and apnea
3. Acute Pain related to frequent heel sticks for glucose monitoring

C. Planning
1. Provide frequent glucose assessment.
2. Provide feedings or IV glucose to maintain levels greater than 50 mg per day.
3. Protect CNS from effects of low glucose levels.

D. Implementation
1. Evaluate for lethargy, poor muscle tone, jitteriness, tremors, and irritability.
2. Monitor glucose at or before 1 hr of age; if hypoglycemic, monitor every 4 hr for 24 hr and frequently until stable.
3. Feed early (before 1 hr of age) to prevent decreases in blood sugars; normal calorie intake to gain weight 15 to 30 g (0.5 to 1 oz) per day is 90 to 120 cal/kg per day.
4. Assess need for IV glucose of D10W at 4 to 6 mg/kg per minute; start at 80 ml/kg per day.
5. Maintain neutral thermal zone to avoid cold stress.
6. Evaluate for lethargy and poor muscle tone.

E. Evaluation
   1. Infant's CNS remains protected with adequate glucose.
   2. Infant has adequate nutrition and maintains glucose greater than 50 mg/dl.
   3. Infant exhibits respiratory, cardiac, temperature, and neurologic stability.

CN

III. Client needs
A. Physiologic adaptation
   1. Glucose of 20 to 25 mg/dl is treated with parenteral glucose, regardless of gestational age.
   2. Glucose levels for the full-term neonate is lowest 30 to 90 min after birth.
   3. Glucose production in a term neonate is approximately 4 to 6 mg/kg per minute.
   4. Pathophysiology of hypoglycemia differs for each neonatal classification: increased utilization of glucose; hyperinsulinism or decreased production/stores; there may be a combination of the two.
B. Management of care: Care of the neonate requires critical thinking skills and knowledge of assessment, and teaching and evaluation methods unique to the RN role. The following skills cannot be delegated to an LPN or UAP.
   1. Monitor glucose levels every 30 min to 1 hr until greater than 50 mg/dl on two consecutive tests, then every 3 to 4 hr until stable.
   2. Provide adequate glucose by oral intake or IV glucose.
C. Safety and infection control: Use correct measures to perform heel stick.
   1. Select site that has not been previously punctured to decrease the risk of infection.
   2. Choose lateral heel to decrease risk of damage to posterior tibial nerve and artery and plantar artery.
   3. Use only an approved microlancet to minimize injury.
   4. Clean site before puncture as directed by hospital policy.
   5. Apply pressure to puncture site after sample obtained.
D. Health promotion and maintenance: Maintain neutral thermal regulation to minimize metabolic demands.
E. Psychologic integrity: Provide parental teaching regarding importance of adequate and timely feedings to maintain blood sugars.
F. Basic care and comfort
   1. Warm heel before heel stick puncture.
   2. Provide nonpharmacologic pain management such as swaddling and nonnutritive sucking.
   3. Consider Sweet-Ease for pain management.
   4. Assess pain level after heel stick procedure.
G. Reduction of risk potential: Assess for potential risks (see analysis section).
H. Pharmacologic and parenteral therapies
   1. Maintain fluid balance.
   2. Maintain glucose balance.

Infant of Diabetic Mother

I. Definition: An infant of a diabetic mother (IDM) is a neonate born to a mother who has an abnormal utilization or production of insulin.

II. Nursing process
A. Assessment
   1. Physical appearance: Macrosomia, ruddy in color, and generous supply of adipose tissue; large size related to exposure of high levels of maternal glucose and the neonate's responses with increased insulin production; insulin has a growth hormone effect on the neonate
   2. Appropriate gestational age assessment: Large neonates may give the impression they are physically and neurologically more mature. Base plan of care on accurate gestational age assessment; this is an indicator of neonatal behavior and functioning
   3. Glucose monitoring: Neonate continues to produce insulin at an increased rate, which depletes glucose stores within a few hours of birth
   4. Hypoglycemia symptoms: Include jitteriness, tremors (which also may be a sign of hypocalcemia), cyanosis, apnea, temperature instability, poor feeding, hypotonia, and seizures
   5. Ability to take feedings: Glucose is available for CNS function; high insulin levels keep glucose levels low
   6. Respiratory status: May have respiratory distress related to inadequate surfactant production and decreased amounts of lecithin production
   7. Polycythemia: Results from increased fetal oxygen consumption, leading to fetal hypoxia; the tissue hypoxia stimulates erythropoietin production, which increases hematocrit
   8. Hyperbilirubinemia: Increased risk from polycythemia
   9. Congenital heart defects: IDMs have increased risk for transposition of the great vessels, ventricular septal defect, and ventricular wall hypertrophy

10. Presence of congenital anomalies, especially if neonate is SGA
11. For LGA birth injuries (see Neonate Large for Gestational Age)

B. Analysis
   1. Imbalanced Nutrition: Less Than Body Requirements related to increased glucose metabolism secondary to increased insulin production
   2. Impaired Gas Exchange related to inadequate surfactant production
   3. Risk for injury and Impaired Calcium Homeostasis related to inappropriate parathyroid response
   4. Risk for injury from Birth Trauma related to macrosomia
   5. Risk for Imbalanced Fluid Volume and hyperbilirubinemia related to polycythemia
   6. Increased Incidence of Congenital Heart Disease related to poor maternal glucose control
   7. Alteration in Hematologic Status: Polycythemia, related to fetal hypoxia

C. Planning
   1. Provide nutrients to maintain stable glucose.
   2. Provide respiratory support as necessary.
   3. Provide measures to decrease bilirubin levels.

D. Implementation
   1. Monitor glucose levels at 30 min to 1 hr of life, hourly during the first 4 hr of life, then every 4 hr for the first 24 hr of life or until stable.
   2. Initiate early feedings (breast or bottle) for glucoses less than 50 mg/dl.
   3. If glucose levels can not be maintained or neonate is too ill for enteral feeding, start IV glucose of D10W at a rate of 4 to 6 mg/kg per minute; once glucose is stable for 24 hr, the infusion is decreased and enteral feedings are increased.
   4. Monitor hematocrit for polycythemia.
   5. Monitor bilirubin level for hyperbilirubinemia.
   6. Monitor for respiratory distress and congenital heart defects.

E. Evaluation
   1. Infant has a glucose level greater than 50 mg/dl.
   2. Infant's calcium levels remain 8 to 10 mg/dl.
   3. Infant takes nutrition to maintain glucose level.
   4. Infant exhibits stable respiratory and cardiac status.
   5. Infant's bilirubin level remains within normal limits.

CN

III. Client needs

A. Physiologic adaptation
   1. Organomegaly—related to hyperinsulinism
   2. Respiratory distress syndrome (hyaline membrane disease)—related to decreased surfactant production
   3. Congenital heart disease—unknown etiology
   4. Hypocalcemia—related to prematurity and hypoparathyroidism

B. Management of care: Care of the IDM requires critical thinking skills and knowledge of assessment, and teaching and evaluation methods unique to the RN role. The following skills cannot be delegated to an LPN or UAP.
   1. Monitor glucose levels to detect low glucose levels.
   2. Monitor glucose closely until stable.
   3. Initiate early feeding.
   4. Support respiratory distress, if present.
   5. Provide thermoregulation.

C. Safety and infection control (see management of care)

D. Health promotion and maintenance: Assess for gestational age and support at appropriate age; IDM may be LGA and not as developmentally mature as size may indicate.

E. Psychologic integrity: Instruct parents on the need for heel sticks and rationale for treatment.

F. Basic care and comfort: See hypoglycemia

G. Reduction of risk potential: Provide careful assessments for the following risk factors for which the IDM is at increased risk:
   1. Hypoglycemia
   2. Hyperbilirubinemia
   3. Birth trauma
   4. Polycythemia
   5. Respiratory distress syndrome
   6. Congenital birth defects

H. Pharmacologic and parenteral therapies: Administer oxygen, fluids, and electrolytes as ordered.

Hyperbilirubinemia

I. Definition: Hyperbilirubinemia is commonly known as jaundice, which is a deposit of bilirubin in lipid tissue; a serum level of bilirubin of 4 to 6 mg/dl exhibits jaundice.

A. Types
   1. Physiologic hyperbilirubinemia—increased levels are not seen in the first 24 hr of life; peak levels appear approximately 3 to 5 days of life in term neonates, 5 to 7 days in the preterm neonate; caused by increased fetal RBC destruction and impaired conjugation of bilirubin, increased bilirubin reabsorption from the intestinal tract; this is a normal physiologic response in the newborn because of:
      a. Increased RBC mass
      b. Shorter red cell life span

c. Slower uptake by liver
d. Lack of intestinal bacteria
e. Poor feeding and/or hydration

2. Pathologic hyperbilirubinemia—consider if the following are true:
   a. Jaundice is evident in the first 24 hr of life
   b. Greater than 5 mg/dl rise in serum bilirubin concentrations per day
   c. Levels greater than 15 mg/dl of total serum bilirubin in term neonates
   d. Conjugated bilirubin level grater than 2 mg/dl or more than 20% of total serum bilirubin concentrations

II. Nursing process

A. Assessment: 50% of term neonates and 80% of preterm neonates exhibit physiologic jaundice on the second to third day of life.
   1. Assess physical appearance: Press skin over bony area such as the forehead, nose, chin, or sternum; if icterus occurs, jaundice is pronounced.
   2. Assess for risk factors that cause increased RBC destruction such as ABO incompatibility, Rh incompatibility, or tissue injury such as bruising from birth trauma or heel sticks.

B. Analysis
   1. Risk for Altered Acid/Base Balance related to cold stress
   2. Imbalanced Nutrition: Less Than Body Requirements related to decreased caloric and volume intake
   3. Risk for Injury related to use of phototherapy

C. Planning
   1. Support thermoregulation.
   2. Provide early and frequent feeding.
   3. Prevent injury related to use of phototherapy.

D. Implementation
   1. Maintain temperature in neutral thermal zone—cold stress results in acidosis; acidosis reduces available serum albumin binding sites.
   2. Encourage early breast-feeding—colostrum has a laxative effect and increases the number of stools and excretion of bilirubin.
   3. Monitor number of voids and number of stools to ensure adequate hydration to encourage excretion of bilirubin.
   4. Encourage feedings to maintain adequate hydration.
   5. Monitor neonate with phototherapy for cold stress or overheating.
   6. Maintain placement of eye patches to provide protection for phototherapy lights.
   7. Keep genitals covered while phototherapy is in use.

E. Evaluation
   1. Infant has normal bilirubin level appropriate for age.
   2. Infant is free from injury related to increased bilirubin levels.
   3. Infant is well nourished and hydrated.

CN

III. Client needs

A. Physiologic adaptation
   1. Neonatal liver is immature and has difficulty keeping up with the normal RBC death and release of bilirubin that occurs after birth.
   2. Fetal or neonatal asphyxia decreases the binding affinity of bilirubin to albumin.
   3. Hypothermia and hypoglycemia release free fatty acids that dislocate bilirubin from albumin.
   4. Indomethacin decreases albumin binding.
   5. Maternal sulfa and salicylates compete with bilirubin for these sites while neonate is still in utero.
   6. Premature neonates have less albumin available for binding with bilirubin.

B. Management of care: If bilirubin level reaches above 20 mg/dl in term neonates, an exchange transfusion may be necessary; in ill or premature neonates, the exchange level may be lower based on gestational age.

C. Safety and infection control: If client is receiving phototherapy care, monitor for:
   1. Thermoregulation
   2. Placement of eye patches to cover eyes to prevent damage
   3. Genitals covered while phototherapy is in place

D. Health promotion and maintenance: Phototherapy enhances the uptake of bilirubin; can use a single, double, or triple light source; types include:
   1. Bank of bili lights
   2. Bili blankets
   3. Bili spots

E. Psychologic integrity: Encourage parents to participate in care, feeding, holding, and diapering.

F. Basic care and comfort: Provide early and frequent feeding to:
   1. Encourage gastric empting and increase in peristalsis, thus reducing hyperbilirubinemia risk.
   2. Encourage stooling and thus the excretion of bound bilirubin.
   3. Help ensure adequate hydration.

G. Reduction of risk potential
   1. Place eye patches and provide genital protection during phototherapy.
   2. Provide thermoregulation.

H. Pharmacologic and parenteral therapies: Administer as ordered.

Respiratory Distress

I. Definition: Respiratory distress occurs in the neonate when respiratory adaptation to extrauterine life fails or is incomplete.

A. Can occur with aspiration at delivery, decreased surfactant, retained lung fluid, or with infection as in pneumonia

B. Manifestations of respiratory distress in a neonate include:
   1. Respiratory distress syndrome
   2. Transient tachypnea of the neonate
   3. Meconium aspiration syndrome
   4. Pneumonia
   5. Persistent pulmonary hypertension of the neonate
   6. Pneumothorax
   7. Bronchopulmonary dysplasia/chronic lung disease
   8. Cardiac causes for respiratory distress

II. Nursing process

A. Assessment
   1. Respiratory distress (note: as gestational age decreases, respiratory distress syndrome increases because of limited surfactant production)—assess neonate for respiratory rate, rhythm, work of breathing, and breath sounds; nasal flaring; grunting; retractions (use of accessory muscles—intercostal, subcostal, substernal, and suprasternal—as neonates attempt to increase lung compliance); apnea—no breathing for greater than 20 s
   2. Color: May be pale/pallor; mottled, cyanotic (cyanosis-circumoral and/or central versus acrocyanosis), or jaundiced
   3. Chest:
      a. Movement (symmetrical)
      b. Size and shape
      c. Heart rate (presence/absence of murmur)
      d. Point of maximal impulse (may shift with air leaks)
      e. Breath sounds (may be decreased or absent, may hear rales, rhonchi, or crackles)
   4. Additional assessments include vital signs, PO_2; complete physical assessment; and assessment of fluid status—retained fluid can increase respiratory distress.
   5. Obtain diagnostic tests: CBC with differential and platelets, blood cultures, metabolic panel

B. Analysis
   1. Impaired Gas Exchange related to inadequate surfactant production; aspiration of meconium; amniotic fluid or pneumonia
   2. Imbalanced Nutrition: Less Than Body Requirements related to increased metabolic need and decreased ability to take oral nutrition efficiently
   3. Risk for Ineffective Thermoregulation related to increased metabolic demands

C. Planning
   1. Support respiratory effort.
   2. Provide nutrition for brain and tissue growth.
   3. Support temperature to allow use of calories for growth and tissue repair.

D. Implementation
   1. Assess respiratory rate and rhythm by auscultation (normal rate is 30 to 60 breaths per minute).
   2. Assess quality, quantity, and location of breath sounds.
   3. Assess respiratory effort—nonlabored easy respirations; lack of retractions (intercostal, subcostal, substernal, suprasternal).
   4. Assess skin color and mucous membranes.
   5. Assess capillary refill.
   6. Provide adequate oxygenation and ventilation.
   7. Provide adequate nutritional support.
   8. Maintain fluid and electrolyte balance.
   9. Provide for thermoregulation.

E. Evaluation
   1. Infant's respirations are nonlabored.
   2. Infant's resting respiratory rate is 30 to 60 breaths per minute.
   3. Infant has clear and equal breath sounds in all lobes.
   4. Infant is free from respiratory and metabolic acidosis or alkalosis.
   5. Parent's verbalize rationale for treatment of their infant.
   6. Infant has adequate nutrition to support normal brain and tissue growth.
   7. Infant has temperature stability.

CN

III. Client needs

A. Physiologic adaptation
   1. Alveolar instability leads to atelectasis.
   2. Atelectasis leads to hypoxia, which then can lead to acidosis.
   3. Acidosis and decreased gas exchange limits surfactant production and can cause pulmonary vasoconstriction.

4. Alveolar instability then leads to decreased PO_2 (hypoxemia), increased PCO_2 (hypercarbia), and decreased pH (acidemia).
5. This series of events can lead to respiratory failure.
6. Prevention of prematurity with appropriate prenatal care is ideal.
7. Antenatal steroids (glucocorticoids) enhance fetal lung development.

B. Management of care: Care of the neonate experiencing respiratory distress requires critical thinking skills and knowledge of assessment, and teaching and evaluation methods unique to the RN role. The following skills cannot be delegated to an LPN or UAP.
1. Obtain chest x-rays to help with diagnosis.
2. Evaluate blood gases.
3. Maintain adequate PO_2 by providing oxygen support and preventing hypoxia.
4. Maintain a normal pH by providing for adequate ventilation and a normal PCO_2.
5. Prevent metabolic acidosis by providing aerobic metabolism.
6. Provide oxygen support to level of neonatal needs using mask, nasal cannula, neonatal head hood, CPAP, ventilator support (conventional or high frequency), or extracorporeal membrane oxygenation.
7. Initiate surfactant replacement therapy.
8. Obtain and review diagnostic tests (see assessment section).
9. Assess for home health care needs and discharge follow-up.

C. Safety and infection control
1. Monitor oxygen saturation in blood via pulse oximetry.
2. Monitor carbon dioxide.
3. Protect from infection (meticulous hand hygiene).
4. Remove central lines as soon as medically possible.
5. Place neonate on a cardiac/apnea monitor for continuous assessment.
6. Assess venous access devices hourly for patency and accuracy of infusion.

D. Health promotion and maintenance: Provide thermoregulation to prevent cold stress or overheating.

E. Psychologic integrity
1. Provide parental teaching related to infants condition, handling restrictions, monitoring devices, and equipment.
2. Allow for parent caregiving as soon as possible; assistance with feeding, diapering, and daily hygiene.

F. Basic care and comfort
1. Provide for adequate nutrition for growth and tissue repair.
2. Humidify and heat oxygen source.
3. Maintain proper positioning.
4. Maintain skin integrity by keeping linens clean and dry; rotate monitoring devices such as pulse oximeter on each shift.
5. Use analgesics and sedatives to prevent neonate from working against the ventilator support and, therefore, decreasing the risk of lung injury.
6. Position neonate to decrease work of breathing.

G. Reduction of risk potential
1. Maintain oxygen source with blender and analyzer at bedside.
2. Maintain suction at bedside.

H. Pharmacologic and parenteral therapies: Client family will state the purpose for and associated side effects of all medications used for respiratory distress.
1. Surfactants—lipoprotein that coats the interior surface of the alveolar membrane
   a. Produced by type II alveolar cells beginning about 22 to 24 weeks' gestation
   b. Can be given artificially; commercially made; administered via the endotracheal tube
   c. Decreases alveolar surface tension
   d. Allows for increased lung compliance, decreases work of breathing
   e. Allows for increased gas exchange
2. Fentanyl (Sublimaze)—dose 1 to 4 mcg/kg per dose; used for sedation and analgesia; monitor for respiratory rate, abdominal distention, loss of bowel sounds, and muscle rigidity
3. Midazolam (Versed)—dose 0.05 to 0.15 mg/kg over at least 5 min, usually repeated every 2 to 4 hr; used as a sedative; monitor for respiratory depression and decrease in BP; monitor hepatic function
4. Lorazepam (Ativan)—dose 0.05 to 0.1 mg/kg IV slow push; used as an anticonvulsant; monitor for respiratory depression and CNS depression

Infection and Sepsis

I. Definition: Infection and sepsis occur in neonates because the neonate has an immature physical response necessary to fight infectious pathogens. The greater the prematurity, the greater the risk is for infection. Infection and sepsis affect

1 to 5 per 1,000 live births. Pathogens can be acquired prenatally, during labor and delivery, or postnatally.

II. Nursing process
  A. Assessment
    1. Perform a comprehensive physical assessment; assess for signs and symptoms.
      a. Poor hypothalamic response—fever is a poor indicator of infection; presentation is often hypothermia as the neonate is unable to maintain temperature in a neutral thermal environment.
      b. Lethargic or irritable
      c. Decreased interest in feeding
      d. Temperature instability
      e. Increased respiratory rate and effort
      f. Hyperbilirubinemia
      g. Color change (pale, mottled, cyanotic)
    2. Obtain diagnostic tests.
      a. Blood cultures before the start of antibiotics, if possible
      b. Septic workup includes: CBC with differential, platelets, blood cultures, lumbar puncture, urine culture, and other cultures as necessary
      c. X-ray to aid in diagnosis
  B. Analysis
    1. Risk for Infection related to immature immunologic system
    2. Imbalanced Nutrition: Less Than Body Requirements related to decreased interest or ability to eat
    3. Ineffective Breathing Pattern related to pathogens and fluid in lungs
    4. Ineffective Coping related to neonatal illness and prolonged hospital stay
  C. Planning
    1. Provide for thermoregulation.
    2. Support increased respiratory effort.
    3. Prevent infection.
    4. Provide adequate nutrition for growth and development.
  D. Implementation
    1. Obtain diagnostic tests (see assessment).
    2. Monitor vital signs, especially BP, watching for decreased cardiac output.
    3. Administer antibiotic therapy—important to start promptly after obtaining blood cultures; administer within 1 hr of suspected sepsis diagnosis.
    4. Provide respiratory support as necessary.
    5. Provide IV glucose and nutritional support.
  E. Evaluation
    1. Infant is free from infection.
    2. Infant has adequate respiratory and nutritional support.
    3. Infant experiences no lasting effects from infection.
    4. Parents verbalize plan of care.

CN

III. Client needs
  A Physiologic adaptation: Immunologic system is immature in the neonate. Premature neonates are at greater risk for infection. Invasive procedures, umbilical catheters, intubation, ventilatory support, and parenteral support increase risk.
    1. Glucose—use of and needs increase
    2. Shock—support BP from decreased cardiac output
    3. Oxygen—requirements increase from greater demand to provide oxygen to brain and tissues.
  B. Management of care: Care of the neonate with infection or sepsis requires critical thinking skills and knowledge of assessment, and teaching and evaluation methods unique to the RN role. The following skills cannot be delegated to an LPN or UAP.
    1. Obtain cultures—blood, sputum, nares, rectal, skin to determine source of infection.
    2. Provide respiratory management.
    3. Provide system support—multisystem organ failure.
    4. Provide follow-up care—increased risk of cerebral palsy in neonate who has had septicemia.
  C. Safety and infection control
    1. Practice strict hand hygiene.
    2. Separate equipment for each neonate.
    3. Use standard precautions; keep each infant isolated.
    4. Use strict aseptic practices with IV tubing changes, and changes in IV fluids every 24 to 48 hr according to hospital policy.
    5. Remove IV lines, central lines, and assistive devices as soon as possible.
  D. Health promotion and maintenance
    1. Support temperature—use warm, humidified oxygen, use double-wall incubator or heat shield, avoid placing neonate in contact with cold surfaces, keep skin dry, use radiant warmers and incubators with servo control, keep crib warmer and incubators away from drafts and direct sources of sunlight.
    2. Assess for increased bilirubin and cell destruction.
  E. Psychologic integrity: Discuss with parents the need to limit handling of a critically ill neonate due to increased oxygen consumption and requirements.
  F. Basic care and comfort
    1. Give glucose to provide CNS protection. Glucose is used at a high rate and glucose

stores are depleted quickly; may need to administer glucose intravenously as the neonate may not have energy for oral feeding. Observe infant for increased respiratory rate; increased risk of aspiration when feeding.

2. Document accurate intake and output.
3. Position and limit handling for increased comfort.

G. Reduction of risk potential
1. Perform good hand hygiene or use hand-cleansing foams before and after providing neonatal care; no rings, watches, fake nails, or nail polish.
2. Follow isolation practices.

H. Pharmacologic and parenteral therapies: Client family will state the purpose of and associate side effects for all medications used to treat infection or sepsis.
1. Ampicillin—dose 100 to 150 mg/kg per dose usually every 12 hr; broad-spectrum antibiotic, stable only 1 hr after mixing into solution
2. Gentamicin—4 mg/kg per dose; varies on gestational age; usually between once every 24 and 48 hr; treatment of aerobic gram-negative bacilli, levels are monitored because of renal effects and ototoxicity.

HIV and AIDS

I. Definition: HIV/AIDS may be transmitted across the placenta, during labor and delivery through contaminated blood or through breast milk; vertical transmission can be decreased if the mother takes zidovudine during the pregnancy.

II. Nursing process

A. Assessment
1. Perform comprehensive physical assessment; assess for signs and symptoms.
   a. Large spleen
   b. Enlarged liver
   c. Swollen glands
   d. Respiratory infections
   e. Rhinorrhea
   f. Interstitial pneumonia
   g. Diarrhea and poor weight gain
   h. Candidiasis infections
   i. Missed developmental milestones
2. Obtain diagnostic tests.
   a. HIV DNA polymerase chain reaction—preferred test; drawn within the first 48 hr of life, repeated at 1 to 2 months of life, and again at 4 to 6 months.
   b. ELISA and Western blot—unable to tell the difference between maternal and fetal antibodies; not appropriate for neonates less than 15 months of age.

B. Analysis
1. Imbalanced Nutrition: Less Than Body Requirements related to inadequate calorie intake
2. Risk for Impaired Skin Integrity related to frequent stooling secondary to diarrhea
3. Risk for Impaired Growth and Development related to decreased parental interaction and stimulation
4. Risk for Infection related to pathogens secondary to suppressed immunoregulation

C. Planning
1. Provide adequate nutrition for brain and tissue growth.
2. Prevent opportunistic infection.
3. Encourage growth and development, and attachment.

D. Implementation (see management of care)

E. Evaluation
1. Infant is free from opportunistic infection.
2. Infant has adequate nutrition for growth and meeting developmental milestones.
3. Parents are prepared to provide care to the best of their abilities and expectations of client outcome are realistic.

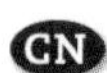

III. Client needs

A. Physiologic adaptation
1. Increased risk for gram-negative sepsis
2. May suffer from severe immunodeficiency

B. Management of care: Care of the neonate of an HIV-positive mother requires critical thinking skills and knowledge of assessment, and teaching and evaluation methods unique to the RN role. The following measures are used by the RN and all health care personnel:
1. Use standard precautions for protection from blood-borne infections.
2. Use gloves for all invasive procedures, diaper changes, and feedings.
3. Provide frequent diaper changes to prevent skin breakdown.
4. Use meticulous hand hygiene.
5. Remove all maternal blood before performing vein punctures or heel sticks.
6. Include parents in neonatal care such as feeding and bathing.

C. Safety and infection control
1. Wash laundry in hot sudsy water with household bleach.
2. Separate food preparation and serving from diaper-changing area.
3. Clean diaper changing area with 1:10 bleach solution after each diaper change.

4. Prevent sharing of toys with other children; inspect toys for sharp edges to prevent cuts and scrapes.
5. Avoid live polio vaccine; continue all other immunizations on normal schedule.
6. Determine neonate's HIV status before permitting circumcision.

D. Health promotion and maintenance: Play music or recordings of parents' voices to increase auditory stimuli.

E. Psychologic integrity
1. Encourage rooming-in with mother to promote interaction and attachment.
2. Provide parents with social support system through public health nursing or social service.
3. Provide support for the financial impact of HIV.

F. Basic care and comfort
1. Encourage holding neonate while feeding.
2. Increase neonate stimulation through frequent gentle touching and handling.
3. Administer small frequent feedings with possible supplementation to increase calories.
4. Provide parental teaching regarding feeding intolerance, vomiting, abdominal distention, and frequent instances of watery stools.
5. Avoid placing neonate in bed with bottles because of potential bacterial grow.
6. Instruct the HIV-positive mother that breast-feeding is contraindicated because of the possible transmission of the virus through breast milk.

G. Reduction of risk potential
1. Teach caregivers the importance of meticulous hand hygiene.
2. Stress importance of medication compliance.

H. Pharmacologic and parenteral therapies: Neonates of HIV-positive mothers are given antiretroviral drugs (zidovudine is most commonly used); this starts at 8 to 12 hr of life and continues for 6 months. The nurse also promotes adequate health care for the mother (see Chapter 29).

Drug-Exposed Neonate

I. Definition: Because many drugs freely cross the placenta, a neonate is at risk of becoming exposed to those drugs while in utero. Maternal use of tobacco products, cocaine, methamphetamines, marijuana, heroin, methadone, phencyclidine, and inhalants result in a drug-exposed neonate. Drugs can be teratogenic and result in congenital anomalies. The neonate is at risk for IUGR and SGA related to intrauterine asphyxia, infections (especially sexually transmitted diseases, HIV, and hepatitis), respiratory distress, and behavioral abnormalities.

II. Nursing process

A. Assessment
1. Obtain a detailed maternal health history, including history of drugs used and last drug usage.
2. Perform comprehensive physical assessments of neonate—may have poor state organization, may overreact to auditory and visual stimuli, and may experience feeding intolerance and GI disturbances in addition to congenital malformations. Assess for the following signs and symptoms:
   a. Level of irritability
   b. Hyperactivity
   c. Hypertonicity
   d. Presence of respiratory distress
   e. Vomiting and diarrhea
   f. Sneezing
   g. High-pitched cry
   h. Poor feeding
   i. Excessive sucking

B. Analysis
1. Impaired Parenting related to ineffective coping skills of mother secondary to drug abuse
2. Imbalanced Nutrition related to irritable GI system with vomiting and diarrhea, and poor suck-swallow coordination
3. Disturbed Sleep Pattern related to CNS irritability secondary to drug withdrawal

C. Planning
1. Aid neonate through the withdrawal process.
2. Provide nutritional and respiratory support.
3. Provide consoling and developmental support during withdrawal.
4. Provide pharmacologic support as needed.

D. Implementation
1. Provide for adequate nutrition and hydration; IV therapy may be necessary.
2. Provide for respiratory support if necessary.
3. Monitor intake and output.
4. Provide swaddling and quiet, dim environment.

E. Evaluation
1. Infant demonstrates adequate growth and development.
2. Infant exhibits respiratory and CNS stability.

3. Parents demonstrate ability to provide comfort and care.
4. Parents demonstrate appropriate coping skills.

CN

III. Client needs
A. Physiologic adaptation
1. Monitor vital signs for stability.
2. Assess for apnea.

B. Management of care: Care of the drug-exposed neonate requires critical thinking skills and knowledge of assessment, and teaching and evaluation methods unique to the RN role. The following skills cannot be delegated to an LPN or UAP.
1. Assess maternal drug habits carefully before administration of a narcotic antagonist (naloxone [Narcan]) to neonate—the use of this drug is contraindicated for respiratory distress in the neonate whose mother uses narcotics because of acute withdrawal.
2. Promote follow-up with public health nurse and social services in discharge planning. Symptoms of withdrawal may appear 24 to 48 hr after birth, but may not be seen until after discharge (up to 2 weeks of life). Assess the need for social services to follow-up at home setting to observe for possible neglect and abuse if mother is still using drugs. Foster placement for the neonate may be a necessary action.

C. Safety and infection control: Provide safe environment in case of seizure activity—raise side rails on crib or warmer; close port holes in incubator; keep suction and oxygen with Ambu bag at bedside.

D. Health promotion and maintenance: Provide parental teaching about caring for infant—education on infant care and normal newborn behavior is critical to prevent abuse and failure to thrive (see psychologic integrity and basic care and comfort).

E. Psychologic integrity
1. Refer family and mother to drug-treatment program.
2. Provide parental teaching on coping strategies to deal with irritable neonate, including decreasing stimulation, gentle rocking, swaddling, and nonnutritive sucking.
3. Instruct parents to expect jitteriness, irritability, and possible disorganized sleep pattern.

F. Basic care and comfort
1. Place in low-traffic, dimly lighted, quiet area of nursery.
2. Console neonate with gentle rocking.
3. Swaddle to reduce increased motor activity; leave hands where nonnutritive sucking can occur.
4. Offer pacifier for nonnutritive sucking.
5. Change diaper frequently to prevent skin excoriation from frequent stooling.
6. Offer small, frequent feedings.
7. Anticipate possible disorganized or poor ability to suck, swallow, and breathe in a coordinated manner, and instruct caregivers to be patient as the newborn becomes more coordinated.

G. Reduction of risk potential
1. Assess maternal history for STDs, HIV, and hepatitis, which are more common in women with substance addiction.
2. Teach family about SIDS and proper sleep positions—neonates with drug exposure have a high rate of death from SIDS; home monitor may be necessary.

H. Pharmacologic and parenteral therapies: Client family will state the purpose for and associated side effects of all medications.
1. Morphine—dose 0.05 to 0.2 mg/kg IV over 5 min, usually repeated every 4 hr; used for analgesia, sedation, and treatment of opioid withdrawal. Monitor for decreased respiratory effort, decreased bowel function. Assess bladder for urinary retention if output is decreased.
2. Methadone—dose 0.125 to 0.5 mg/kg every 8 to 12 hr; wean as tolerated.

Fetal Alcohol Spectrum Disorder

I. Definition: Fetal alcohol spectrum disorder is a condition caused by maternal alcohol use during pregnancy and resulting in permanent physical and mental disabilities in the neonate. Fetal alcohol spectrum disorder occurs in 5 in 1,000 live births.

II. Nursing process
A. Assessment
1. Obtain a detailed maternal health history, including history of alcohol use and history of use of nicotine, marijuana, and caffeine.
2. Assess neonate's physical appearance, including growth deficiencies (e.g., SGA) and facial features—the greater the facial abnormities, the lower the neonate's IQ. Assessment includes:
a. Microcephaly
b. Facial dysmorphology
c. Short palpebral fissures
d. Epicanthal folds
e. Broad nasal bridge

f. Flattened midfacies
g. Short, upturned or beaklike nose
h. Micrognathia
i. Hypoplastic maxilla
j. Thin upper lip and smooth philtrum

3. Assess for associated anomalies such as septal and valvular defects; eyes; kidneys; and skeletal system.
4. Assess social and family environment.
5. Assess neurologic coordination, especially related to feeding; suck may be weak; may be hypotonic and have increased placidity; may exhibit CNS irritability.
6. Assess intelligence, which may range from normal to severely mentally retarded.

B. Analysis
1. Imbalanced Nutrition: Less Than Body Requirements related to disorganized and delayed suck-swallow coordination
2. Delayed Growth and Development related to alteration in neurodevelopmental status related to CNS anomalies
3. Risk for Ineffective Coping related to substance-dependent mother and possible dysfunctional family

C. Planning
1. Provide nutritional support for brain and tissue growth.
2. Support developmental needs.
3. Promote CNS stability.

D. Implementation
1. Provide thermoregulation.
2. Assure adequate nutrition—might require extra time and patience for feeding.
3. Reduce environmental stimuli.
4. Provide a quiet environment and dim light.
5. Assess vital signs closely for CNS irritability and respiratory distress.

E. Evaluation
1. Infant has weight gain and feeding tolerance.
2. Infant has controlled irritability.
3. Parents provide adequate and safe care.
4. Infant demonstrates growth and developmental milestones.

CN

III. Client needs

A. Physiologic adaptation
1. Failure to thrive—caused by delayed oral feeding progression as result of weak suck; may have persistent vomiting until 6 to 7 months of life
2. Hypotonicity
3. Increased placidity
4. Decreased ability to habituate repetitive stimuli

B. Management of care: Care of the neonate with fetal alcohol spectrum disorder during the first week of life requires critical thinking skills and knowledge of assessment, and teaching and evaluation methods unique to the RN role. The following skills cannot be delegated to an LPN or UAP.
1. Plan care for sleeplessness, excessive crying, hyperactivity state, jitteriness, hyperactive rooting and increased nonnutritive sucking, increased agitation, and alertness with the inability to interact with the environment.
2. Refer parents to social service or public health nurse to help strengthen parenting and feeding skills.

C. Safety and infection control: Protect neonate from injury and infection.

D. Health promotion and maintenance: Provide parental and caregiver teaching regarding how to care for the newborn in relation to developmental needs (see psychologic integrity).

E. Psychologic integrity: Provide parental and caregiver teaching regarding the following topics:
1. Dependence—physiologic; signs and symptoms of withdrawal may begin within 6 to 12 hr of life
2. CNS dysfunction
3. Severe mental retardation in relation to normal intelligence
4. Possible difficulty with impulsivity and cognitive impairment (follow-up care necessary)
5. Possible speech and language abnormalities
6. Possible learning disabilities, ADHD and behavioral issues (may not be evident until child becomes of school age)

F. Basic care and comfort: Instruct caregivers how to feed neonate (neonate may have difficulty feeding because of decreased motor coordination).

G. Reduction of risk potential: Promote safety and provide adequate nutrition.

H. Pharmacologic and parenteral therapies: Administer medications and fluids as ordered. Client family will state purpose for and associated side effects of all medications used to manage fetal alcohol spectrum disorder.

Bibliography

Developmental Tasks for the Individual and Family. Retrieved May 6, 2008 from: http://faculty.ccri.edu/rarchambault/Developmental-TasksfortheIndividualandtheFamily.rtf

Duvall, E. M. (1977). *Marriage and family development.* Philadelphia: Lippincott.

Hogan, M. A., Glazebrook, R., Brancato, V., & Rodgers, J. (2007). *Maternal-newborn nursing reviews and rationales.* Philadelphia: Pearson Prentice Hall.

Klossner, N. J., & Hatfield, N. (2005). *Introduction to maternity and pediatric nursing.* Philadelphia: Lippincott Williams & Wilkins.

Pillitteri, A. (2006). *Maternal & child health nursing: Care of the childbearing and childrearing family* (5th ed.). Philadelphia: Lippincott Williams & Wilkins.

Ricci, S. S. (2007). *Essentials of maternity, newborn and women's health nursing*. Philadelphia: Lippincott, Williams & Wilkins.

Simpson, K. R., & Creehan, P. A. (2007). *AWHONN's perinatal nursing* (3rd ed.). Philadelphia: Lippincott Williams & Wilkins.

Witt, C. (2007). *Advances in neonatal care*. Philadelphia: Lippincott Williams & Wilkins.

CHAPTER 8

Practice Test

Healthy Neonate

1. After delivery of a neonate, the nurse's first action is to:
- □ 1. Administer vitamin K injection.
- □ 2. Encourage the mother to breast-feed.
- □ 3. Place the neonate in the warmer.
- □ 4. Establish an airway.

2. The nurse is assigning a 1-min Apgar score to a neonate. The neonate has a pink body and blue feet. The nurse should assign which score for color to this neonate?
- □ 1. 1.
- □ 2. 2.
- □ 3. 3.
- □ 4. 4.

3. The nurse is assessing a newborn. When auscultating the lungs, which of the following is a normal sound?
- □ 1. Vesicular.
- □ 2. Resonance.
- □ 3. Wheezes.
- □ 4. Crackles.

4. The nurse is performing an initial assessment on a neonate in the delivery room. When attempting to suction the infant's nares, the nurse is unable to pass the suction catheter through to the nasopharynx. The nurse should first:
- □ 1. Wait until the infant stops crying and attempt to suction again.
- □ 2. Suction using a bulb syringe.
- □ 3. Record the finding.
- □ 4. Notify the physician.

5. AF A newborn delivered by cesarean section has a birth weight of 7 lb 6 oz. The infant is weighed each night at midnight, during the mother's surgical recovery. The nurse is reviewing the progress notes as noted below.

PROGRESS NOTES

Date	Time	Weight
11/05/2009	0700	7 lb 6 oz
11/06/2009	0715	7 lb 0 oz
11/07/2009	0710	6 lb 14 oz
11/08/2009	0700	6 lb 12 oz
11/09/2009	0720	6 lb 14 oz

The weight loss of this infant is:
- □ 1. More than expected.
- □ 2. As expected.
- □ 3. Less than expected.
- □ 4. Indicative of the need to notify an HCP.

6. A woman is holding her newborn and exploring his body. She tells the nurse, "While I was stroking his head, I felt a swelling over the back of his head." The nurse explains that: "The swelling is:
- □ 1. the anterior fontanelle."
- □ 2. the posterior fontanelle."
- □ 3. scalp edema called a *caput succedaneum*."
- □ 4. bleeding between the scalp and the skull, called a *cephalhematoma*."

7. AF The benefits of breast-feeding for the infant include the lowered risk of which of the following? Select all that apply.
- □ 1. Allergies (asthma, eczema).
- □ 2. Childhood and adolescent obesity.
- □ 3. Ear infections.
- □ 4. Juvenile onset diabetes.
- □ 5. SIDS.

8. The nurse is applying erythromycin ointment to a neonate who was born 20 min ago. The expected outcome of the ointment is prevention of which of the following?
- □ 1. Hemorrhagic disease of the newborn.
- □ 2. Hepatis B.
- □ 3. Ophthalmia neonatorum.
- □ 4. Hyperbilirubinemia.

9. AF The nurse is teaching a mother about care for her new infant boy's uncircumcised genitals. The nurse should instruct the mother to do which of the following? Select all that apply.
- □ 1. Inspect the genital area for irritated skin.
- □ 2. Palpate if testes are descended into the scrotal sac.
- □ 3. Inspect if the urethral opening is at the end of the penis.
- □ 4. Retract the foreskin over the glans to assess for secretions.
- □ 5. Report phimosis to the HCP.

10. The nurse instructs parents to do which of the following to care for the umbilical cord?
- □ 1. Keep umbilical cord dry.
- □ 2. Wash umbilical cord with soap and water daily.
- □ 3. Apply petroleum jelly to umbilical cord daily.
- □ 4. Cover umbilical cord with dry gauze.

Neonates With Variations in Size: Postterm Neonate, Neonate Small for Gestational Age, and Neonate Large for Gestational Age

11. The nurse is plotting a neonate's weight on an intrauterine growth chart. The neonate's weight is above the ninetieth percentile for any given gestational age and assessed as:
- □ 1. Small for gestational age.
- □ 2. Average for gestational age.
- □ 3. Large for gestational age.
- □ 4. Postterm.

12. Parents of a neonate who is 32 week's of age ask the nurse, "Why does he have to have a feeding tube in his nose?" The best nursing response is:
- □ 1. The sucking, swallowing, and breathing are not coordinated.
- □ 2. There is no sucking reflex at this gestational age.
- □ 3. The stomach cannot digest formula or breast milk at this time.
- □ 4. The infant needs extra fluids to prevent dehydration.

13. A neonate who is 28 week's of age is experiencing apnea. The first nursing action is to perform which of the following measures?
- □ 1. Begin oxygen via mask.
- □ 2. Begin cardiopulmonary resuscitation.
- □ 3. Obtain blood gas.
- □ 4. Ensure a patent airway.

14. The primary goal of care for a preterm neonate who is 25 week's of age is to prevent:
- □ 1. Infection.
- □ 2. Weight loss.
- □ 3. Pain.
- □ 4. Hyperglycemia.

Neonates With Health Problems

15. AF The nurse is caring for a newborn whose mother has insulin-dependent diabetes mellitus. The chart indicates that during the prenatal period the woman had frequent episodes of hyperglycemia. The nurse should assess the newborn for which of the following? Select all that apply.
- □ 1. Macrosomia.
- □ 2. Birth injury.
- □ 3. Hyperglycemia.
- □ 4. Congenital defects.
- □ 5. Respiratory distress.
- □ 6. Postterm birth.
- □ 7. SGA infant.

16. The nurse is taking care of a neonate who is receiving phototherapy. The parents ask about the effects of phototherapy. Which statement by the parents after teaching indicates need for additional information?
- □ 1. "Our baby may have diarrhea because of the light therapy."
- □ 2. "Our baby needs frequent feeding to prevent dehydration during light therapy."
- □ 3. "Our baby may have darker skin from the light therapy."
- □ 4. "Our baby may have weight gain from retaining water."

17. AF The nurse is caring for a newborn who is experiencing opioid withdrawal. To calm the infant, the nurse should do which of the following? Select all that apply.
- □ 1. Swaddle the infant in a blanket.
- □ 2. Rock the infant in a slow, rhythmic manner.
- □ 3. Place the infant's crib in a darkened area of the nursery.
- □ 4. Avoid the use of pacifiers.
- □ 5. Plan care activities around infant cues.
- □ 6. Observe for distress signals (arching, gaze aversion).
- □ 7. Hold infant in sitting position with head flexed for feeding.

18. A neonate is admitted to the nursery. While reviewing the maternal history the nurse notes that the mother is diabetic. The nurse should plan which of the following as a priority when coordinating care for this neonate?

- □ 1. Phototherapy.
- □ 2. A RhoGAM workup.
- □ 3. Early protein feeding.
- □ 4. Care for dry, cracking skin.

19. A neonate who is 1 hr of age is found to be jittery, tachypneic, pale, and lethargic. The nurse should first:

- □ 1. Begin oxygen per mask.
- □ 2. Provide feeding.
- □ 3. Place under a radiant warmer.
- □ 4. Check glucose.

20. A neonate is having difficulty breathing. To establish a patent airway, the nurse should first:

- □ 1. Place neonate in Trendelenburg position.
- □ 2. Insert a nasal cannula in neonate's nose and start oxygen.
- □ 3. Position neonate on the back with the head slightly extended.
- □ 4. Pull neonate's tongue down and forward.

Answers and Rationales

1. 4 The nurse's first action is to establish an airway. If an airway is not established, gas exchange cannot take place. All other nursing actions may follow airway establishment. (S)

2. 1 The assignment of a score of 1 for color indicates a pink body with blue feet and hands. A cyanotic or pale body receives a score of 0 for color. A score of 2 is given if the neonate's body is pink, including hands and feet. (A)

3. 4 The newborn's lungs may still contain amniotic fluid and fine crackles are commonly heard over the lung fields. The infant's chest is small; bronchovesicular, rather than vesicular, sounds predominate. Resonance is a percussed, not an auscultated sound. Wheezes are secondary to narrow airway disease such as asthma. (A)

4. 4 The nurse notifies the physician as the inability to pass a catheter is a finding consistent with choanal atresia, which is a medical emergency. Suctioning the nares with a bulb syringe will be ineffective. If the neonate stops crying, the neonate will revert to obligate nasal breathing and may have a cardiac arrest. Recording the finding is not sufficient; the nurse informs the HCP. (M)

5. 2 Infants are expected to lose up to 10% of their birth weight. This infant lost 10 oz and he could lose 11.8 oz. (S)

6. 3 The caput succedaneum is scalp edema as a result of labor. The anterior fontanelle is not located at the back of the head. The posterior fontanelle is a triangular "soft spot" at the occiput; it is not easily palpated when a caput succedaneum is present because of the scalp edema. A cephalhematoma is bleeding between the infant's skull and the periosteum because of the pressures on the head during labor and birth. (M)

7. 1, 2, 3, 5 Benefits of breast-feeding to infant are lower risk of allergies, childhood and adolescent obesity, chronic inflammatory bowel disorders (Crohn disease and ulcerative colitis), infections (URI, ear, meningitis, and diarrhea), childhood cancers (Hodgkin lymphoma and leukemia), SIDS, orthodontia, and cavities. Breast-feeding does not lower the risk for juvenile-onset diabetes. (H)

8. 3 Erythromycin is used to prevent ophthalmia neonatorum. Vitamin K injections are used to prevent hemorrhagic disease of the newborn. Hepatis B vaccine is used to prevent the hepatis B virus. Hyperbilirubinemia is not affected by the use of erythromycin. (S)

9. 1, 2, 3 The nurse instructs the mother to inspect her boy's uncircumcised genitals for skin integrity, urethral opening, and testes descent. Phimosis is a normal finding. Retraction of foreskin over the glans may cause trauma and should not be attempted in the neonatal period. (C)

10. 1 Keeping the umbilical cord dry is the current recommendation for cord care. It will dry and slough off in 7 to 10 days. Washing the cord, applying petroleum jelly, and keeping it covered with gauze will only keep it moist and delay sloughing and increase the risk of infection. (S)

11. 3 LGA neonates are above the ninetieth percentile for any given gestational age. Neonates that are between the ninetieth and tenth percentile are average for gestational age. Those that are below the tenth percentile are SGA. Postterm neonates are those that are greater than 42 weeks' gestation. (H)

12. 1 At 32 weeks' gestation, a neonate has limited ability to coordinate sucking, swallowing, and breathing. The sucking reflex is present at 32 weeks' gestation, but the neonate cannot coordinate the reflex with swallowing and breathing. The stomach has the capacity for digestion at this gestational age. There are no indications that this neonate is dehydrated. (C)

13. 4 Apnea may be caused by an occluded airway. Oxygen and cardiopulmonary resuscitation are not effective if the airway is not patent. Establishing breathing is a priority before obtaining a blood gas. (A)

14. 1 Infection is a great risk of a very premature neonate. Preterm infants do not have the ability to produce the neutrophils to fight infection. Weight loss up to 15% is expected in a preterm neonate. Pain management and hyperglycemia are of nursing concern, but preventing infection is the primary goal. (A)

15. 1, 2, 4, 5 Infants of mothers with insulin-dependent diabetes mellitus who do not maintain glucose levels between 100 and 120 mg/dl are at risk for macrosomia, birth injury, hypoglycemia, congenital defects, and respiratory distress. (A)

16. 4 Babies often have increased weight loss from the birth weight. Weight gain may be delayed after light therapy is discontinued. Bilirubin is lost through the loose, green stools. The skin of the infant may become "bronzed" from the light therapy. Insensible water loss is increased during light therapy. (S)

17. 1, 2, 3, 5, 6, 7 Swaddling, vertical rocking, reducing environmental stimuli, using pacifiers, and planning care around infant cues helps drug-exposed infants to exhibit age-appropriate state modulation. The remaining interventions are effective in reducing the infant's withdrawal symptoms. (C)

18. 3 The nurse provides early protein feeding to prevent a drop in glucose due to hyperinsulinism in infants of diabetic mothers. Phototherapy is indicated if bilirubin levels are elevated. RhoGAM workups are indicated with Rh-negative mothers. Cracked and dry skin is seen most frequently in postterm neonates. (M)

19. 4 This neonate is exhibiting signs of hypoglycemia. The nurse first checks the blood sugar and then promotes breast- or bottle-feeding for the neonate. Feeding will increase the glucose level and diminish the symptoms. (C)

20. 3 The head in the sniffing position with the neck slightly extended is the proper position for opening a neonatal airway. Position is important for opening the soft airway of the neonate. It is not necessary to start oxygen at this time. (R)

SECTION 1

Practice Test

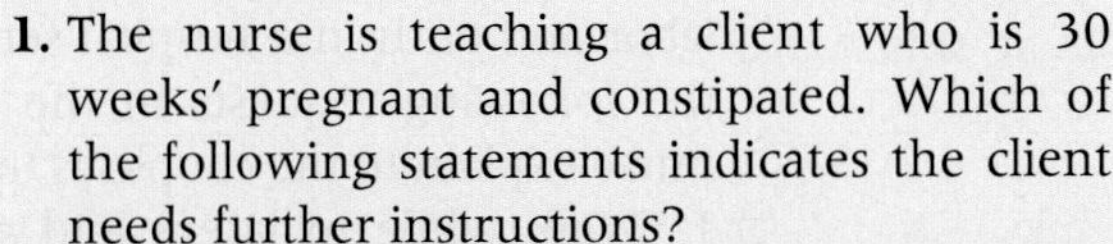

1. The nurse is teaching a client who is 30 weeks' pregnant and constipated. Which of the following statements indicates the client needs further instructions?

□ 1. "I should drink six to eight glasses of water a day."
□ 2. "I should increase my dietary fiber to 25 to 30 g a day."
□ 3. "I should engage in daily physical activity."
□ 4. "I should discontinue my iron if I continue to be constipated."

2. AF A pregnant client is A-negative. After which of the following procedures will the woman need a RhoGAM (Rh immune globulin) injection? Select all that apply.

□ 1. Abortion/miscarriage.
□ 2. Amniocentesis.
□ 3. Biophysical profile.
□ 4. Chorionic villi sampling.
□ 5. Delivery.
□ 6. Ectopic pregnancy.

3. Which of the following is a sign of infection in a neonate?

□ 1. Hyperthermia.
□ 2. Lethargy.
□ 3. Hyperactivity.
□ 4. Daily weight loss of 1 oz.

4. The nurse is conducting a telephone triage at a prenatal clinic. Which of the following clients should the nurse call first?

□ 1. Client who is at 10 weeks' gestation who says, "I have vomited my breakfast 3 times this week."
□ 2. Client who is at 16 weeks' gestation who says, "I have brown spots on my forehead, cheeks, and nose."
□ 3. Client who is at 20 weeks' gestation who says, "I have increased discharge from my vagina."
□ 4. Client who is at 37 weeks' gestation who says, "I have a bad headache and light hurts my eyes."

5. A physician tells the mother that she is carrying a fetus with Down syndrome. After the physician leaves the room, she asks the nurse, "What will the baby be like?" The nurse explains that the fetus will likely have mental retardation and:

□ 1. Close-set eyes, low-set ears, and immature genitals.
□ 2. A protruding tongue, up-slanted eyes, and congenital heart defects.
□ 3. A typical mewing cry, microcephaly, and malformed facial features.
□ 4. Microcephaly, face and limb defects, and behavior and growth problems.

6. The nurse is teaching a pregnant client with hypothyroidism about taking her L-thyroxine. Additional instruction is needed if the client says: "I should take my thyroid medicine with:

□ 1. iron."
□ 2. milk."
□ 3. tea."
□ 4. chocolate."

7. A pregnant client who is at 36 weeks' gestation is admitted to the intrapartum unit. The physician performs an amniocentesis to evaluate fetal lung maturity by measuring the lecithin/sphingomyelin (L/S) ratio. Which of the following values reflects fetal lung maturity?

□ 1. 1:2.
□ 2. 1:4.

- ☐ 3. 1:8.
- ☐ 4. 2:1.

8. The nurse in the intrapartum unit performs Leopold maneuvers to find the PMI of the FHR. The nurse finds a round, hard structure in the uterine fundus, a smooth surface on the maternal left side, and an irregular surface on the maternal right side. Given this information, the nurse should place the fetal monitor ultrasound transducer in the:

- ☐ 1. RUQ.
- ☐ 2. LUQ.
- ☐ 3. RLQ.
- ☐ 4. LLQ.

9. AF A client has just learned she is 8 weeks pregnant. The nurse is reviewing the client's history and physical data as noted in the chart. Which of the following data requires the nurse's immediate intervention at this prenatal visit?

HISTORY AND PHYSICAL

Blood type O Rh-negative
History of premature labor
Inadequate nutritional intake
Marijuana use

- ☐ 1. Blood type O Rh-negative
- ☐ 2. History of premature labor
- ☐ 3. Inadequate nutritional intake
- ☐ 4. Marijuana use

10. The nurse is assessing a female neonate. The nurse should report which of the following observations to the HCP?

- ☐ 1. Regurgitating 7 ml following nursing.
- ☐ 2. Presence of erythema toxicum.
- ☐ 3. Bloody discharge from the vagina.
- ☐ 4. Lack of flexion in left arm.

11. The laboring client receives meperidine (Demerol) IV for labor pain at 5 cm dilation. The nurse should expect the medication to make the client more comfortable in:

- ☐ 1. 30 to 60 s with peak effect in 5 to 7 min.
- ☐ 2. 2 min with peak effect in 2 to 5 min.
- ☐ 3. 2 to 3 min with peak effect in 15 min.
- ☐ 4. 10 to 15 min with peak effect in 30 to 50 min.

12. A nulliparous client at 40 weeks' gestation is admitted to the intrapartum unit in the latent phase of labor. The course of her pregnancy has been uncomplicated. The nurse completes assessments on this client, including BP, pulse, respiration, contraction pattern, and FHR according to which of the following schedules?

- ☐ 1. Every 4 hr.
- ☐ 2. Every 2 hr.
- ☐ 3. Every hr.
- ☐ 4. Every half hr.

13. While reviewing maternal history, the nurse notes a history of monilial infection. In planning for discharge of the infant, the nurse instructs the parents to notify the HCP about which of the following?

- ☐ 1. Milia across nose.
- ☐ 2. Brick orange discoloration in diaper.
- ☐ 3. White patches in cheeks of mouth.
- ☐ 4. Mongolian spots.

14. A pregnant client and her husband attend a childbirth education class. They show the nurse a birth plan that they would like to use during labor and birth in a hospital setting. Which of the following requests in the plan does the nurse explain to the couple as unrealistic?

- ☐ 1. Walk while in latent and active labor as long as she is comfortable.
- ☐ 2. Use hypnobirthing techniques for pain relief in labor.
- ☐ 3. Use no forceps or vacuum extractor or episiotomy to achieve birth.
- ☐ 4. Have their daughter who is 5 years of age visit in the birth room when the infant is stable.

15. AF The HCP orders magnesium sulfate IV for a pregnant client with pre-eclampsia. The order reads: After administering a loading dose of 4 g magnesium sulfate in 100 ml of normal saline over 30 min, hang 1,000 ml of Ringer lactate with 40 g of magnesium sulfate added and infuse 2 g per hr. The nurse should adjust the infusion rate to run at how many milliliters per hr? ______________ ml per hr.

16. A gravid client who is at 32 weeks' gestation with twins tells the nurse, "My abdomen is so large, I cannot sleep well at night." The best nurse response is:

- ☐ 1. "Can you nap during the day?"
- ☐ 2. "Drink hot chocolate or green tea before you go to bed."
- ☐ 3. "Have you asked you physician for a prescription for sleeping pills?"
- ☐ 4. "It may be helpful to use pillows to help support your abdomen and legs."

17. The nurse is preparing to administer a rubella immunization to a woman who has just delivered her first infant and had a prenatal rubella titer of 1:8. The nurse's instructions must be repeated if the mother says:

- ☐ 1. "I should not take the immunization if I am allergic to duck eggs."

□ 2. "After the immunization, I may have some joint pain."
□ 3. "I should use a reliable contraceptive for 3 months."
□ 4. "If I develop a rash, I will contact my health care provider."

18. The postpartum client complains to the nurse that she is urinating "lots and lots and I don't understand why." The nurse should explain that:
□ 1. "The oxytocin (Pitocin) you received in labor is a diuretic causing loss of water through urine."
□ 2. "While you are pregnant, the kidney filtering rate is decreased. Now that you have delivered, the kidneys are at full function."
□ 3. "While you are pregnant, your blood volume increases by more than one-third; you are losing that extra volume."
□ 4. "Because you are bottle-feeding you are losing the fluid you body does not need for breast-feeding."

19. The primigravid client at 26 weeks' gestation tells the nurse her gums are bleeding when she brushes her teeth. The nurse should inform the client of which of the following?
□ 1. "You may be experiencing a vitamin deficiency."
□ 2. "You may need to take supplemental vitamin K injections."
□ 3. "You need to go to the dentist immediately."
□ 4. "You need to use a mouthwash before and after brushing."

20. The nurse is completing the initial newborn assessment. During the assessment, the nurse notes that the BP is 10 mmHg higher in the upper extremities than the BP in the lower extremities. The nurse should first:
□ 1. Notify the HCP.
□ 2. Document the findings.
□ 3. Palpate the femoral pulses.
□ 4. Auscultate for a heart murmur.

21. AF The nurse reviews the following laboratory reports for a client who had a vaginal delivery of a healthy neonate 24 hr ago. The nurse should notify the HCP about which of the following data?

LABORATORY RESULTS

Test	Result
Hematocrit	38%
Hemoglobin	10.0 g/dl
RBC	4,500,000/mm3
WBC	8,000 mm3

□ 1. Hematocrit
□ 2. Hemoglobin
□ 3. RBC
□ 4. WBC

22. AF The nurse is assessing the infant of a mother who is a heroin addict. The nurse should assess for which of the following? Select all that apply.
□ 1. Increased Moro reflex.
□ 2. Jitteriness, hyperactivity.
□ 3. Lethargy.
□ 4. Poor feeding.
□ 5. Shrill, persistent cry.
□ 6. Sneezing, yawning.

23. The nurse is completing the nursing history on the newly admitted client in labor. The client has a history of illegal drug use. At this time, the nurse should gather additional information about this drug use so that the nurse can:
□ 1. Prevent withdrawal symptoms.
□ 2. Alert Child Protective Services.
□ 3. Initiate a referral to a rehabilitation program.
□ 4. Reduce potential drug to drug interaction.

24. A nurse working on a postpartum unit is planning care for a group of clients. The nurse should first make rounds on which of the following clients?
□ 1. Client with a seronegative rubella result.
□ 2. Client who had a prolapsed umbilical cord.
□ 3. Client who had prolonged rupture of membranes.
□ 4. Client who smokes half a pack per day.

25. A client delivered a 10-lb infant 2 hr ago. She is receiving an IV infusion of 20 units oxytocin (Pitocin). Which of the following assessments indicate the drug is having the desired effect?
□ 1. BP is 120/70.
□ 2. Lochia is rubra.
□ 3. Pain is decreased.
□ 4. Uterus is firm.

26. A woman complains of severe perineal pain 6 hr after delivery. Further assessment by the nurse reveals a perineal hematoma. The nurse should first:
□ 1. Administer narcotic pain medication.
□ 2. Apply anesthetic spray to the perineum.
□ 3. Apply an ice pack to the perineum.
□ 4. Place the client in a warm sitz bath.

27. AF The nurse is assigned to care for four postpartum clients from 3 p.m. to 11 p.m. today. In which order of priority does the nurse assess the following clients?
_____ 1. Client who is 25 years of age, 2 days postpartum, and who had a urinary output of 2,400 ml during the last 24 hr.

_____ 2. Primipara who had after-pains at the 6 a.m. breast-feeding session today.

_____ 3. Multipara who is 3 days postpartum and has an oral temperature of 101°F.

_____ 4. Client who is 16 years of age who had a cesarean section yesterday, and placed her infant up for adoption.

28. The nurse is completing the fourth recovery check 1 hr after delivery. When preparing to assess fundal height, the nurse should:

- □ 1. Discontinue IV fluids.
- □ 2. Have the client void.
- □ 3. Provide perineal care.
- □ 4. Put on sterile gloves.

29. Following delivery, a client is refusing to breast-feed her 2-day-old infant stating "I'm not going to do this any more, the cramps are awful." The nurse's most appropriate response is:

- □ 1. "I'll get you some pain medication and you can try again in 30 min."
- □ 2. "That's fine; you are the one who needs to make this decision."
- □ 3. "The pain will stop once your milk comes in."
- □ 4. "Try formula feeding and see if that is better for you."

30. The nurse is providing care for a newborn of a woman who had no prenatal care. The HCP has ordered erythromycin ophthalmic ointment 0.5%. The nurse should apply the ointment to the neonate's eyes:

- □ 1. When the mother's gonococcal and chlamydial culture results are available.
- □ 2. Immediately after delivery or within 1 to 2 hr of birth.
- □ 3. Because the mother did not receive prenatal care.
- □ 4. If the mother was treated for gonococcal or chlamydial STIs during pregnancy.

31. A newborn with jaundice is receiving phototherapy. The parents ask about the purpose of the phototherapy. The nurse explains that the phototherapy will:

- □ 1. Help the body change bilirubin to a fat-soluble material eliminated in the stool.
- □ 2. Help the body change bilirubin to a water-soluble material eliminated in the stool.
- □ 3. Help the body slow the RBC destruction causing the jaundice.
- □ 4. Increase the liver's production of an enzyme that breaks down bilirubin.

32. A client in labor has a history of opioid dependence and took prescribed methadone (Dolophine) during pregnancy. She plans an unmedicated labor because she is not a candidate for epidural anesthesia. At 5 cm, the client requests medication for pain. Which of the following standing orders on the physician's admission orders would cause this client to experience abstinence syndrome?

- □ 1. Meperidine (Demerol), 50 mg IV every 3 to 4 hr as needed for pain.
- □ 2. Morphine, 10 mg IV every 3 to 4 hr as needed for pain.
- □ 3. Fentanyl (Sublimaze), 25 mcg IV every 3 hr for pain.
- □ 4. Butorphanol tartrate (Stadol), 1 mg IV every 3 to 4 hr for pain.

33. The nurse is providing prenatal teaching for a client who is 28 weeks' gestation. The nurse instructs this client about which of the following?

- □ 1. Drugs that cause malformations.
- □ 2. Remedies for morning sickness.
- □ 3. Birth control options.
- □ 4. Childbirth education.

34. After completing the urine pregnancy test, the nurse gives the client the results, "Your pregnancy test is positive." The client looks surprised and begins to cry. The nurse's most appropriate response is:

- □ 1. "Is the timing of this pregnancy unexpected?"
- □ 2. "You weren't ready for this, were you?
- □ 3. "It's common to feel unsure at this time."
- □ 4. "Can I offer you a referral to a counselor?"

35. The nurse is assisting a mother as she bathes her 2-day-old neonate. Which of the following comments would be the most appropriate in regard to thermoregulation?

- □ 1. "You can completely undress your infant and bathe him quickly to keep him from getting cold."
- □ 2. "Since the infant is now 24 hr old, he can control his temperature well."
- □ 3. "Uncover only the portion of the infant you are bathing at that time."
- □ 4. "Since your infant is well, you don't have to worry that he will get cold."

36. AF A client who is pregnant and has four children reports the following obstetric history: a stillbirth at 32 weeks' gestation; triplets (two sons and a daughter) born by cesarean section at 34 weeks' gestation; and a daughter born vaginally at 39 weeks' gestation. What is the client's obstetric history using the GTPAL (gravity, term, preterm, abortion, live birth; five-digit) system?

____

37. AF A woman in her third trimester of pregnancy is being admitted to the hospital for observation. The nurse reviews the history and physical examination record. Which finding from the following chart does the nurse immediately report to the HCP?

HISTORY AND PHYSICAL

Ankle edema 2+

Urine protein 3+

Fetal heart tones 160, LLQ

Deep tendon reflexes 2+, ankle clonus negative

- ☐ 1. Ankle edema
- ☐ 2. Urine protein
- ☐ 3. Fetal heart tones
- ☐ 4. Deep tendon reflexes

38. In teaching a mother about her newborn's jaundice, the nurse instructs the mother that physiologic jaundice occurs:

- ☐ 1. In the first 24 hr of life.
- ☐ 2. When a neonate receives phototherapy.
- ☐ 3. With a positive direct Coombs test.
- ☐ 4. On the second or third day of life.

39. A client who is 8 months' pregnant is admitted to the hospital because of hypertension. The client is receiving a magnesium sulfate infusion. Three hours after the initiation of the magnesium sulfate therapy the nurse assesses the client. The nurse should report which of the following findings to the HCP?

- ☐ 1. Clonus, negative.
- ☐ 2. Urine output, 30 ml per hr.
- ☐ 3. Deep tendon reflexes, 1+.
- ☐ 4. Respirations, 10.

40. The nurse is administering an injection of vitamin K to a neonate. The expected outcome of vitamin K is to:

- ☐ 1. Reduce bilirubin levels.
- ☐ 2. Increase the production of RBCs.
- ☐ 3. Facilitate colonization of the bowel.
- ☐ 4. Prevent neonatal hemorrhagic disorder.

41. Expectant parents ask the nurse how to prepare their daughter who is 3 years of age for the infant. After discussing this issue with the parents, which statement by the parents indicates that they need additional teaching?

- ☐ 1. "We should tell our daughter about the new baby when her mom looks pregnant."
- ☐ 2. "We should bring our daughter to a prenatal visit when an ultrasound will show her the baby."
- ☐ 3. "We should enroll our daughter in a sibling support class a month before the baby is due."
- ☐ 4. "We should move our daughter to her new bedroom just before the baby is due."

42. In discussing stool patterns with a new breastfeeding mother, the nurse should provide which of the following instructions?

- ☐ 1. Typical stool patterns go from meconium to bright green to yellow.
- ☐ 2. Antidiarrheal agents will need to be administered if the stools are not formed.
- ☐ 3. Stools will need to be cultured if they are loose and seedy.
- ☐ 4. A normal stool pattern for a breast-fed neonate is to only stool one time per week.

43. The nurse is teaching the client how to use an oral contraceptive. The nurse evaluates that the client needs additional teaching when the client says, "I should:

- ☐ 1. take the pill at the same time each day."
- ☐ 2. take the pill at bedtime if I develop nausea after taking it."
- ☐ 3. take a missed pill as soon as I realize I missed it."
- ☐ 4. use a backup method such as foam and condoms if I miss a pill."

44. While reviewing a neonate's history, the nurse notes which of the following data as a risk for hypoglycemia?

- ☐ 1. Labor began with rupture of membranes.
- ☐ 2. Neonate had difficulty establishing respirations at birth.
- ☐ 3. Neonate had marked acrocyanosis of the hands and feet.
- ☐ 4. Mother had chocolate cravings during pregnancy.

45. AF A pregnant client who is at term and whose labor is being induced with oxytocin (Pitocin) is on continuous fetal monitoring. A pattern develops of fetal heart rate tracing characterized by decelerations that begin after the peak of the contraction and return to the baseline after the contraction has passed. In which order does the nurse perform this list of interventions? Place in order from first to last.

_____ 1. Notify the HCP.
_____ 2. Administer oxygen by mask at 8 to 10 L/min.
_____ 3. Turn the client to the left side.
_____ 4. Discontinue the oxytocin.

46. The nurse is planning care for a pregnant client who is admitted to the hospital because of premature rupture of membranes. Which of the following increases the risk of infection and is not included in the plan of care?

- ☐ 1. Increase fluid intake.
- ☐ 2. Ambulate client to the bathroom.
- ☐ 3. Provide vaginal examination.
- ☐ 4. Provide external fetal monitoring.

47. The nurse is assessing a neonate. Which of the following observations is reported to the HCP?
- ☐ 1. Abdomen slightly protuberant (rounded).
- ☐ 2. Liver palpable 2 cm under right costal margin.
- ☐ 3. Bowel sounds present at two to three per minute.
- ☐ 4. Clear drainage at the base of the umbilical cord.

48. A client who is 17 years of age and pregnant smokes a pack of cigarettes a day. Smoking cessation is most likely to be promoted if the nurse discusses that cigarette smoking:
- ☐ 1. Causes stained teeth and bad breath.
- ☐ 2. May decrease fertility.
- ☐ 3. Increases the risk for lung cancer and heart disease.
- ☐ 4. Is associated with SIDS and ear infections.

49. AF The nurse is completing the postpartum discharge plan for a client who had a hemoglobin level of 8 mg/dl the morning after delivery. The nurse instructs the client to include which of the following foods in her diet? Select all that apply.
- ☐ 1. Red meats, poultry, and legumes.
- ☐ 2. Dark green, leafy vegetables.
- ☐ 3. Eggs.
- ☐ 4. Milk, cheese, and yogurt.
- ☐ 5. Citrus fruits.
- ☐ 6. Enriched grains and cereals.

50. The nurse is assessing a neonate for possible developmental hip dysplasia. A finding that suggests this problem is:
- ☐ 1. Limited hip abduction.
- ☐ 2. Crying on straightening the leg.
- ☐ 3. Drawing of the legs under when prone.
- ☐ 4. Inward rotation of the heel.

51. The nurse is teaching a pregnant client about nutrition. The nurse learns that the client is lactose-intolerant. Which of the following does the nurse include in a list of high-calcium foods?
- ☐ 1. Eggs.
- ☐ 2. Sardines.
- ☐ 3. Tuna.
- ☐ 4. Liver and organ meats.

52. AF The nurse is to administer vitamin K to a neonate. Mark an "X" at the correct site for the injection.

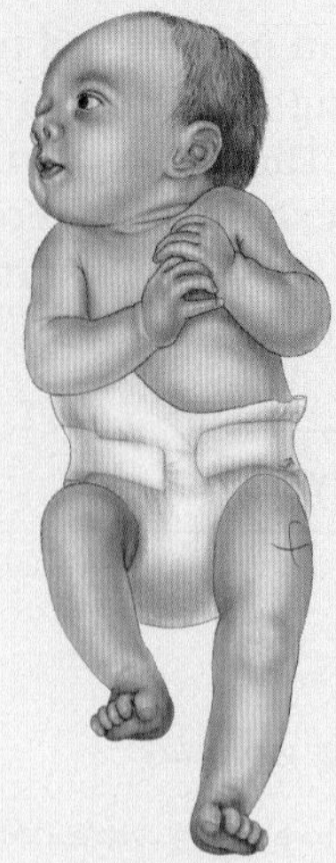

53. The nurse is administering methylergonovine (Methergine) IV to a client following delivery of a healthy neonate. The nurse assesses the client for which of the following adverse effects of this drug?
- ☐ 1. Headache.
- ☐ 2. Hypertension.
- ☐ 3. Tachycardia.
- ☐ 4. Uterine cramping.

54. The nurse has determined that the fetus is in an LOP position. The nurse should assess the client for:
- ☐ 1. Increased pain when placed on her left side.
- ☐ 2. Discomfort in the sacral area.
- ☐ 3. Pressure at the symphysis pubis.
- ☐ 4. Pain across the lower abdomen from fundal-dominant contractions.

55. The nurse is planning care for a client who is 42½ weeks' pregnant and scheduled for induction of labor. The intended outcome of inducing labor in this client is to prevent:
- ☐ 1. Maternal fatigue.
- ☐ 2. Dystotic labor.
- ☐ 3. Reduced placental function.
- ☐ 4. Polyhydramnios.

56. A client is in her third trimester, but not in labor; she has dark red spotting and complains of severe continuous pain on one side of her lower abdomen. The uterus is board-like and tender to touch. The nurse should instruct the woman to:
- ☐ 1. Walk to relieve the pain.
- ☐ 2. Be admitted to the hospital immediately.
- ☐ 3. Rest in bed until she has labor pains.
- ☐ 4. Manage the pain by breathing deeply.

57. The physician ordered IV ampicillin every 6 hr times 2 doses for a woman in early labor. On her chart, the nurse notes that she had vaginal and rectal cultures at 37 weeks' gestation.

The cultures of this woman were most likely positive for:

- □ 1. HIV.
- □ 2. Cytomegalovirus.
- □ 3. Group B streptococcus.
- □ 4. Gonorrhea.

58. The nurse has been providing care for a multipara woman who is 37 weeks' pregnant. She has had ruptured membranes for the past 12 hr, but no contractions. Her pulse has increased over the last 2 hr and the nurse notes that the fetus is also experiencing an increased heart rate of 30 beats above the baseline. These findings are most likely indicative of:

- □ 1. An intrauterine infection.
- □ 2. The beginning of true labor.
- □ 3. Psychologic fear of labor pains.
- □ 4. A prolapsed cord.

59. The nurse is caring for a client following delivery of a health neonate who has eclampsia. During the early postpartum period, (the first 12 to 24 hr) a client with a diagnosis of eclampsia:

- □ 1. May still be at risk for convulsions.
- □ 2. Is more likely to develop an infection.
- □ 3. Should not be encouraged to breast-feed.
- □ 4. Will experience more uterine cramping than most clients in the postpartum period.

60. During pregnancy, which of the following may significantly change a type 1 diabetic woman's insulin requirements?

- □ 1. A large fetus.
- □ 2. A reactive nonstress test.
- □ 3. Anemia.
- □ 4. A UTI.

61. The nurse explains to a woman with type 1 diabetes entering her third trimester that labor may be induced a few weeks before term. When the client asks why this may be necessary, the nurse tells her that early delivery will:

- □ 1. Decrease the chance of congenital anomalies in the newborn.
- □ 2. Decrease the chances of intrauterine fetal damage or death due to placental insufficiency.
- □ 3. Decrease the chances of the infant developing diabetes.
- □ 4. Decrease the infant's chance of developing respiratory distress syndrome after birth.

62. The nurse should screen which of the following women for gestational diabetes?

- □ 1. Client who is 26 years of age who had a positive pregnancy test 3 weeks ago.
- □ 2. Client who is 15 years of age who has a poor diet and has gained 12 lb in the second trimester.
- □ 3. All pregnant clients between 24 and 28 weeks' gestation.
- □ 4. Client who is 40 years of age and pregnant for the fourth time.

63. The nurse is planning care for a client who is in the third trimester of pregnancy. Per diet history, the client is not obtaining adequate nutrition, but weight gain has been within normal limits. The nurse reviews the client's hemoglobin and hematocrit levels at this time because:

- □ 1. The most common type of pathological anemia during pregnancy is iron deficiency anemia.
- □ 2. Undernourished women will develop iron deficiency anemia during pregnancy.
- □ 3. Replenishment of iron stores by oral therapy will be discontinued immediately after delivery.
- □ 4. The normal range for hemoglobin and hematocrit levels is the same for both pregnant and nonpregnant clients.

64. AF The nurse is planning care for a client in the early postpartum period who has cardiac disease. Which of the following activities is included in the plan of care? Select all that apply.

- □ 1. Monitor intake and output.
- □ 2. Encourage ambulation in the first few hours.
- □ 3. Keep the infant in the nursery most of the day.
- □ 4. Give antacids between meals.
- □ 5. Minimize blood loss.
- □ 6. Monitor vital signs closely.

65. A pregnant client has class I heart disease. The nurse should teach the client that she will need to:

- □ 1. Bottle-feed her infant after birth.
- □ 2. Restrict fluid and salt intake in the last trimester.
- □ 3. Stay on complete bed rest throughout the pregnancy.
- □ 4. Avoid exposure to upper respiratory infections.

66. A primigravida client is admitted to the hospital in preterm labor. Vaginal examination reveals that her cervix is 4 cm dilated and 80% effaced. The HCP orders betamethasone (Celestone). The expected outcome of this drug is:

- □ 1. Slowing of uterine contractions.
- □ 2. Absence of chorioamnionitis.
- □ 3. Increase of uteroplacental exchange.
- □ 4. Maturation of fetal lungs.

67. AF A client who is breast-feeding has developed a sore, cracked nipple on the right breast. The nurse is concerned that she will develop mastitis. If the mother develops chills, fever, malaise, and local breast tenderness, the nurse should advise the mother to do which of the following? Select all that apply.

- ☐ 1. Discontinue breast-feeding immediately.
- ☑ 2. Contact the HCP who will likely prescribe an antibiotic.
- ☐ 3. Check the infant for thrush.
- ☐ 4. Wipe the nipple with alcohol.
- ☑ 5. Empty breasts by feeding or pumping if feeding is too uncomfortable.
- ☑ 6. Apply hot or cold compresses to the breast.
- ☑ 7. Wear a good support bra.
- ☐ 8. Take analgesics as needed.

68. The nurse is caring for a gravida 5, para 5, newly delivered client whose infant weighed 9 lb 10 oz. This client is at high risk for:

- ☐ 1. Uterine atony.
- ☐ 2. Altered parenting.
- ☐ 3. Dehydration.
- ☐ 4. Thrombophlebitis.

69. Which one of the following women is at highest risk for a UTI during the postpartum period?

- ☐ 1. Client who is 40 years of age, obese, and having her first child.
- ☐ 2. Client who is 26 years of age who had twins delivered by cesarean delivery.
- ☐ 3. Client who is 22 years of age who had three in-and-out catheterizations during labor.
- ☐ 4. Client who is 16 years of age who has hypertension and a poor diet.

70. Eight hours after delivery, the nurse determines that a new mother is experiencing a postpartum hemorrhage. The first action of the nurse is to:

- ☐ 1. Ask the client to sign a consent for surgery.
- ☐ 2. Massage the uterus.
- ☐ 3. Administer an oxytocic drug.
- ☐ 4. Empty the woman's bladder.

71. A client who recently delivered tells the nurse that she had an untreated monilial infection during her pregnancy. Because the infant is at risk for thrush, the nurse should tell the mother to:

- ☐ 1. Continue her antibiotics until they are all finished.
- ☐ 2. Discontinue breast-feeding until she is treated.
- ☐ 3. Perform adequate hand hygiene after she changes the infant's diaper.
- ☐ 4. Observe the infant for white patches in the mouth that adhere to the tongue.

72. A client who is 39 weeks' pregnant and G1P0 tells the nurse she has noticed an increase in vaginal mucus discharge that also has a small amount of blood in it. The nurse informs the client:

- ☐ 1. She will be in labor soon; cervical effacement and dilation are complete.
- ☐ 2. She has a vaginal infection and should be tested now.
- ☐ 3. There is a possibility of hemorrhage and to go to the hospital.
- ☐ 4. The blood is from rupture of small cervical capillaries and is normal.

73. The nurse is providing care for a woman in the fourth stage of labor. Which of the following is an appropriate goal?

- ☐ 1. Promote parent-infant bonding.
- ☐ 2. Prepare for discharge from the hospital.
- ☐ 3. Give neonate the first bath.
- ☐ 4. Teach mother about neonatal care.

74. A pregnant client has been in stage 2 of labor for 15 min. The nurse should instruct the woman to:

- ☐ 1. Push during the contractions and rest between them.
- ☐ 2. Sip a glass of juice for energy.
- ☐ 3. Stop pushing for two contractions to rest.
- ☐ 4. Take a mild analgesic for discomfort.

75. A primigravida who is 6 weeks' pregnant is having morning sickness each day. The nurse should instruct the client to:

- ☐ 1. Avoid lying down after meals.
- ☐ 2. Eat saltine crackers before rising from bed.
- ☐ 3. Refrain from eating until noon.
- ☐ 4. Take an antacid at bedtime.

Answers and Rationales

1. 4 Constipation in pregnancy is related to hormonally caused physiologic changes (hypoperistalsis with resultant increased reabsorption of water from stool in the colon). Other causes of constipation include food choices, lack of fluids, decreased physical activity, abdominal distention by the pregnant uterus, and displacement and compression of the intestines. Although iron supplementation may contribute to constipation, discontinuation of iron supplementation in the third trimester may place the woman at risk for anemia. (H)

2. 1, 2, 4, 5, 6 RhoGAM (Rh immune globulin) is administered to prevent isoimmunization after birth, miscarriage/pregnancy termination, abdominal trauma, ectopic pregnancy, or invasive procedures such as amniocentesis, version or chorionic villi sampling. A biophysical profile does not present a risk of isoimmunization. (D)

3. 2 A neonate with an infection may show signs of lethargy and irritability. Infected neonates usually will not have the energy to have exhibit hyperactivity. Because of the immaturity of the neonate, hypothermia is the usual response seen in neonatal infections. Expected weight loss in a neonate is 10% to 15% of birth weight. One ounce would fall in the normal, expected weight loss range. (M)

4. 4 The nurse first calls the client experiencing severe headache and photophobia, and blind spots (scotomata); these are signs of progressing pre-eclampsia. The client who has brown spots on her face is experiencing melasma (chloasma) or hyperpigmentation caused by increased melanotropin (a pituitary hormone). The client who has increased vaginal discharge is experiencing a common discomfort of pregnancy, leukorrhea, caused by hyperstimulated cervical mucous glands and requires hygiene education (i.e., wearing panties with cotton crotch). The client who vomited breakfast 3 times is experiencing morning sickness, a common discomfort of pregnancy that requires nutritional education (eat dry carbohydrate snack before arising). (M)

5. 2 The characteristics of Down syndrome are mental retardation, a protruding tongue, up-slanting eyes, and congenital heart malformations (commonly, septal defects). The first choice describes Turner syndrome. The third choice describes cri-du-Chat syndrome and choice 4 describes fetal alcohol syndrome. (M)

6. 1 Iron interferes with absorption of L-thyroxine. The nurse instructs the woman to take the L-thyroxine on an empty stomach. Milk, tea, and chocolate do not interfere with L-thyroxine absorption. (D)

7. 4 The lecithin/sphingomyelin ratio increases after 24 weeks of gestation. Lecithin increases in the amniotic fluid, while sphingomyelin remains constant. When the ratio reaches 2:1, the lungs are considered mature. (M)

8. 2 The Leopold maneuvers reveal the fetal head in the fundus, fetal back on the maternal left side, and fetal small parts on the maternal right side. The the PMI is located over the fetal back or shoulder in the LUQ. (M)

9. 4 Any substance abuse or use during pregnancy places the mother and fetus in jeopardy. The nurse offers the client information on community resources to help her with her substance abuse. Because the client is Rh-negative she will need to receive an RhoGAM injection at 28 weeks' gestation. Inadequate nutritional intake at this time in the gestation is considered a normal variance of pregnancy. The history of preterm labor is not an urgent topic at this time. However, there could be a correlation between preterm labor and substance abuse, which warrants further investigation at the next prenatal visit. (M)

10. 4 Lack of symmetrical movement or lack of flexion in left arm is an abnormal finding. This might be an indicator of birth trauma or injury. Regurgitation, erythema toxicum, and pseudomenstruation are normal findings. (M)

11. 3 Meperidine (Demerol) acts in 30 to 60 s when administered IV. Fentanyl (Sublimaze) acts in 2 min. Demerol takes effect in 10 to 15 min when administered IM. Nalbuphine (Nubain) takes effect in 2 to 3 min when administered IV and in 15 min when given IM. (D)

12. 3 When a woman is in labor without complications and is in the latent phase of labor, BP, pulse, respirations, contraction pattern, and FHR are assessed hourly until a change in status occurs. Temperature is assessed every 4 hr as long as the fetal membranes are intact; temperature is measured every 2 hr after the membranes rupture. Vaginal examinations are limited to reduce the risk of infection and are performed when there is evidence of progress in labor or after membranes rupture to assess for cord prolapse, if indicated. (M)

13. 3 White patches in the cheeks or the mouth may be an indication of *Candida albicans*, which can be contracted from a maternal monilial infection. Milia are a result of clogged sebaceous glands and are a normal finding. Brick orange discoloration, or "brick dust," is pyruvic acid crystals and a normal finding. Mongolian spots are dark blue to blue green discoloration usually found on the back, buttocks, or thighs, and are a normal skin variance. (M)

14. 3 The parents cannot limit the HCP's options for providing for a safe birth. The use of ambulation in latent or active labor is safe as is the use of hypnobirthing. The presence of the daughter who is 5 years of age after the infant is stable is safe, and may facilitate sibling attachment. (M)

15. 25 ml per hour (D)
40 g:1,000 ml/hr = 2 g × ml/hr
X = 25 ml/hr

16. 4 Pillows are effective in providing support and comfort to the gravid abdomen and legs while reclining, thus promoting a more restful atmosphere and sleep. Asking the client to nap during the day is not addressing the problem of comfort and rest. As pregnancy advances and the uterus enlarges with the twin gestation, drinking beverages prior to going to bed will increase the chance of disturbing sleep to get up to void. Expecting the physician to provide a prescription for sleeping pills is not addressing the problem of comfort and rest. (C)

17. 4 A rash is a common side effect of the immunization and does not require notification of an HCP. Rubella vaccine is a known teratogen, and pregnancy is avoided for 3 months after an immunization. The vaccine is cultured in duck eggs, so persons allergic to duck eggs may not receive the vaccine. Transient arthralgia is also a side effect of the immunization. (D)

18. 3 Blood volume increases 30% to 50% during pregnancy; after birth, the extra volume is no longer needed. Oxytocin (Pitocin) is an antidiuretic and causes water retention. During pregnancy, the GFR increases 50%. The body does not retain fluid for milk production. (M)

19. 1 Requirements for both fat-soluble and water-soluble vitamins increase during pregnancy to support the growth of new fetal cells. Although vitamin needs do increase during pregnancy, most of the vitamin intake requirements are met by eating a healthy diet with plenty of fruits and vegetables. The nurse cautions the clients to avoid taking megadoses of vitamins. Megadoses of vitamin C may cause withdrawal scurvy in the newborn at birth. Vitamin K injections are offered to the client experiencing severe hematologic dysfunction. The client is not in need of immediate dental treatment, nor will using a mouthwash before and after brushing be effective. (H)

20. 3 The nurse palpates the femoral pulses. Absent or weak femoral pulses and BP higher in the arms than in the legs are classic signs of coarctation of the aorta; the nurse notifies the HCP when both findings are recognized. Auscultating for a heart murmur is appropriate when assessing for a patent ductus; a patent ductus does not influence the BP or the pulses. It is not sufficient to document the findings; the nurse gathers additional information and provides a complete report to the HCP. (M)

21. 2 Normal reference ranges for female hemoglobin level is 12 to 16 g/dl. If hemoglobin is lower than 10 g/dl, the HCP will likely order supplemental iron. Because the client is also at risk for vertigo on rising, the nurse assists the client move from a lying or sitting position to a standing position. Normal reference ranges for hematocrit are 37% to 47%; for RBCs, 4 to 5.5 mm^3; and for WBCs, 4,500 to 10,000 mm^3. (A)

22. 2, 4, 5 Opioid withdrawal in the newborn is accompanied by jittery, hyperactivity; shrill, persistent cry; yawning and sneezing; increased deep tendon reflexes and decreased Moro reflex. The newborn will have difficulty sucking and feeding and may have vomiting and diarrhea. The newborn will also have a disrupted sleep cycle with no quiet sleep and disturbance of active sleep. (M)

23. 4 Using a nonjudgmental manner, the nurse assesses clients who are in labor for potential substance abuse. Medications given during labor may interact with any recently used illegal drug, and place the client and unborn fetus at risk. Knowing what withdrawal symptoms might be experienced, referring the client into a rehabilitation program, and notifying Child Protective Services are not immediate interventions for the laboring client. (R)

24. 3 The chance for postpartum infection is great for the client with prolonged rupture of membranes; the nurse assesses this client first. The client with a seronegative rubella result requires the rubella vaccine, but the nurse administers that later. The client that had a prolapsed umbilical cord was at greatest risk during labor and delivery, but is not at risk in the postpartum period. The client who smokes is encouraged to reduce her risk factors through smoking cessation, and the nurse can plan to discuss this with the client later in the shift. (S)

25. 4 Oxytocin (Pitocin) is used to stimulate uterine contractions, decreasing the risk for postpartum bleeding. Pitocin will not be effective in controlling BP, lochia color, or decreasing pain. (D)

26. 3 For the first 24 hr after delivery, ice (covered with a towel to prevent thermal injury to the skin) is used to manage postpartum discomforts from a hematoma. If needed, the nurse administers a mild analgesic, as ordered for pain, not narcotic. Anesthetic spray is not recommended. A warm sitz bath may benefit the client after 24 hr if the hematoma has not been ligated. (R)

27. 3, 4, 1, 2 The nurse first assesses the client with an oral temperature of 101°F. A temperature of more than 100.4° F, excluding the first 24-hr postpartum period, is considered to be febrile, and a postpartum infection may be present. Next, the nurse assesses the client who is 16 years of age who had a cesarean section and may need psychosocial support after making her decision regarding adoption. The client with diuresis is responding as expected; fluid shifts naturally occur during the postpartum period. The nurse continues to monitor intake and output. The nurse assesses the client with afterpains last. Afterpains are common discomforts associated with breast-feeding, and disappear as the uterus regains tone. (M)

28. 2 To facilitate assessment of fundal height, it is best if the client's bladder is empty. A full bladder can cause the uterus to be displaced, and bleeding to be increased. IV fluids are maintained until the client has voided. Perineal care is essential for client comfort and reducing infection, but not necessary to assess fundal height. Sterile gloves are not required. (A)

29. 1 Breast-feeding causes the release of oxytocin, and the client may feel tugging or cramping in her lower pelvis during the first few days of breast-feeding. Providing a mild analgesic prior to feeding may help decrease this discomfort and allow the client the opportunity to continue breast-feeding. The nurse is not being supportive with her responses regarding the client's decision and regarding when the milk comes in. Breast-feeding has many advantages, and the nurse assists the client who wishes to breast-feed; analgesics usually sufficiently relieve cramping and are encouraged as the first intervention. (M)

30. 2 Neonatal eye prophylaxis is performed as soon after delivery as possible or in the nursery, if monitoring ensures that all infants receive prophylaxis there. State law requires eye prophylaxis in the majority of states, irrespective of results of blood cultures or amount of prenatal care. (S)

31. 2 Exposure of the skin to ultraviolet light converts the poorly soluble indirect bilirubin into water-soluble chemical groups that can be excreted into bile without conjugation. Phototherapy does not change bilirubin into fat-soluble material, prevent RBC destruction, or increase liver production of enzymes. (A)

32. 4 The client who has an opioid dependency does not receive opioid agonist analgesics. Stadol is an opioid agonist. The client is safely medicated with the other standing orders. (D)

33. 4 When planning education for a client who is at 28 weeks' gestation, the nurse focuses on client needs of the third trimester. Teratogens are a threat in the first trimester. Morning sickness is a first and early-second trimester complaint. Birth control options are commonly discussed after delivery. (H)

34. 3 Ambivalence is a common reaction to pregnancy. Recognize that ambivalence does not mean rejection of the child, but reflects a reaction of all the changes associated with pregnancy and parenthood. Asking closed-ended questions (1, 2, and 3) is not therapeutic when a client is experiencing an emotional challenge. (P)

35. 3 Thermoregulation is a concern for neonates. Well neonates, when exposed and wet, have a great risk of cold stress related to exposure and evaporation. Keeping the neonate covered while bathing will prevent cold stress and will help the neonate to maintain body temperature. (S)

36. 5, 1, 2, 0, 4 The client has been pregnant four times and is now pregnant; she is a gravida 5. She has had two preterm births (one set of triplets at 32 weeks' gestation and a stillbirth at 32 weeks' gestation). She had no abortions. She has four children. (A)

37. 2 The urine protein is a sign of a potential hypertensive disorder. Ankle edema is an expected finding in the third trimester. The fetal heart tones are within normal range. The deep tendon reflexes are normal and ankle clonus should be negative. (M)

38. 4 Physiologic jaundice appears on the second or third day of life as the liver is unable to keep up with the increased demand of bilirubin conjugation. Jaundice that appears in the first 24 hr or is a result of a positive direct Coombs test is considered pathologic jaundice. Phototherapy is a treatment for hyperbilirubinemia, not a cause. (A)

39. 4 Signs of magnesium toxicity include respirations less than 12, absence of reflexes, urine output less than 30 ml per hour, and a significant drop in maternal pulse or BP. The nurse notifies the HCP of the indicators of toxicity. (D)

40. 3 The GI track of neonates initially does not have sufficient bacteria to contribute to the synthesis of vitamin K, and blood coagulability is temporarily decreased. Vitamin K is administered at birth to prevent bleeding. Phototherapy is used to reduce bilirubin levels. Vitamin K will not increase RBC production or facilitate colonization in the bowel. (A)

41. 4 Moving the daughter to a new bedroom just before the birth is a major change and could result in greater emotional turmoil for the daughter. The other actions will help to prepare her for the new sibling. (P)

42. 1 The typical stool transition is from meconium to a bright green to yellow. Breast milk stools are loose and seedy; no intervention is necessary. The normal stool pattern for a breast-fed neonate is more frequent that once per week. Typical stooling may be 3 to 4 times a day. (A)

43. 4 Using a backup method such as foam and condoms is only needed when more than two pills have been missed in succession. The client is instructed to take the pill daily, and at the same time; taking at bedtime allows the client to "sleep" through nausea, and making up pills is done as soon as the client remembers that she did not take it. (H)

44. 2 Difficulty establishing respirations at birth is a sign of stress. Glucose is used at a greater rate in a stressed neonate. Normal labor, beginning with rupture of membranes and acrocyanosis, has no impact on glucose utilization. Cravings in the mother during pregnancy will have no impact in the neonate. (A)

45. 4, 3, 2, 1 The nurse first discontinues the oxytocin (Pitocin), and then turns the client to her left side. Next, the nurse administers oxygen at 8 to 10 L/min, and then notifies the HCP. (M)

46. 3 Vaginal examinations increase the risk of infection in clients who experience premature rupture of membranes. Increasing fluids, ambulating to the bathroom, and external fetal monitoring do not increase infection risk. (R)

47. 4 Clear drainage at the base of the umbilical cord is evaluated for a possible urachus. Abdominal roundness, a liver palpable 2 cm below the right costal margin, and presence of bowel sounds are normal findings. (S)

48. 1 Adolescents respond to smoking cessation information that focuses on their appearance or desirability. Appealing to future health problems, while important to discuss, may not be as effective. Fertility and the infant's health are not concerns for the client at this time. (H)

49. 1, 2, 3, 6 Red meats, poultry, and legumes; dark green, leafy vegetables; eggs; and enriched grains and cereals are iron-rich foods. Milk, cheese, and yogurt, and citrus fruits are not sources of iron. (H)

50. 1 Limited hip abduction is a sign of possible hip dysplasia. Drawing the legs under the body while prone is a normal behavior of a term neonate. Crying while straightening of the legs and inward rotation of feet are usually positional issues. Inward rotation of the heel is a sign of talipes equinovarus. (A)

51. 2 Sardines and other fish including bones are a high source of calcium. Eggs, tuna, and organ meats are high in iron. (H)

52. The vastus lateralis is the appropriate muscle for injections in neonates. The gluteus maximus, ventrogluteal, and deltoid muscles are generally too small. (S)

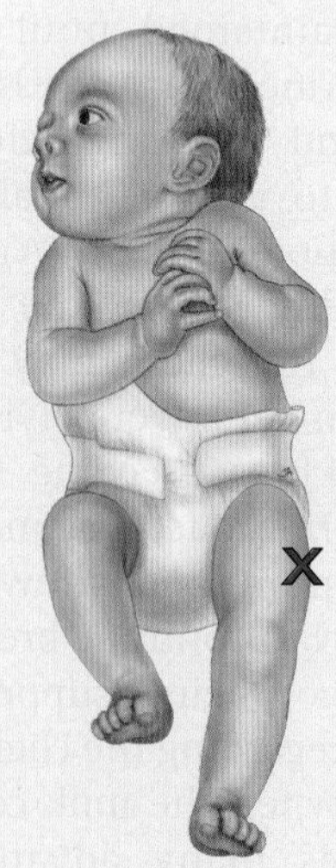

53. 2 Severe hypertensive episodes, bradycardia, and nausea and vomiting can result after giving methylergonovine (Methergine). There is no indication that headache is associated with receiving Methergine. Uterine cramping is a desired effect. (D)

54. 2 The chief complaint of pain in a woman whose fetus is in an LOP position is discomfort in the sacral area or lower back. The back of the infant's head is in the posterior of the pelvis, and because of the shape of the head, there is pressure on the nerves of the spine. Placing the mother on her side may relieve her pain somewhat. Pain from fundal-dominant contractions is not related to the infant's position. Pressure on the symphysis is felt mostly when the head emerges from the birth canal. (C)

55. 3 After 40 to 42 weeks' gestation, placental profusion may decrease, causing the fetus to get less oxygen and nutrition. Therefore, it is safer to deliver the infant if the pregnancy goes beyond 40 to 42 weeks. Usually there is less amniotic fluid (polyhydramnios) after 40 weeks' gestation. The chance of dystotic labor is not related to the length of the pregnancy. Maternal fatigue is not a reason for an induced labor. (R)

56. 2 Dark red spotting or frank bleeding, a boardlike uterus, and continuous pain are symptomatic of abruptio placenta. The client is admitted to the hospital immediately for evaluation by ultrasound and a possible emergency delivery. (R)

57. 3 Two doses of ampicillin or another appropriate antibiotic given during labor 6 hr apart is used to treat group B streptococcus. Women with vaginal and rectal colonization of streptococcus are usually asymptomatic and unaware they are carrying the infection. If the infant contracts a streptococcus infection when it passes through the birth canal, it can develop sepsis, a condition that can be fatal. Gonorrhea would be treated prenatally as soon as the infection is diagnosed and again in the infant after birth. HIV and cytomegalovirus are not treated with antibiotics during labor. (D)

58. 1 Tachycardia in the fetus and an increased pulse in the mother are indicative of an intrauterine infection, especially in light of the prolonged ruptured membranes. With no contractions, active labor has not begun. A prolapsed cord would cause fetal bradycardia but would not affect the mother's pulse rate. Fear can cause an increased pulse in the mother but would not affect the fetus. (R)

59. 1 After birth it is common for the symptoms of pre-eclampsia and eclampsia to resolve quickly, usually within 48 hr. However, symptoms may occur up to 2 weeks after birth, even in women who did not have symptoms of pre-eclampsia before delivery. Even if no convulsions occurred before the birth, they may occur within this period. For this reason, magnesium sulfate infusions are usually continued 12 to 24 hr after the birth, and careful assessment of BP and other signs of worsening pre-eclampsia need to continue. Infection risk does not change. Because of the affect of the magnesium sulfate on smooth muscles, uterine relaxation and excessive bleeding, rather than cramping, are likely. Breast-feeding is encouraged if the mother is able, but she may need additional help. (R)

60. 4 Any type of infection will affect insulin requirements. The size of the fetus and anemia are not related to insulin dose. A nonstress test is an important assessment during the last month of the pregnancy to monitor placental functioning in the diabetic woman, but is not related to insulin needs. (M)

61. 2 Early delivery is elected for diabetic mothers because of the possibility of fetal damage or death because of placental insufficiency. Congenital anomalies occur very early in pregnancy. The infant may suffer from hypoglycemia after delivery and require treatment, but that condition is unrelated to time of delivery. The infant is also unlikely to develop respiratory distress syndrome after 36 weeks unless conditions other than diabetes are present. However, even if the infant is at risk for developing respiratory distress syndrome, it may be better to deliver the infant early and treat the respiratory problems after delivery rather than risk fetal damage or death by continuing the pregnancy in light of poor placental functioning. (R)

62. 3 All pregnant women are tested for gestational diabetes between 24 and 28 weeks' gestation. Some women may be more likely than others to develop gestational diabetes but all women should be screened. (H)

63. 1 Because of hemodilution during pregnancy, blood loss during delivery, and iron needs of the fetus, the most common type of anemia seen during pregnancy and in the postpartum period is iron deficiency anemia. Without iron therapy, even pregnant women with excellent nutrition will end their pregnancy with an iron deficit. At least 20% of women will be anemic. The normal hematocrit for nonpregnant women is between 38% and 45%. However, normal values for pregnant women with adequate iron stores may be as low as 34%. (R)

64. 1, 5, 6 Because of the fluid shifts during the early postpartum period, the plan of care for a woman with cardiac disease includes careful monitoring of vital signs and intake and output. Blood loss is kept to a minimum to prevent strain on the heart from anemia. Bed rest is maintained for the early postpartum period to prevent further strain on the heart from increased activity. The infant can remain with the mother as long as there is assistance with feedings and infant care, as needed. Antacids are not an essential part of her care because of her cardiac disease, but they may be given for other reasons. (M)

65. 4 According to the New York Heart Association functional classification of organic heart disease, women with class I heart disease are asymptomatic with normal activities. However, any change in their situation that puts additional stress on the woman's heart can cause symptoms. An upper respiratory infection decreases the functioning of the lungs, makes breathing more difficult, and can cause a strain on the heart. Bed rest, restricting fluids and sodium, and the avoidance of breast-feeding are recommendations for women with class III or IV heart disease. (H)

66. 4 Betamethasone is used to rapidly mature the fetus's lungs when premature delivery is anticipated. It has no affect on contractions, risk for infection, or uteroplacental function. (D)

67. 2, 5, 6, 7, 8 If a mother develops mastitis, she is instructed to contact her HCP because she will need an antibiotic. The nurse advises the client to support her breasts with a good supportive bra, apply hot or cold compresses, whichever make her the most comfortable, and take analgesics as needed. She does not have to discontinue breast-feeding because it is the tissue of the breast that is infected, not the milk; however, breast-feeding may be too painful and she may need to pump her breasts to maintain the milk supply. She can give the infant her milk. Wiping the nipple with alcohol will be painful and will dry the tissue, causing more breakdown of skin. Thrush is more likely if the mother had a yeast infection and the infant was exposed to the organism when it passed through the birth canal. (C)

68. 1 Because this client has had five children and a large neonate, her uterine muscles have been overstretched, making her prone to uterine atony (relaxation of the smooth muscles of the uterus). She is not at higher risk for dehydration, altered parenting, or thrombophlebitis. (S)

69. 3 Although all of the women are at risk, the woman who was catheterized three times during labor is the most at risk for a urinary track infection because of the opportunity for introducing pathogens when the catheter was inserted. (S)

70. 2 The nurse's first action when there is uterine muscle relaxation causing a postpartum hemorrhage is to massage the uterine fundus and express any clots retained in the uterus. If the uterus does not become firm, other actions after the initial action are to empty the bladder and give one of several oxytocic drugs such as Pitocin IV or IM as ordered. Surgery may be necessary to control excessive bleeding if all other measures fail. (M)

71. 4 A neonate who passes through the birth canal of a mother who has an untreated monilia infection at the time of delivery is at risk for thrush. Sites for thrush in the neonate are the tongue and mouth; white patches that adhere to the tongue (unlike curds of milk) are a symptom of thrush in a neonate. Antibiotics are not used to treat thrush; they may actually cause the development of a yeast infection. The drug used to treat thrush is nystatin (Mycostatin). It is not necessary to stop breast-feeding but it is possible to transfer the yeast infection to the mother's breast and reinfect the neonate if both are not treated. Careful hand hygiene after a diaper change is always appropriate. However, hand hygiene does not reduce the risk for thrush. (R)

72. 4 As the cervix softens and ripens, the cervical canal mucous plug is expelled. The cervical capillaries seep blood as a result of pressure exerted by the fetus. The blood, mixed with mucus, takes on a pink tinge and is referred to as *bloody show*. Cervical effacement and dilation is a process of labor; when complete, the cervix is 100% effaced and dilation is 10 cm. There is no indication the client has an infection, nor is this indication of hemorrhage. (M)

73. 1 Encouraging the parent-infant bonding is an important nursing intervention during the fourth stage of labor. Infants are in a quiet, alert stage for approximately 2 hr after delivery. This is an excellent time for parents-infant bonding. The discharge teaching, and teaching mother about newborn care are tasks for the following day. The newborn is given the first bath after the immediate 2-hr recovery period. (M)

74. 1 The client in stage two of labor is pushing. The client is instructed to push when the contraction occurs and to rest between the contractions. Pushing without contractions is ineffective and will tire the mother and fetus. The client is not given juice for energy at this stage in the labor process; the digestive tract is slowed during labor and this could cause her to have nausea and vomiting, or the client could have to have a cesarean section and should remain NPO. The goal of pushing is to push with each contraction, pushing 3 times and holding each for 10 s. If stage two is prolonged, the client may be instructed to stop pushing for a while to allow the infant to "labor down." The client is not advised to take a mild analgesic for discomfort; this could potentially place the infant at risk for respiratory depression if delivery occurs rapidly. (C)

75. 2 Increasing carbohydrate intake relieves nausea better than any other food. Consuming dry saltine crackers prior to rising relieves nausea for most women. Because the GI system is slower in pregnancy, the client is instructed to avoid lying down after meals and to not go longer than 12 hr between meals during pregnancy to prevent hypoglycemia. The nurse cautions clients about self-medicating for nausea by taking antacids; excessive use of antacids can cause fluid retention. (A)

SECTION 2

Nursing Care of Children

chapter 9

Introduction to Nursing Care of Children

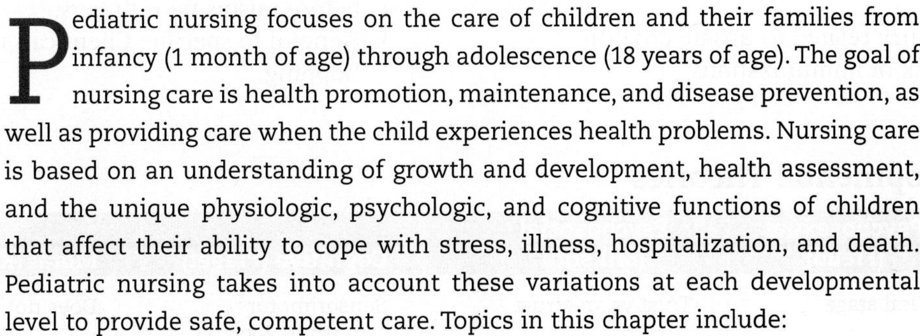

Pediatric nursing focuses on the care of children and their families from infancy (1 month of age) through adolescence (18 years of age). The goal of nursing care is health promotion, maintenance, and disease prevention, as well as providing care when the child experiences health problems. Nursing care is based on an understanding of growth and development, health assessment, and the unique physiologic, psychologic, and cognitive functions of children that affect their ability to cope with stress, illness, hospitalization, and death. Pediatric nursing takes into account these variations at each developmental level to provide safe, competent care. Topics in this chapter include:

- Background Information: Growth and Development
- Health Assessment
- Health Promotion
- Principles of Nursing Care Management

Background Information: Growth and Development

I. Definition
   A. Growth is an indicator of an increase in height, weight, and head circumference.
   B. Development is the predictable, progressive acquisition of motor and cognitive skills.
   C. There are several theories of growth and development related to cognition, psychosexual development, moral behavior, and psychosocial development. Tables 9-1 and 9-2 provide a summary of developmental theories.

II. Nursing process
   A. Assessment
      1. Assess for age-appropriate growth and development (see Table 9-4).
         a. Chronologic age
         b. Mental age: Cognitive level
         c. Developmental stage, using Denver Developmental Screening Test (Denver II)
            (1) For birth to 6 years of age
            (2) Assesses gross motor, fine motor, language, and social development
      2. Assess parent's level of understanding of developmental and physical needs.
   B. Analysis
      1. Risk for Delayed Growth and Development related to parental lack of knowledge
      2. Risk for Deficient Knowledge related to lack of information about age-appropriate growth and development
      3. Risk for Infection related to lack of immunizations
      4. Risk for Injury related to unsafe environment or lack of immunizations
   C. Planning
      1. Identify reason for health visit.
      2. Assess growth and development.
      3. Provide health teaching to child and parents.
      4. Provide anticipatory guidance.
      5. Provide written information sheets.
   D. Implementation
      1. Provide parents with information and guidance about each developmental stage and ways to promote progression.
      2. Assess and promote normal growth and development.
      3. Teach parents about safety issues.
      4. Ensure adequate immunization compliance.
   E. Evaluation
      1. Child exhibits normal, predictive patterns of growth and development.
      2. Parents verbalize understanding of normal growth and development and ways to promote progression.
      3. Parents verbalize an understanding of developmental safety issues as evidenced by choosing age-appropriate toys.
      4. Child receives all recommended immunizations, and communicable diseases and injuries are prevented.

CN

III. Client needs
   A. Physiologic adaptation: Growth progresses in a predictable pattern.
      1. Head to toe (cephalocaudal): Client can hold head up before sitting up.
      2. Center of body to fingertips (proximodistal): Client can grasp rattle with hand before raisins with fingers.
      3. General to specific: Client can walk before hopping.

Table 9-1 Developmental Theories

Age Group	Psychosexual (Freud)	Psychosocial (Erikson)	Cognitive (Piaget)	Moral (Kohlberg)
Infant (birth to 1 year)	Oral stage	Trust vs. mistrust	Sensorimotor (birth to 2 years)	Does not apply
Toddler (1 to 3 years)	Anal stage	Autonomy vs. shame and doubt	Sensorimotor to preoperational	Preconventional level
Preschool (3 to 6 years)	Phallic stage	Initiative vs. guilt	Preoperational (2 to 7 years)	Preconventional level
School age (6 to 12 years)	Latency stage	Industry vs. inferiority	Concrete operations (7 to 11 years)	Conventional level
Adolescent (12 to 18 years)	Genital stage	Identity vs. role confusion	Formal operations (12 to 15 years)	Postconventional level

Table 9-2 Characteristics of Developmental Theories

Age Group	Psychosexual (Freud)	Psychosocial (Erikson)	Cognitive (Piaget)	Moral (Kohlberg)
Infant	Oral activity brings pleasure	Develops trust as needs are met	Moves from reflex to imitative behavior; object permanence develops	Does not apply
Toddler	Controls through toilet training	Learns to control body functions	Egocentric; magical thinking	Morals are external
Preschool	Interested in genitalia; fears genital mutilation	Begins to learn through play; conscience	Egocentric; magical thinking	Morals are external
School Age	Playing and learning	Wants to succeed; develops friends; seeks praise	Thought is logical; inductive reasoning	Conformity and loyalty
Adolescent	Genital organs become a source of tension; interested in friends	Peers important; establishes identity and independence	Thought flexible; reasoning abstract	Defines moral values and principles

B. Management of care: Care of the child and family needing anticipatory guidance requires critical thinking skills and knowledge of assessment, teaching and evaluation unique to the RN role. The following skills cannot be delegated to an LPN or UAP.
   1. Provide child and family teaching about the following:
      a. Purpose, dosage, and timing of scheduled immunizations (see pharmacologic and parenteral therapies)
      b. Risks and benefits of vaccines
      c. Vaccine side effects and how to manage with acetaminophen (Tylenol) and ice to injection site
   2. Document immunizations.
   3. Administer atraumatically.
   4. Delegate responsibly those activities that can be delegated, including measurements, oral intake and urine output, and vital signs. All monitoring information is reported to the RN.

C. Safety and infection control
   1. Provide parents with information about normal developmental expectations.
   2. Provide anticipatory guidance for injury prevention (see Table 9-1).
   3. Teach parents to provide developmentally appropriate and safe toys (Table 9-3).
   4. Provide parents with adequate information and support to maintain immunization schedule.

D. Health promotion and maintenance: Assist parents in understanding and identifying stages of growth and development, including physical, gross and fine motor development, language, and play. Table 9-4 provides a summary of growth and development.

E. Psychologic integrity
   1. Offer encouragement and support for maintaining and promoting child's health.
   2. Allow opportunities for child and family to express developmental concerns, fears, and to ask questions.

F. Basic care and comfort: Provide consistent nurse caregiver to establish trust.

G. Reduction of risk potential
   1. Monitor health supervision schedule.
      a. Head circumference until 2 years of age
      b. Height and weight yearly until 18 years of age

Table 9-3 Developmentally Safe Toys

Age	Toys
Birth to 6 Months	Mobiles and musical mobiles; small-handled rattle; stuffed animal; infant swing
6 to 12 Months	Colorful blocks; cup and spoon; teething toys; squeeze toys
1 to 3 Years	Push-pull toys; rocking horse; sand box toys; housekeeping toys (such as play kitchens, dishes, or child-sized garden tools)
3 to 5 Years	Tricycle; dress-up clothes; jigsaw puzzles; blackboard, chalk; grooming toys

Table 9-4 Stages of Growth and Development

Age	Physical	Gross Motor	Fine Motor	Language	Play
0 to 4 Months	Posterior fontanel closes at 2 months; obligatory nose breather	Lifts head when prone; primitive reflexes begin to fade by 4 months; rolls from back to side at 4 months	By 4 months, can grasp object and bring to mouth	By 4 months, laughs and babbles	Smiles at 2 months; shows excitement with body
4 to 8 Months	Birth weight doubles by 6 months; teeth eruption beginning	Head control; can turn from back to abdomen; can sit unsupported by 8 months	Moves from palmar grasp to beginning pincer grasp	Begins to imitate sounds; can make a few vowel and consonant sounds	Begins to recognize strangers; object permanence beginning; plays peek-a-boo
8 to 12 Months	Birth weight triples by 12 months; head and chest circumference equal; may have six to eight teeth	Begins to creep on knees; by 12 months can walk with hand held; can sit from standing position	By 12 months can release object, can turn pages of book	Can say three to five words in addition to "mama" or "dada;" understands simple commands	Has object permanence; has transitional object such as security blanket
12 to 15 Months	Steady growth	Walks alone	Builds tower with two cubes; uses cup well	Says four to six words; points to express wants	Imitates housework; begins to manage spoon; has temper tantrums
15 to 24 Months	Physiologic anorexia; anterior fontanel closed by 18 months	Runs but falls; throws ball overhand	Builds tower with three to four cubes; release and reach developed	Says 10 words; can identify object by pointing	Uses spoon well; begins to take off clothes
2 Years	One-half adult height	Goes up and down stairs; runs with wide stance	Builds tower of six to seven cubes; can unscrew lids	Has vocabulary of 300 words; uses two- and three-word phrases	Parallel play; dresses in simple clothes
3 to 4 Years	Has 20 teeth; has bladder and bowel control	Jumps; rides tricycle; can skip and hop on one foot by 4 years	Builds tower of 9 to 10 blocks; can copy and circle	By 4 years has 1,500-word vocabulary; begins to name colors	Dresses and feeds self; fears are beginning; play becomes associative; imaginary playmates emerge
5 to 6 Years	May lose first tooth; permanent teeth begin; hand dominance established	Skips and hops on either foot; jumps rope; walks backward heel to toe; can count	Ties shoelaces; uses scissors and pencil; uses knife to spread jam	Vocabulary of 2,100 words; uses six- to eight-word sentences with all grammar parts	Fears are decreasing; begins to use rules; manners developing

(Continued)

Table 9-4 Stages of Growth and Development *(Continued)*

Age	Physical	Gross Motor	Fine Motor	Language	Play
7 to 9 Years	Begins to grow 5 cm per year	Concept of time developed; describes objects; begins to collect	Uses table knife to cut; helps with routine housework	Reads books	Group play; more social; very modest
10 to 12 Years	Boys: Growth slows Girls: May begin pubescent changes	Uses telephone; writes stories; understands there is a world outside of home	Cooks or sews; can care for pet; can perform own grooming	Reads for practical information; enjoys library books	Friends important; more diplomatic; demonstrates affection
12 to 18 Years	Rapid acceleration in growth; mature growth by 17 to 20 years; develops secondary sex characteristics	Motor skills mature	Fine motor skills mature	Abstract thought; enjoys intellectual ideas	Acceptance by peers important; seeks identity

c. BP screening beginning at 2 years of age
d. Hip dislocation assessment until 1 year of age
e. Vision screening beginning at birth and then again at 2 years of age
f. Dental visits beginning at 30 months of age

2. Provide child and family teaching.
   a. Common side effects: Redness and swelling at injection site; drowsiness, fever, rash, and diarrhea
   b. Contraindications to administer vaccine, including:
      (1) High fever
      (2) Immunosuppression from chemotherapy or long-term steroid use: No live virus vaccines such as measles, mumps, rubella, and varicella
      (3) Allergies to vaccine contents (e.g., eggs)

H. Pharmacologic and parenteral therapies: Table 9-5 shows the 2007 general immunization guidelines approved by the American Academy of Pediatrics, Advisory Committee on Immunization Practices (http://www.cdc.gov/nip/recs/child-schedule.htm). Review the Web site for updated information as needed. Scheduled immunizations include the following:
1. Hepatitis A vaccine
2. Hepatitis B vaccine
3. Diphtheria and tetanus toxoid and acellular pertussis vaccine (DTaP) or tetanus toxoid and diphtheria and acellular pertussis (Tdap)
4. *Haemophilus influenzae* type B (HIB) vaccine
5. Inactivated poliovirus vaccine (IPV)
6. Measles, mumps, rubella (MMR) vaccine
7. Varicella virus vaccine
8. Pneumococcal vaccine
9. Rotavirus vaccine

Table 9-5 Immunization Guidelines

Age	Immunization
Birth	Hepatitis B
1 to 4 Months	Hepatitis B
2 Months	DTaP, HIB, IPV, pneumococcal (PCV), rotavirus
4 Months	DTaP, HIB, IPV, pneumococcal (PCV), rotavirus
6 Months	DTaP, pneumococcal (PCV), rotavirus
6 to 18 Months	Hepatitis B, IPV, influenzae (yearly)
12 to 15 Months	HIB, MMR, pneumococcal (PCV), hepatitis A, varicella
15 to 18 Months	DTaP
4 to 6 Years	DTaP, IPV, MMR, varicella
11 to 18 Years	Tdap, meningococcal vaccine (MCV4), HPV

10. Human papilloma virus vaccine (HPV)
11. Meningococcal virus vaccine (MCV)

Health Assessment

I. Definition: Health assessment is completed on a regular schedule to ensure optimum wellness and illness prevention for children. The head-to-toe sequence of health and physical assessment is altered to meet the child's developmental needs.

II. Nursing process
   A. Assessment
      1. Obtain a detailed health history of family and child, including allergies, cognitive level, developmental stage, and immunization schedule.
      2. Assess vital signs, weight and height, body mass index (BMI), head circumference for infants up to 2 years, and complete a comprehensive physical assessment including:
         a. Growth measurements
         b. Physiologic measurements
         c. General appearance
         d. Head-to-toe assessment
      3. Obtain diagnostic tests.
         a. Hemoglobin and hematocrit
         b. Lead level
         c. Urinalysis
         d. Tuberculosis screening
         e. Vision and hearing screening
   B. Analysis: Health-Seeking Behaviors: Wellness visit related to parental desire for ongoing screening
   C. Planning
      1. Complete assessment; provide parental feedback and teaching.
      2. Reduce anxiety.
      3. Promote trust.
   D. Implementation (see management of care)
   E. Evaluation
      1. Child cooperates with the examination as a result of approach to assessment.
      2. Parents understand reasons for health assessments.

CN

III. Client needs
   A. Physiologic adaptation: Physical assessment is completed without producing stress for the child, and obtaining reliable and accurate data.
   B. Management of care: Care of the child and family needing anticipatory guidance requires critical thinking skills and knowledge of assessment, teaching and evaluation unique to the RN role. These skills cannot be delegated to an LPN or UAP.
      1. Perform comprehensive physical assessment (see assessment section).
      2. Provide parents with feedback and anticipatory guidance.
      3. Delegate responsibly those activities that can be delegated, including measurements, oral intake and urine output, and vital signs. All monitoring information is reported to the RN.
   C. Safety and infection control
      1. Keep temperature device in place long enough to obtain accurate measurement.
      2. Assess apical pulse for infants and small children, and radial pulse in children over 2 years of age.
      3. Assure correct size of BP cuff—for child: Three-fourths the size of the extremity.
      4. Monitor child response to examination of ears (can be very traumatic); position and restrain if necessary.
   D. Health promotion and maintenance (see psychologic integrity)
   E. Psychologic integrity
      1. Alter sequence of the physical assessment to minimize stress and anxiety (e.g., complete invasive and painful procedures last) and promote compliance; foster trust to obtain reliable information.
      2. Observe child for cues to readiness.
      3. Examine child in secure position, such as parent's lap.
      4. Reassure child throughout assessment.
      5. Praise child for cooperation.
      6. Use dolls, stuffed animals, or games.
      7. Provide privacy for older children.
   F. Basic care and comfort: Provide consistent nurse caregiver to develop trust.
   G. Reduction of risk potential: Maintain a schedule of health visits for early identification of deviations from normal growth and development.

Health Promotion

I. Definition: Health promotion seeks to promote growth and prevent problems in children through education and anticipatory guidance. Health promotion also includes involving the family in education.

II. Nursing process
   A. Assessment: Health promotion begins with an assessment of strengths and problems related to development, nutrition, immunizations, safety, socialization, and family relationships. Assessment for health promotion behaviors includes observing the following:
      1. Feeding habits
      2. Sleep-wake patterns

3. Dental care and hygiene
4. Play
5. Safety interventions
6. Wellness visits

B. Analysis
   1. Risk for Impaired Parent/Infant/Child Attachment related to developmental delays
   2. Readiness for Enhanced Family Coping related to improved health promotion
   3. Health-Seeking Behaviors: Wellness visit related to parental desire for health promotion
   4. Risk for Injury related to developmental age and stage
   5. Risk for Imbalanced Nutrition: More Than Body Requirements related to poor eating habits

C. Planning
   1. Provide parental teaching.
   2. Provide anticipatory guidance.

D. Implementation (see management of care)

E. Evaluation
   1. Parents verbalize an understanding of health promotion needs for the child.
   2. Child remains free of injury as evidenced by practicing age-appropriate safety such as car and bike safety.
   3. Child maintains appropriate growth for age.

CN

III. Client needs

A. Physiologic adaptation: Ethnic practices are adapted to child's health needs.

B. Management of care: Care of the child and family needing anticipatory guidance requires critical thinking skills and knowledge of assessment, and teaching and evaluation methods unique to the RN role. These skills cannot be delegated to an LPN or UAP.
   1. Delegate responsibly those activities that can be delegated, including measurements, oral intake and urine output, vital signs, and reporting child's subjective data. All monitoring information is reported to the RN.
   2. Provide parental teaching about nutritional needs, dental care, sleep patterns, safety interventions, discipline, and health care visits.
   3. Provide health promotion interventions to:
      a. Identify teaching needs.
      b. Attain and maintain health.
      c. Provide family-centered care.
      d. Provide culturally appropriate care.
      e. Assure health-appropriate forage, stage of development, and cognitive level.

C. Safety and infection control
   1. Teach parents about car safety: Appropriate car seat, use of restraints, and placement in car.
   2. Teach parents about behavioral changes that may occur and how to manage them.
   3. Teach parents how to implement home safety.

D. Health promotion and maintenance
   1. Assess influences on health promotion.
      a. Cultural influences, including health beliefs, health practices, family relationship, and communication
      b. Religious influences, including beliefs about life, food practices, and medical care
      c. Socioeconomic influences, including social class and economic level
      d. Family influences, including structure, function, roles, and parenting abilities
      e. Hereditary influences, including genetics and disorders
   2. Promote health through:
      a. Nutrition (Table 9-6)
      b. Sleep and activity
      c. Dental health
      d. Immunizations
      e. Injury prevention
      f. Anticipatory guidance

E. Psychologic integrity
   1. Allow parents the opportunity to express fears, fatigue, frustration, and anger about childrearing and health maintenance.
   2. Provide parents with ideas, suggestions, and information related to discipline.

F. Basic care and comfort
   1. Provide consistent caregiver that fosters trust for child and family.
   2. Perform history and physical assessment in age-appropriate ways.
      a. Infant: Suggest infant remain on parent's lap
      b. Toddler: Engage toddler with distracting toys; may remain on parent's lap
      c. Preschool: May want parents close by
      d. School-aged child: Allow privacy and participation
      e. Adolescent: May want parents to leave

G. Reduction of risk potential
   1. Provide culturally competent care of children.
   2. Understand the influences on health promotion.
   3. Perform prenatal screening to identify children at risk.
   4. Screen at each visit to identify children at risk.
   5. Promote genetic counseling.

Table 9-6 Nutritional Needs and Anticipatory Guidance

Age Group	Nutrition	Injury Prevention
Infant	• Breast vs. bottle: Breast-fed needs iron supplement after 4 months • Foods introduced one at a time for 4 to 7 days • At 1 year, whole milk until age 2	• No propping of bottles • Proper car seats • Crib rails up • Check bath temperature • Check formula temperature • Do not microwave breast milk • Cover outlets • No walkers
Toddler	• Give finger foods • Avoid foods such as hot dogs, nuts, and candy that may be aspirated • Physiologic anorexia • No more than 24 oz of milk/day • Ritualistic, wants same cup and bowl	• Switch to bed if climbing out of crib • Locks on cabinets with hazardous materials • Never leave near water, such as pool or bath • Toys should have no small parts • Gates on stairs
Preschool	• Food preferences • Begin to use food pyramid for nutrition • Limit fruit juices • Manners develop	• Street and bicycle safety: Use of helmets; car seats • Parents should practice good safety, children imitate • Stranger safety • Animal safety
School Age	• Caloric needs decrease • Balanced diet • Teach how to choose healthy diet	• Proper use of seat belts • Safety apparel for sports • Teach to swim • Fire safety • Cooking safety • Stranger safety
Adolescent	• Accelerated growth • Double needs for calcium, zinc, and protein • Obesity can be an issue	• Car safety • Sex education • Smoking, drug, and alcohol education

Principles of Nursing Care Management

I. Definition: Approaching and preparing children for procedures is an integral part of pediatric nursing. Preparation of children is achieved with consideration to developmental and cognitive abilities, coping strategies, and previous health care experiences.

II. Nursing process

A. Assessment
1. Assess parents' and child's understanding of procedure.
2. Assess developmental and cognitive level of child.
3. Complete detailed health history and physical assessment.

B. Analysis
1. Anxiety related to fears and strange environment
2. Health-Seeking Behaviors: Procedures, related to altered health status
3. Deficient Knowledge: Procedures, related to lack of information about procedure
4. Risk for Noncompliance related to lack of information or fears about procedure

C. Planning: Prepare children for procedures with the following goals:
1. Decrease anxiety.
2. Maintain coping skills.
3. Elicit cooperation.
4. Provide information.
5. Promote compliance.

D. Implementation (see management of care)

E. Evaluation
1. Child has decreased anxiety as evidenced by cooperation during procedure.
2. Child and family verbalize an understanding of procedure and possible outcomes.

CN

III. Client needs

A. Physiologic adaptation: Child and family are adequately prepared for procedure using age-appropriate and developmentally appropriate techniques to reduce anxiety, develop trust, promote cooperation, and enhance coping skills.

B. Management of care: Care of the child and family needing anticipatory guidance requires critical thinking skills and knowledge of assessment, and teaching and evaluation methods unique to the RN role. These skills cannot be delegated to an LPN or UAP.

1. Delegate responsibly those activities that can be delegated, including measurements, oral intake and urine output, and vital signs. All monitoring information must be reported to the RN.
2. Provide child and family teaching.
3. Provide appropriate emotional support and comfort during and after the procedure.

C. Safety and infection control
1. Provide teaching based on child's level of understanding, developmental age, and cognitive level.
2. Provide teaching in an age-appropriate time frame, using concrete terms and visual aides.
3. Emphasize the sensory component, such as feeling cold, and techniques for coping, such as counting.
4. Allow child to handle miniatures of equipment or actual equipment (if appropriate) to practice techniques.

D. Health promotion and maintenance: Prepare children for procedures and provide health teaching based on developmental stage. Table 9-7 provides a summary of developmentally appropriate techniques.
1. To promote ambulation:
   a. Provide a push toy.
   b. Take doll for walk.
2. To increase fluid intake:
   a. Use small medicine cups.
   b. Play games such as having a tea party.
3. To encourage deep breathing and coughing:
   a. Blow bubbles or whistles.
   b. Practice blowing out birthday candles.

Table 9-7 Preparation of Children for Health Teaching According to Developmental Stage

Age	Reduce Anxiety	Thought	Fears	Control	Psychosocial Stage
Infant	Use sensory soothing.	Older infants have memory: Avoid performing painful procedures in crib (maintains safe place). Touch is helpful.	Recognizes strangers at 9 months. Keep frightening objects away from view. Advance slowly.	May need to restrain.	Involve parent or consistent caregiver.
Toddler	Use distraction. Use firm approach.	Explain what child will see, hear, smell, feel at time of procedure. Give permission to cry.	Keep frightening objects away from view.	May resist; try distraction.	Allow choices and participation.
Preschool	Praise for helping.	Explain in simple terms. Use neutral words. Use play to demonstrate.	Keep frightening objects away from view. Bandage over puncture sites.	Allow to wear underpants if possible.	Give choices and praise to reinforce that procedure or treatment is not punishment.
School Age	Offer praise. Allow for questions. Provide privacy.	Use correct language. Explain reasons. Allow handling of equipment.	Fears being unsuccessful. Tell what to expect.	Encourage deep breathing or relaxation.	Include in decisions and allow to participate.
Adolescent	Provide privacy. Encourage questions.	Understands death and disability. Explain outcomes. Encourage questions.	Discuss body image changes. Explain benefits of procedure.	Try to minimize restrictions. Allow a sense of control.	Encourage talking with peers who have had same procedure. Involve in decisions.

4. For range of motion exercises:
   a. Throw soft foam balls.
   b. Ride tricycle.
   c. Pull doll in wagon.
5. To obtain cooperation with injections or IV starts:
   a. Let child play with syringe (no needles).
   b. Teach to count through injection.
   c. Let practice injecting doll or stuffed animal.

E. Psychologic integrity
1. Allow parents at bedside during procedure, if appropriate.
2. Do not lie: Offer information on painful or anxiety-provoking issues such as starting IV last.
3. Encourage expression of fears, anxieties, and concerns and offer opportunities to ask questions.
4. Reinforce positive aspects such as not being ill any more.
5. Offer praise to reinforce self-esteem.

F. Basic care and comfort
1. Provide consistent nurse caregiver to promote trust and cooperation.
2. Use appropriate sedation and analgesia.

Bibliography

American Academy of Pediatrics, Advisory Committee on Immunization Practices. Retrieved from: http://www.cdc.gov/nip/recs/child-schedule.htm. Retrieved May 6, 2008.

Hatfield, N. (2006). *Broadribb's introductory pediatric nursing.* Philadelphia: Lippincott Williams & Wilkins.

Pillitteri, A. (2006). *Maternal & child health nursing: Care of the childbearing and childrearing family* (5th ed.). Philadelphia: Lippincott Williams & Wilkins.

Wong, D. L., et al. (2006). *Maternal child nursing care.* St. Louis: Mosby.

CHAPTER 9

Practice Test

Growth and Development

1. Two toddlers are playing with a stuffed animal when one child suddenly grabs the toy from the other child. The nurse should:
- □ 1. Find a second, similar toy for the toddlers to play with.
- □ 2. Take no action. Let the toddlers work it out.
- □ 3. Remove the stuffed toy.
- □ 4. Refer the child who grabs to a clinical psychologist.

2. The nurse is assessing a child who is 5 years of age. The child is able to draw a person with only six body parts, can draw a square, but can name only six colors. The child is able to walk well, hop using both feet, but is unable to balance on each foot for 3 s. The nurse should:
- □ 1. Document the findings as normal.
- □ 2. Notify the physician because gross motor skills are delayed.
- □ 3. Provide activities that will enhance the delayed gross motor skills.
- □ 4. Refer the infant to an early childhood development program.

3. A client who is 16 years of age and who has been confined to a wheelchair since early childhood has lately been acting rebellious and rude. Her parents ask the nurse, "Are all adolescents like this?" The nurse should respond with which of the following statements?
- □ 1. "Yes, although your daughter's behaviors are more like those of an adolescent boy."
- □ 2. "No. Your daughter must need some help in dealing with her feelings."
- □ 3. "Your daughter's behavior seems to be typical adolescent behavior. Let's talk more about it."
- □ 4. "Your daughter's behavior results from feelings about her disability: ignore them."

4. The parents of an adolescent boy are concerned about the amount of sleep he seems to require. The nurse should advise the parents:
- □ 1. "As long as he seems otherwise well, this sounds like a typical teenager."
- □ 2. "Adolescents need only 8 hours of sleep a night; anything over this is excessive."
- □ 3. "Your son is probably engaged in too many activities and is wearing himself out."
- □ 4. "Your son may be taking drugs; the side effect of many drugs is to cause sleepiness."

5. The nurse is conducting a health assessment on an infant who is 2 months of age. The infant smiles and laughs out loud, is able to lift the head to 45 degrees when in a prone position, but is unable to lift the head to 90 degrees. The infant is also unable to roll from a prone position to a supine position. The nurse should:

- □ 1. Document the findings as normal.
- □ 2. Notify the health care provider (HCP) because gross motor skills are delayed.
- □ 3. Suggest the parents provide activities that will enhance the delayed fine motor skills.
- □ 4. Refer the infant to the community's early childhood development program.

6. The nurse is assessing the growth and development of a child who is 13 months of age. The nurse determines that the child is able to wave "bye-bye," bang two cubes together when held in the hands, and can cruise along furniture. However, the child does not say any other words other than "mama" and "dada" and is unable to walk. The nurse should:

- □ 1. Document the findings as normal.
- □ 2. Notify the HCP because gross motor skills are delayed.
- □ 3. Provide activities that will enhance the delayed fine motor skills.
- □ 4. Refer the child to an early childhood development program.

Health Assessment

7. A mother brings her infant who is 6 months of age to the clinic for a well-child visit. The infant's birth weight was 8 lb 3 oz. The nurse weighs the infant and finds that the infant now weighs 11 lb 8 oz. The nurse should:

- □ 1. Notify the HCP.
- □ 2. Document the weight, as it is normal.
- □ 3. Discuss appropriate finger foods that the infant can eat.
- □ 4. Notify the parents that this infant weighs more than expected.

8. The nurse is assessing a 3-month-old infant with a head injury for increased intracranial pressure. On palpation of the fontanels, the nurse notes that the anterior fontanel has not closed and is soft and flat. The nurse should first:

- □ 1. Document the finding.
- □ 2. Notify the physician.
- □ 3. Increase oral fluids.
- □ 4. Elevate the head of the bed.

9. The nurse is conducting a health assessment of a child who is 15 months of age. The child has two teeth present in the mouth, which are pearly white and in the upper central incisor position. The nurse should:

- □ 1. Document the finding.
- □ 2. Instruct parents on proper oral care.
- □ 3. Refer the child to the HCP.
- □ 4. Stress the importance of drinking whole milk at this age.

10. The nurse is conducting neurologic assessment on a hospitalized client who is 8 months of age. The child has a positive plantar grasp reflex, but the Moro response, palmar grasp, and the tonic neck response are absent. The nurse should:

- □ 1. Do nothing; this is an expected finding.
- □ 2. Notify the HCP.
- □ 3. Include the findings in the next shift report.
- □ 4. Reassess the infant in 2 hr.

11. AF For the most accurate measurement of height for a child younger than 24 months of age, the nurse measures the child in which of the following ways? Select all that apply.

- □ 1. Supine position.
- □ 2. Prone position.
- □ 3. Standing position.
- □ 4. Shoes removed.
- □ 5. Clothes removed.
- □ 6. Fully extending the body.
- □ 7. Body in an upright position with shoes on.

12. AF The nurse is to obtain a urine specimen from a child who is 2 years of age and hospitalized with a urinary tract infection. In what order should the nurse perform the following steps? Place in order from first to last.

_____ 1. Cleanse the genital area.
_____ 2. Apply gloves.
_____ 3. Offer fluids.
_____ 4. Apply collection bag.

Health Promotion

13. The nurse is developing an education program for school-aged children. Which of the following topics is appropriate for this age group?

- □ 1. The importance of crossing streets safely.
- □ 2. The value of having immunizations.
- □ 3. How to prevent communicable disease.
- □ 4. The need to participate in exercise programs.

14. The nurse is teaching a group of children who are 8 years of age about eating well-balanced meals. Which of the following strategies will be most effective with this group of children?

- □ 1. Explain the basics of the food pyramid and give a short quiz to be sure the children understand.

- □ 2. Ask the children to make a list of what they had to eat during the week and check the foods that are not healthy.
- □ 3. Have the children draw their favorite foods and then follow up with what foods are healthy.
- □ 4. Use visual aids to demonstrate basic food groups and ask the children to match the foods with the food group.

15. The nurse is counseling an overweight child who is 10 years of age about weight loss. The nurse should instruct the child about which of the following?

- □ 1. The importance of diet and exercise to her future health.
- □ 2. The components of a high-protein, low-carbohydrate diet.
- □ 3. Ways to reduce calories and increase exercise.
- □ 4. The makeup of a vegetarian diet.

16. AF The parents of a child who is 10 years of age are concerned because the child does not eat breakfast before leaving for school. The nurse should advise the parents to do which of the following? Select all that apply.

- □ 1. Provide high-protein food that the child could take for breakfast, to be eaten on the school bus.
- □ 2. Limit privileges if a complete breakfast is not eaten.
- □ 3. Act as role models by eating breakfast themselves.
- □ 4. Encourage the child to collect prizes from cereal she eats.
- □ 5. Have the child set the alarm clock earlier so there is time for breakfast.

Principles of Nursing Care Management

17. A nurse is planning care for a hospitalized child who is 10 years of age, and is delegating care to a pediatric care assistant. When a nurse delegates a task to a UAP, which of the following is most important?

- □ 1. The nurse has observed the UAP perform the task.
- □ 2. The child and UAP have established a positive relationship.
- □ 3. The task is appropriate for that individual's preparation.
- □ 4. The UAP has previously performed the task.

18. Which technique is most effective in encouraging a preschooler to take fluids by mouth?

- □ 1. Develop a chart for her to check off after she has taken five glasses of fluid.
- □ 2. Promise a reward for complying with drinking fluids.
- □ 3. Leave her favorite drink at the bedside to drink when thirsty.
- □ 4. Play "tea party" and drinking "tea" with imaginary friends.

19. AF A child who is 4 years of age is admitted to the hospital for surgery. The parents are visiting prior to surgery. Before administering the preoperative medicine, the nurse identifies the client by doing which of the following? Select all that apply.

- □ 1. Call the child's name and see if he answers.
- □ 2. Read the child's name on the armband.
- □ 3. Ask the child to state his name.
- □ 4. Ask the parents to verify the type of surgery he is to have.
- □ 5. Check the child's medical record number against the number on his armband.

20. A preschooler becomes very frightened when nursing staff approaches to change the dressing over an open appendectomy incision. What response by the nurse is most correct?

- □ 1. Allow the preschooler to participate in the dressing change.
- □ 2. Provide details regarding the surgical procedure so the child has a better understanding.
- □ 3. Discuss with the child some of the possible fears that he may be having.
- □ 4. Ask one to two other staff members to help restrain the child during the procedure.

Answers and Rationales

1. 1 The solitary play of infancy progresses to *parallel* play in which the toddler plays alongside, not with, other children. The toddler will tend to inspect the toy, talk to it, test its strength, and will often invent several uses for it. Toddlers are egocentric at this time so taking items from peers can be considered normal. Toddlers like to play with "like" toys next to each other; they do not necessarily like to interact with each other, but prefer to observe how the other is playing. Preschoolers enjoy *associative* play, which focuses on group play in similar activities but without strict rules. (A)

2. 3 A child who is 5 years of age can be expected to draw a person with six body parts (90% by 5½ years old) and to draw a square. Naming six colors is appropriate for this age. That this child can walk well and hop is developmentally appropriate. Most children (90% by 5 years of age) can balance on each foot for 3 s. This delay is not overly significant, but gross motor activities such as skipping, hopping, and running should be discussed with the parents because these activities will strengthen the large muscles of the lower extremities. (H)

3. 3 It is normal behavior for adolescents to assert independence and begin to separate from their parents; the behavior is not changed by their daughter's disability, nor is it unique to a girl. The nurse offers reassurance to the parents and then opens the conversation for additional discussion. (H)

4. 1 Many teenagers feel fatigued from a combination of fast-food diets, many activities, and a rapid growth spurt; this is normal behavior and the nurse should explain possible reasons for the sleep pattern. Adolescents may need more than 8 hr of sleep. There are no data to suggest that activities are tiring this teenager. It is not appropriate to suggest the child is taking drugs based on the question the parents are asking the nurse. (H)

5. 1 At 2 months of age, the nurse can expect an infant to laugh, smile, turn the head from side to side when prone, and lift the head momentarily from a surface to 45 degrees. Lifting the head to 90 degrees is expected by 90% of infants by 4 months of age. The infant is not expected to roll from stomach to back until approximately 4 months of age, and then back to stomach at 5 months of age. (H)

6. 1 Some children will walk well by 11 months of age, while others may not walk well until almost 15 months of age; this is considered normal. At 13 months of age, it is still normal to only be saying mama and dada (specific to the parents). Ninety percent of toddlers will have added at least one other word than mama and dada to their vocabulary by 15 months of age, while some 13-month-olds will have six words at this age; again, this is considered normal. (H)

7. 1 The nurse notifies the HCP because this infant's weight is below the 5th percentile rile on the growth chart. This child fits the criteria for failure to thrive (FTT). The nurse can expect the infant's birth weight to double by approximately 6 months of age and to approximately triple by 1 year of age. Finger foods are not appropriate until the pincer grasp is present, which typically happens closer to 9 months of age. (H)

8. 1 The anterior fontanel typically closes between 12 and 18 months of age. The nurse expects the normal finding to be flat and soft. A bulging, firm fontanel may suggest an increase in the intracranial pressure or fluid overload. A sunken, depressed fontanel may suggest dehydration for the infant. (M)

9. 3 The age of tooth eruption shows considerable variation among children, but the order of the eruption is relatively regular and predictable. The first teeth to erupt are the lower central incisors; this occurs between 6 and 10 months of age. The upper central incisors erupt between 8 to 12 months of age. The lower lateral incisors erupt between 10 and 16 months of age. The upper lateral incisors erupt between 9 and 13 months of age. The order of eruption is more important than the exact months of eruption. This child is missing the expected lower central incisors; therefore, the HCP is notified because an early dental consult may be warranted. Some reasons for missing lower central incisors include a cyst may be blocking the eruption, there may not be teeth present to erupt, or a congenital syndrome may be present that is linked to the absence of dentition. (H)

10. 1 The newborn infant has many primitive reflexes. The times at which the reflexes appear and disappear reflect the maturity of the developing nervous system. The plantar grasp is expected to be present at 8 months of age. The Moro response is absent by 6 months of age if neurologic maturation is not delayed. The tonic neck response disappears by 3 to 4 months of age. The palmar grasp lessens by 3 to 4 months of age. (H)

11. 1, 4, 6 Until children are 24 months of age (36 months of age if the birth-to-36-month chart is used), measure recumbent length. Because of the normally flexed position during infancy, fully extend the body by holding the head in midline, grasping the knees together gently, and pushing down on the knees until the legs are fully extended and flat against the table. Shoes should be removed. Clothes do not need to be removed to assess an accurate height. Normally, height is less if measured in the afternoon than in the morning. To minimize this occurrence, place modest pressure under the jaw or the mastoid processes behind the ears. (H)

12. 3, 2, 1, 4 When obtaining a urine specimen from an infant, the nurse assists the client to drink fluids 30 to 60 min prior to specimen collection so the client voids as soon as possible after the collection bag is applied. Next, the nurse applies gloves, and then cleanses the genital area with sterile water to prevent contamination of the urine. Finally, the nurse applies the collection bag and then removes the bag when the specimen is obtained. (M)

13. 1 Motor vehicle accidents are a leading cause of death among school-aged children. Immunizations should have been administered during early childhood. This age group is not at high risk for communicable diseases, particularly if they have had immunizations. Exercise, while important to preventing childhood obesity, is not the highest health risk for this group. (S)

14. 4 School-aged children are concrete thinkers so they respond best to concrete examples such as visual aids and matching. The children in this age group will not learn from a quiz, and likely cannot recall the foods they had to eat during the week. Having the children draw, while an active strategy, does not provide the needed information about health foods. (H)

15. 3 The best approach to maintaining weight and preventing excessive weight gain is to both reduce calories and increase exercise. The nurse also assists the child to learn specific strategies that will be realistic for the child to implement. The other instructions are too general and will not contribute to the intended outcome of weight loss. (H)

16. 1, 3, 5 There are several ways that the parents can help a child have breakfast before going to school. The child can take a nutrition bar or other high-protein snack to eat on the bus. Role modeling is also important in building good nutritional habits, as other aspects of the child's life, and the parents should serve and eat a breakfast. The parents can also encourage the child to have sufficient time in the morning to eat. The other options reinforce inappropriate eating habits. (H)

17. 3 Tasks that the UAP can undertake vary greatly. The nurse must be aware of the scope of the UAP's preparation and the policies of the health care agency. The important consideration is that the task is appropriate for that individual and is within the guidelines for practice at the health care agency. The UAP can perform complicated tasks within the scope of the preparation. Although the nurse observes the UAP and evaluates the UAP on his or her ability to perform the task, the most important aspect of delegation is to delegate within the UAP's educational preparation. A positive relationship with clients, while desirable, is not essential to delegation. Delegation involves giving clear directions and following up after the task has been delegated. (M)

18. 4 Preschoolers have active imaginations and can be enticed to take fluids by playing games. Preschoolers are not able to count effectively or take responsibility for drinking on their own. Offering rewards for this behavior (drinking fluid) teaches the child to expect rewards for other behaviors. (C)

19. 2, 5 Prior to administering medications, the nurse uses two sources of identification. The best sources are the name band and the chart record number on the armband. Children may answer to the wrong name to please an adult. Asking the parents about the surgery does not confirm that this is the correct client, as several children may be having the same surgery. (S)

20. 3 Despite their advances in body-image development, preschoolers have poorly defined body boundaries and little knowledge of their internal anatomy. Intrusive experiences are frightening, particularly those that disrupt skin integrity, such as injections and surgery. The nurse, therefore, discusses and explores possible fears that this child may be having. Some preschoolers mistakenly believe that their "insides" will spill out of their body if there is a break in the skin. This type of a dressing change with an "open" wound involves sterile technique, and therefore a preschooler is developmentally unable to participate. Details of a surgical procedure are appropriate for older school-aged children. Information for preschoolers is limited to what they will hear, feel, and see. Restraining a preschooler during a sterile dressing change is avoided because this compromises the sterile field. (S)

chapter 10

The Child With Common Health Problems

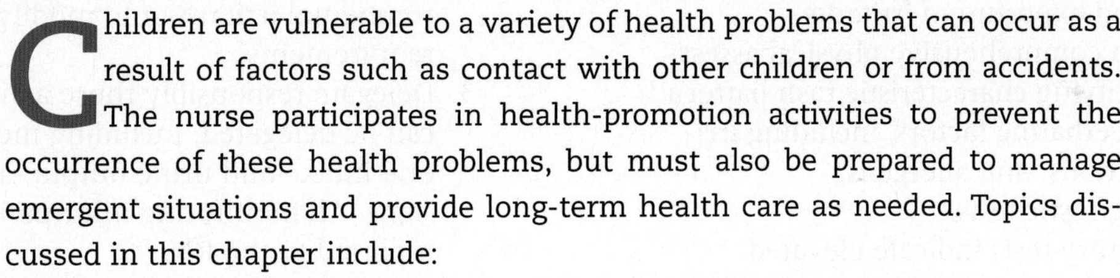

Children are vulnerable to a variety of health problems that can occur as a result of factors such as contact with other children or from accidents. The nurse participates in health-promotion activities to prevent the occurrence of these health problems, but must also be prepared to manage emergent situations and provide long-term health care as needed. Topics discussed in this chapter include:

- Atopic Dermatitis (Eczema)
- Scabies
- Head Lice
- Otitis Media
- Foreign Body Aspiration
- Accidents and Unintentional Injuries
- Poisonings
- Child Abuse
- Burns

Atopic Dermatitis (Eczema)

I. Definition: Atopic dermatitis (eczema) is a chronic condition of the skin easily identified by superficial inflammation and itching.
   A. Etiology of eczema is unknown but it has been theorized that there is a metabolic relationship to elevated serum IgE levels or impaired T-cell functioning. Occurrence is often related to allergies, especially milk.
   B. Types
      1. Infantile: Diagnosed between 2 and 6 months of age and remits by 3 years of age
      2. Childhood: Occurs between 2 and 3 years of age
      3. Preadolescent and adolescent: Occurs at 12 years of age and continues indefinitely

II. Nursing process
   A. Assessment
      1. Assess child for classic signs and symptoms of eczema—begins on cheeks and then found in creases of elbows, wrists, and knees:
         a. Erythema
         b. Pruritus
         c. Small papules and vesicles
         d. Lesions (weep and crust)
      2. Obtain a detailed health history, including allergies and exposure to irritants.
      3. Complete a comprehensive physical assessment identifying characteristic rash pattern.
      4. Assess exacerbating factors, including irritants, infections, and allergens.
      5. Obtain diagnostic tests.
         a. Laboratory tests indicate elevated serum IgE levels and eosinophilia
         b. Possible allergy testing to identify triggers
   B. Analysis
      1. Disturbed Body Image related to itching and weeping of lesions
      2. Impaired Skin Integrity related to vasoconstriction and pruritus
      3. Risk for Infection related to pruritus
   C. Planning
      1. Relieve itching.
      2. Prevent secondary infections.
      3. Promote compliance with drug therapy.
      4. Promote psychologic adaptation to chronic illness.
   D. Implementation (see management of care)
   E. Evaluation
      1. Child's inflammation and pruritus are decreased as evidenced by a decrease in itching.
      2. Child's lesions are improved through effectiveness of topical corticosteroids, antipruritics, and antihistamines.
      3. Child is compliant with drug therapies, and secondary infection from scratching is avoided.
      4. Child and family identify exacerbating factors and methods to prevent recurrence.

CN

III. Client needs
   A. Physiologic adaptation: Eczema is controlled with medication and child's compliance with drug therapies; and with comfort measures such as superfatted soap, emollients, and cotton clothing.
      1. Secondary infection may occur—signs and symptoms include honey-colored crusts with increasing areas of erythema.
      2. Allergy testing results may reveal exacerbating irritants that warrant preparation for dietary or lifestyle changes.
   B. Management of care: The care of the child with eczema requires critical thinking skills and knowledge of assessment, teaching and evaluation unique to the RN role. These skills cannot be delegated to an LPN or UAP.
      1. Perform comprehensive physical assessments and provide care appropriate to the child with eczema.
      2. Assess home needs such as reducing environmental irritants and modifying dietary requirements.
      3. Delegate responsibly those activities that can be delegated, including measurements, oral intake and urine output, and vital signs. All monitoring information is reported to the RN.
   C. Safety and infection control
      1. Prevent infection.
         a. Discourage child from scratching.
            (1) Keep fingernails short.
            (2) Use one-piece clothing over affected area.
         b. Recognize signs and symptoms of secondary infection.
         c. Teach parents and child how to recognize signs and symptoms of secondary infection.
      2. Teach parents about potential irritants and how to avoid contact.
      3. Maintain the six rights of medication administration.
   D. Health promotion and maintenance: Instruct child and family to maintain skin integrity using the following methods:
      1. Use of only water and unscented soap for daily bathing for 10 min
      2. Use of some type of skin cream to seal in moisture within 3 min of bathing

E. Psychologic integrity
   1. Offer support to the child and family coping with chronic illness.
   2. Encourage the child to verbalize anxiety and fears related to body image issues and chronic illness.
F. Basic care and comfort
   1. Ease illness.
      a. Provide skin care.
      b. Control allergens.
      c. Administer drug therapy (see pharmacologic and parenteral therapies).
   2. Decrease inflammation and pruritus.
      a. Avoid wool clothing and blankets; use cotton.
      b. Avoid rough material and stuffed animals that are furred.
      c. Avoid heat and sweating.
      d. Keep child dry.
      e. Bathe daily for 10 min.
      f. Use emollient on skin within 3 min after bathing.
      g. Keep nails trimmed; use mitts on infants if needed.
      h. Use mild laundry detergents and put through rinse cycle twice.
      i. Humidify home environment.
G. Reduction of risk potential
   1. Assist child and family to recognize exacerbating factors for eczema, including irritants and allergens.
   2. Instruct child and family to be alert for secondary infections.
   3. Instruct child and family to identify and avoid potential allergens.
   4. If food allergens have been identified, monitor nutritional status of child.
   5. Wash new clothes, towels, and linens before use.
   6. Encourage use of sunscreen with at least a sun protection factor of 15.
H. Pharmacologic and parenteral therapies: Child and family will state the purpose, dosage, timing, and side effects of all medications used to treat eczema.
   1. Common topical corticosteroids: Fluocinolone acetonide (Synalar):
      a. Outcome: For relief of the inflammatory and pruritic symptoms of dermatic conditions; assess for improvement in skin lesions
      b. Reduction of risk potential: Implement the six rights of medication administration; not for use in children under the age of 2 because of increased risk of toxicity; assess the skin for petechiae and ecchymosis
      c. Management of care: Apply after bathing when skin is still damp; apply gently because of fragility of skin
   2. Antipruritics and antihistamines: Hydroxyzine (Atarax):
      a. Outcome: Used in the management of pruritus; assess child for reduction in itching
      b. Reduction of risk potential: Implement the six rights of medication administration; assess for drowsiness; assess oral mucosa daily for breakdown from side effect of dryness
      c. Management of care: Use frequent warm water rinses to relieve dry mouth; increase fluid intake; avoid irritation of oral mucosa

Scabies

I. Definition: Scabies is a contagious skin disorder caused by the parasite *Sarcoptes scabiei* (itch mite) and is spread by prolonged person-to-person contact. On contact, the itch mite burrows under the skin, causing pruritus after sensitization occurs. Dead mites and their byproducts cause an inflammatory response of the skin in infested areas.

II. Nursing process
A. Assessment
   1. Assess for signs and symptoms of scabies, including intense pruritus, especially during the night.
   2. Assess for burrows (fine grayish red lines on the skin).
   3. Assess child in the most common sites for scabies.
      a. Infants: Head and neck
      b. Children: Wrists, axilla, genitalia
   4. Obtain a detailed health history, including possible contact with scabies.
   5. Obtain diagnostic tests.
      a. Burrow scraping—identifies mites, eggs, or feces
      b. Punch biopsy—confirms diagnosis
      c. Wound culture—for secondary infection
B. Analysis
   1. Impaired Skin Integrity related to pruritus
   2. Disturbed Sleep Pattern related to nighttime pruritus
   3. Risk for Infection related to pruritus
C. Planning
   1. Prevent transmission to other children or family members.
   2. Improve pruritus.
   3. Prevent secondary infection.

D. Implementation
 1. Provide interventions to treat infestation, including drug therapy with scabicide or pediculicide.
 2. Provide interventions to treat pruritus, including drug therapy with antipruritic.
 3. Provide interventions to treat secondary infections, including drug therapy with systemic antibiotics.
 4. Provide interventions to prevent secondary infection.

E. Evaluation
 1. Child affirms reduction in pruritic symptoms.
 2. Child and family describe methods of transmission and factors to prevent recurrence.
 3. Child does not develop any secondary infections.

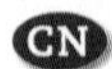

III. Client needs

A. Physiologic adaptation: Scabies is treated with medication, and client compliance with drug therapies prevents transmission to others.
 1. Evaluate the effectiveness of topical medications and antipruritics to treat scabies and itching and prevent secondary infection from scratching.
 2. Recognize the signs and symptoms that may alert the nurse to a potential secondary infection.

B. Management of care: The care of the child with scabies requires critical thinking skills and knowledge of assessment, teaching and evaluation unique to the RN role. These skills cannot be delegated to an LPN or UAP.
 1. Perform comprehensive physical assessments and provide care appropriate to the child with scabies.
 2. Delegate responsibly those activities that can be delegated, including measurements, oral intake and urine output, and vital signs. All monitoring information is reported to the RN.

C. Safety and infection control
 1. Teach child and family that scabies is infectious during the course of the infestation.
 2. Teach child and family that scabies is transmitted for 48 hr by close personal contact or contact with contaminated articles such as combs, hats, clothing, towels, or bedding.
 3. Teach child and family signs and symptoms of secondary bacterial infections or abscess formation such as papules, vesicles, crusting, and cellulitis.
 4. Maintain the six rights of medication administration.

D. Health promotion and maintenance: Identify and educate high-risk groups including school-aged children.

E. Psychologic integrity: Encourage child and family to verbalize anxiety and fears about transmission and infestation with scabies.

F. Basic care and comfort: Apply scabicide.
 1. Precede application with warm soap and water bath.
 2. Assure skin is cool and dry before application.
 3. Apply lotion in thin layer and repeat in 1 week.
 4. Assure lotion remains on skin for 8 to 14 hr before bathing.

G. Reduction of risk potential
 1. Teach child and family methods to prevent secondary bacterial infections, including maintaining short fingernails, and good hand hygiene.
 2. Teach child and family methods to prevent transmission of scabies.
  a. Isolate child until treatment is completed.
  b. Wash all clothing and bedding in hot water with laundry detergent on a daily basis. Drying in a hot dryer is encouraged.
  c. Tightly seal in plastic bags for a minimum of 4 days any toys or other items such as combs and brushes that are unable to be washed.
  d. Treat family members and close contacts prophylactically.
  e. Notify child's school.
  f. If child is hospitalized, disinfect room and sterilize blood pressure equipment.

H. Pharmacologic and parenteral therapies: Child and family state the purpose, dosage, timing, and side effects of scabies medications (Table 10-1).

Head Lice

I. Definition: Pediculosis capitis (head lice) is the contagious infestation of the hair and scalp with lice (Anoplura).

A. Itching from lice is a result of the toxins injected into the scalp after the insect bites into the skin. Repeated biting can lead to increasing sensitization and increasing inflammation.

B. Most common sites for infestation are the occipital region of the scalp, the eyebrows, and eyelashes.

Table 10-1 Treatment for Scabies

Classification	Generic/ Trade Name	Outcome	Reduction of Risk	Management of Care
Scabicide antipruritic	Crotamiton (Eurax)	Treats and eradicates scabies. Treats and reduces symptoms related to pruritus.	Monitor for and report skin irritation.	Apply over entire body, including soles of feet; bathe 48 hr after application to remove drug.
Pediculicide	Permethrin (Nix) (Elimite, Acticin)	Treats scabies and prevents burrowing.	Monitor and report transient tingling.	Apply over entire body, including soles of feet. Avoid contact with eyes.
Scabicide	Lindane cream (Kwell)	Treats and eradicates scabies infestation.	Contraindicated in children less than 2 because of risk of neurotoxicity and seizures. Avoid contact with eyes. Shampoo is effective in treatment of combs and brushes.	Person applying needs to wear gloves. Apply over entire body, including soles of feet.

II. Nursing process

A. Assessment

1. Assess for signs and symptoms of lice.
   a. Scalp pruritus
   b. Appearance of white flecks attached to the hair shaft
2. Obtain diagnostic tests: Visual examination is sufficient for diagnosis.

B. Analysis: Impaired Skin Integrity related to pruritus

C. Planning

1. Restore skin integrity by eradicating lice.
2. Prevent transmission of contagious infestation to peers or family members.

D. Implementation

1. Provide interventions to treat lice.
   a. Remove lice and eggs with specialized fine-tooth comb.
   b. Treat with scabicides or pediculicides.
2. Provide child and family teaching on the prevention of transmission of lice—spread by close contact and sharing of clothing or hair articles such as hats and combs.

E. Evaluation

1. Child's lice are eradicated as evidence by lack of nits and eggs on hair shaft after appropriate treatment with topical medication.
2. Child and family verbalize treatment and prevention of transmission of lice.

CN

III. Client needs

A. Physiologic adaptation: Lice are treated and not transmitted with application of topical medication—evaluate the effectiveness of treatment with pediculicides to eradicate lice and prevent transmission.

B. Management of care: Care of the child with lice requires critical thinking skills and knowledge of assessment, teaching and evaluation unique to the RN role. These skills cannot be delegated to an LPN or UAP.

1. Perform comprehensive physical assessments and provide care appropriate to the child with lice.
2. Assess home needs and availability of a washer and dryer to clean household items.
3. Delegate responsibly those activities that can be delegated, including measurements, oral intake and urine output, and vital signs. All monitoring information is reported to the RN.

C. Safety and infection control

1. Teach child and family methods to prevent transmission, including completing entire course of treatment, and repeating in 7 to 12 days to ensure that all eggs are destroyed.
2. Maintain the six rights of medication administration.

D. Health promotion and maintenance: Instruct child and family methods to prevent infestation, including avoiding sharing of clothing, especially hats, and combs and brushes.

E. Psychologic integrity: Allow child and family to verbalize fears and feelings related to contracting lice.

F. Basic care and comfort: Provide child with diversional activities during treatment and/or hospitalization to promote growth and development.

G. Reduction of risk potential: Provide child and family teaching about treatment.
  1. Apply and remove medications according to drug company directions to avoid neurotoxicity.
  2. Wash in hot water with laundry detergent all bed linens, clothing, combs, brushes, and furniture that have come in contact with the hair of the infected child. Dry items in hot dryer for a minimum of 20 min.
  3. Soak in hot water (130°F) plastic combs and hairbrushes that cannot be placed in the washer.
  4. Seal all toys that cannot be washed in plastic bags for 2 weeks.

H. Pharmacologic and parenteral therapies: Child and family will state the purpose, dosage, timing, and side effects of pediculicides, including pyrethrins (RID).
  1. Outcome: Controls and eradicates head lice and eggs
  2. Reduction of Risk: Avoid contact with mucosal surfaces of eyes and mucosa
  3. Management of Care: Flush eyes with water if experience contact with medication

Otitis Media

I. Definition: Otitis media is an acute or chronic inflammation of the middle ear most commonly caused by blockage of the eustachian tube or bacterial colonization. It is a common complication of upper respiratory infections in children.

II. Nursing process

A. Assessment
  1. Assess for risk factors.
    a. Allergies
    b. Respiratory tract infections
    c. Nasotracheal intubation
    d. Cleft palate
    e. Secondary smoke
    f. Nighttime bottle in bed
  2. Assess predisposing factors—eustachian tubes are wider, shorter, and more horizontal in children.
  3. Assess for signs and symptoms.
    a. Fever
    b. Irritability
    c. Anorexia
    d. Complaints of earache or pain
    e. Infants may tug, pull, or rub at the ear
    f. Infants and young children may roll their head side to side
    g. Evidence of hearing loss
    h. Purulent drainage from the ear
    i. Nausea and vomiting
  4. Obtain a detailed health history, including history of allergies and respiratory infections, and past history of otitis media.
  5. Obtain diagnostic tests.
    a. Otoscopic examination—reveals a bulging erythematous tympanic membrane
    b. Culture of ear drainage—identifies cause
    c. Tympanometry

B. Analysis
  1. Acute Pain related to tympanic membrane pressure
  2. Risk for Infection related to bacterial invasion of middle ear
  3. Hyperthermia related to infectious processes
  4. Risk for Deficient Fluid Volume related to hyperthermia

C. Planning
  1. Relieve pain.
  2. Reduce fever.
  3. Prevent hearing loss.
  4. Reduce anxiety.
  5. Encourage compliance with medication regimen.

D. Implementation
  1. Provide interventions to manage pain.
    a. Administer analgesics such as benzocaine (Auralgan Otic).
    b. Provide local heat.
    c. Position child on affected ear.
    d. Instruct to avoid chewing during acute period because this increases discomfort.
    e. Note that child may have a possible myringotomy for severe bulging tympanic membrane.
  2. Provide interventions to manage infectious process: Antibiotic therapy.

E. Evaluation
  1. Child affirms reduction of ear pain and the ability to sleep.
  2. Child and family are able to verbalize understanding of medication regimen of antibiotics.
  3. Child and family verbalize understanding of myringotomy and tympanoplasty.

CN

III. Client needs

A. Physiologic adaptation: Otitis media is treated with antibiotic therapy.
  1. Evaluate effectiveness of antibiotics to treat infection and prevent hearing loss evidenced by reduction in fever and pain.
  2. Recognize the signs and symptoms that would alert the nurse to a ruptured tympanic membrane: Immediate relief of pain,

decrease in temperature, and visible purulent drainage in the canal.

B. Management of care: Care of the child with otitis media requires critical thinking skills and knowledge of assessment, teaching and evaluation unique to the RN role. These skills cannot be delegated to an LPN or UAP.
   1. Perform comprehensive physical assessments and provide care appropriate to the child with otitis media.
   2. Provide follow-up care to identify compliance with drug regimen and assess for complication such as hearing loss.
   3. Delegate responsibly those activities that can be delegated, including measurements, oral intake and urine output, and vital signs. All monitoring information is reported to the RN.

C. Safety and infection control
   1. Teach child and family how to prevent upper respiratory infections.
   2. Teach child and family the importance of completing the antibiotic regimen to reduce the risk of recurrence.
   3. Assist family in identifying hearing loss.
   4. Maintain the six rights of medication administration.

D. Health promotion and maintenance
   1. Teach family to feed the child in an upright position and not to place bottles in bed.
   2. Assist family in early identification and treatment of allergies.
   3. Teach family to prevent water from entering child's ears if child has tube placement.

E. Psychologic integrity
   1. Assist child in coping with pain.
   2. Encourage child to express anxiety and feelings of fear.
   3. Promote appropriate growth and development.

F. Basic care and comfort
   1. Teach family about the correct instillation of ear drops, if ordered.
      a. Under 3 years of age—external ear (pinna) is pulled down and back
      b. Over 3 years of age—external ear (pinna) is pulled up and out
   2. Assess and manage pain.
      a. Use age-appropriate pain scale to assess severity of pain.
      b. Medicate child for pain with prescribed analgesic such as benzocaine (Auralgan Otic).
      c. Apply local heat or cold for pain relief.
   3. Encourage fluid intake to compensate for fever.

G. Reduction of risk potential
   1. Prevent otitis media through child and family teaching regarding importance of early management of upper respiratory infections.
   2. Encourage parents to maintain immunization schedule.

H. Pharmacologic and parenteral therapies: Child and family will state the purpose, dosage, timing, and side effects of medications used to treat otitis media.
   1. Antipyretics or analgesics—Acetaminophen (Tylenol); to manage pain and fever
      a. Outcome: For fever reduction and treatment of mild-to-moderate pain
      b. Reduction of risk: Maintain the six rights of medication administration; use with caution in children less than 3 years of age; monitor for hepatotoxicity
      c. Management of care: Instruct parents to monitor administration with any other over-the-counter medication that might contain acetaminophen.
   2. Antibiotics—Amoxicillin (Amoxil); to manage infection
      a. Outcome: For treatment of infections of the ear
      b. Reduction of risk: Assess for hypersensitivity to penicillins or cephalosporins, which may cause diarrhea, nausea, or vomiting; monitor for maculopapular rash; monitor for symptoms of superinfection
      c. Management of care: Place drops in child's mouth or mix with juice or formula.

Foreign Body Aspiration

I. Definition: Foreign body aspiration is defined as the lodging of a foreign body in the mainstem or lobar bronchus.
   A. Severity of aspiration is determined by the location, type of object, and degree of obstruction.
   B. Health problem is most common in older infants and children up to 3 years of age.
   C. Most common items aspirated are round foods including hot dogs, round candy, nuts, and grapes; and nonfood items smaller than the diameter of a toilet paper roll (including small toys parts and coins).

II. Nursing process
   A. Assessment
      1. Assess for risk factors.
         a. Sedation
         b. Seizure disorder

c. Central nervous system disorder
d. Narrowed airways of infants and young children

2. Assess for signs and symptoms indicating aspiration of foreign body.
   a. Choking, gagging, and coughing ("brassy" sounding)
   b. Wheezing
   c. Stridor
   d. Dyspnea
   e. Visualization of foreign body on examination
3. Obtain a detailed health history related to developmental stage and ability to ingest foreign body.
4. Perform a comprehensive physical assessment, including vital signs, and SpO_2.
5. Obtain diagnostic tests: Based on history and physical signs.
   a. Radiograph(s)—assist in viewing opaque objects
   b. Bronchoscopy—needed to view objects in the larynx and trachea
   c. Endoscopy—can be diagnostic and therapeutic in the removal of the foreign body

B. Analysis
1. Ineffective Airway Clearance related to laryngeal edema, partial obstruction, and/or inflammation
2. Risk for Aspiration related to ingestion of obstructing object
3. Ineffective Breathing Pattern related to impaired oxygenation
4. Fear related to decreased oxygenation and ability to breathe
5. Impaired Gas Exchange related to obstruction of bronchus
6. Risk for Injury related to developmental curiosity

C. Planning
1. Restore oxygenation and ventilation.
2. Prevent life-threatening obstruction.
3. Reduce fear and anxiety.
4. Promote parental coping.
5. Teach developmental expectations.

D. Implementation
1. Provide interventions for emergency management of airway obstruction.
   a. For children less than 1 year of age: Back blows and chest thrusts
   b. For children older than 1 year of age: Abdominal thrusts; no finger sweeps into mouth
   c. Provide immediate removal of foreign body by endoscopy; if endoscopy is unable to remove foreign body, thoracotomy is necessary.
2. Provide interventions after foreign body removed.
   a. Promote high-humidity environment.
   b. Observe for signs of airway edema.
   c. Treat secondary infections with antibiotics.

E. Evaluation
1. Child's airway remains patent and no respiratory distress or airway edema develops.
2. Child and family describe risk factors for foreign body aspiration and methods to prevent recurrence.
3. Parents state the procedure for treating choking in infant or child.

CN

III. Client needs

A. Physiologic adaptation: Foreign body removed by endoscopy; if endoscopy is unable to remove foreign body, thoracotomy is necessary.
1. Recognize signs and symptoms that would alert the nurse to decreased oxygenation: change in level of consciousness, cyanosis, use of accessory muscles, nasal flaring, grunting, SpO_2 less than 95.
2. Evaluate effectiveness of bronchoscopy and reduction in symptoms of aspiration.
3. Promote tracheotomy on inability to immediately relieve obstruction.

B. Management of care: Care of the child with a foreign body aspiration requires critical thinking skills and knowledge of assessment, teaching and evaluation unique to the RN role. These skills cannot be delegated to an LPN or UAP.
1. Perform comprehensive physical assessments and provide care appropriate to the child with a foreign body aspiration.
2. Provide follow-up care to identify compliance with parental understanding of risk factors and developmental norms for the child.
3. Assess home needs for potential modification to ensure a safe environment.
4. Delegate responsibly those activities that can be delegated, including measurements, oral intake and urine output, and vital signs. All monitoring information is reported to the RN.

C. Safety and infection control: Institute emergency management for a child with a foreign body aspiration, including:
1. Heimlich maneuver
2. Possible endoscopy
3. Possible tracheotomy

D. Health promotion and maintenance
1. Recognize that older infants and children may gag and cough while eating but not be choking.

2. Provide child and family teaching about preventing future foreign body aspiration.

E. Psychologic integrity
1. Allow parents to express anger and guilt over accidental aspiration.
2. Assist parents with coping.
3. Allow child to express fears and anxieties.

F. Basic care and comfort
1. After emergency situation resolved, allow child quiet environment and promote rest.
2. After gag reflex returns, encourage fluid intake.
3. Encourage family to bring security object to calm child.

G. Reduction of risk potential
1. Teach parents about not allowing child access to small objects. High-risk objects include:
   a. Rubber balloons
   b. Small bandages
   c. Price tags
   d. Aluminum or plastic tabs from containers
   e. Coins
2. Teach parents about developmental hazards related to the age of child and imitative behavior such as seeing parent hold pens, pins, or toothpick in mouth.
3. Monitor child for respiratory distress after foreign body removed.

Accidents and Unintentional Injuries

I. Definition: Accidents and unintentional injuries are the leading cause of death in children and typically occur in or near the home environment. Most common accidents and unintentional injuries include falls, ingestions, drowning, and bicycle and motor vehicle injury.

II. Nursing process

A. Assessment: Assess for parental understanding of developmental risk factors including:
1. Curiosity of child.
2. Ability of child to reach, climb, or walk to hazards.
3. Child has inadequate understanding of risk.

B. Analysis
1. Risk for Aspiration related to inadequate knowledge of dangers
2. Risk for Falls related to inability to assess risk and curiosity
3. Risk for Injury related to developmental risk factors
4. Deficient Knowledge of Risk Factors (of parent or child): Related to lack of understanding of development and risk behaviors
5. Risk for Poisoning related to pica or sensorimotor developmental stage

C. Planning
1. Prevent injury.
2. Promote hospital safety for the child.

D. Implementation
1. Provide child and family teaching about safety and childproofing techniques.
   a. Offer education classes in the hospital and on an outpatient basis.
   b. Provide handouts reinforcing teaching goals.
   c. Allow parents an avenue to ask questions.
2. Provide interventions to promote hospital safety, including modifying environment for child's developmental level.

E. Evaluation
1. Child remains free from injury.
2. Child does not experience injury as a result of effective teaching plans.
3. Parents verbalize understanding of developmental expectations of child and what injuries or accidents can be prevented.

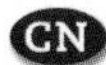

III. Client needs

A. Physiologic adaptation: Infants and children are prone to accidents based on their cognitive functioning, mental capacity, and developmental level. Most accidents and unintentional injuries can be prevented through appropriate parental and community education.

B. Management of care: Childhood accidents and unintentional injuries can be an emergency situation and require critical thinking skills and knowledge of assessment, teaching and evaluation unique to the RN role. These skills cannot be delegated to an LPN or UAP.
1. Perform comprehensive physical assessments and provide care appropriate to the child at risk for accidents/unintentional injuries.
2. Provide follow-up care to identify compliance with parental understanding of risk factors, developmental norms for the child, and childproofing of the home.
3. Assess home needs and environment to ensure home has been adequately modified for safety.
4. Delegate responsibly those activities that can be delegated, including measurements, oral intake and urine output, and vital signs. All monitoring information is reported to the RN.

C. Safety and infection control: Maintain hospital safety.
   1. Modify hospital environment based on child's cognitive, developmental, and physical level.
   2. Provide safety through side rails or netted or bubble top crib at all times.
   3. Permit only Mylar balloons in room; if child is in intensive care, balloons are prohibited, including Mylar, because of oxygen use and flammability.
   4. Avoid leaving small objects at bedside, including syringes.
   5. Follow restraint protocol when necessary to prevent injury.

D. Health promotion and maintenance
   1. Teach parents developmental norms for their child and develop plans to childproof their home and environment.
   2. Provide child with toys and activities that promote health growth and development while ensuring safety.

E. Psychologic integrity
   1. Encourage parents to verbalize feelings of guilt over accidental/unintentional injury.
   2. Support child during recovery from injury and allow play activities that promote expression of feelings.

F. Basic care and comfort
   1. Provide child with security object such as favorite toy or blanket.
   2. Provide consistent nurse caregiver to reduce stress.
   3. Provide developmentally appropriate play opportunities.

G. Reduction of risk potential
   1. Develop teaching plans for parents to promote safety in and around the home environment. Instruct parents and children (as appropriate) to:
      a. Evaluate toys for sharp edges, small pieces.
      b. Understand child's age, motor skills, and where the child can reach.
      c. Evaluate car seat and proper use.
      d. Observe pool or water safety.
      e. Observe bicycle or skate board safety, including helmets, knee and elbow pads.
      f. Evaluate methods to childproof home: Medications and chemical agents, including toxic cleaning products, must be in locked cabinet in original containers.
      g. Manage hanging electrical cords and plants to keep out of child's reach and prevent climbing or ingestion.
      h. Block electrical outlets.
      i. Acknowledge risks for motor vehicle accidents (for adolescent drivers).
      j. Observe firearm safety.
   2. Instruct parents on emergency procedures following an accident/unintentional injury.
      a. Call 911.
      b. Keep emergency phone numbers (e.g., Poison Control Center) by all phones.

H. Pharmacologic and parenteral therapies: Pharmacologic therapies are individualized based on the accident. See topic on poisonings within this chapter.

Poisonings

I. Definition: Poisoning is an accidental ingestion of a substance that can result in harm to the child. Most poisonings occur in children under 6 years of age, and within in the home setting from items such as cosmetics, household products, and medications. Most poisonings are managed in the home setting after parents call the Poison Control Center (PCC). If parents are unable to identify the quantity or toxin ingested, then hospitalization is suggested.

II. Nursing process
   A. Assessment
      1. Assess immediate need for life support.
         a. Vital signs
         b. Signs of shock from corrosive ingestion
      2. Assess seriousness of ingestion, including the amount ingested and length of time before treatment is initiated. Common ingestions include prescription medications and over-the-counter supplements such as iron.
         a. Acetaminophen (Tylenol), assess for:
            (1) Early symptoms of nausea and vomiting, diaphoresis and pallor
            (2) Late symptoms of hepatic involvement including right upper quadrant abdominal pain, jaundice, and confusion
         b. Acetylsalicylic acid (Aspirin), assess for:
            (1) Presence of GI symptoms such as nausea, vomiting, and thirst
            (2) Central nervous system for symptoms of tinnitus, confusion, hyperpnea; elevated temperature, and diaphoresis
            (3) Bleeding (hematopoietic symptom)
      3. Obtain a detailed health history, including possible availability and accessibility to poisoning agents.
      4. Perform a comprehensive physical assessment, including vital signs and fluid and electrolyte status.

B. Analysis
  1. Risk for Injury related to developmental risk factors
  2. Deficient Knowledge of Risk Factors (of parent or child) related to lack of understanding of development and risk behaviors
  3. Risk for Poisoning related to pica or sensorimotor developmental stage

C. Planning
  1. Maintain hemodynamic status during acute ingestion phase.
  2. Promote safety through parental teaching after acute ingestion phase.
  3. Prevent injury by educating parents on childproofing techniques.

D. Implementation: In addition to educating parents about safety techniques, implementation involves interventions for acute poisoning including:
  1. Terminate exposure.
  2. Identify the poison.
     a. Look at the environment for clues.
     b. Question child and witness.
     c. Save all evidence of poison.
  3. Initiate gastric decontamination to remove poison or prevent absorption: Do not induce vomiting; instead use:
     a. Cathartics
     b. Absorbing agent: Activated charcoal
     c. Gastric lavage

E. Evaluation
  1. Child is successfully managed at home on an outpatient basis.
  2. Child has no sequelae from accidental ingestion.
  3. Parents verbalize understanding of active and passive measures to ensure child's safety from future ingestion.

CN

III. Client needs

A. Physiologic adaptation: Infants and children are prone to poisoning because of their cognitive functioning, mental capacity, and developmental level. Most poisonings can be prevented through appropriate parental and community education.

B. Management of care: Childhood poisoning can be an emergency situation and require critical thinking skills and knowledge of assessment, teaching and evaluation unique to the RN role. These skills cannot be delegated to an LPN or UAP.
  1. Perform comprehensive physical assessments and provide care appropriate to the child who has been poisoned.
  2. Provide follow-up care to identify compliance with parental understanding of risk factors, developmental norms for the child, and childproofing of the home.
  3. Assess home for modification to ensure safety.
  4. Delegate responsibly those activities that can be delegated, including measurements, oral intake and urine output, and vital signs. All monitoring information is reported to the RN.

C. Safety and infection control: Treat child before the poison is absorbed to ensure adequate life support. Gastric decontamination removes the poison or prevents absorption.
  1. To remove poison—gastric lavage:
     a. For young infants
     b. For comatose or convulsing children
     c. For rapidly absorbed toxins
  2. To absorb poison—activated charcoal (when mixed with water resembles a black mud; is flavorless): Mix with diet soda and place in an opaque cup with a straw
  3. To diminish intestinal absorption of poison—cathartics: Magnesium citrate is used to evacuate the bowel and prevent or decrease absorption of the poison
  4. Poison antidotes—there are a few antidotes for a minority of poisonings: *N*-acetylcysteine (Mucomyst) for acetaminophen (Tylenol) poisoning

D. Health promotion and maintenance
  1. Teach parents about developmental expectations for their child to assist with their understanding about present and future concerns for safety.
  2. Assist the parents in identifying their home and child's risk factors for accidental poisoning (see reduction of risk potential).

E. Psychologic integrity
  1. Allow parents to verbalize anxiety and guilt over child's ingestion.
  2. Allow child to verbalize anxiety and fear over ingestion and possible hospitalization.
  3. Encourage parental dialog about difficulty with childrearing and monitoring child for safety.

F. Basic care and comfort
  1. If vomiting was induced, allow child a rest period and then encourage oral fluids to prevent dehydration.
  2. Allow family to bring favorite security toy or blanket to reduce anxiety.

G. Reduction of risk potential
  1. Develop teaching plans for parents to promote safety in and around the home environment; this involves preventing injury recurrence.

Table 10-2 Treatment for Poisoning

Classification	Generic/Trade Name	Expected Outcome	Reduction of Risk Potential	Management of Care
Emetic (no longer recommended by American Academy of Pediatrics)	Ipecac syrup	Removes ingested agent through induced vomiting.	Contraindicated for ingestion of corrosives or petroleum distillates.	Vomiting occurs within 15 minutes.
Adsorbing agents	Activated charcoal (Actidose)	Binds toxic substances.	May cause vomiting and diarrhea.	Record and observe stools, which may appear black.
Cathartics	Magnesium citrate (Citroma)	Eliminates stool from the intestine.	May induce cramps, nausea, and fluid and electrolyte disturbance. Assess for hypokalemia.	Monitor for dehydration.
Antidotes	Acetylcysteine (Mucomyst)	Prevents acetaminophen breakdown products from binding with liver cells.	Cautious use in children with asthma because can cause bronchospasm. Causes nausea and dizziness.	Monitor for respiratory distress.

a. Understand injury prevention.
b. Identify risk factors (by completing home assessment and questioning parents about predisposing factors).
c. Identify emergency contacts (e.g., PPC), and place near each telephone.

2. Instruct parents about safe storage of medications and toxins.
   a. Use warning labels on bottles.
   b. Use bottles with childproof closures.
   c. Store toxins and medications in locked cabinet.
3. Instruct parents on emergency procedures following an accident.
   a. Call 911.
   b. Call Poison Control Center.

H. Pharmacologic and parenteral therapies: Child and family will state the purpose, dosage, timing, and side effects of medications for the treatment of poisonings (Table 10-2).

Child Abuse

I. Definition: Child abuse involves the intentional emotional, physical, and sexual abuse or exploitation of a child. Child neglect is the omission of meeting basic needs, usually a result of altered parental ability to cope or provide for the child (see also Chapter 39). High-risk children include those born prematurely or with some defined mental or physical disability. Infants and toddlers are more prone to be physically abused, while school-aged and adolescent children are more commonly the victims of emotional or sexual abuse.

II. Nursing process

A. Assessment: Classic key to suspecting child abuse is inconsistency between the injuries and the history of the accident. Diagnosis is based on a combination of physical and psychologic factors.
1. Interview child and parents separately to clearly identify inconsistencies. Careful verbatim documentation is important.
2. Assess child for physical signs of abuse.
   a. Unusual bruises, burns, fractures, bite marks, unusual mouth injuries
   b. Severe abdominal or central nervous system injury
3. Gather detailed health history, especially for frequency of injury, and if child is dressed in concealing clothing.
4. Gather psychosocial history noting a history of behavior problems, excessive shyness, fearful when parents are near, and/or avoidance of physical contact.

B. Analysis
1. Risk for Injury related to parental anxiety
2. Impaired Skin Integrity related to burns or fractures
3. Compromised Family Coping related to unrealistic developmental expectations
4. Compromised Family Coping related to physical abuse

C. Planning
   1. Ensure child's immediate safety.
   2. Reduce anxiety and fear related to hospitalization.
   3. Promote positive parent-child interaction.
   4. Assist family in obtaining appropriate counseling.
   5. Meet child's immediate physical needs.
D. Implementation
   1. Provide interventions to meet child's immediate physical needs.
      a. Obtain x-rays as indicated.
      b. Manage trauma or injury.
      c. Initiate hospitalization as needed.
   2. Provide interventions to meet child's psychologic needs.
      a. Uncover inconsistencies between the history and injuries.
      b. Protect the child.
      c. Provide emotional support.
      d. Observe parent-child interactions.
      e. Report the abuse as mandated by law.
E. Evaluation
   1. Child's physical needs are met immediately.
   2. Child sustains no further injury because of an affective means of reporting abuse through appropriate channels.
   3. Parents verbalize need for counseling and support.

III. Client needs
A. Physiologic adaptation: Recognize physical and psychologic signs and symptoms that alert potential child abuse.
B. Management of care: Care of the abused child requires critical thinking skills and knowledge of assessment, teaching and evaluation unique to the RN role. These skills cannot be delegated to an LPN or UAP.
   1. Report abuse.
      a. All 50 states mandate reporting. Abuse is reported per facility policy; follow chain of command for reporting.
      b. Child Abuse Prevention and Treatment Act protects the nurse from liability.
   2. Document abuse.
      a. Factually describe every bruise, burn, welt, and stage of healing.
      b. Assess the presenting injury or symptom for consistencies with the description.
      c. Discover if there was any delay in seeking medical care.
   3. Assess for home health needs, especially related to protection of the child.
   4. Delegate responsibly those activities that can be delegated, including measurements, oral intake and urine output, and vital signs. All monitoring information is reported to the RN.
   5. Evaluate community resources for family support.
      a. Promote program that includes both parents, and focuses on strengthening families and family relationships.
      b. Work with diverse populations.
      c. Introduce respite care.
C. Safety and infection control
   1. Place child in a safe environment.
   2. Protect child and prevent further abuse.
   3. Treat injuries.
   4. Avoid interrogating child with multiple questions.
   5. Explain all treatments and procedures.
D. Health promotion and maintenance
   1. Report and document instance of abuse according to facility policy (see management of care).
   2. Provide parents with anticipatory guidance and teach normal developmental expectations, especially in the areas of safety, discipline, and age-appropriate behavior.
   3. Provide parents with positive feedback and encourage participation in care of child.
E. Psychologic integrity
   1. Do not examine the child alone (include parents or other health care personnel).
   2. Engage the child in play that allows for expression of anxiety, fear, and emotions.
   3. Identify parent and child stressors and coping mechanisms.
   4. Refer parents for counseling to Parents Anonymous or other appropriate mental health treatment program.
   5. Use forensic nurses in institutions, when available.
F. Basic care and comfort
   1. Meet basic physical and psychologic needs.
   2. Provide consistent nurse caregiver.
   3. Treat parents nonjudgmentally.
G. Reduction of risk potential
   1. Assess parents' normal coping mechanisms, stressors, developmental expectations of the child, and support systems.
   2. Assist family in identifying strengths, stressors, normal developmental expectations, and support systems.

Burns

I. Definition: Burns are most commonly the result of exposure to an extreme heat source, but may also result from exposure to chemicals, electricity, and cold. (See Chapter 34 for additional information about burns and nursing care for clients with burns.)

A. Children less than 5 years of age are at highest risk for burn injuries and usually sustain second- and third-degree burns because of the thinness and fragility of their skin.

B. The American Burn Association has established criteria for determining the severity of burn injuries and the need for transport to specialized centers.

C. Burn injuries cause both local and systemic responses.

II. Nursing process

A. Assessment

1. Assess child for extent, depth, and severity of injury.

a. Extent

(1) Expressed as percentage of total body surface area (TBSA)

(2) Modified rule of nines used as the child grows

(3) Lund and Browder chart used for infants and children (Figure 10-1).

AREA OF BODY	RELATIVE PERCENTAGE OF BODY SURFACE (VARIES BY AGE)					ESTIMATED PERCENTAGE OF BODY AREA WITH:	
	0-1 year	1-4 years	5-9 years	10-15 years	Adult	2nd-degree burns	3rd- and 4th-degree burns
Head	19	17	13	10	7		
Neck	2	2	2	2	2		
Anterior trunk	13	13	13	13	13		
Posterior trunk	13	13	13	13	13		
Right buttock	2	2	2	2	2		
Left buttock	2	2	2	2	2		
Genitalia	1	1	1	1	1		
Right upper arm	4	4	4	4	4		
Left upper arm	4	4	4	4	4		
Right lower arm	3	3	3	3	3		
Left lower arm	3	3	3	3	3		
Right hand	2	2	2	2	2		
Left hand	2	2	2	2	2		
Right thigh	5	6	8	8	9		
Left thigh	5	6	8	8	9		
Right lower leg	5	5	5	6	7		
Left lower leg	5	5	5	6	7		
Right foor	3	3	3	3	3		
Left foot	3	3	3	3	3		
					TOTALS:	+	=

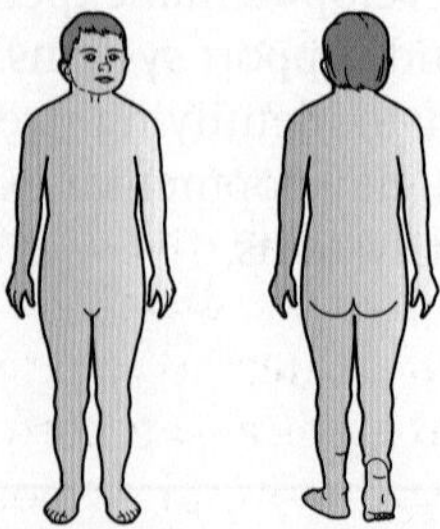

Figure 10-1. The Lund and Browder chart is used to determine the extent of burns in children because it is based on age, thus compensating for changes based on growth.

b. Depth
   (1) First-degree burn (superficial)—dry, painful, red
   (2) Second-degree burn (partial thickness)—edema present, weeping blisters; very painful
   (3) Third-degree burn (full thickness)—skin dry, pale; no pain; fluid shift, causing hypovolemia and shock
c. Severity
   (1) Major—greater than 20% of body surface area burned; requires specialized burn center
   (2) Moderate—10% to 20% of body surface area burned; requires hospitalization
   (3) Minor—less than 10% of body surface area burned; treated on an outpatient basis

2. Assess child for burn complications.
   a. Respiratory complications from inhalation injury—Assess patency of airway in addition to:
      (1) Facial indications—burns on the face and lips; burned nasal hairs, laryngeal edema
      (2) Pulmonary symptoms—hoarseness, wheezing, moist crackles, and increasing secretions
   b. Cardiovascular complications related to the high proportion of body fluid to mass lead to decreased cardiac output: Assess for hypovolemia.
3. Perform a comprehensive physical assessment.
4. Obtain a detailed health history, including history of tetanus toxoid immunization. Determine burn source.
5. Obtain diagnostic tests.
   a. Laboratory tests
      (1) Arterial blood gases—assess level of hypoxia
      (2) Complete blood count—indicates bleeding
      (3) Electrolyte status—monitors fluid shifts
      (4) Blood urea nitrogen (BUN) and creatinine—monitors renal status
      (5) Glucose—may be depleted from lack of stored glycogen
      (6) Carboxyhemoglobin levels—assess for elevated levels
   b. Chest x-ray
   c. Electrocardiogram
   d. Bronchoscopy

B. Analysis
   1. Ineffective Airway Clearance related to increased secretions
   2. Impaired Skin Integrity related to damaged tissues from thermal injury
   3. Acute Pain related to tissue injury and impaired perfusion
   4. Risk for Impaired Tissue Perfusion related to compression from burn injury
   5. Ineffective Breathing Pattern related to impaired respiratory muscles, edema, and pain
   6. Risk for Aspiration related to increased airway secretions
   7. Anxiety related to pain, fear, and separation from parents
   8. Decreased Cardiac Output related to decreased circulating fluid volume
   9. Deficient Fluid Volume related to ongoing losses
   10. Impaired Gas Exchange related to edema
   11. Risk for Infection related to compromised immune response and impaired skin integrity
   12. Imbalanced Nutrition: Less Than Body Requirements related to increased catabolism
   13. Disturbed Body Image related to altered skin appearance

C. Planning
   1. Maintain patent airway.
   2. Maintain hemodynamic stability.
   3. Prevent hypoxia.
   4. Restore fluid and electrolyte balance.
   5. Relieve pain.
   6. Reduce anxiety and fear.
   7. Provide nutritional support.
   8. Manage complications.

D. Implementation
   1. Provide interventions for minor burn—emergency care.
      a. Stop the burning process.
      b. Assess child's condition.
      c. Cover burn with a clean cloth.
      d. Transport child for medical care.
      e. Provide child and family with support.
   2. Provide interventions for minor burns—nonemergency care.
      a. Cleanse with mild soap and water.
      b. Cover with antibacterial ointment and fine-mesh gauze dressing.
      c. Wash and redress as ordered and return to medical care for reassessment.
   3. Provide interventions for major burns.
      a. Establish airway.
      b. Institute fluid resuscitation.
      c. Provide nutritional support.

d. Administer medication: Sedation and analgesia.
e. Provide wound management.

E. Evaluation
1. Child's burns sites heal without damage.
2. Child's tissue perfusion below burn sites is maintained.
3. Child verbalizes reduction in pain.
4. Child's burn wounds do not become infected.
5. Child's tissue perfusion is adequate and urine output is maintained, demonstrating adequate fluid resuscitation.
6. Child's nutritional status is maintained and catabolic state is reversed.
7. Child demonstrates minimal regression to earlier developmental stage.
8. Child and family verbalize feelings and concerns about injury and life changes.
9. Child and family participate in care, including wound management.

CN

III. Client needs

A. Physiologic adaptation: Children are at increased risk for fluid and electrolyte loss, hypothermia, dehydration, and metabolic acidosis. Any burn over 10% of the child's body surface area requires some form of fluid resuscitation.
1. Small muscle mass and lack of body fat puts infants at increased risk for nutritional deficiencies.
2. Immature immune system puts children at increased risk for the development of infections.
3. Signs and symptoms that indicate potential fluid shift, hypovolemia, and a decrease in cardiac output include change in level of consciousness, hypotension, tachycardia, decreased peripheral pulses, and cool, pale skin.

B. Management of care: The care of the child with a burn injury requires critical thinking skills and knowledge of assessment, teaching and evaluation unique to the RN role. These skills cannot be delegated to an LPN or UAP.
1. Assess for home health needs for supplies related to wound care, modification of the home related to smoke alarms and sprinklers, childproof lighters, and water tap temperature regulators.
2. Evaluate community resources for family support in the practice, use, and effectiveness of fire escape plans and other aspects of evacuation; the presence and use of appropriate fire extinguishers; the existence of functioning smoke alarms in appropriate areas of the home, and how to reach the local fire department.
3. Delegate responsibly those activities that can be delegated, including measurements, oral intake and urine output, and vital signs. All monitoring information is reported to the RN.

C. Safety and infection control
1. Respond to immediate safety issues.
   a. Stop the burn source.
   b. Obtain a patent airway.
   c. Remove any rings or constrictive items such as anklets, belts, and necklaces.
2. Prevent infection
   a. Avoid use of antibiotics prophylactically but initiate when a causative agent has been identified.
   b. Assess wounds for change in color or odor.
   c. Provide protective isolation as needed.
   d. Provide wound care with topical agents to prevent bacterial or fungal infections.
   e. Practice sterile technique for dressing changes.
3. Provide parental teaching about pain management, wound care, and means to prevent infection.

D. Health promotion and maintenance
1. Optimize child's functional capacity after the burn injury through interventions and rehabilitation based on individualized and developmental assessments.
2. Recognize that children vary in their physiologic and psychologic responses to burn injury and require treatment adjustment toward these needs.
3. Assist child and family in home care of the wound, including dressing changes, application of medication, physical therapy, and nutritional and psychologic needs.
4. Promote growth and development by determining the child's needs and setting realistic goals.

E. Psychologic integrity
1. Support cultural and spiritual needs of the child and family during the acute and rehabilitative stages of the burn injury.
2. Provide child diversional activity along with pain management to ensure compliance with burn therapies.
3. Prepare child and family for coping with developmental regression.
4. Offer counseling and support groups.
5. Allow child and family to participate in burn therapies.

F. Basic care and comfort
  1. Manage pain.
    a. Assess for pain and administer analgesics, especially for burn-related procedures.
    b. Place child in position of comfort.
    c. Place bed cradle over painful body parts.
    d. Determine child's past experiences with pain.
    e. Use alternative techniques to manage pain, such as distraction, imagery, and relaxation techniques.
  2. Provide a high-protein, high-calorie diet or total parenteral nutrition if child cannot eat.

G. Reduction of risk potential: Identify and prevent complications.
  1. Prevent heat loss by maintaining body temperature.
    a. Keep child covered.
    b. Warm solutions before use.
    c. Use radiant warmer.
  2. Prevent infection: Assess for signs of sepsis.
    a. Temperature instability
    b. Hyperventilation
    c. Ileus
  3. Prevent contractures through:
    a. Positioning
    b. Splinting
    c. Active and passive range of motion
    d. Physical therapy

H. Pharmacologic and parenteral therapies: For a description of medications used to treat burns, see Chapter 34 regarding adult burn management.
  1. Pharmacologic therapies are individualized in children based on severity of burn, child's weight, and body surface area; these include:
    a. Prophylaxis of tetanus toxoid
    b. Analgesics
    c. Antianxiety agents
    d. Topical agents to prevent and/or treat infections
    e. Debriding agents
  2. Fluid resuscitation is regulated to maintain minimal urine output at 1 to 2 ml/kg/hr for children weighing less than 30 kg, and 30 to 50 ml/hr for children weighing more than 30 kg. Parkland formula is used to determine fluid resuscitation needs; Ringer lactate solution is used most frequently.

Bibliography

Hatfield, N. (2006). *Broadribb's introductory pediatric nursing.* Philadelphia: Lippincott Williams & Wilkins.

Pillitteri, A. (2006). *Maternal & child health nursing: Care of the childbearing and childrearing family* (5th ed.). Philadelphia: Lippincott Williams & Wilkins.

Wong, D. L., et al. (2006). *Maternal child nursing care.* St. Louis: Mosby.

CHAPTER 10

Practice Test

Atopic Dermatitis (Eczema)

1. AF A client who is 6 months of age is diagnosed as having acute atopic dermatitis. The nurse is evaluating the parents' understanding of care for their child. Which of these comments indicates that the parents need additional health teaching? Select all that apply.

☐ 1. "We should give a daily bath in tepid water without using soap."
☐ 2. "We should give the child oral Benadryl to relieve itching."
☐ 3. "We should apply hydrocortisone cream to the lesions."
☐ 4. "We should apply alcohol to the lesions daily."
☐ 5. "We should cover the involved areas with a dry dressing."

2. Which of the following outcomes results from the use of hydrocortisone cream as a treatment for atopic dermatitis in a client who is 2 years of age?

☐ 1. Atopic dermatitis shows up as asthma when the child becomes a teenager.
☐ 2. Use of the hydrocortisone cream leads to kidney disease.
☐ 3. Flare-ups of lesions follow therapy.
☐ 4. Atopic dermatitis recurs following a streptococcal infection.

Scabies

3. A teenager with scabies is being treated with permethrin (Elimite) cream. Which of the following client statements indicates a need for further teaching about disease management?
- □ 1. "I think it is really disgusting that they left eggs and feces in my skin."
- □ 2. "I am so glad that after I apply the Elimite cream, the itching will go away."
- □ 3. "Well, at least I will only have to apply one dose of the Elimite."
- □ 4. "I will apply the Elimite cream all over my body, not just where it itches."

4. **AF** A child with scabies is being treated with permethrin 5% cream (Elimite). The nurse should instruct the parents to apply the cream in which of the following ways? Select all that apply.
- □ 1. Apply cream in the morning before the child goes to school.
- □ 2. Apply cream only on the affected areas.
- □ 3. Bathe the child to remove all cream before reapplying the cream.
- □ 4. Apply cream all over the body before bedtime and leave undisturbed throughout the night.
- □ 5. Keep the child out of the sun.

Head Lice

5. Which statement by a parent whose child was just diagnosed with pediculosis capitis (head lice) demonstrates an understanding of the safety and efficacy of the common medications used to treat the infection?
- □ 1. "I am going to request a prescription for Lindane since it works the best."
- □ 2. "After I apply the RID cream I will use the special comb to get the nits out."
- □ 3. "I want to get some Nix cream since it is 100% effective at killing all the eggs."
- □ 4. "I like the RID cream because it won't cause brain toxicity in my child."

6. **AF** An adolescent is being treated for head lice. The nurse should instruct the client to do which of the following? Select all that apply.
- □ 1. Soak combs, brushes, and hair accessories in boiling water for 10 min.
- □ 2. Machine-wash all washable items in cold water.
- □ 3. Dry clothes in a hot dryer for at least 20 min.
- □ 4. Seal items that can not be washed, vacuumed, or dry cleaned in plastic bags for 14 days.
- □ 5. Stay home from school until the nits are gone.

Otitis Media

7. A child who is 5 years of age is diagnosed with acute otitis media. The primary goal of treatment is to:
- □ 1. Relieve pain.
- □ 2. Prevent hearing loss.
- □ 3. Have the child avoid pulling on his ear.
- □ 4. Keep the child from blowing his nose.

8. A child with chronic otitis media is having myringotomy tubes placed. The child asks, "When will the tubes be removed?" The nurse responds with which of the following statements?
- □ 1. "You will have them replaced every 2 months until you reach age 18."
- □ 2. "The tubes remain in place for 6 months and then are absorbed."
- □ 3. "The tubes remain in place for 6 to 12 months until they come out by themselves."
- □ 4. "The tubes are not removed; they grow permanently into place."

9. A toddler with acute otitis media (AOM) is taking amoxicillin. The nurse should instruct the parents about which of the following?
- □ 1. If the AOM does not resolve with amoxicillin, a myringotomy will be necessary.
- □ 2. If the child is older than 24 months, a shorter course of antibiotics is sufficient.
- □ 3. If the child improves clinically, continue the entire duration of antibiotics (10 to 14 days).
- □ 4. If the child experiences ear pain, alternate acetaminophen (Tylenol) and ibuprofen for pain control.

Foreign Body Aspiration

10. An infant aspirates a small toy and begins coughing, turns cyanotic, and is unable to make a sound. The nurse's first action is to:
- □ 1. Perform a chest thrust.
- □ 2. Turn the infant prone and administer back blows.
- □ 3. Stimulate further coughing with a tongue blade.
- □ 4. Verbally encourage the infant to continue coughing.

Accidents and Unintentional Injuries

11. The nurse is teaching a mother regarding potential choking hazards in her toddler. Which of the following statements indicates the mother needs additional follow-up instruction?
- □ 1. "I will buy my child a Mylar balloon to help brighten the room."

- ☐ 2. "I like to give my child teaspoons dipped in peanut butter."
- ☐ 3. "I cut hot dogs length wise to make them easier to pick up."
- ☐ 4. "I take off the aluminum tabs when I give my child a soda."

12. AF The nurse is teaching a group of parents about potential choking hazards for small children. Instructions state that small children should avoid eating which of the following foods until they are older? Select all that apply.

- ☐ 1. Peanuts.
- ☐ 2. Bananas.
- ☐ 3. Wheat bread.
- ☐ 4. Grapes.
- ☐ 5. Strawberries.
- ☐ 6. Popcorn.

Poisonings

13. When making a home visit, the nurse observes a child who is 2 years of age eating paint from a windowsill. The mother tells the nurse this is the first time the child has eaten the paint. Because the house is old, the nurse should tell the parents to:

- ☐ 1. Administer ipecac syrup the next time they see the child eat paint.
- ☐ 2. Teach the child that paint is not an edible substance.
- ☐ 3. Cover the windowsills to prevent the child's access to them.
- ☐ 4. Take the child to a health care facility for testing.

14. AF Parents bring their child who is 2 years of age to the emergency department because the child has ingested approximately 15 acetaminophen tablets 30 min ago. The nurse should do which of the following in priority order? Place the actions in order of first to last.

_____ 1. Administer activated charcoal.
_____ 2. Establish an airway.
_____ 3. Administer *N*-acetylcysteine (Mucomyst).
_____ 4. Assess vital signs.

Child Abuse

15. The nurse is assessing an infant for normal growth and development. Which of the following findings is most likely to indicate abuse?

- ☐ 1. A tall, thin appearance.
- ☐ 2. A scald burn on the chest.
- ☐ 3. Linear abrasions on the ankles and wrists.
- ☐ 4. A maculopapular rash on the buttocks.

16. A child who is 18 months of age is brought to the emergency department by her babysitter. The babysitter states, "She fell from the sofa an hour ago and has not been herself since." On questioning, the babysitter appears to be unsure of time and other facts about the incident. Which question below would be most effective in obtaining more information about the child's injuries?

- ☐ 1. "Why did you leave the child alone on the couch?"
- ☐ 2. "Have you taken a course in safe babysitting?"
- ☐ 3. "Tell me what was happening before she fell."
- ☐ 4. "Where are her parents? Do they know this happened?"

Burns

17. A mother calls the emergency department to report her 18-month-old child has a scald burn on his abdomen from hot coffee. The triage nurse should instruct the mother to do which of the following first?

- ☐ 1. Pour cool water over the scalded skin area.
- ☐ 2. Remove the shirt and apply burn ointment.
- ☐ 3. Bring him to the emergency department.
- ☐ 4. Cover the area with a loose gauze dressing.

18. A child is brought alone by ambulance to the emergency department with second-degree burns from a house fire. After assuring an adequate airway and fluid volume status, the priority nursing goal is to:

- ☐ 1. Decrease anxiety about procedures.
- ☐ 2. Prevent infection.
- ☐ 3. Relieve pain.
- ☐ 4. Locate family members.

19. When a child with extensive burns starts eating after being burned, it is particularly important that the diet have a high content of:

- ☐ 1. Fats.
- ☐ 2. Proteins.
- ☐ 3. Minerals.
- ☐ 4. Carbohydrates.

20. AF A child with 20% second- and third-degree burns is admitted to the burn center. The child weighs 20 kg. The nurse has started an IV infusion of lactated Ringer solution and inserted an indwelling catheter. Which of the following is an indication that the child is going into shock? Select all that apply.

- ☐ 1. Urinary output is 30 ml/hr.
- ☐ 2. Specific gravity is within normal limits.
- ☐ 3. Pain is 7 on a pain scale of 1 to 10.
- ☐ 4. Heart rate is elevated.
- ☐ 5. BP is dropping.

Answers and Rationales

1. 1, 2, 3 Goals of treatment for acute atopic dermatitis are to use moist dressings, avoid allergens, and prevent secondary infection. Bathing the child, using oral diphenhydramine (Benadryl) and applying steroid cream are appropriate actions. Using alcohol is painful with open lesions; the nurse assures dressings are clean and moist. (H)

2. 3 Atopic dermatitis is believed to be caused by an abnormal immune response to allergens in children who are genetically susceptible. Atopic dermatitis may reoccur when the child is again exposed to the substance to which he or she is allergic, but usually resolves by the time the child is a teenager. The nurse instructs parents to use the prescribed steroid cream as directed, usually for 1 to 3 weeks; kidney disease is not an outcome of the use of steroid cream. Atopic dermatitis is not associated with a streptococcal infection. (D)

3. 2 The nurse informs the client and family that although the mite that causes scabies is killed with the permethrin (Elimite) treatment, the rash and the itch is not eliminated until the stratum corneum is replaced in approximately 2 to 3 weeks. Soothing ointments or lotions can be applied for the itching. Lesions are formed as the impregnated female burrows into the statum corneum of the epidermis to deposit eggs and feces. Permethrin 5% cream (Elimite) is applied to all skin surfaces, not just where the rash is present. Only one dose of Elimite is required. (D)

4. 3, 4 Permethrin (Elimite) is applied thoroughly all over the body at night and then left undisturbed for 8 to 14 hr. The cream is then removed by thorough bathing. (D)

5. 2 The makers of many of the pediculicides (including Nix) recommend manual removal of the nits following treatment with an extra–fine-tooth comb. None of the pediculicides are 100% effective in killing all the eggs. The FDA has issued a warning regarding the use of lindane because of the potential for neurotoxicity. Clients are treated with lindane only when the benefits outweigh the risks. (D)

6. 1, 3, 4 To get rid of the lice the nurse teaches the client to machine-wash all washable clothing, towels, and bed linens in hot water; then dry in a hot dryer for at least 20 min. Combs and brushes are boiled for at least 10 min or soaked in permethrin (RID or Nix) for 1 hr. The nurse instructs the client to seal items that cannot be washed, dry cleaned, or vacuumed in a tight garbage bag for at least 14 days. It is not necessary for the child to stay home from school as "no nit" policies at schools do not reduce the transmission of lice. (H)

7. 1 Acute otitis media is painful. Children need pain relief until the inflammation is treated, usually with antibiotics. The child will tend to pull on his or her ear, but this does not damage the middle ear. If the child also has a runny nose, he or she can wipe the nose, but is told to avoid "blowing" in order to prevent pressure on the middle ear. The child can also sleep with the head elevated to facilitate drainage and use warm compresses on the external ear to reduce the inflammation and pain. (H)

8. 3 Because myringotomy tubes are foreign objects, the tympanic membrane will extrude them after a time. The tubes do not need to be replaced. The tubes are not absorbed, nor do they grow into place. (H)

9. 3 The recommendation for the duration of antibiotic therapy for AOMs is 10 to 14 days; in children 6 years of age and older, shorter courses may be sufficient. Amoxicillin is the treatment of choice for AOM and is a first-line drug, thus a myringotomy would not be considered this early. Acetaminophen (Tylenol) and ibuprofen are only alternated for pain control in select situations in which the parent is very clear about dosing schedules as the risk of error is too significant. (D)

10. 2 Chest thrusts can rupture liver tissue in infants; instead, back blows in a prone position are recommended. The toy has obstructed the airway and coughing will likely not dislodge it. (S)

11. 2 The nurse instructs that peanut butter, a staple in the diet of children, is never given to a child unless it is spread thinly on bread or a cracker. A spoonful of peanut butter can obstruct the airway and stick to mucous membranes, becoming difficult or impossible for the child to dislodge. Peanut butter is also high in fat and can add the risk of a lipoid pneumonia. Mylar balloons are the only safe variety of balloon for children. Although soda is not a recommended drink for children, of particular concern is the aluminum tab that can become a foreign body. Hot dogs are a potential choking hazard when cut in short chunks, but by cutting them into lengthwise sticks they can more easily be chewed into tiny pieces. (S)

12. 1, 4, 5, 6 Small children explore matter with their mouths and are prone to aspirate a foreign body (FB). FB aspiration can occur at any age but is most common in children 1 to 3 years of age. The nurse instructs parents to offer food that requires the child to bite or chew; if the child attempts to swallow without chewing, the item is too large to lodge in the throat (e.g., bananas, bread, strawberries). The high fat content of potato chips and peanuts increase the risk of lipoid pneumonia. "Fun foods" are the worst offenders (e.g., hot dogs cut in small pieces, round candy, peanuts, and grapes); popcorn contains a seed that does not dissolve and may swell and cause additional problems. (S)

13. 3 The paint in older homes has a high lead base and can cause lead poisoning. The child is too young to understand directions about not eating paint, so the nurse instructs parents to remove access to the paint by covering the windowsills. Ipecac is not used to induce vomiting for paint ingestion. The parents are instructed to bring the child for testing if he or she continues to eat paint. (H)

14. 2, 4, 1, 3 The nurse follows the ABCs (airway, breathing, circulation). First, the nurse establishes an airway and then assesses vital signs for breathing and circulation. Next the nurse administers the activated charcoal because ingestion has occurred within 6 hr. Finally, the nurse administers *N*-acetylcysteine, which is an antidote for the acetaminophen; this is administered PO or IV, depending on the status of the client. (S)

15. 3 Linear abrasions at the ankles and wrists suggest a restraint was used to tie the child to a bed. A scald burn to the chest can happen from an accidental spill of hot fluid. A variety of diseases could be the cause of the rash on the buttocks. The child's height and appearance may be normal and are not associated with abuse. (P)

16. 3 An open-ended question is apt to supply more information when a person is under stress and easily susceptible to being influenced by the question. The other questions are direct and only require an answer with limited information. (S)

17. 1 The nurse instructs the mother to pour cool water over the involved area to prevent further burning, and then bring the child to the emergency department for further assessment. Nothing else (ointment, dressing) is used until the child has been assessed by health care professionals. (A)

18. 3 Second-degree burns are extremely painful, so pain relief is a priority. Next, the nurse locates the child's family and explains procedures. Preventing infection is a longer-term goal for this child. (A)

19. 2 Protein is needed for rebuilding all the tissue that has been destroyed by the burn. It is also important for the child to consume sufficient calories from fats and to balance protein intake with carbohydrates. If the child eats a well-balanced diet he or she should obtain sufficient minerals. (H)

20. 4, 5 The child is observed for shock that can occur following a severe burn. Shock is noted by the increasing heart rate and dropping BP. This child has an adequate urine output (more than 1 ml/kg body weight) and the specific gravity is within normal range. Pain is expected and is not an indicator of shock. (A)

chapter 11

The Child With Respiratory Health Problems

Respiratory health problems are common in children. Although most health problems can be treated without hospitalization and by the family caregivers at home, other problems (such as bronchiolitis or epiglottitis) may require emergency care and hospitalization. Chronic conditions such as cystic fibrosis are managed throughout the child's life. The nurse plans and coordinates care with the child, family, community, and health care team to prevent, treat, and care for these health problems. Topics in this chapter include:

- Tonsillitis
- Bronchiolitis
- Epiglottitis
- Asthma
- Pneumonia
- Cystic Fibrosis
- Sudden Infant Death Syndrome

Tonsillitis

I. Definition: Tonsillitis is the inflammation of the tonsils in the pharyngeal cavity, and can be caused by either a bacteria (streptococcus) or virus (adenovirus). The condition is often associated with pharyngitis.

II. Nursing process
 A. Assessment
  1. Assess child for signs and symptoms of inflammation from tonsillitis, including edema of the tonsils, which causes them to meet (kiss) midline.
   a. Difficulty swallowing
   b. Mouth breaths
   c. Nasal and/or muffled voice
  2. Assess child for symptoms of acute infection.
   a. Complaints of sore throat
   b. Fever
   c. Anorexia
   d. Referred ear pain
  3. Obtain a detailed health history, including history of allergies and previous history of tonsillitis or upper respiratory infection.
  4. Obtain diagnostic tests.
   a. Throat culture
   b. Visual examination of the throat
 B. Analysis
  1. Ineffective Breathing Pattern related to airway edema
  2. Anxiety related to inability to breathe effectively
  3. Acute Pain related to inflammatory process
  4. Impaired Swallowing related to pain and inflammation
 C. Planning
  1. Maintain respiratory function.
  2. Maintain oxygen supply and demand.
  3. Reduce anxiety.
  4. Treat pain to eliminate or reduce symptoms to a tolerable level.
  5. Prevent aspiration.
 D. Implementation
  1. Treat bacterial infections with antibiotics.
  2. Manage throat pain.
   a. Analgesics
   b. Throat lozenges, when age-appropriate
  3. Provide surgical management for tonsillectomy if repeated episodes of chronic tonsillitis lead to febrile seizures or airway obstruction.
 E. Evaluation
  1. Child has no increased work of breathing evidenced by unlabored respirations and oxygen saturation more than 95%.
  2. Child demonstrates reduction in pain to tolerable level as evidenced by ability to be comforted or ability to indicate reduction of pain on age-appropriate pain scale.
  3. Child participates in age-appropriate activities.

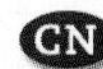

III. Client needs
 A. Physiologic adaptation
  1. Tonsillitis is managed with antibiotics and analgesics on an outpatient basis.
  2. Tonsillectomy is controversial and may be warranted in situations of recurrent febrile seizures and airway obstruction.
 B. Management of care: Care of the child with tonsillitis requires critical thinking skills, knowledge of assessment, and teaching and evaluation methods unique to the RN role. These skills cannot be delegated to an LPN or UAP.
  1. Perform a comprehensive physical assessment and provide care appropriate to the child with tonsillitis.
  2. Delegate responsibly those activities that can be delegated, including measurements, oral intake and urine output, and vital signs. All monitoring information is reported to the RN.
 C. Safety and infection control
  1. Teach child and family the importance of compliance with the antibiotic regimen to prevent complications.
  2. Postoperative tonsillectomy
   a. Prevent bleeding.
    (1) Avoid straws.
    (2) Minimize crying or coughing.
   b. Assess for bleeding.
    (1) Monitor vital signs for hypotension and tachycardia.
    (2) Observe for frequent swallowing.
 D. Health promotion and maintenance
  1. Provide consistent nurse caregiver.
  2. Promote normal growth and development.
 E. Psychologic integrity
  1. Encourage family participation in care of child.
  2. Encourage age appropriate activities to promote growth and development.
  3. Prepare family for the possibility of a needed tonsillectomy.
 F. Basic care and comfort: Manage associated throat discomfort.
  1. Soft liquid diet; encourage fluid intake
  2. Cool mist vaporizer
  3. Warm, salt water gargles
  4. Throat lozenges, when age-appropriate
  5. Analgesics such as acetaminophen (Tylenol)
 G. Reduction of risk potential: Assist the family in understanding and complying with medication regimen to prevent complications.

H. Pharmacologic and parenteral therapies involve use of comfort measures as noted in previous basic care and comfort measures section.

Bronchiolitis

I. Definition: Bronchiolitis is an inflammation of the bronchioles, causing increased production of thick mucus that obstructs the bronchiole tubes and small bronchi. The health problem is considered an infection of the lower respiratory tract, most commonly caused by respiratory syncytial virus (RSV).

II. Nursing process

A. Assessment

1. Assess child for early symptoms of the disease.
   a. Rhinorrhea
   b. Conjunctivitis
   c. Low-grade fever, poor feeding, irritability
   d. Cough
2. Assess for typical symptoms of a lower respiratory tract infection.
   a. Air hunger
   b. Increased coughing and wheezing
   c. Tachypnea
   d. Nasal flaring and retractions
   e. Cyanosis
3. Obtain a detailed health history including birth history, immunization schedule, and possible exposure to RSV.
4. Evaluate treatment through noninvasive blood gas monitoring and blood gas monitoring.
5. Obtain diagnostic tests.
   a. Nasopharyngeal secretions tested for RSV antigen
   b. Chest radiograph

B. Analysis

1. Ineffective Airway Clearance related to copious thick secretions
2. Anxiety related to air hunger and strange environment
3. Ineffective Breathing Pattern related to airway edema and increased work of breathing
4. Fatigue related to increased work of breathing
5. Imbalanced Nutrition: Less Than Body Requirements related to increased work of breathing

C. Planning

1. Maintain respiratory function.
2. Maintain oxygen supply and demand.
3. Reduce anxiety.
4. Decrease work of breathing.
5. Improve nutritional status.

D. Implementation: Provide interventions to assist with increased work of breathing.

1. Maintain patent airway.
2. Place child in 30- to 40-degree angle with head slightly extended.
3. Provide cool, humidified oxygen.
4. Provide for rest.
5. Instill normal saline into nares and implement bulb suctioning before feeding.
6. Promote fluid intake; IV fluids preferred route during acute period.
7. Administer medications—most traditional respiratory medications such as bronchodilators are controversial in their use.
   a. Administer antiviral agent on confirmation of RSV diagnosis.
   b. Use immune globulin for high-risk infants.

E. Evaluation

1. Child's symptoms related to increased work of breathing are diminished.
2. Child's respirations return to within normal limits and child breathes without difficulty.
3. Child's oxygen saturation remains more than 95%.
4. Parents remain with and comfort child to diminish anxiety.
5. Child rests quietly.

CN

III. Client needs

A. Physiologic adaptation

1. Promote contact isolation—respiratory syncytial virus is highly contagious and is spread by direct contact.
2. Evaluate effectiveness of treatment in prevention of respiratory distress.

B. Management of care: Care of the child with bronchiolitis requires critical thinking skills, knowledge of assessment, and teaching and evaluation methods unique to the RN role. These skills cannot be delegated to an LPN or UAP.

1. Do not assign nurses caring for these clients to care for clients who are at high risk for RSV exposure.
2. Perform comprehensive physical assessments and provide care appropriate to the child with bronchiolitis.
3. Delegate responsibly those activities that can be delegated, including measurements, oral intake and urine output, and vital signs. All monitoring information is reported to the RN.

C. Safety and infection control

1. Prevent spread of disease, which occurs through direct contact.
   a. Isolate or group child with other children with RSV.
   b. Practice good hand hygiene and use gloves, mask, and gown.

Table 11-1 Management of RSV

Classification	Generic/Trade Name	Expected Outcomes	Reduction of Risk Potential	Management of Care
Antiviral	Ribavirin (Virazole)	Treats severe lower respiratory tract infections.	Assess for symptoms of cardiac arrest. Assess for hypotension.	Administer via hood, tent, or mask. Assess lungs and signs of increased work of breathing.
Immune globulin	Respiratory syncytial virus immune globulin (RespiGam)	Prevents RSV in high-risk infants.	Not for infants with congenital heart disease. Assess for anaphylactic reaction. Avoid live virus vaccines for 9 months after administration of RespiGam. Monitor blood chemistry.	Assess vital signs and respiratory rate before, during, and after infusion. Teach family to observe for signs and symptoms of aseptic meningitis.

2. Teach family and all employees that may be exposed to RSV and/or ribavirin about precautions.
3. Teach parents signs and symptoms of respiratory distress and the need to seek medical care.
4. Teach family about medications used during hospitalization (see pharmacologic and parenteral therapies).
5. Maintain the six rights of medication administration.

D. Health promotion and maintenance
1. Provide child with a transitional, comfort object.
2. Try and meet oral sucking needs for infants.
3. Provide nurse caregiver.
4. Recognize that children may regress developmentally when ill or stressed.

E. Psychologic integrity
1. Provide child and family with emotional support and the ability to verbalize feelings of fear.
2. Provide child with age-appropriate toys that will promote quiet play and sustain growth and development.

F. Basic care and comfort: Ease and aid breathing.
1. Assist child into a position of comfort: Head of bed elevated 30 to 40 degrees, or in an infant seat.
2. Provide humidified oxygen environment; keep parents at bedside, if possible.

G. Reduction of risk potential
1. Immunize high-risk children with immune globulin Palivizumab (Synagis) during high-risk season, November through April.
2. Provide toys that can be in an aerosolized or humidified environment.
3. Protect staff exposed to ribavirin.
   a. Prohibit pregnant staff.
   b. Cover contact lenses with goggles.
4. Reduce risk of aspiration—do not feed orally when tachypneic (respiratory rate more than 60/min) and there is evidence of increased work of breathing.

H. Pharmacologic and parenteral therapies: Child and family will state the purpose, dosage, timing, and side effects of medications to treat RSV (Table 11-1).

Epiglottitis

I. Definition: Epiglottitis is a bacterial form of croup, and is an inflammatory, obstructive problem.
A. *Croup* is a generic term applied to a group of symptoms characterized by hoarseness, a cough described as "barking," and some degree of stridor and respiratory distress.
B. Epiglottitis is most commonly caused by *Haemophilus influenzae* type b (Hib). This inflammation and edema of the epiglottis result in laryngeal obstruction.
C. Infants and children experience problems with the larynx because of their narrowed airways.

II. Nursing process
A. Assessment
1. Assess for early signs and symptoms.
   a. Sore throat
   b. Pain on swallowing
   c. Absence of cough
   d. Drooling
   e. Agitation
2. Assess for indicators of progression.
   a. Fever, and child appears "sicker" than symptoms indicate
   b. Position of preference is sitting upright, leaning forward, with mouth open (tripod position)

c. Excessive drooling
d. Irritable, anxious
e. Voice is muffled, and froglike croaking is heard on inspiration
f. Retractions noted
g. Tachycardia and tachypnea
3. Obtain a detailed health history, including early asymptomatic period.
4. Obtain diagnostic tests.
a. Portable lateral neck x-ray with child sitting quietly in parent's lap
b. Blood culture
c. Arterial blood gas

B. Analysis
1. Ineffective Airway Clearance related to increased airway edema and increased secretions
2. Ineffective Breathing Pattern related to airway edema
3. Fear related to hypoxia and strange environment
4. Impaired Swallowing related to inflammation and edema of airway
5. Risk for Suffocation related to airway obstruction

C. Planning
1. Maintain respiratory function.
2. Maintain oxygen supply and demand.
3. Reduce anxiety.
4. Decrease work of breathing.
5. Prevent complete airway obstruction and increased respiratory distress.

D. Implementation
1. Initiate emergency endotracheal intubation or tracheotomy, if needed.
2. Provide cool, humidified oxygen environment.
3. Administer IV fluids.
4. Administer parenteral antibiotic regimen.

E. Evaluation
1. Child's symptoms related to increased work of breathing are diminished, as evidenced by age-appropriate respiratory rate and effort.
2. Child's oxygen saturation remains more than 95%.
3. Parents remain with and comfort child to diminish anxiety.
4. Child rests quietly.
5. Child does not require tracheal intubation or tracheotomy, as evidenced by results of lateral neck x-ray.

CN

III. Client needs

A. Physiologic adaptation
1. Onset of epiglottitis is abrupt and is considered an emergency situation, with complete obstruction occurring in 2 to 5 hr.
2. Signs and symptoms of increasing respiratory distress and obstruction of the airway include decreased muscle tone, decreased level of consciousness, pallor to cyanosis, nasal flaring, head bobbing, and grunting.

B. Management of care: Care of the child with epiglottitis requires critical thinking skills, knowledge of assessment, and teaching and evaluation methods unique to the RN role. These skills cannot be delegated to an LPN or UAP.
1. Perform comprehensive physical assessments and provide care appropriate to the child with epiglottitis (see implementation).
2. Delegate responsibly those activities that can be delegated, including measurements, oral intake and urine output, and vital signs. All monitoring information is reported to the RN.

C. Safety and infection control
1. Protect airway
a. Do not inspect the throat with a tongue blade or obtain a throat culture unless:
(1) Immediate tracheal intubation is available
(2) Child is in a medical facility and emergency personnel are available
b. Allow child to remain calmly in parent's lap for any procedures in order to reduce anxiety and ease breathing.
2. Assess temperature axillary, not orally.
3. Maintain NPO status until airway edema subsides.
4. Do not force child into lying position.
5. Maintain the six rights of medication administration.

D. Health promotion and maintenance
1. Encourage maintenance of immunization schedule.
2. Teach family about the importance of following entire antibiotic regimen.

E. Psychologic integrity
1. Maintain quiet, calm environment to reduce anxiety.
2. Minimize personnel examining child to provide consistent care and reduce anxiety.
3. Support child and family during the emergency phase.
4. Allow parents to stay with child throughout hospitalization.

F. Basic care and comfort
1. Ease breathing and decrease airway edema.
a. Assist child into a position of comfort to ease and aid breathing (e.g., sitting up with chin thrust forward).
b. Provide cool mist oxygen.
c. Assure high humidity.
d. Keep parents at child's bedside, if possible.

2. After emergency phase, provide child with transitional comfort object.
3. Provide consistent nurse caregiver.
4. Provide pain and fever control: Administer analgesics and antipyretics.
5. While in high humidity environment provide:
   a. Cotton pajamas
   b. Frequent linen changes
   c. No fuzzy stuffed animals

G. Reduction of risk potential
1. Have resuscitation equipment at bedside.
2. Maintain IV fluids until risk of airway obstruction has passed.
3. Provide immunization with *H. influenzae* type B conjugate vaccine beginning at 2 months of age.

H. Pharmacologic and parenteral therapies: Child and parents will state purpose for and associated side effects of all medications used to treat epiglottitis.
1. 10-day course of parenteral antibiotics or combination of parenteral and oral antibiotics for 10 days
2. Antibiotics are usually cephalosporins—if child has penicillin allergies, quinolone (for children more than 18 months of age) or sulfa drug used

Asthma

I. Definition: Asthma is a chronic inflammatory disease of the airway, resulting from a complex interaction of inflammatory cells. Inflammation results in an increase in smooth muscle response of the airways and bronchial hypersensitivity. The pattern of response moves from inflammation and edema to an increase in mucus secretions, followed by spasm of the bronchi and bronchioles.

II. Nursing process

A. Assessment
1. Assess for modifiable risk factors, including allergens; irritants such as tobacco smoke, exercise, infections, and some medications such as nonsteroidal anti-inflammatory drugs; and strong emotions.
2. Assess for nonmodifiable risk factors, including age, heredity, gender, and ethnicity.
3. Assess for classic signs and symptoms of asthma, including dyspnea, wheezing, and coughing (cough at night and during sleep without presence of infection).
4. Assess for signs and symptoms of a more severe episode.
   a. Dyspnea with a prolonged expiratory phase associated with audible wheezing
   b. Pallor with malar (cheek) flushing
   c. Circumoral and nail bed cyanosis
   d. Restless, irritable
   e. Position of comfort is tripod for young children and upright with hands resting on something to aid in breathing
   f. Breath sounds are coarse; crackles and coarse rhonchi heard and retractions noted
5. Obtain a detailed health history, including exposure to one or more risk factors for precipitating an attack. Include known allergies, history of hospitalizations, and any family history of allergies and asthma.
6. Obtain diagnostic tests: Classified based on an index of clinical and symptomatic severity that guide pharmacotherapies and treatment regimen.
   a. Radiographics rule out disease
   b. Pulmonary function tests (PFTs)
   c. Peak expiratory flow rate (PEFR)
   d. Pulse oximetry and arterial blood gas analysis
   e. Skin testing for allergies

B. Analysis
1. Ineffective Airway Clearance related to increased tenacious mucus production
2. Anxiety related to hypoxia, procedures, and strange environment
3. Ineffective Breathing Pattern related to inflammation and edema
4. Risk for Infection related to increased mucus production
5. Ineffective Tissue Perfusion: Cardiopulmonary, related to hypoxia

C. Planning
1. Maintain respiratory function.
2. Restore oxygen supply and demand.
3. Reduce anxiety.
4. Improve ventilation capacity.
5. Prevent respiratory infection.
6. Promote tissue perfusion and oxygenation.
7. Promote growth and development.

D. Implementation
1. Prevent exacerbation. Instruct child and family to:
   a. Avoid irritants such as tobacco smoke; instruct family and caregivers to assure a smoke-free environment.
   b. Identify and avoids allergens.
   c. Adhere to preventive use of medications.
   d. Monitor for increased symptoms of disease.
2. Reduce inflammation.
   a. Instruct child and family on use of long-term medications.

b. Provide IV fluids to thin tenacious secretions.

E. Evaluation
1. Child and family state exacerbating factors and methods to prevent asthma attack.
2. Child and family identify environmental allergens.
3. Child and family verbalize understanding of home maintenance including medication regimen for acute and long-term management.
4. Child and family verbalize early symptoms and management of asthma attack.
5. Child is free of infection.
6. Child has improved ventilatory capacity without dyspnea.

CN

III. Client needs
A. Physiologic adaptation: Allergic airway reaction can precipitate an early and immediate asthma attack followed by a late obstruction within several hours.
1. Asthma is controlled with medication and environmental adaptation on an outpatient basis. Corticosteroids, mast cell stabilizers, β_2–adrenergic agents, and bronchodilators improve ventilatory capacity and prevent asthma attacks.
2. Signs and symptoms may indicate potential status asthmaticus and potential respiratory failure and death: Decreased pO_2, respiratory acidosis, breath sounds absent, and tachypnea.

B. Management of care: Care of the child with asthma requires critical thinking skills, knowledge of assessment, and teaching and evaluation methods unique to the RN role. These skills cannot be delegated to an LPN or UAP.
1. Perform a comprehensive physical assessment and provide care appropriate to the child with asthma.
2. Provide follow-up management of home care and environment by reducing allergens.
a. Remove wall-to-wall carpeting and replace with wooden or linoleum flooring.
b. Cover furnace or air conditioner outlets with glass fiber or cheesecloth filters.
c. Clean wall or floor heating units weekly.
d. Keep only one bed in a room; cover pillows, mattress, and box spring (which should be scrubbed) with dust-proof casings.
e. Use cotton or synthetic blankets (not quilts or comforters).
f. Launder sheets and pillowcases in hot water (150°F).
g. Evaluate how the home is heated.
h. Reduce or remove any possible smoke from the home.
i. Remove pets from environment.
j. Evaluate home for presence of mold, roaches, and rodents.
3. Assess community resources for child and family, such as community asthma-prevention classes.
4. Delegate responsibly those activities that can be delegated, including measurements, oral intake and urine output, and vital signs. All monitoring information is reported to the RN.

C. Safety and infection control
1. Provide child and family teaching.
a. Modify home environment to remove allergens.
b. Reduce risk for an exacerbation.
(1) Avoid cold or windy weather.
(2) Modify diet: Remove foods containing MSG and sulfites, and yellow dye.
(3) Do not administer aspirin.
c. Recognize early signs and symptoms of bronchospasm.
(1) Rhinorrhea, cough, itching, low-grade fever
(2) Alterations in peak flow rates
d. Use a metered dose inhaler for medication administration.
2. Anticipate care measures for event of asthma attack.
a. Allow child to sit in position of comfort to breath.
b. Provide humidified oxygen.
c. Administer quick-relief medication.
d. Provide IV therapy to prevent dehydration and correct acidosis.
e. Monitor vital signs to detect signs of respiratory or cardiac failure.
f. Monitor peak flow rates and arterial blood gases.
g. Monitor effectiveness of medication: If medications do not work, there is high risk for status asthmaticus.
h. Monitor breath sounds: If diminishing, this can be a warning sign of impending respiratory failure.
3. Maintain the six rights of medication administration.

D. Health promotion and maintenance
1. Instruct child and family about use of peak expiratory flow meter to assess and monitor pulmonary function: Use for children over 5 years of age.
2. Protect from respiratory infections.

3. Keep all respiratory equipment clean.
4. Teach breathing exercises such as diaphragmatic breathing.
5. Provide rest, sleep, and nutritional diet.
6. Provide adequate fluids for liquefaction of secretions.

E. Psychologic integrity
1. Provide child and family with information on community resources such as asthma camps.
2. Promote self-care and self-management.
3. Provide support to child and family.
4. Provide opportunities for child and family to express fears, concerns, and to ask questions.

F. Basic care and comfort
1. Teach child to rinse mouth after inhaling medication to promote comfort and reduce mouth irritation and infection.
2. Provide transition object if in hospital.
3. Act as consistent nurse caregiver.
4. Keep parents at bedside.
5. Provide quiet, age-appropriate activity when child is resting.

G. Reduction of risk potential
1. Recommend influenza vaccine.
2. Discuss allergen control.
a. Maintain home humidity under 50%.
b. Prevent and treat home for cockroaches.
c. Eliminate mice from home.
d. Avoid household smoke.
e. Eliminate carpet and stuffed toys from home, if possible.
f. Cover pillows and mattresses with allergen-proof covers.
3. Provide drug therapy for management of acute exacerbation and long-term control. Type and amount of medication are dictated by severity of asthma.
4. Encourage physical and mental relaxation, including chest physiotherapy (CPT; but not during acute exacerbation), and physical therapy.
5. Prevent asthma attacks through exercise management, which involves taking medications before exercising (e.g., β_2–adrenergic blocker).

H. Pharmacologic and parenteral therapies: Child and family will state the purpose, use, dosage, timing, and side effects of medications for asthma (Tables 11-2 and 11-3).

Table 11-2 Long-term Management of Asthma

Classification	Generic/Trade Name	Expected Outcomes	Reduction of Risk Potential	Management of Care
Inhaled corticosteroids	Budesonide (Pulmicort Turbuhaler) Beclomethasone (Beclovent)	Oral inhalation to control asthma.	Observe for mild cough or wheezing. Use cautiously if taking oral steroids.	Teach client to: • Avoid grapefruit • Avoid infection • Use inhaler • Wash parts of inhaler with water daily
Nonsteroidal anti-inflammatory Mast cell stabilizer	Cromolyn sodium (Intal) Nedocromil sodium (Tilade)	Blocks reaction to allergens. Inhibits response to inhaled allergens.	Assess for bronchospasm.	Teach client to gargle or use throat lozenge after treatment.
Bronchodilator	Salmeterol xinafoate (Serevent)	Prevents nocturnal and exercise symptoms.	Not for children less than 4 years of age. Assess for bronchospasm. May cause tachycardia.	Teach client to use 30–60 min before exercise but not to use again for 12 hr.
Leukotriene modifiers	Montelukast (Singulair)	Diminishes airway spasm and blocks inflammation.	Assess for dizziness and headache.	Teach parents to administer in the evening.
Long-acting β_2–agonist agents	Omalizumab (Xolair)	Mediates allergic response.	Assess for nausea, vomiting, injection site reaction, and diarrhea.	Do not administer live virus vaccines. Teach family to monitor for bleeding and bruising.

Table 11-3 Short-term Management of Asthma Exacerbation

Classification	Generic/Trade Name	Expected Outcomes	Reduction of Risk Potential	Management of Care
β_2-adrenergic agents	Albuterol (Proventil) Metaproterenol Terbutaline	Provides quick relief of exacerbation.	Avoid inhalation of medications (causes tremors, insomnia, irritability, and tachycardia).	Teach parents to reduce child's mouth irritation by rinsing mouth or using lozenges after medication administration.
Anticholinergics	Ipratropium bromide (Atrovent)	Treats bronchospasm from irritants.	Given along with short-acting inhaled β_2-agonists. May precipitate wheezing.	Monitor respiratory status before and after medication administration.
Systemic corticosteroids	Prednisone (Deltasone)	Primarily used short term to control severe asthma episodes and help speed recovery.	Educate about side effects including weight gain, increased appetite, "moon face," mood swings, and increased BP. Used for short-term dosing (<14 days).	Encourage varicella vaccine. Encourage taking with food. Avoid infection.

Pneumonia

I. Definition: Pneumonia is inflammation of the alveoli caused by a variety of agents, and is introduced either through inhalation or through the bloodstream. *Streptococcus pneumoniae* is the most common bacteria causing pneumonia. The inflammatory process causes edema of the lungs and fluid in the alveoli, which leads to hypoxia.

II. Nursing process

A. Assessment
   1. Assess child for typical signs and symptoms of pneumonia.
      a. High fever
      b. Unproductive to productive cough
      c. Dyspnea and tachypnea
      d. Tachycardia
      e. Pleuritic pain
      f. Retractions and nasal flaring
      g. Breath sounds: Fine crackles to rhonchi
   2. Obtain a detailed health history, including recent upper respiratory infection, exposure to RSV, immunization history, immunosuppression, and living environment.
   3. Obtain diagnostic tests.
      a. Chest radiograph
      b. Culture and gram stain of sputum, nasopharyngeal secretions
      c. Blood cultures and complete blood count
      d. Lung biopsy

B. Analysis
   1. Ineffective Airway Clearance related to increased pulmonary fluid
   2. Anxiety related to hypoxia, procedures, and strange environment
   3. Ineffective Breathing Pattern related to inflammation and edema
   4. Risk for Infection related to increased pulmonary fluid
   5. Ineffective Tissue Perfusion: Cardiopulmonary, related to hypoxia

C. Planning
   1. Maintain respiratory function.
   2. Restore oxygen supply and demand.
   3. Reduce anxiety.
   4. Improve ventilation capacity.
   5. Resolve respiratory infection.
   6. Promote tissue perfusion and oxygenation.
   7. Promote growth and development.

D. Implementation: Provide interventions to treat pneumonia.
   1. Provide antimicrobial therapy.
   2. Provide oxygen therapy.
   3. Promote humidified environment.
   4. Maintain patent airway: Suction as needed.
   5. Provide chest physiotherapy.
   6. Increase fluid intake.

7. Administer antipyretics and analgesics for fever and pain.

E. Evaluation
1. Child's symptoms related to increased work of breathing are diminished.
2. Child's oxygen saturation remains more than 95%.
3. Child's parents remain with and comfort child to diminish anxiety.
4. Child rests quietly.
5. Child is free of infection.
6. Child experiences improved ventilatory capacity without dyspnea.

CN

III. Client needs

A. Physiologic adaptation: Prognosis for a child with pneumonia is good, with recovery rapid when treated early. Most children can be managed on an outpatient basis.
1. Antimicrobials, oxygen, fluids, and humidified environment resolve pneumonia and prevent respiratory failure.
2. Thoracentesis may be needed because of potential development of pneumothorax or presence of purulent fluid.

B. Management of care: Care of the child with pneumonia requires critical thinking skills, knowledge of assessment, and teaching and evaluation methods unique to the RN role. These skills cannot be delegated to an LPN or UAP.
1. Perform comprehensive physical assessments and provide care appropriate to the child with pneumonia.
2. Delegate responsibly those activities that can be delegated, including measurements, oral intake and urine output, and vital signs. All monitoring information is reported to the RN.

C. Safety and infection control
1. Provide isolation, if necessary, for pneumococcal or staphylococcal pneumonia.
2. Teach child and family rationale, side effects, and importance of following medication regimen.
3. Teach child and family about disease, treatments, and outcomes.
4. Maintain the six rights of medication administration.

D. Health promotion and maintenance
1. Provide child with a transitional comfort object.
2. Act as consistent nurse caregiver to promote trust.
3. Recognize that children may regress developmentally when ill or stressed.

E. Psychologic integrity
1. Provide child and family with emotional support and the ability to verbalize feelings of fear.
2. Provide child with age-appropriate toys that will promote quiet play and sustain growth and development.
3. Involve family in care of child.
4. Encourage questions from child and family to promote communication.
5. Use strategies to reduce anxiety.

F. Basic care and comfort
1. Reduce anxiety to ease respiratory efforts.
2. Allow for rest to conserve energy.
3. Ease respiratory efforts through cool mist tent and promoting client's lying on affected side.
4. Splint chest wall and decrease pleural pain.

G. Reduction of risk potential
1. Prevent dehydration and liquefy secretions.
   a. Administer IV fluids during the acute phase.
   b. Administer oral fluids with caution if child is dyspneic or tachypneic.
2. Provide immunization with pneumococcal polysaccharide vaccine for high-risk children.

H. Pharmacologic and parenteral therapies
1. Antimicrobials such as amoxicillin clavulanate (Augmentin) or erythromycin are commonly administered orally for the child maintained at home.
2. Ampicillin sulbactam (Unasyn) may be given parenterally for the hospitalized child.

Cystic Fibrosis

I. Definition: Cystic fibrosis (CF) is a chronic disease of the exocrine system, affecting multiple systems including the respiratory and GI systems.

A. Etiology
1. Autosomal recessive trait is inherited from both parents, leading to abnormal transport of sodium and chloride; this results in increased thickness of mucous gland secretions.
2. Thickened mucus causes obstruction in small passageways such as the bronchioles and entrance to pancreas.

B. Clinical symptoms are caused by pancreatic enzyme deficiency, chronic obstructive lung disease and infection, and sweat gland malfunction.

II. Nursing process

A. Assessment
1. Assess for respiratory signs and symptoms.
   a. Wheezing, dry nonproductive cough (initially)

b. Chronic cough with dyspnea and barrel-shaped chest
c. Chronic hypoxia
(1) Clubbing of fingers and toes
(2) Cyanosis
2. Assess for GI signs and symptoms.
a. Meconium ileus (earliest manifestation)
b. Frothy, bulky, foul-smelling stools
c. Inability to absorb fat-soluble vitamins
(1) Bleeds easily
(2) Anemia
d. Prolapsed rectum
e. Thin arms and legs, but distended abdomen
f. Failure to thrive
3. Assess for reproductive signs and symptoms.
a. Delayed puberty
b. Diminished fertility
4. Obtain a detailed health history, including failure to pass meconium, family history of CF, recurrent pulmonary infections, failure to thrive and grow despite adequate intake, parent's indication that the child tastes "salty".
5. Obtain diagnostic tests.
a. Quantitative sweat chloride test
b. Chest radiograph
c. Pulmonary function tests
d. Stool fat or enzyme analysis
e. DNA testing for defective gene
f. Blood analysis: Liver enzymes, serum albumin levels, and electrolytes
g. Sputum culture

B. Analysis
1. Risk for Activity Intolerance related to chronic cough, fatigue, and malnutrition
2. Ineffective Airway Clearance related to tenacious secretions
3. Anxiety related to hypoxia and multiple procedures
4. Ineffective Breathing Pattern related to tenacious secretions
5. Risk for Delayed Development related to malnutrition and multiple hospitalizations
6. Interrupted Family Processes related to multiple health needs of the child
7. Risk for Infection related to stasis of thick pulmonary secretions
8. Fear related to hypoxia and increased mortality rates of disease
9. Impaired Gas Exchange related to tenacious secretions
10. Imbalanced Nutrition: Less Than Body Requirements related to multiple bulky stools

C. Planning
1. Prevent and treat pulmonary infection.
2. Maintain and improve oxygenation and ventilation.
3. Improve airway clearance.
4. Reduce anxiety and fear.
5. Provide child and family teaching about disease, treatments, and complications.
6. Promote self-management of care, such as self-physiotherapy.

D. Implementation
1. Treat disease and prevent complications.
a. Oral pancreatic enzymes (with food intake)
b. Fat-soluble vitamins
c. Respiratory treatments
d. Pulmonary enzymes
2. Treat infections.
a. Antibiotics
b. Oxygen

E. Evaluation
1. Child does not develop pulmonary infections or caregivers recognize symptoms and seek immediate treatment.
2. Child has increased activity tolerance.
3. Child is able to clear airways with appropriate respiratory treatment and support.
4. Child and family explain behavior that promotes respiratory function, such as exercise, respiratory treatments, and adequate fluid intake.
5. Child and family state purpose, dose, timing, and side effects of medications for treatment.

CN

III. Client needs

A. Physiologic adaptation: CF is characterized by airway obstruction from mucus and decreased pancreatic functioning.
1. Diet, medications, and respiratory treatments control CF, promote growth and development, and prevent pulmonary infections.
2. Therapeutic regimen improves gas exchange, promotes airway clearance, improves exercise tolerance, and improves nutritional status.

B. Management of care: Care of the child with CF requires critical thinking skills, knowledge of assessment, and teaching and evaluation methods unique to the RN role. These skills cannot be delegated to an LPN or UAP.
1. Perform comprehensive physical assessments and provide care appropriate to the child with CF.
2. Provide follow-up management of home care and environment, including specialized respiratory equipment such as nebulizers.
3. Assess community resources for child and family, including transportation needs, local chapter of the CF Foundation, camps, and respite care.

4. Delegate responsibly those activities that can be delegated, including measurements, oral intake and urine output, and vital signs. All monitoring information is reported to the RN.

C. Safety and infection control
   1. Provide child and family teaching:
      a. Explanation of disease, signs and symptoms, and complications
      b. Pulmonary regimen of physical activity, chest physiotherapy, postural drainage, percussion, vibration, and coughing
      c. Dietary needs: High-calorie, high-protein, with pancreatic enzymes taken with all food and snacks
      d. Medication regimen and side effects
   2. Prevent pulmonary infection through:
      a. CPT—in morning and evening but not before or just after meals
      b. Postural drainage and percussion
      c. Exercise, deep breathing, and coughing
      d. Bronchodilators
      e. FLUTTER mucus clearance device
      f. ThAIRapy Vest
      g. Aerosolized medication: Dornase alfa (Pulmozyme)
   3. Treat pulmonary infections through high-dose IV or aerosolized antibiotics at home.
   4. Monitor for bleeding, especially hemoptysis more than 300 ml every 24 hr—encourage bed rest, cough suppressants, antibiotics, and vitamin K.
   5. Maintain the six rights of medication administration.

D. Health promotion and maintenance
   1. Provide nutritional support and maintenance.
      a. Pancreatic enzymes with all meals and snacks (do not crush or chew)
      b. High-calorie, high-protein up to 150% of RDA
      c. For infants: Hydrolysate formula with enzymes placed in fruits and cereals
      d. Water miscible vitamins A, D, E, and K along with multivitamins
   2. Refer to the CF Foundation for support.

E. Psychologic integrity
   1. Provide infant with support, transitional comfort object, and consistent nurse caregiver.
   2. Provide complete explanations of all procedures for older children.
   3. Anticipate developmental regression in a frightened and stressed child.
   4. Assist parents in accepting and verbalizing guilt over transmission of disease.
   5. Provide support and encouragement to child and family.
   6. Involve family in all aspects of care.
   7. Offer anticipatory guidance to cope with complex aspects of chronic illness.

F. Basic care and comfort
   1. Provide skin care and repositioning to protect bony prominences.
   2. Provide moisture barriers to aid skin that contacts frequent stools.
   3. Choose injection sites carefully and rotate sites frequently.

G. Reduction of risk potential
   1. Use oxygen cautiously to prevent oxygen narcosis.
   2. Provide genetic counseling for parents.
   3. Do not restrict salt and ensure adequate fluids, especially during warm weather.
   4. Teach parents to avoid OTC cough suppressant that could inhibit expectoration of mucus.
   5. Administer influenza vaccine beginning at 6 months, and pneumococcal vaccine for some children.

H. Pharmacologic and parenteral therapies: Child and family will state the purpose, dosage, timing, and side effects of all medications used to treat CF.
   1. Aerosolized respiratory medication: Mucolytic—dornase alfa (Pulmozyme).
      a. Expected outcome: Medication reduces frequency of respiratory infection and improves pulmonary function.
      b. Reduction of risk potential: Assess for hoarseness, sore throat, and cough; note improvement in dyspnea and sputum clearance.
      c. Management of care: Instruct family to report rash or itching.
   2. Pancreatic enzymes: Pancrelipase (Pancrease)—enzyme replacement.
      a. Expected outcome: Replacement therapy by malabsorption.
      b. Reduction of risk potential: Do not crush or chew enteric-coated tablets; follow with full glass of water or juice. May cause mucous membrane irritation.
      c. Management of care: Instruct proper timing; monitor for weight loss, which may indicate need for higher dosage.

Sudden Infant Death Syndrome

I. Definition: Sudden infant death syndrome (SIDS) is the unexpected death of a healthy infant under

1 year of age without definitive cause of death recorded in autopsy. SIDS most frequently occurs in infants between 2 and 4 months of age during the winter and during sleep.

II. Nursing process

A. Assessment

1. Assess infant for modifiable risk factors.
   a. Sleep position (should be supine)
   b. Type of bedding
   c. Environmental temperature
   d. Sleep space (alone or with an adult)
2. Assess infant for nonmodifiable risk factors.
   a. Gender (more common in males)
   b. Ethnic origin
3. Assess appearance of SIDS victim when found.
   a. Apneic and cyanotic
   b. Frothy, blood-tinged fluid in mouth
   c. Bed is disturbed, blankets over head
4. Obtain a detailed history and family history related to determining risk factors for SIDS.
   a. Siblings
   b. Preterm infant with low birth weight
   c. Infant of drug-addicted mother
   d. Infant of mother who smoked during pregnancy
5. Obtain diagnostic tests (completed on autopsy).
   a. Pulmonary edema
   b. Petechiae within thorax

B. Analysis

1. Risk for SIDS related to increased risk factors such as prone sleep position
2. Interrupted Family Processes related to devastating emotional loss
3. Anticipatory Grieving related to known risk factors for SIDS
4. Impaired Parenting related to guilt over loss of child

C. Planning

1. Provide family with emotional support.
2. Reduce parental guilt and anxiety.
3. Prevent SIDS by providing parental teaching.

D. Implementation

1. Prevent SIDS.
   a. Modify home and sleep environment.
   b. Recognize infants at high risk.
   c. Promote prenatal care.
2. Provide emergency care for suspected SIDS, including resuscitation with current infant CPR regulations.
3. Provide home management if infant is successfully resuscitated.
   a. Provide apnea monitor.
   b. Assess need for possible respiratory stimulant medication.

E. Evaluation

1. Parents verbalize risk factors for the development of SIDS.
2. Parents verbalize feelings of grief and loss.

CN

III. Client needs

A. Physiologic adaptation: The main belief related to SIDS is the possible abnormality in the infant's neurologic regulation of the cardiopulmonary system.

B. Management of care: Care of the child with SIDS and the family requires critical thinking skills, knowledge of assessment, and teaching and evaluation methods unique to the RN role. These skills cannot be delegated to an LPN or UAP.

1. Perform comprehensive physical assessments and provide care appropriate to the child with SIDS.
2. Facilitate home visit for parents to assess home environment for infant at risk or after loss of child, such as purchasing an appropriate firm sleep surface and sleep environment that is not overheated.
3. Evaluate community resources for parents related to grieving and loss.
4. Delegate responsibly those activities that can be delegated, including measurements, oral intake and urine output, and vital signs. All monitoring information is reported to the RN.

C. Safety and infection control

1. Teach parents use of apnea monitor.
2. Teach parents CPR.
3. Assess need for respiratory stimulant medication.

D. Health promotion and maintenance: Teach parents methods to prevent possibility of SIDS.

E. Psychologic integrity

1. Provide family with a private room and staff member to stay with them.
2. Allow parents to express their feelings of guilt and anger.
3. Prepare parents for infant's appearance.
4. Allow parents to touch and hold infant.
5. Prepare parents for needed autopsy.
6. Refer parents to local SIDS organization.

F. Basic care and comfort

1. Do not leave family alone.
2. Reassure parents that occurrence of SIDS is not their fault.

G. Reduction of risk potential: Instruct parents to modify home environment to prevent SIDS.

1. Place infant in supine position to sleep.
2. Avoid soft mattress and bedding.
3. Avoid bed sharing, especially with an adult.
4. Prohibit stuffed animals in bed.
5. Avoid having room too warm or infant overbundled.
6. Encourage good prenatal care and reduction in smoking behavior.

Bibliography

American Lung Association. http://www.lungusa.org

Asthma and Allergy Foundation of America. http://www.aafa.org

Hatfield, N. (2006). *Broadribb's introductory pediatric nursing.* Philadelphia: Lippincott Williams & Wilkins.

Pillitteri, A. (2006). *Maternal & child health nursing: Care of the childbearing and childrearing family* (5th ed.). Philadelphia: Lippincott Williams & Wilkins.

Wong, D. L., et al. (2006). *Maternal child nursing care.* St. Louis: Mosby.

CHAPTER 11

Practice Test

Tonsillitis

1. A child has had a tonsillectomy. Immediately after surgery the nurse should position the child until fully awake in which of the following positions?

☐ 1. On the side, with the head elevated.
☐ 2. On the abdomen, with a pillow under the chest.
☐ 3. On the abdomen, with warm compresses applied to the throat.
☐ 4. On the side, with 30% oxygen by prongs running continuously.

2. Immediately after a tonsillectomy, a child is spitting up small amounts of blood. The nurse's first action is to:

☐ 1. Suction the back of the throat.
☐ 2. Encourage coughing.
☐ 3. Assess for bleeding.
☐ 4. Notify the HCP.

Bronchiolitis

3. A toddler has been hospitalized for laryngotracheobronchitis (LTB). The child is receiving a cool mist vaporizer directed toward the head while in a sitting or upright position. The toddler is in moderate-to-severe respiratory distress. The nurse should first:

☐ 1. Provide parents with needed reassurance.
☐ 2. Assess respiratory function.
☐ 3. Offer beverages to help liquefy secretions.
☐ 4. Give the child age-appropriate play activities.

4. An LPN is caring for an infant with bronchiolitis. The respiratory rate is greater than 60 breaths per minute. The RN intervenes if the LPN plans to:

☐ 1. Give the client a bottle of formula.
☐ 2. Increase the prescribed oxygen.
☐ 3. Elevate the head of the bed.
☐ 4. Calm the infant by sitting in a rocking chair.

Epiglottitis

5. A mother is calling the emergency department at 1:00 a.m. The mother states that her toddler has a barking cough and a very hoarse cry and is turning "a little blue around the mouth" with the coughing fits but otherwise is pink in color. The child has had a recent upper respiratory tract infection. The nurse should tell the mother to:

☐ 1. Bring the child to the emergency department.
☐ 2. Take the child into a steamy bathroom.
☐ 3. Administer a decongestant.
☐ 4. Use chest percussion over the child's back.

6. A child is hospitalized with epiglottitis. Which of the following will be most effective in improving the oxygen status of this child?

☐ 1. Centering the child in a croup tent with oxygen.
☐ 2. Placing the child in an upright position with oxygen via mask.
☐ 3. Administering a flavored cough drop to ease throat pain.
☐ 4. Positioning the child in a semi-Fowler position in a quiet room.

7. AF The experienced LPN under the supervision of the RN team leader is providing nursing care for an infant with respiratory syncytial virus (RSV). Which of the following actions are appropriate for the RN to delegate to the LPN? Select all that apply.

□ 1. Auscultate breath sounds.
□ 2. Administer prescribed aerosolized medications.
□ 3. Initiate nursing care plan.
□ 4. Check oxygen saturation using pulse oximetry.
□ 5. Complete in-depth admission assessment.
□ 6. Evaluate the parent's ability to administer aerosolized medications.

8. A child who is 5 years of age has an abrupt onset of high fever, stridor, drooling, tachypnea, and severe throat pain. Ten liters of oxygen has been applied via mask. The nurse should next:
□ 1. Elevate the head of the bed at a 15-degree angle to ease the "work of breathing."
□ 2. Assess the back of the throat using a flashlight and tongue depressor.
□ 3. Prepare for possible intubation.
□ 4. Place the child in a supine position with his or her head turned to the side.

Asthma

9. AF The nurse is teaching a parent of a preschooler who was recently diagnosed with asthma. The nurse includes which of the following in the teaching plan? Select all that apply.
□ 1. Avoid potential indoor allergens such as mold and dust.
□ 2. Wash all bedding in cold water to reduce and destroy dust mites.
□ 3. Keep the humidity in the house at 50% to 60%.
□ 4. Be sure the child wears warm clothing in cold weather.
□ 5. Avoid foods prepared with sulfite preservatives.

10. AF A child with asthma lives in a home in which both parents smoke. The nurse should encourage the family to establish which of the following "house rules" for smoking? Select all that apply.
□ 1. Do not allow visitors to smoke in the home.
□ 2. Roll car windows down when smoking in the car.
□ 3. Maintain a smoke-free home.
□ 4. Do not smoke around children.
□ 5. Wear one consistent piece of clothing (smoking jacket) when outside.
□ 6. Pick one room in the house to reserve for smoking (the parents' bedroom).
□ 7. When smoking with children nearby, blow smoke away from the child.

11. AF The nurse is instructing a 12-year-old child with asthma to self-administer albuterol through a metered-dose inhaler with a spacer. After attaching the inhaler to the spacer, in which order does the nurse instruct the client to do the following? Place the steps from first to last.
_____ 1. Hold breath for 2 to 3 s and exhale.
_____ 2. Shake the canister.
_____ 3. Place the mouthpiece of the spacer in the mouth and inhale.
_____ 4. Press the canister on the inhaler to put medicine in the holding chamber.

Pneumonia

12. A child is being discharged following hospitalization for pneumococcal pneumonia. The child is to take amoxicillin 250 mg every 8 hr. The nurse instructs the parents to administer the amoxicillin as follows:
□ 1. At 10 a.m., 2 p.m., and 11 p.m.
□ 2. When the child wakes up, at lunch, and as the child goes to bed.
□ 3. At breakfast, lunch, and dinner.
□ 4. At 7 a.m., 3 p.m. and 11 p.m.

13. A child has been admitted to the hospital with pneumococcal pneumonia. To help meet the nutritional needs of this child while preserving the child's energy and maintaining adequate oxygenation, the nurse should:
□ 1. Limit fluid intake.
□ 2. Offer six small meals.
□ 3. Provide three meals.
□ 4. Suggest enteral tube feedings.

14. A child is admitted to the hospital with pneumococcal pneumonia. The nursing goal is to promote effective airway clearance. Which of the following nursing actions is most appropriate to meet this goal?
□ 1. Change positions to prevent pooling of secretions.
□ 2. Promote activity as tolerated to keep lungs aerated.
□ 3. Maintain bed rest to prevent exhaustion.
□ 4. Place in supine position to facilitate lung expansion.

15. A child being treated for bacterial pneumonia is receiving antibiotics, bronchodilators, and acetaminophen (Tylenol). Which of the following is the best indicator of the desired outcome from treatment for ineffective airway clearance?
□ 1. Intake and output are equal.
□ 2. Oxygen saturation is 95%.

☐ 3. Temperature has been less than 99°F for 24 hr.
☐ 4. The child has a productive cough.

Cystic Fibrosis

16. The nurse is instructing a child with cystic fibrosis regarding the use of pancreatic enzyme capsules. The nurse should include the following information?
☐ 1. Do not open capsules and sprinkle on food.
☐ 2. The same number of capsules is taken with all meals.
☐ 3. Capsules are taken with all meals and snacks.
☐ 4. Capsules are taken 30 min after meals to digest nutrients.

17. An infant who failed the newborn screen test for CF has just finished a sweat chloride test to confirm the diagnosis. The laboratory report states that there was 20 mEq of NaCl in the sweat collected. The nurse understands this to mean:
☐ 1. The child will need a 72-hr fecal fat test to confirm the diagnosis.
☐ 2. The child most likely does not have cystic fibrosis.
☐ 3. The child most likely is positive for cystic fibrosis.
☐ 4. The child will need to repeat the newborn screen test.

18. A school-aged child with cystic fibrosis is taking pancreatic enzymes. The nurse should instruct the parents to report which of the following to the HCP?
☐ 1. Weight loss of 0.5 kg in 24 hr.
☐ 2. Formed stool passed 2 days ago.
☐ 3. Weight gain of 0.5 kg within 24 hr.
☐ 4. Frothy, foul-smelling stool passed today.

Sudden Infant Death Syndrome

19. Which of the following infants is at the least risk for SIDS?
☐ 1. Infant placed in side-lying position on a soft sheepskin.
☐ 2. Infant placed in supine position on a firm mattress and sharing a bed with the parent or caregiver.
☐ 3. Infant placed in prone position with a quilted comforter blanket.
☐ 4. Infant placed in supine position on a firm mattress and covered with a thin blanket.

20. When providing teaching regarding the risks for SIDS, the nurse should tell the parents that the peak age for a SIDS event is when the infant is?
☐ 1. Less than 1 month of age.
☐ 2. 2 to 4 months of age.
☐ 3. 4 to 6 months of age.
☐ 4. 6 to 12 months of age.

Answers and Rationales

1. 2 Lowering the child's head slightly and positioning the child on the abdomen allows mouth and throat secretions to flow out, avoiding possible aspiration and allowing for better assessment of bleeding from the surgery site. The other positions do not promote drainage. (A)

2. 3 Children will have a small amount of blood mixed with saliva following a tonsillectomy. Suctioning or coughing could irritate the surgical site and cause hemorrhage. The nurse continues to assess for bleeding. It is not necessary to notify the physician of these normal findings. (R)

3. 2 The most important nursing function in the care of children with LTB is continuous, vigilant observation and accurate assessment of respiratory status. Cardiorespiratory monitoring and noninvasive pulse oximetry equipment supplement visual observations. The trend away from early intubation of children with LTB stresses the importance of nursing assessments and the ability to judge impending respiratory failure so that intubation can be initiated without delay, if needed. (R).

4. 1 Infants with severe respiratory distress (traditionally, a respiratory rate greater than 60 breaths per minute for infants) are not given anything by mouth to prevent aspiration and decrease the work of breathing. Increasing oxygen, elevating the head of the bed, and calming the infant will help to ease the work of breathing. (S)

5. 2 This child has croup, a general term applied to a symptom complex characterized by hoarseness, a cough described as "barking" or "brassy" (croupy), and varying degrees of respiratory distress from swelling in the region of the larynx. Parents can alleviate some symptoms of croup by providing humidified oxygen via a cool mist vaporizer. If this is not available, exposure to a steamed bathroom or the cool night air may alleviate some symptoms. The nurse instructs the parents to bring the child to the emergency department if the child does not respond, or worsens. Antihistamines and decongestants will not help a child with upper airway constriction. Chest percussion is typically useful only when a child needs help expelling thick mucus, as in the instance of cystic fibrosis. (M)

6. 2 The child with epiglottitis is kept in an upright position with oxygen applied. The child with epiglottitis will be irritable and extremely restless, with a frightened expression. A croup tent and the separation it requires from the caregivers will cause more distress for the child. The nurse does not put anything in a child's mouth (e.g., cough drop) with suspected epiglottitis because this may cause the child to gag or cough, which can precipitate further obstruction. Semi-Fowler position does not provide sufficient support for chest expansion. (S)

7. 1, 2, 4 The experienced LPN is capable of gathering data and observations including breath sounds and pulse oximetry. Administering medications, such as aerosolized medications, is within the scope of practice for the LPN/LVN. The actions that are within the scope of practice for the professional RN include independently completing the admission assessment, initiating the nursing care plan, and evaluating a parent's abilities, as these activities require additional education and skills. (M)

8. 3 Endotracheal intubation or tracheostomy is usually considered for epiglottitis with severe respiratory distress. The epiglottal swelling typically will not improve until after 24 hr of antibiotic therapy, and the epiglottis is nearly normal by the third day. Visualizing the back of the throat with a tongue depressor can illicit a gag response, increase swelling of the epiglottis, and cause complete airway obstruction. The child will feel more distress in a supine position or at a low angle such as 15 degrees. The child is kept in an upright position, preferably sitting in parent's arms. (S)

9. 1, 3, 4, 5 Bedding is washed in hot water to destroy dust mites. All of the other points are accurate and appropriate to a teaching plan for a child with a new diagnosis of asthma. (R)

10. 1, 3, 4, 5 The nurse teaches families in which one or more members smokes that "house rules" need to be established for reducing smoke in the child's environment. Maintaining a smoke-free home is a priority. Smoking should not be permitted in the home, car, or when children are present. A "smoking jacket" used by a smoker while smoking outside (when children are not present) can help contain the asthma triggers within the fabric of the jacket, which can help prevent a respiratory reaction. Suggesting that the parents roll down windows, smoke in only one room of the house, or to blow smoke away from their children is giving the parents permission to smoke when their children are nearby. (H)

11. 2, 4, 3, 1 To effectively use a metered-dose inhaler with a spacer, the nurse instructs the client to first shake the canister to mix the medication and then press the canister to release the medication into the holding chamber. Next, the client is instructed to place the spacer into the mouth, inhale and hold the medication for 2 to 3 s, and then exhale. (D)

12. 4 The drug is administered 3 times in 24 hr at evenly spaced intervals. The drug is scheduled at times that are also practical for the family to administer. Although the drug should be given with food to enhance absorption, following typical meal time schedules may not space the drug at every 8 hr. (D)

13. 2 Eating frequent small meals prevents children with pneumonia from tiring, and reduces pressure on the lungs from a distended stomach. Children with pneumonia need a high-fluid intake to keep respiratory secretions moist. Eating large meals will distend the abdomen and put pressure on the lungs. The child does not need to be fed with tube feedings. (A)

14. 1 Children with pneumonia feel exhausted but need to change positions to prevent pooling of lung secretions. The child will not have energy to have continuous activity, and remaining in a supine position promotes pooling. The child does not need to be on complete bed rest, although the child should have frequent rest periods to prevent exhaustion. (A)

15. 2 The best indicator of airway management is oxygen saturation in normal ranges. Intake and output reflect dehydration status; body temperature indicates a response to antibiotics; a productive cough is desirable, but is related to hydration status, resolving infection, and use of bronchodilators. (A)

16. 3 The principle treatment for pancreatic insufficiency is replacement of pancreatic enzymes, which are administered with meals and snacks to ensure that digestive enzymes are mixed with food in the duodenum. Enteric-coated products prevent the neutralization of enzymes by gastric acids, thus allowing activation to occur in the alkaline environment of the small bowel. Usually one to five capsules are administered with a meal and a smaller amount is taken with snacks. Capsules can be swallowed whole or taken apart and sprinkled on a small amount of the food taken at the beginning of the meal. The amount of enzyme is adjusted to achieve normal growth and a decrease in the number of stools to one or two per day. (D)

17. 2 The nurse understands that this infant most likely does not have cystic fibrosis. For diagnostic purposes, the quantitative sweat chloride test is performed on sweat obtained by iontophoresis of pilocarpine. Normally, the sweat chloride content is less than 40 mEq/L; a chloride concentration greater than 60 mEq/L is diagnostic of CF. In infants, a value greater than 40 mEq/L is highly suggestive of CF. (A)

18. 4 Disturbed GI function in a child with cystic fibrosis is reflected in bulky stools that are frothy from undigested fat (*steatorrhea*) and foul smelling from putrefied protein (*azotorrhea*). This finding may signify that the replacement pancreatic enzymes are not being administered correctly or are not sufficient in quantity to aid digestion of fat and protein. (D)

19. 4 To prevent SIDS, the nurse instructs caregivers to place the infant in the supine position during sleep. Evidence exists that a firm mattress, minimal coverings while sleeping (no thick comforters, pillows, sheepskins, etc.), and a smoke-free home can reduce the incidence of SIDS. Some SIDS risk factors include prone or side-lying positions, overheating, and bed-sharing. (S)

20. 2 SIDS is defined as the sudden, unexpected death of an apparently healthy infant that is less than 1 year of age. The death remains unexplained after a complete postmortem examination, review of the case history, and an investigation of the death scene. Peak age for SIDS is 2 to 4 months of age. (S)

chapter

12

The Child With Cardiovascular Health Problems

Common cardiovascular health problems in children include both congenital disease, such as heart defects, as well as acquired disease, such as rheumatic fever. Nursing care is directed toward planning care for the child undergoing diagnostic or surgical interventional strategies to correct defects, and assisting the child to attain and maintain health. Topics in this chapter include:

- Congenital Heart Defects
- Rheumatic Fever
- Kawasaki Disease
- Systemic Hypertension
- Diagnostic and Interventional Strategies: Cardiac Catheterization

Congenital Heart Defects

I. Definition: Congenital heart defects are anatomic abnormalities of the heart that are present at birth and impair cardiac circulation or function.
   A. Defects are classified based on hemodynamic characteristics or blood flow patterns. Table 12-1 provides a summary of common congenital cardiac defects.
      1. Increased pulmonary blood flow
         a. Atrial septal defect (ASD)
         b. Ventricular septal defect (VSD)
         c. Patent ductus arteriosus (PDA)
      2. Decreased pulmonary blood flow: Tetralogy of Fallot
      3. Obstruction of blood flow out of the heart: Coarctation of the aorta
      4. Mixed blood flow between oxygenated and deoxygenated: Transposition of the great vessels
   B. Etiology of most congenital heart defects is unknown. Some contributing factors may include genetic predisposition, maternal rubella, alcoholism, maternal age greater than 40 years, and maternal diabetes.
   C. Two main clinical manifestations result from the severity of the defect and the altered hemodynamics; these include:
      1. Heart failure
      2. Hypoxemia—arterial oxygen tension that is less than normal, identified by decreased PaO_2

II. Nursing process
   A. Assessment
      1. Obtain a detailed health history of pregnancy, feeding problems, siblings, family history of congenital defects, and respiratory difficulties.
      2. Assess for general symptoms of congenital heart defects (symptoms vary based on defect).
         a. Signs related to respiratory distress, including tachypnea, sweating, and poor feeding and weight gain
         b. Growth problems
         c. Edema

Table 12-1 Congenital Cardiac Defects

Defect	Pathophysiology	Assessment	Treatment	Prognosis
Atrial Septal Defect (ASD)	Abnormal opening between atria	Murmur may be only symptom	May close spontaneously. Interventional catheter. Surgical patch.	Very good
Ventricular Septal Defect (VSD)	Abnormal opening between ventricles	Murmur, signs of CHF	Interventional catheter. Surgical patch.	Good
Patent Ductus Arteriosus (PDA)	Connection between pulmonary artery and aorta	Murmur, signs of CHF, wide pulse pressure	Indomethacin for premature newborns. Interventional catheter or surgical ligation for those unresponsive to medication.	Very good
Tetralogy of Fallot	Four defects: 1. VSD 2. Pulmonic stenosis 3. Overriding aorta 4. Right ventricular hypertrophy	Mild to severe cyanosis, murmur, CHF, and symptoms related to hypoxia	Staged repair: Palliative shunt then two to three staged surgical repairs.	Good
Coarctation of the Aorta	Narrowing of the aorta at the ductus insertion	BP and pulses bounding proximal to the defect and weak distal to the defect Epistaxis in older children	Balloon angioplasty or resection of coarctation.	Very good
Transposition of the Great Vessels	Pulmonary artery exits left ventricle and aorta exits right ventricle with no communication	Severe cyanosis and depressed newborn	Balloon atrial septostomy at birth, then arterial switch procedure.	Good, but long-term complications

d. Cyanosis
e. Tachycardia
f. Murmurs

3. Assess for signs and symptoms of chronic hypoxemia.
   a. Polycythemia—increased number of RBCs produced in the presence of chronic hypoxia (reduced tissue oxygenation); may cause increased viscosity of blood
   b. Clubbing—tips of fingers and toes thicken and flatten
   c. Squatting in toddlers and children
   d. Hypercyanotic spells—occur from increased oxygen demands; child becomes cyanotic and flaccid
   e. Cerebral vascular accident (CVA)—increased risk because of increased blood viscosity
4. Obtain diagnostic tests.
   a. Chest radiograph
   b. ECG
   c. Echocardiography
   d. Cardiac catheterization
   e. Laboratory findings
      (1) Increased hematocrit (polycythemia)
      (2) Increased hemoglobin, increased erythrocyte count
      (3) Altered arterial blood gases

B. Analysis
   1. Activity Intolerance related to decreased tissue oxygenation
   2. Anxiety related to hypoxia, multiple procedures, and strange environment
   3. Decreased Cardiac Output related to cardiac blood flow impairment or increased cardiac workload
   4. Delayed Growth and Development related to chronic hypoxia and poor feeding
   5. Excess Fluid Volume related to increased pulmonary edema
   6. Impaired Gas Exchange related to hypoxia
   7. Ineffective Breathing Pattern related to increased pulmonary blood flow
   8. Risk for Infection related to pulmonary stasis
   9. Interrupted Family Processes related to chronic and life-threatening illness
   10. Ineffective Tissue Perfusion: Cardiopulmonary, related to hypoxia

C. Planning
   1. Improve cardiac output.
   2. Decrease cardiac workload and demands.
   3. Improve oxygenation and respiratory effort.
   4. Maintain adequate nutrition.
   5. Remove or reduce excess fluid.
   6. Reduce fear and anxiety.
   7. Provide child and family teaching.
   8. Provide emotional support for child and family.

D. Implementation
   1. Re-establish pulmonary blood flow at birth: Prostaglandin E (Alprostadil)—causes vasodilation and smooth muscle relaxation; can be used to keep open ductus arteriosus and to maintain pulmonary blood flow; used to stabilize infant and then diagnose defects.
   2. Close patent ductus arteriosus: Indomethacin (Indocin) IV—causes closure of patent ductus arteriosus by inhibiting prostaglandins synthesis, which increases sensitivity of ductus to the dilating effects of prostaglandins.
   3. Treat hypercyanotic spells.
      a. Place child in knee-chest position.
      b. Administer 100% oxygen by face mask.
      c. Administer morphine sulfate.
   4. Treat cyanosis.
      a. Maintain hydration.
      b. Provide iron supplements.
      c. Initiate blood transfusion as ordered.
      d. Prevent infections and treat aggressively.
   5. Treat congenital cardiac defects.
      a. Surgery
         (1) Palliative (does not cure)
         (2) Corrective
      b. Interventional cardiac catheterization

E. Evaluation
   1. Child's cardiac output is increased as evidenced by a decrease in symptoms, improved growth, and increased activity tolerance.
   2. Child's respiratory efforts are improved and child exhibits increased exercise tolerance and ability to eat.
   3. Child's nutritional status is maintained or improved and child shows evidence of improved growth and development.
   4. Child's anxiety is reduced regarding procedures and child is compliant.
   5. Child's sleep/wake patterns are maintained.
   6. Child and family describe outpatient management of cardiac regimen.
   7. Child and family state the purpose, dosage, timing, and side effects of the medications prescribed to manage cardiac problems.

CN

III. Client needs

A. Physiologic adaptation: Congenital heart disease is managed with interventional cardiac catheterization or surgical intervention to repair the anatomic defects. Positive findings from cardiac catheterization may warrant the child's preparation for surgery.

1. Cardiac glycosides, diuretics, and surgery improve cardiac output, decrease respiratory effort, and decrease myocardial workload (as evidenced by absence of congestive heart failure, improved growth and development, and absence of complications).
2. Child's therapeutic levels and compliance with home management are evidenced by digoxin levels, arterial blood gases, and oxygen saturation.

B. Management of care: Care of the child with a congenital cardiac defect requires critical thinking skills and knowledge of assessment, and teaching and evaluation methods unique to the RN role. These skills cannot be delegated to an LPN or UAP.

1. Perform a comprehensive physical assessment and provide care to the child with congenital heart defect.
2. Assess for home health needs, including specialized equipment for feeding issues and treatment of heart failure, if present.
3. Evaluate community resources for family support, such as possible transportation needs, local support groups for parents and child, location of camps, and respite care.
4. Delegate responsibly those activities that can be delegated, including measurements, oral intake and urine output, vital signs and reporting child's subjective data. All monitoring information is reported to the RN.

C. Safety and infection control

1. Provide child and family teaching about home care following cardiac surgery.
   a. Possible dietary restrictions
   b. Fluid needs
   c. Activity needs and restrictions
   d. Operative care management
   e. Medication regimen
   f. Home management
   g. Follow-up care
   h. Developmental needs
2. Identify children at high risk for the development of bacterial endocarditis.
3. Maintain the six rights of medication administration.

D. Health promotion and maintenance

1. Foster parent-child attachment.
2. Provide anticipatory guidance to prevent overdependency.
3. Provide opportunities for socialization of the child.
4. Promote normal growth and development.
5. Provide age-appropriate toys.

E. Psychologic integrity

1. Provide emotional support to child and family coping with severe illness.
2. Recommend counseling and support groups to assist with coping, such as Kids with Heart National Association for Children's Heart Disorders.
3. Identify family stressors such as physical exhaustion, financial strain, guilt, fear, and lack of support.

F. Basic care and comfort

1. Provide constant support and reassurance for child undergoing multiple procedures.
2. Provide for consistent sleep/wake patterns.
3. Provide transitional comfort object.
4. Provide consistent nurse caregiver.

G. Reduction of risk potential

1. Institute bacterial endocarditis prophylaxis for high-risk children.
2. Manage polycythemia to prevent cerebrovascular accidents.
   a. Aggressively treat all infections to prevent dehydration.
   b. Administer fluids PO or parenterally.
3. Provide MedicAlert bracelets, if needed, if the child has a pacemaker, heart transplant, or is taking anticoagulants.

H. Pharmacologic and parenteral therapies: Child and family will state the purpose, dosage, timing, and side effects of cardiac glycosides: Digoxin (Lanoxin).

1. Expected outcome—used to increase the force of contraction, decrease heart rate, and enhance diuresis; observe for improved cardiac output and relief of edema
2. Reduction of risk potential
   a. Withhold drug if heart rate is below 90 to 110 beats per minute in infants and young children, and below 70 beats per minute in older children.
   b. Assess for prolonged P-R interval.
   c. Monitor serum potassium level.
3. Management of care
   a. Correct administration: Count apical heart rate for one full minute.
   b. Assess for and teach family signs of toxicity.
      (1) Bradycardia
      (2) Nausea and vomiting
      (3) Visual disturbances
   c. Teach parents about dosing.
      (1) If dose missed and less than 4 hr—administer.
      (2) If dose missed and more than 4 hr—skip and resume with next scheduled dose.

(3) If child vomits—skip dose.
(4) If more than two doses are missed—notify HCP.

Rheumatic Fever

I. Definition: Acute rheumatic fever is an inflammatory, autoimmune disease caused by group A ß-hemolytic streptococcal infection. The disease affects the connective tissue in the body, primarily the heart, joints, subcutaneous tissues, and small vessels in the central nervous system. The most serious complication is rheumatic heart disease, which affects the mitral valve.

II. Nursing process

A. Assessment

1. Assess for general signs and symptoms.
   a. Low-grade fever
   b. Epistaxis
   c. Arthralgia
   d. Pallor
   e. Anorexia
   f. Fatigue
2. Assess for specific signs and symptoms.
   a. Carditis
      (1) Tachycardia
      (2) Cardiomegaly
      (3) Murmur
      (4) ECG changes
   b. Polyarthritis
      (1) Swollen, hot painful joints
      (2) Joint changes
   c. Erythema marginatum: Macule on trunk and extremities
   d. Subcutaneous nodules: Nontender swelling over bony prominences
   e. Chorea
      (1) Irregular movements of extremities
      (2) Facial grimace
      (3) Muscle weakness
3. Obtain a detailed health history, including history of recent streptococcal infection and allergies.
4. Obtain diagnostic tests.
   a. Presence of Aschoff bodies: Hemorrhagic lesions
   b. Jones criteria
   c. Elevated antistreptolysin O titer
   d. Positive throat culture for the presence of strep
   e. Elevated sedimentation rate
   f. ECG shows prolonged P-R interval

B. Analysis

1. Risk for Decreased Cardiac Output related to inflammatory process
2. Hyperthermia related to inflammatory process
3. Risk for Injury related to unstable gait
4. Acute Pain related to painful, joint inflammation
5. Impaired Physical Mobility related to painful, joint inflammation

C. Planning

1. Reduce incidence of cardiac sequelae.
2. Reduce pain to tolerable level.
3. Protect from injury.
4. Reduce fear and anxiety.
5. Provide child and family teaching.
6. Provide emotional support for child and family.
7. Promote family compliance with medication regimen.

D. Implementation

1. Encourage compliance with medication regimen.
2. Palliate symptoms and promote recovery.
   a. Penicillin, PO or IM, for 10 days
   b. Salicylates for fever and inflammation
   c. Sedation for chorea
   d. Corticosteroids for myocardial inflammation
3. Prevent recurrence.
   a. Screening
   b. Prophylaxis

E. Evaluation

1. Child and family state understanding and importance of compliance with medication regimen.
2. Child and family state the purpose, dosage, timing, and side effects of the medications prescribed to treat the disease and prevent cardiac problems.
3. Child and family verbalize understanding of secondary prophylaxis and treatment before invasive procedures.

CN

III. Client needs

A. Physiologic adaptation

1. Aschoff bodies are hemorrhagic lesions found in all patients.
2. Infection, is indicated by carditis—chest pain, dyspnea, tachycardia, and friction rub.

B. Management of care: Care of the child with acute rheumatic fever requires critical thinking skills and knowledge of assessment, and teaching and evaluation methods unique to the RN role. These skills cannot be delegated to an LPN or UAP.

1. Perform a comprehensive physical assessment and provide care to the child with rheumatic fever.

2. Assess for home health needs such as ability to obtain and administer antibiotics, including appropriate equipment.
3. Evaluate community resources for family support for transportation, and possible home health nurses to administer medications.
4. Delegate responsibly those activities that can be delegated, including measurements, oral intake and urine output, vital signs, and reporting child's subjective data. All monitoring information is reported to the RN.

C. Safety and infection control
   1. Promote recovery and prevent injury.
      a. Promote bed rest during acute phase.
      b. Limit exercise with carditis.
      c. Protect from symptoms of chorea.
         (1) Prevent child's handling of sharp implements such as forks.
         (2) Assist with ambulation.
         (3) Provide a calm, quiet environment.
         (4) Initiate seizure precautions.
      d. Monitor for penicillin allergy.
      e. Avoid use of salicylates until diagnosis is confirmed.
   2. Teach parents to recognize signs of recurrence—upper respiratory infection, increased temperature, and joint pain.
   3. Maintain the six rights of medication administration.

D. Health promotion and maintenance
   1. Provide opportunities for socialization for the child.
   2. Promote normal growth and development with diversified age-appropriate activities.

E. Psychologic integrity
   1. Allow child to verbalize feelings about disease and manifestations, especially chorea symptoms.
   2. Provide transitional comfort object for child if hospitalized.
   3. Provide consistent nurse caregiver.

F. Basic care and comfort: Provide passive stimulation to promote growth and development, and managing pain.
   1. Assess pain using age-appropriate scale.
   2. Administer analgesics and anti-inflammatory medications.
   3. Promote bed rest during acute phase.
   4. Elevate extremities above level of heart.
   5. Change position every 2 hr.
   6. Handle child gently.
   7. Treat joint pain with massage, and alternating hot and cold application.

G. Reduction of risk potential:
   1. For children with a history of rheumatic fever or cardiac disease—provide antibiotic prophylaxis for invasive procedures, dental work, and infection.
   2. Prevent rheumatic fever—screening for group A streptococcal pharyngitis.
   3. Prevent recurrence—secondary prophylaxis:
      a. Begin immediately after initial antibiotic treatment.
      b. Continue for 5 to 10 years with PO or IM penicillin.
      c. Severe valvular damage or valve surgery requires lifetime prophylaxis.

H. Pharmacologic and parenteral therapies: Child and family will state the purpose, dosage, timing, and side effects of cardiac glycosides: Penicillin V potassium (Pen-Vee K)—anti-infective.
   1. Expected outcome: Used for infections due to streptococci and as prophylaxis in rheumatic fever.
   2. Reduction of risk potential: Watch for cross sensitivity to cephalosporins; observe for nausea, diarrhea, and flushing.
   3. Management of care: Instruct family to administer until entire course of medication is completed.

Kawasaki Disease

I. Definition: Kawasaki disease, also known as mucocutaneous lymph node syndrome, is an acute systemic vasculitis of unknown etiology. The disease is self-limiting in 6 to 8 weeks, but without treatment more than 25% of children will develop cardiac sequelae that especially can damage the coronary arteries or cause aneurysm formation, resulting in a systemic inflammation of the small to medium-sized blood vessels. Incidence is most common in children under 5 years of age, specifically toddlers.

II. Nursing process
   A. Assessment
      1. Assess for signs and symptoms of acute phase.
         a. Sudden onset of high fever
         b. Conjunctiva become red
         c. Pharyngeal redness with classic "strawberry" tongue
         d. Hands and feet edematous, and palms and soles develop redness
         e. Red rash of hands and feet may desquamate
         f. Cervical lymphadenopathy
         g. Extreme irritability
      2. Assess for signs and symptoms of subacute phase.
         a. Fever resolves and other clinical symptoms disappear

b. Arthritis appears
c. Irritability continues
3. Assess for signs and symptoms of the convalescent phase.
a. All clinical symptoms resolved
b. Arthritis may continue
c. Laboratory values remain abnormal
4. Assess for signs and symptoms of cardiac sequelae: Myocardial infarction from aneurysm formation.
a. Classic symptom is abdominal pain
b. Vomiting
c. Restlessness
d. Pallor and shock
5. Obtain a detailed health history, including allergies.
6. Obtain vital signs and perform comprehensive physical assessment.
7. Obtain diagnostic tests: Based on clinical findings and related laboratory tests; must have had fever that is unresponsive to antipyretics for more than 5 days.
a. Must have at least four of the five diagnostic criteria:
(1) Bilateral conjunctival redness
(2) Changes in the oral mucus membranes
(3) Extremity changes
(4) Rash, especially in the perineum
(5) Cervical lymphadenopathy
b. Laboratory findings
(1) Leukocytosis with shift to left
(2) Elevated erythrocyte sedimentation rate
(3) Elevated liver enzymes
c. Echocardiogram

B. Analysis
1. Activity Intolerance related to high fever, irritability, and joint pain
2. Anxiety related to strange environment and separation from family
3. Hyperthermia related to inflammatory process
4. Acute Pain related to joint inflammation, skin and oral mucous membrane inflammation
5. Impaired Skin Integrity related to desquamation of palms and soles of feet
6. Risk for Impaired Tissue Perfusion: Myocardial, related to coronary artery damage

C. Planning
1. Reduce fever.
2. Prevent cardiac damage.
3. Relieve anxiety.
4. Reduce incidence of cardiac sequelae.
5. Reduce pain to tolerable level.
6. Provide child and family teaching.
7. Provide emotional support for child and family.
8. Promote family compliance with medication regimen.

D. Implementation: Provide the following interventions during acute phase:
1. Administer high-dose IV immune globulin within the first 10 days of illness.
2. Provide salicylate therapy.
a. Aspirin 100 mg/kg/day in divided doses—for fever and inflammation
b. Aspirin 3 to 5 mg/kg/day for 6 to 8 weeks—when afebrile for 48 to 72 hr
3. Monitor vital signs frequently.
4. Monitor heart sounds, rate, and rhythm.

E. Evaluation
1. Child and family state understanding and importance of compliance with medication regimen.
2. Child and family state purpose, dosage, timing, and side effects of medications prescribed to treat the disease and prevent cardiac problems.
3. Child and family verbalize understanding of follow-up visits and testing.

CN

III. Client needs

A. Physiologic adaptation: Inflammation of the small and medium-sized blood vessels, including coronary arteries.
1. Damage may lead to myocardial ischemia and myocardial infarction (MI).
2. Infants at increased risk of cardiac sequelae.
3. Potential for development of heart failure; signs and symptoms include tachycardia, respiratory distress, urine output less than 1 to 2 ml/kg per hour.
4. Potential for development of aspirin toxicity; signs and symptoms include tinnitus, headache, and dizziness.

B. Management of care: Care of the child with Kawasaki disease requires critical thinking skills and knowledge of assessment, and teaching and evaluation methods unique to the registered nurse role. These skills cannot be delegated to an LPN or UAP.
1. Perform a comprehensive physical assessment and provide care to the child with Kawasaki disease.
2. Assess for home health needs, such as follow-up care with medication administration and monitoring child's health status.
3. Evaluate community resources for family support.
4. Delegate responsibly those activities that can be delegated, including measurements,

oral intake and urine output, and vital signs. All monitoring information is reported to the RN.

C. Safety and infection control
   1. Administer salicylates indefinitely if there is coronary artery damage.
   2. Assess for symptoms of CHF.
   3. Provide ECG monitoring during IV gamma globulin infusion.
   4. Teach parents the predictive course of the disease, follow-up care, and monitoring of temperature for several days after discharge.
   5. Teach parents signs and symptoms of salicylates toxicity and to report to health care practitioner.
   6. Teach parents signs and symptoms of myocardial infarction and report immediately to call 911.

D. Health promotion and maintenance
   1. Provide opportunities for socialization for the child when less irritable.
   2. Promote normal growth and development with diversified age-appropriate activities.
   3. Provide consistent nurse caregiver.

E. Psychologic integrity
   1. Allow child and family to verbalize feelings about disease and manifestations, especially desquamation.
   2. Provide transitional comfort object for child if hospitalized.

F. Basic care and comfort
   1. Monitor intake and output.
   2. Monitor daily weights.
   3. Treat skin discomfort.
      a. Cool baths
      b. Unscented lotion
      c. Loose pajamas
   4. Encourage mouth care through clear fluids and soft foods.
   5. Promote passive range of motion exercises for joints.
   6. Provide a quiet environment.

G. Reduction of risk potential
   1. Do not begin salicylate therapy until definitive diagnosis is made.
   2. Continue low-dose aspirin until platelet count is normal.
   3. Perform periodic ECG and echocardiogram.
   4. During IV gamma globulin:
      a. Check vital signs frequently.
      b. Assess for allergic reaction.
      c. Avoid measles, mumps, rubella (MMR) immunization for 11 months after IV gamma globulin.
   5. Stop aspirin and notify HCP if child is exposed to chicken pox or influenza.
   6. Instruct avoidance of contact sports if taking low-dose aspirin.
   7. Promote yearly influenza vaccine.

H. Pharmacologic and parenteral therapies: Child and family will state the purpose, dosage, timing, and side effects of IV immune gamma globulin (Gammagard): Immunoglobulin.
   1. Expected outcome: Reduces inflammation and protects coronary arteries in acute phase of Kawasaki disease.
   2. Reduction of risk potential: Assess for allergic response and stop if noted.
   3. Management of care: Monitor IV infusion and site; assess cardiac status for fluid overload; assess for allergic reaction. Instruct parents not to have child receive MMR for 11 months after infusion.

Systemic Hypertension

I. Definition: Systemic hypertension is the consistent elevation of BP beyond the upper limits of normal for that age. Hypertension may be described as primary or secondary.
   A. Essential or primary hypertension—has no identifiable cause and is primarily seen in adolescents.
   B. Secondary hypertension—hypertension in young children as possible result of a structural abnormality or underlying pathology.

II. Nursing process
   A. Assessment
      1. Assess for nonmodifiable risk factors.
         a. Family history of hypertension
         b. Cultural background (e.g., African American)
      2. Assess for modifiable risk factors.
         a. High-fat, high-salt diet
         b. Smoking
         c. Obesity
         d. Stress
      3. Assess for general complaints, including headache, dizziness, and visual changes.
      4. Obtain a detailed health history, including family history, and history of risk factors, height, and weight.
      5. Obtain vital signs, including BP, and perform comprehensive physical assessment.
      6. Obtain diagnostic tests.
         a. Three separate BP measurements—classification:
            (1) Prehypertension—BP greater than 90th percentile for age and height
            (2) Stage 1 hypertension—BP between 95th and 99th percentile for age and height

(3) Stage 2 hypertension—BP persistently at or above the 99th percentile in addition to 5 mmHg for age, sex, and height

b. Laboratory tests

(1) Urinalysis and renal function tests

(2) Complete blood count, electrolytes, and lipid profile

B. Analysis

1. Anxiety related to lifestyle changes and fear
2. Ineffective Health Maintenance related to lack of knowledge of hypertension, risk factors, and lifestyle influences
3. Deficient Knowledge of Pharmacologic and Nonpharmacologic Management related to new information

C. Planning

1. Manage and reduce BP to normotensive state.
2. Reduce anxiety.
3. Provide child and family teaching about hypertension, including risk factors, lifestyle changes, and medication.
4. Assist child in identifying own risk factors for hypertension, and behaviors that contribute to its development.
5. Promote self-care behaviors such as diet control, home BP monitoring, and exercise program.

D. Implementation: Provide interventions for essential hypertension.

1. Nonpharmacologic
   a. Diet modification, including limiting salt intake
   b. Lifestyle modification, including weight control, exercise, stress reduction, and behavior modification of risk factors such as smoking
2. Pharmacologic
   a. ACE inhibitors
   b. Beta blockers

E. Evaluation

1. Child achieves a normotensive state.
2. Child describes risk factors for the development of hypertension.
3. Child explains health behaviors to promote an improved lifestyle.
4. Child's anxiety is reduced.
5. Child is compliant with hypertensive regimen.

CN

III. Client needs

A. Physiologic adaptation: Essential hypertension is controlled with nonpharmacologic and pharmacologic interventions on an outpatient basis.

1. BP is reduced and complications prevented by ACE inhibitors or beta blockers.
2. Diet is further modified as evidenced by lipid profile.

B. Management of care: Care of the child with essential hypertension requires critical thinking skills and knowledge of assessment, and teaching and evaluation methods unique to the RN role. These skills cannot be delegated to an LPN or UAP.

1. Perform a comprehensive physical assessment and provide care to the child with essential hypertension.
2. Assess for home health needs such as ability to obtain appropriate foods for diet modification.
3. Evaluate community resources for family support such as local gymnasiums or parks for exercise and support groups for life and diet modification.
4. Delegate responsibly those activities that can be delegated, including measurements, oral intake and urine output, and vital signs. All monitoring information is reported to the RN.

C. Safety and infection control

1. Correctly fit BP cuff.
2. Repeat any borderline measurement in standing, sitting, and lying positions.
3. Promote child and family compliance by teaching about lifestyle management and long-term issues related to complications.
4. Teach child and family about medication administration, including rationale, dose, timing and side effects.
5. Maintain the six rights of medication administration.

D. Health promotion and maintenance: Promote self-management.

1. Instruct child and parents to assess BP at home.
2. Assist child to identify personal risk factors and tailor education to those needs.

E. Psychologic integrity

1. Provide support and encouragement throughout diagnosis.
2. Teach stress reduction strategies such as biofeedback.
3. Identify stressors that may interfere with compliance.
4. Promote support groups for weight loss or smoking cessation.

F. Basic care and comfort

1. Provide calm, quiet environment.
2. Promote growth and development through individualizing teaching to meet child's developmental and cognitive needs.

G. Reduction of risk potential

1. Instruct child to stop taking oral contraceptives, if applicable.
2. Acknowledge calcium channel blocker as controversial.

Table 12-2 Drugs Used for Systemic Hypertension in Children

Classification	Generic/ Trade Name	Expected Outcome	Reduction of Risk Potential	Management of Care
ACE Inhibitors	Lisinopril (Prinivil, Zestril) Captopril (Capoten) Enalapril (Vasotec)	Interferes with the production of angiotensin II	Monitor BP and pulse. Monitor electrolytes.	Teach child to avoid rapid position changes. Report signs of infection.
Beta Blockers	Propranolol (Inderal)	Blocks response to beta stimulation and reduces BP	May cause lipid changes and mood problems. Monitor BP and pulse.	Teach family to observe child for signs of depression. May cause impotence.
Vasodilators	Hydralazine (Apresoline)	Acts on smooth muscle, causes arterial vasodilation	May cause drowsiness.	Teach family to administer with meals. Report signs of infection. Caution if client is driving.

3. Promote screening programs to identify high-risk child.

H. Pharmacologic and parenteral therapies: Child and family state the purpose, dosage, timing, and side effects of medications (Table 12-2). Drugs are introduced one at a time.

Diagnostic and Interventional Strategies: Cardiac Catheterization

I. Definition: For this procedure, a radiopaque catheter is inserted into a distal vein or artery and threaded into the heart. Information gathered from the catheterization includes oxygen saturation, pressure changes, cardiac output, and anatomic abnormalities.

II. Nursing process

A. Assessment
1. Assess purpose for cardiac catheterization.
   a. Interventional
   b. Diagnostic
   c. Electrophysiologic
2. Assess child and family for knowledge base regarding the rationale for the test, understanding of preparation, and postprocedural guidelines.
3. Complete a comprehensive physical assessment, including baseline vital signs, height, weight, and evidence of infection, such as diaper rash.
4. Obtain a detailed health history, including history of allergies.
5. Assess all pulses below the procedure site.
6. Obtain diagnostic tests.
   a. Baseline oxygen saturation
   b. Chest radiograph
   c. Complete blood count
   d. Coagulation studies
   e. Arterial blood gas
   f. ECG

B. Analysis
1. Anxiety related to separation from parent and strange environment
2. Risk for Decreased Cardiac Output related to structural defect and risk for hemorrhage
3. Risk for Acute Pain related to invasive procedures
4. Risk for Deficient Fluid Volume related to blood loss and diuretic effect of contrast medium

C. Planning
1. Maintain hemodynamic stability.
2. Reduce anxiety.
3. Prevent dysrhythmias and complications.

D. Implementation
1. Preprocedure preparation
   a. Establish baseline vital signs, height and weight, presence of infection, assess peripheral pulses.
   b. Provide child and family teaching.
   c. Maintain NPO status unless polycythemic, then IV fluids to prevent dehydration.
2. Postprocedure care
   a. Observe for complications—neurovascular assessments
   b. Prevent bleeding

(1) Frequent vital signs to detect bleeding and arrhythmias
(2) Venous: Flat for 4 to 6 hr with extremity straight
(3) Arterial: Flat for 6 to 8 hr with extremity straight
(4) Occlusive waterproof dressing for 24 hr

c. Begin clear liquids and advance as tolerated.
d. Manage pain with analgesics.

E. Evaluation
1. Child's peripheral perfusion is adequate as evidenced by stable vital signs, palpable peripheral pulses, and capillary refill in less than 2 to 3 s.
2. Child and parents demonstrate understanding and need for procedure.
3. Child and family anxiety is reduced.

CN

III. Client needs

A. Physiologic adaptation: When there is an abnormal connection between heart chambers or vessels, blood flows from higher to lower pressure. Most cardiac defects are left to right shunts.
1. Increased blood flow causes hypertrophy of the tissues.
2. Risk for decreased cardiac output from postprocedure complication such as hemorrhage. Signs and symptoms include change in level of consciousness, tachycardia, hypotension, decreased peripheral perfusion, and bleeding at catheter insertion site.

B. Management of care: Care of the child undergoing a cardiac catheterization requires critical thinking skills and knowledge of assessment, and teaching and evaluation methods unique to the RN role. These skills cannot be delegated to an LPN or UAP.
1. Assess for home health needs, including possible environment modification if child cannot climb steps.
2. Evaluate community resources for family support such as a local chapter of the Kids with Heart National Association for Children's Heart Disorders.
3. Delegate responsibly those activities that can be delegated, including measurements, oral intake and urine output, and vital signs. All monitoring information is reported to the RN.

C. Safety and infection control
1. Teach child and family about the procedure, including what the child will see, hear, smell, and feel.
   a. Prepare child for procedure at appropriate developmental level.
   b. Include picture books, videos, and tours of the catheterization laboratory.
2. Prepare child for procedure.
   a. Assure NPO status for 4 to 6 hr.
   b. Protect catheterization site from laboratory draws.
3. Perform postprocedure care.
   a. Promote bed rest with extremity straight for 6 hr.
   b. Manage pressure dressing on catheterization site: Apply direct pressure 2.5 cm (1 in.) above catheter insertion site if bleeding occurs.
   c. Assess neurovascular status (pulses weaker for first few hours).
   d. Assess for presence of hypotension.
      (1) May indicate bleeding
      (2) May be reaction from dye
   e. Assess for arrhythmias, hypothermia, or hyperthermia, and increased output from mercurial dyes.
4. Teach parents to avoid tub baths for at least 3 days.

D. Health promotion and maintenance
1. Provide a transitional comfort object for child to take into procedure.
2. Provide age-appropriate diversional activities.
3. Involve family in all aspects of care.

E. Psychologic integrity
1. Encourage and answer all questions at child's cognitive level.
2. Act as consistent nurse caregiver.
3. Allow parents to stay at bedside.

F. Basic care and comfort (see pharmacologic and parenteral therapies)

G. Reduction of risk potential: Teach parents signs and symptoms of site infection and bleeding and to notify HCP. For infants also at risk for hypoglycemia, instruct parents to:
1. Provide dextrose-containing IV fluids.
2. Assess glucose levels.

H. Pharmacologic and parenteral therapies: Child and family will state the purpose of acetaminophen (Tylenol)—to manage pain.

Bibliography

Hatfield, N. (2006). *Broadribb's introductory pediatric nursing.* Philadelphia: Lippincott Williams & Wilkins.

Pillitteri, A. (2006). *Maternal & child health nursing: Care of the childbearing and childrearing family* (5th ed.). Philadelphia: Lippincott Williams & Wilkins.

Wong, D. L., et al. (2006). *Maternal child nursing care.* St. Louis: Mosby.

CHAPTER 12
Practice Test

Congenital Heart Defects

1. The nurse is assessing an infant with congenital heart disease. To assess this infant for cyanosis, the nurse should assess the:
- □ 1. Soles of the feet and the toes.
- □ 2. Tongue and buccal membrane.
- □ 3. Lips and the circumoral area.
- □ 4. Fingertips and palms of the hands.

2. The nurse is teaching a mother of an infant with tetralogy of Fallot. The nurse instructs the mother to place the infant in which of the following positions if the infant suddenly becomes cyanotic and dyspneic?
- □ 1. Semi-Fowler position in an infant seat.
- □ 2. Supine, with the head turned to one side.
- □ 3. Prone, being sure he or she can breathe easily.
- □ 4. In a knee-chest position.

3. The nurse is feeding an infant who has a congenital heart defect. Which of the following nursing measures will improve the caloric intake of this infant?
- □ 1. Feed the infant 20 cal/oz infant formula in amounts as desired by the infant.
- □ 2. Offer frequent, high-calorie formula feedings (24 cal/oz) every 3 hr.
- □ 3. Instruct parents to start the infant on solids by 4 to 5 months of age.
- □ 4. Allow the infant to sleep through the night to decrease fatigue.

4. When auscultating a child's heart with a stethoscope, the nurse identifies a murmur. The murmur is characterized as being "soft," of medium intensity, heard immediately, and without a thrill present. The nurse documents the grade of this murmur as:
- □ 1. Grade I/VI.
- □ 2. Grade II/VI.
- □ 3. Grade IV/VI.
- □ 4. Grade V/VI.

5. AF The nurse is caring for an infant who is hospitalized prior to surgery for tetralogy of Fallot. The infant has a cyanotic episode. The nurse should do the following in priority order?

_____ 1. Administer oxygen.
_____ 2. Calm and soothe the infant.
_____ 3. Put in knee-chest position.
_____ 4. Hold in an upright position.

6. The nurse is caring for a child who is 2 years of age who has had surgery to repair a ventricular-septal defect (VSD). The nurse should report which of the following to the surgeon?
- □ 1. Crackles bilaterally in the lungs.
- □ 2. Weight gain of 1 kg from preoperative weight.
- □ 3. BP of 104/76.
- □ 4. Oxygenation of 95% on 0.5 L of oxygen.

7. The nurse administers prostaglandin E to an infant born with transposition of the great vessels. What is the expected effect of this drug?
- □ 1. Ductus arteriosus remains open, allowing blood to mix.
- □ 2. Ventricular septal defect closes.
- □ 3. Arterial switch procedure has fewer complications.
- □ 4. Ductus arteriosus closes, allowing for better oxygenation.

8. A premature infant has a patent ductus arteriosus (PDA). What are the expected effects following administration of indomethacin (Indocin)?
- □ 1. Ductus arteriosus remains open.
- □ 2. Ventricular septal defect closes.
- □ 3. Atrial septal defect remains open.
- □ 4. Ductus arteriosus closes.

9. AF A hospitalized infant who is 2 months of age with tricuspid atresia has been receiving digoxin for 3 days. Prior to administering the drug, the nurse checks the infant's apical heart

NURSE'S FULL SIGNATURE, STATUS, AND INITIALS

	INIT.		INIT.
Belinda Thomas, RN	BT		

DIAGNOSIS: Tricuspid atresia, heart failure

ALLERGIES: None — DIET: 2GM sodium

ROUTINE/DAILY ORDERS/FINGERSTICKS/ INSULIN COVERAGE			DATE: 5/11/09		DATE: 5/12/09		DATE: 5/13/09		DATE:	
ORDER DATE	MEDICATIONS, DOSE, ROUTE, FREQUENCY	TIME	SITE	INIT.	SITE	INIT.	SITE	INIT.	SITE	INIT.
4/11/09	Digoxin, 50 mcg IV	0900		BT HR = 120		BT HR = 125		BT HR = 127		

rate. The heart rate is 88 beats per minute. After checking the medication record (see preceding page), the nurse should perform which of the following interventions?
- □ 1. Administer the scheduled digoxin.
- □ 2. Administer the scheduled digoxin; recheck heart rate in 30 min.
- □ 3. Hold the scheduled dose and notify the HCP.
- □ 4. Recheck the heart rate radially, and if it is more than 60, administer the dose.

10. The nurse is administering prescribed digoxin to an infant. Within 10 min, the infant vomits. The nurse should:
- □ 1. Administer a repeat dose because this medication is essential to cardiac function.
- □ 2. Hold repeat dose; administer next dose at the regular time.
- □ 3. Administer a repeat dose that is half the prescribed dose.
- □ 4. Hold a repeat dose for 1 hr and then administer the full prescribed dose.

Rheumatic Fever

11. The nurse is instructing the family and a child who has been diagnosed with rheumatic fever (RF). Which of the following is included in the teaching plan?
- □ 1. Diagnosis of rheumatic fever provides lifelong immunity for further infections.
- □ 2. Child will need antibiotic prophylaxis for invasive procedures.
- □ 3. Child will recover fully, requiring no further treatment in the future.
- □ 4. Management for complications of hypertension.

12. An adolescent is admitted to the hospital with RF. Nursing assessment reveals that the client has a sore throat, painful swollen joints, and a rash on his trunks. He has random movements of his extremities. The temperature is 99°F, respirations are 25, apical heart rate is 150, and BP is 120/82. The nurse should first:
- □ 1. Administer an antipyretic.
- □ 2. Splint the joints.
- □ 3. Notify the HCP.
- □ 4. Apply lotion to the rash.

Kawasaki Disease

13. A preschooler is admitted to the hospital with stage 1 Kawasaki disease. Nursing assessment reveals the child has had a temperature of 102°F for 4 days. He has bilateral conjunctival infection, a "strawberry" tongue, and fissures on the lips. The child has peripheral edema of the hands and feet, and cervical lymphadenopathy. The child is receiving 100 mg/kg of aspirin per day. The nurse should document which of the following as an intended outcome of aspirin therapy?
- □ 1. Absence of conjunctival infection.
- □ 2. Normal body temperature.
- □ 3. No signs of coronary thrombosis.
- □ 4. Fissures on lips healed.

14. A preschooler who has been diagnosed with Kawasaki disease is to receive a high-dose IV gamma globulin. Which of the following is a desired effect of this drug?
- □ 1. Decreases incidence of a rash.
- □ 2. Decreases incidence of peripheral edema.
- □ 3. Decreases incidence of lymphadenopathy.
- □ 4. Decreases incidence of coronary aneurysms.

Systemic Hypertension

15. Which of the following individuals is at greatest risk for systemic hypertension?
- □ 1. African American child who is 14 years of age and obese.
- □ 2. Asian child who is 18 years of age and follows a vegetarian diet.
- □ 3. Native American child who is 12 years of age with a slightly elevated BP on initial assessment.
- □ 4. White child who is 10 years of age and consumes a high-fat diet.

16. A child who is 15 years of age with systemic hypertension is taking propranolol (Inderal) for systemic hypertension. The nurse instructs the child and family to report which of the following to the HCP?
- □ 1. Elevated temperature.
- □ 2. Tachycardia.
- □ 3. Increased appetite.
- □ 4. Depression.

Diagnostic and Interventional Strategies: Cardiac Catheterization

17. AF A child who is 3 years of age has a cardiac catheterization with access through the femoral vein. The child has returned to the nursing unit. While assuring the child that the procedure is over, the nurse should do which of the following? Put the actions in order from highest priority to lowest priority.
- ____ 1. Remind the child to remain flat in bed.
- ____ 2. Inspect the dressing for bleeding.
- ____ 3. Palpate pedal pulses.
- ____ 4. Obtain heart rate.

18. After cardiac surgery, a child has chest tubes inserted that are attached to a water-seal drainage system. The tubing to the water-seal

drainage container becomes disconnected. The nurse should do which of the following first?
- □ 1. Reinsert the tube under the water level.
- □ 2. Clamp the tube near the chest.
- □ 3. Cover the ends of both tubes with sterile dressings and notify the physician.
- □ 4. Place a dressing with petroleum jelly on the insertion site at the chest.

19. The nurse is teamed with an LPN in caring for a group of cardiac patients on a pediatric unit. Which action by the LPN indicates the nurse should intervene immediately?
- □ 1. LPN assists child to the bathroom 2 hr after a cardiac catheterization.
- □ 2. LPN places infant having a cyanotic episode in a knee-chest position.
- □ 3. LPN checks a child's apical heart rate prior to administering digoxin.
- □ 4. LPN brings breakfast to a child who is scheduled for an electrocardiogram.

20. A preschooler has just returned to his hospital room from the cardiac catheterization recovery room. He is vomiting and bleeding; anxious, pale, crying, and sitting in a puddle of blood and emesis. The nurse should first:
- □ 1. Call the pediatric cardiologist and report the incident.
- □ 2. Elevate the head of the bed and place oxygen on the child.
- □ 3. Apply direct continuous pressure 1 in. above the percutaneous site.
- □ 4. Provide emotional comfort measures to this crying child.

Answers and Rationales

1. 2 Children's tongues and buccal membranes are often the most sensitive indicators of cyanosis in children of all ethnic backgrounds. (A)

2. 4 Placing an infant in a knee-chest or squatting position traps blood in the legs, allowing the child to better oxygenate the blood remaining in the torso. The other positions do not facilitate breathing for this child. (A)

3. 2 An infant with cardiac disease has caloric needs that are greater than those of the average infant because of the increased metabolic rate, yet the ability to take in adequate calories is hampered by fatigue. A 3-hr feeding schedule works the best because it allows for a sufficient number of calories, but also provides sufficient rest periods between feeds. (H)

4. 2. A grade II/VI murmur is characteristically soft, but is heard very quickly after placing the stethoscope on the chest. Grade I/VI murmurs are difficult to hear for the untrained ear. Grade IV/VI murmurs will have a murmur present and be loud, with a thrill present. Grade V/VI murmurs are so loud that the stethoscope may only need to "hover" above the chest to be able to hear it. (M)

5. 3, 4, 2, 1 The nurse first places the infant in the knee-chest position to create blood flow resistance to the peripheral extremities and shunt blood to the major organs. This position provides more available oxygen to the heart. Next, the nurse holds the infant in an upright position to facilitate air exchange and attempts to quiet the distressed infant through use of soothing techniques. If none of these measures improves oxygenation status quickly enough, the nurse administers oxygen. Frequently, the first three actions provide the appropriate relief. (M)

6. 1 Crackles in the lungs is a sign of heart failure and requires medical intervention; the nurse notifies the surgeon of this finding. The slight elevation in BP, oxygenation level, and 1 kg weight gain are all within normal limits following surgery to repair a VSD. (M)

7. 1 Prostaglandin E is administered to provide intracardiac blood mixing. Prostaglandin E keeps open the ductus arteriosus, allowing oxygenated blood to be shunted to the right side of the heart where it can be pumped out through the transposed aorta. A cardiac catheterization may also take place in which a balloon atrial septostomy (Rashkind procedure) is performed, increasing the mixing of oxygenated blood and maintaining cardiac output over a longer period. (D)

8. 4 The administration of indomethacin has proved successful in closing a patent ductus in premature infants and some newborns. The drug is not used for other defects. (D)

9. 3 Digoxin is a potentially dangerous drug because the margin of safety of therapeutic, toxic, and lethal doses is very narrow, particularly in children. As a general rule, the drug is not given if the pulse is below 90 to 110 beats per minutes in infants and young children or below 70 beats per minute in older children (the cutoff point for adults is 60 beats per minute). (D)

10. 2 If the child vomits a prescribed dose of digoxin, the nurse administers the next dose at the scheduled time. The nurse does not administer a second dose. If more than two consecutive doses are missed (vomited), notify the HCP. (D)

11. 2 Children who have had acute RF are susceptible to recurrent affects of the disease for the rest of their lives and are followed medically for at least 5 years. Children and families are made aware of the need for continuing antibiotic prophylaxis for invasive procedures. Having one episode of RF does not confirm immunity. The child may fully recover from this episode, but will require continued monitoring. Children with RF are not at risk for hypertension. (H)

12. 3 The nurse first notifies the HCP about the increased heart rate. The elevated heart rate is an indicator of carditis, which can cause significant heart damage. Splinting the joints will not relieve the underlying inflammation that is causing the pain; the pain will subside in time. The temperature is normal and the client does not need an antipyretic at this time. Lotion may be applied to the rash, but after the nurse has notified the HCP. (M)

13. 2 Aspirin is administered initially at a dose to reduce the inflammation and to control the fever. After the fever has subsided, aspirin is continued at a lower dose, for 6 to 8 weeks to prevent coronary thrombosis. The nurse provides care for the infection in the eye by instilling artificial tears and using cool compresses. The nurse provides mouth care every 4 hr and uses petroleum on the lip fissures as needed. (D)

14. 4 The current treatment of KD includes high-dose IV gamma globulin. Gamma globulin has been demonstrated to be effective at reducing the incidence of coronary artery abnormalities if given within the first 10 days of the illness. Gamma globulin is not used to treat the rash, peripheral edema, or lymphadenopathy. (D)

15. 1 Systemic hypertension involves a consistently elevated BP in children. Persons at risk include adolescents and African Americans; clients with a family history; and clients who are obese, consume a high-fat diet, and have BPs elevated above normal on several readings. Thus, the child who is 14 years of age, obese, and African American is at greatest risk for systemic hypertension; the nurse continues to assess this high-risk client and develops a plan for risk reduction. (H)

16. 4 Depression is a potential side effect of propranolol use. The nurse teaches the family and client to report signs of depression to the HCP. Side effects of propranolol do not typically include fever; the drug may cause bradycardia, rather than tachycardia, and nausea, vomiting, and diarrhea, rather than increased appetite. (D)

17. 2, 3, 4, 1 The nurse first assesses the insertion site for bleeding or the presence of a hematoma. Next, the nurse palpates the pedal pulses because insertion of a catheter into the femoral vein can cause vessel spasm, interfering with circulation to the leg. Assessing pedal pulses ensures that circulation distal to the insertion site is adequate. The nurse then obtains other vital signs. The child is instructed to remain flat for 6 to 8 hr after the procedure to prevent pressure on the insertion site. The nurse also reassures the child and offers explanations about ongoing procedures. (S)

18. 2 A disconnected chest tube allows air to enter the chest cavity, causing a pneumothorax; the nurse immediately clamps the chest tube exiting the chest. The other actions do not prevent air from entering the chest cavity. (S)

19. 1 Because the femoral artery is usually used as the access site during a cardiac catheterization, children are required to remain on bed rest (with the head only slightly elevated) for several hours after the procedure to avoid arterial bleeding at the site. A knee-chest position is the correct position for an infant during a cyanotic episode as it will create peripheral resistance to the extremities, shunting blood to the heart. The apical heart rate is assessed prior to administering this medication; administration can be performed by an experienced LPN, although medication is checked with the RN prior to administration. Because echocardiography is noninvasive, there is no need to withhold meals before this procedure. (S)

20. 3 Depending on hospital policy, the child may be kept in bed with the affected extremity maintained straight for 6 to 8 hr following arterial catheterization to facilitate healing and prevent bleeding. When this child sat up to vomit, the percutaneous site began to bleed. The risks related to blood loss and hypovolemia are the priority situation that needs to be addressed first. (A)

chapter

13

The Child With Hematologic Health Problems

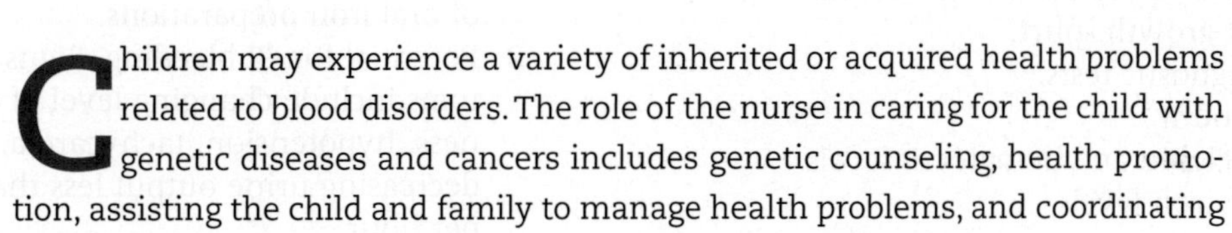

Children may experience a variety of inherited or acquired health problems related to blood disorders. The role of the nurse in caring for the child with genetic diseases and cancers includes genetic counseling, health promotion, assisting the child and family to manage health problems, and coordinating end of life care. The following topics are included in this chapter:

- Iron Deficiency Anemia
- Sickle Cell Anemia
- Hemophilia
- Leukemia
- β-Thalassemia (Cooley Anemia)
- End-of-Life Care

Iron Deficiency Anemia

I. Definition: Iron deficiency anemia is an inadequate supply of iron for production of hemoglobin in RBCs. Insufficient reserves of iron lead to decreased hemoglobin concentration, decreased oxygen-carrying capacity of the blood, and depleted RBC mass. Iron deficiency anemia is most commonly caused by blood loss, malabsorption of iron, or inadequate iron intake.

II. Nursing process

A. Assessment

1. Assess child for signs and symptoms of anemia—symptoms appear late because of slow progression of anemia.
   a. Dyspnea on exertion
   b. Fatigue
   c. Irritability
   d. Pallor
   e. Tachycardia
2. Assess child for signs and symptoms of chronic anemia.
   a. Paresthesia in extremities
   b. Smooth tongue
   c. Spoon-shaped nails
   d. Neuralgic pain
3. Obtain detailed health history, diet history, and recent growth spurt.
4. Obtain diagnostic tests.
   a. RBC count
   b. Hemoglobin and hematocrit levels
   c. Serum iron levels
   d. Transferrin levels
   e. Bone marrow aspiration

B. Analysis

1. Activity Intolerance related to tissue hypoxia and fatigue
2. Ineffective Health Maintenance related to lack of knowledge about appropriate diet
3. Imbalanced Nutrition: Less Than Body Requirements related to inadequate intake, increased growth, or body losses

C. Planning

1. Restore iron losses.
2. Improve activity tolerance.
3. Improve tissue oxygenation.
4. Prevent infection and bleeding.
5. Promote health behavior modifications of diet.

D. Implementation: Provide family teaching about medication administration and side effects (see pharmacologic and parenteral therapies) in addition to providing interventions for iron deficiency anemia.

1. Increase intake of iron by eating iron-rich foods.
2. Administer medications that may be used to treat iron deficiency anemia.
   a. Oral iron preparations
   b. Vitamin supplementation if intrinsic factor is depleted
   c. Chelation, if needed, for hemochromatosis
3. Instruct family about diet.

E. Evaluation

1. Child's vital signs are stable, and no signs of tachycardia are present.
2. Child exhibits increased activity tolerance with decreased fatigue.
3. Child and family verbalize understanding of increased dietary intake of iron.
4. Child and family verbalize correct method to for administration of oral iron preparations.
5. Child's serum values for return to normal levels.

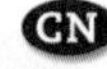

III. Client needs

A. Physiologic adaptation: Anemia is controlled with increased dietary intake of iron and oral iron preparations.

1. Tissue oxygenation is improved and myocardial workload is decreased as result of oral iron preparations.
2. Potential for GI bleeding. Signs and symptoms include changing level of consciousness, hypotension, tachycardia, pallor, and decreasing urine output less than 1 ml/kg per hour.

B. Management of care: Care of the child with iron deficiency anemia requires critical thinking skills and knowledge of assessment, and teaching and evaluation methods unique to the RN role. These skills cannot be delegated to an LPN or UAP.

1. Assess for home health needs, including evaluation of resources to purchase iron supplements, formulas, or appropriate foods.
2. Evaluate community resources for family support such as availability of supplemental nutrition programs such as Women, Infants, and Children (WIC).
3. Delegate responsibly those activities that can be delegated, including measurements, oral intake and urine output, vital signs, and reporting child's subjective data. All monitoring information is reported to the RN.

C. Safety and infection control

1. Teach child and family about signs and symptoms of chronic anemia, bleeding, and infection.

2. Teach child and family about medications, including correct administration and side effects.
3. Maintain the six rights of medication administration.

D. Health promotion and maintenance: Provide child and family teaching.
 1. Prepare foods high in iron: Dark green leafy vegetables, whole grains, liver, raisins, egg yolks, and meats. For infants, instruct iron-fortified formula and cereals.
 2. Administer oral iron preparations: Serve between meals, with fruit juice containing vitamin C to enhance iron absorption (provide straw to protect teeth). For infants, serve iron preparations with a syringe.
 3. Prepare foods high in vitamin B_{12}, including vitamin-fortified cereals, organ meats, dairy products, crab, and clams.
 4. Acknowledge side effects of medication, such as constipation.

E. Psychologic integrity
 1. Assist child and family in coping with dietary and lifestyle changes.
 2. Provide passive stimulation for the infant or child during times of fatigue.

F. Basic care and comfort
 1. Elevate head of bed to decrease oxygen demands.
 2. Allow frequent periods of rest.
 3. Provide small, frequent feedings.
 4. Brush teeth after iron administration.

G. Reduction of risk potential: Assess for guaiac results (oral iron preparations may cause false-positive results on test) in addition to providing parent teaching.
 1. Avoid giving iron preparations with milk products (may interfere with absorption).
 2. Store iron safely out of child's reach.
 3. Assess for normal stool characteristics (black, tarry).

H. Pharmacologic and parenteral therapies: Child and family will state the purpose, dosage, timing, and side effects of medications used to manage iron deficiency anemia:
 1. Ferrous sulfate (Feosol): Iron preparation
  a. Expected outcome: Replaces iron stores and improves hemoglobin and hematocrit levels.
  b. Reduction of risk potential: Assess for nausea, constipation, black, tarry stools; monitor hemoglobin and hematocrit.
  c. Management of care: Instruct parents to watch for constipation and change in stool color.
 2. Iron dextran (DexFerrum): Iron preparation
  a. Expected outcome: Used when PO preparations are ineffective or contraindicated; IM or IV route preferred.
  b. Reduction of risk potential: Z-track method of administration; observe for rash, headache, flushing.
   (1) Notify HCP of backache, chills, or fever.
   (2) Monitor hemoglobin and hematocrit.
  c. Management of care: Teach parents not to administer if on oral iron preparations.
 3. Cyanocobalamin (vitamin B_{12})
  a. Expected outcome: Used for malabsorption when intrinsic factor is depleted.
  b. Reduction of risk potential: Observe for mild diarrhea, rash, flushing; monitor hemoglobin, hematocrit, folate, and reticulocyte levels.
  c. Management of care: Teach parents to observe for injection-site tenderness.

Sickle Cell Anemia

I. Definition: Sickle cell anemia is a hereditary group of diseases in which hemoglobin A is partially or completely replaced by abnormal hemoglobin S. Hemoglobin S is very sensitive to the oxygen-carrying capacity of the RBCs. During periods of hypoxia, cells assume the classic sickle shape, become rigid, and clump together in the microcirculation. Sickling causes hemolysis, which increases blood viscosity, obstruction, and infarctions. Acute disease exacerbation results in sickle cell crises; these may vary in frequency and severity. Table 13-1 lists the three types of crises, along with causes and symptoms.

Table 13-1 Sickle Cell Crises

Crises	Cause	Symptoms
Vaso-occlusive: Most Common	Stasis of blood, ischemia, infarction	Pain, fever, and ischemia of tissues
Aplastic	Diminished production and increased destruction of RBCs	Pallor, lethargy, dyspnea
Sequestration	Pooling of blood in the spleen	Lethargy, pallor, hypovolemic shock

II. Nursing process
 A. Assessment
  1. Assess for factors that precipitate sickling, including dehydration, stress, infection, high altitude, and acidosis.
  2. Assess for signs and symptoms of sickling crisis.
   a. Infants—colic from abdominal infarction, splenomegaly
   b. Toddlers and preschoolers—pain at site of vaso-occlusive crisis
   c. School-aged children and adolescents—delayed growth, enuresis, pain at site of vaso-occlusive crisis
  3. Complete a detailed health history of prior hospitalizations and developmental level.
  4. Obtain diagnostic tests.
   a. Hemoglobin electrophoresis
   b. Sickle-turbidity test (Sickledex)—presence of more than 50% hemoglobin S is indicative of disease; lower levels indicate trait
   c. Sickling test (sickle cell preparation)—shape of RBCs is crescent or sickle-shaped
 B. Analysis
  1. Activity Intolerance related to impaired tissue perfusion and fatigue
  2. Anxiety related to pain and fear
  3. Excess Fluid Volume related to hydration regimen for treatment of crisis
  4. Acute Pain related to impaired tissue perfusion
  5. Risk for Impaired Urinary Elimination related to increased fluid intake to prevent dehydration
 C. Planning
  1. Improve hydration to restore circulation.
  2. Relieve vaso-occlusive crisis pain.
  3. Improve activity tolerance.
  4. Prevent infection.
  5. Prevent anemia.
  6. Reduce anxiety.
 D. Implementation: Prevent crises by maintaining hydration and preventing infection. For vaso-occlusive crisis:
  1. Promote bed rest.
  2. Instruct avoidance of stress.
  3. Maintain hydration at 1½ normal.
  4. Provide brief oxygen therapy.
  5. Initiate transfusions as needed.
  6. Administer medications.
   a. Analgesics
   b. Antineoplastics
   c. Anti-infectives
   d. Vaccines: Pneumococcal, *Haemophilus influenzae* type b and meningococcal
  7. Provide child and family teaching about crisis prevention, side effects of crisis prevention, and medication management.
 E. Evaluation
  1. Child demonstrates reduction in pain as evidenced by ability to be comforted, and vital signs within normal limits.
  2. Child and family verbalize understanding of crisis prevention.
  3. Child and family identify potential complications of crisis.
  4. Child and family verbalize correct method for administration of pain medication.

CN

III. Client needs
 A. Physiologic adaptation: Sickle cell anemia is controlled through prevention techniques of hydration, and avoidance of infection, high altitude, and stressful situations. Clumping of cells in the microcirculation is reduced as a result of vaso-occlusive crisis management.
  1. Risk for system involvement indicating infarction and complications of crisis. Symptoms include tachycardia, dyspnea, or hypotension.
  2. Risk for pulmonary infarction: Acute chest syndrome. Symptoms include chest pain, fever, cough, tachypnea, and wheezing.
 B. Management of care: Care of the child with sickle cell anemia requires critical thinking skills and knowledge of assessment, and teaching and evaluation methods unique to the RN role. These skills cannot be delegated to an LPN or UAP.
  1. Assess for home health needs.
   a. Evaluate home options such as a primary care pediatrician versus a comprehensive sickle cell program.
   b. Stress the need for coordinated care and communication among the family, pediatrician, and subspecialists.
   c. Assess availability of specialized medical equipment.
  2. Evaluate community resources for family support.
   a. Patient support groups and community-based organizations can be important resources.
   b. Relevant issues include health insurance coverage, transportation for health care, and education of school personnel.
  3. Delegate responsibly those activities that can be delegated, including measurements, oral intake and urine output, vital signs,

and reporting child's subjective data. All monitoring information is reported to the RN.

C. Safety and infection control
   1. Provide skin care to prevent breakdown.
   2. Protect child from sources of infection.
   3. Teach child and family about preventing infection.
   4. Maintain the six rights of medication administration.
D. Health promotion and maintenance
   1. Optimize functional ability and prevent complications through interventions that prevent and manage sickle cell crises.
   2. Teach child and family methods to prevent infection.
   3. Provide family with genetic counseling.
E. Psychologic integrity
   1. Assist child and family in coping with life-long illness.
   2. Identify stressors that may precipitate a crisis or impact recovery.
   3. Teach child relaxation techniques to reduce anxiety and stress.
   4. Assist child and family in coping with enuresis as a side effect of hydration management.
F. Basic care and comfort
   1. Assist child into a position of comfort with extremities extended.
   2. Elevate head of bed 30 degrees.
   3. Reduce stress on joints.
   4. Maintain normal body temperature.
   5. Encourage high-calorie, high-protein diet.
   6. Encourage folic acid supplements.
   7. Teach relaxation techniques to reduce stress.
   8. Reduce energy expenditure to improve oxygenation, including bed rest and administration of pain medication to promote comfort.
   9. Promote PO and IV fluid intake to prevent dehydration.
G. Reduction of risk potential
   1. Remove tight clothing that may impede circulation.
   2. Do not raise knee gatch of bed (places stress on joints).
   3. Avoid administration of meperidine (Demerol) for pain management because of risk for seizures.
   4. Promote pneumococcal vaccine and prophylactic penicillin to prevent disease.
   5. Assist child and family in identifying activities that precipitate a vaso-occlusive crisis.
H. Pharmacologic and parenteral therapies: Child and family will verbalize the purpose, timing, and side effects of medication used to manage sickle cell anemia and vaso-occlusive crisis.
   1. IV normal saline
      a. Expected outcome: Promotes hemodilution and hydration
      b. Reduction of risk potential: Prevents sickling and vaso-oclusive crisis
      c. Management of care: Monitor infusion
   2. Hydroxyurea (Hydrea): Antineoplastics
      a. Expected outcome: Promotes the production of fetal hemoglobin.
      b. Reduction of risk potential: Assess for anorexia, nausea, and bone marrow suppression.
         (1) Monitor CBCs—therapy is discontinued if WBC count is less than 2,500/mm^3 or platelets less than 100,000/mm^3
         (2) Monitor intake and output
      c. Management of care: Instruct parents to watch for decreased urine output or early signs of infection.
   3. Folic acid (folacin): Vitamin supplement
      a. Expected outcome: For treatment of anemia by stimulating RBC and platelet production.
      b. Reduction of risk potential: Assess for slight flushing.
      c. Management of care: Instruct parents on importance of giving child supplement daily.

Hemophilia

I. Definition: Hemophilia is a hereditary bleeding disorder characterized by a deficiency in one of the factors necessary for coagulation. Two major classifications of X-linked recessive hemophilia include deficiency of factor VIII (classic hemophilia A) or deficiency of factor IX (Christmas disease; hemophilia B) or factor XI. Abnormal bleeding occurs because a stable fibrin clot is not produced as a result of missing clotting factor.

II. Nursing process
   A. Assessment
      1. Complete a detailed health history, including prior hospitalizations, prior episodes of bleeding, and developmental level.
      2. Assess child for bleeding.
         a. Bleeding from any trauma—especially in the mouth, throat, and thorax
         b. Hemarthrosis—resulting in pain, tenderness, swelling, and impaired range of motion in the joints
         c. Ecchymosis without petechiae

d. Peripheral neuropathy
e. Epistaxis
3. Obtain diagnostic tests.
a. Factor VIII or IX assay showing deficiency
b. Prolonged PTT
c. Normal bleeding time, PT, and platelet count

B. Analysis
1. Risk for Injury: Bleeding, related to hypoprothrombinemia
2. Risk for Acute Pain related to bleeding and hemarthrosis
3. Impaired Physical Mobility related to hemarthrosis
4. Risk for Social Isolation related to restricted activity
5. Ineffective Tissue Perfusion: cardiopulmonary related to bleeding

C. Planning
1. Maintain hemodynamic stability.
2. Prevent bleeding episodes.
3. Recognize bleeding symptoms.
4. Maintain joint mobility.
5. Promote growth and development.

D. Implementation
1. Prevent bleeding.
a. Administer fresh-frozen plasma.
b. Administer hemostatic agent: Desmopressin (DDAVP).
c. Administer antihemophilic factor.
d. Avoid medications that interfere with platelet aggregation such as aspirin and most nonsteroidal anti-inflammatories.
2. Manage bleeding.
a. Initiate blood transfusions as ordered.
b. Maintain pressure on bleeding sites.
c. Administer fibrinolysis inhibitor: Aminocaproic acid.
3. Manage hemarthrosis.
a. Encourage rest, ice, and elevation during acute bleeding.
b. Promote range of motion exercise 48 hr after acute bleeding.
c. Maintain normal body weight.
d. Provide analgesics.

E. Evaluation
1. Child and family are compliant with administration of antihemophilic factor.
2. Child and family verbalize methods to prevent and manage episodes of bleeding.
3. Child maintains joint mobility.
4. Child tolerates limited activity, frequent transfusions, and hospitalization.

CN

III. Client needs

A. Physiologic adaptation: Bleeding is controlled through medication management on an outpatient basis.
1. Antihemophilic factor is effective in reducing bleeding episodes, reducing joint damage, and preventing organ damage.
2. Acute bleeding is indicated by tachycardia, hypotension, change in level of consciousness.

B. Management of care: Care of the child with hemophilia requires critical thinking skills and knowledge of assessment, and teaching and evaluation methods unique to the RN role. These skills cannot be delegated to an LPN or UAP.
1. Assess for home health needs.
a. Prevent injury by modifying home environment.
b. Administer antihemophilic factor using appropriate IV equipment.
2. Evaluate community resources for family support, including a local chapter of a hemophilia support group, transportation for frequent medical or physical therapy appointments, and education of the school.
3. Delegate responsibly those activities that can be delegated, including measurements, oral intake and urine output, vital signs, and reporting child's subjective data. All monitoring information is reported to the RN.

C. Safety and infection control
1. Recognize signs of internal bleeding such as:
a. Headache or changes in neurologic status—indicate intracranial bleeding.
b. Vomiting frank blood or coffee ground material.
c. Backache or flank pain—may indicate internal bleeding.
d. Urine that is dark or smoky color.
e. Unexplained increase in pulse rate or decrease in BP.
f. Joint pain.
2. Prevent injury.
a. Pad toys and other objects.
b. Discourage activity that may result in injury.
c. Recommend use of protective head gear, knee pads, and elbow pads.
d. Avoid IM injection.
3. Control and manage bleeding.
a. Apply pressure to site for 10 to 15 min.
b. Suture, if necessary, for deeper cuts.
c. Administer deficient factor or plasma.
d. Immobilize and elevate extremity.
e. Avoid range of motion during acute bleeding.
f. Apply cold compresses or ice bags.
g. Restrict activity for 48 hr after injury.
4. Teach child and family how to assess for and manage bleeding at home.

Table 13-2 Drugs Used to Manage Hemophilia

Classification	Generic/Trade Name	Expected Outcome	Reduction of Risk Potential	Management of Care
Analgesics	Oxycodone and acetaminophen (Percocet)	Used for analgesia because contains acetaminophen, which does not interfere with platelet aggregation.	Monitor for nausea, constipation, and sedation.	Teach parents to promote fluid intake.
Antihemophilic Factor	Desmopressin acetate (DDVAP)	Used to increase factor VIII activity in children with mild hemophilia.	Monitor fluid intake and output to avoid water retention and sodium depletion. Weigh daily. Monitor for headache, sleepiness, and nausea.	Instruct parents to encourage fluids and avoid dehydration. Report weight gain.
Antihemophilic Factor	Cryoprecipitated antihemophilic factor (AHF)	Used to promote the coagulation process and decrease bleeding episodes.	Monitor for anaphylactic reactions to infusion and discontinue immediately.	Instruct parents about side effects such as dizziness, headache, sore throat, urticaria, nausea, vomiting, and fatigue.
Fibrinolysis Inhibitor	Aminocaproic acid (Amicar)	Used to control excessive bleeding or prevent bleeding during dental procedures for hemophiliacs.	Monitor dizziness, headache, and hypotension. Monitor and report signs and symptoms of muscle weakness, fever, oliguria, or thrombophlebitis.	Instruct parents to report reddish-brown urine, chest pain, or difficulty breathing.

5. Maintain the six rights of medication administration.

D. Health promotion and maintenance
1. Promote optimal functional capability through interventions that prevent or immediately treat bleeding episodes.
2. Assist child in identifying activities that promote growth and development but prevent injury.
3. Teach child and family management of hemarthrosis.
4. Assist child in administering own antihemophilic factor when developmentally capable.

E. Psychologic integrity
1. Assist child and family in coping with lifelong illness.
2. Encourage participation in support groups.
3. Encourage verbalization of fears.
4. Understand cultural diversity in expression of fear, lack of knowledge, manifestation of pain, and regimen compliance.
5. Understand developmental variations.

F. Basic care and comfort: Provide rest periods and administer analgesics for pain.

G. Reduction of risk potential: Provide medic alert bracelet in addition to teaching child and family how to prevent bleeding episodes.
1. Use electric razor.
2. Avoid IM injections.
3. Use soft toothbrush or water irrigating device.
4. Avoid constipation.

H. Pharmacologic and parenteral therapies: Child and family will state purpose, route, and side effects of analgesics, antihemophilic factor, and fibrinolysis inhibitor for treatment of pain associated with bleeding episodes. See Table 13-2 for drugs used to manage hemophilia.

Leukemia

I. Definition: Leukemia is the abnormal, uncontrolled proliferation of WBCs in bone marrow. The most common type of leukemia in children is acute lymphocytic leukemia (ALL), affecting children between the ages of 3 and 7. Bone marrow alteration occurs because of the rapid production of immature cells (blast cells). This proliferation of

WBCs prevents normal cells from receiving nutrients. Ultimately, the bone marrow atrophies, causing anemia, bleeding, and infection.

II. Nursing process

A. Assessment
1. Complete a detailed health history, including family history of cancer, and exposure to viruses, ionizing radiation, and chemicals.
2. Perform a comprehensive physical examination.
3. Assess for signs and symptoms of bone marrow infiltration.
   a. High fever
   b. Abdominal or bone pain
   c. Pallor, petechiae, and ecchymosis
   d. Abnormal bleeding such as nosebleeds
4. Assess for signs and symptoms of CNS infiltration.
   a. Headache
   b. Vomiting
   c. Irritability
   d. Papilledema
5. Obtain diagnostic tests.
   a. Before treatment: CBC—leukocytosis, 15,000 to 500,000/mm^3
   b. After treatment:
      (1) Thrombocytopenia
      (2) Neutropenia
      (3) Anemia
   c. Bone marrow aspiration

B. Analysis
1. Activity Intolerance related to bone marrow suppression and fever
2. Anxiety related to situational crisis, painful procedures, and strange environment
3. Risk for Ineffective Coping related to situational crisis and lack of coping mechanism
4. Risk for Infection related to altered immune response and immunosuppression
5. Risk for Injury: Anemia and bleeding related to bone marrow suppression
6. Deficient Knowledge: Treatment, related to lack of knowledge of disease and treatment
7. Ineffective Protection related to bone marrow suppression

C. Planning
1. Prevent infection.
2. Prevent dehydration.
3. Provide adequate fluids and nutrition.
4. Assess and prevent bleeding.
5. Control pain.
6. Assess for CNS involvement.
7. Manage chemotherapy side effects.
8. Provide emotional support and family teaching.

D. Implementation: Manage leukemia
1. Systemic chemotherapy
2. Intrathecal chemotherapy
3. Anti-infectives
4. Granulocyte medications
5. Transfusions
6. Possible bone marrow transplant

E. Evaluation
1. Child and family demonstrate positive coping mechanisms as evidenced by expression of feelings, goal setting, and use of resources.
2. Child is free from infection and bleeding as evidenced by being afebrile, having clear lungs, no petechiae and normal laboratory values.
3. Child and family verbalize understanding of treatment, procedures, and chemotherapy-induced side effects.

CN

III. Client needs

A. Physiologic adaptation
1. Assess child's tolerance for activity.
2. Evaluate leukocyte count for severe infection leading to life-threatening complications such as septicemia.
3. Evaluate for thrombocytopenia accompanied by fatigue, lethargy, and hemorrhage.
4. Recognize signs and symptoms that would alert the nurse to CNS system invasion: Headache, confusion, and seizures.
5. Assess for tissue or structure compression from organ enlargement.
6. Institute protective isolation and neutropenic precautions when the absolute neutrophil count (ANC) is less than 500 cells/mm^3.
7. Institute bleeding precautions when platelet count drops below 50,000/mm^3.

B. Management of care: Care of the child with leukemia requires critical thinking skills and knowledge of assessment, and teaching and evaluation methods unique to the RN role. These skills cannot be delegated to an LPN or UAP.
1. Assess bleeding and infection.
2. Provide teaching about chemotherapy.
3. Assess for home health needs such as specialized equipment for treatment of side effects of chemotherapy, infusion therapy, and possible physical care.
4. Evaluate community resources for family support.
   a. Availability of home nursing care
   b. Durable medical equipment
   c. Delivery services for food, equipment, and medication

   d. Transportation for multiple medical care visits
   e. Local chapter of the Leukemia & Lymphoma Society for family and child support
5. Assign staff and roommates as appropriate if child is neutropenic.
6. Delegate responsibly those activities that can be delegated, including measurements, oral intake and urine output, vital signs, and reporting child's subjective data. All monitoring information is reported to the RN.

C. Safety and infection control
1. Prevent infection.
   a. Provide private room (protective isolation).
   b. Promote frequent hand hygiene.
   c. Use aseptic technique for all procedures.
   d. Inspect mouth and skin frequently.
   e. Institute neutropenic precautions when appropriate.
      (1) No raw fruits and vegetables
      (2) No fresh flowers
      (3) No standing water
      (4) Drinking water must be less than 15 min old
2. Assess for signs and symptoms of infection.
   a. Monitor CBC.
   b. Avoid constipation to minimize rectal trauma.
   c. Avoid invasive procedures.
   d. Administer antibiotics, antivirals, or granulocyte factors as ordered.
   e. Teach parents about avoiding live virus immunization.
3. Provide fluids and nutrition.
   a. Increase fluids to promote excretion of chemotherapy.
   b. Provide a high-protein, high-calorie, bland diet.
   c. Administer antiemetics to promote appetite.
4. Assess and prevent bleeding.
   a. Touch child gently, and pad side rails.
   b. Inspect for bleeding—petechiae, bruising, bleeding.
   c. Assess all body fluids and stool for bleeding.
   d. Measure abdominal circumference to detect occult bleeding.
   e. Avoid injections; hold gentle pressure for 10 min.
   f. No rectal temperatures.
   g. Soft toothbrush or water irrigating device.
   h. Assess CBC—monitor for occult and spontaneous bleeding when platelet count less than 20,000/mm^3.
5. Manage pain.
6. Assess for CNS involvement—confusion, lethargy, and headache.
7. Manage chemotherapy side effects.
   a. Monitor for nausea and vomiting; give antiemetics.
   b. Monitor for signs of dehydration.
   c. Monitor for bone marrow suppression.
   d. Monitor for hemorrhagic cystitis.
   e. Assess mouth and provide oral rinses such as Peridex.
      (1) Nystatin mouthwash
      (2) Local anesthetic such as benzocaine (Orabase)
      (3) Avoid lemon glycerin mouth swabs
   f. Encourage bland, soft diet, and avoidance of spicy, hot, cold, and acidic foods and fluids.
   g. Teach parents and child about hair loss; care of central venous access; side effects of chemotherapy.

D. Health promotion and maintenance: Instruct parents and child about chemotherapy and side effects.
1. Manage side effects.
2. Prevent infection—avoid crowds; avoid others with infections.
3. Recognize signs and symptoms of bleeding.
4. Avoid medications that might induce bleeding such as nonsteroidal anti-inflammatory drugs and any drugs containing aspirin.
5. Acknowledge possibility for bone marrow transplant.

E. Psychologic integrity
1. Refer to support groups such as American Cancer Society.
2. Encourage verbalization of fears, concerns, guilt, anger, and opportunity to ask questions.
3. Understand cultural diversity in expression of fear, lack of knowledge, manifestation of pain, dietary needs, death and dying rituals.
4. Understand developmental variations.

F. Basic care and comfort
1. Medicate for pain.
2. Provide antiemetic, bland, cool diet, and promote hydration for nausea and vomiting.
3. Provide pain relief, oral mouth rinses, and acupressure for stomatitis.
4. Act as consistent nurse caregiver.
5. Provide transitional, comfort object at bedside.

Table 13-3 Drugs Used to Treat Leukemias

Classification	Generic/Trade Name	Expected Outcome	Reduction of Risk Potential	Management of Care
Antibiotics	Ampicillin sodium (Ampicin) Cefotaxime sodium (Claforan)	Treats or prevents infection.	Determine sensitivity to penicillin.	Inspect skin for rashes indicating sensitivity to ampicillin. Monitor and manage diarrhea.
Chemotherapy	Vincristine (Oncovin) High-dose cytarabine (Cytosar-U) Daunorubicin (Cerubidine)	Treats cancer by arresting abnormal cell growth.	Monitor for bleeding and infection. Monitor serum electrolytes.	Instruct parents how to manage side effects including nausea, vomiting, alopecia, and stomatitis.
Steroids	Prednisone (Deltasone)	Used in conjunction with chemotherapy.	Monitor BP for ascension. Assess for delayed wound healing.	Monitor weight. Assess wounds for signs of infection. Monitor for complaints of headache.
Granulocyte Colony Stimulating Factors	Epoetin alfa (Epogen) Filgrastim (Neupogen)	Elevates hematocrit and decreases neutropenia.	Monitor CBC, aPTT, and INR. Monitor for hypertensive encephalopathy.	Assess child for bone pain, headache, and hypertension.
Narcotic Analgesics	Morphine sulfate (Roxanol)	Provides symptomatic relief of severe pain.	Provide continuous monitoring for respiratory depression.	Monitor respiratory rate. Assess for pain relief.
Antiemetics	Ondansetron hydrochloride (Zofran)	Prevents nausea and vomiting from chemotherapy.	Monitor fluid and electrolyte status.	Assess and manage diarrhea. Monitor for headache.

G. Reduction of risk potential
   1. Teach parents and child side effects of all medications.
   2. Teach parents and child how to monitor and prevent infection and bleeding.
   3. Monitor WBC count for infection.
   4. Monitor platelet count for increased risk for bleeding.

H. Pharmacologic and parenteral therapies: Child and family will state the purpose, dosage, timing, and side effects of medications used to manage leukemia, as well as side effects of treatment. See Table 13-3 for drugs used to treat leukemias.

β-Thalassemia (Cooley Anemia)

I. Definition: Thalassemia major is a hereditary group of hemolytic anemias characterized by a reduction in the production of one of the globin chains in the synthesis of hemoglobin. Deficiency in the polypeptide chain impairs hemoglobin synthesis, causing RBCs to be hypochromic and microcytotic. Thalassemia most commonly occurs in children of Mediterranean origin, but has been seen in children of Southeast Asian Chinese, African and Philippine descent.

II. Nursing process
   A. Assessment
      1. Complete a detailed health history, including prior hospitalizations and developmental level.
      2. Assess child for signs and symptoms of altered hemoglobin synthesis.
         a. Severe anemia
         b. Failure to thrive (see Chapter 15)
         c. Bone abnormalities such as frontal bossing or prominent maxilla
         d. Flattened bridge of nose
         e. Pallor and jaundice
         f. Splenomegaly and hepatomegaly
         g. Bleeding tendencies, especially epistaxis

3. Obtain diagnostic tests.
   a. CBC
   b. Reticulocyte count
   c. Radiograph of the skull and long bones

B. Analysis
   1. Fatigue related to severe anemia
   2. Delayed Growth and Development related to inadequate tissue oxygenation
   3. Anticipatory Grieving related to need for frequent hospitalizations and family separations
   4. Impaired Tissue Integrity related to hemochromatosis
   5. Ineffective Tissue Perfusion: cardiopulmonary related to severe anemia

C. Planning
   1. Improve tissue oxygenation.
   2. Improve activity tolerance.
   3. Minimize complications from iron overload.
   4. Promote growth and development.

D. Implementation
   1. Prevent iron overload.
      a. Administer chelating agents.
      b. Avoid iron-rich foods; iron supplements contraindicated.
   2. Treat severe anemia.
      a. Transfuse with packed red blood cells (PRBCs) every 3 to 4 weeks.
      b. Prepare for possible splenectomy.

E. Evaluation
   1. Child and family verbalize an understanding of therapeutic regimen.
   2. Child and family describe iron-rich foods to avoid.
   3. Child and family verbalize an understanding of the signs and symptoms of transfusion reaction.
   4. Child is compliant with therapeutic regimen.

CN

III. Client needs

A. Physiologic adaptation: Anemia is controlled with multiple transfusions of PRBCs.
   1. Evaluate hemoglobin and hematocrit.
   2. Evaluate the effectiveness of chelating agents to remove excess iron, leading to reduced tissue damage.
   3. Recognize the need for splenectomy related to severe splenomegaly and abdominal distention and pressure.

B. Management of care: Care of the child with thalassemia major requires critical thinking skills and knowledge of assessment, and teaching and evaluation methods unique to the RN role. These skills cannot be delegated to an LPN or UAP.
   1. Assess for home health needs, including setting up a home transfusion and chelation program.
   2. Evaluate community resources for family support.
      a. Availability of home nursing care
      b. Durable medical equipment
      c. Delivery services for food, equipment, and medication
      d. Transportation for multiple medical care visits
      e. Local chapter of a thalassemia group for family and child support
   3. Delegate responsibly those activities that can be delegated, including measurements, oral intake and urine output, vital signs, and reporting child's subjective data. All monitoring information is reported to the RN.

C. Safety and infection control
   1. Teach family signs and symptoms of increased risk for infection after splenectomy.
   2. Monitor vital signs for signs of infection, including increased temperature and heart rate.
   3. Teach family about need for frequent transfusions, possible reactions, and hospitalizations.
   4. Maintain the six rights of medication administration.

D. Health promotion and maintenance
   1. Optimize functional ability and prevent complications through interventions that prevent and manage severe anemia and hemochromatosis.
   2. Provide family with genetic counseling.
   3. Instruct avoidance of strenuous exercise.

E. Psychologic integrity
   1. Assist child and family in coping with life-long illness.
   2. Prepare child and family for a possible splenectomy.
   3. Prepare child and family for a possible bone marrow transplant.

F. Basic care and comfort: Anticipate possible premedication before multiple transfusions with acetaminophen (Tylenol) and diphenhydramine (Benadryl).

G. Reduction of risk potential
   1. Teach parents and child side effects of all medications.
   2. Teach parents and child how to monitor and prevent infection and bleeding.
   3. Monitor WBC count for infection.
   4. Monitor for increased iron levels.

H. Pharmacologic and parenteral therapies: Child and family will verbalize understanding of the

purpose, route, and side effects of chelating agent: Deferoxamine mesylate (Desferal).
1. Expected outcome: Used to bind with iron in the management of hemochromatosis and hemosiderosis.
2. Reduction of risk potential: Monitor for rash, diarrhea, dysuria, and blurred vision.
3. Management of care: Monitor injection site for induration and pain; monitor urine for reddish color.

End-of-Life Care

I. Definition: End-of-life care for children is affected by language and cognitive development in addition to cultural, religious, and ethnic factors. Nursing care involves eliciting knowledge, providing information, and allowing the child to ask questions.

II. Nursing process
   A. Assessment: Assess for presence of cultural, religious, and ethnic factors in relation to developmental stage in order to understand child's concept of death. Table 13-4 depicts concepts of death by developmental stage.
   B. Analysis
      1. Anxiety related to loss of control and separation from parents
      2. Risk for Hopelessness related to hospitalizations and illness
      3. Anticipatory Grieving related to fear and lack of knowledge about disease outcome
   C. Planning
      1. Maintain family dynamics through involvement in child's care.
      2. Minimize anxiety and fear.
      3. Encourage verbalization of fear.
   D. Implementation: Provide interventions related to end-of-life issues.
      1. Act as consistent nurse caregiver.
      2. Try not to allow child to be alone if death is imminent.

Table 13-4 Concept of Death

Age Group	Concept of Death
Toddler	No concept of time. Primary fear is separation.
Preschooler	Temporary. Responds with guilt and punishment.
School Age	Understands permanence. Fears pain and abandonment. Curious.
Adolescent	Anger of loss of independence. Risk-taker.

      3. Encourage touching.
      4. Allow child to discuss life events.
      5. Be aware of regression.
      6. Include siblings in dying process.
   E. Evaluation
      1. Child verbalizes fears and concerns.
      2. Child's family participates in dying process.
      3. Child's family verbalizes fears and anxieties.

CN

III. Client needs
   A. Physiologic adaptation: Adaptation to end of life will be influenced by cultural, religious, ethnic, developmental, and cognitive factors.
   B. Management of care: Care of the dying child requires critical thinking skills and knowledge of assessment, and teaching and evaluation methods unique to the RN role. These skills cannot be delegated to an LPN or UAP.
      1. Assess for home health needs including any environmental modification for the child.
      2. Evaluate community resources for family support.
         a. Availability of hospice
         b. Durable medical equipment
         c. Bereavement support for child and family
      3. Delegate responsibly those activities that can be delegated, including measurements, oral intake and urine output, vital signs, and reporting child's subjective data. All monitoring information is reported to the RN.
   C. Safety and infection control: Promote a protective environment.
      1. Reduce exposure to infection.
      2. Maintain hand hygiene.
      3. Monitor child if receiving narcotics.
   D. Health promotion and maintenance
      1. Provide family with comprehensive teaching about child's needs.
      2. Inform family of formal bereavement programs.
      3. Promote healthy grieving.
   E. Psychologic integrity
      1. Provide clergy, if requested.
      2. Encourage play therapy.
      3. Assist child and family with emotional issues related to the dying process.
      4. Provide emotional support for the parents.
      5. Assist family in identifying and using coping mechanisms.
   F. Basic care and comfort
      1. Encourage quiet play.
      2. Meet all needs for basic comfort.
      3. Provide quiet, nonstimulating environment.
   G. Reduction of risk potential: Monitor child for hypotension if on narcotics and antianxiety medications.

H. Pharmacologic and parenteral therapies: Child and family will verbalize understanding of the purpose for and side effects of medications.
   1. Antianxiety medications: Lorazepam (Ativan)
      a. Expected outcome: Reduces anxiety.
      b. Reduction of risk potential: Monitor for drowsiness; do not abruptly discontinue medication; not for use in children less than 12 years of age.
      c. Management of care: Offer emotional support, monitor for hypotension.
   2. Narcotics: Morphine sulfate
      a. Expected outcome: Alters pain perception.
      b. Reduction of risk potential: Do not crush, break, or dissolve extended-release form of medication.
      c. Management of care: Assess reduction in pain, assess for respiratory depression, and assess for voiding difficulty.

Bibliography

Hatfield, N. (2006). *Broadribb's introductory pediatric nursing.* Philadelphia: Lippincott Williams & Wilkins.

Pillitteri, A. (2006). *Maternal & child health nursing: Care of the childbearing and childrearing family* (5th ed.). Philadelphia: Lippincott Williams & Wilkins.

Wong, D. L., et al. (2006). *Maternal child nursing care.* St. Louis: Mosby.

CHAPTER 13

Practice Test

Iron Deficiency Anemia

1. The nurse is assessing children in an ambulatory clinic. Which child is most likely to have iron deficiency anemia?
- □ 1. Male child who is 3 months of age and receives only breast-feedings.
- □ 2. Female child who is 15 years of age and has heavy menstrual periods.
- □ 3. Female child who is 8 years of age and brings a sandwich and fruit to school for lunch.
- □ 4. Male child who is 12 months of age and eats table food.

2. A male child who is 9 months of age with iron deficiency anemia is given ferrous sulfate therapy. Which of the following indicates that he is actually taking the medication daily?
- □ 1. His reticulocyte count is decreased.
- □ 2. He develops diarrhea.
- □ 3. His stools appear black.
- □ 4. He is less irritable than he was at his last visit.

Sickle Cell Anemia

3. AF A school-aged child is admitted to the hospital with a vaso-occlusive sickle cell crisis. The nurse should do which of the following in priority order? Place in order of highest priority to lowest priority.
- _____ 1. Administer morphine for the pain.
- _____ 2. Start oxygen per nasal cannula.
- _____ 3. Start an IV infusion.
- _____ 4. Draw blood for electrolyte and pH balance.

4. The nurse is planning care for a child with sickle cell disease (SCD). Which of the following is the primary goal of care for this child?
- □ 1. Prevent bleeding.
- □ 2. Prevent respiratory infection.
- □ 3. Prevent fluid loss.
- □ 4. Prevent iron deficiency.

5. To prevent sickle cell crisis, the nurse instructs the parents of a child with sickle cell anemia to:
- □ 1. Notify HCP if child develops an upper respiratory infection.
- □ 2. Prevent child from drinking an excessive amount of fluids per day.
- □ 3. Encourage child to participate in strength-training activities.
- □ 4. Administer an iron supplement.

6. A preschooler with sickle cell disease is hospitalized with severe pain in the arms and legs, preceded by 3 days of upper respiratory infection. The vital signs are temperature = 101.3°F, heart rate = 136 beats per minute, respiratory rate = 34 breaths per minute, BP = 90/65 mmHg, and oxygen saturation = 89%. The child has dusky mucous membranes, clubbed fingernails, cough, and delayed capillary refill. Which of the following is the priority for nursing care for this child?
- □ 1. Control pain.
- □ 2. Ensure adequate IV fluid intake.

□ 3. Provide bronchodilator respiratory treatments.
□ 4. Initiate oxygen therapy.

7. The nurse is providing genetic counseling to parents about their risk for having a child with sickle cell disease. The wife has sickle cell trait; the husband has sickle cell disease. What is the chance that their child will have sickle cell disease?
□ 1. 25%.
□ 2. 50%.
□ 3. 75%.
□ 4. 100%.

Hemophilia

8. A male child who is 10 years of age with hemophilia has slipped on the ice at school and bumped his knee. The nurse should:
□ 1. Apply a tourniquet to decrease blood flow to the area.
□ 2. Begin an IV infusion of factor VIII.
□ 3. Have the child walk to increase circulation and prevent swelling.
□ 4. Apply a warm compress to increase blood absorption.

9. The nurse is caring for a hospitalized child with hemophilia who has severe joint pain. Which of the following will be most effective in relieving the child's joint pain?
□ 1. Applying a heating pad.
□ 2. Providing passive range of motion exercises.
□ 3. Applying an ice pack.
□ 4. Administering salicylates.

10. A child with hemophilia receives factor VIII concentrate. The nurse should instruct the child and family to report which of the following to the HCP?
□ 1. Periorbital edema.
□ 2. Jaundice.
□ 3. Diarrhea.
□ 4. Fatigue.

11. A child with hemophilia wants to join the basketball team. The nurse should advise the parents to do which of the following?
□ 1. Encourage the child's choice.
□ 2. Provide the team trainer with factor VIII concentrate.
□ 3. Explore the possibility of joining the swim team.
□ 4. Suggest the child participate in gymnastics instead.

Leukemia

12. The nurse is planning care for a preschooler who is hospitalized with a diagnosis of acute lymphocytic leukemia (ALL). The nurse should establish which of the following as the primary goal of care?
□ 1. Protect from injury.
□ 2. Maintain hydration.
□ 3. Manage bleeding episodes
□ 4. Prevent infection.

13. A preschooler is to have a bone marrow aspiration. When preparing this child for the procedure, the nurse should?
□ 1. Provide sufficient details about the procedure.
□ 2. Tell the child the procedure will not hurt.
□ 3. Provide details on expected sights, smells, sensations, and sounds.
□ 4. Explain the function of the bone marrow and how it will be removed.

14. AF A child with leukemia is receiving cyclophosphamide (Cytoxan). The nurse assesses the child for which of the following adverse effects? Select all that apply.
□ 1. Cardiac arrhythmias.
□ 2. Mouth ulcers.
□ 3. Alopecia.
□ 4. Double vision.
□ 5. Cystitis.
□ 6. Abdominal pain.

15. An adolescent with leukemia is experiencing severe nausea. The nurse offers which of the following drinks to help the child relieve the nausea, while meeting fluid and nutrition needs?
□ 1. Orange juice.
□ 2. Milkshake.
□ 3. Carbonated soft drink.
□ 4. Water.

16. A child is hospitalized with acute lymphocytic leukemia and has a temperature of 101.1°F. The child is lethargic and fatigued. Nursing assessment reveals petechiae, cervical lymphadenopathy, and an enlarged spleen. The nurse plans care to manage which of the following first?
□ 1. Petechiae.
□ 2. Enlarged lymph nodes.
□ 3. Fatigue.
□ 4. Enlarged spleen.

β-Thalassemia (Cooley Anemia)

17. An infant with thalassemia major is hospitalized and receiving PRBCs. The nurse is assessing the effectiveness of this intervention. Which of the following indicates that the PRBCs have had intended effects?
□ 1. Iron levels are elevated.
□ 2. WBC count is normal.

□ 3. Hemoglobin is 12 g/dl.
□ 4. Reticulocyte count is low.

End-of-Life Care

18. The parents of a child who is near death visit infrequently and when they are present they spend much of their time talking to other parents. It is important for the nurse to understand that the parents' behavior is:
□ 1. Typical for parents of a child with a terminal disease.
□ 2. Related to the fact that their other children also require their time.
□ 3. Indicative of the stage of grief they are experiencing.
□ 4. A reflection of a weak parent-child relationship.

19. A child with leukemia had been in remission for several years, but death is now imminent. The nurse is assisting the parents as they prepare for the child's death. Which of the following approaches will be most helpful?
□ 1. Reflect to the parents that the death of a child is more difficult than that of an adult.
□ 2. Help parents understand that grief is stronger when preceded by hope.
□ 3. Recognize that the parents have been prepared for this death since the time of diagnosis.
□ 4. Understand the parent's trust in the health care system will be undermined by the death of their child.

20. A child with leukemia who is 12 years of age has hospice home care. His twin sister, who spends most of her time with her brother, is crying and tells the nurse, "It's not fair; I wish it was me who is dying. I don't know how I can live without him." The nurse should respond by saying:
□ 1. "This is hard for you, but you will need to be strong for your brother right now."
□ 2. "Let's talk about how you can best cope with your life when your brother dies."
□ 3. "You seem sad and scared when you think about life without your brother."
□ 4. "Maybe it would be helpful for you to spend less time with your brother right now."

Answers and Rationales

1. 2 Adolescents with heavy menstrual flows lose enough blood each month to cause iron deficiency anemia. The nurse refers the child to have a CBC to detect the anemia. The child who is 3 months of age still has maternal stores of iron. The child who is 8 years of age likely has an adequate iron intake if eating iron-fortified bread in the sandwich. The child who is 12 months of age child will likely be obtaining iron-fortified milk and cereals. (H)

2. 3 Ferrous sulfate therapy causes stools to appear black in color. The nurse instructs the parents to expect this side effect. (H)

3. 3, 2, 1, 4 The nurse first starts an IV as dehydration increases sickling of cells; maintaining fluid balance is a priority. The nurse next starts oxygen and then administers morphine for pain; these actions are followed by obtaining a blood sample for laboratory studies. (A)

4. 3 Nursing care for the child with sickle cell disease (SCD) is directed at preventing fluid loss because fluid loss will further exacerbate a sickling crisis, because the RBCs will not be "full" and plump and will more likely be in a sickled shape, increasing the potential of "log jams" within the small arterial capillaries of the major organs. Infection in a child with SCD can lead to an exacerbation of the disease, particularly of a respiratory origin; however, this will be addressed after volume levels have been corrected. Administration of pneumococcal and meningococcal vaccines is recommended for these children because of their susceptibility to infection as a result of a functional asplenia. Oral penicillin prophylaxis is often administered by 2 months of age. Bleeding is not a major risk factor from SCD. Iron deficiency will be present when children have SCD; however, the treatment will not take priority over fluid loss or prevention of infection. (A)

5. 1 Reduction of oxygen and dehydration both lead to increased sickling of cells. Instruct parents to seek health care if child develops an upper respiratory infection. Provide adequate fluid intake to prevent dehydration. Children with sickle cell disease can participate in most sports and activities that do not decrease oxygen levels, (e.g., high-altitude mountain climbing), but strength training in and of itself will not prevent a sickle cell crisis. Iron supplements are contraindicated in sickle cell disease. (H)

6. 4 The priority nursing intervention is to initiate oxygen therapy because the sickling crises will continue until oxygenation is improved. Pain control and IV hydration are important, but oxygen is the first priority for this child. (C)

7. 2 The chance for this couple to have a child with sickle cell disease is 50% because one person has the trait and the other the disease. The risk for this couple for having a child with sickle cell trait is also 50%. If both parents have sickle cell disease, the chance for having a child with sickle cell disease is 100%. (A)

8. 2 Immediately replacing the clotting factor that is missing (factor VIII) best restores coagulation ability. The tourniquet will not totally stop the bleeding in this child. The child should not increase circulation until the bleeding is controlled. Warm compresses cannot be used until the bleeding is stopped; ice is commonly used first to prevent swelling. (D)

9. 3 Bleeding episodes into a child's joints can lead to significant pain. Applying an ice pack will help to alleviate this discomfort. A heating pad, passive range of motion, and salicylates may aggravate the pain. (C)

10. 2 The nurse instructs the family to inform the HCP about indications of jaundice such as yellow-tinged skin or sclera because factor VIII concentrate is derived from human plasma, which may have a risk of carrying hepatitis. Periorbital edema, diarrhea, and fatigue are not indications of problems with using factor VIII concentrate. (H)

11. 3 Advise children with hemophilia to avoid contact sports such as basketball. Swimming is an appropriate sport because the child can participate in a team sport that is competitive without risking bleeding episodes. It is unlikely that the school will assume responsibility for administering medications, and the parents should not risk having the child participate in a contact sport. Children who participate in gymnastics often have muscle and joint injuries, which could precipitate a bleeding episode for this child. (H)

12. 4 In ALL, lymphoblasts crowd the bone marrow and there is suppression of the formed elements of the blood, particularly WBCs, placing the child at risk for infection; therefore, the priority nursing action is to prevent infection. Encourage all personnel to practice good hand hygiene and avoid having anyone with an infection be in the room with this client. Prevention and management of bleeding and protection from injury are important, but the primary goal is to prevent infection. Children with ALL normally are not hypovolemic and require additional measures to maintain hydration. (S)

13. 3 Preschoolers have vivid imaginations and are magical thinkers. Details on sights, smells, sensations, and sounds will help to decrease fears. Details and explanations or physiologic functions should be reserved for older school-aged children. Telling the child that he or she will not experience pain may not be true for this child. (M)

14. 2, 3, 5, 6 Cyclophosphamide (Cytoxan) has side effects that involve most body systems. Assess the child for nausea, vomiting, ulcers in the mouth, hair loss, depressed WBC, and cystitis. The child is susceptible to infections; report the earliest sign of an elevated temperature to the health care provider. Cardiac arrhythmias and double vision are not typical side effects of Cytoxan. Side effects disappear or are reversed once the drug is discontinued. (D)

15. 3 Carbonated drinks are best tolerated by clients with nausea; the drink also provides needed calories and fluids. Orange juice is acidic and is not well tolerated by clients with nausea. The milkshake, although high in nutrients, may be too difficult to swallow and digest. Water does not relieve nausea and offers no nutritional value. (C)

16. 1 The petechiae are a result of suppressed production of thrombocytes, and the child is at risk for bleeding. The nurse first initiates safety precautions. Although protecting the child from injury is important, the enlarged lymph nodes and spleen are not nursing priorities. Fatigue is a result of RBC suppression and will be managed by transfusions of PRBCs. (R)

17. 3 PRBCs are given to treat the anemia; hemoglobin levels of 10 g/dl and above are desired. Increased iron levels accompany the disease, and the ultimate goal is to decrease iron levels through iron chelation therapy. The WBC count is usually not affected by the disease if treated early; a low reticulocyte is decreased because of the disease and will improve once the disease is managed. (D)

18. 3 Parents who begin a stage of anticipatory grief may "pull away" from their child as if the child has already died. Families may find that talking and sharing with other parents of critically ill children is helpful and therapeutic. (P)

19. 2 Parents often experience greater grief when they have experienced the hope provided by the remission of their child's disease. The nurse allows the parents to express this grief. Reactions to death of a family member are not based on the age of the dying family member. No matter how well prepared the parents may be for the death of their child, it will not make coping with death easier. Family members may displace anger and frustration on the health care system and health care providers, but death does not necessarily undermine trust. (P)

20. 3 Active listening is a helping response that communicates caring and understanding. Informing the sister that she needs to be strong does not acknowledge her feelings. Now is not the time for the nurse to refocus the sister's thinking about the future; the nurse can be most helpful by listening to her feelings at the present time. Suggesting that the sister spend less time with her brother neither helps her deal with her feelings nor gives her an opportunity to be with her brother at a time when they may need to be together. (P)

chapter

14

The Child With Health Problems of the Gastrointestinal Tract

Health problems of the GI tract in pediatric clients are relatively infrequent, and are typically noted in the neonate or infant. Problems with fluid and electrolyte imbalance such as vomiting and diarrhea are often secondary to other health problems, while defects in physical development and GI dysfunction present as primary health problems. The nurse plans care with the child, family, and the health care team to promote and restore health. Topics in this chapter include:

- Diarrhea and Gastroenteritis
- Vomiting
- Cleft Lip and Cleft Palate
- Esophageal Atresia and Tracheoesophageal Fistula
- Appendicitis
- Pyloric Stenosis
- Intussusception
- Hirschsprung Disease

Diarrhea and Gastroenteritis

I. Definition: Diarrhea is the increased frequency in association with the decreased consistency of stool, and is often the result of a virus, bacteria, or parasite. Gastroenteritis includes an inflammation of the intestines.

II. Nursing process
   A. Assessment
      1. Complete a detailed health history, including recent travel experiences, ingestion of foreign substances, parasites, medications, and food allergies.
      2. Perform a comprehensive physical assessment; assess for signs and symptoms of diarrhea.
         a. Increased number of loose, watery stools
         b. Abdominal pain and cramping
         c. Dehydration
         d. Fluid and electrolyte abnormalities
         e. Metabolic acidosis
      3. Obtain diagnostic tests.
         a. Stool cultures
         b. Blood cultures
         c. Serum electrolytes
         d. Arterial blood gas analysis
   B. Analysis
      1. Deficient Fluid Volume related to ongoing GI losses and anorexia
      2. Fear related to separation from parents and strange environment
      3. Imbalanced Nutrition: Less Than Body Requirements related to ongoing GI losses
      4. Risk for Impaired Skin Integrity related to irritation from frequent stooling
   C. Planning
      1. Restore fluid volume and prevent dehydration.
      2. Reduce fear.
      3. Improve nutritional intake.
      4. Maintain skin integrity.
   D. Implementation
      1. Treat diarrhea.
         a. Rest
         b. Nutritional supplement
         c. Fluid replacement
         d. Assessment of fluid and electrolyte imbalance
      2. Treat dehydration.
         a. Fluid and electrolyte replacement
         b. Intake and output measurement
         c. Daily weights
   E. Evaluation
      1. Child exhibits signs of adequate hydration as evidenced by improved skin turgor and urine output.
      2. Child exhibits diminished fear and improved comfort.
      3. Child gains weight and begins to consume regular diet.
      4. Child does not experience skin breakdown.

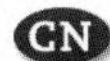

III. Client needs
   A. Physiologic adaptation: Diarrhea is managed with oral rehydration solutions and dehydration prevented on an outpatient basis.
      1. Recognize risk for dehydration, fluid and electrolyte imbalance, and metabolic acidosis—indicated by percentage loss of body weight, irritability, poor skin turgor, prolonged capillary refill 2 s or more, tachycardia, deep rapid respirations, absent tears, dry mucus membranes, plasma pH less than 7.33, and decreased plasma HCO_3.
      2. Recognize risk for hypokalemia—indicated by muscle weakness, hypotension, drowsiness, ECG: Flattened T waves, presence of U wave, serum potassium 3.5 mEq/L or less.
   B. Management of care: Care of the child with diarrhea and possible dehydration requires critical thinking skills and knowledge of assessment, and teaching and evaluation methods unique to the RN role. These skills cannot be delegated to an LPN or UAP.
      1. Perform comprehensive physical assessments and provide care appropriate to the child with diarrhea and possible dehydration.
      2. Delegate responsibly those activities that can be delegated, including measurements, oral intake and urine output, vital signs, and reporting child's subjective data. All monitoring information is reported to the RN.
   C. Safety and infection control
      1. Provide safe management of diarrhea.
         a. Provide enteric isolation as required.
         b. Practice good hand hygiene.
         c. Monitor electrolytes—replace potassium after kidney function is established.
         d. Monitor daily weight and promote strict intake and output.
         e. Provide oral rehydration with electrolyte solution.
         f. Monitor skin integrity.
         g. Avoid rectal temperature.
      2. Teach parents to manage child with mild-to-moderate diarrhea and dehydration in home setting.
         a. Practice good hand hygiene technique.
         b. Wear rubber gloves when changing diapers.

c. Provide oral rehydrating solutions.
d. Avoid fluids high in sodium such as milk, carbonated fluids, and concentrated sweets.
e. Reintroduce regular diet when child is rehydrated.
3. Provide safe management of child with severe diarrhea and dehydration.
a. Maintain NPO status.
b. Initiate IV fluids and electrolyte replacement.
c. Provide IV potassium.

D. Health promotion and maintenance
1. Encourage family to visit and participate in care.
2. Instruct breast-feeding may continue along with additional rehydration solutions.
3. Provide stimulation with age-appropriate toys and activities to enhance growth and development.

E. Psychologic integrity
1. Explain to family about the illness, management, and home care to promote compliance.
2. Allow family the opportunity to express feelings, fears, concerns, and to ask questions.
3. Reduce stress by touching, holding, and comforting the child.

F. Basic care and comfort
1. Provide consistent nurse caregiving.
2. Allow parents at bedside.
3. Use ointment around anus.

G. Reduction of risk potential
1. Monitor ECG when hypokalemic.
2. Ensure child has voided before administering IV potassium replacement.

H. Pharmacologic and parenteral therapies: Oral rehydration and IV infusions of fluids and electrolytes are used as needed to manage diarrhea and gastroenteritis.

Vomiting

I. Definition: Vomiting is the forceful loss of stomach contents via the mouth; also known as *emesis*. There are multiple causative agents including infection, increased intracranial pressure, food, and other allergies, and psychologic aversion.

II. Nursing process

A. Assessment
1. Complete a detailed health history, including age, patterns of vomiting, allergies, recent infections, and food intolerance.
2. Perform a comprehensive physical assessment; assess for signs and symptoms associated with vomiting.
a. Character of vomitus such as blood, undigested food contents, or presence of bile
b. Abdominal pain and cramping
c. Nausea
d. Dehydration
e. Fluid and electrolyte imbalance
f. Metabolic alkalosis
3. Obtain diagnostic tests.
a. History and physical examination
b. Urinalysis
c. Serum electrolytes
d. Radiographs of chest or abdomen

B. Analysis
1. Risk for Aspiration related to vomiting
2. Deficient Fluid Volume related to ongoing GI losses and nausea
3. Fear related to separation from parents and strange environment
4. Imbalanced Nutrition: Less Than Body Requirements related to ongoing GI losses

C. Planning
1. Restore fluid volume and prevent dehydration.
2. Reduce fear.
3. Improve nutritional intake.
4. Prevent complications.

D. Implementation
1. Detect and treat cause.
2. Prevent complications by treating fluid and electrolyte loss.
3. Administer antiemetics, if needed.

E. Evaluation
1. Child exhibits signs of adequate hydration as evidenced by improved skin turgor and urine output.
2. Child exhibits diminished fear and improved comfort.
3. Child gains weight and begins to consume regular diet.
4. Child does not become dehydrated.

CN

III. Client needs

A. Physiologic adaptation: Vomiting is managed by administering antiemetics and replacing fluids and electrolytes as needed.
1. Recognize risk for potential dehydration, fluid and electrolyte imbalance, and metabolic alkalosis—indicated by percentage loss of body weight, irritability, poor skin turgor, prolonged capillary refill 2 s or more, tachycardia, absent tears, dry mucous membranes, elevated urine pH, and elevated plasma HCO_3.
2. Recognize risk for potential hypokalemia—indicate by muscle weakness, hypotension, drowsiness, ECG: Flattened T waves,

presence of U wave, serum potassium 3.5 mEq/L or less.

B. Management of care: Care of the child with vomiting and possible dehydration requires critical thinking skills and knowledge of assessment, and teaching and evaluation methods unique to the RN role. These skills cannot be delegated to an LPN or UAP.
   1. Perform comprehensive physical assessments and provide care appropriate to the infant/child with vomiting and possible dehydration.
   2. Delegate responsibly those activities that can be delegated, including measurements, oral intake and urine output, vital signs, and reporting child's subjective data. All monitoring information is reported to the RN.

C. Safety and infection control: Provide safe management of vomiting
   1. Maintain patent airway.
   2. Position on side to prevent aspiration.
   3. Measure daily weights and strict intake and output.
   4. Monitor urine specific gravity.
   5. Monitor electrolytes—replace potassium.
   6. Provide oral rehydration.

D. Health promotion and maintenance
   1. Encourage family to visit and participate in care.
   2. Provide stimulation with age-appropriate toys and activities to enhance growth and development.

E. Psychologic integrity
   1. Explain to family about the illness, management, and home care to promote compliance.
   2. Allow family the opportunity to express feelings, fears, concerns, and to ask questions.
   3. Touch, hold, and comfort the child to reduce stress.

F. Basic care and comfort
   1. Provide consistent nurse caregiver.
   2. Allow parents at bedside.
   3. Provide skin and oral care after vomiting.

G. Reduction of risk potential
   1. Monitor ECG when hypokalemic.
   2. Ensure child has voided before administering IV potassium replacement.

H. Pharmacologic and parenteral therapies: Child and family will state the purpose, dosage, timing, and side effects of antiemetic medication: Ondansetron (Zofran).
   1. Expected outcome: Prevents nausea and vomiting.
   2. Reduction of risk potential: Observe for sedation, diarrhea, and headache; monitor fluid and electrolytes.
   3. Management of care: Teach parents signs and symptoms of dehydration and to notify health care practitioner; administer acetaminophen (Tylenol) for headache.

Cleft Lip and Cleft Palate

I. Definition: Cleft lip and cleft palate are congenital anomalies that result in first trimester failure of the lip and/or palate to fuse in utero. Multiple complications may result such as speech difficulty, dentition problems, and hearing deficits.

II. Nursing process

A. Assessment
   1. Complete a detailed health history, including prenatal risk factors such as maternal rubella virus.
   2. Perform a comprehensive physical assessment; assess for signs and symptoms of presence of cleft lip/palate.
      a. Physical notch or separation in lip, either unilateral or bilateral.
      b. Presence of opening in palate, with possible nasal deviation.
   3. Obtain diagnostic tests: Prenatal ultrasound.

B. Analysis
   1. Risk for Aspiration related to excess secretions and altered eating patterns
   2. Interrupted Family Processes related to an infant with a birth defect and frequent hospitalization
   3. Imbalanced Nutrition: Less Than Body Requirements related to defect that impairs eating
   4. Risk for Trauma related to impaired swallowing and surgical intervention

C. Planning
   1. Prevent aspiration.
   2. Provide adequate nutrition.
   3. Provide parental teaching about anomaly to promote acceptance of infant.
   4. Provide child and family with preoperative teaching.
   5. Promote postoperative prevention of trauma to surgical site: Lip and/or palate.

D. Implementation (see management of care)

E. Evaluation
   1. Child consumes adequate nutrition for growth without aspirating.
   2. Child's family accepts child and demonstrates adequate parenting skills.
   3. Child's operative site is free of trauma and infection.

III. Client needs

A. Physiologic adaptation: Cleft lip is repaired shortly after birth, and cleft palate is repaired

between the ages of 12 and 18 months to allow normal growth of palate.
1. For cleft lip: Cheiloplasty repair
2. For cleft palate: Staphylorrhaphy

B. Management of care: Care of the infant or child with a cleft lip/palate requires critical thinking skills and knowledge of assessment, and teaching and evaluation methods unique to the RN role. These skills cannot be delegated to an LPN or UAP.
1. Perform comprehensive physical assessments and provide care appropriate to the infant or child with a cleft lip/palate.
2. Facilitate outpatient follow-up care including dental visits.
3. Assess for home health needs and obtain necessary equipment for feeding preoperatively.
4. Delegate responsibly those activities that can be delegated, including measurements, oral intake and urine output, vital signs, and reporting child's subjective data. All monitoring information is reported to the RN.

C. Safety and infection control
1. Teach parents successful feeding techniques.
   a. Maintain head in upright position.
   b. Use special nipples such as the cleft lip/cleft palate nurser.
   c. Provide for frequent burping.
   d. Use a feeding device (NUK nipple, Haberman Feeder) for infants who cannot suck.
   e. Use ESSR method of feeding—enlarge the nipple, stimulate sucking, swallow, and rest.
2. Provide preoperative care.
   a. Promote nutritional and fluid status.
   b. Monitor baseline vital signs, weight, intake and output, and sleep-wake patterns.
   c. Assess infant's ability to swallow and handle secretions.
   d. Provide parents with instruction about postoperative management, including appropriate feeding methods.
3. Provide postoperative cleft lip care.
   a. Apply lip protective device.
   b. Apply elbow restraints.
   c. Position child on back or side.
   d. Provide analgesia for pain and sedation.
   e. Promote clear liquids, then progress diet.
   f. Provide cup feeding.
   g. Cleanse suture line and apply thin coat of antibiotic ointment.
   h. Monitor for bleeding and infection.
4. Provide postoperative cleft palate care.
   a. Monitor for bleeding and infection.
   b. Position prone to promote drainage.
   c. Resume postoperative feeding with cup or breast.
   d. Maintain NPO status, if needed, to protect surgical site.
   e. Avoid hard cookies and foods.
   f. Begin speech training.
5. Maintain the six rights of medication administration.

D. Health promotion and maintenance
1. Encourage family to visit and participate in care.
2. Provide stimulation with age-appropriate toys and activities to enhance growth and development.

E. Psychologic integrity
1. Encourage parental expression of grief, and promote attachment.
2. Allow parents to participate in care.
3. Provide postoperative photos to encourage hope and acceptance.
4. Refer to support groups such as American Cleft Palate Craniofacial Association.

F. Basic care and comfort
1. Provide consistent nurse caregiver.
2. Provide analgesia for postoperative pain.
3. Provide soft toys.

G. Reduction of risk potential: Identify children at risk for the development of complications and refer appropriately.

H. Pharmacologic and parenteral therapies: Pharmacologic therapies are rarely required.

Esophageal Atresia and Tracheoesophageal Fistula

I. Definition: Esophageal atresia (EA) is an embryonic failure of the esophagus to develop a continuous feeding tube from the pharynx to the stomach. Tracheoesophageal fistula (TEF) occurs during fetal development when an abnormal connection (fistula) develops, causing a connection between the esophagus and the trachea. Surgical intervention prevents aspiration pneumonia and respiratory distress.

II. Nursing process

A. Assessment
1. Complete a detailed health history, including prenatal risk factors and birth weight.
2. Perform a comprehensive physical assessment; assess for signs and symptoms of TEF.
   a. Frothy saliva in the mouth
   b. Drooling

c. Classic three "Cs": coughing, choking (especially during feeding), and cyanosis
d. Vomiting
e. Abdominal distention
3. Obtain diagnostic tests.
a. Failure to pass nasogastric/orogastric tube into the esophagus
b. Prenatal polyhydramnios on ultrasound

B. Analysis
1. Risk for Aspiration related to excess volume and inability to swallow secretions
2. Ineffective Airway Clearance related to swallowing obstruction
3. Interrupted Family Processes related to newborn defect and immediate hospitalization
4. Impaired Swallowing related to excess secretions and swallowing obstruction

C. Planning
1. Prevent or reduce respiratory distress.
2. Provide adequate calories and nutrition for growth.
3. Prevent respiratory complications.
4. Reduce anxiety and promote family functioning.

D. Implementation
1. Maintain patient airway.
2. Prevent aspiration and pneumonia.
3. Decompress esophageal pouch.
4. Implement care following surgical repair.

E. Evaluation
1. Child's respiratory status shows absence of respiratory distress.
2. Child maintains weight gain.
3. Child sleeps and rests as appropriate and is comforted.
4. Child's family demonstrates positive parenting skills and care measures.

CN

III. Client needs

A. Physiologic adaptation: TEF is managed with surgical repair and introduction of postoperative oral feedings.
1. Monitor respiratory status to maintain airway and prevent aspiration.
2. Recognize risk for anastomosis leak—indicated by purulent drainage, increased temperature, and leukocytosis.
3. Evaluate postoperative barium swallow to confirm absence of anastomosis leak and begin feeding with sterile water.

B. Management of care: Care of the child with TEF or EA requires critical thinking skills and knowledge of assessment, and teaching and evaluation methods unique to the RN role. These skills cannot be delegated to an LPN or UAP.
1. Perform comprehensive physical assessments and provide care.
2. Facilitate outpatient follow-up care to ensure adequate growth and development.
3. Assess for home health needs and obtain necessary equipment if child requires gastrostomy feedings or other special feeding techniques or suctioning.
4. Delegate responsibly those activities that can be delegated, including measurements, oral intake and urine output, vital signs, and reporting child's subjective data. All monitoring information is reported to the RN.

C. Safety and infection control
1. Provide preoperative interventions.
a. Maintain NPO status.
b. Suction upper airway as appropriate.
c. Provide humidified oxygen.
d. Decompress esophageal pouch using catheter set to low suction.
e. Provide IV fluids.
f. Place in infant seat with head elevated at least 30 degrees.
g. Place gastrostomy tube.
h. Administer prophylactic antibiotics.
i. Teach parents about home care needs for suctioning, recognizing signs and symptoms of respiratory distress, and intolerance to gastrostomy feeding.
2. Provide postoperative interventions.
a. Inspect surgical incision.
b. Assess for symptoms of dehydration.
c. Place gastrostomy tube to low suction.
d. Perform barium swallow 5 to 7 days postoperatively before beginning oral feeding.
(1) Begin feeding with sterile water.
(2) If unable to begin oral feedings, institute gastrostomy feedings.
e. Teach family about postoperative home management, including appropriate feeding techniques, evidence of respiratory distress, and infant CPR.

D. Health promotion and maintenance
1. Provide tactile stimulation to promote development, and comfort infant.
2. Encourage family to visit and participate in care.
3. Provide stimulation with age-appropriate toys and activities to enhance growth and development.

E. Psychologic integrity: Foster parent-child attachment by encouraging visitation, participation in care, and expression of feelings.

F. Basic care and comfort
  1. Offer pacifier for nonnutritive sucking.
  2. Provide mouth care.
  3. Administer analgesics for postoperative discomfort.
G. Reduction of risk potential
  1. Initiate follow-up care for careful long-term assessment of complications such as anastomotic leak, esophageal strictures, and feeding difficulties.
  2. Teach caregivers infant CPR.
H. Pharmacologic and parenteral therapies: IV fluids may be used until gastrostomy feedings are initiated.

Appendicitis

I. Definition: Appendicitis is the inflammation of the vermiform appendix. The lumen becomes obstructed with mucus causing increased pressure, inflammatory changes, and bacteremia. If undiagnosed and untreated, appendicitis rapidly progresses to perforation and ultimately peritonitis. The condition is uncommon in children under 2 years of age.

II. Nursing process
A. Assessment
  1. Complete a detailed health history, including dietary habits and history of constipation.
  2. Perform a comprehensive physical assessment; assess for signs and symptoms of acute appendicitis.
    a. Crampy, abdominal pain, especially periumbilical
    b. Focal abdominal tenderness at McBurney point
    c. Rovsing signs
    d. Rebound tenderness
    e. Nausea, vomiting, anorexia
    f. Low-grade fever
  3. Initiate preoperative assessments.
    a. Fluid status, intake and output, skin turgor, capillary refill
    b. Vital signs, height, and weight
  4. Obtain diagnostic tests.
    a. History and physical examination
    b. CBC
    c. Urinalysis
    d. Ultrasound and CT scan
B. Analysis
  1. Risk for Deficient Fluid Volume related to vomiting and anorexia
  2. Fear and Anxiety related to pain, procedures, and strange environment
  3. Risk for Infection related to possibility of rupture and peritonitis
  4. Acute Pain related to inflammation of appendix
C. Planning
  1. Prevent dehydration and provide hydration.
  2. Reduce fear and anxiety.
  3. Prevent infection and complications.
  4. Reduce pain to tolerable level.
  5. Prepare for surgery.
D. Implementation
  1. Preoperative interventions.
    a. Administer antibiotics.
    b. Provide IV fluids.
    c. Provide IV electrolytes.
  2. Postoperative interventions.
    a. Provide IV fluids.
    b. Promote pain management.
E. Evaluation
  1. Child receives adequate hydration to replace ongoing fluid loss.
  2. Child exhibits signs of adequate hydration as evidenced by urine output of 1 to 2 ml/kg per hour.
  3. Child's fear and anxiety are reduced as evidenced by child verbalizing fears and asking questions.
  4. Child's pain is reduced to a tolerable level.
  5. Child and family verbalize understanding of preoperative teaching.

III. Client needs
A. Physiologic adaptation: Appendicitis is adequately diagnosed and surgical intervention (appendectomy) prevents perforation and peritonitis. Increased risk of infection from perforation is indicated by high fever and pain that immediately resolves but then becomes more diffuse.
B. Management of care: Care of the child with appendicitis requires critical thinking skills and knowledge of assessment, and teaching and evaluation methods unique to the RN role. These skills cannot be delegated to an LPN or UAP.
  1. Perform comprehensive physical assessments and provide care appropriate to the child with appendicitis.
  2. Delegate responsibly those activities that can be delegated, including measurements, oral intake and urine output, vital signs, and reporting child's subjective data. All monitoring information is reported to the RN.
C. Safety and infection control
  1. Preoperative interventions
    a. Position child in semi-Fowler or right side-lying position.
    b. Maintain NPO status.

c. Provide pain management including application of ice packs for 20 min/hr, if ordered.
d. Administer IV fluids, electrolytes, and antibiotics.
e. Monitor for signs and symptoms of dehydration.
f. Monitor for signs and symptoms of perforation.
2. Postoperative interventions
a. Continue pain management.
b. Resume diet when bowel sounds return.
c. Teach parents signs and symptoms of incisional infection.

D. Health promotion and maintenance
1. Encourage family to visit and participate in care.
2. Provide stimulation with age-appropriate toys and activities to enhance growth and development.

E. Psychologic integrity
1. Provide child and family opportunities to express fears, concerns, and to ask questions.
2. Allow transitional comfort object from home.

F. Basic care and comfort
1. Promote right side-lying or low to semi-Fowler position for preoperative comfort.
2. Provide preoperative and postoperative skin and mouth care.
3. Act as consistent nurse caregiver.

G. Reduction of risk potential
1. Promote early identification and differential diagnosis to prevent complications and reduce mortality.
2. Never apply heat to right lower abdomen; this increases risk of perforation.

H. Pharmacologic and parenteral therapies: IV fluids are used as needed to prevent dehydration. Antibiotics are used if there is peritonitis. Child and family will state the purpose for and associated side effects of all medications.

Pyloric Stenosis

I. Definition: Pyloric stenosis is the narrowing of the pyloric canal from hypertrophied muscles of the pylorus. The problem is identified in the first weeks of life because of continuous projective vomiting with feeding.

II. Nursing process
A. Assessment
1. Complete a detailed health history, including feeding history, vomiting, and failure to grow.
2. Perform a comprehensive physical assessment; assess for signs and symptoms of pyloric stenosis.
a. Mild regurgitation that progresses to projectile vomiting
b. Absence of bile in vomitus
c. Irritability and hunger after vomiting
d. Left to right visible peristaltic waves
e. Olive-shaped mass to the right of umbilicus
f. Dehydration, fluid and electrolyte imbalance, and metabolic alkalosis
3. Obtain diagnostic tests.
a. History and physical examination
b. Presence of olive-shaped mass
c. Abdominal ultrasound
d. Serum electrolytes

B. Analysis
1. Risk for Aspiration related to vomiting
2. Deficient Fluid Volume related to ongoing GI losses and vomiting
3. Fear related to separation from parents and strange environment
4. Imbalanced Nutrition: Less Than Body Requirements related to ongoing vomiting

C. Planning
1. Restore fluid volume and prevent dehydration.
2. Reduce fear.
3. Improve nutritional intake.
4. Prevent postoperative complications.

D. Implementation
1. Preoperative interventions
a. Monitor hydration, fluid and electrolyte balance, and rehydrate with IV fluids—administer IV sodium and potassium as indicated by laboratory findings.
b. Monitor weight, intake and output, and urine specific gravity.
c. Insert nasogastric tube for decompression.
d. Maintain NPO status.
2. Postoperative (pyloromyotomy) interventions
a. Maintain fluid and electrolyte balance.
b. Begin oral feedings in 4 to 6 hr with glucose or electrolyte solution.

E. Evaluation
1. Child exhibits signs of adequate hydration as evidenced by improved skin turgor and urine output.
2. Child exhibits diminished fear and improved comfort.
3. Child gains weight and begins to consume regular diet.
4. Child does not become dehydrated.

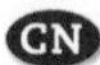

III. Client needs

A. Physiologic adaptation: Pyloric stenosis is managed with preoperative fluid and electrolyte maintenance and restoration and surgical intervention.
   1. Recognize risk for dehydration and metabolic alkalosis—indicated by percentage loss of body weight, irritability, poor skin turgor, prolonged capillary refill 2 s or more, tachycardia, absent tears, dry mucus membranes, elevated urine pH, and elevated plasma HCO_3.
   2. Recognize risk for hypokalemia—indicated by muscle weakness, hypotension, drowsiness, ECG: Flattened T waves, presence of U wave, serum potassium 3.5 mEq/L or more.

B. Management of care: Care of the child with pyloric stenosis requires critical thinking skills and knowledge of assessment, and teaching and evaluation methods unique to the RN role. These skills cannot be delegated to an LPN or UAP.
   1. Perform comprehensive physical assessments and provide care appropriate to the infant with a pyloric stenosis.
   2. Facilitate outpatient postoperative follow-up care.
   3. Delegate responsibly those activities that can be delegated, including measurements, oral intake and urine output, vital signs, and reporting child's subjective data. All monitoring information is reported to the RN.

C. Safety and infection control
   1. Preoperative interventions
      a. Maintain NPO status.
      b. If using oral feedings, position infant on right side to facilitate gastric emptying.
      c. Initiate decompression of stomach with nasogastric tube.
      d. Administer IV fluids.
      e. Position infant with head elevated 30 to 80 degrees using an infant seat or propped mattress.
   2. Postoperative interventions
      a. Inspect surgical incision.
      b. Assess for symptoms of dehydration because vomiting is not uncommon.
      c. Teach parents about home care needs for promoting nutrition and monitoring incision site for infection.
      d. After feeding, position the infant with the head and shoulders elevated 30 to 80 degrees and turned slightly to the right side; infant should remain in this position for 45 to 60 min after feeding.

D. Health promotion and maintenance
   1. Encourage family to visit and participate in care.
   2. Provide stimulation with age-appropriate toys and activities to enhance growth and development.

E. Psychologic integrity
   1. Explain pyloric stenosis to family, as well as management and home care to promote recovery and nutrition.
   2. Allow family the opportunity to express feelings, fears, concerns, and to ask questions.
   3. Touch, hold, and comfort the child to reduce stress.
   4. Provide parental reassurance that problem can be corrected.
   5. Encourage parents to visit and participate in care.

F. Basic care and comfort
   1. Provide consistent nurse caregiving.
   2. Provide skin and mouth care for dehydrated infants.

G. Reduction of risk potential
   1. Monitor ECG when hypokalemic.
   2. Ensure child has voided before administering IV potassium replacement.

H. Pharmacologic and parenteral therapies: IV fluids and electrolytes are used to maintain hydration and electrolyte balance.

Intussusception

I. Definition: Intussusception is the telescoping of one proximal portion of the bowel into a distal portion. The telescoping causes edema and pressure to increase, resulting in ischemia and leaking of blood and mucus into the intestine.

II. Nursing process

A. Assessment
   1. Complete a detailed health history, including history of pain and character of stool and vomiting.
   2. Perform a comprehensive physical assessment; assess for signs and symptoms of intestinal telescoping.
      a. Sudden crampy abdominal pain
      b. Periods without pain
      c. Palpable sausage-shaped mass in the abdomen
      d. Currant jelly stools
      e. Vomiting
   3. Obtain diagnostic tests: Barium enema after abdominal radiograph.

B. Analysis
 1. Deficient Fluid Volume related to pain and vomiting
 2. Fear related to separation from parents and strange environment
 3. Risk for Imbalanced Nutrition: Less Than Body Requirements related to vomiting and pain
 4. Acute Pain related to edema and telescoping of intestines

C. Planning
 1. Restore fluid volume and prevent dehydration.
 2. Reduce fear.
 3. Improve nutritional intake.
 4. Manage pain.

D. Implementation (see management of care)

E. Evaluation
 1. Child exhibits signs of adequate hydration as evidenced by improved skin turgor and urine output.
 2. Child exhibits diminished fear and improved comfort.
 3. Child begins to consume regular diet and gains weight.
 4. Child does not become dehydrated.
 5. Child's pain is reduced to a tolerable level.

CN

III. Client needs

A. Physiologic adaptation: Intussusception is managed with preoperative fluid and electrolyte maintenance, nonsurgical hydrostatic reduction using an air or barium enema, and possible surgery if hydrostatic reduction is not successful.
 1. Recognize risk for dehydration and metabolic acidosis—indicated by percentage loss of body weight, irritability, poor skin turgor, prolonged capillary refill 2 s or more, tachycardia, deep rapid respirations, absent tears, dry mucous membranes, plasma pH less than 7.33, and decreased plasma HCO_3.
 2. Recognize risk for hypokalemia—indicated by muscle weakness, hypotension, drowsiness, ECG: Flattened T waves, presence of U wave, serum potassium 3.5 mEq/L or more.

B. Management of care: Care of the infant with intussusception requires critical thinking skills and knowledge of assessment, and teaching and evaluation methods unique to the RN role. These skills cannot be delegated to an LPN or UAP.
 1. Perform comprehensive physical assessments and provide care appropriate to the infant with intussusception.
 2. Facilitate outpatient postoperative follow-up care.
 3. Delegate responsibly those activities that can be delegated, including measurements, oral intake and urine output, vital signs, and reporting child's subjective data. All monitoring information is reported to the RN.

C. Safety and infection control
 1. Examine all stools before any procedure or surgery—report any brown stool to physician; indicative of a reduction in intussusception.
 2. Monitor for signs and symptoms of dehydration, weight, intake and output.
 3. Prepare parents for nonsurgical procedures and their success at reducing the telescoping: Nonsurgical approaches involve administering an air or barium enema; success rate is 70% to 90%. A surgeon should be present during the administration of the enema as there is a risk of perforation.
 4. Prepare parents for surgical procedures.

D. Health promotion and maintenance
 1. Encourage family to visit and participate in care.
 2. Provide stimulation with age-appropriate toys and activities to enhance growth and development.

E. Psychologic integrity
 1. Maintain parent child attachment by encouraging parents to stay with infant.
 2. Offer parents the opportunity to express fears and concerns and answer all questions.
 3. Explain to family about the illness, management, and home care.
 4. Touch, hold, and comfort the child to reduce stress.

F. Basic care and comfort
 1. Provide consistent nurse caregiver.
 2. Allow parents at bedside.
 3. Position infant or child for comfort.

G. Reduction of risk potential: Instruct parents about risk of recurrence and high risk for death if treatment is not sought within 24 hr.

H. Pharmacologic and parenteral therapies: IV fluids may be administered to prevent dehydration.

Hirschsprung Disease

I. Definition: Hirschsprung disease (congenital aganglionic megacolon) is a congenital absence of the ganglion cells in the rectum and lower colon, which decreases the ability of the internal sphincter to relax, along with lack of peristalsis.

II. Nursing process

A. Assessment
 1. Complete a detailed health history, including history of chronic constipation.

2. Perform a comprehensive physical assessment; assess for signs and symptoms of abnormal peristalsis in infants.
   a. Abdominal distention
   b. Vomiting
   c. Failure to pass meconium within 48 hr of birth
3. Assess for signs and symptoms of abnormal peristalsis in older infants and children.
   a. Constipation with stools described as ribbonlike
   b. Vomiting
   c. Abdominal distention
   d. Failure to thrive
4. Obtain diagnostic tests.
   a. Barium enema
   b. Rectal biopsy
   c. Anorectal manometry

B. Analysis
1. Deficient Fluid Volume related to vomiting and abdominal distention
2. Fear related to separation from parents and strange environment
3. Imbalanced Nutrition: Less Than Body Requirements related to vomiting
4. Risk for Impaired Skin Integrity related to colostomy contents near skin
5. Interrupted Family Processes related to an infant with a congenital anomaly and frequent hospitalization

C. Planning
1. Restore fluid volume and prevent dehydration.
2. Reduce fear.
3. Improve nutritional intake.
4. Maintain skin integrity.
5. Provide child and family teaching.

D. Implementation
1. Promote fluid and electrolyte management.
2. Prepare child and parents for surgical intervention.

E. Evaluation
1. Child receives adequate hydration to replace ongoing fluid loss.
2. Child exhibits signs of adequate hydration as evidenced by urine output of 1 to 2 ml/kg per hour.
3. Child's fear and anxiety are reduced as evidenced by child verbalizing fears and asking questions.
4. Child maintains nutritional intake and continues to grow.
5. Child and family verbalize understanding of preoperative teaching.

CN

III. Client needs

A. Physiologic adaptation: Hirschsprung disease is managed with temporary colostomy and corrective surgery: Soave endorectal pull-through procedure.
1. Recognize risk for life-threatening complication of enterocolitis—indicated by severe diarrhea, fever, GI bleeding, and hypovolemia.
2. Recognize risk for dehydration and metabolic acidosis—indicated by percentage loss of body weight, irritability, poor skin turgor, prolonged capillary refill 2 s or more, tachycardia, deep rapid respirations, absent tears, dry mucous membranes, plasma pH less than 7.33, and decreased plasma HCO_3.
3. Recognize risk for hypokalemia—indicated by muscle weakness, hypotension, drowsiness, ECG: Flattened T waves, presence of U wave, serum potassium 3.5 mEq/L or more.

B. Management of care: Care of the infant/child with Hirschsprung disease requires critical thinking skills and knowledge of assessment, and teaching and evaluation methods unique to the RN role. These skills cannot be delegated to an LPN or UAP.
1. Perform comprehensive physical assessments and provide care appropriate to the infant/child with Hirschsprung disease.
2. Facilitate outpatient postoperative follow-up care.
3. Assist with preparation for home care, including colostomy equipment.
4. Delegate responsibly those activities that can be delegated, including measurements, oral intake and urine output, vital signs, and reporting child's subjective data. All monitoring information is reported to the RN.

C. Safety and infection control
1. Provide preoperative interventions.
   a. Provide bowel preparation, including antibiotics.
   b. Assess abdominal circumference.
   c. Maintain fluid and electrolyte status.
   d. Monitor vital signs for evidence of enterocolitis.
   e. Avoid taking rectal temperature.
   f. Provide age-appropriate teaching about surgery and colostomy.
   g. Prepare parents by teaching them about the diagnosis, management, and care of a colostomy.
2. Provide postoperative interventions.
   a. Initiate nasogastric decompression.
   b. Monitor fluid and electrolyte losses via nasogastric tube, intake and output, and stool from ostomy.
   c. Monitor ostomy.
      (1) Prevent urine contamination of ostomy.
      (2) Assess ostomy for bleeding or breakdown.

d. Assess abdomen for return of bowel sounds and correct functioning of the colostomy.
e. Assess fluid and electrolyte status.
f. Assess for pain.

D. Health promotion and maintenance
1. Promote self-care through child and family teaching about colostomy care.
2. Provide stimulation through touch and age-appropriate toys and activities.
3. Provide transitional comfort object.

E. Psychologic integrity
1. Assist parents in adjusting to congenital disorder.
2. Promote parent-child attachment.
3. Refer to enterostomal therapist for support and teaching needs.

F. Basic care and comfort
1. Manage postoperative discomfort.
2. Provide consistent nurse caregiver.
3. Provide skin care around colostomy.
4. Provide mouth care when NPO.

G. Reduction of risk potential
1. Avoid rectal thermometers or suppositories before or after surgical correction.
2. Monitor ECG when hypokalemic.
3. Ensure child has voided before administering IV potassium replacement.

H. Pharmacologic and parenteral therapies: IV fluids are used to prevent dehydration. Antibiotics are used to manage infection. Child and family will state the purpose for and associated side effects of all medications.

Bibliography

Hatfield, N. (2006). *Broadribb's introductory pediatric nursing.* Philadelphia: Lippincott Williams & Wilkins.

Pillitteri, A. (2006). *Maternal & child health nursing: Care of the childbearing and childrearing family* (5th ed.). Philadelphia: Lippincott Williams & Wilkins.

Wong, D. L., et al. (2006). *Maternal child nursing care.* St. Louis: Mosby.

CHAPTER 14

Practice Test

Diarrhea and Gastroenteritis

1. An infant who is 2 months of age is admitted to the emergency department with severe diarrhea. Before adding potassium to the IV fluids, the nurse documents on the chart that the infant:

□ 1. Has voided.
□ 2. Cries with tears.
□ 3. Has arm restraints applied.
□ 4. Has a temperature of 98.2°F.

2. AF Which of the following suggests that an infant with diarrhea is dehydrated? Select all that apply.

□ 1. Tacky mucous membranes.
□ 2. Sunken fontanelles.
□ 3. Salty saliva.
□ 4. Restlessness.
□ 5. Increased urine output.

3. Which of the following statements by a parent of an infant with diarrhea indicates that the parents understand the correct action for treating diarrhea in their infant?

□ 1. "I should restrict foods and fluids as long as my child has loose stools."
□ 2. "I could give Kaopectate as long as I follow the directions on the bottle."
□ 3. "I should offer milk after each episode of diarrhea."
□ 4. "I should take the baby's temperature and call our doctor."

4. AF A child who is 3 years of age has been admitted with diarrhea. He has mild dehydration (less than 5%). The nurse is reviewing the laboratory report of the stool specimen, below. Based on the review of the laboratory report from the stool specimen, the nurse should do which of the following first?

LABORATORY RESULTS

Test	Result
WBC	Mildly elevated
RBC	Few
Bacteria	Positive for *E. coli*
Ova and Parasites	Negative

☐ 1. Start an IV infusion.
☐ 2. Institute enteric precautions.
☐ 3. Instruct the family to wash all family bed linens in hot water.
☐ 4. Cleanse and protect the anal area.

Vomiting

5. The nurse is planning postoperative care for an infant who had surgical correction for pyloric stenosis. The infant has been vomiting for 24 hr after surgery. The nurse should first:
☐ 1. Continue IV fluids, recording intake and output.
☐ 2. Notify the surgeon because this much vomiting is a potential emergency.
☐ 3. Place the infant in a prone position to prevent aspiration.
☐ 4. Add infant cereal to the feedings to decrease the emesis.

Cleft Lip and Cleft Palate

6. An infant is hospitalized for repair of a cleft lip and palate. The priority nursing goal of care for this client prior to surgery is to prevent:
☐ 1. Pneumonia.
☐ 2. Oral infection.
☐ 3. Dehydration.
☐ 4. Muscle atrophy.

7. An infant is hospitalized following surgical repair of a cleft lip. The primary goal of nursing care during the first postoperative days is to:
☐ 1. Protect the infant's tongue from swelling.
☐ 2. Prevent the infant from vomiting.
☐ 3. Prevent crust formation on the suture line.
☐ 4. Keep the infant in a prone position.

8. A child who is 18 months of age has had a cleft palate repair. The nurse is instructing the mother about feeding the child a liquid diet. Which statement by the mother indicates that she understands how to feed her child?
☐ 1. "I will teach him to use a straw so that drinking is fun."
☐ 2. "I will feed him small sips at a time from a spoon."
☐ 3. "I will offer him small glasses of fluid at a time."
☐ 4. "I will give him large glasses of fluid so that he drinks more."

9. AF The nurse is providing care for an infant who had a surgical repair of a cleft palate. Which of the following nursing actions is appropriate in the immediate postoperative period? Select all that apply.
☐ 1. Place the infant in a prone position.
☐ 2. Use spoons and straws for liquids.
☐ 3. Apply elbow restraints.
☐ 4. Use tongue depressors to visualize the palate.
☐ 5. Have the child drink from spill-proof sippy cups.
☐ 6. Offer a diet of toast and peanut butter.
☐ 7. Administer opioids to relieve pain.

10. AF The nurse is discussing the care plan with the parents of a child who is 3 years of age who is being discharged following cleft palate surgery. The nurse should instruct the parents to report which of the following to an HCP? Select all that apply.
☐ 1. Otitis media.
☐ 2. Lack of weight gain.
☐ 3. Hyperactivity.
☐ 4. Speech delays.
☐ 5. Fighting with siblings.

Esophageal Atresia and Tracheoesophageal Fistula

11. A neonate is born with a TEF. The nurse should instruct the parents to place the infant in which of the following positions?
☐ 1. Prone, allowing oral secretions to drain from the mouth.
☐ 2. Side-lying, relieving respiratory distress.
☐ 3. Supine, with head of bed at a 30 degree incline, minimizing reflux.
☐ 4. Supine, with bed flat, to decrease intracranial pressure.

12. AF The nurse is caring for an infant with EA and TEF. Which of the following nursing actions is appropriate in the plan of care for this infant? Select all that apply.
☐ 1. Stop oral feedings.
☐ 2. Feed small, frequent amounts.
☐ 3. Place in supine position with head of bed elevated.
☐ 4. Start on IV fluids.
☐ 5. Administer prescribed broad-spectrum antibiotics.
☐ 6. Thicken formula with rice.
☐ 7. Suction mouth frequently.

13. A newborn is suspected of having a TEF. Which of the following is the safest way to detect this fistula in a newborn?
☐ 1. Offer a diluted commercial formula and observe for choking.
☐ 2. Assess the infant for gag and swallowing reflexes.
☐ 3. Offer the infant a pacifier after feeding.

□ 4. Pass a nasogastric catheter and aspirate stomach contents.

Appendicitis

14. The nurse is assessing an adolescent who is admitted to the hospital with appendicitis. The nurse should report which of the following to the HCP?
- □ 1. Change of pain rating of 7 to 8 on a 10-point pain scale.
- □ 2. Sudden relief of sharp pain, shifting to diffuse pain.
- □ 3. Shallow breathing with normal vital signs.
- □ 4. Decrease of pain rating from 8 to 6 when parents visit.

15. A school-aged child has an emergency appendectomy. The nurse should report which of the following to the HCP if noted in the immediate postoperative period?
- □ 1. Abdominal pain.
- □ 2. "Tugging" at the incision line.
- □ 3. Thirst.
- □ 4. A rigid abdomen.

Pyloric Stenosis

16. Following surgery for pyloric stenosis, the nurse instructs the parents that when feeding the infant they should burp the child following feedings to prevent:
- □ 1. Pressure on the incision line.
- □ 2. Abdominal discomfort.
- □ 3. Flatulence.
- □ 4. Intestinal obstruction.

17. Which of the following suggests that a child's postoperative feeding schedule following pyloric stenosis surgery should be slowed?
- □ 1. Flatulence.
- □ 2. Vomiting.
- □ 3. Semiformed bowel movements.
- □ 4. The infant falls asleep at each feeding.

Intussusception

18. The nurse is planning care for a child hospitalized for diagnosis of an intussusception. The nurse should report which of the following information to the surgeon?
- □ 1. Passage of a normal brown stool.
- □ 2. Anorexia and weight loss.
- □ 3. Abdominal pain and vomiting.
- □ 4. Passage of a currant jelly stool.

Hirschsprung Disease

19. The nurse is assessing a child who is 10 years of age and is admitted for diagnosis of congenital aganglionic megacolon (Hirschsprung disease). What type of stool is characteristic for a school-aged child who is suspected of having Hirschsprung disease?
- □ 1. Explosive, watery diarrhea.
- □ 2. Currant jelly stools.
- □ 3. Ribbonlike, foul-smelling stools.
- □ 4. Frothy, floating, foul-smelling stools.

20. AF The nurse is inserting a nasogastric tube into an infant who is having surgery to repair a congenital aganglionic megacolon. Identify the correct placement of the nasogastric tube with an "X".

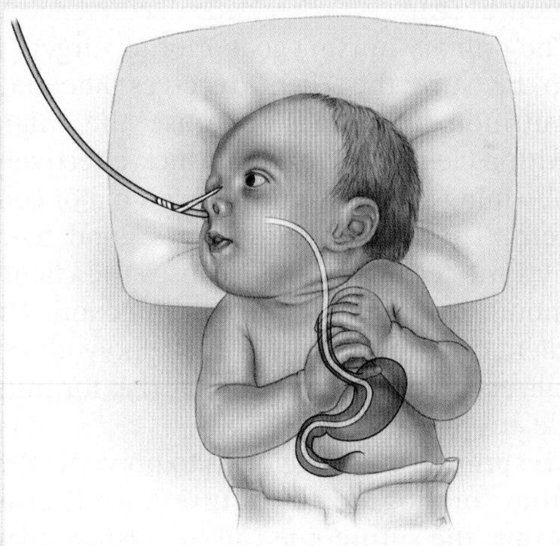

Answers and Rationales

1. 1 With severe diarrhea, kidney function may fail. The nurse documents that kidney function is intact before adding potassium to prevent hyperkalemia. Voiding indicates appropriate renal function. Presence of tears is indicative of improvement in dehydration, but is less critical than voiding. Restraints are not necessary. A temperature of 98.2°F is normal. (A)

2. 1, 2, 4 Diarrhea in infants is a serious condition as it can proceed rapidly to dehydration. Clinical signs of dehydration are irritability and restlessness, weakness, stupor, loss of body weight, poor skin turgor, and sunken fontanelles. The urine output is decreased in dehydrated infants. The saliva decreases with dehydration and is not salty. (A)

3. 4 Diarrhea is potentially dangerous in infants because it can rapidly lead to dehydration and death. The parents should understand early signs of dehydration such as a low-grade fever (100°F) and to report the findings to their HCP. The parents should offer oral rehydration solutions to prevent dehydration. Kaopectate does not treat the underlying cause of the diarrhea; milk is not added to the diet until the child can tolerate clear liquids. (A)

4. 2 The stool specimen indicates the client has *E. coli* in his stool. The nurse institutes enteric precautions, and ensures those who come in contact with the child perform good hand hygiene and wear a gown to prevent spread of infection. Restoring fluid balance is a goal of therapy, but because the dehydration is mild, oral rehydration is the first choice for replacing fluids. The nurse also cleanses and protects the anal area from irritation from the diarrhea, but on an ongoing basis and not as the priority for care. It is not necessary for the family to wash all of their bed linens, as only those in contact with the client are contaminated. (S)

5. 1 Postoperative vomiting may occur and most infants, even with successful surgery, exhibit some vomiting during the first 24 to 48 hr. IV fluids are administered until the infant can retain adequate amounts by mouth. (A)

6. 3 The primary nursing goal prior to surgery is to be sure the client receives adequate nutrition and fluids. Because the infant with a cleft lip is unable to suck effectively, obtaining adequate nutrition is a major concern. The nurse also observes good hand hygiene technique and cleanses the client's mouth frequently to prevent infection. The client can move freely, even if elbow immobilizers are used, and is not at risk for muscle atrophy. (S)

7. 3 The primary nursing goal is to prevent crust from forming on the suture line. If crust forms, the suture line can be pushed apart and a large scar could result. The nurse should not place the infant in a prone position to avoid pressure on the suture line. Swelling of the tongue is not common. If the infant vomits, the nurse prevents aspiration and consults with the HCP about use of antiemetic drugs. (R)

8. 3 Toddlers generally do better with small rather than large amounts of fluids. Using a straw or spoon could injure the suture line. The nurse can continue to offer positive reinforcement to the mother. (C)

9. 1, 3, 7 After a palatoplasty, the child is allowed to lie on the abdomen as the risk for disturbing the incision line (inside the mouth) is low. Elbow restraints are applied for an infant who is 4 to 6 weeks of age. Opioids are administered initially for pain, and acetaminophen may be given as needed thereafter. Avoid the use of suction or other objects in the mouth, such as tongue depressors, thermometers, spoons, or straws. Hard food items are avoided because they can damage the repaired palate (toast, hard cookies, potato chips, and pretzels). (S)

10. 1, 2, 4 Surgery for cleft palate changes the slant of the eustachian tube, allowing bacteria from the posterior throat to enter the middle ear easily, which may cause the child to experience frequent bouts with otitis media. The child should be able to eat, so weight loss is a concern. Speech delays also follow cleft palate repair; therefore, parents are taught to observe speech patterns and report differences for early identification and treatment. Fighting among siblings is typical and, unless unusual or persistent, does not need to be reported to the HCP. (H)

11. 3 When a newborn has a TEF, the most desirable position is supine with the head elevated on an inclined plane of at least 30 degrees. This position minimizes the reflux of gastric secretions up the distal esophagus into the trachea and bronchi. The other positions do not minimize gastric reflux. (A)

12. 1, 3, 5, 7 When infants have EA/TEF, the nurse maintains NPO status and initiates IV fluids. The nurse places the infant in a supine position with the head of the bed elevated at least 30 degrees and removes secretions from the mouth and upper pouch with frequent suctioning. Because aspiration pneumonia is almost inevitable and appears early, broad-spectrum antibiotics are often started. The nurse avoids feeding the infant any solid foods and thickening of formula with rice. (S)

13. 4 If a nasogastric tube will not pass to the stomach, it is likely that there is an obstruction in the esophagus. Offering formula is not safe. The presence of the ability of the infant to suck, gag, or swallow does not confirm the presence of the fistula. (A)

14. 2 The nurse notifies the HCP if the client has sudden relief of sharp pain and on presence of more diffuse pain. This change in the pain indicates the appendix has ruptured. The diffuse pain is typically accompanied by rigid guarding of the abdomen, progressive abdominal distention, tachycardia, pallor, chills, and irritability. The slight increase in pain can be expected; the decrease in pain when parents visit may be attributed to being distracted from the pain. Shallow breathing is likely due to the pain and is insignificant when the other vital signs are normal. (S)

15. 4 The nurse notifies the HCP about presence of a tense, rigid abdomen because it is an early symptom of peritonitis. The other findings are expected in the immediate postoperative period. (A)

16. 1 Burping an infant prevents pressure in the stomach from air that was swallowed during the feeding. Burping may minimize abdominal discomfort and flatulence, but the primary reason is to prevent pressure on the incision line. Burping does not prevent intestinal obstruction. (A)

17. 2 Vomiting after a feeding suggests the pyloric valve is not yet able to accommodate feedings well, possibly from edema. Return of bowel activity after surgery may result in passing of flatus, and is normal. Semiformed bowel movements are normal after feedings are resumed. The infant falling asleep at feedings may be because of drowsiness secondary to analgesia or anesthesia. (A)

18. 1 Passage of a normal brown stool usually indicates that the intussusception has reduced itself. The nurse reports this finding to the surgeon, who may choose to alter the plan of care (surgery/diagnostic procedures). The classic signs of intussusception are colicky abdominal pain with vomiting and currant jelly stools. A more chronic picture is characterized by diarrhea, anorexia, weight loss, occasional vomiting, and periodic pain. (A)

19. 3 An older child with Hirschsprung disease will experience ribbonlike, foul-smelling stools as a result of aganglionic portion of the colon. Explosive watery stools may be indicative of gastroenteritis; current jelly stools are seen in clients with intussusception; frothy, foul-smelling stools may indicate malabsorption. (A)

20. The nasogastric tube is placed in the infant's stomach. (S)

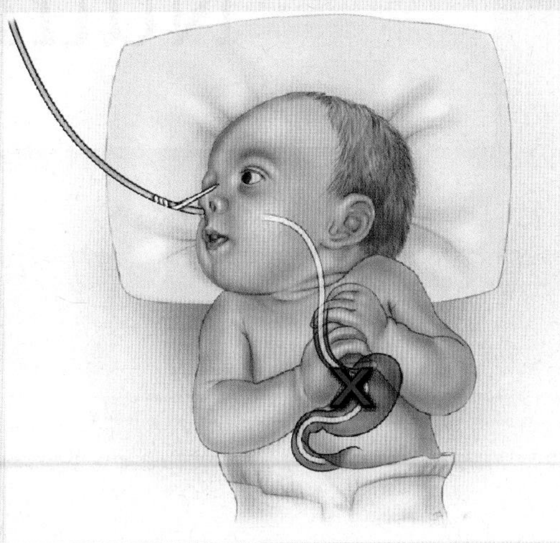

chapter 15

The Child With Health Problems Involving Ingestion, Nutrition, or Diet

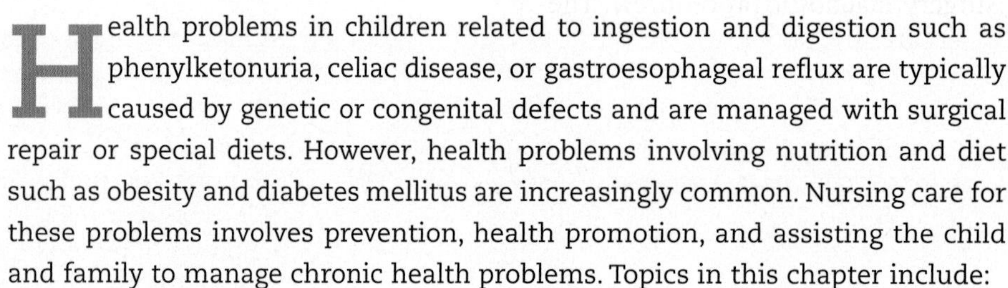

Health problems in children related to ingestion and digestion such as phenylketonuria, celiac disease, or gastroesophageal reflux are typically caused by genetic or congenital defects and are managed with surgical repair or special diets. However, health problems involving nutrition and diet such as obesity and diabetes mellitus are increasingly common. Nursing care for these problems involves prevention, health promotion, and assisting the child and family to manage chronic health problems. Topics in this chapter include:

- Phenylketonuria
- Failure to Thrive
- Obesity
- Gastroesophageal Reflux
- Celiac Disease
- Diabetes Mellitus

Phenylketonuria

I. Definition: Inborn errors of metabolism include a large number of inherited disorders characterized by a lack of an enzyme necessary for metabolism. They are primarily problems with fat, protein, or carbohydrate metabolism. Phenylketonuria (PKU) is an inborn error of metabolism characterized by a lack of the enzyme necessary for the metabolism of phenylalanine.

A. Phenylalanine is found in all natural food proteins.

B. Phenylalanine cannot convert to tyrosine. Excess phenylalanine leads to defective myelinization and ultimately to mental retardation and other neurologic sequelae.

II. Nursing process

A. Assessment

1. Complete a detailed health history, including history of allergies, and whether newborn has been screened at birth for PKU.
2. Complete a detailed history of growth and development and a physical examination including baseline vital signs, height, and weight.
3. Assess child and family for their knowledge base about the rationale for PKU test, understanding of preparation, and possible lifestyle modifications based on test results.
4. Assess for signs and symptoms of PKU.
   a. Infant: Failure to thrive, vomiting, irritability, and possible hyperactive behaviors
   b. Older child: Bizarre, psychiatric behaviors including head banging, screaming, inappropriate or lack of response to stimuli, and seizures
5. Obtain diagnostic tests.
   a. Newborn screening—Guthrie blood test: Fresh heel blood (not cord blood) is used for accurate results
   b. Electroencephalograph (EEG) for infant and older child

B. Analysis

1. Delayed Growth and Development related to inadequate protein intake
2. Imbalanced Nutrition: Less Than Body Requirements related to strict restrictions in protein intake
3. Deficient Parental Knowledge: Disease and treatment, related to complexity of dietary management

C. Planning

1. Develop dietary plan that restricts phenylalanine but includes protein nutrition for growth.
2. Prevent intellectual, physical, and neurologic complications.
3. Provide child and family teaching about the disease, dietary restrictions, and frequent monitoring.
4. Promote early self-care behaviors such as dietary calculation of phenylalanine.

D. Implementation

1. Promote dietary restriction of protein.
2. Provide medium chain triglycerides (MCT) and glucose polymers (Polycose).
3. Promote possible breast-feeding with monitoring.

E. Evaluation

1. Child exhibits tolerance to low-phenylalanine formula.
2. Parents verbalize understanding of dietary management and can identify appropriate foods to allow.
3. Child's phenylalanine levels are in safe range, 2 to 8 mg/dl.

CN

III. Client needs

A. Physiologic adaptation: Phenylalanine levels are controlled through rigorous dietary restriction of protein and monitoring of phenylalanine and tyrosine levels. The following are assessed:

1. Tolerance of diet restrictions
2. Alterations in intellectual, physical, or neurologic status

B. Management of care: Care of the child with phenylketonuria requires critical thinking skills and knowledge of assessment, and teaching and evaluation methods unique to the RN role. These skills cannot be delegated to an LPN or UAP.

1. Perform comprehensive physical assessments and provide care appropriate to the child with phenylketonuria.
2. Assess for home health needs such as availability of gram scale to prepare formula.
3. Evaluate community resources for family support such as specialty food stores, availability of a PKU express pack for parents, and local PKU support groups.
4. Delegate responsibly those activities that can be delegated, including measurements, oral intake and urine output, vital signs, and reporting child's subjective data. All monitoring information is reported to the RN.

C. Safety and infection control

1. Perform Guthrie blood test after a source of protein is ingested; repeat if positive.
2. Restrict dietary protein to maintain phenylalanine levels in safe range.
   a. Provide milk substitutes for infants—Lofenalac formula.

b. Avoid highest sources of phenylalanine—aspartame, milk, eggs, and meat.
3. Monitor intellectual and neurologic development.
4. Teach family about the disease, dietary management, reading food labels, and frequent monitoring. Provide food sources low in phenylalanine, such as orange juice, bananas, lettuce, and potatoes.

D. Health promotion and maintenance: Encourage participation in self-management as early as preschool age.

E. Psychologic integrity
1. Offer family support and opportunity to ask questions.
2. Provide older child with opportunity to verbalize feelings and issues related to strict dietary control.
3. Encourage special camps for adolescents.
4. Encourage support groups for parents.

F. Basic care and comfort
1. Encourage and answer all questions at child's cognitive level.
2. Provide consistent nurse caregiver if child is hospitalized.
3. Allow parents to stay at bedside.
4. Provide age-appropriate activities to stimulate developmental and cognitive level.

G. Reduction of risk potential
1. Provide health care practitioner follow-up because of early discharge.
2. Provide screening for infants discharged early or born at home.
3. Reduce and maintain phenylalanine at safe levels—protein amounts calculated daily based on:
a. Phenylalanine and tyrosine levels
b. Growth needs and spurts
4. Instruct family and child about the need to maintain low-phenylalanine diet for life.
5. Encourage genetic counseling and prenatal testing of pregnant adolescents with PKU.

H. Pharmacologic and parenteral therapies: Rarely used because health problem is managed by dietary control.

Failure to Thrive

I. Definition: Failure to thrive is the inability to obtain or use calories and results in lack of growth. Consistently falling below the fifth percentile for age alerts health care practitioners.

A. Organic failure to thrive has a pathophysiologic basis. There can be a variety of underlying causes, including genetic abnormalities, loss of nutrients through malabsorption, endocrine disorders, chronic urinary tract infections, or congenital heart disease.

B. Nonorganic failure to thrive (which accounts for 50% of failure to thrive) is an outcome of varied psychosocial factors such as difficult parent-child interactions, psychologic deprivation, and economic conditions of the family.

II. Nursing process

A. Assessment
1. Assess for risk factors for the development of failure to thrive.
a. Physical causes such as congenital heart disease
b. Altered parent-child interaction such as neglect
c. Health beliefs such as prolonged diet of formula
d. Finances
e. Insufficient production of breast milk
f. Lack of parental knowledge about feeding and nutritional needs
g. Feeding resistance (may develop with high-risk infants)
2. Assess for characteristic findings.
a. Infant factors: Difficult temperament, avoids physical contact, avoids face-to-face contact
b. Parental factors: Lack of parenting knowledge, teen parent with poor support system
3. Complete a comprehensive physical assessment including baseline vital signs, height, weight, allergies, and patterns of weight gain.
4. Obtain a detailed health history including dietary patterns, cultural beliefs, and developmental and family assessment—includes history of difficult feeding, lack of stimulation, family stressors, and vomiting after eating.
5. Obtain diagnostic tests: Condition based on failure to grow; tests rule out organic from nonorganic cause.

B. Analysis
1. Risk for Impaired Parent/Infant Attachment related to inability to meet emotional or physical needs
2. Delayed Growth and Development related to inadequate intake of calories
3. Imbalanced Nutrition: Less Than Body Requirements related to impaired dyad relationship
4. Deficient Knowledge: Infant Feeding, Bonding, or Developmental Needs, related to stress, psychosocial issues, or cognitive impairment
5. Risk for Impaired Parenting related to parental age, lack of support, insufficient knowledge of needs

C. Planning
   1. Promote growth and development.
   2. Identify parental factors contributing to failure to thrive.
   3. Assist parents in identifying risk factors related to attachment.
   4. Provide child and family teaching.

D. Implementation
   1. Reverse malnutrition; provide infant with sufficient calories for growth.
      a. Correct nutritional deficiencies
      b. Treat underlying physical problems
      c. Modify feeding-resistance issues
   2. Provide family support and teaching about nutritional needs, feeding methods and times, and specific food preparation.
   3. Provide child and family teaching about normal developmental expectations and parenting skills.

E. Evaluation
   1. Child receives enough calories to promote growth.
   2. Parents develop positive coping strategies and improved parenting skills.
   3. Parents identify methods to promote nutrition for child.

CN

III. Client needs
   A. Physiologic adaptation: Failure to thrive is resolved through a multidisciplinary approach including health care practitioners, nutritional specialists, and mental health professionals. Evaluate the effectiveness of parent education through home care visits and follow-up to ensure continued growth and development.
   B. Management of care: Care of the child with failure to thrive requires critical thinking skills and knowledge of assessment, and teaching and evaluation methods unique to the RN role. These skills cannot be delegated to an LPN or UAP.
      1. Perform comprehensive physical assessments and provide care appropriate to the infant/child with failure to thrive.
      2. Assess for home health needs such as home health nursing visits.
      3. Evaluate community resources for family support such as education programs for parents, infant stimulation programs, and availability of local pediatricians for follow-up.
      4. Delegate responsibly those activities that can be delegated, including measurements, oral intake and urine output, vital signs, and reporting child's subjective data. All monitoring information is reported to the RN.
   C. Safety and infection control
      1. Measure initial weight and then monitor daily weights.
      2. Assess food intake—use feeding checklist.
      3. Observe parent interaction, including feeding behavior.
   D. Health promotion and maintenance
      1. Plan program of play to stimulate child and promote growth and development.
      2. Optimize plan of care through tailored interventions based on an individualized child and family assessments of teaching needs.
   E. Psychologic integrity
      1. Provide a positive feeding environment for the parent and child.
      2. Provide opportunities for parents to express concerns, fears, anxieties, or to ask questions.
      3. Use behavior modification to diminish food aversion and promote positive feeding patterns.
      4. Promote parental self-esteem through teaching about positive parenting strategies.
   F. Basic care and comfort
      1. Encourage and answer all questions at child's cognitive level.
      2. Provide consistent nurse caregiver.
      3. Allow parents to stay at bedside.
      4. Provide age-appropriate activities to stimulate developmental and cognitive level.
   G. Reduction of risk potential: Avoid sweets and juices.
   H. Pharmacologic and parenteral therapies: Used as needed to maintain adequate fluid and nutrition. Child and family will state the purpose for and associated side effects of all medications.

Obesity

I. Definition: Obesity is a result of consistent caloric intake beyond the body's needs and expenditures. For children 6 to 11 years of age, obesity is defined by the sex- and age-specific 95th percentile cutoff points of the revised NCHS/CDC growth charts.

II. Nursing process
   A. Assessment
      1. Assess child for nonmodifiable risk factors, including genetics, and disease state such as hypothyroidism.
      2. Assess child for modifiable risk factors, such as diet, physical activity, and stressors.
      3. Obtain a detailed health history, including family history of obesity, type 2 diabetes, and/or cardiovascular risk factors, as well as history of type and amount of physical activity.

4. Complete a comprehensive physical assessment, including baseline vital signs, height, and weight—measure and plot height, weight, and body mass index (BMI) on growth charts.
5. Perform a nutritional assessment to determine dietary practices, 3-day diet history, types and quantity of foods consumed, preparation techniques, and cultural food preferences. Evaluate the importance of food to identify use as a coping mechanism.
6. Obtain diagnostic tests: Based on body mass index and body weight; other tests for endocrine or other diseases may be used to rule out physiologic cause or identify comorbidities.

B. Analysis
1. Risk for Disturbed Body Image related to excess weight
2. Deficient Knowledge: Diet, Exercise, and Weight Loss Techniques related to emotional state or unfamiliarity with methods to control weight
3. Imbalanced Nutrition: More Than Body Requirements related to poor dietary habits, lack of knowledge of weight control, use of food as coping mechanism

C. Planning
1. Reduce weight.
2. Improve activity tolerance.
3. Prevent complications of obesity.
4. Assist child and family in identifying risk factors for obesity.
5. Promote health behavior modification of risk factors, improved healthy lifestyle, and coping mechanisms.

D. Implementation: Provide interventions to manage obesity.
1. Encourage diet.
2. Promote physical activity.
3. Promote behavior modification.
4. Encourage support programs.

E. Evaluation
1. Child verbalizes methods to achieve weight reduction or maintain current weight during growth.
2. Child and family verbalize understanding of dietary changes, exercise options, and consequences of obesity.
3. Child attains optimum weight.

CN

III. Client needs

A. Physiologic adaptation: Obesity is reduced with traditional techniques of diet and physical activity on an outpatient basis.

B. Management of care: Care of the child with obesity requires critical thinking skills and knowledge of assessment, and teaching and evaluation methods unique to the RN role. These skills cannot be delegated to an LPN or UAP.
1. Perform comprehensive physical assessments and provide care appropriate to the infant/child with obesity.
2. Assess for home health needs including the ability to purchase and prepare nutritious and low-calorie foods and opportunity to increase physical activity.
3. Evaluate community resources for family support such as local weight-loss program and public parks with bike or walking trails.
4. Delegate responsibly those activities that can be delegated, including measurements, oral intake and urine output, vital signs, and reporting child's subjective data. All monitoring information is reported to the RN.

C. Safety and infection control: Provide child and family teaching.
1. Maintain nutrition appropriate to growth and developmental needs.
2. Read nutrition labels.
3. Plan meals that include all four food groups.
4. Observe for problems related to comorbidities (e.g., sleep apnea).

D. Health promotion and maintenance
1. Assist child and family in identifying risk factors for complications of obesity, such as hypercholesterolemia, and provide teaching to promote healthy behaviors.
2. Teach child self-management such as assisting with meal planning and preparation.
3. Teach child and family about need for increasing age-appropriate physical activity.

E. Psychologic integrity
1. Encourage child to verbalize feelings about being overweight.
2. Assist child in realistic goal setting.
3. Support and acknowledge difficulty in altering lifestyle.
4. Refer to commercial weight-loss program.
5. Encourage family intervention to promote family change.

F. Basic care and comfort
1. Promote skin care, especially in warm weather.
2. Provide age-appropriate toys and activities to stimulate growth and development.

G. Reduction of risk potential: In addition to early identification of children at risk for obesity, prevent obesity through early childhood education about healthy eating habits and regular exercise programs.

H. Pharmacologic and parenteral therapies: Used as needed to treat related health problems such as diabetes. Child and family will state the purpose for and associated side effects of all medications.

Gastroesophageal Reflux

I. Definition: Gastroesophageal reflux (GER) is the return of gastric contents into the esophagus as a result of a poorly functioning lower esophageal or cardiac sphincter. Complications such as aspiration, pneumonia, and esophagitis indicate that the child has developed gastroesophageal reflux disease with associated tissue damage.

II. Nursing process

A. Assessment
1. Assess risk for developing GER.
   a. Premature infants
   b. Presence of asthma, cystic fibrosis, or cerebral palsy
   c. Presence of long-term nasogastric intubation
2. Assess for signs and symptoms of reflux.
   a. Passive regurgitation
   b. Esophagitis with bleeding noted in stool or emesis
   c. Poor weight gain
   d. Obstructive apnea in infants
   e. Heartburn in older children
   f. Anemia
3. Obtain a detailed history, including history of vomiting, irritability, or refusal to eat.
4. Perform a comprehensive physical assessment including baseline vital signs, height, and weight.
5. Obtain diagnostic tests.
   a. Stool for guaiac
   b. Barium swallow
   c. Upper GI series
   d. Esophageal pH monitoring
   e. Endoscopy with biopsy

B. Analysis
1. Risk for Aspiration related to frequent vomiting
2. Delayed Growth and Development related to refusal to eat, vomiting, and pain
3. Risk for Injury related to reflux of gastric acid into esophagus
4. Risk for Acute Pain related to tissue erosion of esophagus

C. Planning
1. Maintain growth and development.
2. Reduce esophageal irritation.
3. Provide parental teaching for home care about positioning, diet, and medications.
4. Assist parents in identifying risk factors that precipitate reflux.

D. Implementation
1. Promote positioning.
   a. Infants younger than 1 year of age are positioned prone while awake and supine when sleeping.
   b. Children older than 1 year of age are positioned with the head of the bed elevated and the child turned to the left side, particularly after eating.
2. Promote diet modification (see safety and infection control).
3. Promote medication regimen (see pharmacologic and parenteral therapies).
4. Provide interventions for surgery for severe complications.

E. Evaluation
1. Child's symptoms of reflux are reduced as evidenced by improved growth and development.
2. Parents are compliant with therapeutic regimen.
3. Parents identify risk factors for reflux and methods to reduce them.
4. Child follows prescribed low-fat, low-acidic diet.

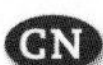

III. Client needs

A. Physiologic adaptation: GER is controlled with diet and medication administration on an outpatient basis.
1. Evaluate the effectiveness of prokinetic agents, proton pump inhibitors, and H_2 blockers in the management of reflux, reduction of pain, and promotion of growth.
2. Recognize risk for decrease in tissue perfusion from dehydration—indicated by sunken fontanels, dry mucous membranes, absence of tears, poor skin turgor, and urine output of less than 1 to 2 ml/kg per hour.

B. Management of care: Care of the child with gastroesophageal reflux requires critical thinking skills and knowledge of assessment, and teaching and evaluation methods unique to the RN role. These skills cannot be delegated to an LPN or UAP.
1. Perform comprehensive physical assessments and provide care appropriate to the infant/child with gastroesophageal reflux.
2. Assess for home health needs and facilitate follow-up care such as appropriate equipment, including infant seat for placement after feeding.
3. Evaluate community resources for family support such as GER support groups,

availability of local pediatricians for follow-up, and sources for alternative formulas.
4. Delegate responsibly those activities that can be delegated, including measurements, oral intake and urine output, vital signs, and reporting child's subjective data. All monitoring information is reported to the RN.

C. Safety and infection control
1. Provide parental teaching about GER, its causes, signs and symptoms, and risk to safety.
2. Manage diet and feeding to prevent complications.
   a. Monitor emesis for causative factors, amount, character, presence of blood.
   b. Determine the relationship of vomiting to feeding and activity.
   c. Monitor for signs and symptoms of dehydration.
   d. Keep suction equipment at bedside.
3. Teach parents about diet, and foods to avoid feeding child such as foods high in fat and acidity, and those that are spicy, caffeinated, and carbonated.
4. Teach methods to reduce reflux by positioning the infant after feeding (see implementation).

D. Health promotion and maintenance
1. Provide age-appropriate toys and activities to stimulate growth and development.
2. Provide parent teaching about developmental expectations.

E. Psychologic integrity
1. Reassure parents about prone position for children under 1 year while they are awake and its safety. The risk of SIDS must be considered and the child should sleep in the supine position.
2. Allow parents opportunity to ask questions.
3. Provide appropriate level of teaching to child and family to meet developmental, cognitive, and emotional needs.

F. Basic care and comfort
1. Provide small, frequent feedings; thickened with cereal.
2. Enlarge nipple.
3. Promote frequent burping during feeding.
4. Promote appropriate positioning after feeding.
5. Administer acetaminophen (Tylenol) for pain.

G. Reduction of risk potential: Provide correct positioning depending on age of child (see implementation).

H. Pharmacologic and parenteral therapies: Child and family will state the purpose, dosage, timing, and side effects of medications used to treat GER (Table 15-1).

Celiac Disease

I. Definition: Celiac disease is a dietary intolerance to gluten, which is the main protein component in barley, rye, oats, and wheat (BROW). The intolerance

Table 15-1 Medications Used to Treat GER

Classification	Generic/Trade Name	Expected Outcome	Reduction of Risk Potential	Management of Care
Histamine receptor antagonists	Ranitidine (Zantac)	Provides symptomatic treatment of reflux.	Monitor serum creatinine.	Teach parents that additional antacids can be given 2 hr before or after medication. Administer medication before feeding.
Proton pump inhibitors	Omeprazole (Prilosec)	Treats esophagitis.	Monitor urinalysis and liver function tests. Observe for nausea, vomiting, and abdominal pain.	Teach parents to give before food. Teach parents to observe for severe diarrhea.
Prokinetic agents	Metoclopramide (Reglan)	Provides symptomatic treatment of reflux.	Verify correct concentration and infusion rate (multiple infusion line incompatibilities). Observe for extrapyramidal symptoms. Monitor electrolyte levels.	Teach parents to report symptoms of facial grimacing and trembling hands.

to gluten leads to an accumulation of glutamine, causing intestinal villi to atrophy.

II. Nursing process

A. Assessment

1. Assess for signs and symptoms of gluten intolerance when solid foods are introduced into diet.
   a. Watery diarrhea along with steatorrhea
   b. Anorexia and vomiting
   c. Abdominal pain and distention
   d. Failure to thrive
2. Obtain a detailed history, including history of diarrhea, irritability, or refusal to eat.
3. Perform a comprehensive physical assessment including baseline vital signs, height, and weight.
4. Obtain diagnostic tests: In addition to assessing for full remission of symptoms when gluten removed from diet, diagnostic tests include monitoring IgG and IgA antibodies (disappear when gluten is removed from diet).

B. Analysis

1. Diarrhea related to intestinal mucosa irritation
2. Risk for Deficient Fluid Volume related to diarrhea
3. Imbalanced Nutrition: Less Than Body Requirements related to diarrhea and malabsorption of nutrients
4. Risk for Acute Pain related to toxic irritation of intestinal mucosa and diarrhea

C. Planning

1. Restore nutritional status.
2. Maintain hydration.
3. Reduce risk for pain.
4. Provide dietary teaching about gluten products.

D. Implementation

1. Manage diet (gluten-free diet).
2. Provide vitamin supplements as needed.

E. Evaluation

1. Child affirms reduction in abdominal pain, reduction in diarrhea, and tolerance of diet.
2. Child identifies foods that contribute to malabsorption and chooses appropriate alternatives.

CN

III. Client needs

A. Physiologic adaptation: Celiac disease is controlled with lifelong dietary modification and vitamin supplements. Child is at risk for celiac crisis leading to electrolyte imbalance and acidosis—indicated by distended abdomen, decreased bowel sounds, paralytic ileus, and metabolic disturbances such as hypokalemia and hypocalcemia.

B. Management of care: Care of the child with celiac disease requires critical thinking skills and knowledge of assessment, and teaching and evaluation methods unique to the RN role. These skills cannot be delegated to an LPN or UAP.

1. Perform comprehensive physical assessments and provide care appropriate to the child with celiac disease.
2. Assess for community resources such as the availability of grocery stores with a wide range of gluten-free foods and referral to the Celiac Sprue Association/United States of America, Inc.
3. Delegate responsibly those activities that can be delegated, including measurements, oral intake and urine output, vital signs, and reporting child's subjective data. All monitoring information is reported to the RN.

C. Safety and infection control: In addition to monitoring for a celiac crisis, teach child and family basics of gluten-free diet.

1. Foods permitted—fresh protein sources such as meat and eggs; dairy products; fruits and vegetables, rice, and corn.
2. Foods avoided—any food containing hydrolyzed vegetable protein such as commercially prepared ice cream; any food or fluid containing barley, rye, oats, and wheat.

D. Health promotion and maintenance

1. Provide age-appropriate toys and activities to promote growth and development.
2. Allow child to participate in diet management to promote self-management and treatment efficacy.

E. Psychologic integrity

1. Assist child with issues related to compliance with diet.
2. Allow child and family the opportunity to express fears, concerns, and to ask questions.
3. Offer support groups such as the Celiac Sprue Association/United States of America, Inc.

F. Basic care and comfort

1. Provide consistent nurse caregiver.
2. Allow parents to stay with child.
3. Provide skin care to prevent breakdown from diarrhea.

G. Reduction of risk potential

1. Teach child and family how to read food labels to identify hydrolyzed vegetable protein.
2. Teach child and family how to prevent celiac crisis by following diet plan.

H. Provide pharmacologic and parenteral therapies. Celiac disease is managed by diet; parenteral therapies are used to manage electrolyte and fluid imbalances of celiac crisis.

Diabetes Mellitus

I. Definition: Diabetes mellitus (DM) is a chronic metabolic disorder resulting from a partial or complete lack of insulin. Insulin supports CHO, fat, and protein metabolism, and is necessary for glucose transport into muscle and fat cells and storage of glycogen in the liver. Without insulin, glucose cannot enter the cell so it concentrates in the bloodstream. DM may be characterized as type 1 or type 2. (For information about gestational diabetes and diabetes in neonates see Section 1, Chapters 5 and 8. For information about diabetes in adults see Section 3, Chapter 27.)

A. Type 1: Characterized by destruction of the pancreatic beta cells leading to absolute insulin deficiency. Onset is rapid and the child will require lifetime management with insulin replacement.

B. Type 2: Arises because of insulin resistance when the body fails to use insulin properly, combined with some insulin deficiency. The incidence of type 2 diabetes is increasing from increased childhood obesity along with sedentary lifestyle and poor nutrition. The disease usually occurs in adolescence and requires lifetime management. (See also Chapter 27.)

II. Nursing process

A. Assessment

1. Assess child for risk factors for development of DM.
   a. Type 1: Usually an autoimmune disease occurring along with a genetic predisposition; viral infections have been implicated as precipitating events in the autoimmune response.
   b. Type 2: Risk factors include obesity, genetic predisposition, and insulin resistance.
2. Assess for signs and symptoms.
   a. Type 1: Chemical events produce hyperglycemia and ketoacidosis leading to weight loss and polyphagia, polydipsia, and polyuria—may be indicated by abdominal pain, dry skin, fatigue, blurred vision, and increased risk for infection.
   b. Type 2: May be indicated by obesity, fatigue, and increased risk for infection. The child may also present with polyphagia, polydipsia, and polyuria.
3. Complete a detailed history and physical assessment including baseline vital signs, height, weight, presenting symptoms, and family history of diabetes.
4. Obtain diagnostic tests.
   a. Random blood glucose: Level of 200 mg/dl or more on two occasions
   b. 8-hr fasting blood glucose: Level of 126 mg/dl or more
   c. Oral glucose tolerance test: Level 200 mg/dl or more in a the 2-hr sample
   d. Positive urinalysis for glucose needs follow-up
   e. Evaluate HgA_{1c} in the control of glucose levels (6.5% to 8% acceptable range in children)

B. Analysis

1. Risk for Injury related to deficiency in insulin and hypoglycemia
2. Deficient Knowledge: New Diagnosis, related to complex care needs
3. Risk for Ineffective Therapeutic Regimen Management related to complex medical regimen

C. Planning

1. Provide thorough teaching to child and family.
2. Restore blood glucose levels to normal range.
3. Relieve fear and anxiety.
4. Promote self-care behaviors such as monitoring of glucose levels.

D. Implementation

1. Provide glycemic control: Exogenous insulin.
   a. Maintain glucose levels at nearly normal.
   b. Prevent complications.
2. Promote dietary management, including three meals per day and two snacks.
   a. Base calories on age and growth needs.
   b. Discourage concentrated sweets.
3. Promote adequate exercise: Instruct child and family to learn to adjust food intake and insulin administration based on blood glucose levels. With assistance, most children can participate in sports and learn to maintain glucose levels.

E. Evaluation

1. Child has a normal blood glucose level.
2. Child and family verbalize understanding of disease, diagnosis, and management.
3. Child and family describe risk factors for the development of complications such as hypoglycemia.

CN

III. Client needs

A. Physiologic adaptation: DM is managed and complications prevented with a combination of insulin, diet, and exercise. Risk for development of hypoglycemia is indicated by increased insulin use from infection, excessive exercise, or not eating. Risk for hyperglycemia and ketoacidosis is indicated by hyperglycemia, polyuria, polydipsia, dehydration, nausea, vomiting, fruity breath, and loss of consciousness.

B. Management of care: Care of the child with diabetes requires critical thinking skills and knowledge of assessment, and teaching and evaluation methods unique to the RN role. These skills cannot be delegated to an LPN or UAP.
   1. Perform comprehensive physical assessments and provide care appropriate to the infant/child with diabetes.
   2. Assess for home health needs and facilitate follow-up care such as presence of all diabetic supplies, record-keeping tools, and appropriate foods.
   3. Evaluate community resources for family support such as local parent groups and local American Diabetes Association, and availability of diabetes equipment.
   4. Delegate responsibly those activities that can be delegated, including measurements, oral intake and urine output, vital signs, and reporting child's subjective data. All monitoring information must be reported to the RN.
   5. Provide multidisciplinary approach to care including health care provider (HCP), nurse, dietician, social worker, child, and family.

C. Safety and infection control
   1. Monitor blood glucose levels.
      a. Teach home glucose monitoring.
      b. Monitor glycosylated hemoglobin.
      c. Use urine only when blood glucose is 240 mg/dl or more.
   2. Monitor for and manage complication of hypoglycemia.
      a. Monitor for hypoglycemia: Indicated by change in behavior, such as confusion; tachycardia; diaphoretic; shakiness; and glucose levels less than 60 mg/dl.
      b. Manage hypoglycemia.
         (1) Offer 10- to 15-g simple carbohydrate such as fruit juice or IM glucagon for the unconscious child—place child in side-lying position after administration of glucagons to prevent aspiration in case vomiting occurs.
         (2) Follow with complex carbohydrate and protein.
         (3) Teach child and family to carry hard candy.
   3. Monitor for and manage complication of hyperglycemia.
      a. Monitor for hyperglycemia:
         (1) Respirations are deep and rapid (Kussmaul)
         (2) Breath is described as fruity/acetonelike
         (3) Reflexes are diminished
         (4) Glucose levels more than 240 mg/dl
      b. Manage hyperglycemia: Provide IV fluids and insulin replacement.
   4. Protect from injury and infection.
      a. Assess skin integrity, especially legs and feet.
      b. Provide skin care.
      c. Remove any tight clothes, shoes, socks, and linens.
   5. Provide extensive child and family teaching about disease, diagnosis, and management.
      a. Promote medication use, dose, timing, injection sites, and side effects (see pharmacologic and parenteral therapies).
      b. Teach how to recognize and manage signs and symptoms of hypoglycemia and hyperglycemia.
      c. Encourage dietary management.
      d. Develop exercise plan that reflects balance of food intake and insulin (see implementation).
      e. Promote illness management and teach needs for altered insulin dosing amounts.
      f. Instruct correct blood glucose monitoring.
      g. Provide guidelines for monitoring urine for ketones.

D. Health promotion and maintenance
   1. Teach child and family about the need for regular exercise individualized to developmental level.
   2. Promote self-management at early ages by allowing child to assist with blood glucose testing, diet management, and insulin administration.
   3. Prepare child for return to school.
   4. Prepare school for child's return.

E. Psychologic integrity
   1. Assess family and child's developmental, emotional, and psychologic readiness to receive in-depth information about disease.
   2. Allow child and family to verbalize feelings and ask questions.
   3. Encourage support groups for child and family such as the American Diabetes Association and Children with Diabetes.
   4. Suggest summer camps for diabetic children.
   5. Assist child and family in recognizing strategies to cope with lifestyle changes.

Table 15-2 Antidiabetic Agents

Classification	Generic/Trade Name	Expected Outcome	Reduction of Risk Potential	Management of Care
Antidiabetic agent: Rapid-acting	Lispro (Humalog)	Control hyperglycemia in diabetic child. **Onset: 15 min** **Peak: 30–90 min** **Duration: 5 hr**	Assess for signs and symptoms of hypoglycemia. Monitor glucose levels.	Know onset and peak times of insulin to manage food intake and assess for complications.
Antidiabetic agent: Short-acting	Humulin R Iletin II Regular	Control hyperglycemia in diabetic child. **Onset: 30 min** **Peak: 2–4 hr** **Duration: 5–7 hr**	Assess for signs and symptoms of hypoglycemia. Monitor glucose levels.	Know onset and peak times of insulin to manage food intake and assess for complications.
Antidiabetic agent: Intermediate-acting	Humulin N Humulin L	Control hyperglycemia in diabetic child. **Onset: 1–2 hr** **Peak: 6–14 hr** **Duration: 20–24 hr**	Assess for signs and symptoms of hypoglycemia. Monitor glucose levels.	Know onset and peak times of insulin to manage food intake and assess for complications.
Antidiabetic agent: Long-acting	Lantus Humulin U Ultralente	Control hyperglycemia in diabetic child. **Onset: 6–14 hr** **Peak: 10–16 hr** **Duration: 20–24 hr**	Assess for signs and symptoms of hypoglycemia. Monitor glucose levels.	Know onset and peak times of insulin to manage food intake and assess for complications.

F. Basic care and comfort
   1. Encourage and answer all questions at child's cognitive level.
   2. Provide consistent nurse caregiver.
   3. Allow parents to stay at bedside.
   4. Provide age-appropriate activities to stimulate developmental and cognitive level.

G. Reduction of risk potential
   1. Monitor glycosylated hemoglobin (HgA_{1C} levels) every 3 months.
   2. Treat complications—if cannot determine if child is experiencing hypoglycemia versus hyperglycemia, treat for hypoglycemia.
   3. Manage insulin during infection, stress, or illness by holding insulin and testing glucose levels every 3 to 4 hr.
   4. Promote exercise management.
      a. Increase food with physical activity.
      b. Encourage snacking 30 min before team sport activity.
   5. Teach parents about complications and relationship to disease control; provide guidelines for screening, including ophthalmologic examinations.
   6. Encourage use of medic-alert bracelet.

H. Pharmacologic and parenteral therapies: Child and family will state the purpose, dosage, timing, and side effects of insulin preparations. Table 15-2 contains a list of antidiabetic agents.

Bibliography

Hatfield, N. (2006). *Broadribb's introductory pediatric nursing.* Philadelphia: Lippincott Williams & Wilkins.

Pillitteri, A. (2006). *Maternal & child health nursing: Care of the childbearing and childrearing family* (5th ed.). Philadelphia: Lippincott Williams & Wilkins.

Wong, D. L., et al. (2006). *Maternal child nursing care.* St. Louis: Mosby.

CHAPTER 15

Practice Test

Phenylketonuria

1. The nurse is observing a mother of a child who is 3 years of age with PKU as she makes food choices from a menu. Choosing which of the following foods indicates that the child and his mother are not following the prescribed diet?
   - □ 1. A dish of pears.
   - □ 2. Chocolate pudding.
   - □ 3. Lettuce leaves.
   - □ 4. Orange juice.
2. The nurse is assessing children at risk for PKU. Which one of the following children is at greatest risk?
   - □ 1. Blond, blue-eyed, fair-skinned child with eczema.
   - □ 2. African American, dark-eyed child with asthma.
   - □ 3. Child with dark complexion who is overweight and has labile personalities.
   - □ 4. Red-headed child who experiences frequent contact dermatitis.

Failure to Thrive

3. The nurse is caring for an infant with nonorganic failure to thrive (NFTT). Which of the following nursing actions is most important when feeding the child?
   - □ 1. Have the same person feed the infant.
   - □ 2. Provide a calm and quiet atmosphere.
   - □ 3. Continue to offer feeding in spite of the infant's refusal to eat or drink.
   - □ 4. Maintain a face-to-face posture with the infant.
4. AF The nurse is assessing an infant who has NFTT. Which of the following findings typical of NFTT will assist the nurse plan of care for this infant? Select all that apply.
   - □ 1. Frequent smiling.
   - □ 2. Flaccid and unresponsive posture.
   - □ 3. Accelerated development.
   - □ 4. Weight and height below 15th percentile.
   - □ 5. No fear of strangers when typically expected.
   - □ 6. Continual scan of environment ("radar gaze").
   - □ 7. Feeding disorders such as vomiting or anorexia.

Obesity

5. The nurse is providing nutrition counseling for an obese adolescent. The most effective method for the nurse to obtain a nutrition history from this client is to:
   - □ 1. Ask her what she knows about good nutrition.
   - □ 2. Tell her to list what she plans to eat for the next 24 hr.
   - □ 3. Ask her what she ate yesterday if it was a typical day.
   - □ 4. Telephone her mother and ask her what she ate yesterday.
6. The nurse is providing information about weight-management programs to a group of school-aged children and their parents. Which weight-management program is most appropriate for school-aged children?
   - □ 1. Jenny Craig.
   - □ 2. Weight Watchers.
   - □ 3. Weight maintenance over time.
   - □ 4. Atkins diet.

Gastroesophageal Reflux

7. A premature infant who has complications from GER had a Nissen fundoplication. The nurse is assessing the infant following surgery. Which of the following is an expected outcome from the surgery?
   - □ 1. A stomach pH level more than 7.5.
   - □ 2. Decreased irritability following feedings.
   - □ 3. A stomach pH level less than 7.5.
   - □ 4. Increased appetite.
8. The nurse is instructing the parents of a neonate with GER about home care for their infant. The nurse should instruct the parents to place their child in which of the following positions following eating?
   - □ 1. Supine.
   - □ 2. Prone.
   - □ 3. High Fowler.
   - □ 4. Side-lying on right side.

Celiac Disease

9. The nurse is teaching the mother of a preschool-aged child with celiac disease about a gluten-free diet. The nurse determines that

the mother understands the diet if she tells the nurse she will prepare:
- □ 1. Eggs and orange juice.
- □ 2. Wheat toast and grape jelly.
- □ 3. Cheerios (oat cereal) and skim milk.
- □ 4. Rye toast and peanut butter.

Diabetes Mellitus

10. The nurse is instructing a school-aged child about managing his DM. Which of the following situations is likely to precipitate a hypoglycemic reaction in a child with DM?
- □ 1. Participation in a soccer game.
- □ 2. Eating a high-carbohydrate lunch.
- □ 3. Developing an upper respiratory infection.
- □ 4. Forgetting to take insulin.

11. The nurse is showing a child with type 1 DM how to administer her own insulin. The child is receiving a combination of short-acting and long-acting insulin. She has appropriately learned the technique when she:
- □ 1. Administers the insulin into a doll at a 30-degree angle.
- □ 2. Draws up the regular insulin into the syringe first.
- □ 3. Wipes off the needle with an alcohol swab.
- □ 4. Administers the insulin IM into rotating sites.

12. The nurse is assessing a school-aged child with type 1 DM. The nurse should report which of the following information to the HCP?
- □ 1. A great toe that is red and edematous.
- □ 2. A cut on lower shin of the child's leg.
- □ 3. A respiratory rate of 30, with deep inspirations.
- □ 4. A mother who has no knowledge of her child's medications.

13. A diabetic child is admitted to the emergency department with hot and dry skin, rapid and deep respirations, and a fruity odor to her breath. Which task, when performed by a new-graduate RN, requires the RN preceptor to intervene?
- □ 1. Assessment of child's vital signs every 15 min.
- □ 2. Verification of child's order for sliding-scale insulin.
- □ 3. Providing encouragement to the child to drink some orange juice.
- □ 4. Verification of child's glucose by fingerstick.

14. The nurse is caring for a hospitalized child who is 10 years of age. The child has type 1 DM and is developing diabetic ketoacidosis (DKA). Which of the following tasks does the nurse delegate?
- □ 1. Unit clerk to page the physician to come to the unit.
- □ 2. LPN to administer IV push insulin according to the sliding scale.
- □ 3. Nursing assistant to check the patient's level of consciousness.
- □ 4. Student nurse extern to give the child a glass of orange juice.

15. A child who is 7 years of age with autism is diagnosed with type 1 DM. His mother, who is 27 years of age, is his primary caregiver and has a mental age of a client who is 13 years of age. Which of the following instructions about type 1 DM should be deferred until the diabetic educator can complete the needed teaching in their home?
- □ 1. Urine ketone testing.
- □ 2. Blood glucose monitoring.
- □ 3. Signs of hyperglycemia and hypoglycemia.
- □ 4. Glucagon administration.

16. AF The nurse is preparing to teach the signs and symptoms of hypoglycemia to a family whose toddler was recently diagnosed with type 1 DM. The nurse should teach the family about which of the following clinical signs of hypoglycemia? Select all that apply.
- □ 1. Fruity breath.
- □ 2. Sweaty, pale skin.
- □ 3. Flushed, dry skin.
- □ 4. Dizziness.
- □ 5. Nausea and vomiting.
- □ 6. Normal breath odor.
- □ 7. Dilated pupils.

17. The nurse has just administered glucagon to a child with type 1 DM who is unresponsive because of hypoglycemia. What should the nurse do next?
- □ 1. Have child drink a glass of orange juice.
- □ 2. Check child's blood sugar.
- □ 3. Place child in a side-lying position.
- □ 4. Administer prescribed sliding-scale insulin.

18. The nurse is planning care for a group of clients with type 1 DM. Which child would the nurse expect to have the most difficulty adjusting to the diagnosis of type 1 DM?
- □ 1. A toddler.
- □ 2. A preschooler.
- □ 3. A school-aged child.
- □ 4. A teenager.

19. A school-aged child has been diagnosed with type 1 DM. Which statement by the child can the nurse evaluate as demonstrating good understanding of his insulin therapy?
- □ 1. "I like the fact that my lispro insulin will last all day."

□ 2. "It is amazing that my ultralente insulin stays in my blood for 24 hours."
□ 3. "My lispro insulin is my intermediate-acting insulin."
□ 4. "If I take my ultralente insulin it will peak within 15 minutes."

20. The nurse is providing teaching to the parent of a child with type 1 DM. The nurse determines the parent understands when urine ketone testing should occur when the parent says which of the following? "I will check for ketones:
□ 1. When my child's blood sugar drops less than 70 mg/dl."
□ 2. Before meals and before bedtime."
□ 3. Every morning when my child gets up."
□ 4. When my child's sugars are high or when he is sick."

Answers and Rationales

1. 2 The nurse instructs clients with PKU to avoid food that is high in phenylalanine. Milk is high in phenylalanine. Milk and milk products from which the chocolate pudding is made are contraindicated on this diet. Fruits and vegetables are low in phenylalanine and can be included in the diet. (H)

2. 1 Infants with PKU are usually blond, blue-eyed, and fair, and often have eczema. The other physical assessment findings are not typically found in children with PKU. (A)

3. 3 Perseverance is one of the most important actions in feeding an infant with NFTT. Parents or nursing staff often give up when a child begins negative feeding behavior. Calm perseverance through lengthy meals of food refusal will gradually decrease the negative behavior. The same person (parent or nursing staff) feeds the infant to the extent possible, in a quiet atmosphere, and while holding the infant in a face-to-face position and talking to the child as is appropriate; however, the most important aspect of feeding this child with NFTT is to continue with the feeding. (C)

4. 2, 5, 6, 7 Common clinical manifestations of NFTT are an unresponsive posture, growth failure (below the 5th percentile in weight only or weight and height), no fear of strangers, wide-eyed gaze and continual scan of the environment ("radar gaze"), feeding or eating disorders, delayed developmental milestones, and poor hygiene. The child with NFTT does not smile and has delayed development. (A)

5. 3 A 24-hr recall history is the best method to obtain a dietary history from an adolescent. Open-ended questions tend not to provide sufficient details for a nutrition history. By asking what the client plans to eat in the future gives the client an opportunity to report the "right" answer. The nurse obtains the information directly from the client; asking the mother has the potential to undermine trust. (H)

6. 3 Allowing a child the opportunity to maintain a steady weight while increasing height as they get older has proven to be one of the safest ways for children to fight weight issues. Weight loss is not stressed, rather the child is encouraged to maintain the present weight or lose weight very slowly. The child will gradually become thinner as he or she gets taller. Diet programs have not proven to be successful with the general pediatric population. Because obesity is often a lifelong problem, the nurse provides children, adolescents, and their families with a diet that fosters healthier eating habits. (H)

7. 2 The Nissen fundoplication is the most common surgical procedure for GER. This surgery involves passage of the gastric fundus behind the esophagus to encircle the distal esophagus, preventing stomach acid from entering the esophagus. Infants with GER are often irritable following feedings, most likely from the burning sensation in the esophagus; following surgery they are much less irritable. The surgery will not affect the pH of the stomach; however, the pH noted in the esophagus should be less acidic. The child's appetite will not be greatly affected. (A)

8. 2 Current recommendations indicate that children under 1 year of age be placed in the prone position, particularly following eating. Unless the risk of death from GER outweighs the risk of SIDS, the child is positioned in a supine position to sleep. The neonate is placed at 30-degree elevation (low Fowler) as long as there is straight alignment. The goal of positioning is to avoid increasing the intra-abdominal pressure. Children older than 1 year of age are positioned with the head of the bed elevated at 30 degrees, with the child placed on the left side. (H)

9. 1 Children with celiac disease cannot digest the protein in common grains such as wheat, rye, and oats. Eggs and orange juice would be appropriate foods. (H)

10. 1 Exercise uses glucose. The nurse instructs the child that unless the amount of insulin administered is reduced, hypoglycemia can result. Eating a high-carbohydrate lunch increases the need for insulin; not taking the insulin leads to hyperglycemia. Infection increases the child's insulin requirements. (H)

11. 2 Drawing up the regular insulin first prevents mixing a long-acting form into the vial of regular insulin. This keeps the regular insulin for an emergency. Insulin is given subcutaneously. (H)

12. 3 Rapid, deep respirations (Kussmaul) are symptomatic of diabetic ketoacidosis (DKA). A red and edematous toe and deep cut to a shin are significant because of the increased risk of infection; however, they will not take priority over a potential DKA situation. The knowledge deficit for a mother who has a child with type 1 DM is significant, but is not a priority over DKA. (R)

13. 3 The client is exhibiting symptoms that are consistent with hyperglycemia. The RN does not give any additional glucose. All of the other interventions are appropriate for this patient. The new-graduate RN notifies the physician about the assessment findings. (S)

14. 1 During this situation, the RN does not leave the patient. The nurse calls the unit clerk and asks him or her to page the physician. LPNs generally do not administer IV push medications. Assessing level of consciousness is not within the scope of practice of a nursing assistant. Children with DKA already have a high glucose level and do not need orange juice. (M)

15. 1 Teaching a family about type 1 DM is a complex process that can be very confusing, and is particularly challenging for a family member who is cognitively compromised. The nurse begins teaching the mother about blood glucose monitoring, then teaches the family about the signs and symptoms of hyper- and hypoglycemia. Glucagon administration is vital because this can be a lifesaving measure should the child's blood sugar drop dangerously low; the nurse assures that the family knows how to do this prior to discharge. Although urine ketone testing is easy to teach it does require careful technique and is deferred until the family is in their home setting and has had time to settle into their new routine. (M)

16. 2, 4, 6, 7 The clinical findings that are commonly seen in a child with hypoglycemia include sweaty skin, pallor, dizziness, normal breath odor, and dilated pupils. Fruity breath, flushed, dry skin, and nausea and vomiting are commonly found with hyperglycemia. (H)

17. 3 Vomiting may occur after administration of glucagons. The nurse places the child on his side to prevent aspiration in case the child vomits. The nurse does not have the child drink anything, and does not administer sliding-scale insulin as the blood sugar is already low. It is too soon to check the blood sugar. (S)

18. 4 Adolescents appear to have the most difficulty in adjusting to type 1 DM or any other chronic illness. Adolescence is a time when there is much stress to be "perfect" and to be like peers. If the adolescent can accept that difference is a part of life and that each person is different in some way, then with adequate family support he or she can adjust well. With toddlers and preschoolers, insulin injections and glucose testing may be difficult at first. However, they usually accept the procedures when the parents use a matter-of-fact approach without calling attention to the "hurt." School-aged children tend to accept their condition more easily than adolescents because they can understand the basic concepts related to their disease and treatment. (P)

19. 2 Ultralente is a long-acting insulin. It takes 6 to 14 hr to start working. It has no peak or a very small peak 10 to 16 hr after injection, and stays in the blood for 20 to 24 hr. Lispro is a rapid-acting insulin that peaks at 30 to 90 min and lasts about 5 hr. (D)

20. 4 Urine ketone testing is easily taught, but requires careful attention to technique. The test strip must be used accurately and the test timed precisely. Testing for ketones is recommended during times of illness or when glucose readings are high. (M)

chapter 16

The Child With Health Problems of the Genitourinary System

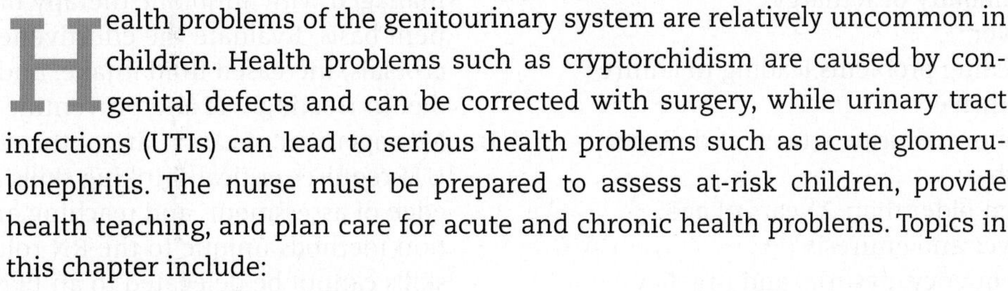

Health problems of the genitourinary system are relatively uncommon in children. Health problems such as cryptorchidism are caused by congenital defects and can be corrected with surgery, while urinary tract infections (UTIs) can lead to serious health problems such as acute glomerulonephritis. The nurse must be prepared to assess at-risk children, provide health teaching, and plan care for acute and chronic health problems. Topics in this chapter include:

- Urinary Tract Infection
- Cryptorchidism
- Hypospadias and Epispadias
- Wilms Tumor
- Glomerulonephritis
- Nephrotic Syndrome
- Acute Renal Failure

Urinary Tract Infection

I. Definition: Urinary tract infection (UTI) is a clinical state that may involve the structures of the lower and upper urinary tract, including the bladder, ureters, and kidney. Reflux from the ureters into the kidney is the leading cause of infection. Infection causes inflammation of the bladder from a variety of organisms, the most common of which is *Escherichia coli.*

II. Nursing process
 A. Assessment
  1. Complete a detailed health history and physical assessment, including voiding behaviors, constipation, and irritability.
  2. Assess for risk factors.
   a. Female: Urethra 2 cm in length
   b. Male: Uncircumcised, or improper cleaning of circumcision site
   c. Male and female risk factors include:
    (1) Urinary stasis
     (a) Constipation
     (b) Reflux
    (2) Presence of indwelling Foley catheter
    (3) Use of tight clothing or diapers
    (4) Use of bubble bath products
  3. Assess for signs and symptoms.
   a. Infants and children younger than 2 years of age:
    (1) Vomiting and diarrhea
    (2) Irritability or lethargy
    (3) Fever
    (4) Feeding problems leading to failure to thrive
    (5) Abnormal urine stream and diaper rash
   b. Children older than 2 years of age:
    (1) Fever and enuresis
    (2) Frequency, dysuria, and urgency
    (3) Strong or foul-smelling urine
    (4) Frequency, dysuria, hematuria
    (5) Upper urinary tract: Flank pain, fever and chills
  4. Obtain diagnostic tests.
   a. Urinalysis and culture
   b. Dipstick urine for presence of nitrates and WBCs
 B. Analysis
  1. Fear and Anxiety related to pain, strange environment, and procedures
  2. Infection related to urinary stasis
  3. Acute Pain related to infection and inflammation
  4. Risk for Ineffective Therapeutic Regimen related to inadequate knowledge of treatment
 C. Planning
  1. Eliminate infection.
  2. Promote hydration.
  3. Relieve pain or reduce pain to a tolerable level.
  4. Reduce fear and anxiety.
  5. Promote parental compliance with treatment regimen.
  6. Prevent recurrence.
 D. Implementation
  1. Eliminate infection—provide antibiotic therapy.
  2. Identify cause and risk factors.
  3. Prevent recurrent infections.
 E. Evaluation
  1. Child is free of infection and related symptoms.
  2. Child has reduced fear and anxiety as evidenced by ability to rest quietly and compliance with care.
  3. Child's pain is reduced as evidenced by verbal affirmation or infant's ability to rest and eat.
  4. Parents verbalize understanding of therapeutic regimen and importance of compliance.
  5. Parents identify risk factors for recurrence and methods to prevent future UTIs.

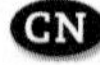

III. Client needs
 A. Physiologic adaptation: UTIs are identified and managed with antibiotic therapy on an outpatient basis. Evaluate the effectiveness of antimicrobials, increased fluid intake, and acid-ash diet in treating UTI and preventing recurrence.
 B. Management of care: Care of the child with a UTI requires critical thinking skills and knowledge of assessment, and teaching and evaluation methods unique to the RN role. These skills cannot be delegated to an LPN or UAP.
  1. Perform comprehensive physical assessments and provide care appropriate to the child with a UTI.
  2. Provide follow-up care to identify compliance with drug regimen and assess for complications such as glomerulonephritis.
  3. Delegate responsibly those activities that can be delegated, including oral intake and urine output, vital signs, and reporting child's subjective data. All monitoring information is reported to the RN.
 C. Safety and infection control
  1. Obtain clean-catch urine from female child sitting on toilet facing the tank.
  2. Assess frequency of urination in infants to identify infection—change diaper every 30 min.

Table 16-1 Drugs Used With Urinary Tract Infections

Classification	Generic/Trade Name	Expected Outcome	Reduction of Risk Potential	Management of Care
Anti-infective	Trimethoprim/ sulfamethoxazole (Bactrim, Septra)	Treats bacterial UTIs.	Monitor for rash, nausea, photosensitivity, and urticaria. Not to be used if child has asthma.	Teach parents to promote fluid intake and use sunscreen.
Urinary Tract Anti-infective	Nitrofurantoin (Macrodantin)	Treats UTI caused by susceptible organism.	Monitor for nausea and oliguria. Monitor for superinfections.	Teach parents to give with milk or food. Urine may turn orange or brown.
Prokinetic Agents	Ceftazidime (Fortaz)	Treats UTIs.	Monitor kidney function. Monitor creatinine level. Contraindicated if allergic to penicillin.	Teach parents to monitor for diarrhea and report immediately.

3. Promote fluid intake of clear liquids up to 100 ml/kg daily.
4. Teach child and family to avoid caffeinated and carbonated beverages.
5. Teach parents about anti-infectives, dosage, timing, suggestions on how to administer, and importance of compliance with complete regimen.
6. Maintain the six rights of medication administration.

D. Health promotion and maintenance
1. Provide a transitional comfort object for child to take into procedure.
2. Provide age-appropriate diversional activities.
3. Involve family in all aspects of care.

E. Psychologic integrity
1. Provide child with explanation of procedure and treatment; use pictures or dolls when developmentally appropriate.
2. Encourage the child and family to express fears, concerns, and to ask questions.

F. Basic care and comfort
1. Promote fluid intake.
2. Provide perineal care.
3. Provide consistent nurse caregiver.

G. Reduction of risk potential
1. Perform urinalysis during routine wellness visits.
2. Teach parents methods to prevent recurrence.
   a. Provide good perineal hygiene.
   b. Use cotton underwear.
   c. Encourage complete emptying of bladder.
   d. Increase fluid intake.
   e. Encourage child to void every 2 hr.
   f. Acidify urine through diet high in acid-ash: Meat, fish, cheese; bread and whole grains; eggs; cranberries, prunes, and tomatoes.

H. Pharmacologic and parenteral therapies: Child and family will state the purpose, dosage, timing, and side effects of medications used to treat UTIs (Table 16-1).

Cryptorchidism

I. Definition: Cryptorchidism (undescended testes) is the failure of one or both testes to descend through the inguinal canal into the scrotum in utero.

II. Nursing process

A. Assessment
1. Complete a detailed health history and physical assessment, including history of prematurity.
2. Assess for signs and symptoms: One or both testes are not palpable in the scrotum.
3. Obtain diagnostic tests.
   a. Palpation
   b. Ultrasound
   c. Laparoscopy

B. Analysis
1. Anxiety related to procedures and strange environment
2. Risk for Disturbed Body Image related to difference in physical appearance
3. Risk for Trauma related to potential surgical intervention

C. Planning
1. Reduce anxiety.
2. Prevent body image disturbance.

3. Provide child and family teaching about procedure and surgery.

D. Implementation (see management of care)

E. Evaluation

1. Child's fear and anxiety are reduced evidenced by ability to rest quietly and compliance with care.
2. Parents verbalize understanding of therapeutic regimen and importance of compliance.

CN

III. Client needs

A. Physiologic adaptation: Cryptorchidism is managed with luteinizing hormone spray or human chorionic gonadotropin injection until the child is 1 year of age and followed by surgical intervention (orchiopexy) to prevent complications such as infertility, testicular cancer, testicular torsion, and psychologic problems.

1. Assess the effectiveness of hormone therapy in promoting testicular descent and reducing need for surgery.
2. Recognize risk for impaired tissue perfusion from testicular torsion—indicated by nausea, vomiting, and abdominal pain, as well as testes that are red, warm, and edematous.

B. Management of care: Care of the child with cryptorchidism requires critical thinking skills and knowledge of assessment, and teaching and evaluation methods unique to the RN role. These skills cannot be delegated to an LPN or UAP.

1. Perform comprehensive physical assessments and provide care appropriate to the child with cryptorchidism.
2. Provide follow-up care to identify that testes have descended or at risk for postoperative infection.
3. Delegate responsibly those activities that can be delegated, including measurements, oral intake and urine output, vital signs, and reporting child's subjective data. All monitoring information is reported to the RN.

C. Safety and infection control: Teach parents the importance of surgical treatment to avoid complications (see physiologic adaptation), as well as postoperative care for child in the home environment.

1. Teach signs and symptoms of infection.
2. Provide pain management with analgesics, as needed.

D. Health promotion and maintenance

1. Provide a transitional comfort object for child to take into surgery.
2. Provide age-appropriate diversional activities.
3. Involve family in all aspects of care.

E. Psychologic integrity: Provide parents with explanation of procedure and treatment, and encourage expression of fears, concerns, and asking of questions.

F. Basic care and comfort

1. Allow parents at bedside.
2. Provide consistent nurse caregiver.
3. Administer analgesic for postoperative pain.

G. Reduction of risk potential: Perform surgery when child is less than 24 months of age to reduce risk of infertility.

H. Pharmacologic and parenteral therapies are used to manage pain as previously noted. Child and family will state the purpose for and associated risk factors for all medications.

Hypospadias and Epispadias

I. Definition: Hypospadias and epispadias are abnormally positioned urethral openings. They are often associated with other abnormalities of the urinary tract.

A. Hypospadias is a congenital defect in which the urethral opening is located below the glans penis or anywhere along the ventral surface of the penile shaft.

B. Epispadias is when the urethral opening is on the dorsal surface of the penis and is usually associated with the complex problem, bladder exstrophy (externalization of the bladder).

II. Nursing process

A. Assessment

1. Complete a detailed health history and physical assessment, including vital signs, height and weight, and developmental level.
2. Obtain diagnostic tests: Diagnosis based on visual examination.

B. Analysis

1. Risk for Disturbed Body Image related to malplaced urethra and shortened penis
2. Risk for Infection related to bacterial contamination of urine
3. Impaired Urinary Elimination related to malplaced urethra

C. Planning

1. Improve voiding ability.
2. Improve physical appearance.
3. Preserve renal function.
4. Instruct parents about surgery and need to delay circumcision.

D. Implementation: Provide interventions for surgical reconstruction of congenital defect (see physiologic adaptation).

E. Evaluation

1. Child demonstrates ability to void appropriately.

2. Child's physical appearance is normal or near-normal to reduce psychologic problems and enhance body image.
3. Child is free from complications such as UTIs.
4. Parents verbalize understanding of therapeutic regimen and importance of compliance.

CN

III. Client needs

A. Physiologic adaptation: Congenital defect is managed with surgery and follow-up care. Recognize increased risk for infection—indicated by fever, restlessness, dysuria, frequency, abnormal urinary stream, foul-smelling urine.
   1. Hypospadias: Surgical management for reconstruction, usually performed between the ages of 6 and 18 months of age.
   2. Epispadias/exstrophy: Surgical management to attain urinary control, prevent UTI, preserve genitalia, and prevent psychologic complications.

B. Management of care: Care of the child with hypospadias or epispadias requires critical thinking skills and knowledge of assessment, and teaching and evaluation methods unique to the RN role. These skills cannot be delegated to an LPN or UAP.
   1. Perform comprehensive physical assessments and provide care appropriate to the child with hypospadias or epispadias.
   2. Provide parental teaching about the defect, surgical treatment and cosmetic outcome, and home management.
   3. Provide follow-up care to identify risk for postoperative infection.
   4. Delegate responsibly those activities that can be delegated, including measurements, oral intake and urine output, vital signs, and reporting child's subjective data. All monitoring information is reported to the RN.

C. Safety and infection control
   1. Avoid circumcision if defect is suspected at birth.
   2. Provide postoperative safety management.
      a. Manage pressure dressing and possible urinary stent.
      b. Promote fluid intake.
      c. Monitor intake and output and characteristics of urine.
   3. Provide parents with discharge teaching.
      a. Apply antibiotic ointment to penis following voiding.
      b. Recognize signs and symptoms of UTI.
      c. Avoid tub baths, swimming, playing near sand, and rough play activity.
      d. Provide care of the stent.
      e. Follow-up with care within 4 days for dressing removal.

D. Health promotion and maintenance
   1. Provide a transitional comfort object for child to take into surgery.
   2. Provide age-appropriate diversional activities.
   3. Involve family in all aspects of care.

E. Psychologic integrity
   1. Encourage parents to express fears, guilt, concerns, and to ask questions.
   2. Assist parents to cope with the possibility of an inadequate sexual organ if exstrophy of the bladder is associated with epispadias.

F. Basic care and comfort: Control pain with analgesics.

G. Reduction of risk potential
   1. Administer brief course of testosterone preoperatively to enhance penis size and facilitate surgery.
   2. Use prophylactic antibiotics as appropriate.

H. Pharmacologic and parenteral therapies: Administer analgesics for pain, and testosterone, as previously noted. Child and family will state the purpose for and associated side effects of all medications.

Wilms Tumor

I. Definition: Wilms tumor (nephroblastoma) is a unilateral or bilateral tumor usually found encapsulated on the left kidney. Nephroblastoma is the most common intra-abdominal tumor in children.

II. Nursing process

A. Assessment
   1. Complete a detailed health history, including family history of cancer, congenital anomalies, or evidence of malignancy.
   2. Complete a detailed physical assessment, including vital signs, height and weight, and developmental level.
   3. Assess for signs and symptoms of tumor.
      a. Nontender, firm abdominal mass that does not cross midline
      b. Distended abdomen
      c. Occasional hypertension
      d. Anemia—pallor, anorexia, lethargy
      e. Urinary retention and hematuria
   4. Obtain diagnostic tests: Abdominal ultrasound and CT scan.

B. Analysis
   1. Activity Intolerance related to anemia
   2. Anxiety related to procedures, fearful environment, and rapid treatment
   3. Anticipatory Grieving related to unknown diagnosis outcome

4. Risk for Infection related to surgery and immunosuppression from chemotherapy
5. Risk for Acute Pain related to procedures and surgical intervention
6. Risk for Ineffective Therapeutic Regimen Management related to rapid diagnosis and treatment

C. Planning
1. Prevent tumor rupture by preventing abdominal palpation.
2. Provide adequate fluids and nutrition.
3. Control pain.
4. Manage side effects of chemotherapy.
5. Offer emotional support to child and family.
6. Reduce fear and anxiety.

D. Implementation (see management of care)

E. Evaluation
1. Child and family demonstrate understanding of therapeutic regimen.
2. Child is free from infection and bleeding.
3. Child and family understand treatment of chemotherapy-induced side effects.
4. Child's pain is reduced to a tolerable level.
5. Child's anxiety is reduced as evidenced by compliance with care.

CN

III. Client needs

A. Physiologic adaptation: Wilms tumor is managed with surgical intervention, nephrectomy, to remove tumor, kidney, and adrenal gland; and chemotherapy and radiation (depending on stage and histology).
1. Recognize risk for possible alteration in tissue perfusion: Paralytic ileus—indicated by abdominal distention, absent bowel sounds, and vomiting.
2. Initiate child and family preparation for radiation therapy based on findings from histologic exam.

B. Management of care: Care of the child with a Wilms tumor requires critical thinking skills and knowledge of assessment, and teaching and evaluation methods unique to the RN role. These skills cannot be delegated to an LPN or UAP.
1. Perform a comprehensive physical assessment and provide care appropriate to the child with Wilms tumor.
2. Provide preoperative and postoperative interventions for the management of Wilms tumor (see safety and infection control).
3. Provide follow-up care to identify risk for postoperative infection and side effects of chemotherapy.
4. Evaluate community resources such as local support groups for parents, availability of respite care, and possible transportation for chemotherapy.
5. Delegate responsibly those activities that can be delegated, including measurements, oral intake and urine output, vital signs, and reporting child's subjective data. All monitoring information is reported to the RN.

C. Safety and infection control
1. Provide preoperative management.
   a. Monitor vital signs, especially BP.
   b. Do not allow abdominal palpation; include sign over bed.
   c. Measure abdominal girth.
   d. Maintain careful physical handling of child.
   e. Provide preoperative preparation of child at developmental level.
      (1) Tour the OR, PACU, and ICU.
      (2) Touch and see equipment such as incentive spirometer.
2. Provide postoperative management.
   a. Continue to monitor vital signs.
   b. Assess for hemorrhage and infection.
   c. Monitor for paralytic ileus.
   d. Monitor remaining kidney output carefully.
      (1) Intake and output
      (2) Daily weight
   e. Prepare child and family for chemotherapy: Purpose, dosage, timing, and management of side effects.

D. Health promotion and maintenance
1. Provide a transitional comfort object for child to take into surgery.
2. Provide age-appropriate diversional activities.
3. Involve family in all aspects of care.

E. Psychologic integrity: Diagnosis and treatment begin within 24 to 48 hr—encourage parents to express fears, concerns, guilt, and anger, and to begin to ask questions. Additional care involves the following:
1. Promote play therapy for child to allow for expression of feelings and coping with side effects of chemotherapy such as alopecia.
2. Understand cultural diversity in expression of fear, lack of knowledge, manifestation of pain, dietary needs, and death and dying rituals.

F. Basic care and comfort
1. Administer pain medication.
2. Manage nausea and vomiting—provide antiemetic, bland and cool diet, and promote hydration.
3. Treat stomatitis—pain relief, oral mouth rinses, and acupressure.

G. Reduction of risk potential
 1. Do not allow anyone to palpate tumor preoperatively.
 2. Promote postoperative lifetime prevention of injury from contact sports or high-impact activity.
 3. Prevent UTIs.

H. Pharmacologic and parenteral therapies: For information about chemotherapy see Chapter 32.

Glomerulonephritis

I. Definition: Glomerulonephritis is an immune complex disease usually caused by group A β-hemolytic streptococcus such as pharyngitis or impetigo. The disease can be acute or chronic. Acute glomerulonephritis is used to describe disease processes that cause damage to the glomeruli. Chronic glomerulonephritis is an advanced stage of the disease, characterized by progressive destruction of the glomeruli. The cause of glomerulonephritis is an antigen-antibody reaction produced by an infection. The most common form of glomerulonephritis is acute poststreptococcal glomerulonephritis (APSGN). Beginning with antigen-reaction, glomeruli become edematous and infiltrated with leukocytes; there is a decrease in glomerular filtration, resulting in excessive accumulation of water and retention of sodium. This causes increased fluid volume and this leads to edema and circulatory congestion.

II. Nursing process

A. Assessment
 1. Obtain a detailed health history, including recent history of pharyngitis or tonsillitis, or a skin infection such as impetigo.
 2. Complete a detailed physical assessment including vital signs, height and weight, and developmental level.
 3. Assess for signs and symptoms of glomerular damage.
  a. Periorbital edema
  b. Urine is cloudy, tea colored
  c. Oliguria
  d. Pale and lethargic
  e. Hypertensive
  f. Edema may last from 4 days to 3 weeks, then diuresis
  g. Hematuria, proteinuria, and azotemia
 4. Obtain diagnostic tests.
  a. Urinalysis
  b. Serum blood urea nitrogen (BUN) and creatinine
  c. Pharynx cultures
  d. Chest radiograph

B. Analysis
 1. Anxiety related to multiple procedures and strange environment
 2. Excess Fluid Volume related to compromised regulatory mechanism
 3. Risk for Injury: Hypertension, related to increased hyperperfusion of the brain and edema
 4. Deficient Knowledge: Disease Process, related to multiple new physical needs
 5. Imbalanced Nutrition: Less Than Body Requirements related to anorexia
 6. Risk for Ineffective Therapeutic Regimen Management related to complexity of disease and treatment regimen
 7. Impaired Urinary Elimination: Altered patterns, related to glomerular damage

C. Planning
 1. Reduce anxiety.
 2. Reduce fluid overload and improve urinary output.
 3. Prevent complications associated with hypertension and excess fluid.
 4. Provide child and family teaching about procedures, treatment, and outcome.
 5. Maintain and improve nutritional status.

D. Implementation.
 1. Teach home management if mild disease.
 2. Monitor fluid balance.
  a. Possible sodium and water restriction
  b. Possible diuretics
 3. Manage hypertension.
  a. Loop diuretics
  b. Antihypertensives for severe hypertension
 4. Promote diet management.
 5. Monitor for complications—hypertensive encephalopathy: Headache, dizziness, abdominal pain; cardiac decompensation from hypervolemia; and acute renal failure.

E. Evaluation
 1. Child achieves improved urinary output as evidenced by output 1 ml to 2 ml/kg per hour.
 2. Child has normal fluid balance as evidenced by decreasing edema, clear lung fields, and vital signs within range for age.
 3. Child has an improved nutritional state as evidenced by increased caloric intake and normal serum albumin level.
 4. Child is free from complications from hypertension or edema through ongoing assessment and early treatment.
 5. Child and family verbalize understanding of disease, treatment, and outcomes.

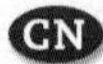

III. Client needs

A. Physiologic adaptation: Acute glomerulonephritis is identified early and managed supportively to prevent complications and restore near-normal to normal kidney function.
1. Recognize risk for crisis—indicated by hypertensive encephalopathy: Headache, dizziness, abdominal pain, and vomiting.
2. Evaluate the effectiveness of diuretics and sodium and water restriction in controlling edema and hypertension.

B. Management of care: Care of the child with acute glomerulonephritis requires critical thinking skills and knowledge of assessment, and teaching and evaluation methods unique to the RN role. These skills cannot be delegated to an LPN or UAP.
1. Perform comprehensive physical assessments and provide care appropriate to the child with acute glomerulonephritis.
2. Provide follow-up care to monitor for return of normal kidney function.
3. Delegate responsibly those activities that can be delegated, including measurements, oral intake and urine output, vital signs, and reporting child's subjective data. All monitoring information is reported to the RN.

C. Safety and infection control
1. Monitor edema and urine output.
   a. Maintain strict intake and output: Note volume and character of urine.
   b. Monitor daily weight.
   c. Measure urine specific gravity and protein levels.
2. Provide nutrition and diet appropriate to electrolyte levels.
   a. Refrain from adding salt.
   b. Restrict sodium in foods, as needed.
   c. Restrict potassium during oliguric phase.
   d. Restrict protein if child is azotemic.
   e. Restrict fluids when urine output is significantly reduced.
3. Monitor for complications: Hypertension.
   a. Monitor vital signs.
   b. Administer loop diuretics (see pharmacologic and parenteral therapies).
   c. Administer antihypertensives as indicated.
   d. Initiate seizure precautions.
4. Teach parents to report signs and symptoms of hematuria, headache, or increasing edema.
5. Teach child and parents to identify and avoid foods high in sodium, potassium, and protein.
   a. Sodium: Seafood, meat, chicken, canned and processed foods
   b. Potassium: Bananas, citrus fruit, meat, fish, peanut butter, potatoes, and coca cola
   c. Protein: Animal sources such as meat, chicken, and fish
6. Teach parents about home maintenance including activity, diet, and identification and prevention of infection.
7. Maintain the six rights of medication administration.

D. Health promotion and maintenance
1. Involve child in care to promote compliance with multiple procedures and therapeutic regimen.
2. Encourage child to participate in diet choices to promote nutritional intake.
3. Assist child and family in identifying need for follow-up, especially if home managed.
4. Teach child and family about procedures and treatment regimen.

E. Psychologic integrity
1. Provide diversional and recreational activities when energy is improved and edema subsides.
2. Offer parents and child a constant opportunity to express fears and concerns in coping with disease.
3. Provide parents with ongoing information about the child's progress.

F. Basic care and comfort
1. Provide consistent nurse caregiver.
2. Provide transitional comfort object if hospitalized.
3. Encourage parents to stay at bedside and participate in care.

G. Reduction of risk potential
1. Provide prompt and complete treatment of sore throats and impetigo.
2. Avoid medications that are nephrotoxic.

H. Pharmacologic and parenteral therapies: Child and family will state the purpose, dosage, timing, and side effects of loop diuretics: Furosemide (Lasix).
1. Expected outcome: Treats edema and manages hypertension.
2. Reduction of risk potential: Monitor potassium level, evaluate for U wave on ECG.
3. Management of care: Monitor vital signs and symptoms of hypokalemia; monitor intake and output.

Nephrotic Syndrome

I. Definition: Nephrotic syndrome is glomerular injury resulting in increased glomeruli permeability to protein resulting in massive proteinuria, hypoalbuminemia, and edema. The syndrome can be attributed to congenital, primary (idiopathic), or secondary types.

The most common form is minimal-change nephrotic syndrome. The syndrome typically is seen in preschool children through adolescence.

II. Nursing process

A. Assessment

1. Obtain a detailed health history, including recent viral upper respiratory illness.
2. Complete a detailed physical assessment, including vital signs, height and weight, and developmental level.
3. Assess for signs and symptoms of the onset of nephrotic syndrome.
   a. Weight gain
   b. Edema
      (1) Periorbital
      (2) Ascites
      (3) Legs and ankle edema
      (4) Labial or scrotal edema
      (5) Diarrhea and anorexia
   c. Urine dark, frothy, and decreased in amount
   d. Pallor
   e. Irritable
   f. BP normal
4. Obtain diagnostic tests.
   a. History and clinical findings
   b. Urinalysis
   c. Serum protein levels
   d. Serum sodium levels

B. Analysis

1. Fear related to procedures and strange environment
2. Interrupted Family Processes related to knowledge deficit about disease and management
3. Excess Fluid Volume related to compromised regulatory mechanism
4. Risk for Infection related to decreased immune response
5. Risk for Impaired Skin Integrity related to edema
6. Impaired Urinary Elimination: Altered patterns related to glomerular damage

C. Planning

1. Decrease edema.
2. Prevent infection.
3. Reduce fear.
4. Maintain skin integrity and prevent skin breakdown.
5. Improve urinary output.
6. Instruct parents about disease and treatment.

D. Implementation: Provide interventions to reduce excretion of protein.

1. Offer diet low in sodium, fat, and sugar; offer nutritional supplements, if needed.
2. Administer corticosteroids per dosing schedule as ordered. Prednisone is drug of choice. Drugs must be discontinued slowly over 6 to 8 weeks' time.
3. Administer immunosuppressants such as cyclophosphamide (Cytoxan) as ordered; used when child becomes steroid-resistant or has frequent relapses.
4. Administer diuretics.

E. Evaluation

1. Child's urinary elimination is optimized as evidenced by decreased edema and urine output of at least 1 to 2 ml/kg per hour.
2. Child's fear is reduced as evidenced by child's ability to sleep, be comforted, and compliant with treatment.
3. Child's skin integrity is maintained as evidenced by no areas of breakdown.
4. Parents verbalize understanding of treatment regimen and are involved in care.

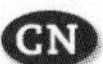

III. Client needs

A. Physiologic adaptation: Nephrotic syndrome is managed with diet, steroids, and immunosuppressants with complete remission, urine maintained protein-free, and no evidence of exacerbation.

1. Evaluate effectiveness of corticosteroids and immunosuppressants to reduce edema, reduce proteinuria, increase urine output, and restore renal function evidenced by absence of edema, return of normal urine output, and protein-free urine.
2. Recognize risk for decrease in tissue perfusion—indicated by kidney leading to end-stage renal disease: Nausea, decreasing urine output to 50 ml or less per 24 hr, azotemia, and metabolic acidosis.
3. Evaluate CBC and electrolytes to monitor for infection and electrolyte abnormalities.

B. Management of care: Care of the child with nephrotic syndrome requires critical thinking skills and knowledge of assessment, and teaching and evaluation methods unique to the RN role. These skills cannot be delegated to an LPN or UAP.

1. Perform comprehensive physical assessments and provide care appropriate to the child with nephrotic syndrome.
2. Select roommates carefully for child that is edematous and taking corticosteroids.
3. Provide follow-up care to identify exacerbations and initiate treatment.
4. Assess for home needs such as urine tests for protein.
5. Delegate responsibly those activities that can be delegated, including measurements, oral intake and urine output, vital signs, and reporting child's subjective data. All

monitoring information must be reported to the RN.

C. Safety and infection control
   1. Monitor urine status and edema.
      a. Monitor intake and output.
      b. Monitor daily weights.
      c. Monitor urine for albumin and specific gravity: Test first morning specimen—high specific indicates ongoing disease process.
      d. Measure abdominal girth.
   2. Manage edema.
      a. Provide skin care and frequent repositioning.
      b. Support edematous legs or scrotum.
      c. Avoid use of adhesive on skin.
      d. Cleanse opposing skin areas—use antiseptic powder or cotton.
   3. Institute regular diet with no added salt—restrict salt for massive edema.
   4. Observe for signs and symptoms of infection; treat infection with antibiotics.
   5. Teach parents to anticipate diuresis in 1 to 3 weeks and how to manage.
   6. Teach parents about discharge management at home.
      a. Test urine for albumin.
      b. Administer medications.
         (1) Administer corticosteroids until urine is protein-free for 10 days to 2 weeks.
         (2) Administer immunosuppressants to reduce relapse and promote long-term remission.
      c. Observe for side effects of medications.
      d. Observe for signs and symptoms of infection.
      e. Monitor for signs of relapse (discuss when to seek medical attention).
   7. Maintain the six rights of medication administration.

D. Health promotion and maintenance
   1. Involve child in care to promote compliance with long therapeutic regimen.
   2. Encourage child to participate in diet choices to promote nutritional intake.
   3. Assist child and family in identifying relapse symptoms and need for immediate health care.
   4. Teach child self-care at home, such as monitoring urine testing.

E. Psychologic integrity
   1. Encourage diversional and recreational activities when energy is improved and edema subsides.
   2. Offer parents and child a constant opportunity to express fears and concerns in coping with disease.

F. Basic care and comfort
   1. Provide consistent nurse caregiver.
   2. Provide transitional comfort object if hospitalized.
   3. Encourage parents to stay at bedside and participate in care.

G. Reduction of risk potential
   1. While taking corticosteroids and immunosuppressants:
      a. Avoid others who are infectious.
      b. Advise about high risk of sterility.
   2. Promote bed rest and hydration during diuresis phase.

H. Pharmacologic and parenteral therapies: Child and family will state the purpose, dosage, timing, and side effects of the following:
   1. Corticosteroids: Prednisone (Deltasone)
      a. Expected outcome: Treats inflammatory conditions.
      b. Reduction of risk potential: Monitor BP for ascension; assess for delayed wound healing; monitor weight.
      c. Management of care: Teach parents to weigh daily; monitor for gastric distress; avoid use of aspirin-containing products.
   2. Immunosuppressant: Cyclophosphamide (Cytoxan)
      a. Expected outcome: Treats nephrotic syndrome to suppress inflammatory response.
      b. Reduction of risk potential: Monitor for bleeding; monitor for infection.
      c. Management of care: Teach about side effects—nausea, vomiting, stomatitis, alopecia.

Acute Renal Failure

I. Definition: Acute renal failure is the sudden loss of kidney function resulting from the inability of the kidneys to regulate the composition of urine in response to the child's physiologic needs. Causes are defined as prerenal (related to hypovolemia such as dehydration, burns, or shock); intrarenal (caused by vascular disorders, tubular nephropathy, or nephritis, resulting in decreased glomerular filtration); and postrenal (caused by obstruction to flow of urine). The most common cause for acute renal failure in children is hypoperfusion of the kidneys as a result of dehydration, but the disorder can occur as a result of injury or other conditions. Progression occurs in four phases: Initiating phase (when kidney is injured and lasts from hours to days), oliguric phase (8 to 15 days), diuresis phase, and recovery phase (1 to 2 years). (See also Chapter 28.)

II. Nursing process
  A. Assessment
    1. Obtain a detailed health history, including present illness; medications, particularly those that are nephrotoxic such as penicillins, sulphonamides, antineoplastic drugs; exposure to toxins; and recent blood loss.
    2. Perform a detailed physical assessment including vital signs, height and weight, and developmental level.
    3. Assess for signs and symptoms during oliguric phase.
      a. Oligoanuria: Less than 1 ml/kg per hour or 300 ml/m^2
      b. Edema
      c. Sleepiness
      d. Anorexia, nausea, and vomiting
      e. Hypertension
      f. Symptoms of congestive heart failure
      g. Dysrhythmias
      h. Acidosis
    4. Assess for signs and symptoms during diuresis phase.
      a. Urine output increases over several days
      b. Tachycardia and hypotension
      c. Child is less sleepy
    5. Assess for signs and symptoms during recovery phase.
      a. Urine output normal
      b. Normal level of consciousness
      c. Child's strength improves
    6. Obtain diagnostic tests.
      a. History and physical examination
      b. Serum electrolytes
      c. Arterial blood gas analysis
      d. Urinalysis
  B. Analysis
    1. Anxiety related to declining level of consciousness, procedures, and critical care environment
    2. Risk for Decreased Cardiac Output related to fluid overload and dysrhythmias
    3. Excess Fluid Volume related to compromised regulatory mechanism
    4. Risk for Injury: Anemia, related to increased hemolysis
    5. Risk for Infection related to decreased immune response and poor nutrition
    6. Deficient Knowledge: Disease Process, related to multiple new physical needs
    7. Imbalanced Nutrition: Less Than Body Requirements related to anorexia and vomiting
    8. Risk for Ineffective Family Therapeutic Regimen Management related to complexity of disease and treatment regimen
    9. Impaired Urinary Elimination: Altered patterns, related to kidney hypoperfusion
  C. Planning
    1. Reduce anxiety.
    2. Reduce fluid overload and improve urinary output.
    3. Prevent complications associated with anemia, infection, and electrolyte disturbance.
    4. Provide child and family teaching about procedures, treatment, and outcome.
    5. Maintain and improve nutritional status.
  D. Implementation: Provide interventions to manage acute renal failure.
    1. Manage underlying cause.
    2. Provide supportive care.
    3. Prevent and manage complications.
  E. Evaluation
    1. Child achieves improved urinary output as evidenced by output 1 ml to 2 ml/kg per hour.
    2. Child has normal fluid balance as evidenced by decreasing circulatory congestion, clear lung fields, and vital signs within range for age.
    3. Child has normal cardiac output as evidenced by strong peripheral pulses, absence of dysrhythmias, and normal BP for age.
    4. Child has an improved nutritional state as evidenced by increased caloric intake and normal serum albumin level.
    5. Child is free from complications from anemia, electrolyte disturbance, or infection as a result of ongoing assessment and early treatment.
    6. Child and family verbalize understanding of disease, treatment, and outcomes.

CN

III. Client needs
  A. Physiologic adaptation: Acute renal failure is identified early and managed supportively to prevent complications and restore near-normal to normal kidney function.
    1. Recognize risk for decrease in cardiac output—indicated by decreased level of consciousness, hypotension, tachycardia, presence of S_3, crackles, decreased peripheral pulses, jugular vein distention.
    2. Recognize risk for electrolyte abnormality: Hyponatremia—indicated by nausea and vomiting, lethargy, serum sodium 115 mEq/L or less.
    3. Recognize risk for electrolyte abnormality: Hyperkalemia—indicated by bradycardia, elevated T wave, prolonged P-R interval, serum potassium 5.5 mEq/L or more.
    4. Recognize risk for dehydration and metabolic acidosis—indicated by percentage loss of body weight, irritability, poor skin

turgor, prolonged capillary refill 2 s or more, tachycardia, deep rapid respirations, absent tears, dry mucous membranes, plasma pH less than 7.33, and decreased plasma HCO_3.

B. Management of care: Care of the child with acute renal failure requires critical thinking skills and knowledge of assessment, and teaching and evaluation methods unique to the RN role. These skills cannot be delegated to an LPN or UAP.
   1. Perform comprehensive physical assessments and provide care appropriate to the child with acute renal failure.
   2. Provide follow-up care to monitor for return of normal kidney function.
   3. Follow careful assignment protocol: No staff, visitors, or roommates that may be infectious.
   4. Delegate responsibly those activities that can be delegated, including measurements, oral intake and urine output, vital signs, and reporting child's subjective data. All monitoring information is reported to the RN.

C. Safety and infection control
   1. Monitor urine output and edema.
      a. Monitor intake and output hourly.
      b. Monitor daily weight: 1 kg of weight gain equals 1 liter of fluid retained.
      c. Monitor specific gravity.
      d. Monitor for signs of congestive heart failure.
         (1) Assess lung sounds.
         (2) Assess heart sounds.
   2. Monitor blood and urine laboratory tests.
      a. Sodium
      b. Potassium
      c. Calcium
      d. BUN and creatinine
      e. Blood gas
   3. Monitor vital signs and manage hypertension.
      a. Maintain fluid and sodium restriction.
      b. Administer diuretics and antihypertensives, as needed.
   4. Manage hyperkalemia.
      a. Administer medications to shift potassium into cell.
         (1) IV sodium bicarbonate
         (2) IV calcium gluconate
         (3) IV glucose, 50% and insulin drip
      b. Administer medication to bind with potassium and remove from body: Potassium exchange resins—sodium polystyrene sulfonate (Kayexalate).
      c. Remove potassium from body: Renal replacement therapy.
   5. Manage anemia.
      a. Monitor serum BUN.
      b. Administer iron supplements.
      c. Administer epoetin alfa (Epogen).
   6. Protect from infection.
      a. Assess all sites such as IV, Foley, and pulmonary.
      b. Monitor vital signs, especially temperature.
      c. Monitor WBC count.
      d. Provide strict skin and perineal care.
      e. Practice good hand hygiene and aseptic technique.
      f. Select appropriate roommate or caregiver.
   7. Provide diet appropriate to appetite, age, and electrolyte status.
      a. Promote diet high in carbohydrates, low in protein.
      b. Restrict potassium, sodium, and phosphorous.
      c. Administer fluids based on urine output, and regulate hourly—maintain zero water balance.
   8. Prepare child and family for treatment regimen.
      a. Evaluate education, cognitive, and developmental level.
      b. Explain all tests, procedures, and evaluate understanding.
      c. Explain renal replacement therapy.
      d. Discuss need for and importance of follow-up.
   9. Maintain the six rights of medication administration.

D. Health promotion and maintenance
   1. Involve child in care to promote compliance with multiple procedures and long therapeutic regimen.
   2. Encourage child to participate in diet choices to promote nutritional intake.
   3. Assist child and family in identifying need for follow-up for 1 to 2 years.
   4. Teach child and family about procedures and treatment regimen.

E. Psychologic integrity
   1. Provide diversional and recreational activities when energy is improved and edema subsides.
   2. Offer parents and child a constant opportunity to express fears and concerns in coping with disease.
   3. Provide parents with ongoing information about the child's progress.

F. Basic care and comfort
   1. Provide consistent nurse caregiver.
   2. Provide transitional comfort object if hospitalized.

Table 16-2 Drugs Used to Treat Complications of Acute Renal Failure

Classification	Generic/Trade Name	Expected Outcome	Reduction of Risk Potential	Management of Care
Fluid and Electrolyte Agent	Calcium gluconate (Kalcinate)	Treats cardiac toxicity from hyperkalemia.	Monitor for tingling, hypotension, and bradycardia. Monitor ECG for decreased QT interval. Monitor serum calcium levels.	Observe for symptoms of hypocalcemia and hypercalcemia.
Ion Exchange Resin	Sodium polystyrene sulfonate (Kayexalate)	Cation exchange resin binds with intestinal potassium and removes from body.	Monitor for diarrhea, vomiting, and anorexia. Monitor serum potassium levels.	Manage diarrhea and prevent skin breakdown.
Hematopoietic Growth Factor	Epoetin alfa (Epogen)	Elevates hematocrit.	Monitor activated partial thromboplastin time (aPTT) and initialized normal ration (INR). Monitor hematocrit levels.	Monitor closely for hypertension. Monitor for neurologic symptoms such as complaints of an aura.

3. Encourage parents to stay at bedside and participate in care.

G. Reduction of risk potential
1. Identify children at high risk and provide early interventions.
2. Use caution when administering nephrotoxic drugs.
3. Monitor for fixed specific gravity of urine, indicating further kidney damage.

H. Pharmacologic and parenteral therapies: Child and family will state the purpose, dosage, timing, and side effects of medications to treat complications of acute renal failure (Table 16-2).

Bibliography

Hatfield, N. (2006). *Broadribb's introductory pediatric nursing.* Philadelphia: Lippincott Williams & Wilkins.

Pillitteri, A. (2006). *Maternal & child health nursing: Care of the childbearing and childrearing family* (5th ed.). Philadelphia: Lippincott Williams & Wilkins.

Wong, D. L., et al. (2006). *Maternal child nursing care.* St. Louis: Mosby.

CHAPTER 16
Practice Test

Urinary Tract Infection

1. Which one of the following infants is most at risk for a UTI?
- □ 1. Female infant who has a twin.
- □ 2. Male infant who was circumcised.
- □ 3. Female infant who delivered at 37 weeks' gestation.
- □ 4. Male infant who remains uncircumcised.

2. AF A female client who is 4 years of age has had three UTIs in the last 6 months. To prevent further UTIs, the nurse should teach the mother to do which of the following? Select all that apply.
- □ 1. Encourage the child to be more active to increase urine output.
- □ 2. Offer fluids frequently throughout the day.
- □ 3. Have the child take tub baths to clean her perineal area.
- □ 4. Avoid use of public toilets.
- □ 5. Teach her to wipe her perineum front to back after voiding.

3. The nurse is teaching a child who is 4 years of age about having a urinary catheterization procedure. Which approach will be most effective in teaching this child about the procedure?
- □ 1. Demonstrate the procedure using an age-appropriate doll.
- □ 2. Explain where the catheter will be inserted.
- □ 3. Draw a diagram of the urinary tract system and catheter.
- □ 4. Tell a story about a child having a catheterization.

4. AF The nurse is teaching the mother of a child who is taking nitrofurantoin (Macrodantin) for a UTI about how to administer the drug. The nurse should include which of the following in the teaching plan? Select all that apply.
- □ 1. Restrict fluids.
- □ 2. Give with milk.
- □ 3. Report oliguria.
- □ 4. Expect yellow-brown urine.
- □ 5. Apply lotion to rash.

Cryptorchidism

5. While caring for a neonate with cryptorchidism, the nurse tells the parents that the purpose of treatment with orchiopexy is to:
- □ 1. Prevent psychologic disability from the empty scrotum.
- □ 2. Close the inguinal canal.
- □ 3. Avoid torsion of the testicle.
- □ 4. Decrease the incidence of testicular cancer and sterility.

Hypospadias and Epispadias

6. Parents are considering not consenting to surgical repair of their infant's hypospadias. The nurse should be sure that the parents understand which of the following difficulties could be anticipated in the future? Their boy will have:
- □ 1. Painful urination.
- □ 2. Growth delay of the genitals.
- □ 3. Inability to correct the defect in the future.
- □ 4. Difficulty standing to void.

7. A child has had a surgical correction of a hypospadias. Following surgery the nurse should report which of the following to the HCP?
- □ 1. Urine output from catheter is 4 ml/kg per hour.
- □ 2. The child has not voided within 6 hr of removing the catheter.
- □ 3. The child has pain in the penis.
- □ 4. The drainage from the catheter is blood-tinged.

Wilms Tumor

8. The nurse is planning care for a child who has Wilms tumor. Preoperatively, the nurse should post a sign above that bed to remind staff of which of the following?
- □ 1. "Do not examine throat."
- □ 2. "No blood pressures in upper extremities."
- □ 3. "Provide child with frequent rest periods."
- □ 4. "Do not palpate abdomen."

9. The nurse is providing teaching to the parents of a child who is 10 years of age who has had a nephrectomy to remove a Wilms tumor. The nurse should instruct the parents that the child should:
- □ 1. Avoid contact sports.
- □ 2. Reduce fluid intake.
- □ 3. Avoid adding salt to food.
- □ 4. Stay out of swimming pools.

Glomerulonephritis

10. AF The nurse is assessing a child who is 6 years of age with possible APSGN. The nurse should report which of the following to the HCP? Select all that apply.
- □ 1. Orbital edema.
- □ 2. Increased appetite.
- □ 3. Frequent urination.
- □ 4. Loss of appetite.
- □ 5. Dark-colored urine.
- □ 6. Antecedent streptococcal infection.

11. The nurse is helping the parents plan a diet for their child with APSGN. Which of the following diets is most appropriate?
- □ 1. Regular diet with no added salt.
- □ 2. High-protein diet.
- □ 3. Low-carbohydrate diet.
- □ 4. Regular diet with no added sugar.

12. AF A child who is 15 years of age is hospitalized with acute glomerulonephritis. The nurse is reviewing the client's urine chemistry laboratory reports as noted below.

LABORATORY RESULTS

Test	Result
Urine specific gravity	1.030
Protein	8 g/dl
Potassium	35 mEq
Creatinine	2 mg/dl

Which of the findings does the nurse draw to the attention of the HCP?

□ 1. Urine specific gravity.
□ 2. Protein.
□ 3. Potassium.
□ 4. Creatinine.

Nephrotic Syndrome

13. A child who is 4 years of age with nephrotic syndrome is experiencing severe periorbital edema. To reduce periorbital edema the nurse should:
□ 1. Apply cool, sterile soaks to child's head.
□ 2. Encourage child to eat low-protein foods.
□ 3. Apply warm compresses to child's eyes at bedtime.
□ 4. Elevate the head of the bed.

14. The best site to administer an IM injection to a child with nephrotic syndrome is:
□ 1. Deltoid.
□ 2. Dorsal gluteal.
□ 3. Gluteus maximus.
□ 4. Ventral-gluteal.

15. A child who is 8 years of age is admitted to the hospital and diagnosed with nephrotic syndrome. The child is pale and lethargic, and has ascites. To determine if ascites is increasing, the nurse should:
□ 1. Measure abdominal girth.
□ 2. Weigh the child.
□ 3. Track changes in the BP.
□ 4. Assess bowel sounds.

16. A child who is 10 years of age with nephrotic syndrome has ascites. The child's respirations are 28 to 30 per minute and labored. The nurse should do which of the following first?
□ 1. Notify the HCP.
□ 2. Elevate the head of the bed.
□ 3. Restrict fluids to 30 ml/hr.
□ 4. Prepare for an abdominal paracentesis.

Acute Renal Failure

17. AF A teenager with acute renal failure has an arteriovenous shunt in place for hemodialysis. Which of the following activities are appropriate for this client? Select all that apply.
□ 1. Video games.
□ 2. Jogging.
□ 3. Swimming.
□ 4. Roller blading.
□ 5. Soccer.

18. The nurse is assessing an adolescent who is in the oliguric stage of acute renal failure. The child weighs 100 kg. Which of the following indicates that treatment is effective?
□ 1. The child has gained 2 kg.
□ 2. The urine output is 300 ml/hr.
□ 3. The respirations are 14.
□ 4. The heart rate is 100.

19. The nurse is assessing the extent of generalized edema for a child with acute renal failure. Which of the following is the most effective way to assess this child for edema?
□ 1. Document changes in vital signs.
□ 2. Note swelling around the eyes.
□ 3. Measure abdominal girth.
□ 4. Track changes in daily weight.

20. The nurse is planning care for a child with renal failure who is receiving epoetin alfa (Epogen). Which of the following is an expected outcome of this drug?
□ 1. Increased glomerular filtration rate.
□ 2. Increased RBC count.
□ 3. Normal urinary output.
□ 4. Normal potassium levels.

Answers and Rationales

1. 4 Considerable evidence suggests there are fewer UTIs among circumcised male infants than among uncircumcised male infants. However, the difference is not significant enough for the American Academy of Pediatrics to recommend routine circumcision in newborn males. Overall, the incidence of UTIs in newborns is low. (H)

2. 2, 5 *E. coli* is easily spread from the rectum to the urinary meatus and causes UTI; therefore, the nurse instructs the mother to teach the child to wipe her perineum from front to back. Increasing fluid intake increases urinary output and works to flush out bacteria. Being ambulatory does not increase urine output; tub baths are a source of spread of bacteria to the meatus and urinary tract. UTIs are not spread on toilet seats. (H)

3. 1 For preschool-aged children, the procedure is explained using a doll. For those who are older, a simple drawing of the bladder, urethra, ureters, and kidneys makes the procedure more understandable. Precise details of anatomic functions are best reserved for the older school-aged child and/or adolescent, when appropriate. Telling a story may cause the child to imagine the procedure to be more complicated; the doll is a concrete way to explain what the procedure involves. (H)

4. 2, 3, 4 Instruct the mother to give nitrofurantoin with milk or food. The drug may cause oliguria (which is reported to the HCP), as well as a yellow-brown coloring of urine (normal effect). The nurse teaches the mother to provide an adequate fluid intake. Rash is not a common side effect, but if it does occur, instruct the mother to notify the HCP immediately as it may be a sign of an allergic reaction. (D)

5. 4 Cryptorchidism is seen in 3% of full-term infant boys. Infertility and testicular cancer are the biggest risks for a child with cryptorchidism. Children who have had an undiagnosed and untreated cryptorchidism have a 22% increase in testicular cancers compared to the general population. Treatment typically waits until a child reaches 3 years of age because there is still the chance of a spontaneous resolution until that time. The procedure does not prevent psychologic trauma, close the inguinal canal, or avoid torsion of the testicle. (M)

6. 4 Although there are no problems with voiding or growth of the genitals, the boy will have difficulty standing to void because of the location of the urethra on the underside of the penis. Other difficulties include self-concept issues and embarrassment, and delay of surgery may be additionally painful for the male child because of physical maturation. (H)

7. 2 The nurse notifies the HCP if the child has not voided within 6 hr of removing the catheter because the absence of voiding may indicate an obstruction. A urine output of 4 ml/kg per hour is normal; if the urine output is less than 2 ml/kg per hour the nurse notifies the HCP. Drainage from the catheter may be blood-tinged, which is considered normal; the nurse reports the presence of clots. Pain in the penis is normal postoperative pain; the nurse reports bladder distention or bladder spasms. (C)

8. 4 Preoperatively, the most important concern is that the tumor is not palpated unless absolutely necessary because manipulation of the tumor mass may cause dissemination of cancer cells to near and distant organs and sites. The sign for the throat is the most appropriate for a child with epiglottitis. Rest is always important, but not most important. Taking the BP in the upper extremities is not of concern with this client. (M)

9. 1 Because the child has one kidney, the child is instructed to avoid contact sports to prevent injury to the remaining organ. Prompt detection and treatment of any signs of genitourinary infection is also important. The nurse promotes adequate fluid intake and a normal diet. Swimming is an ideal sport for this child as it does not involve body contact or risk for injury. (S)

10. 1, 4, 5, 6 Orbital edema, loss of appetite, dark-colored urine preceded by a streptococcal infection are indications of APSGN. The nurse alerts the HCP to the presence of these symptoms. An increased appetite and frequent urination are not associated with APSGN. (S)

11. 1 With APSGN there is a decrease in plasma filtration, resulting in excessive accumulation of water and retention of sodium that expands plasma and interstitial fluid volumes, leading to circulatory congestion and edema. For most children with APSGN, a regular diet is allowed, but should not contain any added salt. Foods high in sodium and salted treats are eliminated, and parents are advised not to give snacks such as potato chips or pretzels. Typically, the total amount of salt ingested is usually less than prescribed because of the child's poor appetite. Protein loss is not an issue with APSGN. Carbohydrate and sugar content does not require specific attention with APSGN. (H)

12. 1 The nurse verifies that the HCP has noted the elevated specific gravity. Clients with glomerulonephritis have concentrated urine from oliguria caused by the inflammation of the glomeruli. The other laboratory results are in normal range. (A)

13. 4 As edema tends to be dependent, elevating an edematous body part usually reduces swelling. Periorbital edema is the most common location of edema in children with renal problems. Eating low-protein foods will not reduce the swelling. The warm or cool compresses will not reduce the swelling as effectively as elevating the head of the bed. (C)

14. 1 Administering injections into an edematous body part leads to poor drug absorption. Selecting a site high in the body reduces the possibility of edema being present. (D)

15. 1 Ascites is accumulation of fluid in the abdominal cavity and is noted by an increasing abdominal size. Although the child may be gaining weight, weighing the child does not indicate where the fluid is accumulating. The child may have vomiting and diarrhea, but assessing the bowel sounds does not indicate the extent of the increasing ascites. (A)

16. 2 The child is having difficult breathing because of ascites. High Fowler position (sitting upright) allows ascites fluid to settle downward and not press against the diaphragm, compromising breathing. It is not necessary to notify the HCP or restrict fluids, as the dyspnea is a result of the ascites. Diuretics and IV 25% albumin may be ordered to treat the ascites by promoting the fluid shift from the interstitial space into the circulatory system. An abdominal paracentesis is not required. (A)

17. 1, 2, 4 The child with an arteriovenous shunt in place is instructed to avoid sports such as soccer that could accidentally cause the shunt to dislodge, and swimming, which could introduce the possibility of infection at the shunt site. Video games, jogging, and roller blading are appropriate as long as the shunt is protected. (H)

18. 2 During the oliguric stage of acute renal failure, the goal is to increase urine output to 3 to 4 ml/kg per hour. Weight gain does not indicate increased urine output. The respirations and heart rate are within normal limits. (A)

19. 4 Weight gain is the most effective way to monitor edema; a weight gain of 1 kg is equivalent to 1 liter of body fluid. Although the child may have changes in vital signs and edema, the edema is generalized, and changes in the edema are best monitored by changes in weight. (A)

20. 2 Epoetin alfa (Epogen) is used in clients with acute renal failure to correct anemia; the RBC count should increase and the hemoglobin and hematocrit return to normal levels. Epoetin alfa does not affect the glomerular filtration rate, urine concentration, or potassium levels. (D)

chapter

17 The Child With Neurologic Health Problems

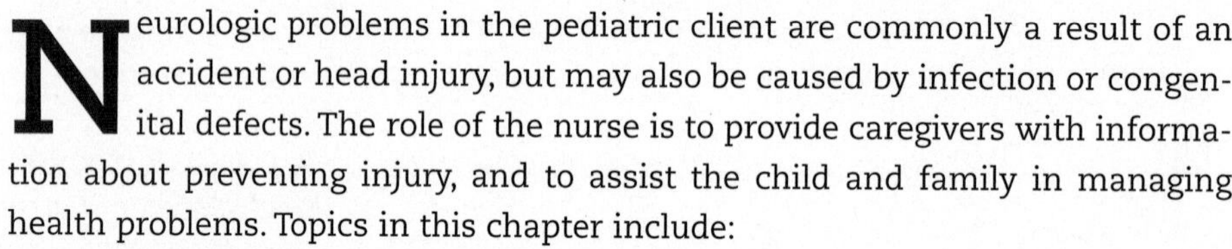

Neurologic problems in the pediatric client are commonly a result of an accident or head injury, but may also be caused by infection or congenital defects. The role of the nurse is to provide caregivers with information about preventing injury, and to assist the child and family in managing health problems. Topics in this chapter include:

- Head Injury
- Myelomeningocele
- Hydrocephalus
- Seizure Disorder
- Meningitis
- Down Syndrome

Head Injury

I. Definition: Head injuries involve traumatic processes causing damage to the scalp, skull, meninges, and/or brain. Types of head injuries include fractures, lacerations, concussions, and contusions. Table 17-1 provides a brief description of each type of head injury. Complications of head injuries are a result of cerebral bleeding, hematomas, fractures, or increased intracranial pressure (ICP), which is a result of head trauma and hemorrhage causing swelling and impeding circulation to the brain.

II. Nursing process

A. Assessment

1. Complete a detailed health history and physical assessment to rule out drug allergies, hemophilia, diabetes mellitus, or epilepsy, which may present with similar symptoms; include in assessment history and description of trauma including falls, motor vehicle and bicycle accidents, and questions about physical abuse.
2. Assess for signs and symptoms of hematomas (usually a result of increased ICP).
   a. Change in level of consciousness (LOC): Restlessness is first sign
   b. Headache, nausea, and vomiting
   c. Pupillary changes and papilledema
   d. Tense, bulging fontanels
   e. Decreased appetite
3. Assess for signs and symptoms of head injury.
   a. Rhinorrhea
   b. Otorrhea
   c. Battle sign
   d. Raccoon eyes
4. Obtain diagnostic tests.
   a. History and physical examination
   b. Pediatric Glasgow coma scale (GCS)
   c. Emergency evaluation in the field
   d. Head radiograph
   e. Lateral neck radiograph
   f. CT scan and MRI of head

B. Analysis

1. Risk for Ineffective Airway Clearance related to decreased LOC or depressed respirations
2. Anxiety related to change in LOC and unfamiliar environment
3. Risk for Deficient Fluid Volume related to vomiting and hyperosmotic agents
4. Risk for Excess Fluid Volume related to free water excess
5. Decreased Intracranial Adaptive Capacity: Altered LOC, related to increased cerebral perfusion
6. Risk for Injury: Seizures, related to intracranial bleeding or hypoxia
7. Deficient Knowledge related to no prior experience with head injury
8. Risk for Imbalanced Nutrition: Less Than Body Requirements related to altered LOC

C. Planning

1. Maintain cerebral perfusion.
2. Prevent complications of cerebral trauma and edema.
3. Reduce anxiety.
4. Maintain fluid volume.
5. Maintain patent airway.
6. Prevent injury.
7. Maintain nutritional intake.
8. Provide child and family teaching and emotional support.
9. Promote growth and development.

D. Implementation

1. Provide interventions to treat head injury.
   a. Mild-to-moderate injury with transient of consciousness is managed in home setting.
   b. For severe injury and loss of consciousness:
      (1) Maintain IV fluids if NPO, vomiting, or unconscious.
      (2) Manage fluid balance: Strict intake and output measurement.
      (3) Administer medications as indicated by type of injury and symptoms.
      (4) Prepare for possible surgical intervention.
2. Provide interventions to treat increased ICP.
   a. Monitor ICP.
   b. Administer osmotic diuretics.

Table 17-1 Types of Head Injuries

Type of Injury	Description
Concussion	Jarring of the brain causing a temporary neurologic dysfunction
Contusion	Bruising injury to the brain with superficial petechial hemorrhage
Epidural hematoma	Rapid, arterial bleeding between dura and skull
Subdural hematoma	Slow, venous bleeding between dura and cerebrum
Intracerebral hemorrhage	Bleeding into brain
Fractures	A disruption of the cranial bones. Needs more force because of cranial flexibility; types include basilar, depressed, and linear.

3. Provide interventions to prevent increased ICP: Minimize crying, limit suctioning, and position child to avoid neck vein compression.

E. Evaluation
1. Child's cerebral perfusion is maintained as evidenced by GCS of greater than 13.
2. Child exhibits no evidence of secondary neurologic damage such as cerebral ischemia, hypoxia, or herniation.
3. Child maintains optimum fluid volume as evidenced by urine output of 1 to 2 ml/kg per hour and urine specific gravity between 1.010 and 1.025.
4. Child's anxiety is reduced as evidenced by ability to rest, be comforted, and tolerate procedures and treatment.
5. Child maintains patent airway as evidenced by normal respirations, clear lung sounds, and normal arterial blood gas.
6. Child is free from injury as evidenced by absence of seizure activity.
7. Child maintains good nutritional intake as evidenced by good skin turgor, normal body weight, and normal serum albumin levels.
8. Child and family verbalize understanding of head injury, treatment, and possible outcome.

III. Client needs

A. Physiologic adaptation: Minor head injury is treated on an outpatient basis with adequate follow-up care. Severe head injury and increased ICP are managed in intensive care with monitoring of neurologic status, reduction of stimuli, and administration of osmotic diuretics to reduce neurologic sequelae.
1. Recognize risk for decreased intracranial adaptive capacity: Potential herniation—indicated by increased BP with widened pulse pressure and bradycardia.
2. Recognize risk for complication of increased ICP: Diabetes insipidus—indicated by urine output more than 200 ml/hr for 2 hr and specific gravity of urine less than 1.005.
3. Recognize risk for child abuse—indicated by subdural hematomas and retinal hemorrhage.
4. Prepare child for surgery on positive assessment findings of asymmetric pupils and declining neurologic status.

B. Management of care: Care of the child with a head injury and increased ICP requires critical thinking skills and knowledge of assessment, and teaching and evaluation methods unique to the RN role. These skills cannot be delegated to an LPN or UAP.
1. Perform comprehensive physical assessments and provide care appropriate to the child with a head injury and increased ICP.
2. Provide follow-up care within 1 to 2 days for children managed in home setting.
3. Assess home needs for the child with neurologic sequelae such as need for modifications to home, need for adaptive devices, and possible wheelchair accessibility of home.
4. Identify community resources such as local support groups for parents, equipment services, and educational support for the child.
5. Delegate responsibly those activities that can be delegated, including measurements, oral intake and urine output, vital signs, and reporting the child's subjective data. All monitoring information is reported to the RN.

C. Safety and infection control
1. Assess and document neurologic status using the pediatric GCS, including pupillary function and speech.
2. Assess neurologic reflexes.
   a. Gag
   b. Babinski
   c. Cough
   d. Startle
3. Monitor for evidence of increased ICP.
   a. Monitor vital signs.
   b. Monitor ICP via intracranial catheter: Normal is less than 15 mmHg.
   c. Calculate cerebral perfusion pressure (CPP): Mean systemic arterial pressure minus ICP—Normal is 80 to 100 mmHg.
   d. Monitor urine output for evidence of decreased CPP: Less than 0.5 ml/kg per hour.
4. Manage increased ICP.
   a. Elevate head of bed 30 degrees.
   b. Maintain child's head in neutral position.
   c. Provide nonstimulating environment.
   d. Hold nursing activities until ICP less than 15 mmHg.
      (1) Avoid suctioning, if possible.
      (2) Avoid repositioning.
      (3) Minimize painful activities.
   e. Administer hyperosmotic agents.
   f. Avoid hip and neck flexion.
   g. Avoid stimulating Valsalva maneuver—avoid suctioning if possible; intervene if child is straining or has constipation.
   h. Hyperoxygenate and hyperventilate: Maintain PCO_2 at 25 to 30 mmHg.

i. Administer short-acting pain medication for painful procedures.
j. Maintain normothermic state—administer antipyretics; provide hypothermia blanket.

5. Maintain cerebral tissue perfusion.
   a. Monitor and record GCS including pupillary reaction and size.
   b. Evaluate presence of protective reflexes such as gag and cough.
   c. Elevate head of bed 30 to 45 degrees.
   d. Reorient as needed.
   e. Administer hyperosmotic medications such as mannitol.
6. Assess and manage cerebrospinal fluid (CSF) leak.
   a. Test for positive response on glucose strip for any clear fluid from nose and ears.
   b. Manage with antibiotics.
   c. Avoid blowing nose or cleaning ear.
   d. Notify physician on indication of CSF leak.
7. Manage fluid volume.
   a. Monitor intake and output.
   b. Assess specific gravity.
   c. Monitor for dehydration or overhydration.
   d. Measure daily weights.
8. Maintain airway.
   a. Monitor lung sounds and quality of respirations.
   b. Monitor arterial blood gases.
   c. Reposition, suction, and oxygen unless at risk for increased ICP.
9. Protect from injury: Seizures.
   a. Observe and record all seizure activity.
   b. Initiate seizure precautions.
10. Provide diet appropriate to appetite, age, and neurologic status.
   a. Monitor albumin, protein, and BUN.
   b. Assess skin turgor.
   c. Observe for evidence of infection.
   d. Administer tube feedings of TPN.
   e. Elevate head of bed 30 degrees.
11. Prepare child and family for treatment regimen.
   a. Evaluate education, cognitive, and developmental level.
   b. Explain all tests, procedures, and evaluate understanding.
   c. Prepare for intensive care unit stay.
   d. Discuss need for and importance of posthospitalization follow-up.
12. Maintain the six rights of medication administration.

D. Health promotion and maintenance
   1. Involve child in care to promote compliance with multiple procedures and involved therapeutic regimen.
   2. Encourage child to participate in fluid and diet choices to promote nutritional intake.
   3. Assist child and family in identifying need for follow-up.
   4. Instruct child and family about procedures and treatment regimen.

E. Psychologic integrity
   1. Provide quiet diversional and recreational activities when energy is improved and edema subsides.
   2. Offer parents and child a constant opportunity to express fears and concerns in coping with injury and possible sequelae.
   3. Provide parents with ongoing information about child's progress.

F. Basic care and comfort
   1. Provide consistent nurse caregiver.
   2. Provide transitional comfort object if child is hospitalized.
   3. Encourage parents to stay at bedside and participate in care.
   4. Administer acetaminophen (Tylenol) for headache (avoid use of narcotic analgesia).

G. Reduction of risk potential
   1. Stabilize neck until lateral neck spinal cord injury is ruled out.
   2. Instruct injury prevention such as use of car seats and seat belts, bike safety, and use of headgear for impact sports.
   3. Initiate tetanus toxoid immunization/booster if presence of scalp lacerations.
   4. Explain risk for postconcussion reinjury.

H. Pharmacologic and parenteral therapies: Child and family will state the purpose, dosage, timing, and side effects of medications to treat complications of increased ICP during hospitalization: Hyperosmotic agent: Mannitol (Osmitrol)
   1. Expected outcome: Increases intravascular pressure by pulling fluid from the interstitial spaces, including the brain cells.
   2. Reduction of risk potential: Monitor for tremor, seizures, altered BP; monitor electrolytes.
   3. Management of care: Monitor for diuresis; assess for symptoms of electrolyte alterations.

Myelomeningocele

I. Definition: Myelomeningocele is the failure of the neural tube to close in utero, externalizing the spinal cord and meninges. The exposed sac is covered by a thin membrane that is fragile and prone to leaking. Myelomeningocele is a type of spina bifida, which is a malformation of the spine in which the laminae of the vertebrae do not close. Associated defects and complications of myelomeningocele include talipes equinovarus (clubfoot) and hydrocephalus.

II. Nursing process
   A. Assessment
      1. Complete a detailed health history to assess prenatal monitoring.
      2. Complete a detailed physical assessment, including birth assessment for size and intact nature of sac, and neurologic assessment including motor function.
      3. Assess for signs and symptoms of myelomeningocele: Signs will depend on level of defect and spinal cord involvement.
         a. Flaccid paralysis of legs below defect
         b. Altered bowel and bladder function
      4. Obtain diagnostic tests.
         a. Prenatal ultrasound
         b. Brain and spinal cord
            (1) CT scan and MRI
            (2) Ultrasound
            (3) Myelography
         c. Urinalysis
         d. Serum BUN and creatinine
   B. Analysis
      1. Risk for Infection related to exposure to organisms, meningeal sac, and reduced immune response
      2. Risk for Injury: Neuromuscular, related to paralysis and constant exposure to latex
      3. Risk for Decreased Intracranial Adaptive Capacity: Altered LOC, related to increased cerebral perfusion
      4. Deficient Knowledge: Parent Education, related to no prior experience with spinal cord defect
      5. Impaired Physical Mobility related to immobility and paralysis of lower extremities
      6. Risk for Impaired Skin Integrity related to continence issues
      7. Risk for Delayed Growth and Development related to altered mobility
      8. Risk for Ineffective Therapeutic Regimen Management related to multiple physical needs
   C. Planning
      1. Reduce risk of infection.
      2. Prevent complications of cerebral perfusion and edema.
      4. Maintain fluid volume.
      5. Maintain skin integrity and reduce skin breakdown.
      6. Prevent injury.
      7. Maintain nutritional intake.
      8. Provide child and family teaching.
      9. Promote growth and development.
   D. Implementation: Provide interventions to manage myelomeningocele.
      1. Prevent infection preoperatively.
      2. Monitor for surgical closure of sac within 12 to 18 hr after birth.
      3. Provide intervention for associated problems.
         a. Initiate shunt procedures for hydrocephalus.
         b. Provide antibiotic therapy for meningitis, UTI, or pneumonia.
         c. Manage orthopaedic issues: Prevent contractures, correct deformity, and protect skin.
         d. Manage genitourinary issues: Preserve renal function and achieve urinary continence.
   E. Evaluation
      1. Child's cerebral perfusion is maintained as evidenced by GCS of greater than 13.
      2. Child exhibits no signs of infection as evidenced by normal temperature, no organisms in urinalysis, and no symptoms of meningitis.
      3. Child maintains optimum fluid volume as evidenced by urine output of 1 to 2 ml/kg per hour and urine specific gravity between 1.010 and 1.025.
      4. Child's anxiety is reduced as evidenced by child's ability to rest, be comforted, and tolerate procedures and treatment.
      5. Child is free from injury as evidenced by reduced risk of hip or lower extremity deformities.
      6. Child maintains good nutritional intake as evidenced by good skin turgor, normal body weight, and normal serum albumin levels.
      7. Child maintains normal bowel functioning as evidenced by normal stool consistency.
      8. Child and family verbalize understanding of myelomeningocele treatment and possible outcomes.

CN

III. Client needs
   A. Physiologic adaptation: Myelomeningocele is managed with surgical closure, prevention of infection, neurologic assessment, and family support with adequate follow-up care to reduce the risk of complications. Hydrocephalus is managed in intensive care with monitoring of neurologic status, reducing stimuli, and surgical shunt placement to reduce neurologic sequelae.
      1. Recognize risk for increased ICP—indicated by tense bulging fontanel, irritability, headache, and nausea.

2. Recognize risk for decreased intracranial adaptive capacity: Potential herniation—indicated by increased BP with widened pulse pressure and bradycardia.
3. Recognize high risk for CNS infection: Meningitis—indicated by elevated temperature, irritability, lethargy, and nuchal rigidity.
4. Recognize high risk for renal infection—indicated by fever, nausea, and vomiting.

B. Management of care: Care of the child with a myelomeningocele and possible hydrocephalus requires critical thinking skills and knowledge of assessment, and teaching and evaluation methods unique to the RN role. These skills cannot be delegated to an LPN or UAP.
   1. Perform comprehensive physical assessments and provide care appropriate to the child with a myelomeningocele.
   2. Provide follow-up care for early detection of shunt malfunction, shunt infection, or urinary complications.
   3. Assess home needs: Obtain necessary equipment and modify home setting.
   4. Identify community resources such as the Spina Bifida Association of America and The National Information Center for Children and Youth with Disabilities, rehabilitation services, and alternative schools.
   5. Delegate responsibly those activities that can be delegated, including measurements, oral intake and urine output, vital signs, and reporting child's subjective data. All monitoring information is reported to the RN.

C. Safety and infection control
   1. Protect sac preoperatively.
      a. Apply sterile, moist, nonadherent normal saline dressing.
      b. Provide dressing change every 2 to 4 hr.
      c. Avoid diapering.
      d. Maintain prone or side-lying position.
      e. Assess sac for redness, tears, drainage, or signs of infection.
      f. Administer antibiotics.
   2. Assess for increased ICP and hydrocephalus.
      a. Provide neurologic assessments.
      b. Measure head circumference.
      c. Assess fontanels.
   3. Assess hip and joint function.
   4. Protect skin.
      a. Avoid rectal temperature.
      b. Promote meticulous perineal skin care.
      c. Obtain pressure-reducing mattress.
      d. Maintain proper placement of braces to reduce breakdown.
   5. Manage orthopaedic problems.
      a. Encourage physical therapy to maintain muscle tone and joint function.
      b. Promote orthoses to provide lower extremity support for possible ambulation.
      c. Promote gentle range of motion exercises.
      d. Obtain wheelchair.
   6. Manage genitourinary issues.
      a. Evaluate urine output for signs of infection.
      b. Perform periodic ultrasound to evaluate structures.
      c. Clean intermittent catheterization with antispasmodics.
   7. Promote bowel control.
      a. Encourage high-fiber diet with adequate fluids.
      b. Encourage bowel training.
      c. Prevent constipation or diarrhea.
   8. Provide parental teaching of intermittent catheterization: Follow-up ultrasound and urinalysis every 3 to 6 months.
   9. Instruct child as young as 6 years of age in self-catheterization.

D. Health promotion and maintenance
   1. Involve child in care to promote compliance with multiple procedures and involved therapeutic regimen.
   2. Encourage child to participate in decision-making to ensure compliance and promote development of self-esteem.
   3. Assist child and family in identifying need for follow-up ultrasound and urinalysis every 3 to 6 months.
   4. Provide child and family teaching about procedures and treatment regimen including positioning, feeding, catheterization, physical exercises, and symptoms of complications.

E. Psychologic integrity
   1. Provide tactile stimulation through touch to promote development and parental attachment.
   2. Offer parents a constant opportunity to express fears, guilt, anger, and concerns in coping with defect and possible sequelae.
   3. Provide parents with ongoing information about child's progress.
   4. Refer parents to support groups such as the Spina Bifida Association of America.

F. Basic care and comfort
   1. Provide consistent nurse caregiver.
   2. Provide transitional comfort object if child is hospitalized.

3. Encourage parents to stay at bedside and participate in care.
4. Provide meticulous skin care.

G. Reduction of risk potential: Promote prenatal reduction of risk.
1. Prenatal folic acid administration for child-bearing woman
2. Prenatal ultrasound
3. Prenatal serum alpha-fetoprotein
4. Cesarean delivery, if needed

H. Pharmacologic and parenteral therapies: Child and family will state the purpose for and side effects of anticholinergics: Oxybutynin chloride (Ditropan).
1. Expected outcome: Relieves symptoms associated with voiding in children with a neurogenic bladder.
2. Reduction of risk potential: Instruct child to watch for signs of UTI such as concentrated urine, pain on urination.
3. Management of care: Instruct parents that sustained-release tablet must not be chewed or crushed; monitor child during hot weather for symptoms of fever and heat stroke.

Hydrocephalus

I. Definition: Hydrocephalus is an imbalance between the production of cerebral spinal fluid (CSF) or absorption of CSF caused by ventricular obstruction or malformations. In communicating hydrocephalus there is excessive production of CSF or failure of the absorption of the CSF. In noncommunicating hydrocephalus, the most common type, there is a block between the ventricles and the subarachnoid space.

II. Nursing process

A. Assessment
1. Complete a detailed health history and physical assessment to rule out intrauterine infection. Include in assessment birth history, recent infections, or head trauma.
2. Assess for signs and symptoms of hydrocephalus in infants.
   a. Increasing head circumference
   b. Widely separated suture lines producing a hollow sound on percussion (Macewen sign)
   c. Tense, bulging, anterior fontanel
   d. Frontal bossing
   e. Sunsetting eyes
3. Assess for signs and symptoms of hydrocephalus in children.
   a. Irritability and complaint of headache on rising
   b. Nausea and vomiting
   c. Ataxia
   d. Nystagmus
4. Obtain diagnostic tests.
   a. Prenatal ultrasound
   b. Angiography, CT scan, and MRI
   c. Transillumination
   d. Skull radiography

B. Analysis
1. Risk for Infection related to surgical intervention and shunt placement
2. Risk for Decreased Intracranial Adaptive Capacity: Altered LOC, related to increased cerebral perfusion
3. Deficient Knowledge: Parent Education, related to no prior experience with spinal cord defect
4. Risk for Impaired Skin Integrity related to immobility
5. Risk for Ineffective Therapeutic Regimen Management related to multiple physical needs
6. Risk for Delayed Growth and Development related to decreased cerebral perfusion

C. Planning
1. Reduce risk of infection.
2. Prevent complications of cerebral perfusion and edema.
3. Maintain fluid volume.
4. Maintain skin integrity and reduce skin breakdown.
5. Prevent injury.
6. Maintain nutritional intake.
7. Provide child and family teaching.
8. Promote growth and development.

D. Implementation: Provide interventions to manage hydrocephalus.
1. Relieve hydrocephalus: Surgical intervention—ventriculoperitoneal (VP) shunt placement or ventriculoatrial shunt in adolescents.
2. Manage complications such as seizures, brain herniation, or developmental delays.

E. Evaluation
1. Child's cerebral perfusion is maintained as evidenced by GCS of greater than 13.
2. Child exhibits no signs of infection as evidenced by normal temperature, no organisms in lumbar puncture, and no symptoms of meningitis.
3. Child exhibits no signs of shunt obstruction as evidenced by absence of headache, vomiting, and diplopia.
4. Child maintains optimum fluid volume as evidenced by urine output of 1 to 2 ml/kg per hour and urine specific gravity between 1.010 and 1.025.

5. Child's anxiety is reduced as evidenced by ability to rest, be comforted, and tolerate procedures and treatment.
6. Child maintains good nutritional intake as evidenced by good skin turgor, normal body weight, and normal serum albumin levels.
7. Parents verbalize understanding of anomaly, treatment, and possible outcome.

CN

III. Client needs
  A. Physiologic adaptation: Hydrocephalus is managed in intensive care with monitoring of neurologic status, reduction of stimuli, and surgical shunt placement to reduce neurologic sequelae.
    1. Recognize risk for shunt malfunction—indicated by fever, inflammation of the shunt site, and abdominal pain.
    2. Recognize risk for cerebrospinal infection—indicated by elevated temperature, vomiting, difficulty feeding, and change in LOC.
  B. Management of care: Care of the infant with a hydrocephalus requires critical thinking skills and knowledge of assessment, and teaching and evaluation methods unique to the RN role. These skills cannot be delegated to an LPN or UAP.
    1. Perform comprehensive physical assessments and provide care appropriate to the infant with hydrocephalus.
    2. Provide follow-up care to optimize functional ability.
    3. Assess home needs for the child with neurologic sequelae such as need to modify the home setting to protect child from injury.
    4. Identify community resources such as local chapters of the National Hydrocephalus Foundation, rehabilitation services, alternative schools, and respite care.
    5. Delegate responsibly those activities that can be delegated, including measurements, oral intake and urine output, vital signs, and reporting child's subjective data. All monitoring information is reported to the RN.
  C. Safety and infection control
    1. Manage child preoperatively.
      a. Monitor external ventricular devices for management of increased ICP.
      b. Measure head circumference daily.
      c. Assess and palpate suture lines and fontanels.
      d. Assess for irritability, feeding difficulty, and altered vital signs.
      e. Administer small, frequent feedings.
    2. Manage child postoperatively.
      a. Assess vital signs and neurologic status; measure head circumference.
      b. Position flat on nonoperative side.
      c. Monitor for signs and symptoms of increased ICP: For increased ICP, elevate head of bed 30 degrees.
      d. Monitor for infection.
      e. Monitor intake and output: Restrict fluids; maintain NPO status for 24 to 48 hr.
    3. Instruct parents how to manage infant/toddler at home and recognize infection or shunt malfunction—indicated by headache, irritability, and loss of appetite.
  D. Health promotion and maintenance
    1. Involve parents in care to promote compliance with multiple procedures and involved therapeutic regimen.
    2. Assist family in identifying need for follow-up.
    3. Provide child and family teaching about procedures and treatment regimen including positioning, feeding, and signs and symptoms of infection and shunt malfunction.
    4. Counsel family about the frequency of shunt blockage and infection.
  E. Psychologic integrity
    1. Provide tactile stimulation through touch to promote development and parental attachment.
    2 Offer parents a constant opportunity to express fears, guilt, anger, and concerns in coping with defect and possible sequelae.
    3. Provide parents with ongoing information about child's progress.
    4. Refer to support groups such as the National Hydrocephalus Foundation.
  F. Basic care and comfort
    1. Provide consistent nurse caregiver.
    2. Provide transitional comfort object if child is hospitalized.
    3. Encourage parents to stay at bedside and participate in care.
    4. Provide meticulous skin care.
  G. Reduction of risk potential: Promote prenatal ultrasound at 14 weeks' gestation.
  H. Pharmacologic and parenteral therapies. IV infusions.
    1. Expected outcome: Maintains fluid balance.
    2. Reduction of risk potential: Monitor infusion to prevent fluid overload.
    3. Management of care: Maintain accurate intake and output records.

Seizure Disorder

I. Definition: A seizure is a sudden, involuntary change in motor function, consciousness, or autonomic function as a result of excessive electrical activity in the brain. Epilepsy is a classification of a group of seizure disorders. Seizures may be referred to as partial or generalized.

A. Partial seizure
   1. Simple: Involves localized motor symptoms.
      a. Aversive—eyes or eyes and head turn away from focus
      b. Rolandic—tonic-clonic movements of face
   2. Complex (psychomotor): Most common in children greater than 3 years of age. Presents with altered behavior, impaired consciousness, purposeless motor movement, and an aura.

B. Generalized seizure
   1. Tonic-clonic: Involves loss of consciousness, symmetric tonic contraction of entire body, and is followed by postictal phase.
   2. Absence: Most common in children 4 to 12 years of age; involves brief loss of consciousness, slight loss of motor control, and minor motor movements of face or hands.
   3. Atonic and akinetic: Common in children 2 to 5 years of age; involves momentary loss of muscle tone.
   4. Myoclonic: Involves brief spasm or contractions of muscles; may result in loss of consciousness.
   5. Infantile spasms: Most common in infants in first 6 to 8 months of life; involves brief, symmetric muscle spasms or contractions.

II. Nursing process

A. Assessment
   1. Complete a detailed health history and physical assessment to rule out intrauterine infection of the fetus and anoxia; genetic history of seizures—include birth history, recent infections, and exposure to toxins, injury, or metabolic alterations.
   2. Obtain a history of seizures including precipitating factors, warning signs, physical sequelae from previous seizures such as falls, oral secretions, incontinence, cyanosis, postictal phase.
   3. Obtain diagnostic tests.
      a. EEG
      b. CT scan or MRI
      c. CBC, electrolytes, glucose, and lead levels

B. Analysis
   1. Risk for Injury: Seizures, related to loss of bodily control
   2. Deficient Knowledge: Disease Process and Safety Behavior, related to lack of exposure to disease and possible misinformation
   3. Risk for Chronic Low Self Esteem related to social isolation and safety limitations
   4. Risk for Ineffective Therapeutic Regimen Management related to multiple physical and safety needs

C. Planning
   1. Prevent injury.
   2. Provide child and family teaching.
   3. Improve child's self-esteem.

D. Implementation: Provide interventions to prevent and treat seizures.
   1. Rule out and treat physiologic source of seizure.
   2. Administer antiepileptics.

E. Evaluation
   1. Child and family verbalize understanding of disease process, procedures, treatment, medications, safety procedures, and need for follow-up.
   2. Child identifies coping strategies for living with seizures.
   3. Child is free from injury as evidenced by no seizure activity.

CN

III. Client needs

A. Physiologic adaptation: Seizure activity is controlled with antiepileptics and dose adjustment on an outpatient basis.
   1. Recognize high risk for injury: Status epilepticus—indicated by a continuous seizure that lasts for more than 30 min or a series of seizures that the child does not emerge from in postictal phase.
   2. Assess child for seizure-free period that would allow for increasing activity, driving, and possible medication adjustment or withdrawal.
   3. Evaluate anticonvulsant levels with seizures.

B. Management of care: Care of the child with seizures requires critical thinking skills and knowledge of assessment, and teaching and evaluation methods unique to the RN role. These skills cannot be delegated to an LPN or UAP.
   1. Perform comprehensive physical assessments and provide care appropriate to the child with seizures.
   2. Provide follow-up care to optimize functional ability and promote safety.
   3. Assess home needs for the child such as protective modification of the home setting.
   4. Identify community resources such as the local chapter of the Epilepsy Foundation.
   5. Delegate responsibly those activities that can be delegated, including measurements,

oral intake and urine output, vital signs, and reporting the child's subjective data. All monitoring information is reported to the RN.

C. Safety and infection control
   1. Identify risk for seizures and protect from injury.
      a. Monitor LOC.
      b. Monitor and record all seizure activity.
      c. Institute seizure precautions.
   2. Manage child during a seizure.
      a. Protect airway.
      b. Administer anticonvulsants such as IV lorazepam (Ativan).
   3. Provide child and family teaching.
      a. Explain seizure type and severity, and method of control.
      b. Instruct about medications, dose, timing, and side effects.
      c. Advise medication follow-up to determine therapeutic levels and identify blood dyscrasias.
      d. Instruct family what to do during a seizure.
         (1) Move furniture away.
         (2) Loosen clothes.
         (3) Do not restrain.
         (4) Roll to side if possible.
         (5) Call 911 for seizure lasting more than 60 s.
   4. Provide teaching to child and family about home safety management.
      a. Observe laws regarding driving—each state has own laws; usually can drive if seizure-free for 6 months to 2 years.
      b. Do not cook or bathe alone.
      c. Do not swim alone.
      d. Avoid climbing.
      e. Wear medic-alert bracelet.
      f. Wear protective body gear during high-impact activities.
   5. Maintain the six rights of medication administration.

D. Health promotion and maintenance: Assess family and child teaching needs, including educational, developmental, and cognitive level, and presence of cultural or religious factors that may influence learning.
   1. Involve parents in care to promote compliance with multiple procedures and involved therapeutic regimen.
   2. Assist family in identifying need for follow-up to monitor drug levels and seizure control.
   3. Instruct family about procedures and treatment regimen including safety, medication side effects, and management (see pharmacologic and parenteral therapies).
   4. Promote growth and development by providing age-appropriate toys and safe activities.
   5. Assist parents in educating school setting about needs and limitations.

E. Psychologic integrity
   1. Offer parents a constant opportunity to express fears, guilt, anger, and concerns in coping with seizures and possible sequelae.
   2. Provide child opportunities to express anger, fears, and concerns.
   3. Promote self-esteem through encouraging self-management and dispelling fears and misconceptions.
   4. Refer to support groups such as the Epilepsy Foundation.

F. Basic care and comfort
   1. Provide consistent nurse caregiver.
   2. Provide transitional comfort object if hospitalized.
   3. Encourage parents to stay at bedside and participate in care.
   4. Provide emotional comfort during postictal phase.

G. Reduction of risk potential
   1. Encourage use of medic-alert bracelet.
   2. Promote pharmacotherapy recommendations for the prevention of seizures: Antiepileptics.
   3. Assist child and family in identifying precursors or warning signs such as auras.
   4. Assist family in understanding the management of side effects of anticonvulsants.
   5. Instruct child and family on steps to take during a seizure (see safety and infection control).

H. Pharmacologic and parenteral therapies: Child and family will state the purpose for and side effects of medications to treat seizures: Antiepileptics. See Table 17-2 for drugs used to treat seizure disorders.

Meningitis

I. Definition: Meningitis involves inflammation of the membranes of the brain or spinal cord and is typically caused by a bacterial or viral infection that invades the CSF. Infection such as otitis media or infection secondary to a basilar skull fracture can occur elsewhere in the body and invade the CNS.

II. Nursing process
   A. Assessment
      1. Complete a detailed health history and physical assessment to rule out intrauterine infection, including recent history of other source of infection.

Table 17-2 Drugs Used to Treat Seizure Disorders

Classification	Generic/Trade Name	Expected Outcome	Reduction of Risk Potential	Management of Care
Antiepileptic	Phenytoin (Dilantin)	Controls partial or secondary seizures.	Monitor drug levels. Monitor CBC. Monitor diabetics for loss of glycemic control.	Teach family to monitor for gingival hyperplasia. Teach child good dental care and follow-up. Urine may turn pink to red-brown color. Increase intake of vitamin D and folic acid. Do not take med with milk.
Antiepileptic	Phenobarbital (Luminal)	Manages all seizure activity, including febrile seizures.	Use with caution in children with diabetes mellitus. Monitor liver enzymes and vitamin D levels.	Monitor for sedation and irritability. Increase intake of vitamin D and folic acid. Do not take med with milk.
Antiepileptic	Valproic acid (Depacon)	Manages primary generalized seizures.	Monitor for nausea, weight gain, and hair loss. Monitor for thrombocytopenia.	Do not administer with carbonated beverage. Give with food. May cause false-positive urine for ketones.
Antiepileptic	Levetiracetam (Keppra)	Manages partial seizures in children over 4 years of age.	Monitor renal studies every 3 months.	Monitor for sedation. Take with food.
Antiepileptic	Topiramate (Topamax)	Treats partial and tonic-clonic seizures.	Monitor renal studies.	Female patient needs to use alternative birth control. Increase fluid intake. Do not break or chew tablet.

2. Assess for presence of meningeal signs and symptoms.
   a. For infants and young children:
      (1) Fever
      (2) Poor feeding
      (3) Irritability
      (4) Tense, bulging fontanel
   b. For adolescents:
      (1) Nuchal rigidity
      (2) Fever, headache
      (3) Photophobia
      (4) Brudzinski or Kernig sign
3. Assess for general signs of infection.
   a. Fever and irritability
   b. Altered LOC
   c. High-pitched cry
   d. Petechiae or purpura
   e. Projectile vomiting
   f. Signs of increased ICP
4. Obtain diagnostic tests.
   a. Lumbar puncture
   b. CBC
   c. Blood culture

B. Analysis
1. Risk for Deficient Fluid Volume related to vomiting and altered LOC
2. Infection related to presence of infectious agent in the brain
3. Risk for Injury: Seizures, related to edema, and meningeal irritation
4. Deficient Knowledge: Disease Process, related to no prior experience with disease process
5. Acute Pain related to meningeal irritation and increased ICP
6. Risk for Ineffective Tissue Perfusion: Cerebral, related to edema and increased ICP
7. Risk for Ineffective Therapeutic Regimen Management related to multiple physical needs

C. Planning
1. Identify infectious agent.
2. Protect from injury: Seizures.
3. Maintain cerebral tissue perfusion.
4. Reduce pain to tolerable level.
5. Maintain fluid intake.
6. Provide developmentally appropriate teaching.

D. Implementation: Provide interventions to treat infection and meningeal irritation.
1. Promote isolation.
2. Administer parenteral antibiotics.

3. Maintain hydration.
4. Reduce increased ICP.
5. Control seizures.
6. Prevent complications such as seizures or increased ICP.
7. Administer analgesics, antipyretics, and corticosteroids.

E. Evaluation
1. Child's infection is identified and managed appropriately.
2. Child does not experience any seizure activity, or early treatment prevents injury.
3. Child's cerebral perfusion is maintained as evidenced by GCS of greater than 13, improved LOC, normal papillary reaction, and absence of meningeal symptoms.
4. Child verbalizes a decrease in pain, rests quietly, and is able to be comforted.
5. Child maintains optimum fluid volume as evidenced by urine output of 1 to 2 ml/kg per hour and urine specific gravity between 1.010 and 1.025.
6. Child and family verbalize understanding of disease, procedures, treatment, and need for follow-up.

CN

III. Client needs

A. Physiologic adaptation: Meningitis is managed with isolation, hospitalization, and IV antibiotics with possible neurologic sequelae.
1. Recognize risk for decreased intracranial adaptive capacity: Increased ICP—indicated by change in LOC, increased BP, bradycardia, and seizures.
2. Recognize risk for decrease in tissue perfusion: Dehydration—indicated by percentage loss of body weight, irritability, poor skin turgor, prolonged capillary refill 2 s or more, tachycardia, deep rapid respirations, absent tears, dry mucus membranes, plasma pH less than 7.33 and decreased plasma HCO_3, urine specific gravity more than 1.025, serum sodium more than 150 mEq/L, BUN more than 18 mg/dl, and creatinine more than 0.4 mg/dl.

B. Management of care: Care of the child with meningitis requires critical thinking skills and knowledge of assessment, and teaching and evaluation methods unique to the RN role. These skills cannot be delegated to an LPN or UAP.
1. Perform comprehensive physical assessments and provide care appropriate to the child with meningitis.
2. Provide follow-up care to optimize child's functional ability.
3. Assess home needs for the child with neurologic sequelae such as home visits, modification of the home setting, nutritional needs, and equipment.
4. Identify community resources for equipment, rehabilitation services, local parental support groups, and alternative schools.
5. Delegate responsibly those activities that can be delegated, including measurements, oral intake and urine output, vital signs, and reporting child's subjective data. All monitoring information is reported to the RN.

C. Safety and infection control
1. Monitor infection.
   a. Monitor vital signs, including temperature.
   b. Monitor results of CBC.
   c. Perform neurologic assessments, including behavior.
2. Manage infection.
   a. Provide isolation as indicated—respiratory precautions for a minimum of 24 hr after antibiotic therapy is initiated.
   b. Administer antibiotics.
   c. Administer antipyretics.
   d. Initiate tepid sponge baths and cooling blankets for temperature more than 39.5°C (103.1°F).
3. Identify risk for seizures and protect from injury.
   a. Monitor LOC.
   b. Monitor and record all seizure activity.
   c. Institute seizure precautions.
   d. During seizure: Protect airway; administer anticonvulsants.
4. Maintain cerebral tissue perfusion.
   a. Monitor and record GCS, including pupillary reaction and size.
   b. Evaluate presence of protective reflexes such as gag and cough.
   c. Assess for meningeal irritation signs: Brudzinski and Kernig signs.
   d. Elevate head of bed 30 to 45 degrees.
   e. Reorient as needed.
   f. Administer hyperosmotic medications such as mannitol.
5. Manage meningeal pain and headache.
   a. Administer analgesics and evaluate response.
   b. Decrease stimuli: Reduce noise and light and limit visitors.
   c. Avoid Valsalva maneuver.
6. Improve hydration and fluid volume.
   a. Promote IV fluids.
   b. Monitor intake and output, weight, and skin turgor.
   c. Monitor electrolytes.

D. Health promotion and maintenance
   1. Provide child and family teaching about disease, procedures, treatment, and follow-up.
      a. Assess family's educational, developmental, and cognitive levels, including cultural or religious factors that may influence learning.
      b. Provide teaching about medications, dose, timing, and side effects (see pharmacologic and parenteral therapies).
      c. Provide teaching about treatments associated with neurologic sequelae.
   2. Involve parents in care to promote compliance with multiple procedures and involved therapeutic regimen.
   3. Assist family in identifying need for follow-up care.
   4. Promote growth and development by providing age-appropriate activities and toys.
   5. Initiate meningococcal vaccine (MCV4) vaccine for all children beginning at 11 to 12 years of age.

E. Psychologic integrity
   1. Offer parents a constant opportunity to express fears, guilt, anger, and concerns in coping with meningitis and possible sequelae.
   2. Provide child opportunities to express anger, fears, and concerns.
   3. Keep parents informed of child's progress.

F. Basic care and comfort
   1. Provide consistent nurse caregiver.
   2. Provide transitional comfort object if child is hospitalized.
   3. Encourage parents to stay at bedside and participate in care.
   4. Administer analgesics for headache and meningeal irritation.

G. Reduction of risk potential
   1. Administer *Haemophilus influenzae* type B vaccine.
   2. Administer pneumococcal conjugate vaccine for infants beginning at 2 months of age.
   3. Administer prophylactic antibiotics for individuals who have had contact with patient.

Down Syndrome

I. Definition: Down syndrome is a genetic congenital condition that is a result of an extra chromosome 21 (trisomy 21). The condition may result in mild to severe developmental delays and is commonly associated with congenital heart defects, hypothyroidism, and other medical conditions.

II. Nursing process

A. Assessment
   1. Complete a detailed health history and physical assessment, including maternal age and family history of Down syndrome.
   2. Assess for characteristic signs and symptoms.
      a. Epicanthal folds
      b. Narrow palate
      c. Short, broad hands
      d. Transpalmar crease (simian)
      e. Depressed nasal bridge
      f. Muscle weakness
      g. Intelligence varies with degrees of developmental delay
   3. Obtain diagnostic tests.
      a. History and physical examination
      b. Karyotype
      c. Fetal ultrasound

B. Analysis
   1. Delayed Growth and Development elated to impaired cognition and motor ability
   2. Risk for Interrupted Family Processes related to complex needs of child

C. Planning
   1. Provide child and family support and teaching.
   2. Promote growth and development potential.

D. Implementation: Provide interventions to manage developmental delay.
   1. Promote growth and development, social development, and motor development.
   2. Treat coexisting conditions.
   3. Provide child and family teaching and support.

E. Evaluation
   1. Child achieves maximum potential growth and development as evidenced by increased cognitive, social, and physical abilities.
   2. Parents are prepared to manage child with long-term needs.

CN

III. Client needs

A. Physiologic adaptation: The child with Down syndrome is managed with a multidisciplinary approach and long-term follow-up care on an outpatient basis. Evaluate effectiveness of treatment regimen in promoting the child's optimum functional capacity.

B. Management of care: Care of the child with Down syndrome requires critical thinking skills and knowledge of assessment, and teaching and evaluation methods unique to the RN role. These skills cannot be delegated to an LPN or UAP.
   1. Perform comprehensive physical assessments and provide care appropriate to the child with Down syndrome.

2. Provide follow-up care to optimize functional ability in home and school.
3. Assess home needs for the child with developmental delay, including modification of the home setting, specialized equipment, and early stimulation programs.
4. Identify community resources such as parent groups, local chapter of the National Down Syndrome Society, early intervention programs, alternative schools, and respite care.
5. Delegate responsibly those activities that can be delegated, including measurements, oral intake and urine output, vital signs, and reporting child's subjective data. All monitoring information is reported to the RN.

C. Safety and infection control: Use behavior modification and modify the home setting to promote safety goals and prevent injury.

D. Health promotion and maintenance
1. Provide toys and activities that promote growth potential.
2. Set realistic goals designed in small steps.
3. Encourage self-management at child's developmental level to promote growth potential.
4. Assist family in identifying need for follow-up.
5. Instruct family about procedures and treatment regimen including safety and medication side effects and management.
6. Promote growth and development by providing age-appropriate activities and toys.
7. Initiate early-intervention school programs and planning.

E. Psychologic integrity
1. Offer parents a constant opportunity to express fears, guilt, anger, and concerns in coping with diagnosis and possible sequelae.
2. Communicate at child's cognitive level to promote compliance with care.
3. Promote parent-child attachment and involvement in care.
4. Refer parents to grief counselor and support groups: National Down Syndrome Society.
5. Provide consideration of cultural variables when providing parent teaching.

F. Basic care and comfort
1. Provide consistent nurse caregiver.
2. Provide a transitional comfort object if child is hospitalized.
3. Encourage parents to stay at bedside and participate in care.

G. Reduction of risk potential
1. Encourage prenatal diagnosis: Ultrasound, amniocentesis, chorionic villus sampling.
2. Encourage genetic counseling.

H. Pharmacologic and parenteral therapies are used to manage related health problems such as seizures, heart disease, or infections.

Bibliography

Hatfield, N. (2006). *Broadribb's introductory pediatric nursing.* Philadelphia: Lippincott Williams & Wilkins.

Pillitteri, A. (2006). *Maternal & child health nursing: Care of the childbearing and childrearing family* (5th ed.). Philadelphia: Lippincott Williams & Wilkins.

Wong, D. L., et al. (2006). *Maternal child nursing care.* St. Louis: Mosby.

CHAPTER 17
Practice Test

Head Injury

1. AF A child who is 9 years of age has suffered a concussion after a fall from a tree and his parents bring him to the emergency department. The nurse is assessing the child. Which of the following indicate increased ICP? Select all that apply.

□ 1. Increased temperature.
□ 2. Decreased respiratory rate.
□ 3. Numbness of fingers.
□ 4. Increased pulse rate.
□ 5. Decreased consciousness.

2. The nurse is assessing a group of clients on a pediatric unit. Which of the following clients has findings that should be reported to the physician?

□ 1. Child who is 7 years of age with a GCS score of 13.
□ 2. Child who is 8 years of age with one fixed and dilated pupil.
□ 3. Child who is 18 months of age with a flat and soft anterior fontanel.
□ 4. Child who is 2 months of age with a positive Moro reflex.

3. The nurse is taking care of a child with a basilar skull fracture. Which of the following findings should the nurse draw to the attention of the physician?
- ☐ 1. Headache and crying.
- ☐ 2. Pupils bilaterally equal and reactive to light.
- ☐ 3. Increased drowsiness and fever.
- ☐ 4. Decreased appetite and nausea.

4. A mother tells the nurse that her son was hit in the head while playing football earlier in the evening. Although the child did not lose consciousness, he is experiencing a headache and has vomited three times in the last hour. The nurse should tell the mother to:
- ☐ 1. Bring her son to the health care facility immediately.
- ☐ 2. Administer acetaminophen every 4 hr as needed for pain.
- ☐ 3. Allow the child to sleep, waking the child every hour to assess consciousness.
- ☐ 4. Give the child saltine crackers to settle the stomach and prevent nausea.

5. Parents of a child who has fallen on his head call the emergency department. The parents report no abrasions or lacerations, but explain that the child is dizzy. The nurse should instruct the parents of a child who has sustained a possible concussion to:
- ☐ 1. Let the child sleep until he feels well enough to be up.
- ☐ 2. Keep the child awake for at least 5 hr after the injury.
- ☐ 3. Monitor the child's vital signs every 30 min.
- ☐ 4. Rouse the child every 1 to 2 hr to check the LOC.

Myelomeningocele

6. The nurse is caring for an infant with myelomeningocele. Prior to surgery, the nurse should:
- ☐ 1. Turn the child from front to back every 2 hr.
- ☐ 2. Change diapers frequently.
- ☐ 3. Administer low-dose continuous pain medication.
- ☐ 4. Encourage high fluid intake.

7. The nurse should place an infant with a myelomeningocele in which position prior to surgery?
- ☐ 1. Semi-Fowler position in an infant chair.
- ☐ 2. On the left side with head dependent.
- ☐ 3. Prone with no pillow.
- ☐ 4. Supine with head elevated.

8. A newborn has surgery for repair of a myelomeningocele. Following surgery, the nurse should do which of the following first?
- ☐ 1. Assess blink reflex.
- ☐ 2. Evaluate paracervical reflux.
- ☐ 3. Record total 24-hr urine output.
- ☐ 4. Measure head circumference.

Hydrocephalus

9. An infant with hydrocephalus had a ventriculoperitoneal shunt inserted. Immediately following the procedure, the nurse should place the infant in which of the following positions?
- ☐ 1. Mid-Fowler position.
- ☐ 2. Sims position with the head of the bed elevated 30 degrees.
- ☐ 3. Trendelenberg position.
- ☐ 4. Supine, with the head of the bed flat.

10. The nurse is caring for a neonate who had a ventriculoarterial shunt placed for hydrocephalus. When assessing the neonate, the nurse notes that the ICP is increasing. The newborn's back is arched and his feet are pointing downward. The IV infusion of normal saline is infusing at a keep-open rate. The nurse should do which of the following first?
- ☐ 1. Reposition the newborn on his side.
- ☐ 2. Increase the IV drip rate.
- ☐ 3. Notify the physician.
- ☐ 4. Open the valve of the shunt.

Seizure Disorder

11. A child who is 8 years of age is diagnosed as having tonic-clonic seizures. The nurse should teach the parents that:
- ☐ 1. Their daughter should maintain an active lifestyle.
- ☐ 2. If their daughter shows symptoms of beginning a seizure, immediately give her medication.
- ☐ 3. Their daughter should carry a padded tongue blade with her at all times.
- ☐ 4. Their daughter should be kept quiet late in the day when she is most likely to have a seizure.

12. A child who is 10 years of age with seizures takes phenytoin sodium (Dilantin), 75 mg 4 times a day. The nurse should teach the child to:
- ☐ 1. Report numbness of the fingers.
- ☐ 2. Brush teeth after each meal.
- ☐ 3. Avoid flashing lights.
- ☐ 4. Stand up slowly to prevent dizziness.

13. A child is in status epilepticus. The physician has ordered 150 mg of IV push phenytoin. The child already has an IV of D5.45NS running at 75 ml/hr. The nurse should:
- ☐ 1. Flush the IV line with saline, administer the drug slowly, then flush with saline.
- ☐ 2. Administer the medication slow IV push over 1-min period.
- ☐ 3. Slow the IV rate to a keep-open rate and administer the phenytoin.

□ 4. Change the infusing fluid to D5W and administer the phenytoin.

14. A child is taking phenobarbital for a seizure disorder. The nurse should teach the child and family to:

□ 1. Inspect the mouth for monilial infection.
□ 2. Do not discontinue the drug abruptly.
□ 3. Never go swimming.
□ 4. Avoid foods containing caffeine.

15. AF A child is hospitalized with a seizure disorder. The child, who is in a bed with padded side rails, has a tonic-clonic seizure. The nurse should do which of the following in priority order? Place the nursing actions in order of first to last.

_____ 1. Loosen clothing around the neck.
_____ 2. Turn the child on the side.
_____ 3. Clear the area around the child.
_____ 4. Suction the airway.

Meningitis

16. AF A child who is 15 years of age is hospitalized with bacterial meningitis. At 5:30 p.m., the client's mother reports her child is "burning up." The nurse is reviewing the client's medication administration records below.

NURSE'S FULL SIGNATURE, STATUS AND INITIALS			
	INIT.		INIT.
Linda Roberts, RN	LR		
Rick Jones, RN	RJ		

DIAGNOSIS: Bacterial meningitis	
ALLERGIES: None	DIET: Regular
ROUTINE/DAILY/ORDERS FINGERSTICKS/ INSULIN COVERAGE	DATE: 4/21/09

ORDER DATE	MEDICATIONS, DOSE, ROUTE, FREQUENCY	TIME	SITE	INIT.
4/21/09	Aspirin 325mg for temperature over 99 °F. every 3 to 4 hours as needed	0910		LR T = 100 °F
		1315		LR T = 99.5 °F
		1610		RJ T = 101 °F

The physician has ordered aspirin 325 mg every 3 to 4 hr for temperature over 99°F. The child's temperature at 17:30 p.m. is 102.5°F. The nurse should do which of the following first?

□ 1. Notify the physician.
□ 2. Initiate tepid sponge baths.
□ 3. Institute seizure precautions.
□ 4. Administer another dose of aspirin.

17. A child is suspected of having bacterial meningitis and is undergoing testing. The nurse can inform the child's parents that which of the following tests is used to provide the definitive diagnosis of the infection?

□ 1. Arterial blood gas.
□ 2. Lumbar puncture.
□ 3. Bone marrow aspiration.
□ 4. Blood culture.

18. A child who is 1 year of age has experienced a febrile seizure. To prevent another seizure, the nurse should teach the parents to:

□ 1. Administer antibiotics when the child exhibits symptoms of a cold.
□ 2. Administer acetaminophen for temperature over 99°F.
□ 3. Administer phenobarbital when the temperature is above 101°F.
□ 4. Place the child in an ice bath for a temperature above 100°F.

Down Syndrome

19. An infant who is 6 months of age was born with Down syndrome and is moderately cognitively impaired. The parents understand the plan of care when they indicate:

□ 1. Their infant will thrive best at a specialized care facility.
□ 2. They will not expose the infant to normal children in school to maintain his self-esteem.
□ 3. The infant will benefit from an early education program.
□ 4. With good schooling, the infant will achieve at an average level.

20. The nurse is teaching the parent of a child with Down syndrome about promoting growth and development. The nurse should instruct the parent to:

□ 1. Provide as much help to the child as possible.
□ 2. Seek professional help for the child's daily needs.
□ 3. Encourage self-care in the child as soon as it is appropriate.
□ 4. Place the child in a home for handicapped children.

Answers and Rationales

1. 1, 2, 5 Increased ICP puts pressure on vital centers, increasing temperature and BP and decreasing respiratory and pulse rates. As the ICP increases, the child will become increasingly restless and then exhibit a decreasing LOC. Numbness of the fingers is not a sign of increased ICP. (A)

2. 2 Widely dilated and fixed pupils suggest paralysis of cranial nerve III secondary to pressure from herniation of the brain. A unilateral fixed pupil usually suggests a lesion on the same side of the brain. A GCS score of 15 is normal; less than 8 suggests coma. The anterior fontanel typically closes between 12 and 18 months of age; flat and soft are normal findings. A positive Moro reflex is expected of an infant who is 2 months of age and is one of the best indicators of neurologic health in infancy. (C)

3. 3 Posttraumatic meningitis is suspected in children with increasing drowsiness and fever who also have basilar skull fractures. The other assessment findings are possible findings of a child with a skull fracture. (S)

4. 1 If a child loses consciousness or vomits more than three times following a head trauma, the nurse immediately advises medical attention. Administering acetaminophen might mask the pain, and giving crackers may settle the stomach, but these methods do not deal with the fact that the child has vomited three times since having a head injury. Because the child has vomited three times, allowing the child to sleep while continuing to assess him is not appropriate. (S)

5. 4 ICP increases without dramatic symptoms, and a decreasing LOC is a good indication that ICP is increasing; therefore, the nurse advises the parents to wake the child to assess the LOC every 1 to 2 hr. The nurse explains to the parents the importance of not letting the child sleep through the night; although it is not necessary to keep the child awake for a long time, the child must be awake enough to assess the LOC. The parents can evaluate the child when they awaken him. (R)

6. 2 Because infants with myelomeningocele do not have innervation to the lower spinal cord and do not have bladder control, they void continually; therefore, the nurse changes the diapers frequently to prevent skin excoriation. The infant is not positioned on his back as that would put pressure on the myelomeningocele, and he does not require continuous pain medication. The infant obtains adequate amounts of fluids to maintain hydration, so it is not necessary to encourage additional fluids. (C)

7. 3 Placing the infant in prone position prevents direct trauma to the lesion and reduces the chance that feces will contaminate the lesion. The other positions put pressure on the myelomeningocele. (R)

8. 4 Following surgical repair of a myelomeningocele, cerebrospinal fluid can accumulate and lead to hydrocephalus; therefore, the nurse measures the newborn's head for increasing size. The client should have a blink reflex once recovered from anesthesia. The nurse maintains intake and output records, but this is not the first thing to do following surgery. (A)

9. 4 Keeping the infant flat prevents gravity from moving more fluid into the shunt than necessary and prevents excessive CSF leak. As the infant becomes stable the nurse can gradually elevate the head of the bed. The other positions immediately following surgery will increase pressure and potentially cause CSF leak. (R)

10. 3 The client has signs of increasing ICP (the ICP and opisthotonic positioning). The nurse notifies the physician and prepares to assist with a ventricular tap. The nurse is prepared to manage the possibility for increasing ICP, which may precipitate respiratory arrest. Repositioning the client does not decrease ICP. Increasing fluids increase circulatory load for the client. It is not the nurse's role to open the valve of the shunt. (A)

11. 1 It is important for children who experience seizures to maintain as near normal a lifestyle as possible to maintain self-esteem and achievement. Most seizure medications must reach a therapeutic level before they are effective and they need to be continued without skipping a dose. Tongue blades are not used during seizures as they can cause injury to the mouth. Parents can alert teachers and nurses at school to the needs of their daughter, who can wear a medical alert tag. (H)

12. 2 A side effect of phenytoin sodium is gingival hypertrophy. Good tooth-brushing helps prevent inflammation under the gum tissue. Numbness of the fingers and postural hypotension are not side effects of phenytoin. Flashing lights do not precipitate seizures in children who are controlled with medication. (D)

13. 1 If IV phenytoin is used, it is administered only with normal saline because phenytoin precipitates when mixed with glucose. When administered, the medication is given slow IV push at a rate that does not exceed 50 mg/min. (D)

14. 2 Phenobarbital is always tapered, not stopped abruptly, or seizures from the child's dependency on the drug can result. If the child is taking phenytoin sodium, it is important to brush the teeth and gums to prevent gingival hypertrophy; phenobarbital does not cause bacterial overgrowth in the mouth and monilial infection is not a side effect of taking the drug. Swimming is an appropriate sport; however, no child should swim alone. Caffeine does not interact with phenobarbital adversely. (D)

15. 3, 1, 2, 4 The goal of care for a client who is having a seizure is to prevent respiratory arrest and aspiration. The nurse first clears the area around the child; next, the nurse loosens clothing around the neck and turns the child on the side. The nurse can then suction the airway and administer oxygen as needed. (R)

16. 1 Because the client's temperature continues to rise in spite of recently administering aspirin, the nurse notifies the physician. After notifying the physician, the nurse can bathe the client with tepid water. If the temperature cannot be lowered shortly, the client is also at risk for seizures; the nurse pads side rails and observes for seizure activity. The nurse cannot administer another dose of aspirin without physician orders. (M)

17. 2 The lumbar puncture is the definitive diagnostic test. Samples are obtained for culture, Gram stain, CBC, and determination of glucose and protein content. The other tests do not confirm bacterial meningitis. (A)

18. 2 The nurse instructs the parents to take the child's temperature when illness is suspected and administer acetaminophen promptly when fever is noted. Ice baths are distressing to the child; phenobarbital is a slow-acting drug and is given in this setting. Antibiotics are only appropriate for bacterial infections. (H)

19. 3 Children with cognitive impairment often benefit from early language and social skill development programs so they can learn slowly but consistently. Children with Down syndrome can function within the home and community and do not need to be placed in a care facility. (H)

20. 3 Encouraging self-care in a cognitively impaired child allows the child to be as independent as possible. Unless the parents are unable to care for the child, the child does not need to be placed in a care facility or have additional help at home. (H)

chapter

18

The Child With Musculoskeletal Health Problems

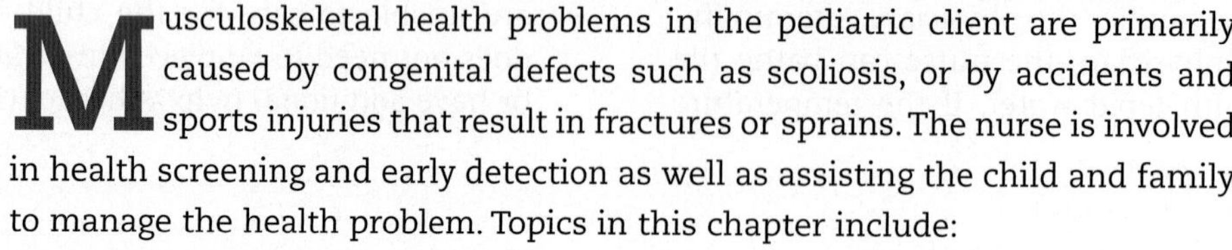

Musculoskeletal health problems in the pediatric client are primarily caused by congenital defects such as scoliosis, or by accidents and sports injuries that result in fractures or sprains. The nurse is involved in health screening and early detection as well as assisting the child and family to manage the health problem. Topics in this chapter include:

- Fracture
- Developmental Dysplasia of the Hip
- Congenital Clubfoot
- Scoliosis
- Juvenile Idiopathic Arthritis
- Pseudohypertrophic (Duchenne) Muscular Dystrophy
- Cerebral Palsy

Fracture

I. Definition: A fracture is a break or disruption of the bone continuity resulting from trauma or demineralization. Causes of fractures in children are usually a result of immature physical and cognitive abilities.

II. Nursing process

A. Assessment

1. Complete a detailed health history and physical assessment including history of injury, talking with parents or other witnesses, and instituting emergency care.
2. Assess for signs and symptoms of a fracture.
   a. Pain at affected area
   b. Loss of motor function
   c. Visible bone deformity
   d. Edema
   e. Muscle spasm
   f. Ecchymosis
3. Assess muscle tone, strength, mobility of joint, and swelling.
4. Obtain diagnostic tests.
   a. Radiography and/or other imaging tests
   b. CBC
   c. Serum alkaline phosphatase, lactic dehydrogenase (LDH), and creatine phosphokinase (CPK)

B. Analysis

1. Risk for Injury: Cast, Immobilizer, or Traction, related to improper maintenance or positioning
2. Deficient Knowledge: Treatment Regimen and Home Management, related to lack of information about treatment of fractures
3. Impaired Physical Mobility related to pain, surgery, or fixation device
4. Acute Pain related to soft tissue damage
5. Risk for Impaired Skin Integrity related to immobility and cast or fixation device
6. Risk for Ineffective Tissue Perfusion related to inflammation and edema

C. Planning

1. Reduce risk of injury.
2. Provide child and family teaching.
3. Manage pain, hemorrhage, and edema.
4. Improve mobility.
5. Reduce risk of skin breakdown.
6. Improve tissue perfusion.

D. Implementation: Provide interventions to manage a fracture.

1. Promote reduction to regain proper alignment.
2. Promote retention of alignment with splint, cast, traction, or fixator devices.
3. Restore function and prevent complications.

E. Evaluation

1. Child has reduced risk of injury as evidenced by maintenance of proper body alignment and cast care.
2. Child and family verbalize understanding of fracture treatment, complications, and home management.
3. Child verbalizes a decrease in pain to tolerable level and evidence supports appearance of comfort.
4. Child maintains mobility appropriate to fracture and treatment.
5. Child's skin remains intact through serial assessment and early intervention.
6. Child has adequate tissue perfusion as evidenced by good skin turgor, good color, capillary refill 2 s or more, equal pulses, and lack of paresthesia.

GN

III. Client needs

A. Physiologic adaptation: Emergency management of a fracture includes immobilization and determining extent of injury using the five "Ps": pain, pulselessness, pallor, paresthesia, and paralysis.

1. Recognize risk for complication of large-bone fractures: Fat embolism—indicated by chest pain, signs of shock such as tachypnea, confusion, hypotension, and petechial rash from neck to below nipple line.
2. Recognize risk for complication of neurovascular compromise: Compartment syndrome—indicated by child complaints of severe pain, peripheral pulses weak to absent, and pain with passive movement.
3. Rule out child abuse as cause of fracture; fractures in infancy are rare.

B. Management of care: Care of the child with a fracture requires critical thinking skills and knowledge of assessment, and teaching and evaluation methods unique to the RN role. These skills cannot be delegated to an LPN or UAP.

1. Perform comprehensive physical assessments and provide care appropriate to the child with a fracture.
2. Provide follow-up care to evaluate cast and plans for removal.
3. Assess home needs for equipment, mobility issues, and accessibility.
4. Identify community resources to support family such as transportation needs and availability of home equipment including crutches or wheelchair, and possible in-home tutoring.
5. Delegate responsibly those activities that can be delegated, including measurements, oral intake and urine output, vital signs, and

reporting child's subjective data. All monitoring information is reported to the RN.

C. Safety and infection control
   1. Assess for and prevent impaired tissue perfusion.
      a. Provide frequent neurovascular assessments—notify physician if capillary refill is more than 4 to 6 s.
      b. Inspect pin sites or incision sites for redness, swelling, and drainage.
      c. Assess vital signs, lung sounds, and review results of arterial blood gases.
   2. Prevent skin breakdown.
      a. Assess skin, wound, or immobilized part every 2 hr.
      b. Remove antiembolic devices every shift to inspect skin.
      c. Reposition every 2 hr, if permitted.
      d. Use pressure-relief mattress.
      e. Use overbed frame and trapeze to assist with mobility and transfers.
      f. Maintain nutrition and hydration.
   3. Maintain and provide child and family teaching about traction.
      a. Explain purpose of skin or skeletal traction.
      b. Maintain proper body alignment—do not remove weights; do not allow child to turn in the direction of the traction.
      c. Assure weights are hanging freely.
      d. Provide frequent neurovascular assessments.
      e. Assess and protect skin.
      f. Assess pin sites, if appropriate.
   4. Provide cast care.
      a. Leave cast open to air until dry.
      b. Touch cast with palm of hands only until dry.
      c. Reposition child every 2 hr.
      d. Avoid soiling of cast with urine or stool.
      e. When dry, petal edges of cast.
   5. Assess and maintain mobility.
      a. Assess child's range of motion.
      b. Assess muscle strength.
      c. Teach isometric exercises and active range of motion.
      d. Encourage flexion and extension exercises of affected part during rehabilitative phase.
      e. Monitor for complications of immobility such as constipation, skin breakdown, atrophy of unused muscles.

D. Health promotion and maintenance
   1. Provide child and family teaching about treatment for and complications of fractures, as well as types of fractures and healing process.
   2. Instruct child and family about home management of fractures, casts, and crutches; involve child in care to promote compliance with multiple procedures and therapeutic regimen.
      a. Teach exercises to be performed daily.
      b. Instruct on appropriate crutch-walking technique.
      c. Identify and report compromised neurovascular status.
      d. Manage pain.
      e. Instruct about cast care and maintenance.
   3. Assist child and family in identifying need for follow-up.
   4. Provide age and developmentally appropriate diversional activities to promote growth and development.

E. Psychologic integrity
   1. Provide quiet diversional and recreational activities when energy is improved and pain subsides.
   2 Offer parents and child a constant opportunity to express fears and concerns in coping with injury and possible home needs.
   3. Provide parents with ongoing information about child's progress.

F. Basic care and comfort
   1. Provide consistent nurse caregiver.
   2. Provide transitional comfort object if child is hospitalized.
   3. Encourage parents to stay at bedside and participate in care.
   4. Manage pain.
      a. Reposition unaffected extremities every 2 hr.
      b. Use distraction techniques.
      c. Apply ice 20 to 30 min every 1 to 2 hr.
      d. Do not allow fractured extremity to hang in a dependent position; provide constant support to the extremity.
   5. Promote good skin care and turning protocol.

G. Reduction of risk potential: Provide child, family, and community with teaching about injury prevention (see also safety and infection control).

H. Pharmacologic and parenteral therapies: Analgesics are used as needed to manage pain. Use age-appropriate pain scale to assess effectiveness of analgesia.

Developmental Dysplasia of the Hip

I. Definition: Developmental dysplasia of the hip (DDH) involves a group of disorders associated with abnormal hip development in utero. Contributing factors include intrauterine position, delivery type, and joint laxity. Types of DDH include subluxation, dysplasia, and dislocation. The main types are the result of either laxity of the supporting capsule or an abnormal acetabulum.

II. Nursing process
   A. Assessment
      1. Complete a detailed health history and physical assessment including history of delivery, especially breech birth.
      2. Assess for signs and symptoms of a hip dysplasia.
         a. Newborn
            (1) Tendency to subluxate (slip) or dislocate
            (2) Ortolani sign ("click")
         b. Child more than 2 to 3 months of age
            (1) Beginning at 6 to 10 weeks of life, affected hip observed as having limited range of motion
            (2) Allis or Galeazzi sign: Lower position of knee of the affected side when knees and hips are flexed
            (3) Asymmetry of gluteal and thigh skinfolds
         c. Child of walking age: Limp or toe walking; lordosis
      3. Obtain diagnostic tests.
         a. Barlow and Ortolani tests; only a useful test until 6 to 10 weeks of life, and then contractures develop and tests unreliable
         b. Ultrasound during newborn period
         c. X-rays useful after 6 months of age
   B. Analysis
      1. Risk for Injury: Abduction Device or Cast Complications, related to improper maintenance or positioning
      2. Deficient Knowledge: Treatment Regimen and Home Management, related to lack of information about treatment of DDH
      3. Impaired Physical Mobility related to pain, surgery, or abduction device
      4. Risk for Impaired Skin Integrity related to immobility and cast or abduction device
      5. Risk for Ineffective Tissue Perfusion related to inflammation and edema associated with surgery, traction, casting, or placement of abduction device
   C. Planning
      1. Reduce risk of injury.
      2. Provide child and family teaching.
      3. Improve mobility.
      4. Reduce risk of skin breakdown.
      5. Improve tissue perfusion.
   D. Implementation: Provide interventions to manage DDH.
      1. For newborn to child 6 months of age: Maintain hip joint—dynamic splinting with abduction device such as Pavlik harness; applied as soon as condition identified.
      2. For child older than 6 months of age:
         a. Home traction for 3 weeks
         b. Closed-reduction surgery
         c. Hip spica cast for 2 to 4 months
   E. Evaluation
      1. Child has reduced risk of injury as evidenced by maintenance of proper body alignment and cast care.
      2. Child and family verbalize understanding of DDH treatment, complications, and home management.
      3. Child maintains mobility appropriate to abduction device or cast.
      4. Child's skin remains intact through use of reduction device or casting.
      5. Child has adequate tissue perfusion as evidenced by good skin turgor, good color, capillary refill 2 s or more, equal pulses, and lack of paresthesia.
      6. Child is free from infection as evidenced by approximated, well-healed surgical site.

CN

III. Client needs
   A. Physiologic adaptation: DDH is managed with abduction devices and/or surgery to prevent hip contractures and promote the development of normal motor skills. Assess sleep patterns, appetite, and achievement of growth and developmental milestones; discuss child's tolerance of abduction device with family.
   B. Management of care: Care of the child with DDH requires critical thinking skills and knowledge of assessment, and teaching and evaluation methods unique to the RN role. These skills cannot be delegated to an LPN or UAP.
      1. Perform comprehensive physical assessments and provide care appropriate to the child with DDH.
      2. Provide follow-up care to evaluate abduction device or cast and plans for removal.
      3. Assess home needs for equipment such as cast care materials or abduction device padding.
      4. Identify community resources such as health department for specialized car seat and transportation for follow-up medica[l] visits.
      5. Delegate responsibly those activi[ties that] can be delegated, including

oral intake and urine output, vital signs, and reporting child's subjective data. All monitoring information is reported to the RN.

C. Safety and infection control
   1. Instruct parents to apply and maintain abduction device.
      a. Place undershirt beneath chest straps; place knee socks beneath extremity pieces.
      b. Check skin under straps two to three times per day.
      c. Massage skin under straps once per day.
      d. Apply diaper beneath straps.
      e. Do not remove harness; bathe by sponge bath.
   2. Provide child and parent teaching about cast care.
      a. Place clothing over cast so food and toys cannot be stuffed into cast.
      b. Avoid soiling of cast through appropriate diaper placement.

D. Health promotion and maintenance
   1. Involve child and family in care to promote compliance with multiple procedures and involved therapeutic regimen.
   2. Encourage child and family to participate in activities of daily living.
   3. Assist child and family in identifying need for follow-up.
   4. Instruct child and family about reduction device or cast and home management (see safety and infection control).
   5. Provide age-appropriate and developmentally appropriate diversional activities to promote growth and development.

E. Psychologic integrity: Offer parents and child a constant opportunity to express fears and concerns in coping with DDH and possible home needs. Provide parents with ongoing information about the child's progress.

F. Basic care and comfort
   1. Provide consistent nurse caregiver.
   2. Provide transitional comfort object if hospitalized; introduce toys that can be used if the child is immobilized.
   3. Encourage parents to stay at bedside and p‐ icipate in care.

'de good skin care and turning protocol.
 of risk potential
t complications through early detec-
DDH.
'e that only appropriately educated
ers may elicit Barlow and
sts.
'opriate car seat if child in
vice.

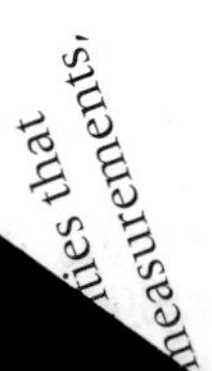

H. Pharmacologic and parenteral therapies are rarely required.

Congenital Clubfoot

I. Definition: Congenital clubfoot is a malformation of the lower extremities. The deformity is named based on the position of the foot (talipes equinovarus, calcaneovalgus, talipes valgus). The most common form is talipes equinovarus.

II. Nursing process

A. Assessment
   1. Complete a detailed health history and physical assessment, including family history.
   2. Assess for signs and symptoms of clubfoot: Visual examination reveals foot plantar flexed and forefoot adducted.
   3. Obtain diagnostic tests: Radiograph and ultrasound for foot and ankle.

B. Analysis
   1. Risk for Delayed Growth and Development related to immobilization
   2. Deficient Knowledge: Treatment/Procedures, related to lack of information about the defect
   3. Impaired Physical Mobility related to musculoskeletal impairment
   4. Risk for Impaired Skin Integrity related to immobilization and cast

C. Planning
   1. Improve physical mobility.
   2. Maintain and promote growth and development.
   3. Reduce risk of skin breakdown.
   4. Provide parent teaching.

D. Implementation
   1. Promote serial manipulation and casting—change casts weekly until clubfoot corrected.
      a. If corrected: Promote maintenance splinting (orthopaedic shoes).
      b. If not corrected by 4 to 9 months of age: Promote surgical intervention; serial surgery may be necessary for severe defects.
   2. Provide follow-up care to prevent recurrence.

E. Evaluation
   1. Child experiences normal growth and development as evidenced by demonstration of developmental tasks.
   2. Child's skin remains intact through use of serial casting.
   3. Child has adequate tissue perfusion and no skin breakdown as evidenced by good skin turgor, good color, capillary refill 2 s or more, equal pulses, and lack of paresthesia.

4. Parents verbalize understanding of congenital clubfoot treatment, complications, and home management.

CN

III. Client needs

A. Physiologic adaptation: Congenital clubfoot is managed with serial casting and/or surgery to promote normal ambulation and the development of normal motor skills. Failure to achieve ankle and foot alignment indicates need for surgical preparation between 4 and 9 months of age.

B. Management of care: Care of the child with congenital clubfoot requires critical thinking skills and knowledge of assessment, and teaching and evaluation methods unique to the RN role. These skills cannot be delegated to an LPN or UAP.

1. Perform comprehensive physical assessments and provide care appropriate to the child with congenital clubfoot.
2. Provide follow-up care to evaluate cast, plans for removal, and prevention of recurrence.
3. Assess home needs for equipment such as cast care materials.
4. Identify community resources for transportation for follow-up and specialized car seat.
5. Delegate responsibly those activities that can be delegated, including measurements, oral intake and urine output, vital signs, and reporting child's subjective data. All monitoring information is reported to the RN.

C. Safety and infection control: Assess and provide cast care.

1. Leave open to air until dry.
2. Touch cast with palm of hands only until dry.
3. Reposition child every 2 hr.
4. Avoid soiling with urine or stool by using diapers as needed and assisting child to void and defecate on a regular basis.
5. Petal edges when cast is dry.

D. Health promotion and maintenance

1. Assess family readiness to learn, and provide teaching about type of clubfoot, its treatment, and complications.
2. Involve family in care to promote compliance with multiple procedures and therapeutic regimen.
3. Assist family in identifying need for follow-up.
4. Teach family about cast and home management.
   a. Perform foot manipulation exercises daily.
   b. Promote serial casting and follow-up care.
   c. Identify and report compromised neurovascular status.
   d. Manage pain.
   e. Perform cast care and maintenance.
   f. Acknowledge possibility of surgical intervention.
5. Provide age-appropriate and developmentally appropriate diversional activities to promote growth and development.

E. Psychologic integrity

1. Promote child-parent bonding.
2. Provide parent teaching about developmental needs and methods to promote needs during casting.
3. Provide quiet diversional and recreational activities appropriate for developmental age.
4. Offer parents a constant opportunity to express fears and concerns in coping with congenital clubfoot and possible home needs.
5. Provide parents with ongoing information about the child's progress.

F. Basic care and comfort

1. Provide consistent nurse caregiver.
2. Provide transitional comfort object if child is hospitalized.
3. Encourage parents to stay at bedside and participate in care.
4. Promote good skin care and turning protocol.

G. Reduction of risk potential: Promote early identification and institution of treatment.

H. Pharmacologic and parenteral therapies are rarely required.

Scoliosis

I. Definition: Scoliosis is a lateral curvature of the spine and may be classified as congenital, neuromuscular, or idiopathic. Idiopathic scoliosis is the predominant type; this occurs in newborns and older children, but most commonly in adolescents between 10 and 18 years of age. The condition is managed based on age of child and severity of curvature.

II. Nursing process

A. Assessment

1. Complete a detailed health history and physical assessment, including family history.
2. Assess for signs and symptoms of spinal curvature.
   a. Shoulders are asymmetrical; when bending forward, rib hump noted in thoracic area

   b. Uneven hips and shoulders; head and hips not in alignment
   c. Uneven waistline, which may be noticed by uneven hemlines of clothing; one hip more prominent than the other
3. Obtain diagnostic tests: Spinal radiographs and Cobb technique for measuring curve.

B. Analysis
1. Disturbed Body Image related to perception of difference in appearance
2. Risk For Injury: Brace, related to orthotic intervention
3. Deficient Knowledge: Treatment Regimen and Home Management, related to lack of information about treatment of scoliosis
4. Acute Pain related to spinal surgery
5. Impaired Physical Mobility related to orthotic intervention or spinal surgery
6. Risk for Impaired Skin Integrity related to orthotic intervention

C. Planning
1. Promote positive body image.
2. Reduce risk of injury.
3. Provide child and family teaching.
4. Manage and improve pain.
5. Improve mobility.
6. Reduce risk of skin breakdown.

D. Implementation
1. Promote bracing and exercise: Boston brace or TLSO (thoracic, lumbar, sacral orthosis).
2. Initiate surgical intervention: Spinal fusion with instrumentation or bone grafts.

E. Evaluation
1. Child has reduced risk of injury as evidenced by maintenance of orthotic regimen and exercise plan.
2. Child and family verbalize understanding of scoliosis, treatment, surgery, and follow-up care.
3. Child verbalizes a decrease in pain to tolerable level and evidence supports appearance of comfort.
4. Child maintains mobility appropriate to brace and surgical intervention.
5. Child's skin remains intact through serial assessment and early intervention.
6. Child verbalizes concerns about body image and demonstrates positive coping mechanisms and expression of self-esteem.

CN

III. Client needs

A. Physiologic adaptation: Treatment decisions for scoliosis are based on type of curve, magnitude, skeletal maturity, and underlying disease.
1. Recognize risk for increase in intra-abdominal pressure: Mesenteric artery syndrome—indicated by vomiting and abdominal distention.
2. Assess for tolerance and compliance with orthotic regimen. Failure of orthotic regimen may warrant child and family preparation for surgery.
3. Monitor for degree of curvature.

B. Management of care: Care of the child with scoliosis requires critical thinking skills and knowledge of assessment, and teaching and evaluation methods unique to the RN role. These skills cannot be delegated to an LPN or UAP.
1. Perform comprehensive physical assessments and provide care appropriate to the child with scoliosis.
2. Provide follow-up care to evaluate effectiveness of orthotic regimen and need for surgery.
3. Assess needs for modification of home setting to accommodate limited mobility, how to accomplish activities of daily living, and need for equipment such as special mattresses.
4. Identify community resources for local chapter of the National Scoliosis Foundation for family support and information, possible transportation for follow-up visits, and arrangement for in-home schooling.
5. Delegate responsibly those activities that can be delegated, including measurements, oral intake and urine output, vital signs, and reporting child's subjective data. All monitoring information is reported to the RN.

C. Safety and infection control
1. Provide postoperative management for spinal fusion and instrumentation.
   a. Log roll to reposition child: Avoid twisting.
   b. Provide neurovascular assessments.
   c. Promote good pulmonary assessments and care: Incentive spirometry, coughing, and repositioning.
   d. Assess and manage pain.
   e. Prepare child for use of TLSO for spinal stabilization after surgery.
2. Provide child and parent teaching about orthotic care and management.
   a. Assure brace is worn 16 to 23 hr per day.
   b. Monitor skin under brace for areas of breakdown.
   c. Avoid lotions and powders under brace.
   d. Promote lightweight, soft clothing under brace (i.e., T-shirt).
   e. Maintain exercise program.

f. Promote positive body image.
g. Use appropriate methods to ambulate and get up and out of chairs and bed.
3. Assess home setting for hazards when wearing orthotic device, including use of handrails, and avoidance of wet, uneven, or slippery surfaces.

D. Health promotion and maintenance
1. Involve child in care to promote compliance with orthotic and exercise regimen.
2. Encourage child to participate in activities of daily living.
3. Assist child and family in identifying the importance of follow-up care.
4. Instruct child and family about orthotic device, surgery, and home management.

E. Psychologic integrity
1. Encourage child to verbalize feelings about wearing brace.
2. Provide quiet diversional and recreational activities when energy is improved and pain subsides.
3. Offer parents and child a constant opportunity to express fears and concerns in coping with scoliosis and possible home needs.
4. Provide parents with ongoing information about child's progress.
5. Address possible school issues and needs related to bracing.
6. Refer to support groups such as National Scoliosis Foundation.

F. Basic care and comfort
1. Provide consistent nurse caregiver.
2. Provide favorite diversional items (e.g., iPod) if hospitalized.
3. Encourage parents to stay at bedside and participate in care.
4. Manage pain.
5. Promote good skin care and log rolling/turning protocol.

G. Reduction of risk potential
1. Screen all children 10 years of age and older during health care visits.
2. Provide long-term monitoring to observe progression of curve.

H. Pharmacologic and parenteral therapies are rarely required.

Juvenile Idiopathic Arthritis

I. Definition: Juvenile idiopathic arthritis (JIA), formerly known as *juvenile rheumatoid arthritis* (JRA), is a chronic, inflammatory disorder of connective tissue, presenting with synovitis of one or more joints. The condition is characterized by remission and exacerbation.

II. Nursing process

A. Assessment
1. Complete a detailed health history and physical assessment, including family history.
2. Assess for signs and symptoms of joint involvement.
   a. Stiffness, swelling, and loss of motion in affected joints
   b. Joints may range from pain-free to tender and painful
   c. Morning stiffness
   d. Uveitis (iridocyclitis)
3. Obtain diagnostic tests.
   a. Erythrocyte sedimentation rate (ESR)
   b. Antinuclear antibodies
   c. Rheumatoid factor
   d. CBC
   e. Synovial fluid culture

B. Analysis
1. Fatigue related to anemia or medication side effects
2. Deficient Knowledge: Disease and Treatment, related to lack of information about treatment regimen
3. Chronic Pain: Joint, related to inflammation and degenerative damage
4. Impaired Physical Mobility related to joint stiffness and pain

C. Planning
1. Improve activity tolerance and reduce fatigue.
2. Provide child and family teaching.
3. Control and manage pain.
4. Improve mobility and reduce stiffness.

D. Implementation
1. Manage pain.
2. Preserve joint function.
3. Minimize inflammatory process.
4. Promote growth and development.
5. Promote early identification of complications, such as uveitis or carditis.

E. Evaluation
1. Child verbalizes improved energy and maintains activity within limitations.
2. Child and family verbalize understanding of disease, treatment, medications, and home management.
3. Child verbalizes a decrease in pain and stiffness as evidenced by participation in activities of daily living.

CN

III. Client needs

A. Physiologic adaptation: Joint inflammation and stiffness is controlled with a complex medication regimen, physical therapy, and heat application to promote joint function and prevent joint deformity. Evaluate effectiveness of medication regimen (salicylates, corticosteroids, cytotoxic medications, immunologic modifiers, biologic agents, nonsteroidal anti-inflammatory drugs, and antirheumatic drugs) in controlling inflammation and relieving pain.

B. Management of care: Care of the child with JIA requires critical thinking skills and knowledge of assessment, and teaching and evaluation methods unique to the RN role. These skills cannot be delegated to an LPN or UAP.
   1. Perform comprehensive physical assessments and provide care appropriate to the child with JIA.
   2. Provide follow-up care to evaluate medication and therapy compliance, joint mobility or deformity, remissions, and exacerbations.
   3. Assess home setting for equipment needs such as adaptive devices and braces for mobility issues related to ambulation, as well as accessibility, if home has multiple levels.
   4. Identify community resources such as community pool for exercise, local chapter of the American Juvenile Arthritis Organization, and possible transportation needs.
   5. Delegate responsibly those activities that can be delegated, including measurements, oral intake and urine output, vital signs, and reporting child's subjective data. All monitoring information is reported to the RN.

C. Safety and infection control
   1. Provide child and family teaching about medication/treatment regimen purpose, side effects, and long-term adverse effects.
   2. Provide written information on all medications and treatments.
   3. Maintain the six rights of medication administration.

D. Health promotion and maintenance
   1. Encourage well-balanced diet to maintain normal weight.
   2. Provide methods to facilitate independence such as modified utensils, elevated toilet seat, and handrails and other such assistive devices for mobility.
   3. Assist child and family to identify factors that exacerbate pain, such as stress, climate, movement, and noncompliance with regimen.

E. Psychologic integrity
   1. Assist child and family to identify coping mechanisms.
   2. Assist child and family in expressing feelings and provide opportunity to discuss concerns.
   3. Include child in decision-making and care plan to promote compliance and success with treatment.
   4. Refer to community agencies such as American Juvenile Arthritis Foundation.

F. Basic care and comfort: Manage joint pain and inflammatory process.
   1. Assess severity of pain, location, stiffness, and precipitating factors such as weight gain, activity level, and presence of fatigue.
   2. Administer medications and monitor effects.
   3. Administer moist warm heat, paraffin baths, or whirlpool baths.
   4. Provide several rest periods.
   5. Promote position of comfort; elevate and support joints.
   6. Promote range of motion exercises.
   7. Encourage stretching exercises.
   8. Encourage nonimpact activities such as swimming.
   9. Apply splints as ordered.
   10. Encourage daily bath with warm water for 10-min period; avoid overactivity and nonpharmacologic pain-relief methods.

G. Reduction of risk potential: Provide child and parent teaching about medication side effects, including adverse effects and the importance of reporting symptoms to prevent toxicity, bleeding, or impaired cardiac or renal function.

H. Pharmacologic and parenteral therapies: Child and family will state the purpose, dosage, timing, and side effects of medications to treat JIA (see Table 18-1).

Pseudohypertrophic (Duchenne) Muscular Dystrophy

I. Definition: Muscular dystrophy is a group of muscle disorders in which there is gradual degeneration of muscle fibers, leading to deformity and disability. Pseudohypertrophic muscular dystrophy, also called *childhood muscular dystrophy* or *Duchenne muscular dystrophy* (DMD), is the most severe form and most common in children. The condition is X-linked recessive, meaning females are carriers and males are affected. Fat and fibrous tissue infiltrates muscles and causes weakness of the myocardium and respiratory muscles. DMD typically results in death before early adulthood.

II. Nursing process
   A. Assessment
      1. Complete a detailed health history and physical assessment, including family history and developmental delays in walking.
      2. Assess for signs and symptoms characteristic of DMD.

Table 18-1 Medications Used to Treat Juvenile Idiopathic Arthritis

Classification	Generic/Trade Name	Expected Outcome	Reduction of Risk Potential	Management of Care
Salicylates	Aspirin (acetylsalicylic acid); salsalate (Arthra-G); choline salicylates (Trilisate)	Relieves mild-to-moderate pain. Acts as anti-inflammatory.	Monitor clotting times. Monitor for toxicity: Tinnitus, confusion, and gastric bleeding.	Teach family to monitor for nausea, reflux, and bleeding: Administer with food or milk; watch color of stools. Report any bleeding or ringing in ears.
Nonsteroidal anti-inflammatory drugs (NSAIDs)	Ibuprofen (Advil); diclofenac (Voltaren)	Acts as anti-inflammatory to treat mild-to-moderate pain.	Evaluate for hypertension, cardiac or renal disease.	Teach family to monitor for mild GI disturbance and to administer with food or milk.
Corticosteroids	Cortisone (Cortone); prednisone (Deltasone); dexamethasone (Decadron)	Acts as anti-inflammatory (for short-term use).	Monitor electrolytes. Monitor adrenal function.	Teach family to monitor weight, edema, and behavior change.
Biologic agent	Etanercept (Enbrel)	Interrupts inflammatory response.	Purified protein derivative (PPD) before treatment. Avoid live virus vaccines.	Monitor for infection. Notify HCP if exposed to varicella.
Chelating agent	Penicillamine (Depen)	Used when other therapy does not work.	Monitor for leucopenia and thrombocytopenia.	Teach child to report any loss of taste. Teach family to monitor for infection and bleeding.
Gold salts	Auranofin (Ridaura)	Slows down cartilage damage.	Use controversial: Monitor BUN and creatinine and serum blood count.	Expect GI disturbance and possibly rash. Teach to expect metallic taste.
Cytotoxic agents	Cyclophosphamide (Cytoxan); methotrexate (Mexate)	Suppresses inflammatory response.	Monitor CBC. Monitor liver enzymes.	Expect GI disturbances. Teach family to protect child from infection and monitor for bleeding.
Antimalarials	Hydroxychloroquine sulfate (Plaquenil)	Treats JIA.	Monitor CBC.	Encourage eye exams to detect retinopathy. Hypotension may occur: Teach to sit before rising. Hair bleaching may occur.
Immunosuppressants	Azathioprine (Imuran)	Used when other treatments are ineffective.	Causes pancytopenia: Monitor all blood counts.	Teach family to protect child from infection.

a. Progressive muscle weakness, atrophy, and contractures
b. Difficulty in running or climbing steps may be first sign
c. Abnormal waddling gait
d. Hypertrophied calf muscles from fatty infiltrates
e. Gower sign: Classic method of rising by "walking" hands up legs
f. Developmental delay: Mild-to-moderate mental impairment

3. Assess for complications of disease progression, including obesity, contractures, infections, and later respiratory or cardiac failure.

4. Obtain diagnostic tests.
    a. Based on clinical examination
    b. Muscle biopsy
    c. EMG
    d. Serum creatinine phosphokinase (CPK)
    e. Serum deoxyribonucleic acid

B. Analysis
1. Anticipatory Grieving related to perceived potential loss of life
2. Risk for Infection related to decrease in pulmonary capacity
3. Risk for Injury: Abduction Device or Cast, related to improper maintenance
4. Deficient Knowledge: Treatment Regimen and Home Management, related to lack of information about treatment of DMD
5. Imbalanced Nutrition: More Than Body Requirements related to muscle weakness and immobility
6. Impaired Physical Mobility related to progressive muscle weakness
7. Risk for Impaired Skin Integrity related to immobility and weakness

C. Planning
1. Promote coping mechanisms and establishment of support systems.
2. Reduce risk of infection.
3. Reduce risk of injury.
4. Provide child and family teaching.
5. Maintain mobility.
6. Reduce risk of skin breakdown.
7. Maintain normal body weight.

D. Implementation
1. Administer corticosteroids for children older than 5 years of age; corticosteroids (usually prednisone) are used to promote strength in children who exhibit extreme muscular weakness.
2. Promote muscle function.
    a. Range of motion exercises
    b. Surgery for contractures
    c. Bracing or splinting

E. Evaluation
1. Child and family verbalize feelings and establish support systems.
2. Child has reduced risk of infection as evidenced by normal vital signs and clear lung fields.
3. Child has reduced risk of injury as evidenced by maintenance of proper body alignment.
4. Child and family verbalize understanding of DMD treatment, complications, home management, and outcome.
5. Child maintains mobility appropriate to deteriorating muscle tone.
6. Child's skin remains intact as evidenced by no areas of breakdown over bony prominences.
7. Child maintains normal body weight.

CN

III. Client needs

A. Physiologic adaptation: There is no definitive treatment for DMD—disorder is managed with supportive care and promotion and maintenance of function as long as possible using a multidisciplinary approach.

B. Management of care: Care of the child with DMD requires critical thinking skills and knowledge of assessment, and teaching and evaluation methods unique to the RN role. These skills cannot be delegated to an LPN or UAP.
1. Perform comprehensive physical assessments and provide care appropriate to the child with DMD.
2. Provide follow-up care to evaluate progress, maintain functional status, and support family.
3. Assess home needs for equipment such as splints, AFOs (ankle-foot orthoses), soft "pressure care" mattresses or wheelchair ramps.
4. Identify community resources such as local chapter of the Muscular Dystrophy Association, transportation needs to physical therapy, and possible home school needs.
5. Delegate responsibly those activities that can be delegated, including measurements, oral intake and urine output, vital signs, and reporting child's subjective data. All monitoring information is reported to the RN.

C. Safety and infection control
1. Provide teaching for child and family about disease, progression, exercise program, supportive care measures, home needs, and support groups.
2. Teach parents early signs and symptoms of respiratory infection and the importance of seeking immediate treatment.
3. Teach parents importance of maintaining normal body weight.

D. Health promotion and maintenance
1. Tailor care to promote growth and development and maintain functional capacity with child and family participation.
2. Involve child in care to promote compliance with physical therapy to assist in improving self-esteem.
3. Encourage child to participate in activities of daily living, up to individual limits.
4. Instruct child and family about supportive measures.

5. Provide age-appropriate and developmentally appropriate diversional activities to promote growth and development.

E. Psychologic integrity
1. Assist child and family in coping with fatal disease. Encourage verbalization of feelings about ultimate disease outcome.
2. Build child's self-esteem through promoting self-management.
3. Refer to support groups such as Muscular Dystrophy Association.

F. Basic care and comfort
1. Provide consistent nurse caregiver.
2. Provide transitional comfort object or preferred diversional activity when energy is improved.
3. Encourage parents to stay at bedside and participate in care.
4. Manage fatigue and muscle weakness with rest and by organizing care activities to allow rest.
5. Promote good skin care and turning protocol.

G. Reduction of risk potential
1. Promote prenatal diagnosis using polymerase chain reaction.
2. Encourage genetic counseling for parents, female siblings, maternal aunts, and their female children.

H. Pharmacologic and parenteral therapies: Pharmacologic needs vary depending on presenting symptomatology, procedures, or surgical interventions. Child and family will state the purpose, dosage, timing, and side effects of medications used to treat health problems caused by DMD; for example, cardiac health problems such as arrhythmias, or respiratory problems such as dyspnea. If child is using corticosteroids, monitor for osteoporosis, infection, poor wound healing, edema of face and abdomen, and elevated blood sugar. If discontinued, drug must be tapered.

Cerebral Palsy

I. Definition: Cerebral palsy (CP) is a nonspecific term applied to disorders characterized by impaired movement and posture, which may be accompanied by language and intellectual deficits. The condition is nonprogressive, with a variety of etiologies and clinical findings. Anoxia from prolonged labor or use of anesthesia during labor can cause vascular occlusion, atrophy, and loss of neurons. CP is classified by clinical type: Spasticity (most common), dysthenia, and ataxia. CP is described by limb involvement: Hemiplegia, diplegia, paraplegia, quadriplegia, monoplegia, and triplegia. CP can also be described by degree of severity: Mild, moderate, and severe.

II. Nursing process

A. Assessment
1. Complete a detailed health history including family history and history of birth to address labor and delivery problems, intrauterine or birth asphyxia, intrauterine infection, birth weight, and presence of neonatal problems.
2. Complete a detailed physical assessment; assess for signs and symptoms of CP.
   a. Poor head control after 3 months of age
   b. Rigid arms and legs
   c. Arching back (opisthotonic)
   d. Floppy or altered muscle tone
   e. Child reflexes present after 6 months of age
   f. Inability to sit by 8 months of age
   g. Failure to smile by 3 months of age
   h. Feeding difficulties
3. Obtain diagnostic tests: Neurologic examination and history.

B. Analysis
1. Risk for Caregiver Role Strain related to complex, lifelong needs
2. Risk for Interrupted Family Processes related to complex, lifelong needs
3. Risk for injury: Accidents, related to cognitive and intellectual impairment
4. Impaired Physical Mobility related to neuromuscular impairment
5. Self-Care Deficit: Bathing/Hygiene, Dressing/Grooming, Feeding, and Toileting, related to intellectual and physical inabilities
6. Impaired Verbal Communication related to cognitive and intellectual impairment

C. Planning
1. Identify family coping mechanisms and support systems.
2. Promote family functioning.
3. Prevent injuries.
4. Promote physical mobility.
5. Promote growth and development.
6. Improve cognitive and intellectual abilities to child's capacity.

D. Implementation: Provide interventions to manage multidisciplinary needs.
1. Promote physical therapy with use of orthotic devices (braces, splints).
2. Promote occupational therapy.
3. Promote speech therapy.
4. Promote special education programs.
5. Administer medications for muscle spasticity.
6. Administer medications for pain, anxiety, and secondary conditions such as seizures.

7. Administer medications for gastrointestinal reflux.
8. Initiate surgical interventions for contractures or deformities.
9. Provide nutritional interventions such as special formulas or tube feedings.

E. Evaluation
1. Parents identify and promote positive coping mechanisms and maintain functional support systems.
2. Child experiences no injuries as a result of safety modifications in home setting.
3. Child participates in activities of daily living within identified capacity.
4. Child learns to communicate needs and wants to family and others.
5. Child reaches growth milestones as evidenced by intake of appropriate diet.
6. Child demonstrates ability for locomotion appropriate to identified capacity.

CN

III. Client needs

A. Physiologic adaptation: CP is a complex problem requiring a multidisciplinary approach to promote and maintain cognitive, intellectual, social, and physical growth (see implementation). Promote ongoing evaluation of child to assess progress and identify complications.

B. Management of care: Care of the child with CP requires critical thinking skills and knowledge of assessment, and teaching and evaluation methods unique to the RN role. These skills cannot be delegated to an LPN or UAP.
1. Perform comprehensive physical assessments and provide care appropriate to the child with CP.
2. Provide follow-up care to evaluate progress, maintain functional status, and support family.
3. Assess needs of home setting, including specialized adaptive equipment and wheelchairs, modification of the environment related to mobility issues, and possible equipment for tube feedings.
4. Identify community resources, including transportation for multidisciplinary health care visits, availability of equipment delivery, possible medication and grocery delivery, specialized schools, need for respite care, and local chapter of United Cerebral Palsy for family information and support.
5. Delegate responsibly those activities that can be delegated, including measurements, oral intake and urine output, vital signs, and reporting child's subjective data. All monitoring information is reported to the RN.

C. Safety and infection control
1. Promote safety in home setting.
   a. Provide padded furniture or high seat.
   b. Keep side rails raised on crib and then on bed.
   c. Avoid area rugs.
   d. Do not polish floors.
   e. Avoid child seats or jumping seats.
2. Instruct parents about providing safe toys that are appropriate to developmental age, not chronological age.
3. Promote rest and good nutrition.
4. Teach appropriate use of car seats and safety harnesses.
5. Instruct use of helmet for ambulatory child.

D. Health promotion and maintenance
1. Provide parent teaching about physical therapy, occupational therapy, speech therapy, special education programs, surgical intervention, medication therapy, and promotion of child's functional capacity.
2. Tailor care to functional capacity with child and family participation; provide frequent rest periods.
3. Involve child in care to promote self-management, compliance with treatment regimen, and improve self-esteem; encourage child to participate in activities of daily living up to individual limits.
4. Provide developmentally appropriate diversional activities to promote growth and development.
5. Arrange special education related to mental and developmental age.

E. Psychologic integrity
1. Encourage family to verbalize fears, concerns, guilt, anger, and feelings about birth outcome.
2. Refer to support groups such as United Cerebral Palsy.

F. Basic care and comfort
1. Provide consistent nurse caregiver.
2. Provide transitional comfort object if child is hospitalized.
3. Encourage parents to stay at bedside and participate in care.

G. Reduction of risk potential
1. Promote early identification and assessment of children at risk.
2. Avoid contact with infected persons.
3. Initiate routine immunizations.

H. Pharmacologic and parenteral therapies: Family will state the purpose, dosage, timing, and side effects of medications.

1. Baclofen (Lioresal)
   a. Expected outcome: Provides symptomatic relief of muscle spasms.
   b. Reduction of risk potential: Monitor BP, weight, serum glucose levels, and hepatic function tests; if child has seizures, monitor for loss of seizure control.
   c. Management of care: Monitor for loss of glycemic control; instruct parents not to abruptly stop medication, and to administer with milk if taking orally.
2. Botulinum toxin type A (Botox)
   a. Expected outcome: Treats muscle spacticity for lower extremities.
   b. Reduction of risk potential: Evaluate at 1 to 2 weeks for effectiveness.
   c. Management of care: Inform practitioner of all medications and herbal supplements before initiating treatment; notify if difficulty breathing or swallowing.
3. Baclofen (Lioresal) pump (used for muscle spacticity not responsive to oral or injectable medication)
   a. Expected outcome: Provides symptomatic relief of muscle spasms causing pain and interfering with activities of daily living.
   b. Reduction of risk potential: For children at least 4 years of age: Monitor BP, weight, serum glucose levels, and hepatic function tests. If child has seizures, monitor for loss of seizure control.
   c. Management of care: Delivered intrathecally by surgically implanted pump; instruct parents not to abruptly stop medication and to avoid extreme temperatures, metal detectors, and MRIs.

Bibilography

Hatfield, N. (2006). *Broadribb's introductory pediatric nursing.* Philadelphia: Lippincott Williams & Wilkins.

Pillitteri, A. (2006). *Maternal & child health nursing: Care of the childbearing and childrearing family* (5th ed.). Philadelphia: Lippincott Williams & Wilkins.

Wong, D. L., et al. (2006). *Maternal child nursing care.* St. Louis: Mosby.

CHAPTER 18 Practice Test

Fracture

1. An adolescent has a full-body plaster cast. When being admitted to the nursing unit, the child immediately becomes diaphoretic and complains of being hot. The nurse should do which of the following first?

□ 1. Assess for signs of infection.
□ 2. Notify the surgeon.
□ 3. Moisten the cast with cool water.
□ 4. Advise the adolescent that this is to be expected.

2. The nurse is assessing a child who is 10 years of age with a fractured femur. Which of the following observations should the nurse report to a HCP?

□ 1. Presence of pulses above the injury site.
□ 2. Pain and tenderness at the site.
□ 3. Paresthesia sensation above the injury site.
□ 4. Bright red color to the skin.

Developmental Dysplasia of the Hip

3. AF The nurse is conducting a health assessment of a neonate. Which of the following should be drawn to the attention of the HCP? Select all that apply.

□ 1. Unequal abduction of the hips.
□ 2. Limbs of equal length.
□ 3. Unequal gluteal folds.
□ 4. Positive Ortolani sign.
□ 5. Startle reflex.

4. Which of the following statements by the parents of a child with DDH indicates an understanding of how to care for their child when using a Pavlik harness?

□ 1. "I will carefully adjust the straps on the harness if they seem too snug."
□ 2. "I will need to bring my child back to the clinic every month for the straps to be adjusted."

☐ 3. "I will remove the Pavlik harness at night and use a triple diaper instead, which is softer on the skin."
☐ 4. "The Pavlik harness will need to stay on around the clock."

Congenital Clubfoot

5. The nurse is teaching the parents of a child with a clubfoot about treatment and expected outcomes. The parents indicate they understand teaching when the mother says:
☐ 1. "Our child will not need treatment because his feet will straighten as they grow."
☐ 2. "Our child may need surgery if the casts do not correct the curvature in the feet."
☐ 3. "Our child will walk with a slight limp due to the unequal foot sizes and the poor muscle development."
☐ 4. "When our child has his clubfoot corrected successfully, he will not have any signs of the defect."

6. The nurse is teaching a parent of a child with a clubfoot about serial casting. The nurse evaluates that the parent understands the procedure when the parent says:
☐ 1. "I will perform the stretching exercises at home until casts are put on at 6 months of age."
☐ 2. "I will have to bring my child back to the clinic every few days for the first 2 weeks for manipulation and casting."
☐ 3. "This is going to be a long commitment in time, since the casting will continue until my baby is 2 years of age."
☐ 4. "I will need to arrange time off from work for the corrective surgery when the baby is 18 months of age."

Scoliosis

7. While an adolescent wears a body brace for scoliosis, the nurse should provide which of the following instructions?
☐ 1. Continue with age-appropriate activities.
☐ 2. Stand absolutely still whenever she is out of the brace.
☐ 3. Wear the brace a maximum of 20 hr each day.
☐ 4. Secondary sex development will stop until the brace is removed.

8. During a screening for scoliosis, the nurse identifies an 8-degree curvature of the spine in a female child who is 12 years of age. The nurse should tell the child and her parents:
☐ 1. "This may only be a postural variation, possibly from carrying a heavy backpack."
☐ 2. "This type of curvature will require exercises and chiropractic treatment."
☐ 3. "Your daughter will need to use a brace to correct the curvature."
☐ 4. "This curve in the spine typically involves realignment and straightening with internal fixation."

9. The nurse is developing a care plan for a female child who is 12 years of age and receiving surgery to correct idiopathic scoliosis. Which postoperative problem is a priority?
☐ 1. Pain.
☐ 2. Hypotension.
☐ 3. Prevention of pressure wounds.
☐ 4. Infection control.

Juvenile Idiopathic Arthritis

10. A child who is 7 years of age and diagnosed with JIA has extreme pain when she wakes in the morning. The nurse can advise the parents to:
☐ 1. Have her take 325 mg of aspirin immediately on waking.
☐ 2. Encourage her to take a warm bath each morning before school.
☐ 3. Have her do isotonic exercises until the pain is relieved.
☐ 4. Encourage her to remain in bed until the pain is gone.

11. Which of the following instructions should the nurse provide while teaching the parents of a female child who is 17 years of age and taking methotrexate for JIA?
☐ 1. The need to avoid becoming pregnant.
☐ 2. That the medication should be taken with food to avoid GI upset.
☐ 3. There may be a temporary allergic reaction at the injection site.
☐ 4. They may notice skin fragility as a possible side effect.

12. The nurse is providing health counseling for an adolescent with JIA who wants to develop an exercise program. Which of the following activities is most appropriate for muscle strengthening and maintaining joint mobility?
☐ 1. Golfing.
☐ 2. Running.
☐ 3. Walking.
☐ 4. Swimming.

Pseudohypertrophic (Duchenne) Muscular Dystrophy

13. The nurse is discussing health promotion with the mother of a child with DMD. The mother asks about the best diet for her child. The nurse should advise the mother that:
☐ 1. There is no special diet necessary for her son.
☐ 2. A high-protein, high-carbohydrate diet may be helpful.

- ☐ 3. Extra creatinine should be added to his diet daily.
- ☐ 4. A moderate-calorie diet will help him remain ambulatory longer.

14. A school-aged child has DMD. Which of the following actions will help this child maintain physical function for as long as possible?
- ☐ 1. Provide occasional rest periods during the school day.
- ☐ 2. Encourage daily exercise on a treadmill for approximately 30 min.
- ☐ 3. Use a wheelchair when the child needs to walk long distances.
- ☐ 4. Encourage normal play activities such as participating on a soccer team.

15. AF Which of the following relatives of a child diagnosed with DMD should the nurse recommend to receive genetic counseling? Select all that apply.
- ☐ 1. The parents.
- ☐ 2. Male siblings.
- ☐ 3. Female siblings.
- ☐ 4. Uncles and their sons.
- ☐ 5. Aunts and their daughters.
- ☐ 6. All first cousins.

Cerebral Palsy

16. The nurse is conducting a health assessment on a child with CP. Which of the following statements made by the mother indicates an appropriate understanding of her child's long-term needs?
- ☐ 1. "I know that once my child begins school she will catch up with other children."
- ☐ 2. "I realize that my child will need all of my attention for the rest of her life."
- ☐ 3. "I understand my child will grow up, and needs to develop as much independence as is appropriate."
- ☐ 4. "I realize that my child will need close supervision once she becomes sexually active."

17. AF The nurse is assessing a child with spastic type CP. The nurse should assess and document which of the following? Select all that apply.
- ☐ 1. Increased muscle tone.
- ☐ 2. Decreased deep tendon reflexes.
- ☐ 3. Extent of contractures.
- ☐ 4. Evidence of scoliosis.
- ☐ 5. Scissoring when walking.
- ☐ 6. Facial grimace.
- ☐ 7. Elbow, wrist, and fingers in flexed position with thumb adducted.

18. A child with spastic type CP had a "test dose" of intrathecal baclofen earlier in the morning. The child is now 4 hr postprocedure. Which of the following will indicate that the child is a candidate for a baclofen pump placement?
- ☐ 1. Relief of spasticity.
- ☐ 2. Increased spasticity.
- ☐ 3. Ability to freely move arms and legs.
- ☐ 4. Ability to walk with stand-by assistance.

19. The nurse is assessing a child who is 8 months of age. The mother reports that the baby smiles readily, uses his tongue to push food back out of the mouth, sits with some support when placed in a high chair, and likes to push away or arch back when held close. The nurse should tell the mother:
- ☐ 1. The child is developing normally.
- ☐ 2. Thicken the child's formula with rice.
- ☐ 3. Notify the HCP.
- ☐ 4. Try bundling the child when he pushes away.

20. A toddler with CP is demonstrating a speech delay. The nurse should advise the caregivers to use which of the following feeding techniques to facilitate the development of speech?
- ☐ 1. Hold the child in a semi-reclining position to make use of gravity flow.
- ☐ 2. Place food in the midcenter of the tongue.
- ☐ 3. Provide manual jaw control with a hand while standing at the child's side.
- ☐ 4. Place food at the side of the tongue, first one side, then the other.

Answers and Rationales

1. 4 Plaster becomes hot as it sets; therefore, the nurse prepares the client to expect being hot and even to sweat. There is no need to notify the surgeon at this time. The cast is not removed for client comfort as the heat will disappear as the cast dries. The cast is not being applied following an open wound such as occurs with compound fractures, so infection is not likely. Moistening the cast will soften the material and delay drying. (C)

2. 2 Pain and point of tenderness is one of the five "Ps" of ischemia related to a vascular injury; therefore, the nurse notifies the HCP. Other indications of ischemia are weak or absent pulses distal to the fracture site, paresthesia distal to the fracture, pallor, and paralysis distal to the fracture site. (R)

3. 1, 3, 4 DDH is indicated when the child is in a prone position and shows unequal gluteal folds and restricted abduction of the hip on the affected side. Shortening of limb on the affected side (Allis sign) and positive Ortolani sign (which is assessed for only by an experienced clinician to prevent further damage to the hip) are also positive signs of DDH. The startle reflex is a normal reflex in neonates. (H)

4. 4 The harness will stay on continuously. The physician may or may not allow for removal during bathing. In general, parents are instructed to avoid adjusting the harness without supervision. The child is examined by the HCP before any adjustment is attempted to make sure the hips are aligned correctly. The former practice of double or triple diapering for DDH is no longer recommended because it promotes hip extension, which worsens the DDH. (H)

5. 2 If the serial casting has not straightened the foot, surgical intervention with pin fixation and the releasing of tight joints and tendons is the next step. A clubfoot will not straighten on its own. In most children there will not be a limp, yet a child's muscle development may be delayed and the foot may be smaller in size. (C)

6. 2 Serial casting is started shortly after birth. Manipulation and casting are repeated frequently (every few days for 1 to 2 weeks, then at 1- to 2-week intervals) to accommodate the rapid growth of early infancy. Failure to achieve normal alignment by 3 months of age indicates the need for surgical intervention, which may take place between 6 and 12 months of age. (H)

7. 1 Wearing a body brace should not interfere with normal activities, which are necessary to maintain adolescent self-esteem. The child can move when not wearing the brace, but should wear the brace for 23 hr a day. The girl will continue to mature while wearing the brace. (H)

8. 1 Not all spinal curvatures are scoliosis. A curve of less than 10 degrees is considered a postural variation. Curves less than 20 degrees are mild and, if nonprogressive, do not require treatment. The nurse encourages the child and her parents to contact their HCP for additional follow-up as needed. (H)

9. 1 Clients typically have considerable pain for the first few days after surgery and require frequent administration of pain medication, preferably the use of opioids administered intravenously on a regular schedule, or patient-controlled analgesia (PCA). The other problems are all possible complications following this type of surgery, but the priority, until noted otherwise, is to provide adequate pain control. (C)

10. 2 Pain and stiffness associated with JIA can be relieved by moist heat, such as a warm bath. The nurse can also help the child and parents plan daily activities to minimize pain. Taking aspirin on an empty stomach could lead to gastric irritation. The child should remain active, not remain in bed until pain is gone. Isometric exercises are to increase muscle strength, and clients with JIA need to improve joint function. (H)

11. 1 The nurse instructs the client and parents about possible side effects of methotrexate, particularly the risk for birth defects; the client must avoid becoming pregnant. NSAIDs cause GI upset and skin fragility. Etanercept is a tumor necrosis factor (inhibitor) alpha receptor blocker and effective drug for JIA, but has a possible side effect of transient allergic reactions at the injection site and increased risks for infection. (D)

12. 4 Swimming is an excellent way for clients with JIA to obtain exercise because the activity strengthens muscles and maintains mobility in larger joints. Running, walking, and golfing do not provide the same musculoskeletal benefits for the child with JIA. (H)

13. 4 Preventing a child from gaining excess weight can allow him to be ambulatory longer. Because of limited mobility, it is easy to gain weight. (H)

14. 4 Maintaining optimal function in all muscles for as long as possible is the primary goal for a child with DMD. It has been found that children who remain as active as possible are able to avoid wheelchair confinement for a longer time. Maintenance of function of muscles includes stretching exercises, muscle training, and breathing exercises. If a child is interested in playing soccer he should be encouraged to participate. He may not be able to keep up at all times, but the aerobic exercise will be very beneficial. Exercising alone on a treadmill is boring and unimaginative for a child. Wheelchairs should be avoided until absolutely necessary. (H)

15. 1, 3, 5 DMD is inherited as an X-linked recessive trait, and the single gene defect is located on the short arm of the X chromosome. Genetic counseling is an important aspect of the care of the family. As in all X-linked disorders, males are affected almost exclusively, and females are carriers of the disorder. Genetic counseling is recommended for parents, female siblings, and maternal aunts and their female offspring. (H)

16. 3 Children with CP need to have as much independence as possible so they can reach their full potential. The other statements by the mother are not realistic and would require nursing intervention. (H)

17. 1, 3, 4, 5, 7 The child with spastic type CP has increased muscle tone, increased deep tendon reflexes, contractures (particularly that of the heel cord, adductor muscles, and knees), and intoeing and scissoring when walking. The elbow, wrist, and fingers are typically found in a flexed position with the thumb adducted. The nurse assesses and documents these findings. The child with spastic type CP does not have a facial grimace. (A)

18. 1 The positive effect of a baclofen test dose is relief of spasticity. The onset of action is usually 30 to 60 min after the administration and will peak within 6 hr. This finding will make the child a potential candidate for a baclofen pump placement. Intrathecal baclofen therapy is best suited for children with severe spasticity that interferes with activities of daily living and ambulation. The benefits of baclofen include fewer systemic side effects, dosage titration for maximizing effects, and reversibility of therapy with the removal of the pump, if desired. (D)

19. 3 This child is demonstrating potential warning signs of CP. After 6 months of age, the tongue should no longer be pushing soft food out of the mouth. Normally, children are sitting without support by 8 months of age. Pushing away or an arching back is a common physical finding of a child with CP. This child should be evaluated by an HCP and considered for a possible therapeutic treatment program that focuses on early intervention for children with CP. (H)

20. 4 Feeding techniques that force the child to use the lips and tongue in eating help facilitate speech development; therefore, placing food at the side of the tongue (first one side and then the other), making the child use the lips to take food from the spoon rather than placing it directly on the tongue, and avoiding using the teeth to remove the food from the utensil will help the child learn to speak. Holding the child in a semi-reclining position does not encourage the use of the lips and tongue. Providing manual jaw control limits the child's mouth movements and will not encourage the child to use the muscles of the tongue and mouth. (H)

SECTION 2

Practice Test

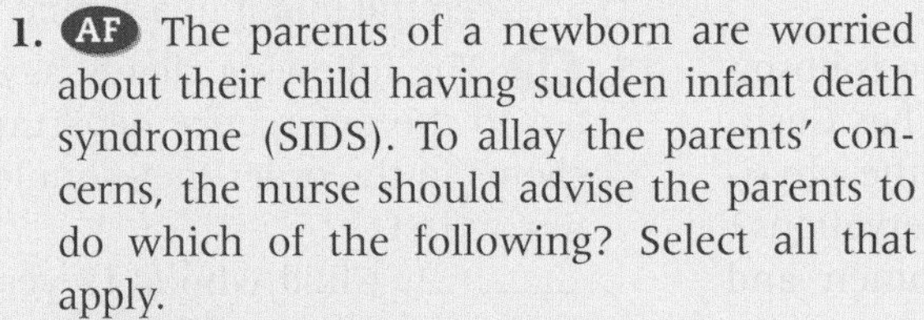

1. AF The parents of a newborn are worried about their child having sudden infant death syndrome (SIDS). To allay the parents' concerns, the nurse should advise the parents to do which of the following? Select all that apply.
   - □ 1. Use a home apnea monitor.
   - □ 2. Place the child in supine position.
   - □ 3. Cover the child with a warm blanket.
   - □ 4. Use a firm mattress.
   - □ 5. Maintain a smoke-free environment.

2. An infant with tetralogy of Fallot has a cyanotic episode. Which of the following is the best position for this infant?
   - □ 1. Prone.
   - □ 2. Knee-chest.
   - □ 3. High Fowler.
   - □ 4. Supine.

3. A neonate is receiving 100 mcg of digoxin. The nurse draws up the prescribed dose in a syringe. There are 2 ml of digoxin to give this neonate. What should the nurse do next?
   - □ 1. Question this dose as being too large.
   - □ 2. Administer the medication in a needleless syringe in the side of the cheek.
   - □ 3. Place the dose in a nipple to ease administration.
   - □ 4. Dilute the dose in a small amount of formula.

4. The nurse finds that a toddler's BP is lower in the right leg than it is in the right arm. Which of the following interventions should the nurse take?
   - □ 1. Document as normal because BP is lower in the legs.
   - □ 2. Document as abnormal because BP is higher in the legs.
   - □ 3. Notify the physician.
   - □ 4. Report the finding to the nurse at the next shift report.

5. To prepare a child who is 6 years of age for a bone marrow aspiration, the nurse should explain that:
   - □ 1. The procedure is performed under general anesthesia.
   - □ 2. A narrow needle is used so the child will not feel pain.
   - □ 3. The child can expect to experience leg pain following the procedure.
   - □ 4. The child will have to lie on his stomach for the aspiration.

6. AF A child who is 9 years of age is admitted to the hospital with a vaso-occlusive sickle cell crisis. The child is having severe pain and is dehydrated. The nurse should do which of the following in priority order? Place in order of highest priority to lowest priority.
   - _____ 1. Administer morphine.
   - _____ 2. Start oxygen per nasal cannula.
   - _____ 3. Start an IV infusion.
   - _____ 4. Draw blood for electrolyte and pH balance.

7. When caring for a child with leukemia, which of the following is a primary nursing goal?
   - □ 1. Meet developmental needs.
   - □ 2. Prevent infections.
   - □ 3. Promote adequate nutrition.
   - □ 4. Provide therapeutic play.

8. The nurse is caring for a child who has a gastrostomy tube in place. Prior to giving a feeding, the nurse observes that the tube is filled with dark brown fluid. The nurse should:
   - □ 1. Give the feeding quickly to keep the tube from plugging.

- □ 2. Assess whether the skin surrounding the tube is bleeding.
- □ 3. Report to the primary health care provider (HCP) that a complication may be occurring.
- □ 4. Assess the drainage for pH; if this is above 7.35, give the feeding.

9. A graduate nurse is drawing up insulin that is U-100 strength into a U-50 syringe. The RN who is the preceptor for the graduate nurse should do which of the following first?

- □ 1. Confirm the correct dosage as this is a high-alert medication.
- □ 2. Observe the graduate nurse administer the insulin to assure safe technique.
- □ 3. Have the graduate nurse redraw the medication into a U-100 syringe.
- □ 4. Check the dosage against the physician's prescription for the insulin.

10. The nurse is assessing a toddler who is hospitalized with an adrenal tumor and has Cushing syndrome. The nurse notifies the physician for which of the following observations?

- □ 1. Purple striae present on abdomen and thighs.
- □ 2. Crackles bilaterally in lower lobes of lungs.
- □ 3. Weight gain of 1 kg since the previous day.
- □ 4. +1 edema in ankles and calves.

11. A child has a history of minimal change nephrotic syndrome (MCNS). What laboratory data are reported to the physician as a potential indication that the child has had a relapse?

- □ 1. Hypoalbuminemia.
- □ 2. Hypoalbuminuria.
- □ 3. Low hemoglobin and hematocrit.
- □ 4. Low platelet count.

12. The nurse is planning care for an infant who has just been diagnosed with Down syndrome. In discussing the plan of care with the parents, the nurse should do which of the following first?

- □ 1. Provide the names of facilities available for caring for children with Down syndrome.
- □ 2. Contact a social worker for the mother to talk to about her feelings.
- □ 3. Urge the parents to obtain a second opinion of the child's neurologic status.
- □ 4. Provide information regarding parent support groups.

13. An infant is diagnosed as having cerebral palsy. The nurse should tell the parents:

- □ 1. Their child will benefit from early interventions to increase his ability for self-care.
- □ 2. Administering an antiacetylcholinergic drug will decrease muscle spasms.
- □ 3. The mother should be tested during future pregnancies in order to determine the presence of another child with cerebral palsy.
- □ 4. Their child's disease will cause progressive brain cell degeneration as the child grows older.

14. AF In caring for a premature infant who is receiving phototherapy, the nurse should do which of the following? Select all that apply.

- □ 1. Monitor temperature every 2 hr.
- □ 2. Apply eye patches.
- □ 3. Cover the genitalia.
- □ 4. Remove infant from under lights for a 1-hr period every 3 hr for feeding and stimulation.
- □ 5. Keep the infant in a supine position.

15. AF The following clients have been admitted to the emergency department. Place the clients in the order they should be seen from first to last.

_____ 1. Child who is 12 years of age with a fractured tibia.
_____ 2. Child who is 8 years of age with lacerations to legs and arms.
_____ 3. Child who is 16 years of age with a "sore throat."
_____ 4. Infant who is 6 months of age with diarrhea and dehydration.

16. The nurse is conducting a health screening for school-aged children. Several children have small white particles on the strands of their hair. The nurse should do which of the following?

- □ 1. Contact the parents and have them obtain treatment.
- □ 2. Inform the principal and advise that the classroom be closed until all children are treated.
- □ 3. Use a comb to remove the particles.
- □ 4. Screen all children before they return to school.

17. A female child who is 3 years of age is in an ambulatory clinic because she has a bad cold. Her mother tells the nurse the girl's problem was caused by her being affected by "mal de ojo." The nurse should:

- □ 1. Tell her mother this is not a legitimate illness.
- □ 2. Teach her mother that colds are caused by viruses.
- □ 3. Ask her mother what symptoms her daughter is experiencing.

□ 4. Explain there is nothing to do for illnesses caused by evil spirits.

18. An infant who is 3 months of age is hospitalized for pneumonia. As the nurse approaches the crib to administer an IV antibiotic, the infant becomes startled and draws in her arms and legs. The nurse should:

□ 1. Notify the HCP.
□ 2. Withhold the antibiotic.
□ 3. Restrain the child before administering the antibiotic.
□ 4. Administer the antibiotic.

19. AF A child who is 10 years of age is scheduled for an appendectomy. Prior to sending the client to surgery, the nurse has the client mark the incision site. Where should the nurse have the client mark the site?

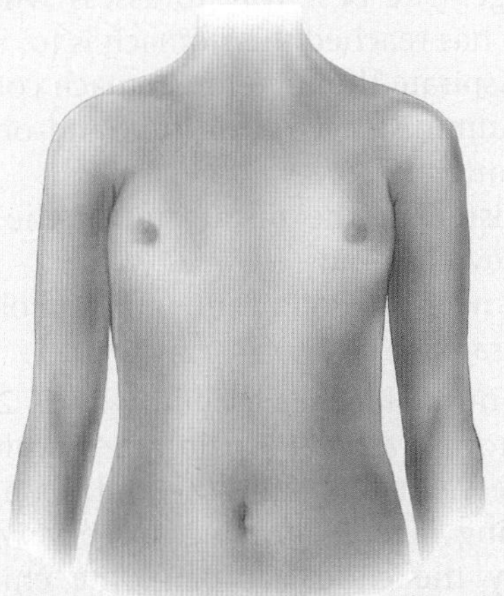

20. An adolescent is prescribed retinoic acid cream as therapy for acne. The nurse should advise the client to:

□ 1. Avoid applying the medication just before bedtime.
□ 2. Apply cream while the face is wet.
□ 3. Avoid being in the sun for extended periods of time.
□ 4. Avoid applying the cream directly on lesions.

21. AF The nurse is to administer 250 ml of D5W intravenously in 3 hr to an infant with dehydration. The infusion set delivers 1 ml/60 gtts. The nurse should set the infusion to deliver how many drops per minute? Round to the nearest whole number.

______________ ml.

22. The nurse is caring for an adolescent hospitalized with a spinal cord injury. The client is paralyzed below the waist. Which of the following activities would best foster the developmental progress for this adolescent?

□ 1. Asking whether the client wants a bath before or after lunch.
□ 2. Watching television on the set in the room.
□ 3. Talking to another adolescent who is in a similar situation.
□ 4. Having a teacher bring school homework to the hospital.

23. An adolescent tells the nurse that she wishes her breasts would grow larger. The nurse should respond:

□ 1. "It is unlikely that your breasts will grow any more. I wouldn't spend time thinking about it."
□ 2. "You look fine to me. Why would you want larger breasts?"
□ 3. "Breast growth usually stops by 16 years of age. What is the reason you were hoping yours would grow more?"
□ 4. "Let's talk about your concern. You know that breast size has nothing to do with ability to reproduce."

24. The nurse is conducting a health assessment of a teenager. The client's height and weight are in normal range and all other findings are within normal limits. The teenager tells the nurse that she has followed one fad diet after another and is still trying to find the right "diet" to follow. The nurse should do which of the following?

□ 1. Refer the child to a dietitian for counseling about appropriate foods for adolescents.
□ 2. Tell the client that eating any type of food as long as it has sufficient calories will help her reach optimum height and weight.
□ 3. Notify the mother and ask her to be sure that her teenager obtains a well-balanced diet.
□ 4. Understand that fad diets are a way of expressing identity; because the client is otherwise healthy, no intervention is necessary.

25. A child who is 9 years of age has a cast removed from a fractured arm. The nurse is teaching the child range of motion exercises. Which of the following would be the best way to evaluate learning?

□ 1. Child consistently practices the exercises.
□ 2. Child can perform a return demonstration of the exercises.
□ 3. Child is eager to learn more exercises.
□ 4. Child explains the importance of the exercises.

26. The nurse is teaching an adolescent to use a four-point crutch gait. When teaching an adolescent, the nurse should recognize that the adolescent:

□ 1. May act as if he knows more than he actually does.
□ 2. Will not be interested in learning something this simple and can figure it out by himself.
□ 3. Will require more explanations about using crutches than adults.
□ 4. Will need few explanations because he has seen friends walk on crutches.

27. AF A child who is 7 years of age is to return to the home setting on a ventilator. Prior to discharge, the nurse evaluates the situation. Which of the following factors is most important in determining effectiveness of home care for this child? Select all that apply.

□ 1. Ambulance service within 5 miles of home.
□ 2. A house with a one-floor plan.
□ 3. A dedicated home care provider.
□ 4. An above-average income.
□ 5. Support for the caregiver.
□ 6. Reliable electricity.

28. AF The nurse is to administer 7.2 mg dexamethasone (Decadron) intravenously. The vial of medication is 4 mg/ml. How much medication should the nurse administer?

______________ ml.

29. The nurse is administering an oral antibiotic to a hospitalized child who is 4 years of age. To gain a preschooler's cooperation to swallow the medication, the nurse should:

□ 1. Offer to play a game with him if he takes the medicine.
□ 2. Tell him it is time to take his medicine.
□ 3. Compare the taste of the medicine to a chocolate bar.
□ 4. Leave the medicine on his stand so he can take it when he is ready.

30. The nurse prepares to administer an IV antibiotic to a child who is 3 years of age with pneumococcal pneumonia, and realizes that he is extremely underweight for his age. The nurse should first:

□ 1. Contact the pharmacist for clarification.
□ 2. Administer the prescribed dose, as dose is determined by type of micro-organism, not by weight.
□ 3. Measure his height and weight and check whether the dose is correct for him.
□ 4. Call the child's physician and discuss the potential dose.

31. AF To administer an IM injection to an infant who is 2 months of age, the nurse uses which site?

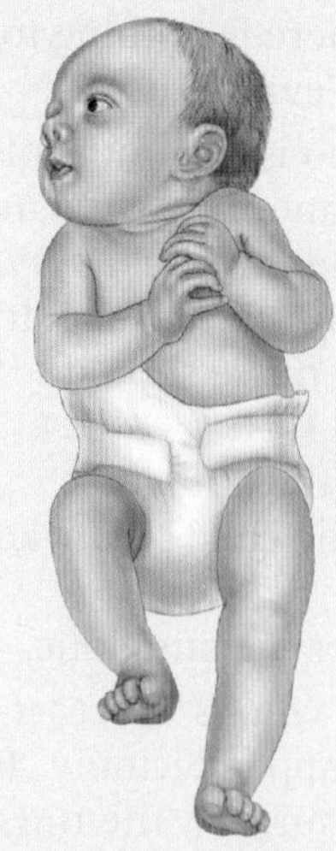

32. The nurse inserted a nasogastric tube for an enteral feeding into an infant who is 6 months of age. The best way to assess whether the tube has reached the stomach is to:

□ 1. Aspirate the tube for stomach contents.
□ 2. Administer 1 ml of fluid and observe for coughing.
□ 3. Listen at the distal end of the tube for bowel sounds.
□ 4. Lower the end of the tube and observe for drainage.

33. The nurse teaches a child who is 2 years of age to use a FACES pain rating scale prior to surgery. At that time the child points to the smiling face. Following surgery when it is likely the child has pain, the child points again to the smiling face. The nurse interprets this as:

□ 1. The child does not have pain.
□ 2. The child is using the scale to indicate how she would like to feel, not what she is currently feeling.
□ 3. The child has difficulty focusing on the right side of the scale.
□ 4. The child cannot differentiate the differences in the "smiles" on the scale.

34. A preschooler is receiving conscious sedation for a surgical procedure. Which nursing action is most important while the child is being sedated?

□ 1. Keep the room absolutely quiet so that the child can sleep.
□ 2. Assess vital signs frequently, as they can become depressed.
□ 3. Ask the child to periodically count from one to ten.
□ 4. Keep the child's head in a dependent position.

35. A child who is 5 years of age is admitted to the emergency department with a high fever of rapid onset, sore throat, coughing with stridor, and retractions. The nurse should make which of the following assessments first?

- ☐ 1. Inspect the epiglottis with a tongue blade.
- ☐ 2. Obtain a throat culture.
- ☐ 3. Monitor oxygen saturation levels.
- ☐ 4. Take the child's temperature.

36. AF A child who is 7 years of age is scheduled for a tonsillectomy. The nurse is reviewing the laboratory studies as shown below.

LABORATORY RESULTS

Test	Result
Urine specific gravity	1.012
White blood cell count	8,500,000/mm^3
Bleeding time	15 minutes
Hemoglobin	13 g/dL

Which of the following laboratory values should be reported to the physician prior to surgery?

- ☐ 1. Specific gravity.
- ☐ 2. WBC count.
- ☐ 3. Bleeding time.
- ☐ 4. Hemoglobin.

37. A child with bacterial pneumonia is receiving oxygen. To prevent drying and thickening of respiratory secretions when oxygen is administered, the nurse should:

- ☐ 1. Restrict fluid intake to 30 ml/hr.
- ☐ 2. Provide frequent postural drainage.
- ☐ 3. Ensure oxygen is warmed and humidified.
- ☐ 4. Remove oxygen periodically to allow normal mucus accumulation.

38. A child is admitted to the hospital with bacterial pneumonia caused by *Haemophilus influenza type b*. The child is started on a course of antibiotics administered intravenously. The nurse places the child in droplet precautions for which of the following time periods?

- ☐ 1. Until the bacterial count is normal.
- ☐ 2. For 24 hr after starting antibiotics.
- ☐ 3. Until the child is discharged from the hospital.
- ☐ 4. When the child no longer has a productive cough.

39. A child is undergoing testing for food allergies. Which of the following would best identify foods to which a child is allergic?

- ☐ 1. Elimination diet.
- ☐ 2. Hyposensitivity testing.
- ☐ 3. Restriction of all protein from the diet.
- ☐ 4. Corticosteroid challenge testing.

40. A child who is 5 years of age with roseola is pruritic and has a temperature of 99.5°F. The nurse should teach the parents to:

- ☐ 1. Dress the child warmly to bring out the rash so that it fades quickly.
- ☐ 2. Apply cool compresses to the skin to stop local itching.
- ☐ 3. Discuss with the child the importance of not scratching lesions.
- ☐ 4. Administer infant aspirin every 4 hr as necessary for comfort.

41. The mother of a child with chicken pox asks the nurse when her child can return to school. The nurse advises the mother that the child can return to school:

- ☐ 1. When all lesions have completely faded.
- ☐ 2. As soon as the temperature is normal.
- ☐ 3. 10 days after the initial lesions appear.
- ☐ 4. As soon as all lesions are crusted.

42. The nurse is teaching a first aid class for a group of grade-school children who are going camping. To prevent Lyme disease, the children should do which of the following?

- ☐ 1. Only drink water from mountain streams.
- ☐ 2. Avoid petting strange animals.
- ☐ 3. Wear long pants tucked inside their socks when in the woods.
- ☐ 4. Avoid contact with leaves or bushes without knowing what kind they are.

43. A nurse is assessing an infant who is receiving antibiotic therapy, and notes the presence of a white membrane on the infant's tongue. The nurse should do which of the following?

- ☐ 1. Advise parents to brush the child's teeth and tongue after each dose of antibiotic.
- ☐ 2. Refer parents to their HCP.
- ☐ 3. Instruct parents to discontinue antibiotic therapy.
- ☐ 4. Inform parents that this is normal and not to worry.

44. A child is hospitalized with bacterial pneumonia. The physician has ordered the following medications: Amoxicillin, nystatin drops, acetaminophen (Tylenol) for temperature over 99°F, racemic ephedrine. When administering nystatin, which of the following administration techniques is best?

- ☐ 1. Administer along with the amoxicillin.
- ☐ 2. Mix with orange juice to disguise the taste.
- ☐ 3. Administer immediately after meals.
- ☐ 4. Administer at the same time as the racemic ephedrine.

45. To alleviate discomfort in a child following an immunization, the nurse should instruct the parents to:

- ☐ 1. Apply a warm compress to the injection site.

□ 2. Administer aspirin (80 mg per year of age).
□ 3. Administer acetaminophen (Tylenol) (80 mg per year of age).
□ 4. Keep the arm in which the injection was given in a dependent position.

46. A toddler is treated for pinworms. In order to prevent reinfection, the nurse should instruct the mother to:
□ 1. Prohibit the child from playing on the floor.
□ 2. Wash bedding of all family members in hot water with bleach.
□ 3. Help the child wash her hands before eating.
□ 4. Increase fluids so the child will void frequently.

47. Which response by a child suggests that she understands about the administration of a prescribed antibiotic for impetigo?
□ 1. "I have to take this until the itchiness stops."
□ 2. "I'll continue the drug until it's all gone."
□ 3. "I'll have to take the drug for at least 4 days."
□ 4. "Taking the drug will prevent itchiness."

48. A child with a urinary catheter receives propantheline bromide (Pro-Banthine) following bladder surgery. The drug is effective if the child:
□ 1. Does not vomit.
□ 2. Is pain-free.
□ 3. Voids within 4 hr.
□ 4. Does not have bladder spasms.

49. A child is taking cyclosporin following a kidney transplant. The expected outcome of this drug is to:
□ 1. Prevent systemic infection.
□ 2. Reduce the possibility of rejection of the new kidney.
□ 3. Prevent hemorrhage at the incision site.
□ 4. Stimulate urine production in his remaining kidney.

50. A client who is 16 years of age has dysmenorrhea. The nurse should advise her to:
□ 1. Take ibuprofen (Motrin) at the earliest onset of pain.
□ 2. Take acetaminophen on the day her menstrual cycle is to start.
□ 3. Restrict fluid intake during her menstrual cycle.
□ 4. Use ice packs to reduce pain.

51. AF The nurse is providing care for an adolescent with type 1 diabetes mellitus who is hospitalized for appendicitis. The nurse notes a fruity odor to the client's breath. The client is weak and nauseated with poor skin turgor; his last meal was lunch, 2 hr earlier. The client uses lispro insulin. In which order should the nurse perform the following interventions? Place in order of first to last.
_____ 1. Obtain a finger stick blood sugar.
_____ 2. Start an IV infusion with normal saline.
_____ 3. Administer lispro insulin.
_____ 4. Notify the physician.

52. The nurse instructs a teenager who has had several episodes of vulvovaginitis to:
□ 1. Apply personal hygiene sprays if vaginal odor develops.
□ 2. Use nylon rather than cotton underpants to decrease moisture.
□ 3. Wipe from front to back after urinating or defecating.
□ 4. Soak in a strong bubble bath solution to maintain hygiene.

53. AF The nurse is planning care for a child with diabetes insipidus. The nurse is reviewing the laboratory results below. Which of the following results indicates that the child is responding favorably to medical therapy?

LABORATORY RESULTS

Test	Result
Urine specific gravity	1.015
24-hour urine output	1750 ml
Number of white cells in urine	Decreased
Serum glucose	100 mg/dL

□ 1. Urine specific gravity.
□ 2. 24-hr urine output.
□ 3. Decrease in the number of white cells.
□ 4. Serum glucose.

54. Both parents of a child who is 7 years of age have type 1 diabetes mellitus (DM). The nurse should advise the parents to immediately notify their HCP if their child exhibits which of the following symptoms?
□ 1. Loss of weight.
□ 2. Craving for sweets.
□ 3. Severe itching.
□ 4. Fatigue.

55. AF A child who is 6 years of age is admitted to the hospital with head trauma 6 hr after a motor vehicle accident. She is receiving an IV infusion of 10% dextrose in water. The nurse should monitor which of the following? Select all that apply.
□ 1. Urinary output.
□ 2. Specific gravity of urine.
□ 3. Pupillary response.
□ 4. Ability to speak.
□ 5. Diarrhea.

56. A client who is 16 years of age has suffered a thoracic level spinal injury from a diving accident. To initiate CPR at the poolside, the rescuer should first:

- □ 1. Hyperextend the victim's neck to clear the airway prior to administering mouth-to-mouth resuscitation.
- □ 2. Administer cardiopulmonary resuscitation in a prone position.
- □ 3. Place a rolled towel under the neck.
- □ 4. Elevate the mandible to assess the victim's airway with the head in a neutral position.

57. Which of the following measures is most effective in aiding bronchodilation in a child with laryngotracheobronchitis?

- □ 1. Urge the child to take oral fluids.
- □ 2. Administer an oral analgesic.
- □ 3. Teach the child to take shallow breaths.
- □ 4. Assist with racemic epinephrine by nebulizer.

58. On the third week of hospitalization following a spinal cord injury, a client has a bright red face and is sweating profusely. The nurse should first:

- □ 1. Administer mouth-to-mouth resuscitation.
- □ 2. Lower the head to increase cerebral circulation.
- □ 3. Massage the lower extremities to cause vasodilation.
- □ 4. Determine if the retention catheter is blocked.

59. During an absence seizure, the nurse should:

- □ 1. Ask the child to hold her breath or count to ten, if possible.
- □ 2. Attempt to distract the child by calling her name.
- □ 3. Ask the child to continue talking to keep attention focused.
- □ 4. Observe the child carefully.

60. A child who is 10 years of age develops bacterial conjunctivitis of the right eye. The eye is inflamed and drains a thick, yellow discharge. The nurse should teach the child to:

- □ 1. Keep the eye covered at all times.
- □ 2. Apply ophthalmic drops for no more than 3 days.
- □ 3. Clean the discharge away from the inner to outer canthus.
- □ 4. Attend school only when the discharge has disappeared.

61. The nurse is assessing school-age children for vision problems. Which child is at greatest risk for deficiency in color perception?

- □ 1. Male child who has had frequent middle ear infections.
- □ 2. Female child who was born prematurely.
- □ 3. Female child whose teacher reports that she rubs her eyes.
- □ 4. Male child who says he does not like television.

62. The nurse is teaching the mother of a child who will have myringotomy tubes inserted. Which statement by a mother indicates that she understands the precautions required for her child after the insertion of myringotomy tubes?

- □ 1. "I will keep him away from all children to prevent infections."
- □ 2. "I will be certain he takes showers, not tub baths."
- □ 3. "I will make him use earplugs when he swims."
- □ 4. "I will not shampoo his hair until the tubes come out."

63. A UAP is assigned to give morning care to a child who is blind. The nurse is observing the UAP approach the child for the first time. The UAP touches the child and then calls him by name. The nurse should do which of the following when giving feedback to the UAP?

- □ 1. Remind the UAP to call the child's name and then touch him.
- □ 2. Thank the UAP for using touch with a blind child.
- □ 3. Explain that the child will soon recognize the UAP's voice and will not need to touch the child.
- □ 4. Tell the UAP to touch the child and then tell him who he or she is.

64. AF The nurse in the emergency department is assigned to triage. There has been a school bus accident and the injured children have been brought to the emergency department. In which order should the nurse assess these children? Place in order of first to last.

_____ 1. Child with abrasions.
_____ 2. Child with a sprained wrist.
_____ 3. Child with a suspected simple fracture.
_____ 4. Child with an elbow fracture.

65. A child with acute epiglottitis has been discharged to home. Which of the following instructions does the nurse provide the parents to help the child breath easier?

- □ 1. Increase room humidity.
- □ 2. Limit fluid intake.
- □ 3. Enforce strict bed rest.
- □ 4. Play "rapid breathing" games with him.

66. Prior to administering edentate calcium disodium (EDTA) to a child with lead poisoning, the nurse should obtain:

- □ 1. Pulse and BP.
- □ 2. Specific gravity of urine.

□ 3. Serum lead level.
□ 4. Patellar reflex.

67. A child is brought to the emergency department by his caregiver after falling off his bike; the child was not wearing a helmet. While assessing the child, the nurse learns that he cannot recall how his accident happened. The nurse should conclude that:
□ 1. The cause of the accident may have been child abuse.
□ 2. Loss of memory has occurred because of a concussion.
□ 3. The child has increasing ICP.
□ 4. The child may feel guilty for being so careless.

68. A preschooler is admitted to the emergency department after sustaining a snake bite that occurred while he was playing unsupervised in a wooded area. What method might be the most effective in determining what type of snake was involved?
□ 1. Ask the child to describe the snake.
□ 2. Ask the child to draw a picture of the snake.
□ 3. Ask the child to identify the snake from a picture.
□ 4. Ask the child if the snake had a stripe on its back.

69. A child is seen in the emergency department with tearing and pain in his right eye. To assess for a foreign body under the upper lid, the nurse should:
□ 1. Catch his attention with a toy so that he looks down.
□ 2. Apply cool water to the lid to cause it to retract.
□ 3. Evert the upper lid over an applicator stick.
□ 4. Apply topical anesthesia to the upper lid.

70. Following surgery, a child is to use an incentive spirometer four times daily. The nurse observes the child is using the spirometer correctly when the child does which of the following?
□ 1. Inhales and blows on the spirometer tube to elevate the balls.
□ 2. Exhales and inhales through the mouthpiece to elevate the balls.
□ 3. Inhales through the mouthpiece, elevates the balls for 1 s, and exhales.
□ 4. Exhales, inhales through the nose, exhales to elevate the balls.

71. The nurse is conducting a health assessment of a male child who is 8 years of age. Which of the following findings requires follow-up?
□ 1. Sleeping for 8 hr at night.
□ 2. A lack of concentration.
□ 3. Intense interest in video games.
□ 4. Unrealistic fears.

72. A child with attention deficit disorder (ADD) is taking methylphenidate HCl (Ritalin). The nurse is assessing the effectiveness of the drug for this child. Which of the following indicates an adverse reaction to the drug?
□ 1. Rapid increase in height.
□ 2. Hypotension.
□ 3. Anorexia.
□ 4. Sleepiness.

73. The nurse is assessing an infant who is 6 months of age with nonorganic failure to thrive. Which of the following requires immediate intervention?
□ 1. The infant stares at the nurse.
□ 2. The infant's weight is below average.
□ 3. The infant does not respond to the mother.
□ 4. The infant has speech delays.

74. The nurse is conducting a health assessment on a child with cerebral palsy. Which of the following statements made by the mother indicates an appropriate understanding of her child's long-term needs?
□ 1. "I know that once my child begins school she will catch up with other children."
□ 2. "I realize that my child will need all of my attention for the rest of her life."
□ 3. "I understand my child will grow up and needs to develop as much independence as is appropriate."
□ 4. "I realize that my child will need close supervision once she becomes sexually active."

75. AF A child has had a kidney transplant. Which of the data from the laboratory report below suggests that the transplanted kidney is not functioning well?

LABORATORY RESULTS

Test	Result
BUN	85 mg/dL
White cell count	14,000/mm^3
Serum potassium	3.8 mEq/L
Red cell count	4,800,000/mm^3

□ 1. BUN.
□ 2. WBC count.
□ 3. Serum potassium.
□ 4. RBC count.

Answers and Rationales

1. 2, 4, 5 To decrease the risk of SIDS, the nurse advises the parents to use a crib with a firm mattress and place the child in a supine position. The nurse also advises that parents maintain a smoke-free environment. There is no evidence to indicate that home monitors are useful as there is not a relationship between apnea and SIDS. Only a lightweight blanket needs to be used to keep the child from becoming overheated. (H)

2. 2 The knee-chest position creates blood flow resistance to the peripheral extremities, shunting blood to the major organs; this provides more available oxygen to the heart. Prone, high Fowler, and supine positions do not promote shunting of the blood, but rather allow the blood to accumulate where it is drawn by gravity, depending on the body position. (A)

3. 1 Infants rarely receive more than 1 ml (50 mcg or 0.05 mg/ml) in one dose; a higher dose is an immediate warning of a dosage error. To ensure safety, compare the calculation with another staff member's calculation before giving the drug. (D)

4. 2 With a coarctation of the aorta (COA), there is localized narrowing near the insertion of the ductus arteriosus, resulting in increased pressure in the head and upper extremities and decreased pressure distal to the obstruction (body and lower extremities). The pulses in the lower extremity would also be weakened. This is an important cardiac assessment as oftentimes there is not an audible murmur, which will alert the physician to the presence of the cardiac defect. (R)

5. 4 The marrow is aspirated from the iliac crest; therefore, the child will have to lie quietly on his stomach. Bone marrow aspiration is rarely done under general anesthesia; instead, conscious sedation is used. The aspiration is painful, and the nurse should not indicate otherwise. (A)

6. 3, 2, 1, 4 Maintaining fluid balance is a priority because dehydration increases sickling of cells. The nurse's first step is to start an IV; next, the nurse starts oxygen and then administers morphine for pain. Last, the nurse obtains a blood sample for laboratory studies. (A)

7. 2 The risk for infection with a child with leukemia is of primary concern. Chemotherapy suppresses normal WBC formation, placing a child at risk for infection, which can potentially delay further rounds of chemotherapy. (S)

8. 3 A potential complication of using a gastrostomy tube is that the tube may migrate through the pyloric valve into the duodenum and cause obstruction. Brown fluid suggests this has happened, as the tube is likely filled with feces. An alkaline pH suggests the complication has occurred, because bowel secretions are alkaline while stomach secretions are acid. (S)

9. 3 Insulin comes dissolved in liquid at different strengths, and the syringe corresponds to the strength of the insulin; therefore, the RN has the graduate nurse discard the dose and redraw the insulin into the correct syringe. The graduate and the preceptor also confirm the dosage, and the preceptor observes the graduate nurse administer the medication unless the graduate has been observed to have safely administered insulin before. (D)

10. 2 The presence of crackles in the patient's lungs indicates excess fluid volume from excess water and sodium reabsorption, and may be a symptom of pulmonary edema, which must be treated rapidly. Striae (stretch marks), weight gain, and dependent edema are common findings in patients with Cushing disease. These findings are monitored, but are not urgent. (M)

11. 1 The glomerular membrane, normally impermeable to albumin and other proteins, becomes permeable to proteins, especially albumin, which leaks through the membrane and are lost in the urine (*hyperalbuminuria*). This reduces the serum albumin level (*hypoalbuminemia*). Hemoglobin and hematocrit are usually normal or elevated as a result of hemoconcentration. The platelet count may be elevated also as a result of hemoconcentration. (R)

12. 4 Parents of cognitively impaired children often need help to adjust to this unexpected event in their life, and parent support groups can help with this adjustment. Providing information about health care facilities conveys a message that that is the choice parents should make. The diagnosis of Down syndrome likely does not require a second opinion and suggesting to the parents to seek one creates an opening for false hope. A referral to a social worker is helpful as the parents seek information about community resources for their child. (H)

13. 1 Parents are encouraged to enroll their child in preschool when old enough in order to increase opportunity for independence, self-care, and socialization with other children. Cerebral palsy is not a progressive disorder and it cannot be identified by tests conducted during pregnancy. Antiacetylcholinergic drugs do not reduce muscle spasms. (H)

14. 1, 2, 3 Because the neonate is at risk for cold stress or overheating from exposure or heat from the lights, assessing temperature is a critical part of care. Applying eye patches and covering genitalia is necessary protection for exposure to the ultraviolet lights. The rate of bilirubin reabsorption is in relation to the time exposed to the ultraviolet lights. The phototherapy is interrupted only for 20 to 30 min for feedings. The nurse turns the infant every 2 hr so the entire body is exposed evenly to the lights. (S).

15. 4, 1, 2, 3 The infant who is 6 months of age and experiencing diarrhea is seen first because of risk for further dehydration; the nurse starts an IV infusion immediately. The child who is 12 years of age is seen next; this child is considered to require urgent care, but can wait several hours. The child who is 8 years of age can be seen next; this child is considered to require nonurgent care, and will respond to assessment and first aid. The nurse cares for the child who is 16 years of age last; a "sore throat" is considered nonurgent, and likely will not require the services of the emergency department. (M)

16. 1 These children have pediculosis capitis (head lice), the eggs of which are revealed as small white particles on hair strands. The nurse refers the children for treatment which will involve topical treatment of the hair. The classroom does not need to be closed, and asking children to be screened before returning to school does not reduce transmission of the lice. Using a comb is not a sufficient method to remove the lice. (S)

17. 3 Respecting cultural values is important in establishing effective nurse-client relationships. By asking about the symptoms, the nurse conveys respect while obtaining helpful information. The other comments deny the mother's belief and do not facilitate the nurse's ability to help the child. (P)

18. 4 The infant is exhibiting a normal startle (Moro) reflex; therefore, the nurse continues to administer the antibiotic. Typically, the Moro reflex lasts until 3 to 4 months, and then disappears. There is no reason to notify the HCP, and it is not necessary to restrain the child to administer IV medications. (A)

19. The incision site for an appendectomy is at McBurney's point. (S)

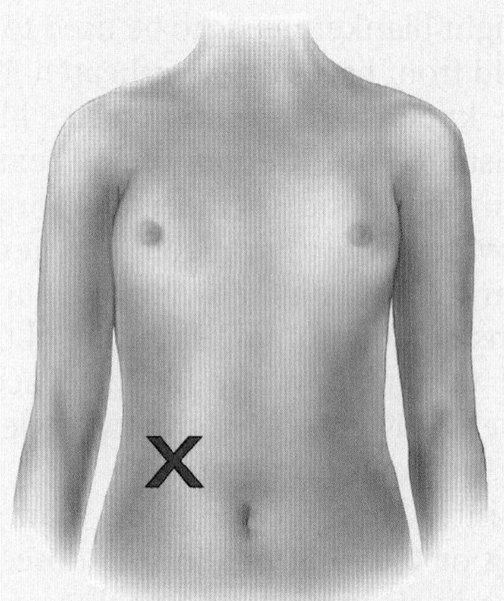

20. 3 The nurse advises the child to stay out of the sun because vitamin A makes the skin more susceptible to ultraviolet rays, thereby increasing the chance for sunburn. The cream can be applied before bedtime and should be applied to lesions. (H)

21. The answer is 83 ml. The drop rate is calculated as follows (D):
250 ml fluid for 3 hr = 83.3 ml/hr
83 ml × 60 drops/ml = 4,980
60 min = 83 gtt/min

22. 3 A developmental task of adolescence is to develop a sense of identity by "trying on" roles and discussing values and goals with others; this is best accomplished with a peer. The other options facilitate nursing care and independence, but do not promote the developing sense of identity. (H)

23. 3 Many adolescents are disappointed about their personal appearance. Promoting discussion about this topic helps them work through their feelings and re-establish self-worth. The other responses by the nurse do not facilitate further communication about the client's concerns. (H)

24. 4 Following diets other than those their parents prefer can be an effective way to express adolescent identity and meet needs for growth and development. Because the client is otherwise healthy, a referral to the dietician is not needed. Fad diets do not help clients achieve optimum height and weight. The nurse should respect the client's confidentiality and trust and not discuss the situation with the mother. (H)

25. 1 Evaluation of learning determines that the child can actually do the exercises, and consistent practicing assures that the child will continue to perform them. It is not sufficient for the child to simply return the demonstration; a return demonstration evaluates immediate recall, not application of the learned information. The child should do the required exercises well before learning others. The fact that the child can explain the exercises does not mean he will perform them. (A)

26. 1 Adolescents may manifest an air of knowing more than they actually do as part of working through a sense of identity; therefore, the nurse develops a teaching plan that supports the child's need for identity while assuring that he can walk safely with the crutches. The nurse adapts the teaching approach to the child's level of understanding. Learning to walk with crutches requires explanation and return demonstrations for both adults and adolescents. (S)

27. 3, 5 Home care is more successful if there is someone able to assume primary care of the child and if there is someone who can provide respite for the caregiver. Although the caregiver should know how to contact emergency response services, it is not necessary to have services within 5 miles. If the family income is not sufficient, the nurse refers the family to social services, which can assist with financial planning. Electricity to run the ventilator is necessary, but the ventilator can also be run with an emergency back up generator. (M)

28. The answer is 1.8 ml. The calculation is as follows (D):

$$\frac{4\text{ mg}}{1\text{ mg}} = \frac{7.2\text{ mg}}{x\text{ ml}}$$

$4x = 7.2$

$x = 7.2/4$

$x = 1.8$ ml

29. 2 Direct communication is the most affective way to obtain the child's cooperation. Bribing is ineffective, and medicine is never compared to candy. Children cannot be depended on to take medicine without supervision. (D)

30. 3 Before administering any medication, confirm that the dose is correct for the child's weight and height and check a drug reference for dosage because of the great variability in the size of children for their age. If there is a discrepancy at that time, the nurse contacts the pharmacist and, as needed, the physician. (D)

31. 2 The gluteus maximus muscle is not well developed in infants until they can walk. Thus, the vastus lateralis muscle is the most appropriate site for IM injections. (D)

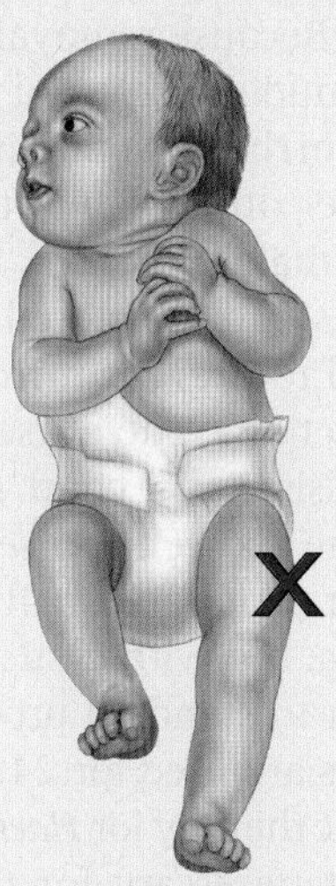

32. 1 If stomach contents can be aspirated, the end of the tube must be in the stomach. Administering fluids can cause aspiration if the tube is misplaced, and the presence of bowel sounds is not sufficient evidence of placement. Drainage from the tube could be coming from the esophagus and does not confirm tube placement. (S)

33. 2 A child who is younger than 3 years of age usually cannot use the FACES scale. In general, preschoolers employ "magical thinking," or believe that what they wish will come true; therefore, they may be using the pain scale to "wish" for a smiling face, rather than to rate their pain. If the child continues to be unable to use the scale, the nurse assesses pain by observing the child and asking the child to talk about the pain. (C)

34. 2 Conscious sedation is the use of a drug such as pentobarbital sodium to induce a conscious but sleepy state. Vital signs are monitored closely to be certain the child's vital centers do not become depressed. The child may count from one to ten as the sedative is being administered, but at most levels of sedation the child is not asked to speak. The usual position for sedation is recumbent. (S)

35. 3 This child may have acute epiglottitis, which is treated as a medical emergency. The most important assessments are related to monitoring oxygen levels and maintaining airway stability. The nurse does not insert a tongue blade or obtain a throat culture as these actions may cause laryngospasm and airway obstruction. Once the airway status and oxygen saturation levels are obtained, the nurse can proceed with additional data gathering, including all vital signs and the client's health history. (S)

36. 3 The chart reveals that bleeding time is abnormal. Because removal of tonsils leaves a large denuded area, not a simple suture line, hemorrhage following surgery can occur. The other laboratory values are within normal limits. (A)

37. 3 Oxygen is administered warmed and humidified to prevent it from drying respiratory secretions. The nurse encourages fluids and assists the child in coughing up mucus. The oxygen is used continuously. Postural drainage is usually not used with pneumonia, but with cystic fibrosis. (C)

38. 2 In addition to standard precautions, droplet precautions are used for 24 hr after the start of antibiotic therapy for *Haemophilus influenza b*. It is not necessary for the nurse to use droplet precautions until the bacterial count is normal or when the cough subsides. It is not necessary to wait until the child is discharged to remove droplet precautions. (S)

39. 1 Elimination diets involve adding foods slowly to a child's diet so foods to which the child is allergic can be identified; protein is not restricted. The other tests are not involved in testing for food allergies. (A)

40. 2 Cool compress can minimize pruritus; warm clothes and warm baths or compresses will cause further pruritus. Aspirin is not given with increased temperature (flulike symptoms) because of the risk of Reye syndrome with viral illnesses. Young children cannot easily refrain from scratching; the nurse can instruct the parents to keep the fingernails cut and, if necessary, discuss the need for a mild antihistamine such as diphenhydramine HCl (Benadryl) if the cool compresses are not effective. (H)

41. 4 Chicken pox lesions are infectious until all of the lesions are dried and crusted. The child remains isolated from others until this occurs. (S)

42. 3 Lyme disease is prevented by reducing the possibility of bites from deer ticks; methods to reduce bites include tucking pant legs into socks, keeping legs and ankles covered, and using insect repellent. Drinking water from unknown sources is a risk for GI diseases caused by bacteria, parasites, or amoebae. Although not related to Lyme disease, the nurse also teaches children to avoid petting strange animals because of the risk of rabies and to avoid touching leaves or bushes because this could produce contact dermatitis such as poison ivy. (H)

43. 2 The child likely has thrush (oral candidiasis), a fungal infection that presents with a white membrane on the tongue or mucous membrane that does not scrape away. Thrush is caused by an overgrowth of bacteria caused by the antibiotic, for which the HCP can prescribe an antifungal agent. The child should continue using the antibiotic. Brushing the teeth and tongue will not remove the infection. (H)

44. 3 The child is receiving nystatin to prevent oral candidiasis (thrush) caused by the antibiotic therapy. Nystatin drops are given after meals to allow it to remain on the tongue for an extended period of time. Nystatin does not need to be given with the amoxicillin or racemic ephedrine, particularly if the child needs to follow that medication with something to drink. Medications are not mixed with juice or milk because it is difficult to be sure all of the medication is taken. (D)

45. 3 The nurse advises parents to avoid administering aspirin because of the risk of Reye syndrome; acetaminophen or ibuprofen are the drugs of choice to relieve the inflammation and associated pain. A warm compress provides only temporary relief. It is not necessary to keep the arm in a dependent position. (H)

46. 3 Pinworm infections are usually spread from the diaper area to the mouth by unwashed hands. It is not necessary to restrict the child from playing on the floor. The pinworms are not spread from bed linens. Voiding frequently does not help in the treatment or prevention of pinworms. (H)

47. 2 Impetigo is a streptococcal skin infection. To reduce the incidence of complications following streptococcal infections, the antibiotic needs to be taken for the entire prescription, usually 10 days. Topical antibiotics, gentle washing of the area, and divisional therapy may help with the itching. The parents should also trim the fingernails to prevent skin injury from scratching. (H)

48. 4 The presence of a bladder catheter can cause painful bladder spasms. A drug such as propantheline bromide (Pro-Banthine) reduces the incidence of bladder spasms. Pro-Banthine does not prevent vomiting or manage pain. When the catheter is removed, the nurse documents the first voiding, which should occur within 2 to 6 hr following removal of the catheter. (D)

49. 2 Cyclosporin is an immunosuppressive drug that helps prevent transplant rejection. Cyclosporin does not prevent infection or hemorrhage, and does not act to stimulate urine production. (D)

50. 1 An anti-inflammatory agent such as ibuprofen (Motrin) reduces discomfort of dysmenorrhea when it is administered at the earliest onset of pain. Acetaminophen can be used for pain as needed, but should not be taken unnecessarily because of the hepatic toxicity associated with acetaminophen excess. The girl should drink fluids as tolerated; heat may be more effective in managing cramps. (C)

51. 2, 1, 4, 3 The client is experiencing ketoacidosis. The first action is to initiate IV fluids to prevent further dehydration. Next, the nurse obtains serum glucose values to report to the physician, who will then order the appropriate dose of insulin. (A)

52. 3 Vulvovaginitis may be caused by spread of *Escherichia coli* from the rectum to the vagina; therefore, the nurse instructs the client to wipe from front to back. The nurse also advises the girl to wear cotton underpants to absorb moisture, but this instruction is secondary. Personal hygiene sprays and bubble baths should be avoided as they are irritating. (H)

53. 4 A normal urine specific gravity (1.003 to 1.030) is assurance that urine concentration is taking place. The 24-hr urine output exceeds normal output; the white cells in the urine do not indicate outcome of medical therapy; the serum glucose is within normal range. (A)

54. 1 This child is at high risk for having DM. The nurse alerts the parents to signs that the child may be affected, such as loss of weight, because lack of insulin reduces the ability of body cells to use glucose, which leads to starvation of cells. The child may have a craving for sweets, itching, or fatigue, but these are not typically signs of the onset of DM and the parents should consider other causes before contacting the HCP. (H)

55. 1, 2, 3, 4 The child is receiving D10W. A 10% solution is hypertonic, so it moves fluid from extravascular spaces into the blood stream. If urinary output is not adequate, heart failure from fluid overload can result. The nurse monitors the urinary output and specific gravity, and speech and pupil response as indications of increasing intracranial pressure. The child will not have diarrhea at this time. (A)

56. 4 CPR procedures must be modified when a spinal injury is suspected. The rescuer should not move the victim's neck to avoid further spinal cord injury; this will necessitate elevating the mandible and keeping the head in a neutral position. (R)

57. 4 Racemic epinephrine can be an effective bronchodilator as this drug acts to increase the lumen of airways. Taking oral fluids or analgesics will not promote bronchodilation. The child should be encouraged to take deep breaths in conjunction with the bronchodilation. (D)

58. 4 Flushing and sweating are typical symptoms of autonomic dysreflexia, a response to an irritating factor such as a full bladder. Relieving the irritation reduces the response. Lowering the client's head could increase intracranial pressure (ICP), and is NOT performed. Massaging of lower extremities is avoided because of risk of deep vein thromboses (DVTs). Mouth-to-mouth resuscitation is not indicated in a client with spontaneous respirations. (A)

59. 4 In absence seizures the child looses contact with the surroundings for just a few seconds. The nurse does not need to intervene, but should observe the child and document the event. The child will not be able to focus, count, or speak during the seizure. When the seizure is over, the child will not be aware of having it. (A)

60. 3 The nurse teaches the child to use the proper technique for cleaning the affected eye to prevent the infection from spreading to the other eye; if both eyes are involved, the child is instructed to use separate cleaning materials and perform good hand hygiene. The eye is not covered. The child should use mediation as prescribed; the course of the medication will be longer than 3 days. The child can return to school 24 hr after starting antibiotic therapy. (H)

61. 4 Color deficiency is a sex-linked trait, so it only occurs in males. Middle ear infections, rubbing eyes, and prematurity are not associated with color deficiency. (H)

62. 3 Myringotomy tubes allow water to enter the middle ear, which can lead to infection. The nurse instructs the caregiver to use earplugs when it is possible that water will enter the ear. It is not necessary to isolate the child. The child should not take showers while the tubes are in place as it is difficult to prevent water from entering the ear. The child can have his hair washed, but care needs to be taken to avoid having water and soap enter the middle ear. (H)

63. 1 Touching a blind person before he or she realizes that someone is present can be frightening. The nurse instructs the UAP to first say the child's name, introduce him or herself, and then touch the child so the child knows the position of the UAP. (M)

64. 4, 3, 1, 2 The child with an elbow fracture is seen first; elbow injuries are particularly dangerous in children because edema can interfere with blood vessels and nerves that pass beside the joint. The child with a simple fracture can be seen next, although not a priority because the skin has not been broken and he is not at risk for infection. The child with abrasions is assessed third, particularly to assess for extent of injury and potential for infection. The child with a sprained wrist is seen last as this child is not in immediate danger. (M)

65. 1 A moist environment helps prevent respiratory secretions from drying and becoming difficult to expectorate. The nurse instructs the parents to maintain an adequate fluid intake for the child to prevent dehydration and to liquefy secretions. The child can participate in quiet play activities, which also promote lung expansion. Respiratory therapy is not necessary. (C)

66. 2 Chelating agents like EDTA evacuate lead through urinary excretion. It is important to assess that urinary function is present before administration. The nurse does not need to document vital signs, reflexes, or serum lead level at this time. (D)

67. 2 One indicator of a concussion is that the person does not remember the circumstances just prior to the accident that caused the injury. The other conclusions are not warranted at this time. (A)

68. 3 Children with limited vocabularies are able to identify a photo of a snake better than they are able to describe a snake. Treatment depends on the type of snake, so it is important to have as accurate a description as possible. (A)

69. 3 Everting the upper lid over an applicator stick offers a full view of the anterior globe. The other strategies do not provide a full view of a potential foreign body. (A)

70. 2 The purpose of incentive spirometry is to make the child take a deep breath to better aerate the lungs. The child should first exhale and then inhale through the mouthpiece to elevate the balls and keep the balls elevated for as long as possible (about 3 s), and then remove the mouthpiece and passively exhale. (A)

71. 2 A child who is 8 years of age should be able to concentrate. Lack of concentration may be indicative of a behavior disorder. The nurse gathers additional information and refers the child to an HCP, if needed. The other findings are normal for a child who is 8 years of age. (H)

72. 3 Ritalin typically causes a loss of appetite. Weighing the child periodically to detect whether this has led to a loss of weight is important. Ritalin does not affect growth, so increased height is not related to the use of the drug. Ritalin can cause insomnia, not sleepiness. Although rare, Ritalin can produce either increase or decrease in BP, but the primary side effect is loss of appetite. (D)

73. 2 The priority goal for an infant with nonorganic failure to thrive is to assure adequate nutrition. The nurse refers the infant to an HCP if his weight is below normal because he is in danger of becoming malnourished. The infant with failure to thrive has difficulty establishing relationships with parents and others and also experiences delays in speech. (A)

74. 3 Children with cerebral palsy need to have as much independence as possible so they can reach their full potential. The other statements by the mother are not realistic and require nursing intervention. (H)

75. 1 An elevated blood urea nitrogen (BUN) indicates the kidney is not excreting nitrogenous wastes from the body; this is an undesirable finding for a client with a recent renal transplant. An elevated WBC count is a sign of an infection. The serum potassium is normal. The RBC count is normal. (A)

SECTION 3

Nursing Care of Adults With Medical-Surgical Health Problems

chapter 19

Introduction to Nursing Care of the Adult Client

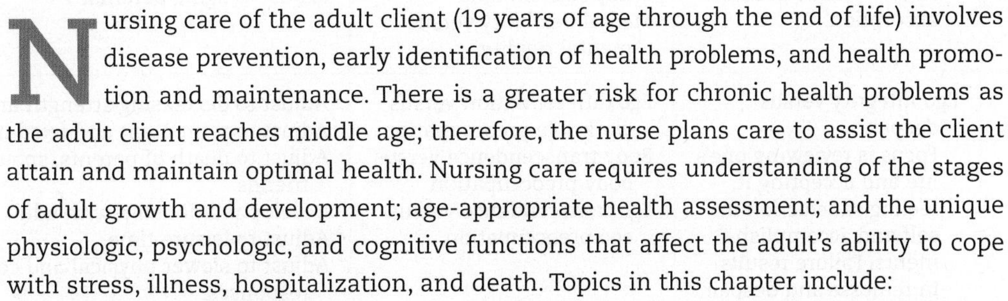

Nursing care of the adult client (19 years of age through the end of life) involves disease prevention, early identification of health problems, and health promotion and maintenance. There is a greater risk for chronic health problems as the adult client reaches middle age; therefore, the nurse plans care to assist the client attain and maintain optimal health. Nursing care requires understanding of the stages of adult growth and development; age-appropriate health assessment; and the unique physiologic, psychologic, and cognitive functions that affect the adult's ability to cope with stress, illness, hospitalization, and death. Topics in this chapter include:

- Background Information: Growth and Development
- Health Assessment
- Health Promotion
- Principles of Nursing Care Management

Background Information: Growth and Development

I. Definition: Adults represent the largest segment of the population in the United States. Because the "baby boomer" generation is approaching 65 years of age, there will be increasing numbers of older adult clients (85 years of age and older) within the next few years.

II. Theories of growth and development: Adults progress through predictable stages of psychosocial, cognitive, and moral development from young adulthood through the end of life. Theorists such as Erikson, Peck, and Havighurst have described adult growth and development in various stages as depicted in Table 19-1.

Health Assessment

I. Definition: Adult clients require a complete health assessment, including physical assessments, cognitive, and emotional assessments, and a detailed risk assessment to ensure optimum health throughout the aging process. The nurse must be skilled in interview techniques and age-related physical assessment techniques. The nurse must also be familiar with current recommendations for age-related screening examinations for cancer, heart disease, and other health problems. Specific information about health assessment related to health problems follows in subsequent chapters in this unit.

A. Young adult client
   1. Physical assessment: Young adults transition from adolescence to attain full height and physical development. There are few physical changes during this period.
   2. Risk assessment: Health risk factors are as follows:
      a. Accidents
         (1) Reinforce motor vehicle safety: Promote use of seat belt when driving and helmet when cycling; defensive driving; and designated

Table 19-1 Adult Growth and Development According to Major Theorists

Age	Erikson	Peck	Havighurst
Young adult (19 to 40 years of age)	Intimacy versus isolation: Need to develop intimate relationships. Failure results in social isolation and loneliness.	N/A	Select a mate. Learn to live with a partner. Start a family. Rear children. Manage a home. Begin occupation. Accept civic responsibility.
Middle age (40 to 65 years of age)	Generativity versus stagnation: Focus moves to meeting needs of others; develop values of charity and consideration. Failure results in self-absorption.	Valuing wisdom versus physical power. Socializing versus sexualizing relationships. Emotional flexibility versus emotional impoverishment. Mental flexibility versus mental rigidity.	Achieve adult civic and social responsibility. Establish standard of living. Assist teens to become responsible adults. Develop leisure activities. Relate to spouse as a person. Adjust to physical changes. Adjust to aging parents.
Younger old age (65 to 75 years of age)	Ego integrity versus despair: Focus is reviewing one's life and accepting it, feeling satisfaction in self and accomplishments. Failure results in remorse and despair.	Ego differentiation versus work role preoccupation. Body transcendence versus body preoccupation. Ego transcendence versus ego preoccupation.	Adjust to decreasing strength and health. Adjust to retirement and fixed income. Adjust to death of parents, spouse, and friends. Develop relationship with adult children. Adjust to leisure time. Adjust to slower physical and cognitive responses. Keep active and involved.
Old age (75 years of age and older)	N/A	N/A	Adapt to living alone. Safeguard physical and mental health. Adjust to possibility of moving into nursing home. Stay in touch with other family members. Find meaning in life. Adjust to one's own eventual death.

drivers if drinking. Check brakes and tires.

(2) Provide teaching related to water safety: Assess depth of pool or lake before diving; supervise backyard pools.

(3) Promote use of workplace safety precautions.

b. Suicide: Screen client for depression; if present, refer client for counseling.

c. Hypertension: Measure BP every 2 years.

d. Substance abuse: Screen for substance abuse; initiate smoking cessation/prevention programs; encourage educational programs; refer for counseling/rehabilitation as indicated.

e. Sexually transmitted diseases (STDs): Provide teaching regarding condom use, safe sex practices, and signs and symptoms of STDs. Encourage regular screenings.

f. Violence: Promote avoidance of dangerous situations; promote anger management counseling as indicated.

g. Abuse of women: Encourage regular screening for indicators of abusive relationships; teach date-rape prevention; refer client to social services and community resources as indicated.

h. Malignancies

(1) Instruct client to avoid ultraviolet rays and perform a monthly self-examination for breast or testicular cancer.

(2) Perform routine Papanicolaou tests when client is sexually active.

(3) Perform skin and oral mucosa examination every 3 years.

(4) Screen for risk factors of cervical cancer according to American Cancer Society guidelines beginning when sexually active and at least by age 21, and then every 2 to 3 years; women over 70 with normal Pap tests no longer need cervical cancer screening.

i. Obesity: Promote healthy eating habits and regular aerobic exercise. Provide teaching related to risks of obesity.

B. Middle-aged client

1. Physical assessment: Physical changes become apparent during middle age. All body systems are affected.

a. Integument: Hair thins and begins to gray; skin turgor and moisture decrease; skin wrinkles appear, especially in areas exposed to sun.

b. Musculoskeletal: Fat is deposited in the abdominal area; intervertebral discs thin; bones lose calcium.

c. Cardiovascular: Blood vessels become less elastic.

d. Sensory: Visual acuity declines (especially near vision); hearing declines (especially high-frequency sounds).

e. GI/genitourinary: Metabolism slows; tone of large intestine slows; glomerular filtration rate decreases; estrogen and testosterone levels decline.

2. Risk assessment: Health risk factors are as follows:

a. Accidents

(1) Encourage visual acuity testing yearly.

(2) Teach precautions for night driving.

(3) Inspect home setting for hazards.

(4) Modify home setting for physical challenges.

(5) Teach safety precautions for use of machinery.

b. Cancer—in addition to teaching client to avoid ultraviolet rays and to perform monthly self-examination for breast or testicular cancer, assess adherence to the following:

(1) Digital rectal examination annually beginning at 40 years of age.

(2) Fecal occult blood test annually beginning at 50 years of age.

(3) Sigmoidoscopy every 5 years or colonoscopy every 10 years beginning at 50 years of age.

(4) Clinical breast examination annually beginning at age 40.

(5) Mammogram annually beginning at 40 years of age, and MRI if high risk.

(6) Papanicolaou test (see previous discussion for cervical cancer).

(7) Pelvic examination annually beginning at 40 years of age.

(8) Per American Cancer Society guidelines, beginning with menopause, women are informed of risk for endometrial cancer and instructed to report bleeding or spotting to the HCP. Biopsy may be done for women at high risk, starting at 35 years of age.

(9) Prostate-specific antigen annually beginning at 50 years of age.

(10) Skin, mouth, and thyroid screening yearly beginning at 40 years of age.

c. Cardiovascular disease—in addition to encouraging smoking cessation programs and recommending regular aerobic exercise, perform the following:
   (1) Obtain/review lipid panel.
   (2) Screen for diabetes.
   (3) Screen for family history of heart disease and early cardiac-related deaths.

d. Obesity: Provide teaching related to risks of obesity; promote healthy eating habits and reduce caloric intake.

e. Alcoholism: Screen for alcohol abuse and provide teaching related to risks of alcoholism. Refer client to Alcoholics Anonymous or rehabilitation as indicated.

f. Mental health alterations: Identify stressors, and screen for anxiety and depression. Refer to support groups as indicated.

C. Older adult client

1. Physical assessment: Physical changes continue throughout the aging process into older adulthood. These changes vary for each individual, but all body systems are affected.
   a. Integument: Skin becomes fragile, pale, and dry; wrinkling continues and tissues sag; lentigo senilis (age spots) appear on exposed body parts; perspiration decreases; nails become thick and ridged; hair continues to thin and gray.
   b. Musculoskeletal: Reaction time slows; joints become stiff; balance becomes impaired.
   c. Sensory: Intolerance to cold develops; sense of smell decreases; sense of taste decreases (especially salt); appearance of arcus senilis around corneas.
   d. Respiratory: Vital capacity is reduced and residual volume is increased; dyspnea with exertion.
   e. Cardiovascular: Systolic and diastolic BP increases; orthostatic hypotension.
   f. GI/genitourinary: Swallowing time delayed; indigestion and constipation increase; renal function reduced; urinary urgency and frequency.
   g. Cognitive: Short-term memory impaired; slow cognitive decline; depression.

2. Risk assessment: Health risk factors are as follows:
   a. Accidents
      (1) Suggest use of assistive devices such as a cane or other walking aid to compensate for impaired balance; promote use of nonskid shoes.
      (2) Encourage participation in exercise programs to improve balance and muscle strength.
      (3) Provide environmental assessment to identify and remove hazards; this includes decluttering the environment, ensuring adequate lighting, installing stair rails, marking edges of doorways and steps, and modifying bathroom with grab bars and raised toilet seat.
      (4) Provide teaching about driving, including: avoid night driving (compensates for increased sensitivity to glare); drive on familiar roads and for short distances (compensates for delayed reaction time); use caution when turning head to view periphery; and participate in older adult driving program.
      (5) Provide teaching regarding fire safety and burn prevention, including: check smoke and carbon monoxide alarms; monitor temperature of hot water to prevent burns.
      (6) Maintain warm environment to prevent hypothermia.
      (7) Recommend use of emergency calling systems, such as Lifeline.
   b. Effects of chronic illnesses: For chronic illnesses, modify home setting to optimize self-care; screen for depression and suicide risk; and refer to community resources as indicated. Chronic illness may include:
      (1) Osteoporosis
      (2) Orthostatic hypotension
      (3) Dyspnea with exertion
      (4) Cancer
      (5) Arthritis
      (6) Stroke
      (7) Heart disease
      (8) Presbycusis (loss of hearing)
      (9) Presbyopia (loss of vision)
   c. Drug use and misuse
      (1) Monitor closely if taking sedatives or analgesics.
      (2) Encourage use of alternative sleep aids.

(3) Provide teaching related to dangers of prescribed medications.
(4) Maintain list of all medications and doses for HCPs.
(5) Review use of over-the-counter (OTC) medications.
(6) Recommend annual medication review.

d. Alcoholism: Screen for alcohol abuse and review interaction between medications and alcohol. Refer to community resources as indicated.

e. Dementia: Provide regular assessment of client and caregiver, in addition to the following:
(1) Suggest use of notes and lists to compensate for short-term memory loss.
(2) Teach caregiver to modify home setting for safety: Control access to poisons and medications; take knobs off kitchen stoves to prevent burns; apply special locks on doors to prevent wandering; consider use of electronic identification devices such as wrist bands, if wanders.
(3) Refer caregiver to support services, such as adult day care and respite care.

f. Elder abuse: Screen for signs of abuse and neglect, and report suspected abuse in accordance with state law. Refer to support services as indicated.

Health Promotion

I. Definition: Health promotion involves taking action to prevent health problems. There are three levels of prevention.

A. Primary prevention: Refers to generalized health promotion and protection against specific diseases focused on healthy individuals.
1. Prevent accidents and falls.
2. Encourage participation in nutrition and exercise programs.
3. Promote stress management.
4. Provide teaching about occupational and recreational safety.
5. Initiate follow-up with immunizations.
6. Assess for risks associated with specific diseases.
7. Promote environmental sanitation.

B. Secondary prevention: Refers to the early detection of disease with prompt intervention for individuals with health problems; includes prevention of complications.
1. Initiate screening for disease.
2. Promote regular medical, dental, and vision examinations.
3. Encourage self-examinations for breast and testicular cancer.
4. Provide nursing interventions to prevent complications associated with disease.
5. Perform delegated medical acts.

C. Tertiary prevention: Refers to the rehabilitation and restoration to optimum level of functioning of an individual with a stabilized or irreversible illness.
1. Refer client to self-help groups as indicated.
2. Provide client and family teaching related to the recognition and prevention of complications.
3. Initiate rehabilitation or restorative care.
4. Provide palliative care.

Principles of Nursing Care Management

I. Definition: Principles of managing care for adult clients include client teaching, using ethical and legal principles to guide care, setting priorities, and delegating care.

A. Client teaching involves a process of assessment, planning, implementing, and evaluating.
1. Assessment—perform comprehensive assessments involving client needs, readiness, and barriers to learning.
a. Assess client needs—prioritize client's learning needs involving gaps in knowledge, previous experience, preferred learning style, and family members or significant others desires to be involved.
b. Assess client readiness related to desire to learn, ability to learn, and support system.
c. Assess client barriers to learning—determine level of understanding; primary language (non-English speaking); and ability to read and write; presence of hearing or visual deficits; level of comfort; and developmental and/or environmental barriers.
2. Planning—develop individualized teaching plan.
a. Establish learning outcomes.
b. Identify relevant content.
c. Select teaching strategies.
d. Obtain teaching aids for reinforcement.
3. Implementation—implement teaching plan.
a. Promote active involvement in learning.
b. Use language suited to client's level of understanding.

c. Involve client's family, if desired.
d. Reduce distractions and provide privacy.
e. Proceed from simple to complex.
f. Promote client comfort and receptiveness.
g. Repeat key concepts and principles.
h. Use multiple methods.
i. Provide culturally sensitive instruction.
j. Provide practice of psychomotor skills.

4. Evaluation—ensure client understands teaching as evidenced by integration of learning into health behaviors on a consistent basis.
   a. Collaborate with client and family to evaluate learning.
   b. Provide client and family teaching about strategies to evaluate learning progress such as return demonstration, quizzes or tests, games, and journaling or keeping diaries.

B. Ethical and legal issues guide the nurse in planning care. Nurse responsibility involves accountability for one's own actions, responsibility for adhering to nurses' code of ethics (see next entry), ethical decision-making, and client advocacy (see also Chapter 40).

1. Ethical principles
   a. Autonomy—observe client's right to make own decisions.
   b. Nonmaleficence—avoid doing harm.
   c. Beneficence—promote doing good.
   d. Justice—provide fair and equal treatment.
   e. Fidelity—keep promises.
   f. Veracity—practice honesty.
2. Legal principles
   a. Regulation of nursing practice per state law
   b. Nurse Practice Act: Regulatory authority of state board of nursing.
      (1) Provides standards of care and outlines nursing responsibilities.
      (2) Functions as implied contract—unwritten agreement with client to provide care.
   c. Client rights—clients have certain rights to privacy and health care choices as specified by federal and state laws and by specific health care agencies; common rights include the following:
      (1) Considerate, respectful care
      (2) Full disclosure and identity/status of health care workers involved in their care
      (3) Participate in plan of care and to refuse treatment
      (4) Privacy and confidentiality
      (5) Have an advance directive, which is honored by the health care facility
      (6) Review own medical record
      (7) Appropriate and medically indicated care
   d. Issues of malpractice/negligence may include:
      (1) Failure to recognize change in condition
      (2) Failure to document care given, observations made, or doctor's calls
      (3) Assault (threat) and battery (physical harm): Physically restraining client without order
      (4) Failure to obtain informed consent: Client not competent to give consent
      (5) Omission of nursing intervention or delegated medical act
      (6) Commission of intervention in negligent manner causing harm
      (7) Failure to monitor unstable client
      (8) Failure to provide discharge/medication instructions that client is able to understand
      (9) Patient abandonment: Leaving client without reporting off to another nurse
      (10) False imprisonment: Preventing client from discharging self against medical advice
      (11) Breach of confidentiality (also a violation of Health Insurance Portability and Accountability Act or HIPAA)
      (12) Failure to delegate or supervise assistive personnel appropriately

C. Setting priorities—priorities are set based on the following:

1. Level of threat
   a. Life-threatening—high priority
   b. Health-threatening—medium priority
   c. Health promotion/anticipatory guidance—low priority
2. Maslow hierarchy
   a. Physiologic needs (air, food, water)
   b. Safety and security
   c. Love and belonging
   d. Self-esteem
   e. Self-actualization
3. Additional factors include client's values and beliefs, client and family preferences for care, and available resources.

D. Delegation—responsibilities performed by the RN only (cannot be delegated) include assessment, analysis of data, determining nursing diagnosis, and client teaching. When delegating tasks, the following must occur:

1. Five rights of delegation
   a. Right task
   b. Right circumstances
   c. Right person
   d. Right direction and communication
   e. Right supervision and evaluation
2. Principles of delegation
   a. RN may delegate task but not responsibility for care.
   b. RN is legally responsible for quality of delegation and supervision.
   c. Client must be medically stable.
   d. Task must be a routine one that does not require substantial knowledge or skill.
   e. Task must have predictable outcome and be safe for client.
   f. Delegation must comply with state statute and agency policy.
   g. RN must assess health care worker's ability to perform task.
   h. RN must provide clear direction, including parameters for reporting information.
   i. RN must monitor performance of delegated act and assess client response.
3. Supervision following delegation
   a. Provide clear direction to caregiver for task completion.
   b. Identify type of data to be reported immediately.
   c. Follow up to determine that task was completed appropriately.
   d. Identify need for additional teaching/training of assistive personnel.
   e. Offer praise appropriately and promptly for good performance.

Bibliography

Altman, G. (2004). *Delmar's fundamental and advanced nursing skills* (2nd ed.) Albany, NY: Delmar.

Ellis, J., & Hartley, C. (2005). *Managing and coordinating nursing care.* Philadelphia: Lippincott Williams & Wilkins.

Karch, A. (2006). *Lippincott's nursing drug guide.* Philadelphia: Lippincott Williams & Wilkins.

Lewis, S., Heitkemper, M., & Dirksen, S. (2004). *Medical-surgical nursing* (6th ed.). St Louis: Mosby.

Purnell, L., & Paulanka, B. (Eds.) (2003). *Transcultural healthcare: A culturally competent approach.* Philadelphia: F.A. Davis.

Smeltzer, B., et al (2006). *Brunner and Suddarth's textbook of medical-surgical nursing* (11th ed.). Philadelphia: Lippincott Williams & Wilkins.

Taylor, C., Lillis, C., LeMone, P., & Lynn, P. (2006). *Fundamentals of nursing.* Philadelphia: Lippincott Williams & Wilkins.

Weber, J. R., & Kelley, J. (2007). *Nurses handbook of health assessment.* Philadelphia: Lippincott Williams & Wilkins.

Yarbro, C. H., Frogge, M., & Goodman, M. (2004). *Cancer symptom management* (3rd ed.). Sudbury, MA: Jones and Bartlett.

CHAPTER 19

Practice Test

Background Information: Growth and Development

1. The nurse is assessing the developmental level of a young adult. The client lives alone, works at home as a computer programmer, and indicates he does not have friends or hobbies, but he indicates his job is very intense and he works long hours. The nurse can plan with the client to work toward fuller development and maturation by suggesting the client:

☐ 1. Include more leisure activities in his life.
☐ 2. Develop relationships with others.
☐ 3. Be more active and involved in the community.
☐ 4. Stay in touch with his family.

2. The nurse is counseling a middle-aged adult who has recently become physically disabled. Which of the following is an expected reaction of this client? The client will:

☐ 1. Experience all stages of grief in order to go on with life.
☐ 2. Progress sequentially through the stages of grief.
☐ 3. Not achieve total acceptance of the disability.
☐ 4. Respond to grief in an individualistic manner.

Health Assessment

3. The most appropriate way for the nurse to assess a client's ability to perform activities of daily living is to:

☐ 1. Ask family members to describe what they've seen.

□ 2. Ask the client what he or she is able to perform or not perform.
□ 3. Review documentation on the client's chart about current activity.
□ 4. Observe client performing varied activities of daily living.

4. AF The nurse is assessing a client's abdomen. In which order, first to last, should the nurse conduct the physical assessment?
_____ 1. Auscultation.
_____ 2. Inspection.
_____ 3. Percussion.
_____ 4. Palpation.

5. The nurse is conducting a health assessment on a client who is 80 years of age. What statement by the client indicates the nurse should investigate further?
□ 1. Client reports an increased incidence of colds.
□ 2. Client can no longer drive the car because of vision problems.
□ 3. Client obtains more than 9 hr of sleep per night.
□ 4. Client has thoughts of mixing acetaminophen (Tylenol) and alcohol.

6. The nurse is reviewing the laboratory reports of a client who is 82 years of age. The client has a WBC count of 3,000/mm^3. The nurse should interpret this finding as being related to which of the following?
□ 1. Normal aging.
□ 2. Polycythemia vera.
□ 3. Stress.
□ 4. Viral infection.

7. AF A client who is 79 years of age is being admitted to the hospital after falling off a 6-foot ladder. In obtaining the health history, the nurse should determine which of the following? Select all that apply.
□ 1. Symptoms at the time of the fall.
□ 2. History of a previous fall.
□ 3. Location of the fall.
□ 4. Activity at the time of the fall.
□ 5. Time of the fall.
□ 6. Trauma postfall.
□ 7. Who was present at the time of the fall.

8. The nurse is conducting a cancer screening program. Which of the following clients has the greatest risk for cancer?
□ 1. White American client who is 70 years of age with urinary retention.
□ 2. Asian client who is 86 years of age with elevated prostate-specific antigen (PSA).
□ 3. African American client who is 45 years of age whose father had prostate cancer.
□ 4. Native American client who is 67 years of age with a history of benign prostate hypertrophy.

Health Promotion

9. AF The nurse is planning care with an adult client who has a hearing loss. Which of the following strategies will be most effective for the nurse to use when communicating with this client? Select all that apply.
□ 1. Complete tasks quickly.
□ 2. Sit in front of the client.
□ 3. Reduce background noise.
□ 4. Speak in a loud voice.
□ 5. Use facial expressions and gestures.
□ 6. Use short sentences.

10. Which of the following would be the most effective method for cleaning the teeth of an immobilized hospitalized client?
□ 1. Assist the client to use lemon and glycerin swabs.
□ 2. Brush with a soft-bristle tooth brush.
□ 3. Rinse the mouth with mouth wash and peroxide.
□ 4. Wipe the mouth and teeth with a sponge stick.

11. The nurse is planning care for an obese female client who is 68 years of age. The client experiences dribbling urine when she coughs, sneezes, and changes positions. The nurse should instruct the client to promote urinary health by encouraging her to:
□ 1. Increase consumption of fluids such as coffee and tea.
□ 2. Use a Foley catheter.
□ 3. Participate in a weight loss program.
□ 4. Perform muscle strength-building exercises.

12. The nurse is planning care with an older adult who is at risk for falling because of postural hypotension. Which of the following will be most effective in preventing falls in this client?
□ 1. Complete a fall diary.
□ 2. Attach a sensor to the client that will alarm when client attempts to get up.
□ 3. Encourage a family member to stay with the client.
□ 4. Instruct the client to sit, obtain balance, dangle legs, and rise slowly.

13. To reduce the risk of osteoporosis, the nurse should advise an older adult to:
□ 1. Obtain three to five servings of red meat per week.

□ 2. Drink at least eight glasses of fluids per day.
□ 3. Eat dairy products and dark, green vegetables.
□ 4. Perform weight-bearing exercises for at least 15 min a day.

14. A nurse is planning a health promotion program for a female client who is 68 years of age who has been diagnosed with high serum lipids. The goal is to increase the amount of exercise this sedentary client currently performs. The most appropriate exercise program would be:
□ 1. Jogging three to five times per week for 30 to 60 min.
□ 2. Playing golf three times per week for 60 min.
□ 3. Walking three to five times per week for 30 to 60 min.
□ 4. Swimming once a week for 30 min.

Principles of Nursing Care Management

15. The nurse is assessing a client's knowledge about his diagnosis of coronary syndrome that he has had for 4 years. When assessing the client's learning needs, the nurse should take which of the following statements into consideration?
□ 1. The client has had his heart condition for 4 years and is probably very knowledgeable about his condition.
□ 2. The client's learning needs may have changed over the course of his illness.
□ 3. The client's condition is presently stable so he will have fewer learning needs.
□ 4. Clients are usually more motivated to learn about their condition when they are hospitalized.

16. The nurse is teaching an older adult client about taking his medications and the expected outcomes of each drug. Which of the following is true about the biological half-life of drugs in older adults? The half-life:
□ 1. Decreases the risk of adverse reactions.
□ 2. Decreases the effectiveness of the drug.
□ 3. Increases the risk of adverse reactions.
□ 4. Increases the effectiveness of the drug.

17. The nurse is caring for a chronically ill client who has not been adhering to his treatment plan. Which of the following will be most helpful to the nurse and client as they discuss ways for the client to follow a treatment plan?
□ 1. The client must follow the plan of care to continue to receive medical treatment.
□ 2. Family members have a responsibility to talk the client into adhering to the plan of care.
□ 3. Many chronically ill clients refuse treatment in order to get more attention from the nursing staff.
□ 4. Clients have the right to make their own decision regarding the health care they receive.

18. AF A client is transferred from the postanesthesia recovery unit to a medical-surgical unit. Which of the following can be delegated to a UAP? Select all that apply.
□ 1. Obtaining the client's admission vital signs.
□ 2. Making sure the client's call light is within reach.
□ 3. Recording the client's urinary output.
□ 4. Obtaining the client's admission assessment.
□ 5. Assessing the client's pain level.
□ 6. Giving the client a cup of ice.

19. The charge nurse is making assignments for a team that includes two RNs and one UAP. One client requires a nurse to perform several complex procedures. The charge nurse should:
□ 1. Assign each complex procedure to a different nurse.
□ 2. Assign the same number of clients to each nurse, but with lower acuity.
□ 3. Assign fewer clients to the nurse managing this client's care.
□ 4. Assign additional unlicensed assistive personnel to assist the nurse.

20. The charge nurse is making assignments for a team of two RNs and one LPN. The nurse should delegate the care of which of the following clients to the LPN?
□ 1. Client with esophageal varices who is having esophageal bleeding.
□ 2. Client who is diagnosed with a seizure disorder who is having a seizure.
□ 3. Client returning from abdominal surgery who is having chest pain.
□ 4. Client returning from the recovery room who is semiconscious.

Answers and Rationales

1. 2 The primary developmental task of a young adult client is to establish intimacy versus isolation; failure to do so can result in social isolation and loneliness. Adding more leisure time is an activity of middle adulthood. Becoming more active in the community is a task of the young older adult. Staying in touch with family is a task for the older adult. (H)

2. 4 Adults respond to the diagnosis of a newly acquired disability in a variety of ways. Clients do not always experience all stages of grief nor do they progress sequentially through the stages of grief. Some but not all clients achieve total acceptance of the disability. (P)

3. 4 In order to assess the client's ability to perform activities of daily living, it is important for the nurse to observe the client actually performing them. This way, the nurse can assess for any problems that are occurring with a specific activity. Asking the client what he is able to do will not always provide reliable information, and documentation on the chart may not reflect if the client has had help in performing specific tasks. Family members can provide some information but are not trained in how to evaluate the client. (H)

4. 2, 1, 3, 4 When assessing a client's abdomen the nurse first inspects the contour and symmetry of the abdomen. Next, the nurse auscultates for bowel sounds; this step is done before percussion and palpation as these can alter the character of the bowel sounds. Percussion and palpation are the last steps of physical assessment of the abdomen. (A)

5. 4 The nurse investigates the client's statement about mixing Tylenol and alcohol, and determines the purpose of mixing the two drugs and whether the client might be having suicidal ideations. The immune system of an older adult declines with aging, so increased incidence of colds may be common; the nurse instructs the client about ways to prevent colds. Inability to drive may contribute to changing from an independent role to a dependent role, resulting in social isolation, which is a risk factor for substance abuse. Generally, 9 hr of sleep is adequate; older adults tend to become anxious and use medications and alcohol when less than 8 hr of sleep is achieved. (A)

6. 4 The aging process results in a decline in the function of WBCs rather than the number of WBCs. Low WBC counts may indicate viral infections, alcoholism, dietary deficient, systemic lupus erythematosus, rheumatoid arthritis, drug toxicity, dietary deficiency, bone marrow failure, and/or liver and spleen disease. Generally, acute infections, inflammatory process, and stress could provoke a rise in WBCs. In addition, trauma, stress, tissue necrosis, and certain chronic medications can also prompt an increase in WBCs. (A)

7. 1, 2, 3, 4, 5, 6 The acronym SPLATT (symptoms, previous fall, location, activity at the time, time, and trauma) can guide the assessment of an older adult who has fallen. It may be helpful to know if there was someone with the person when the fall occurred to present a bystander's perspective, but the information is not necessary and it is more important to get the client to describe in his or her own words what happened. (S)

8. 3 This client presents with three major predisposing factors (45 years of age, race, and family history) associated with prostate cancer. The client who is 70 years of age is at risk because of his age, but not race or the urinary retention. The client who is 86 years of age has a high incidence of cancer, but generally Asians have the lowest incidence. A positive PSA is not a definitive diagnostic tool; the only risk factor present for the client who is 67 years of age is age-related. Native American incidence is not as high risk as African American incidence. BPH is common in most men this age. (H)

9. 2, 3, 5, 6 Individuals who are hard of hearing tend to use lip reading; therefore, the nurse faces the client when talking so the client can see the speaker's face and lips. The nurse avoids overarticulating or shouting at the client. It is not necessary to complete tasks quickly; the nurse remains calm and patient, and uses facial expressions or gestures to support the communication. (H)

10. 2 Mechanical cleansing (brushing) is the most effective method of oral care. Simply rinsing or cleansing with a swab is ineffective; lemon and glycerin swabs can be harmful to tooth enamel. If brushing is impossible, cleanse the teeth with a gauze pad and have the client rinse with an antiseptic mouthwash. (C)

11. 3 The goal is to promote health in this client who has stress incontinence. Participating in a weight loss program or support group may decrease the intra-abdominal pressure contributing to the incontinence. Participating in swimming, bicycling, or low-impact exercise is beneficial to weight loss. Kegel exercises are useful, but not necessary. Clients with urinary stress incontinence are encouraged to avoid drinks with caffeine and alcohol. Perineal care is essential to prevent skin breakdown, but the client does not require a Foley or straight catheter at this time. (H)

12. 4 There are many risk factors for falls in older adults. Postural hypotension is a common risk. The nurse should instruct the client about postural hypotension and provide practical information regarding how to sit on the bed or chair, dangle the legs first and then rise slowly, supported by a walker if necessary. A diary of instances of an individual's falls may predict future falls by tracking the events and behaviors at the time of the fall, but is not the most effective in preventing the fall. Attaching a sensor to the client or bed is reserved for clients who are at a serious risk for injury. (S)

13. 3 Dairy products and dark, green vegetables contain calcium, phosphorus, and vitamin D, which prevent osteoporosis. Red meat contains iron, which helps prevent anemia. Fluids and exercise do not contribute to the prevention of osteoporosis. (H)

14. 3 The nurse first assesses what the client enjoys doing in order to promote following through with the activity on a regular basis. The client will obtain the most benefit from aerobic exercises such as walking, biking, jogging, or swimming. Because the client has been sedentary, the nurse instructs the client to start the exercise program with walking slowly 10 min four times a day and increasing to 30 to 60 min three to five times per week. Jogging is not a realistic exercise at this time. Playing golf is not considered an aerobic activity; therefore, it is not beneficial in lowering serum lipids. To illicit cardiovascular changes, the client would need to swim more than once a week. (H)

15. 2 This client has lived with his diagnosis for 4 years and, depending on the progression of his illness, his learning needs may have changed. He may at this time have more questions about his illness and how to manage it. The nurse does not assume that the client is stable and knowledgeable about his illness because he has been diagnosed for a long period of time; clients are sometimes less likely to want to learn during hospitalization because they are not feeling well enough to learn. (H)

16. 3 Drugs are not filtered in the older adult's body as quickly as in the young adult; therefore, filtration is slow and the drug remains in the older adult for a longer period of time. As a result, there is an increase in the risk of adverse reactions, especially when several different types of medications are prescribed. In this situation, biological half-life has to do with time necessary to be secreted rather than effectiveness. (D)

17. 4 Adult clients have a right to make their own decisions regarding health care and whether or not they want to comply with the treatment plan. Medical treatment cannot be withheld if the client chooses to not follow the treatment plan. It is not appropriate to attempt talking the client into complying with the treatment plan or to assume that he or she will refuse treatment to gain attention from the nursing staff. (M)

18. 1, 2, 3, 6 Tasks within the UAP's scope of practice include obtaining vital signs and recording the urinary output, as well as placing the call light within reach and giving the client a cup of ice. Assessing the client on admission and assessing the client's level of pain are nursing interventions that are in the RN's scope of practice. (M)

19. 3 The charge nurse assigns fewer clients to the RN who will be taking care of the client with high-acuity needs. Even though the RN would be assigned clients with lower acuity in addition to the client with high acuity, the RN will be planning care for more clients. Dividing the care for the high-acuity client among several RNs increases the risk of error. The UAP will not be able to perform the complex procedures required for the high-acuity client. (M)

20. 2 Although a nurse will need to check on the client with the seizure disorder, prevention of injury and airway maintenance is within the scope of practice of an LPN. Management of esophageal bleeding requires complex care that is beyond the LPN scope of practice. The semiconscious client and the client with chest pain require the nurse to assess and make clinical judgments that are based on an advanced level of knowledge. (M)

chapter 20

The Client With Cardiac Health Problems

Heart disease is the leading cause of death for adults in the United States. The death rate is higher for older adults, and incidence of heart disease in women is increasing. Health problems such as acute coronary syndrome (ACS), coronary artery disease (CAD), and shock require hospitalization, and often in technologically sophisticated intensive care units, where nursing care is essential for monitoring client progress and identifying life-threatening changes. Because health problems such as hypertension and heart failure (HF) often require lifestyle changes and long-term care, nurses have an important role in both health teaching and health promotion to assist clients to maintain and restore health. Topics discussed in this chapter include:

- Acute Coronary Syndrome
- Coronary Artery Disease
- Heart Failure and Cardiomyopathy
- Hypertension
- Inflammatory and Valvular Diseases
- Valvular and Cardiac Surgery
- Cardiac Dysrhythmias
- Shock and Multiple Organ Dysfunction Syndrome

Acute Coronary Syndrome

I. Definition: Acute coronary syndrome (ACS) describes the spectrum of clinical presentations of coronary artery disease (CAD).
  A. ACS includes unstable angina (UA), non–ST-segment elevation myocardial infarction (MI) (non-STEMI), and ST-segment elevation MI (STEMI). Diagnostic criteria is as follows:
    1. UA
      a. Chest pain that is not relieved by nitroglycerine or rest
      b. ECG changes suggestive of ischemia (ST-segment depression)
      c. No elevation of serum cardiac markers
    2. Non-STEMI
      a. ECG ischemic ST-segment changes
      b. Elevation of serum cardiac markers
    3. STEMI
      a. ECG changes with ST-segment elevation
      b. Elevation of serum cardiac markers
  B. MI occurs when there is insufficient blood flow, causing lack of oxygen to one or more areas of the heart. The onset of MI can occur suddenly or gradually, evolving over several hr.
    1. Physical changes occur in the heart around 3 to 6 hr after the infarction, when the infarcted area appears blue and swollen.
    2. Infarct turns gray with yellow streaks after 48 hr.
    3. Granulation tissue forms in 8 to 10 days following infarction.
    4. Scar tissue forms in 2 to 3 months following infarction.
  C. Acute MI results from abrupt decrease or total cessation of blood flow to the myocardium as a result of plaque rupture, new coronary artery thrombosis, or coronary artery spasm. Zones of MI include:
    1. Ischemia: The outer area of the infarcted myocardium still has viable tissue but there is a diminished blood supply because of the infarction process. On the ECG, the diminished blood supply is reflected by an inverted T wave and/or ST-segment depression.
    2. Injury: In the zone of injury, cells do not fully repolarize because of decreased blood supply. If perfusion is restored within 6 hr, the condition is reversible. On the ECG, this is reflected by an elevated ST segment.
    3. Infarction: Cellular death and muscle necrosis occurs; as healing takes place, cells in this area are replaced by scar tissue.
  D. Classification of MI
    1. Muscle layers
      a. Transmural or full thickness involves all three layers: endocardium, myocardium, and epicardium.
      b. Nontransmural MI involves partial wall damage (does not infarct the full thickness of the heart muscle).
    2. Location of MI and coronary artery involved:
      a. Anterior wall infarction: Results from occlusion of left anterior descending (LAD)
      b. Septal: Results from occlusion of LAD
      c. Lateral wall infarction: Results from occlusion of the circumflex coronary artery
      d. Inferior wall infarction: Results from occlusion of right coronary artery (RCA)
      e. Posterior wall infarction: Results from occlusion of right coronary artery (RCA) or circumflex
      f. Right ventricle wall infarction: Results from occlusion of right coronary artery (RCA)

II. Nursing process
  A. Assessment (see also assessment for CAD)
    1. Complete a detailed health history and physical assessment, including vital signs.
    2. Assess client for signs and symptoms of MI: Findings will vary with size and extent of the ischemia, injury, or infarction; client's status; and history of CAD and/or previous MI.
      a. Classic symptom: Substernal chest pain described as crushing; may radiate to arms, neck, back, and/or jaw and continue for more than 15 min unrelieved by vasodilators (nitroglycerin). Note that for about 30% of women, chest pain is not the first or classic sign of MI; women may report fatigue, sleep disturbances, nausea, and shortness of breath as first signs. Chest pain in women may be described as "burning in the chest."
      b. Atypical symptoms: May be experienced by older adults, women, and diabetics; includes dyspnea, confusion, weakness, or fainting.
      c. Other signs and symptoms:
        (1) Pale, diaphoretic, cool, clammy skin
        (2) Weakness, light-headedness
        (3) Vagal effects (bradycardia, nausea and vomiting)
        (4) Change in LOC, apprehension, anxiety, fear

(5) Tachypnea and dyspnea
(6) Crackles
(7) Distention of neck veins
(8) Pericardial friction rub
(9) Elevated temperature
(10) Fever occurs within the first 24 hr and may continue for 1 week
(11) Signs of dysrhythmias, shock, HF

3. Assess for risk factors.
   a. Dysrhythmias: Bradycardia, tachycardia, premature ventricular contractions (PVCs)
   b. Hypotension
   c. New mitral regurgitation murmur, S3 crackles
   d. Coronary artery spasm
   e. Severe anemia (decreased oxygen supply)
   f. Severe aortic stenosis
4. Obtain diagnostic tests.
   a. 12-lead electrocardiogram (ECG): Compare with earlier tracing.
      (1) Changes on ECG correlate with the location of ischemia, injury, and infarction
      (2) ST depression or inversion of T wave
      (3) Acute ST elevation
      (4) Abnormal Q wave—more than 0.04 s in duration or one-fourth the size of the R wave; appears within 1 hr of transmural MI
   b. Cardiac markers
      (1) Total CK—elevates in 3 to 6 hr after infarction, peaks at 24 hr, and returns to normal within 72 hr
      (2) CK-MB—elevates in 4 to 6 hr after pain, peaks in 24 hr, and returns to normal within 72 hr; is specific for myocardial damage
      (3) Troponin T (cTnT)—elevates in 3 to 6 hr and remains elevated for 14 to 21 days
      (4) Troponin I (cTnI)—elevates in 7 to 14 hr after MI and remains elevated for 5 to 7 days; is highly specific for myocardial damage
      (5) Myoglobin—rises within 1 hr after cell death, peaks in 4 to 6 hr, and returns to normal within 24 to 36 hr or less
   c. Echocardiography: Assess left ventricular function, wall motion abnormalities, and complications such as ventricular septal defect, aneurysms, mitral regurgitation, and pericardial effusions.
   d. Cardiac catheterization and arteriography: Assess location and extent of coronary artery obstruction for definitive diagnosis.
   e. Thallium scans: Assess for ischemia or necrotic muscle tissue.
   f. Multigated cardiac blood pool imaging scans: Evaluate left ventricular function.
   g. Other laboratory tests: WBC, C-reactive protein (CRP), serum electrolytes, BUN, creatinine, PT/INR, PTT. WBC is elevated on second day of MI and lasts up to a week.
5. Assess signs and symptoms, labs, and ECG to determine whether client is experiencing unstable angina, non-STEMI or STEMI.
   a. Unstable angina
      (1) Symptoms of angina at rest, new-onset angina of ordinary physical activity, and increasing angina
      (2) Symptoms last longer than 20 min
      (3) Ischemic ST-segment changes in two or more contiguous 12 leads: Serum cardiac markers are within normal range.
   b. Non-STEMI
      (1) Pain is unrelieved by rest or nitroglycerine (lasts longer 20 min).
      (2) Ischemic ECG changes in two or more contiguous 12 leads.
      (3) Serum cardiac markers are elevated.
   c. STEMI
      (1) Chest discomfort lasts longer than 20 to 30 min.
      (2) Involves classic symptoms (see previous signs and symptoms); women, older adults, and diabetics may experience atypical symptoms.
      (3) Pain is unrelieved by rest and nitroglycerin.
      (4) ECG changes in two or more contiguous 12 leads, indicating hyperacute T waves (early) and ST-segment elevation of 1 mm (0.1 mV) or greater.
      (5) Serum cardiac markers are elevated.

B. Analysis
1. Acute Pain: Chest, related to ineffective myocardial perfusion
2. Ineffective Tissue Perfusion: Cardiopulmonary, related to decreased myocardial oxygen supply and/or increased myocardial oxygen demand

3. Decreased Cardiac Output related to alterations in preload, afterload, contractility, heart rate
4. Risk for Ineffective Tissue Perfusion: Cardiopulmonary, related to thrombolytic therapy impact on myocardial tissue
5. Ineffective Coping related to situational crisis and personal vulnerability
6. Powerlessness related to lack of control over current situation or disease progression
7. Anxiety related to chest pain, lifestyle change, ineffective coping, fear, and critical care environment
8. Activity Intolerance related to decreased perfusion, tissue hypoxia, fatigue, chest pain
9. Ineffective Health Maintenance related to lack of knowledge of illness, risk factors, and unhealthy lifestyle

C. Planning
1. Maintain hemodynamic stability.
2. Restore the balance between oxygen demand and supply.
3. Improve coronary artery perfusion.
4. Decrease myocardial workload and oxygen demand.
5. Relieve or eliminate angina.
6. Increase activity tolerance.
7. Reduce anxiety.
8. Prevent dysrhythmias and other MI complications.
9. Provide client and family teaching on therapeutic regimen, lifestyle modifications (i.e., smoking cessation, diet, BP control, glucose control).

D. Implementation (see also implementation for CAD)
1. Provide interventions for acute chest pain.
   a. Assess cardiopulmonary status and vital signs; apply oxygen.
   b. Place client in semi- to high Fowler position.
   c. Perform 12-lead ECG.
   d. Administer aspirin (can be chewed).
   e. Administer nitroglycerin: One tablet or spray sublingual; may repeat at 5-min intervals if chest pain continues, for a total of three doses.
   f. Administer morphine IV.
   g. Draw serial cardiac markers—CK-MB, troponin T and I, myoglobin.
   h. Provide continual observation of client: Monitor for recurrent chest pain, symptoms, mental status, vital signs, SpO_2, heart sounds, lung sounds, urine output, and diagnostic findings.
   i. Maintain calm environment and provide emotional support.
2. Provide interventions for UA and non-STEMI.
   a. Monitor continuously for ECG changes within cardiac high-acuity unit.
   b. Provide pain and ischemic management (see pharmacologic and parenteral therapies).
3. Provide interventions for STEMI.
   a. Place client on a monitor and watch closely for dysrhythmias (ventricular fibrillation [VF] is common in early hours of MI).
   b. Obtain 12-lead ECG.
   c. Assess cardiopulmonary status and vital signs; apply oxygen.
   d. Start IV access (AHA/ACC guidelines recommend at least two good IV sites for administration of drugs, volume support, and reperfusion therapy).
   e. Minimize time of onset to time of administration of interventions such as thrombolytic/fibrinolytics, percutaneous coronary intervention (PCI), or surgical intervention.
      (1) PCI
      (2) Thrombolytics/fibrinolytics
      (3) Assess for reperfusion dysrhythmias
      (4) Intra-aortic balloon pump (IABP)
      (5) Coronary artery bypass graft (CABG) surgery
   f. Assess for potential complications, including dysrhythmias and cardiogenic shock.

E. Evaluation
1. Client affirms the absence of angina and associated symptoms.
2. Client has coronary artery flow restored within 30 to 90 min.
3. Client's vital signs are stable, and client experiences normal sinus rhythm or controlled ventricular rate.
4. Client verbalizes knowledge of home care and follow-up requirements.
5. Client explains health behaviors that promote a healthy lifestyle: Smoking cessation, regular physical exercise, low-fat diet, and maintenance of ideal weight.
6. Client describes low-fat diet foods; low-sodium and diabetic diet, if prescribed.
7. Client states the purpose, dosage, timing, and side effects of the medications prescribed for the treatment of angina and MI.
8. Client describes self-care behaviors to monitor at home, including daily weight, BP, pulse, edema, or blood sugar, if needed.

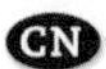

III. Client needs

A. Physiologic adaptation: Stable angina is controlled with medication and dose adjustments on an outpatient basis.
   1. Evaluate the effectiveness of nitrates, beta blocker, and/or calcium channel blocker to improve coronary artery perfusion, restore balance between oxygen demand and supply, and decrease myocardial workload and oxygen demand.
   2. Assess client's cardiac tolerance to increasing levels of activity and exercise.
   3. Recognize risk for decrease in cardiac output—indicated by decreased mental alertness; hypotension (systolic BP less than 90 mmHg); tachycardia; presence of heart murmur, S3, S4; lung crackles; urine output less than 0.5 ml/kg per hour; decreased peripheral pulses; cool, pale, cyanotic, or diaphoretic skin; edema; and jugular venous distention.
   4. Evaluate troponin, CK-MB, and myoglobin with uncontrolled, acute chest pain. Cardiac markers are diagnostic criteria for an acute MI (see ACS) and are not elevated with stable angina.
   5. Prepare client for cardiac catheterization on positive findings from diagnostic stress testing.

B. Management of care: Care of the client with ACS requires critical thinking skills and knowledge of assessment, and teaching and evaluation methods unique to the RN role. These skills cannot be delegated to an LPN or UAP.
   1. Delegate responsibly those activities that can be delegated, including basic care needs and vital sign assessments for the stable client. All monitoring information is reported to the RN.
   2. Perform comprehensive physical assessments and provide care to the client with acute angina and symptoms.
   3. Provide information on changes in client status to the physician and appropriate members of the multidisciplinary team.
   4. Facilitate outpatient follow-up care.
   5. Assess for home health care needs for managing activity restrictions and understanding how to follow health care plan.
   6. Evaluate community resources for continued cardiac education, support groups, smoking cessation, exercise, and rehabilitation.

C. Safety and infection control
   1. Teach client to assess BP and heart rate if client is on a beta blocker, calcium channel blocker, ACE inhibitor, or nitrates.
   2. Teach client to gradually increase exercise activity, always exercise with a friend, avoid temperature extremes, and designate a place to rest if angina should develop.

D. Health promotion and maintenance
   1. Optimize functional capability through tailored interventions based on individualized assessments and needs.
   2. Recognize that the older adult client may have atypical symptoms of angina, and medications may not be as well tolerated.
   3. Assist client in identifying personalized risk factors for angina and provide teaching in these areas to promote health.
   4. Instruct client about self-care behaviors for monitoring at home, such as weight, BP, heart rate, edema, and blood sugar.
   5. Promote nutritional diet including foods that are low-sodium, low-fat, and low-cholesterol; avoid large amounts of caffeine.

E. Psychologic integrity
   1. Assist client and family in coping with risk factor modification and lifestyle changes.
   2. Identify barriers and challenges to goals that may interfere with recovery: Flexible visiting hours can assist in relieving anxiety and other stress that can create a situation promoting pain occurrence (depending on the client's status, need for rest, procedures, and family dynamics).
   3. Identify counseling and support groups to assist the client in reduction of emotional stressors and denial. Address spiritual needs of client and family to assist in allaying anxieties and fears.

F. Basic care and comfort
   1. Promote position changes to avoid pressure ulcers.
   2. Provide pain management.
   3. Administer antiemetics, if needed for nausea and/or vomiting.
   4. Administer anxiolytics, if needed for anxiety.

G. Reduction of risk potential
   1. Teach client side effects of all medications and how to manage them.
   2. Teach the client and family what to expect in the course of recovery and rehabilitation.
   3. Instruct the client on premedication with nitroglycerin for exercise activity or sexual activity, according to physician guidelines.

H. Pharmacologic and parenteral therapies: Client and family will state the purpose, dosage, timing, and side effects of all medications. (See also pharmacologic and parenteral therapies for CAD.)

1. Oxygen: Increases oxygen to myocardium and prevents complications from hypoxemia.
2. Nitroglycerin: Reduces myocardial oxygen consumption, thereby decreasing myocardial ischemia and pain.
3. Analgesics: Decrease pain and anxiety by administering morphine sulfate.
4. Beta-adrenergic blocking agents: Decrease oxygen demand by decreasing heart rate and contractility; reduce morbidity and mortality.
5. Thrombolytic/fibrinolytics: Dissolve blood clots; not appropriate therapy for UA and non-STEMI. Complications include bleeding.
   a. Alteplase (t-PA)—Recombinant form of human tissue plasminogen activator. Heparin required to avoid reocclusion; monitor PTT (goal 50–75 s); administer along with aspirin.
   b. Reteplase (r-PA)
   c. Tenecteplase (TNK-tPA)
   d. Anistreplase (APSAC)
6. Antiplatelet and antithrombotic combination therapy
   a. Aspirin: Diminishes platelet aggregation and has been shown to reduce mortality rates.
   b. Adenosine diphosphate (AD) antagonist (e.g., clopidogrel, ticlopidine): Used for clients unable to take aspirin.
   c. Heparin: Unfractionated heparin (UFH) to prevent conversion of fibrinogen to fibrin; to inactivate thrombin.
   d. Low-molecular-weight heparin (LMWH) to prevent conversion of fibrinogen to fibrin; to inactive thrombin.
   e. Glycoprotein IIb/IIIa blockers and receptor inhibitors (e.g., eptifibatide, tirofiban, abciximab): Treats non-STEMI elevation; prevents platelet aggregation.
7. Calcium channel blocking agents: Prevent and treat vasospasms, which can occur after invasive procedures; may be used if client does not tolerate beta blocker therapy.
8. Angiotensin-converting enzyme inhibitors (ACE-I): Prevent ventricular remodeling (dilation) and preserve ejection fraction.

Coronary Artery Disease

I. Definition: Coronary artery disease (CAD) is a progressive narrowing of one or more of the coronary arteries by atherosclerosis. Atherosclerotic lesions are composed of lipid, cholesterol, calcium, and other blood components form a plaque within the inner lining of the artery and decrease the blood and oxygen supply to the myocardium.

A. Angina is chest pain or discomfort caused by myocardial ischemia. CAD and coronary artery spasm are the major causes of angina.
   1. Stable angina pectoris occurs with exertion, is relieved by rest, and does not increase in frequency or severity.
   2. Variant or Prinzmetal angina is caused by coronary artery spasm.
   3. Silent angina or silent ischemia is asymptomatic myocardial ischemia associated with diabetes mellitus and hypertension.
   4. Unstable angina is classified as an ACS.

B. Collateral circulation can develop over time in response to narrowed coronary arteries. Small branches of the artery form alternate routes of blood flow. The collaterals may not be able to supply enough blood and oxygen to the myocardium, especially during increased exertion.

II. Nursing process

A. Assessment
   1. Assess client for angina: Pain, including quality, level, location, radiation to other locations, and length of time—cardinal symptom of angina is substernal chest pain or discomfort. Pain may radiate to the neck, jaw, back, left shoulder, arms, hands, and may be described as pressure, aching, burning, constrictive, crushing, squeezing, suffocating, tightness, or indigestion.
   2. Assess precipitating factors that trigger angina, including physical exertion, hot or cold temperatures, emotion, heavy meal consumption, smoking, sexual activity, and stimulants (caffeine, cocaine, amphetamines).
   3. Assess for associated symptoms such as palpitations, dyspnea, diaphoresis, fatigue, and nausea and vomiting.
   4. Obtain a detailed health history, including allergies, prior hospitalizations, psychosocial history, and family medical history.
   5. Obtain a comprehensive physical assessment.
      a. Assess vital signs and SpO_2.
      b. Assess fluid status: Intake and output, weight trend, and signs of edema.
   6. Assess risk factors for CAD.
      a. Unmodifiable risk factors: Age, gender, and heredity—risk increased in men over 45 years of age; women over 55 years of age, and clients with a family history of heart disease.

b. Modifiable risk factors: Smoking, diabetes, hypertension, elevated lipid levels, obesity, physical inactivity, and stressful lifestyle.
c. Contributing risk factors: Elevated plasma homocysteine levels and C-reactive protein (CRP), metabolic syndrome, and menopause.

7. Obtain diagnostic tests.
   a. Chest x-ray
   b. 12-lead ECG—compare with earlier tracing
   c. Serum electrolytes, fasting blood glucose, BUN, creatinine, CBC, fasting lipid profile (cholesterol, HDL, LDL, triglycerides), CRP, homocysteine, PT/INR, PTT
   d. Exercise ECG stress test
   e. Pharmacologic stress test if unable to physically exercise
   f. Exercise stress echocardiogram or dobutamine stress echocardiography
   g. Adenosine or dipyridamole myocardial perfusion imaging
   h. Coronary magnetic resonance angiography
   i. Positron emission tomography
   j. Electron beam computerized tomography
   k. Holter or event monitor for dysrhythmia assessment
8. Prepare client for cardiac catheterization and arteriography, if needed.

B. Analysis
   1. Ineffective Tissue Perfusion: Myocardial, related to atherosclerosis
   2. Acute Pain: Chest, related to impaired myocardial perfusion, oxygen demand greater than supply, presence of precipitating factors (increased activity, temperature extreme, emotion, stress, smoking, stimulant)
   3. Risk for Decreased Cardiac Output related to impaired myocardial perfusion
   4. Anxiety related to chest pain, lifestyle change, ineffective coping, and fear
   5. Activity Intolerance related to decreased perfusion, tissue hypoxia, fatigue, chest pain
   6. Ineffective Health Maintenance related to lack of knowledge of CAD, risk factors, and unhealthy lifestyle
   7. Ineffective Therapeutic Regimen Management related to lack of knowledge of medications and self care behaviors

C. Planning (see planning for ACS)

D. Implementation
   1. Provide interventions for chronic, stable angina (see pharmacologic and parenteral therapies): Medications that may be used in the treatment of CAD and angina include:
      a. Nitrates
      b. Antiplatelet therapy
      c. Beta blocker
      d. Calcium channel blocker
      e. Angiotensin converting enzyme inhibitor (ACE inhibitor)
      f. Lipid-lowering agents
   2. Provide client teaching regarding medications and side effects, diet ways to manage modifiable risk factors, and how to promote a healthy lifestyle.

E. Evaluation
   1. Client's vital signs are within normal limits and client exhibits normal sinus rhythm or controlled ventricular rate with chronic atrial fibrillation.
   2. Client affirms absence of angina and associated symptoms.
   3. Client's functional capability is optimized through tailored interventions based on individualized assessments and needs.
   4. Client exhibits tolerance to increasing levels of activity and exercise.
   5. Client verbalizes risk factors for CAD, factors contributing to anginal symptoms, and the procedure to follow to manage acute chest pain in the home setting.
   6. Client states the purpose, dosage, timing, and side effects of the medications prescribed for the treatment of angina and CAD.
   7. Client exhibits control of lipids, indicated by cholesterol less than 200 mg/dl, LDL less than 130 mg/dl, HDL more than 40 mg/dl, and triglycerides less than 150 mg/dl.
   8. Client exhibits control of BP, with reading of less than 140/90 and less than 130/80 with diabetes and chronic kidney disease.
   9. Client demonstrates control of diabetes.

CN

III. Client needs

A. Physiologic adaptation: Stable angina is controlled with medication and dose adjustments on an outpatient basis.
   1. Evaluate the effectiveness of nitrates, beta blocker, and/or calcium channel blocker to improve coronary artery perfusion, restore the balance between oxygen demand and supply, and decrease myocardial workload and oxygen demand.
   2. Assess client's cardiac tolerance to increasing levels of activity and exercise.

3. Recognize risk for decrease in cardiac output: Decreased mental alertness—indicated by hypotension (systolic BP reading less than 90 mmHg); tachycardia; presence of heart murmur, S3, S4; lung crackles; urine output less than 0.5 ml/kg per hour; decreased peripheral pulses; cool, pale, cyanotic, or diaphoretic skin; edema; and jugular venous distention.
4. Evaluate troponin, CK-MB, and myoglobin with uncontrolled, acute chest pain. Cardiac markers are diagnostic criteria for an acute MI (see Acute Coronary Syndrome); cardiac markers are not elevated with stable angina.

B. Management of care: Care of the client with CAD requires critical thinking skills and knowledge of assessment, and teaching and evaluation methods unique to the RN role. These skills cannot be delegated to an LPN or UAP.
1. Delegate responsibly those activities that can be delegated, including basic care needs and assessment of vital signs for the stable client. All monitoring information is reported to the RN.
2. Perform comprehensive physical assessments and provide care to the client with acute angina and symptoms.
3. Provide information on changes in client status to the physician and appropriate members of the multidisciplinary team.
4. Provide interventions for a hospitalized client with acute chest pain. (See ACS for UA and unresolved chest pain.)
5. Prepare client for cardiac catheterization on positive findings from diagnostic stress testing.
   a. Provide precardiac catheterization interventions.
      (1) Assess for allergies to radiopaque dye, iodine, or shellfish.
      (2) Verify that physician obtains written and informed consent.
      (3) Maintain NPO status for 6 to 8 hr prior to procedure.
      (4) Provide adequate hydration.
         (a) IV insertion with fluids as ordered
         (b) Clear liquids up to 4 hr before procedure may be allowed
      (5) Use *N*-acetylcysteine (Mucomyst) prior to and after cardiac catheterization in clients at risk for contrast nephropathy.
      (6) Assess baseline vital signs, SpO_2, and peripheral pulses.
      (7) Describe the pre- and postprocedure routine to the client.
      (8) Explain to client that he or she will be awake and may experience a flushing sensation as dye is injected or a fluttering feeling as the catheter passes through the heart.
   b. Provide postprocedure interventions.
      (1) Maintain strict bed rest for 4 to 6 hr with head of bed elevated 15 degrees, keeping affected extremity straight.
      (2) Provide continuous ECG monitoring.
      (3) Monitor vital signs and SpO_2 per agency protocol.
      (4) Assess peripheral pulses, color, sensation, temperature of extremity, signs of bleeding or hematoma at insertion site with vital signs.
      (5) Maintain pressure dressing at insertion site.
      (6) Maintain IV, encourage oral fluids, and monitor intake and output.
      (7) Report to physician presence of chest pain, dysrhythmias, bleeding, hematoma, and significant changes in vital signs or peripheral pulses.
6. Facilitate outpatient follow-up care.
7. Assess for home health care needs for additional instruction and follow-up with medications, monitoring of PTT and INR, and activity levels.
8. Evaluate community resources for continued cardiac education, support groups, smoking cessation, exercise, and rehabilitation.

C. Safety and infection control
1. Provide teaching about correct administration of medications and associated side effects (see pharmacologic and parenteral therapies).
2. Promote low-fat diet (low-sodium, calorie-reduction, and diabetic diet, if prescribed).
3. Promote gradual increase in exercise as indicated by client ability; this includes walking at a moderate pace at 3 to 5 times per week for 30 to 60 min. Teach client to always exercise with a friend, avoid temperature extremes, designate a place to rest, and to observe warning signals to stop activity and rest (e.g., chest pain, shortness of breath, dizziness, faintness, weakness, or unusual fatigue).
4. Promote self-care behaviors to manage symptoms in home setting.

a. Perform daily monitoring of weight, BP, pulse, edema, or blood sugar, if indicated; assess BP and heart rate if taking a beta blocker, calcium channel blocker, ACE inhibitor, or nitrates.
b. Manage acute chest pain and use of sublingual nitroglycerin: Stop activity; sit or lie down with head elevated; if chest pain does not subside, take one nitroglycerin tablet: Place tablet under tongue or in buccal pouch and allow it to dissolve thoroughly (translingual spray on or under tongue).
(1) If chest pain continues, repeat nitroglycerin every 5 min for a total of three doses. Obtain emergency medical assistance if pain persists after three doses of nitroglycerin over a 15-min period.
(2) Store tablets in a dark glass container away from heat and moisture; replace tablets every 6 months.
(3) Observe common side effects such as mild headache, dizziness, and flushing.

D. Health promotion and maintenance
1. Assist client in identifying personalized risk factors for CAD.
2. Provide teaching on health behaviors that promote a healthy lifestyle, including smoking cessation and avoidance of secondary smoke, maintenance of ideal weight, regular physical exercise, stress management, and reduction or elimination of alcohol intake.
3. Provide client teaching about monitoring self-care behaviors in home setting (see safety and infection control).

E. Psychologic integrity
1. Assist client and family in coping with lifestyle changes.
2. Identify stress factors and anxiety that may interfere with recovery.
3. Introduce counseling and support groups to assist the client with smoking cessation, along with medication management with nicotine replacement or bupropion.
4. Identify gender differences in symptoms of angina: Women may present with fatigue, shortness of breath, indigestion, nausea, and jaw pain.
5. Determine estrogen replacement during menopause, with the physician.
6. Recognize that the older adult may have atypical symptoms of CAD and medications may not be as well tolerated.

F. Basic care and comfort: Provide a quiet, calm environment.

G. Reduction of risk potential
1. Instruct client to notify nurse if experiencing angina symptoms.
2. Assist client in identifying activities that precipitate angina.
3. Instruct client on premedication with nitroglycerin for exercise activity or sexual activity, according to physician guidelines.
4. Consider vitamin B_6, B_{12}, and folic acid for elevated homocysteine levels.

H. Pharmacologic and parenteral therapies: Client will state the purpose, dosage, timing, and side effects of medications for the treatment of chronic, stable angina.
1. Nitrates: For long-term management of angina pectoris. Side effects include headache, flushing, postural hypotension, and tachycardia.
a. Transdermal controlled-release nitrate patch
b. Nitroglycerin ointment
c. Long-acting oral nitrates
(1) Isosorbide dinitrate (Isordil)
(2) Isosorbide mononitrate (Imdur)
2. Antiplatelet therapy: Inhibit platelet aggregation and clotting. Side effects include prolonged bleeding time and bruising.
a. Aspirin 81, 325 mg PO daily
b. Ticlopidine (Ticlid) or clopidogrel (Plavix), if aspirin is contraindicated
3. Lipid-lowering drugs for clients with hyperlipidemia
a. HMG-CoA reductase inhibitors (statins): Atorvastatin (Lipitor), rosuvastatin (Crestor), simvastatin, (Zocor)
(1) Decreases total cholesterol and LDL
(2) Side effects include GI disturbance, headache, myalgia, rash, liver toxicity, and myopathy (skeletal muscle weakness, wasting, histologic changes)
(3) Check baseline and periodic liver function tests (LFTs) and creatine phosphokinase (CK); instruct client to report muscle pain or weakness
b. Fibric acid derivatives (fibrates): Gemfibrozil (Lopid), fenofibrate (TriCor)
(1) Decreases triglycerides and increases HDL
(2) Side effects include GI disturbance, vertigo, fatigue, rash, gallstones, myalgia, myopathy, and liver dysfunction
(3) Check LFTs; myopathy increases with use of statins; instruct client

to report any muscle pain or weakness

c. Nicotinic acid (niacin)
   (1) Causes beneficial effect on all lipid indices.
   (2) Side effects include flushing, itching, GI distress, liver toxicity, increased uric acid, and glucose intolerance.
   (3) Pretreat with ASA 325 mg 30 min before niacin to minimize flushing; give with meals. Use cautiously in clients with gout, diabetes, and peptic ulcer. Perform baseline and periodic assessment of LFTs and blood sugar; uric acid levels with a history of gout.

d. Bile acid sequestrants (resins): Colesevelam (WelChol), cholestyramine (Questran), colestipol (Colestid)
   (1) Decreases total cholesterol and LDL.
   (2) Side effects include GI symptoms of constipation, abdominal pain, heartburn, flatulence, and nausea; as well as decreased absorption of other medications.
   (3) Separate time of administration from other medications. For constipation, increase fluid and dietary fiber intake, consider a bulk laxative or stool softener.

e. Intestinal cholesterol absorption inhibitors: Zetia
   (1) Decreases total cholesterol and LDL.
   (2) Side effects include abdominal pain, fatigue, diarrhea, sinusitis, arthralgia, and greater incidence of liver toxicity when used with statins.
   (3) Check LFTs.

4. Beta blockers, ACE inhibitors, and calcium channel blockers (see Table 20-3: Medications for treatment of chronic hypertension).

Heart Failure and Cardiomyopathy

I. Definition: Heart failure and cardiomyopathy are general terms indicating the failing ability of the heart to pump oxygenated blood to meet metabolic demands of the body.

A. Heart failure (HF), formerly called *congestive HF,* is a clinical syndrome that results from any structural or functional cardiac disorder impairing the ability of the ventricle to eject blood (systolic dysfunction) or fill with blood (diastolic dysfunction). The heart is unable to maintain an adequate cardiac output to meet the metabolic needs of the body.

1. Effective cardiac output is determined by heart rate and the three components of stroke volume:
   a. Preload—degree of myocardial stretch produced by the pressure exerted from the volume of blood in the ventricle, which is influenced by venous return to the heart and ventricular compliance
   b. Afterload—resistance the ventricle has to pump against to eject blood, which is influenced by arterial vasodilation or vasoconstriction
   c. Contractility—contractile force generated by the myocardium
2. Clinically, HF is described as "right-sided" or "left-sided."
   a. Left-sided failure involves congestion in the lungs from blood backing up into the pulmonary veins, causing shortness of breath and dyspnea, which can progress to pulmonary edema.
   b. Right-sided failure involves blood backing up into the veins and capillaries. The client experiences ankle edema and congestion in the abdominal cavity and liver.
3. HF is also described as high-output and low-output.
   a. High-output failure involves more demand for oxygenated blood than the failing heart can provide; its causes include anemia and hyperthyroidism.
   b. Low-output failure occurs as a result of ischemic heart disease, hypertension, and cardiac myopathy.

B. Cardiomyopathy is a disease that affects myocardial structure and impairs cardiac function. There are three types of cardiomyopathy.

1. Dilated cardiomyopathy—dilated ventricles with destruction of myocardial fibers limiting contractility and causing systolic dysfunction
2. Hypertrophic cardiomyopathy—myocardial thickening of the ventricular wall and septum causing a rigid ventricle and diastolic dysfunction
3. Restrictive cardiomyopathy—ventricles become rigid with fibrotic tissue, causing diastolic dysfunction

II. Nursing process

A. Assessment

1. Obtain detailed health history, including allergies, prior hospitalizations, family medical history, and psychosocial history.

2. Perform comprehensive physical assessment.
   a. Assess vital signs and SpO_2.
   b. Assess fluid status—intake and output, daily weight trend, signs of pulmonary crackles or peripheral edema.
   c. Assess ability to perform routine and desired activities of daily living.
   d. Ask client, "How many pillows do you use to sleep at night?"
3. Assess symptom severity as determined by New York Heart Association—functional class (I–IV).
4. Assess HF stage in development and progression (A, B, C, or D).
   a. Stage A and B indicate client at risk for HF.
   b. Stage C and D indicate HF.
5. Assess for cardinal symptoms of HF, including dyspnea, fatigue, exercise intolerance, and fluid retention, which leads to pulmonary congestion and peripheral edema.
6. Assess for signs and symptoms of left-sided HF.
   a. Dyspnea, crackles, orthopnea, paroxysmal nocturnal dyspnea, cough, decreased oxygen saturation, signs of hypoxia
   b. Fatigue
   c. Tachycardiad. Restlessness, mental confusion, decreased memory
   d. S3 heart sound
   e. Weight gain
7. Assess for signs and symptoms of right-sided HF.
   a. Dependent, peripheral edema; check feet, legs, sacrum
   b. Jugular venous distention
   c. Positive hepatojugular reflex
   d. Hepatomegaly and splenomegaly
   e. Ascites
   f. Abdominal discomfort, anorexia, nausea
   g. Fatigue
   h. Weight gain
8. Assess for signs and symptoms of biventricular failure, indicated by signs and symptoms of both right- and left-sided HF.
9. Assess presence of risk factors for HF.
   a. Atherosclerosis/CAD
   b. Hypertension
   c. Valvular heart disease
   d. Cardiomyopathy
   e. Cardiotoxic drugs: Excessive alcohol intake, cocaine, chemotherapy
   f. Diabetes mellitus
   g. Thyroid disorder
   h. Smoking
   i. Obesity
   j. Hyperlipidemia
10. Obtain diagnostic tests.
   a. Chest x-ray
   b. 12-lead ECG
   c. Serum electrolytes (including calcium and magnesium), fasting blood glucose, hemoglobin A_1c, BUN, creatinine, CBC, urinalysis, fasting lipid profile (cholesterol, HDL, LDL, triglycerides), liver function tests, thyroid-stimulating hormone, B-type natriuretic peptide (BNP), arterial blood gas
   d. Echocardiogram with Doppler to assess left ventricular size, wall thickness, ejection fraction, and valvular function
   e. Exercise stress testing or cardiac catheterization/coronary angiography may be performed to evaluate if CAD is contributing to HF
   f. Nuclear ventriculography or multiple gated acquisition (MUGA) scan

B. Analysis
   1. Decreased Cardiac Output related to systolic and/or diastolic dysfunction
   2. Impaired Gas Exchange related to fluid volume excess, pulmonary congestion
   3. Dyspnea related to impaired gas exchange, impaired cardiac output
   4. Ineffective Tissue Perfusion: Peripheral, related to decreased cardiac output
   5. Fatigue related to decreased cardiac output, imbalance between oxygen supply and demand
   6. Activity Intolerance related to decreased cardiac output, imbalance between oxygen supply and demand
   7. Excess Fluid Volume related to impaired cardiac output, decreased renal perfusion
   8. Ineffective Health Maintenance related to lack of knowledge of HF, risk factors, and unhealthy lifestyle
   9. Ineffective Therapeutic Regimen Management related to lack of knowledge of medications, diet, and self-care behaviors to monitor at home
   10. Anxiety related to dyspnea, activity intolerance, poor prognosis, decreased quality of life
   11. Hopelessness related to poor prognosis, decreased role performance, and quality of life

C. Planning
   1. Control or eliminate precipitating cause of HF or acute exacerbation.
   2. Maintain hemodynamic stability and normovolemia.

3. Optimize cardiac function and improve cardiac output.
4. Improve client symptoms and comfort.
5. Reduce anxiety and feeling of hopelessness.
6. Enhance functional capacity and quality of life.
7. Promote adherence to the therapeutic regimen.
8. Reduce hospitalizations.

D. Implementation (see management of care)

E. Evaluation
1. Client's vital signs, SpO_2, and urine output are within targeted range.
2. Client experiences normal sinus rhythm or controlled ventricular rate with supraventricular tachydysrhythmias such as atrial fibrillation.
3. Client affirms improvement or absence of symptoms.
4. Client exhibits absence of pulmonary crackles and peripheral edema.
5. Client exhibits tolerance to increasing levels of activity.
6. Client follows a low-sodium diet.
7. Client's laboratory values are within normal range.
8. Client states the purpose, dosage, timing, and side effects of medications.
9. Client's functional capability is optimized through tailored interventions and self-care behaviors based on individualized assessments and needs.

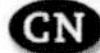

III. Client needs

A. Physiologic adaptation: When the client hospitalized for acute decompensated HF has stabilized, an oral regimen of medications is started to maintain improved symptoms and reduce subsequent risk of decompensation and hospitalization.
1. Administer on weekly to biweekly period during outpatient care: Gradual upward titration of ACE inhibitors (or alternatives), beta blockers, and diuretics to optimum, tolerated doses for the treatment of chronic HF.
2. Assess for resolving symptoms of HF, signs of improved cardiac output, fluid weight loss, and tolerance to increasing levels of activity.

B. Management of care: Care of the client experiencing HF and hemodynamic instability requires critical thinking skills and knowledge of assessment, and teaching and evaluation methods unique to the RN role. These skills cannot be delegated to an LPN or UAP.
1. Delegate responsibly those activities that can be delegated, including basic care needs, measuring and recording of vital signs, daily weights, and intake and output for the stable client. All monitoring information is reported to the RN.
2. Provide interventions to manage acute decompensated HF.
   a. Perform comprehensive physical assessments and provide care to the client with acute HF and hemodynamic instability.
   b. Optimize cardiac output by decreasing preload and afterload, increasing contractility, and attaining normovolemia.
   c. Place client on bed rest, and adjust client into semi- to high Fowler position, as tolerated.
   d. Provide continuous ECG and pulse oximetry monitoring.
   e. Auscultate heart and lung sounds frequently.
   f. Measure systolic BP: 90 mmHg or more and 140 mmHg or less.
   g. Administer medications used for acute exacerbation of HF (see pharmacologic and parenteral therapies).
   h. Administer titrate oxygen to maintain SpO_2 in targeted range: Oxygen, 2 to 6 L via nasal cannula or 40% to 100% via face mask.
      (1) Endotracheal intubation with mechanical ventilation may be required for pulmonary edema or severe hypoxia and hypercapnia.
      (2) Monitor arterial blood gas to evaluate outcome of oxygen administration.
   i. Assess labs and monitor electrolytes closely.
   j. Maintain arterial line for clients on potent vasoactive medications.
   k. Use pulmonary artery catheter to obtain a more comprehensive hemodynamic profile in critically ill clients with refractory HF to guide pharmacologic therapy.
   l. Use bioimpedance cardiography as a noninvasive procedure for obtaining hemodynamics.
   m. Use intra-aortic balloon pump and ventricular assist device for refractory HF unresponsive to pharmacologic therapy.
3. Provide interventions to manage chronic HF.
   a. Administer medications used for chronic, systolic HF (see pharmacologic and parenteral therapies).

b. Monitor hemodynamic changes for improvement of cardiac output and reduction of fluid volume excess. Provide information on changes in client status to physician and appropriate members of the multidisciplinary team.
   (1) Vital signs in targeted range
   (2) Skin pink and warm without pallor; peripheral pulses palpable; apical pulse equal to peripheral pulse
   (3) Resolved or controlled dysrhythmias, normal heart sounds (S_1,S_2)
   (4) Urine output 30 ml/hr or more, based on intake and fluid volume, and weight status
   (5) Improvement in symptoms, mental alertness, and activity tolerance
   (6) Absence of adventitious lung sounds
   (7) SpO_2 in targeted range
   (8) Absence of dependent, pitting peripheral edema
   (9) Daily weights decrease, and then stabilize at targeted dry weight
   (10) Intake equal to or more than output
c. Provide, along with dietician, instruction and reinforcement on a 2-g sodium, healthy heart diet—fluid restriction may be ordered.
d. Provide teaching to the client and family on medications, activity, and self-care behaviors for monitoring at home.
e. Facilitate and reinforce the need for outpatient follow-up care.

4. Discuss treatment options for clients with HF and cardiomyopathy.
   a. Coronary artery revascularization with PTCA or CABG surgery—performed in appropriate clients to improve coronary circulation and cardiac hemodynamics.
   b. Valve replacement or repair surgery—considered for severe mitral or aortic valve stenosis or regurgitation.
   c. Implantable cardioverter defibrillator (ICD)—considered for clients with history of cardiac arrest and at risk for sudden cardiac death from recurrent sustained ventricular tachycardia or ventricular fibrillation.
   d. Cardiac resynchronization therapy—biventricular pacing to provide simultaneous stimulation of the right and left ventricles; restores a synchronous ventricular contraction for improved cardiac function and symptoms in select clients with QRS more than 0.12.
   e. Cardiac-assist device or cardiac transplant—considered in select clients refractory to medical treatment in end-stage HF or dilated cardiomyopathy.
   f. Ventricular septal myotomy/myectomy or septal ablation—considered in clients with obstructive hypertrophic cardiomyopathy.

C. Safety and infection control: Provide client teaching.
   1. Assess heart rate: If client is taking a beta blocker or digoxin—hold medication and contact HCP for further instructions if pulse is less than 60 beats per minute (in select clients, heart rate to 50 beats per minute may be tolerated if the client is asymptomatic).
   2. Assess BP: If client is on an ACE inhibitor or beta blocker—hold medication and contact HCP for further instructions if systolic BP is less than 90 mmHg (in select clients, systolic BP of 85 may be tolerated if client is asymptomatic).
   3. Provide client teaching about gradual increase of exercise activity, and safety precautions (e.g., always exercise with a friend; designate a place to rest; communicate warning signals to stop activity to rest on experience of chest pain, shortness of breath, dizziness, faintness, weakness, or unusual fatigue; avoid temperature extremes).

D. Health promotion and maintenance
   1. Instruct individually tailored, mild-to-moderate exercise such as walking—based on tolerance and capability, walking at a moderate pace at 3 to 5 times per week for 30 to 45 min.
   2. Promote 2-g sodium, healthy heart diet (fluid restriction, calorie reduction, and diabetic diet, if prescribed); reduce or eliminate alcohol; maintain ideal weight; maintain adequate nutritional intake to avoid risk for cardiac cachexia and protein calorie malnutrition.
   3. Promote self-monitoring for signs of fluid volume excess and associated symptoms—monitor daily weight record and assess for edema; self-monitoring of pulse and BP; instruct client about signs and symptoms that require medical attention.
      a. Weight increase of 2 to 3 lb over 1 to 2 days
      b. Symptoms of impending exacerbation: Increased dyspnea, paroxysmal

nocturnal dyspnea, orthopnea, lower extremity edema, increased abdominal girth, early satiety, nausea or vomiting after meals

c. Holding a medication for low pulse or BP

4. Assess for home health care needs and community resources for continued cardiac education, support groups, smoking cessation, and cardiac rehabilitation.

E. Psychologic integrity: HF is the leading cause of hospitalization for clients 65 years of age and older. Hypertrophic cardiomyopathy is a genetic disorder that is a cause of sudden death in young athletes.
   1. Monitor closely the response to ACE inhibitors in African American clients as they may be less effective; addition of isosorbide dinitrate and hydralazine to the standard HF regimen may be more efficacious.
   2. Observe higher incidence of cough in Asian clients treated with an ACE inhibitor
   3. Assist client and family in coping with lifestyle changes.
   4. Distinguish for client and family short-term interventions for acute exacerbations versus prolonged life support in end-stage HF without expected return to good functional capacity.
   5. Instruct client and family about treatment options, living will, and advance directive to determine preferences while the client is able to participate in decisions with end-of-life care.

F. Basic care and comfort
   1. During acute phase: Encourage rest to reduce workload of the heart and organize activities around periods of rest; provide a calm and quiet environment.
   2. During end-of-life management: Assess and manage symptoms to maintain client comfort. Assess and arrange for home health, hospice, or palliative care needs.

G. Reduction of risk potential
   1. Observe medication contraindications and precautions: Positive inotropic drugs are contraindicated in the treatment of hypertrophic cardiomyopathy. Calcium channel blockers are not routinely used in the treatment of HF.
   2. Promote early identification of clients at risk for development of HF (Stage A and B) with periodic evaluation for signs and symptoms of HF.
   3. Manage risk factors leading to the development of HF, including hypertension, diabetes, metabolic syndrome, and atherosclerotic disease; counsel client to avoid behaviors that increase risk of HF (smoking, excessive alcohol consumption, illicit drug use).
   4. Identify factors leading to hospitalization, including sodium retention, noncompliance with medications and diet, dysrhythmias, inadequate or inappropriate drug therapy, pulmonary infections, emotional stress, and thyrotoxicosis.
   5. Monitor clients for electrolyte imbalances and anemia.

H. Pharmacologic and parenteral therapies: Client and family will state the purpose, dosage, timing, and side effects of all medications. See Table 20-1 for medications used for acute exacerbation of HF. Medications used for treatment of chronic, systolic HF follow (see also Table 20-3).
   1. Diuretics (loop diuretics are usually required)
      a. Decrease preload, pulmonary congestion, and peripheral edema
      b. Improve heart failure symptoms
   2. ACE inhibitors
      a. Decrease afterload and BP
      b. Inhibit adverse effects of the rennin-angiotensin-aldosterone system
      c. Reduce mortality, hospitalization, and cardiac remodeling process
      d. Improve HF symptoms, survival, and overall sense of well-being
   3. Alternatives for ACE inhibitors
      a. Angiotensin II receptor blockers (ARBs)—decrease left ventricular afterload and decreases heart rate
      b. Hydralazine (Apresoline) and isosorbide dinitrate (Isordil) combination—hydralazine decreases afterload and Isordil decreases preload
   4. Beta blockers and alpha-beta blockers: Metoprolol (Toprol-XL), bisoprolol (Zebeta), or carvedilol (Coreg)—initiate at low dose, gradual upward weekly titration as tolerated to target dose. Adjustment period may require 2 to 3 months and client may feel worse with decreased exercise tolerance before improving.
      a. Decrease heart rate, contractility, afterload, and BP
      b. Inhibit adverse effects of sympathetic nervous system in HF
      c. Reduce risk of death, symptoms of HF, and risk of MI with long-term use
   5. Aldosterone antagonists (aldosterone receptor blockers)

Table 20-1 Medications for Treatment of Acute Exacerbation, Refractory, or End-Stage Heart Failure (HF)

Classification	Generic/ Trade Name	Expected Outcomes	Reduction of Risk Potential	Management of Care
B-type Natriuretic Peptide	Nesiritide (Natrecor)	Balances venous and arterial dilation with preload and afterload reduction; Natriuresis—sodium and water diuresis.	Contraindicated in systolic BP <90. Monitor for hypotension, angina, dysrhythmias.	Promote IV infusion, short-term treatment. Closely monitor BP and ECG.
Beta-Adrenergic Agonist Inotropic Agent	Dobutamine (Dobutrex); dopamine (Intropin)	Increases contractility; dobutamine also causes mild afterload reduction; dopamine at 1–2 mcg/kg/min increases urine output; dopamine at 3–10 mcg/kg/min causes beta-1 stimulation with increased contractility to improve CO and symptoms; dopamine at >10 mcg/kg/min stimulates alpha receptors, causing arterial and venous vasoconstriction.	Monitor for dysrhythmias, tachycardia, BP changes, and symptoms due to increased myocardial oxygen demand.	Promote IV infusions; monitor ECG; assess need for continuous home infusions for palliation of symptoms and patient comfort with end-stage HF; administer dopamine at 3–10 mcg/kg/min for client with low systolic BP and intolerant to dobutamine in HF.
Calcium Sensitizer Inotropic Drug	Levosimendan (Simdax)	Increases contractility and CO without increased oxygen demand; reduces preload and afterload; improves coronary blood flow.	Monitor for hypotension and headache.	Promote IV infusion: Used for short-term treatment; monitor BP and for improvement of symptoms.
Phosphodiesterase Inhibitor Inotropic Agent	Milrinone (Primacor)	Increases contractility and decreases afterload.	Monitor for tachycardia, ventricular dysrhythmias, thrombocytopenia, and symptoms of increased myocardial oxygen demand.	Promote IV infusion with loading dose; assess need for continuous home infusions for palliation of symptoms and client comfort for end-stage HF.
Peripheral Vasodilator	Nitroglycerin (Tridil); sodium nitroprusside (Nipride)	Decreases preload and afterload: Greater preload reduction with NTG; greater afterload reduction with Nipride.	Monitor for hypotension, dysrhythmias, headache, cyanide toxicity with Nipride.	Promote IV infusions; monitor BP; administer Nipride through arterial line; maintain bed rest.

a. Inhibit fibrosis and cardiac remodeling effects of aldosterone.

b. Reduce mortality and hospitalization.

6. Cardiac glycoside: Digoxin (Lanoxin)—check digoxin level with signs of toxicity; digoxin immune fab is antidote. Assess apical pulse and K^+ prior to administration.

a. Increases contractility, decrease heart rate.

b. Hypokalemia potentiates digoxin toxicity.

c. Side effects include bradycardia, heart blocks, nausea and vomiting, and visual disturbances.

Table 20-2 Classification of Blood Pressure in Adults

Blood Pressure Classification	Systolic BP (mmHg)	Diastolic BP (mmHg)
Normal	<120	And <80
Prehypertension	120–139	Or ≥80–89
Stage 1 Hypertension	140–159	Or ≥90–99
Stage 2 Hypertension	≥160	≥100

From the U.S. Department of Health and Human Services (2004). The seventh report of the Joint National Committee on Prevention, Detection, Evaluation, and Treatment of High Blood Pressure. Available at http://www.nhlbi.nih.gov/guidelines/hypertension/jnc7full.pdf.

Hypertension

I. Definition: Hypertension is a sustained elevation of BP and is defined in adult clients as a systolic BP 140 or more, or diastolic BP 90 or more (Table 20-2). Hypertension is a major risk factor for coronary artery, cerebral, renal, and peripheral disease from the damaging effects on blood vessels. Diagnosis is based on the presence of elevated readings on at least three occasions over several weeks. There are three classifications of hypertension:
   A. Primary hypertension—involves elevated BP from an unknown cause.
   B. Secondary hypertension—develops as a consequence of another condition (see assessment for causes of secondary hypertension).
   C. Hypertensive crisis (malignant hypertension)—involves severe, abrupt increase in BP, and is an acute, life-threatening event requiring emergency treatment to prevent or decrease risk of organ damage.

II. Nursing process
   A. Assessment
      1. Assess for risk factors, including age between 30 and 50 years, smoking, obesity, hyperlipidemia, physical inactivity, family history, diabetes mellitus, and African American descent.
      2. Assess for causes of secondary hypertension.
         a. Chronic kidney disease
         b. Renal artery stenosis
         c. Primary aldosteronism
         d. Chronic steroid therapy and Cushing syndrome
         e. Pheochromocytoma
         f. Coarctation of the aorta
         g. Thyroid or parathyroid disease
         h. Sleep apnea
         i. Drug-induced
      3. Obtain a comprehensive health history and perform a detailed physical assessment to determine the underlying cause and detect complications of hypertension.
         a. Assess vital signs and measure BP with verification in the contralateral arm.
         b. Examine heart, lung, and lower extremities for pulses and edema.
         c. Auscultate for carotid, abdominal, and femoral bruits.
         d. Examine abdomen for abnormal aortic pulsation, masses, and enlarged kidneys.
         e. Perform neurologic assessment and retinal examination.
         f. Palpate thyroid gland.
         g. Measure weight and calculate BMI.
      4. Assess for presence of symptoms: Client may be asymptomatic, but signs and symptoms may include fatigue, palpitation, angina, dyspnea, dizziness, headache, visual disturbance, and weight gain.
      5. Obtain diagnostic tests.
         a. Serum electrolytes, BUN, creatinine, creatinine clearance, blood glucose, CBC, fasting lipid profile, urinalysis
         b. ECG
         c. Echocardiogram
         d. Ambulatory BP monitoring
   B. Analysis
      1. Ineffective Tissue Perfusion: Peripheral, related to increased SVR or decreased cardiac output
      2. Ineffective Health Maintenance related to lack of knowledge of disorder and treatment
      3. Anxiety related to lifestyle changes and possible complications
      4. Ineffective Therapeutic Regimen Management related to lack of knowledge and side effects of medications
   C. Planning
      1. Reduce and control BP at normal range.
      2. Reduce or prevent organ damage.
      3. Provide client and family teaching.
      4. Promote adherence to the therapeutic regimen.
   D. Implementation
      1. Monitor vital signs and laboratory results.
      2. Provide client teaching regarding hypertension, risk factors, BP goal, medications, and associated side effects, diet, management of modifiable risk factors, and self-care behaviors to monitor at home.
   E. Evaluation
      1. Client's BP is controlled at less than 140/90; client with diabetes and chronic

kidney disease maintains BP at less than 130/80.
2. Client describes risk factors contributing to hypertension.
3. Client states the purpose, dosage, timing, and side effects of medications.
4. Client exhibits minimal or no side effects from medications.
5. Client adheres to the therapeutic regimen.

CN

III. Client needs

A. Physiologic adaptation: Hypertension is controlled with medication and dose adjustments on an outpatient basis. Hypertensive crisis requires administration of IV antihypertensive agents and frequent or continuous monitoring of BP with an arterial line in the critical care setting: Oral agents are started with downward titration of IV medications to transition toward long-term oral antihypertensive therapy.
  1. Evaluate the effectiveness of medications in decreasing and controlling BP less than 140/90 without adverse side effects.
  2. Recognize risk for target organ damage—indicated by neurologic dysfunction, cardiovascular complications, HF, retinal damage, or renal insufficiency.

B. Management of care: Care of the client experiencing hypertension requires critical thinking skills and knowledge of assessment, and teaching and evaluation methods unique to the RN role. These skills cannot be delegated to an LPN or UAP.
  1. Delegate responsibly those activities that can be delegated, including basic care needs and assessment of vital signs for the stable client. All monitoring information must be reported to the RN.
  2. Administer medications that may be used in the treatment of hypertension (see pharmacologic and parenteral therapies).
  3. Promote accurate BP assessment for diagnosis and treatment.
     a. Client sitting or supine for 5 min with arm at heart level
     b. Measurement of both arms; use arm with higher reading
     c. Place inflatable bladder of cuff at 80% of upper arm circumference
  4. Provide interventions during hypertensive crisis.
     a. IV administration of direct vasodilator, beta blocker, or ACE inhibitor—IV titration to lower BP to target range and prevent risk for hypotension: Monitor arterial line or automated BP frequently; promote bed rest.
     b. Monitor continuous ECG and SpO_2.
     c. Provide frequent monitoring of vital signs, neurologic, cardiovascular, respiratory, and renal status.
  5. Provide interventions for invasive procedures used to treat certain secondary causes of hypertension, for example:
     a. Angioplasty and stenting or surgery for renal artery stenosis
     b. Surgery for pheochromocytoma adrenal tumor

C. Safety and infection control
  1. Take BP every 2 to 3 min or continuous monitoring via arterial line with initial administration of IV antihypertensive drugs and close vital sign monitoring throughout IV course.
  2. Teach client to rise slowly from bed or chair to reduce postural symptoms from oral antihypertensive drugs.

D. Health promotion and maintenance
  1. Provide client and family teaching about the following:
     a. Medications—schedule medications convenient to a daily routine and link timing with another daily activity to improve adherence.
     b. Diet
        (1) 2-g sodium diet
        (2) DASH diet (dietary approaches to manage hypertension)
        (3) Low-fat, calorie reduction, or diabetic diet, if prescribed
     c. Self-care behaviors for monitoring in home setting
        (1) BP, pulse, daily weight, and edema record
        (2) Blood sugar monitoring, if diabetic
        (3) When to seek medical attention
     d. Health behaviors that promote a healthy lifestyle, including smoking cessation; weight loss, if indicated, and maintenance of ideal weight; regular physical exercise; stress management; and reduction or elimination of alcohol.
  2. Promote regular follow-up care.

E. Psychologic integrity
  1. Monitor for potential reduced effectiveness of treatment in African Americans because of high prevalence and severity of hypertension; this includes monotherapy with beta blockers, ACE-I, and angiotensin receptor blockers. Combination therapy may be required to achieve and maintain target BP.

2. Observe hypertension as common in older adults as they are sensitive to BP changes and orthostatic hypotension.

F. Basic care and comfort: Provide a quiet, calm environment, and encourage client to voice concerns.

G. Reduction of risk potential
1. Control BP to reduce risk of HF, CAD, peripheral vascular disease, stroke, transient ischemic attack, chronic kidney disease, and retinopathy.
2. Monitor for hypotension with antihypertensive medications and electrolyte alterations with diuretics.

H. Pharmacologic and parenteral therapies: Client and family will state the purpose, dosage, timing, and side effects of all medications.
1. See Table 20-3 for medications used to treat chronic hypertension.
2. See Table 20-4 for IV medications used to treat hypertensive crisis.

Inflammatory and Valvular Diseases

I. Definition: Inflammatory heart disease involves inflammation of the layers of the heart. Valvular heart disease occurs when the heart valves do not open completely (stenosis) or close completely (insufficiency or regurgitation).

A. Types of inflammatory heart diseases include:
1. Pericarditis—acute or chronic inflammation of the pericardium.
   a. Acute pericarditis is idiopathic, with coxsackievirus B the most common identified virus; this occurs as a result of infections, noninfections, and hypersensitive or autoimmune causes. Acute pericarditis may occur 48 to 72 hr post MI, or in 2 to 4 weeks (Dresser syndrome).
   b. Chronic pericarditis occurs over an extended time period and can have signs of right-sided HF.
2. Myocarditis—inflammation of the myocardium.
3. Endocarditis—inflammation of the inner lying of the heart and valves. Splenomegaly and embolic complications may occur from vegetation fragments traveling through the circulation.
4. Rheumatic heart disease—primarily affects connective tissue, most often the cardiac valves. Often caused by beta-hemolytic streptococcal bacteria (see also Chapter 12).

B. Types of valvular diseases include mitral valve prolapse, mitral stenosis, mitral insufficiency (regurgitation), aortic stenosis, and aortic insufficiency. Right-sided heart valve problems include tricuspid stenosis, tricuspid insufficiency, pulmonary stenosis, and pulmonary insufficiency (Fig. 20-1).

II. Nursing process

A. Assessment
1. Perform a comprehensive health history and physical assessment.
2. Assess for signs and symptoms of inflammatory heart disease.
   a. Pericarditis: Chest pain, dyspnea, and a pericardial friction rub. Pain is aggravated by lying supine, deep breathing, coughing, or swallowing, and pain is relieved by leaning forward. Chronic pericarditis can have signs of right-sided HF.
   b. Myocarditis: Fever, fatigue, malaise, myalgias, pharyngitis, dyspnea, lymphadenopathy, and nausea and vomiting. Following a viral infection, can see cardiac signs of pericarditis, S3, crackles, jugular venous distention, and peripheral edema.
   c. Endocarditis:
      (1) Signs and symptoms include fever, anorexia, weight loss, fatigue, cardiac murmurs, abdominal discomfort, and clubbing of fingers in subacute forms of endocarditis.
      (2) Vascular manifestations include splinter hemorrhages in the nail beds, Osler nodes (reddish tender lesions) on the fingertips or toes, Janeway lesions (flat, painless, small, red spots) on the palms and soles, and Roth spots (retinal hemorrhage).
   d. Rheumatic heart disease: Precordial chest pain, tachycardia, HF, pericardial friction rub, cardiomegaly, pericardial effusion, palpitations, and migratory joint pain.
3. Assess for signs and symptoms of valvular heart diseases—client may have heart murmurs, cardiac dysrhythmias, hypotension and dizziness, fatigue, dyspnea, and symptoms of right-sided heart failure.
   a. Mitral valve prolapse
   b. Mitral stenosis
   c. Mitral insufficiency (regurgitation)
   d. Aortic stenosis
   e. Aortic insufficiency
   f. Right-sided heart valve problems

Table 20-3 Medications for Treatment of Chronic Hypertension

Classification	Generic/ Trade Name	Expected Outcomes	Reduction of Risk Potential	Management of Care
Thiazide Diuretics	Chlorothiazide (Diuril); chlorthalidone (Thalitone); hydrochlorothiazide (HydroDIURIL, Microzide); polythiazide (Renese); metolazone (Mykrox, Zaroxolyn)	Promotes mild sodium and water excretion. Decreases BP, preload, and fluid retention.	Monitor for electrolyte imbalances, hypotension, hyperglycemia, hyperuricemia, metabolic alkalosis.	Combine with dietary sodium restriction. Monitor for orthostatic hypotension, U/O, I&O, daily weight, and potassium. Take early in day.
Loop Diuretics	Bumetanide (Bumex); furosemide (Lasix); torsemide (Demadex)	Promotes more potent fluid loss than thiazides.	See thiazides; monitor for fluid depletion and renal impairment. Promote slow IVP to prevent ototoxicity.	Same as thiazides; monitor BUN, creatinine, and K^+ closely.
Potassium-sparing Diuretics	Amiloride (Midamor); triamterene (Dyrenium)	Promotes mild sodium and water excretion with less excretion of K^+.	Monitor for hyperkalemia, dizziness, and hypotension.	Contraindicated for clients with renal failure and used cautiously with ACE inhibitors. Stop potassium supplementation if indicated. Provide client teaching to avoid high-potassium foods.
Aldosterone Receptor Blockers	Spironolactone (Aldactone); eplerenone (Inspra)	Inhibits sodium and water retention, and potassium excretion effects of aldosterone.	See potassium-sparing diuretics.	See potassium-sparing diuretics.
Angiotensin Converting Enzyme (ACE) Inhibitors	Benazepril (Lotensin); captopril (Capoten); enalapril (Vasotec); fosinopril (Monopril); lisinopril (Prinivil, Zestril); moexipril (Univasc); perindopril (Aceon); quinapril (Accupril); ramipril (Altace); trandolapril (Mavik)	Promotes afterload reduction and decreased BP.	Not given if history of angioedema, anuric renal failure. Monitor for increase K^+, creatinine, cough, angioedema, symptomatic hypotension.	Assess BP, postural changes, U/O, K^+. Initiate at low dose with gradual increase as tolerated. Avoid NSAIDs.
Angiotensin II Receptor Blockers	Candesartan (Atacand); eprosartan (Teveten); irbesartan (Avapro); losartan (Cozaar); olmesartan (Benicar); telmisartan (Micardis); valsartan (Diovan)	Provides similar effects of ACE-I.	Alternative to ACE inhibitor. Monitor for increase K^+, BUN, and creatinine, symptomatic hypotension.	Assess BP, postural changes, and U/O. Initiate at low dose with gradual upward titration as tolerated.

Classification	Generic/ Trade Name	Expected Outcomes	Reduction of Risk Potential	Management of Care
Alpha-1 Blockers	Doxazosin (Cardura); prazosin (Minipress); terazosin (Hytrin)	Promotes peripheral vasodilation and afterload reduction.	Monitor for syncope, orthostatic hypotension, and reflex tachycardia.	Assess BP and postural changes. Administer at bedtime to reduce risk of orthostatic hypotension.
Beta blockers	Atenolol (Tenormin); betaxolol (Kerlone); bisoprolol (Zebeta); metoprolol (Lopressor, Toprol-XL); nadolol (Corgard); propranolol (Inderal); timolol (Blocadren)	Decreases BP, HR, contractility, and afterload.	Use with caution in clients with asthma or reactive airway disease. Monitor for bradycardia or heart block, hypotension, fluid retention, and fatigue. Avoid abrupt discontinuation: Can cause rebound tachycardia and hypertension.	Assess BP, HR, I&O, and daily weight. Initiate at low dose with gradual upward titration to target dose. Provide counseling for depression or sexual dysfunction.
Combined Alpha-Beta Blocker	Carvedilol (Coreg); labetalol (Normodyne Trandate)	Decreases afterload, BP, HR, and contractility.	Use in stable clients and with extreme caution, or not at all in clients with reactive airway disease. Monitor for bradycardia or heart block, hypotension, fluid retention, and fatigue.	Administer with food; space apart other meds that may decrease BP. Assess BP, HR, I&O, and U/O. Initiate at low dose with gradual upward titration to target dose.
Central Alpha-2 Agonists	Clonidine (Catapres); clonidine patch; methyldopa (Aldomet); reserpine; guanfacine (Tenex)	Promotes peripheral vasodilation, decreased afterload and BP.	Monitor for hypotension, dry mouth, dizziness, sedation, and sexual dysfunction.	Assess BP, promote caution with driving. Transdermal may have fewer side effects and better compliance.
Direct Vasodilators	Hydralazine (Apresoline); minoxidil (Loniten)	Potent peripheral vasodilation; decreases afterload and BP.	Monitor for hypotension and tachycardia.	Assess BP and postural changes. Administer hydralazine PO or IV dosing.
Non-Dihydropyridines Calcium Channel Blockers Dihydropyridines Calcium Channel Blockers	Diltiazem (Cardizem); verapamil (Calan, Isoptin); amlodipine (Norvasc); felodipine (Plendil); isradipine (DynaCirc); nicardipine sustained release (Cardene); nifedipine (Procardia); nisoldipine (Sular)	Decreases afterload and BP; diltiazem and verapamil have antidysrhythmic effect and inhibit coronary artery spasm (also nifedipine).	First generation contraindicated for the treatment of systolic HF. Monitor for hypotension, bradycardia.	Assess HR and BP. Dihydropyridines have more peripheral vascular selectivity.

Table 20-4 Intravenous Medications for Hypertensive Crisis

Classification	Generic/ Trade Name	Expected Outcomes	Reduction of Risk Potential	Management of Care
IV Vasodilators	Diazoxide (Hyperstat) sodium nitroprusside (Nipride); nitroglycerin (Tridil)	Decreases BP: More afterload reduction with Nipride and Hyperstat; more preload reduction with NTG.	Monitor for hypotension, arrhythmias, headache, and cyanide toxicity with Nipride.	Promote IV infusions and close monitoring of BP; administer Nipride with arterial line; maintain bed rest.
IV Beta Blocker	Esmolol (Brevibloc)	Decreases BP, afterload, and HR.	Monitor for hypotension, postural changes, bradycardia, and bronchospasm.	Promote IV infusions and close monitoring of BP. Maintain bed rest.
IV Alpha/Beta Blocker	Labetalol (Normodyne)	Decreases BP, afterload, and HR.	Monitor for hypotension, postural changes, bradycardia, and bronchospasm.	Promote IV infusions and close monitoring of BP. Maintain bed rest.
IV ACE inhibitor	Enalaprilat (Vasotec)	Decreases afterload and BP.	Monitor for hypotension and postural changes.	Promote close monitoring of BP; Check K+. Maintain bed rest.

4. Obtain diagnostic tests.
   a. Pericarditis: ESR, ECG, echocardiogram, hemodynamic monitoring, chest x-ray, CT scan, MRI
   b. Myocarditis: Erythrocyte sedimentation rate (ESR), CBC, antiviral antibodies, ECG, heart biopsy, serum immunoglobulins, cultures and sensitivity
   c. Endocarditis: CBC, immune testing, blood cultures and sensitivity, urine analysis, ECG
   d. Rheumatic fever: CBC, C-reactive protein, erythrocyte sedimentation rate, antistreptolysin titer (ASO) titer
   e. Valvular heart disease: ECGs, echocardiography, cardiac catheterization, chest x-ray

B. Analysis
1. Activity Intolerance related to reduced cardiac reserve and cardiac output
2. Acute Pain related to tissue inflammation
3. Risk for Injury related to dysrhythmias
4. Fear related to life-threatening diagnosis
5. Ineffective Health Maintenance related to lack of knowledge about disease and treatment process

C. Planning
1. Control or eliminate precipitating cause of symptoms.
2. Improve client symptoms and comfort.
3. Reduce anxiety and fear.
4. Prevent cardiac tamponade and complications such as heart failure or dysrhythmias.
5. Promote adherence to therapeutic regimen.
6. Enhance functional capacity and quality of life.

D. Implementation
1. Monitor vital signs with close attention to BP, pulses, heart sounds, and lung sounds.
2. Monitor response to pharmacologic therapy.
3. For acute pericarditis, monitor for signs of cardiac tamponade (pulsus paradoxus, jugular vein distention with clear lung sounds, muffled heart sounds, narrowed pulse pressure, tachycardia, and hypotension).
4. Instruct client about control of symptoms, medications, and associated side effects, monitoring of pulse, and signs and symptoms that require medical attention.
5. Promote administration of prophylactic antibiotics prior to invasive or dental procedures.
6. Prepare client for invasive interventions such as pericardiocentesis or surgical interventions (valvuloplasty, annuloplasty, valve replacement).

E. Evaluation
1. Client verbalizes decrease in, or absence of, pain.
2. Client's vital signs, temperature, and urine output are within targeted range.

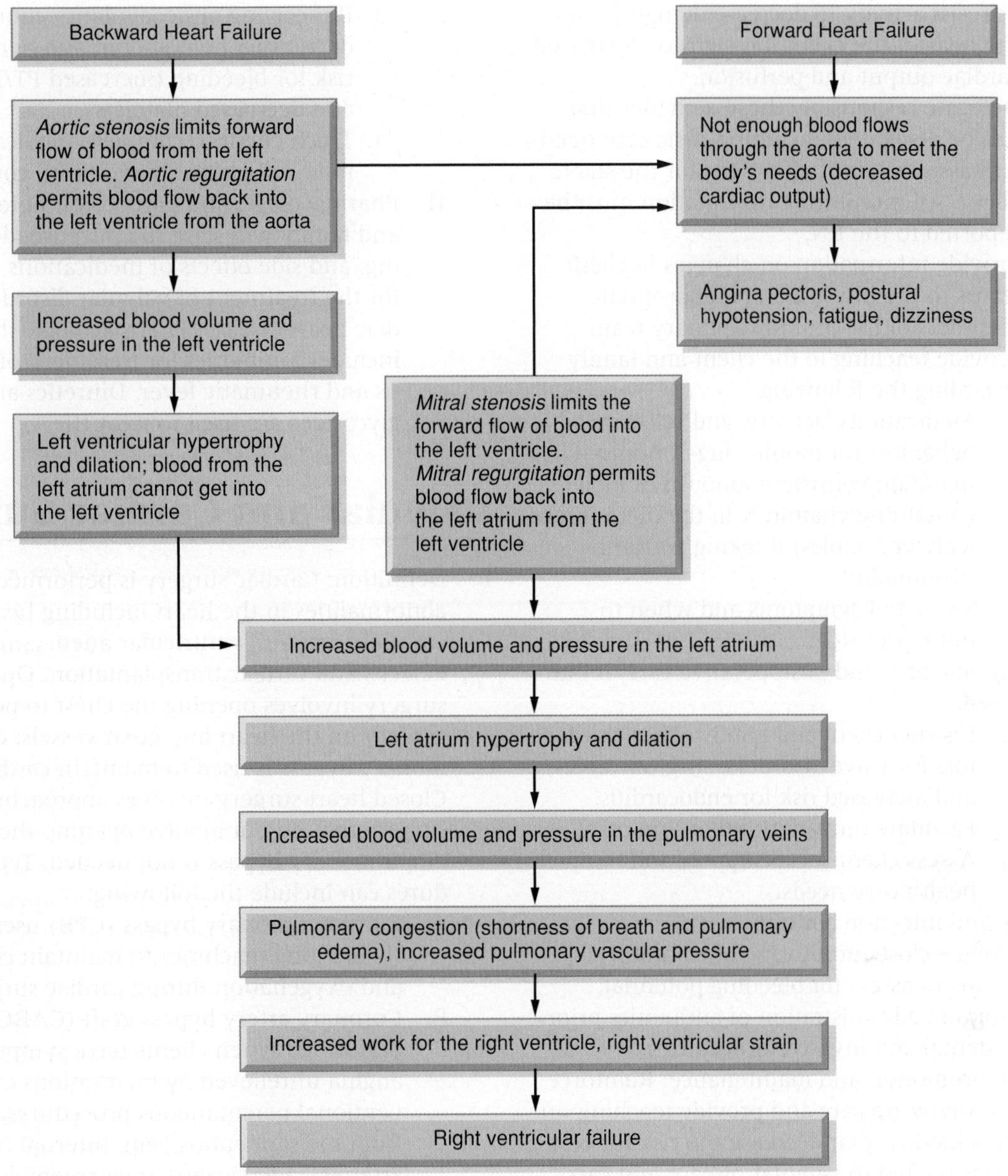

Figure 20-1. Pathophysiology; left-sided heart failure as a result of aortic and mitral valvular heart disease and the development of right ventricular failure. (From Smeltzer, S. C., & Bare, B. G. [2008]. *Brunner & Suddarth's textbook of medical surgical nursing* [11th ed.]. Philadelphia: Lippincott Williams & Wilkins.)

3. Client adheres to therapeutic plan of care and obtains prophylactic antibiotic therapy before invasive procedures.
4. Client affirms absence of symptoms.
5. Client's laboratory values are within normal range.

CN

III. Client needs

A. Physiologic adaptation: Treatment is based on client symptoms and progression of the valve problem, which may vary among clients. Assess client's need for and response to administration of analgesic, nonsteroidal anti-inflammatory drugs, corticosteroids for pain and fever.
   1. Administer antidysrhythmic and anticoagulant therapy if atrial fibrillation is present.
   2. Provide surgical interventions if client is unresponsive to pharmacologic therapy (see Valvular and Cardiac Surgery).
   3. Monitor for onset of severe dyspnea and worsening of symptoms, which could indicate pulmonary edema.

B. Management of care: Care of the client experiencing inflammatory or valvular heart disease requires critical thinking skills and knowledge of assessment, and teaching and evaluation methods unique to the RN role. These skills cannot be delegated to an LPN or UAP.
   1. Perform comprehensive physical assessments and provide care to the client with acute symptoms of valvular heart disease—manage

or resist activity to decrease demands on the heart if the client has signs of decreased cardiac output and perfusion.
2. Delegate responsibly those activities that can be delegated, including basic care needs and assessment of vital signs for the stable client. All monitoring information must be reported to the RN.
3. Provide information on changes in client status to the physician and appropriate members of the multidisciplinary team.
4. Provide teaching to the client and family regarding the following:
   a. Medications, activity, and self-care behaviors for monitoring at home—maintain consistent amount of food containing vitamin K in the diet (green leafy vegetables) if taking warfarin (Coumadin).
   b. Signs and symptoms and when to notify the HCP.
5. Provide pre- and postoperative care, if indicated.
   a. Instruct client and family about risk factors for valve disorders, surgical valves, and increased risk for endocarditis.
   b. Facilitate outpatient follow-up care.
   c. Assess client social support and home health care needs.

C. Safety and infection control
1. Provide close monitoring of laboratory results to assess for bleeding potential.
2. Promote administration of antibiotics prior to dental and invasive procedures.

D. Health promotion and maintenance: Reinforce regular follow-up care and provide teaching on health behaviors that decrease the risk for complications related to valvular disease and cardiac disorders.

E. Psychologic integrity
1. Assist client and family in coping with lifestyle changes.
2. Identify factors, such as anxiety, that may interfere with recovery.
3. Introduce counseling and support groups to assist the client with smoking cessation and medication management, if indicated.

F. Basic care and comfort
1. Provide pain management.
2. Turn and position client every 2 hr while on bed rest.
3. Provide skin care.

G. Reduction of risk potential
1. Instruct client about the importance of good oral mouth care.
2. Assess for and treat signs of decreased cardiac output.
3. If receiving anticoagulants, monitor for decreasing hemoglobin and hematocrit and risk for bleeding (increased PT/INR, APTT, and decreased platelets).
4. Teach client to complete medication regimen, taking antibiotics until completed.

H. Pharmacologic and parenteral therapies: Client and family will state the purpose, dosage, timing, and side effects of medications prescribed for the treatment of valvular disorders and cardiac heart disease. Pharmacologic therapy includes antibiotics for treatment of endocarditis and rheumatic fever. Diuretics and cardiac glycosides are used to treat HF.

Valvular and Cardiac Surgery

I. Definition: Cardiac surgery is performed to correct abnormalities in the heart including heart valves, coronary arteries, ventricular aneurysms, septal defects, and cardiac transplantation. Open heart surgery involves opening the chest to perform surgery on the heart and great vessels; cardiopulmonary bypass is used to maintain cardiac function. Closed heart surgery involves approaches to cardiac surgery that do not involve opening the chest; cardiopulmonary bypass is not needed. Types of procedures can include the following:

A. Cardiopulmonary bypass (CPB) uses a pump (heart/lung machine) to maintain circulation and oxygenation during cardiac surgery.

B. Coronary artery bypass graft (CABG) surgery is performed when clients have symptomatic angina unrelieved by medications and interventional percutaneous procedures. Vessels from the saphenous vein, internal mammary arteries, radial artery or gastroepiploic arteries may be used (Fig. 20-2).

C. Minimally invasive direct coronary artery bypass graft (MIDCAB) is performed through a left anterior thoracotomy incision using a port access and video-assisted technology. Cardiopulmonary bypass is not needed.

D. Port coronary artery bypass graft (PortCAB) is a minimally invasive coronary artery bypass that does not require open heart surgery; rather, the procedure allows the surgeon to access the coronary arteries through a small port. Cardiopulmonary bypass is still required.

E. Percutaneous transluminal coronary angioplasty (PTCA) involves threading a balloon-tipped catheter from an artery (usually femoral) to the coronary artery. The balloon is inflated, which compresses plaque in the artery, dilates the artery, and allows blood to flow freely.

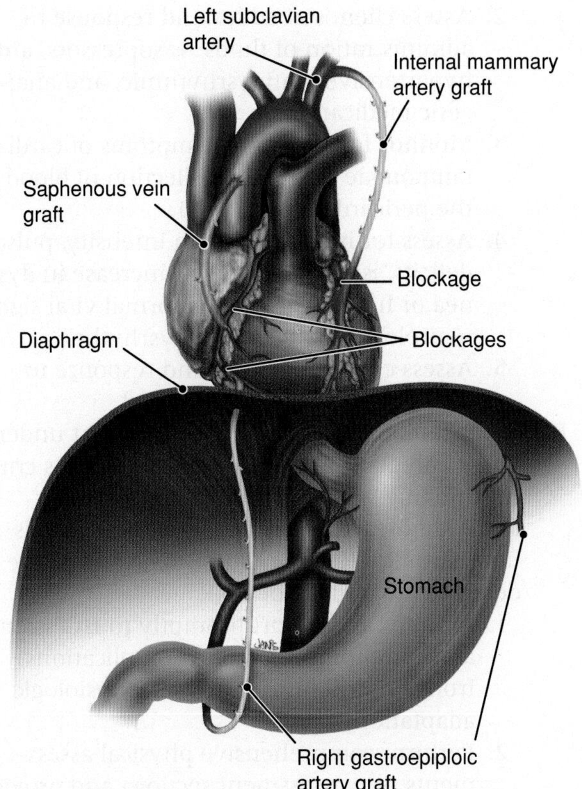

Figure 20-2. Three coronary artery bypass grafts. (From Smeltzer, S. C., & Bare, B. G. [2008]. *Brunner & Suddarth's textbook of medical surgical nursing* [11th ed.]. Philadelphia: Lippincott Williams & Wilkins.)

F. Surgical removal (ablation) of accessory pathways of dysrhythmias, including mapping cardiac electrophysiologic function to locate the source of dysrhythmias, along with other surgical procedures, are involved in heart surgery.

G. Valve repair: Valvuloplasty is reconstruction including repair or removal of calcification or vegetation.

H. Valve replacement
   1. Mechanical valves are more durable and longer-lasting; subject to mechanical failure; require lifetime anticoagulation with warfarin (Coumadin); infections are harder to treat.
   2. Tissue valves may deteriorate and require frequent replacement, but not associated with risk of thrombus formation; no long-term anticoagulation; infections are easier to treat.

I. Annuloplasty is narrowing a dilated valve with a prosthetic ring, purse-string sutures, or enlarging a stenosed valve with a balloon.

II. Nursing process

A. Assessment
   1. Assess for signs and symptoms—symptoms and severity depends on the extent of the valvular dysfunction, heart, and CAD.
   2. Obtain past medical and surgical history; psychosocial and spiritual history.
   3. Perform comprehensive physical assessments.
      a. Preoperative: Assess vital signs; SpO_2, ventilator settings, ABGs, peripheral pulses; capillary refill; color, temperature, sensation, movement of extremity; edema; activity tolerance; and presence and location of pain and discomfort.
      b. Postoperative: Complete assessment of all body systems and intervene appropriately for complications—assessment includes neurologic, cardiac, respiratory, and peripheral vascular, as well as fluid and electrolytes.
   4. Assess hemodynamic monitoring parameters: Preload, afterload, contractility, and heart rate every hour and as needed.
   5. Assess for signs of impaired gas exchange: Restlessness, anxiety, cyanosis of peripheral and mucous membranes, tachycardia, and fighting the ventilator.
   6. Obtain diagnostic tests.
      a. Valvular (see diagnostic tests for inflammation and valvular diseases)
      b. Chest x-ray, K+, Mg+, BUN, creatinine, ABGs, H & H, PT, APTT, drug levels, if appropriate
      c. Hemodynamic profile (pulmonary artery catheter)

B. Analysis
   1. Fear related to the surgical procedure and uncertain outcome
   2. Deficient Knowledge of health problem regarding the surgical procedure and postoperative course
   3. Decreased Cardiac Output related to blood loss, compromised myocardial function, and dysrhythmias
   4. Impaired Gas Exchange related to trauma of extensive chest surgery
   5. Risk for Deficient Fluid Volume and electrolyte imbalance
   6. Disturbed Sensory Perception: Visual and Auditory, related to excessive environmental stimuli, insufficient sleep, and psychologic stress
   7. Acute Pain related to surgical trauma and pleural irritation
   8. Deficient Knowledge: Self-Care Activities, related to changes in activity level

C. Planning
   1. Provide adequate cardiac output and tissue perfusion.
   2. Maintain adequate gas exchange.
   3. Maintain fluid and electrolyte balance.

4. Keep client alert and oriented.
5. Relieve pain.
6. Maintain normal body temperature.
7. Maintain hemodynamic stability.
8. Promote activity tolerance.
9. Reduce anxiety.
10. Prevent dysrhythmias, MI, and other complications.
11. Provide teaching on CAD, risk factors, and the therapeutic regimen.
12. Improve quality of life.

D. Implementation: Interventions are individualized to client's needs—promote drug therapy to maintain adequate cardiac output and tissue perfusion (see pharmacologic and parenteral therapies).

E. Evaluation
1. Client demonstrates reduced fear as evidenced by positive attitude about outcome of surgery.
2. Client learns about the surgical procedure and postoperative course, discusses expected immediate postoperative environment, and demonstrates expected activities to follow surgery (deep breathing and foot exercises).
3. Client shows no evidence of complications and takes medications as prescribed.
4. Client's vital signs are within normal limits and client exhibits normal sinus rhythm or controlled ventricular rate with chronic atrial fibrillation.
5. Client is weaned from ventilator, vasopressor drugs, and affirms the absence of pain and associated symptoms.
6. Client's functional capability is optimized through tailored interventions based on individualized assessments and needs.
7. Client exhibits tolerance to increasing levels of activity and exercise.
8. Client describes risk factors for CAD, factors contributing to anginal symptoms, and the procedure to follow in home setting for acute chest pain.
9. Client states the purpose, dosage, timing, and side effects of the medications prescribed.

CN

III. Client needs

A. Physiologic adaptation: Treatment is based on client symptoms and type of heart problem.
1. Recognize risk for complications from surgical procedure—indicated by altered cardiac output, gas exchange, fluid and electrolyte balance; sensory-perception imbalance, body temperature, and tissue perfusion can result in complications.
2. Assess client's need for and response to administration of fluids, vasopressors, antihypertensive, antidysrhythmic, and analgesic medications.
3. Monitor for signs and symptoms of cardiac tamponade caused by collection of blood in the pericardial sac.
4. Assess for increase in pain intensity, pulse deficits, ischemic changes, increase in dyspnea or heart murmur, abnormal vital signs, neurologic changes, and dysrhythmias.
5. Assess client's need for and response to blood transfusions, if indicated.

B. Management of care: Care of the client undergoing valvular or cardiac surgery requires critical thinking skills and knowledge of assessment, and teaching and evaluation methods unique to the RN role. These skills cannot be delegated to an LPN or UAP.
1. Monitor and report promptly to HCP signs and symptoms related to complications from surgical procedure (see physiologic adaptation).
2. Perform comprehensive physical assessments (see assessment section) and provide care to the client with acute symptoms of an aortic aneurysm.
3. Delegate responsibly those activities that can be delegated, including basic care needs and assessment of vital signs for the stable client. All monitoring information must be reported to the RN.
4. Provide information on changes in client status to the physician and appropriate members of the multidisciplinary team.
5. Provide interventions following open heart surgery.
   a. Monitor vital signs and peripheral pulses every hour.
   b. Provide continuous monitoring of ECG, arterial line BP, and SpO_2.
   c. Monitor heart sounds and lung sounds.
   d. Provide neurologic and neurovascular assessments.
   e. Monitor fluid and electrolytes, hemoglobin, hematocrit, renal function, and coagulation studies.
   f. Assess for hypovolemia; monitor intake and output every hour.
   g. Administer morphine or other prescribed medications to control pain.
   h. Assess wounds and provide incision care per protocol.
   i. Promote deep-breathing exercises or incentive spirometry after extubation.
   j. Encourage initial bed rest and gradual increase in activity.

k. Assess level of understanding of client and family; provide emotional support and teaching about postoperative course.
6. Provide client and family teaching (see health promotion and maintenance).
7. Facilitate outpatient follow-up care.
8. Assess client social support and home health care needs prior to discharge.

C. Safety and infection control
1. Provide close monitoring of BP and heart rate to maintain targeted range.
2. Provide close monitoring of PT and INR if taking warfarin (Coumadin).

D. Health promotion and maintenance
1. Assist client in identifying personalized risk factors for CAD.
2. Provide client and family teaching about the following:
a. Medications and associated side effects.
b. Self-care behaviors for client monitoring.
(1) BP, pulse, symptoms requiring immediate attention
(2) Prophylactic antibiotics prior to invasive procedures and routine dental care
(3) Importance of follow-up for lab tests if taking warfarin (Coumadin) or other types of anticoagulants
c. Health behaviors to promote a healthy lifestyle, including elimination of all forms of tobacco; maintenance of ideal weight, and weight loss, if indicated; regular physical exercise; and stress management.

E. Psychologic integrity
1. Identify any variations in care for older adult clients: Atherosclerosis is more common and occurs earlier in clients with diabetes mellitus; older adults may have deconditioning with less endurance for exercise and resilience with postoperative recovery.
2. Assist client and family in coping with lifestyle changes; identify stress factors and anxiety that may interfere with recovery.
3. Recommend counseling and support groups to assist client with smoking cessation as needed.
4. Assess client's ability to manage independently, social support, and home- and community-based care needs.

F. Basic care and comfort
1. Provide adequate pain management.
2. Turn and position client every 2 hr while on bed rest.
3. Provide skin care.
4. Position client for comfort; elevate head of bed 30 degrees as needed.

G. Reduction of risk potential
1. Assess for and treat hypovolemia.
2. Monitor for decreasing hemoglobin and hematocrit and risk for bleeding (increased PT/INR, APTT, and decreased platelets).
3. Provide teaching on foods to limit with high vitamin K if taking warfarin (Coumadin).

H. Pharmacologic and parenteral therapies: Client and family will state the purpose, dosage, timing, and side effects of all medications. (Also see pharmacologic and parenteral therapies to treat CAD.)
1. Antiplatelets—aspirin, ticlopidine (Ticlid), or clopidogrel (Plavix) to prevent clotting
2. Antidysrhythmias—amiodarone (Cordarone) to manage dysrhythmias
3. Anticoagulant—warfarin (Coumadin) to prevent clotting

Cardiac Dysrhythmias

I. Definition: Dysrhythmia (also referred to as *arrhythmia*) is a disorder of electrical impulse formation and/or impulse conduction in the heart or impulses generated from outside the normal conduction pathway. Types of dysrhythmias include the following:

A. Normal sinus rhythm—regular rhythm; heart rate 60 to 100 beats per minute; PR interval .12 to .20 s; QRS complex .04 to 10 s (Fig. 20-3).
B. Sinus bradycardia—heart rate is less than 60 beats per minute (Fig. 20-4).
C. Sinus tachycardia—heart rate 101 to 150 beats per minute; upper limit 160 to 180 (Fig. 20-5).
D. Premature atrial contraction—early beat from ectopic foci in the atria outside the SA node (Fig. 20-6).
E. Atrial fibrillation—disorganized, multiple, rapid impulses from many foci in the atria; no discernible P waves, with irregular ventricular rate (Fig. 20-7).
F. Atrial flutter—rapid impulses from ectopic foci in the atria; classic saw-tooth appearance; flutter waves (Fig. 20-8).
G. Junctional rhythm—impulse originates from the AV node; P waves can be inverted, absent, or after the QRS complex; ventricular rate is 40 to 60 beats per minute (Fig. 20-9).
H. Premature ventricular contractions (PVCs)—early ventricular contractions that have a wide and bizarre appearance; complexes may be unifocal or multifocal; may occur in repetitive patterns such as bigeminy or trigeminy (Fig. 20-10).

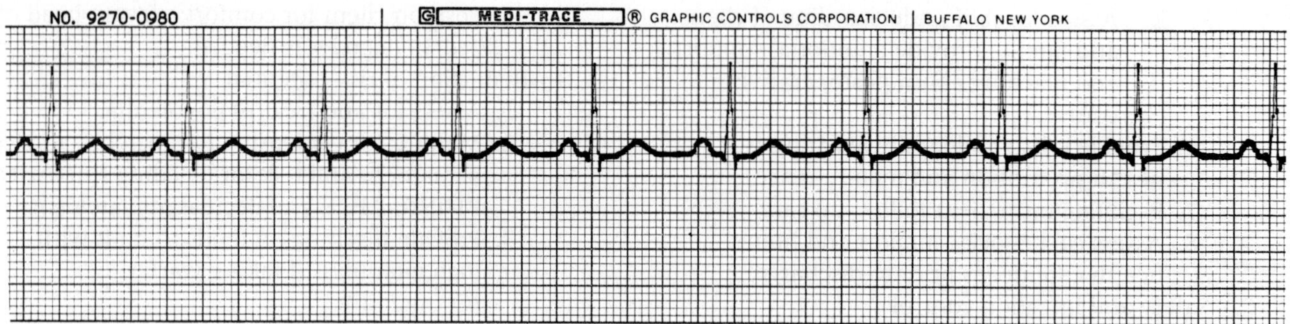

Figure 20-3. Normal sinus rhythm in lead II. (From Smeltzer, S. C., & Bare, B. G. [2008]. *Brunner & Suddarth's textbook of medical surgical nursing* [11th ed.]. Philadelphia: Lippincott Williams & Wilkins.)

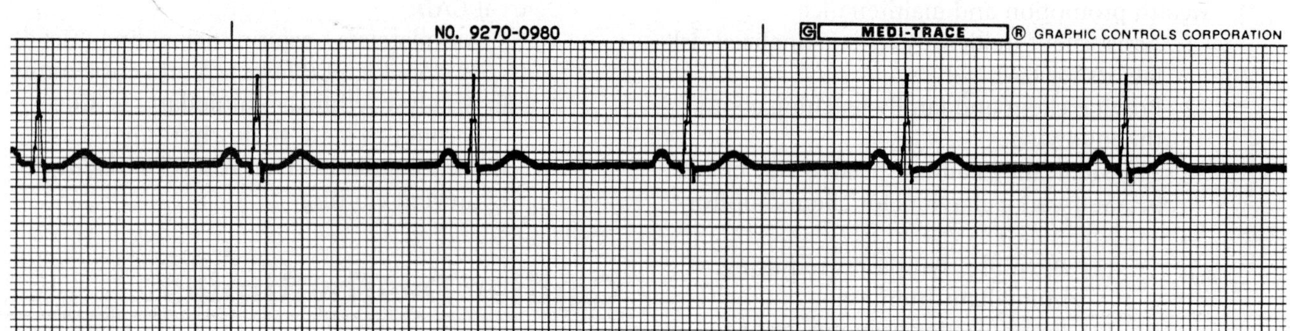

Figure 20-4. Sinus bradycardia in lead II. (From Smeltzer, S. C., & Bare, B. G. [2008]. *Brunner & Suddarth's textbook of medical surgical nursing* [11th ed.]. Philadelphia: Lippincott Williams & Wilkins.)

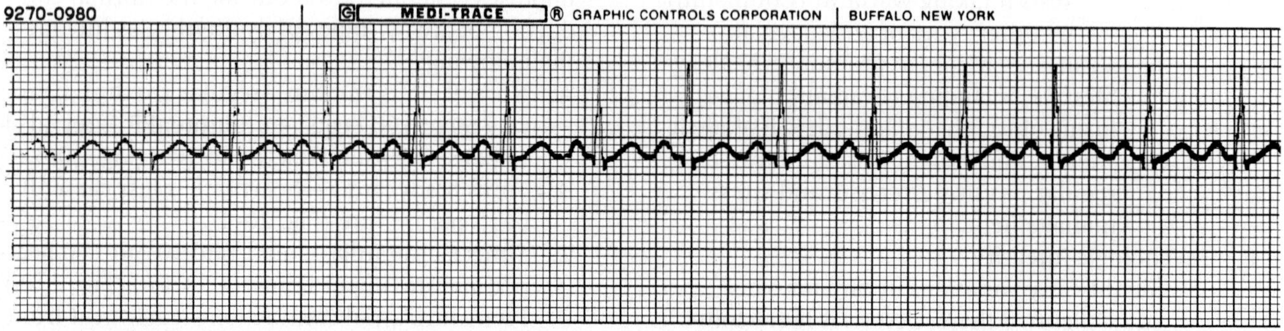

Figure 20-5. Sinus tachycardia in lead II. (From Smeltzer, S. C., & Bare, B. G. [2008]. *Brunner & Suddarth's textbook of medical surgical nursing* [11th ed.]. Philadelphia: Lippincott Williams & Wilkins.)

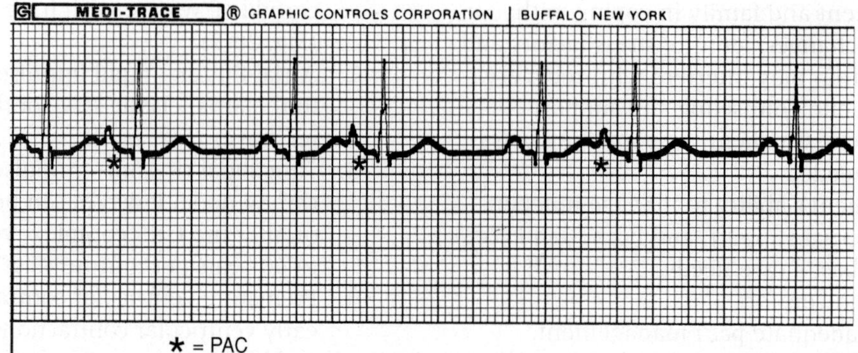

Figure 20-6. Premature atrial complexes (PACs) in lead II. (From Smeltzer, S. C., & Bare, B. G. [2008]. *Brunner & Suddarth's textbook of medical surgical nursing* [11th ed.]. Philadelphia: Lippincott Williams & Wilkins.)

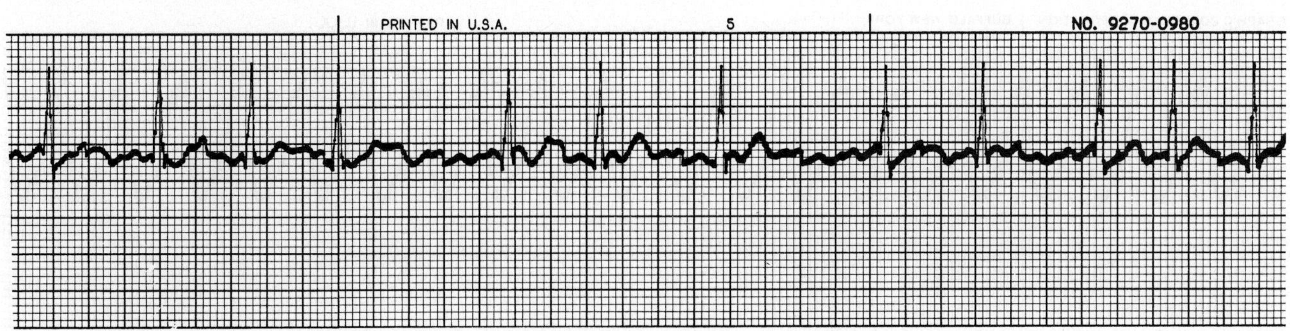

Figure 20-7. Atrial fibrillation in lead II. (From Smeltzer, S. C., & Bare, B. G. [2008]. *Brunner & Suddarth's textbook of medical surgical nursing* [11th ed.]. Philadelphia: Lippincott Williams & Wilkins.)

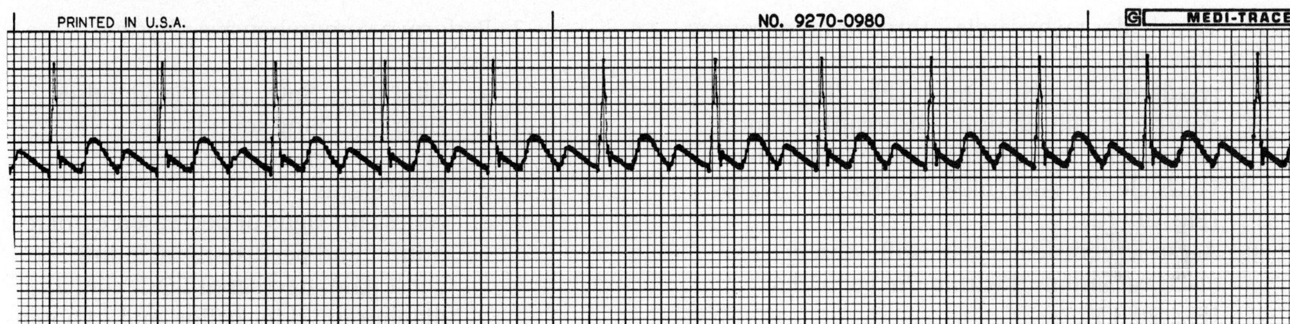

Figure 20-8. Atrial flutter in lead II. (From Smeltzer, S. C., & Bare, B. G. [2008]. *Brunner & Suddarth's textbook of medical surgical nursing* [11th ed.]. Philadelphia: Lippincott Williams & Wilkins.)

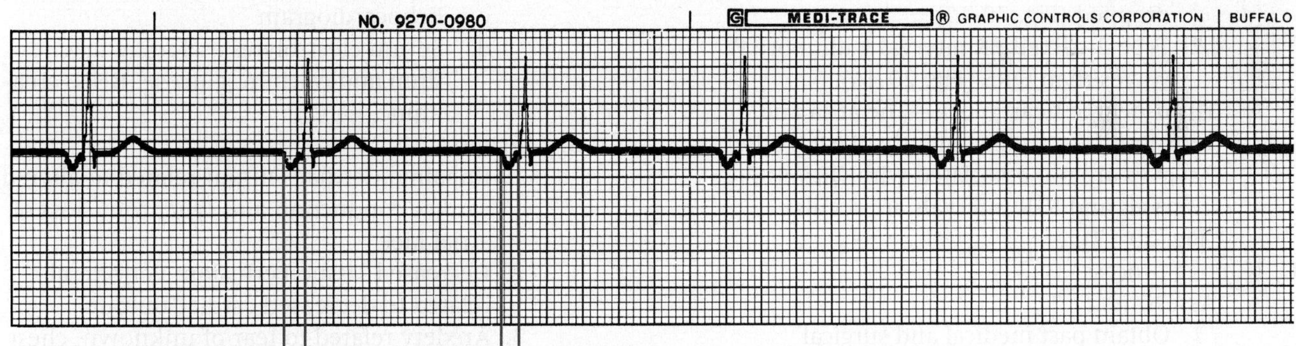

Figure 20-9. Junctional rhythm in lead II. (From Smeltzer, S. C., & Bare, B. G. [2008]. *Brunner & Suddarth's textbook of medical surgical nursing* [11th ed.]. Philadelphia: Lippincott Williams & Wilkins.)

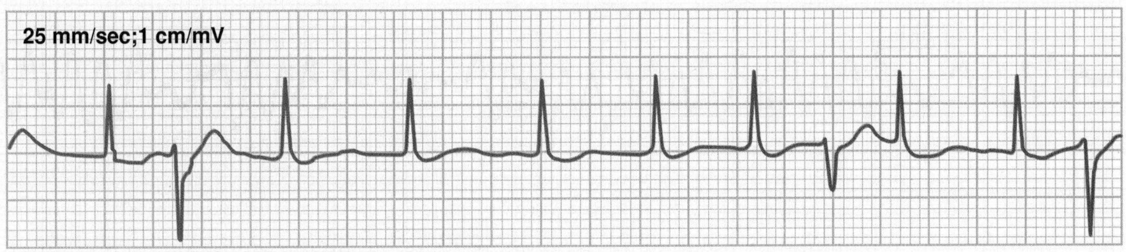

Figure 20-10. Premature ventricular contractions.

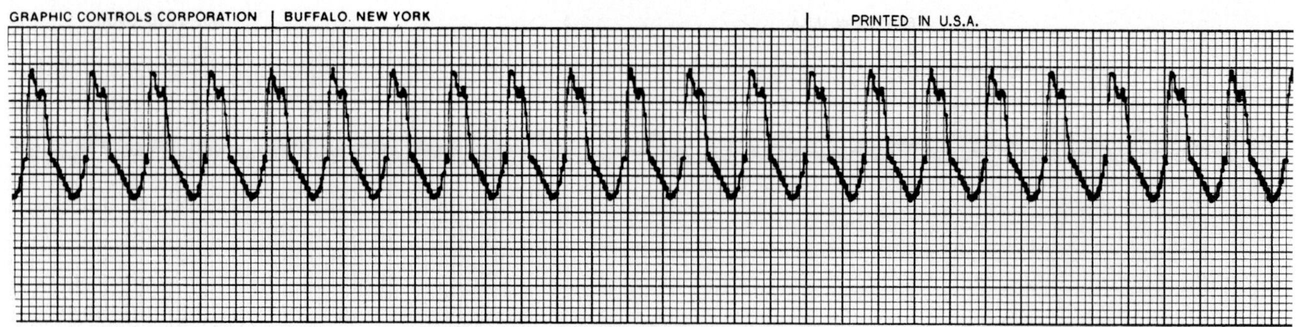

Figure 20-11. Ventricular tachycardia in lead V_1. (From Smeltzer, S. C., & Bare, B. G. [2008]. *Brunner & Suddarth's textbook of medical surgical nursing* [11th ed.]. Philadelphia: Lippincott Williams & Wilkins.)

I. Ventricular tachycardia—three or more consecutive PVCs occurring at a rapid rate; rhythm regular to slightly irregular (Fig. 20-11).

J. Ventricular fibrillation—disorganized, multiple, rapid impulses from many foci in the ventricle; no discernible P, QRS, or T waves (Fig. 20-12).

K. Asystole/ventricular standstill—absence of electrical impulses within the ventricles (Fig. 20-13).

L. First-degree heart block—PR interval is greater than 0.20 s (Fig. 20-14).

M. Second-degree heart block
   1. Type 1—Wenckebach: Steady lengthening of the PR interval until a QRS complex is dropped (Fig. 20-15).
   2. Type 2—fixed PR interval with more P waves than QRS (Fig. 20-16).

N. Third-degree heart block—The atria and ventricles beat independently of each other; P waves are not associated with QRS; P-P intervals and R-R intervals are regular (Fig. 20-17).

II. Nursing process

A. Assessment
   1. Obtain past medical and surgical history.
   2. Perform a comprehensive physical assessment.
      a. Vital signs, SpO_2, peripheral pulses
      b. Heart and lung sounds
      c. Level of consciousness (LOC)
      d. Fluid status
      e. Assess for signs of decreased cardiac output and perfusion, including chest pain, decreased LOC, cool and diaphoretic skin, pallor, and hypotension.
   3. Obtain diagnostic tests (see also diagnostic tests for CAD).
      a. 12-Lead ECG
      b. Chest x-ray
      c. Echocardiogram
      d. Serum electrolytes including magnesium and calcium, glucose, BUN, creatinine, CBC

B. Analysis
   1. Impaired Cardiac Output related to altered cardiac conduction and synchrony, loss of atrial kick
   2. Decreased Tissue Perfusion: Peripheral, related to decreased cardiac output
   3. Anxiety related to fear of unknown, chest pain, abnormal chest sensation

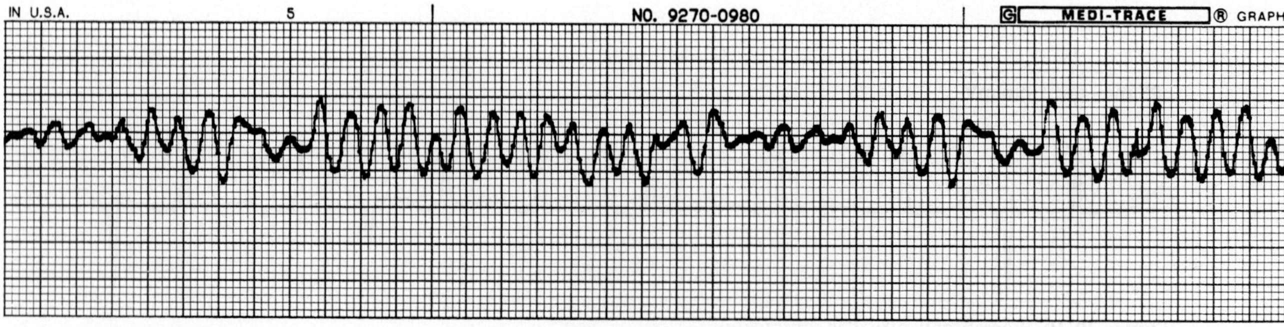

Figure 20-12. Ventricular fibrillation in lead II. (From Smeltzer, S. C., & Bare, B. G. [2008]. *Brunner & Suddarth's textbook of medical surgical nursing* [11th ed.]. Philadelphia: Lippincott Williams & Wilkins.)

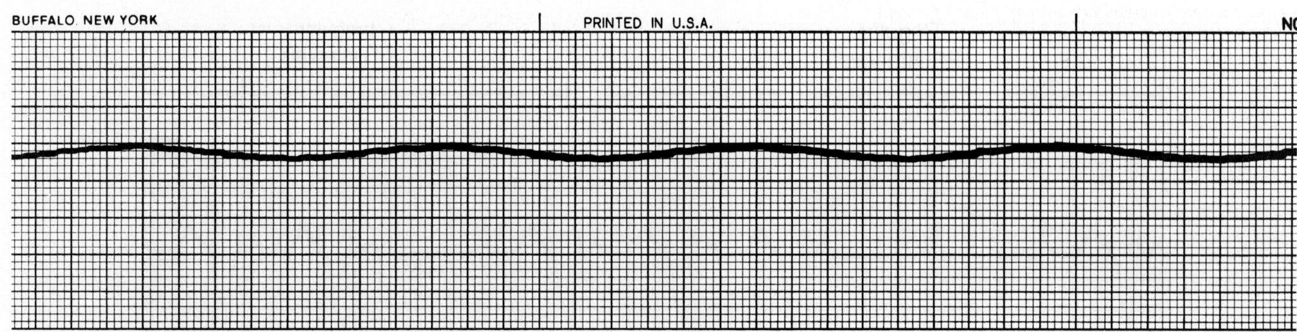

Figure 20-13. Asystole. Always check two different leads to confirm rhythm. (From Smeltzer, S. C., & Bare, B. G. [2008]. *Brunner & Suddarth's textbook of medical surgical nursing* [11th ed.]. Philadelphia: Lippincott Williams & Wilkins.)

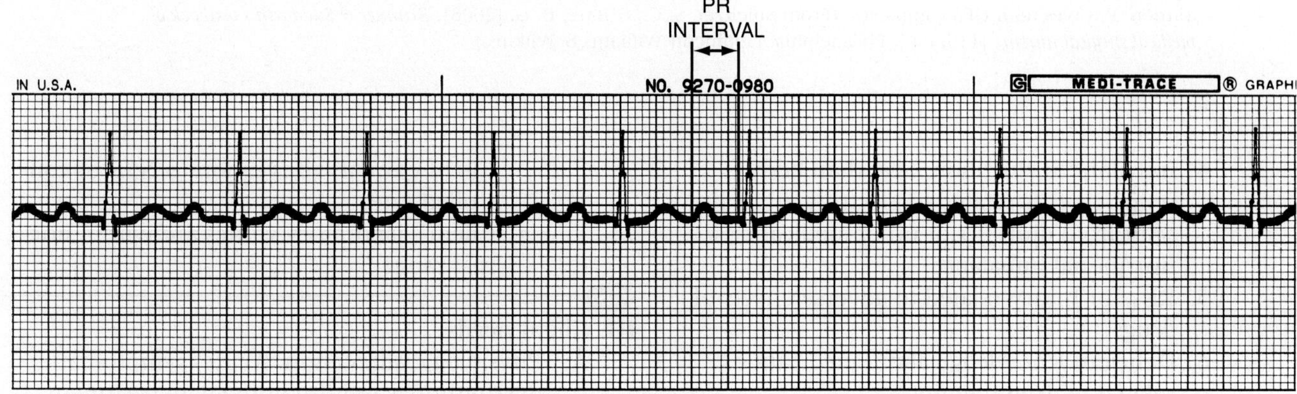

Figure 20-14. Sinus rhythm with first-degree AV block in lead II. Note that PR is constant but greater than 0.20 seconds. (From Smeltzer, S. C., & Bare, B. G. [2008]. *Brunner & Suddarth's textbook of medical surgical nursing* [11th ed.]. Philadelphia: Lippincott Williams & Wilkins.)

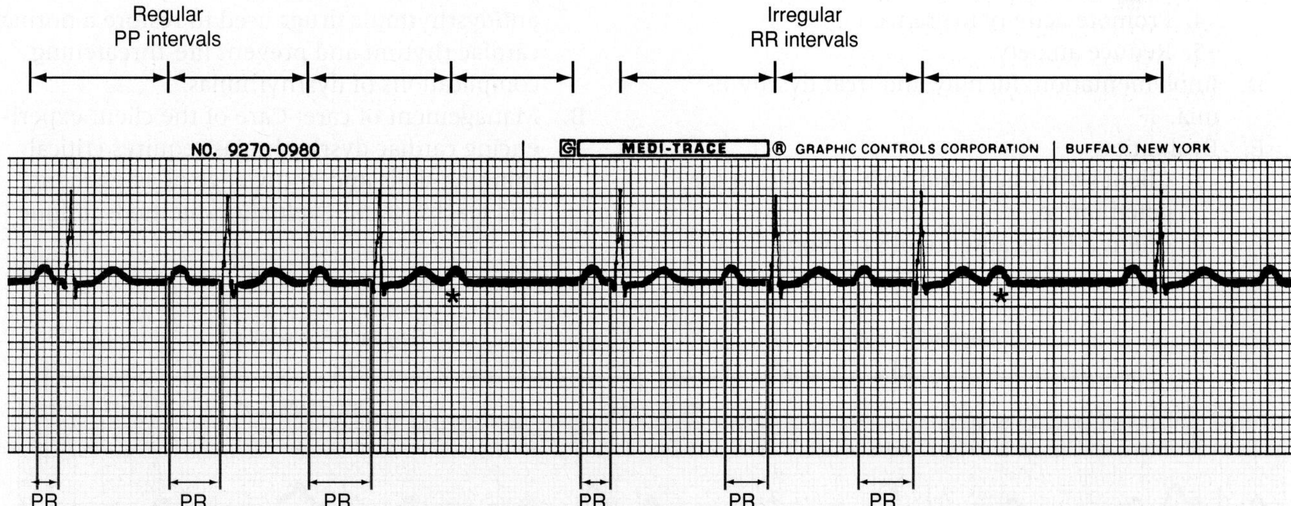

Figure 20-15. Sinus rhythm with second-degree AV block, type I in lead II. Note progressively longer PR durations until there is a nonconducted P wave, indicated by the *asterisk*. (From Smeltzer, S. C., & Bare, B. G. [2008]. *Brunner & Suddarth's textbook of medical surgical nursing* [11th ed.]. Philadelphia: Lippincott Williams & Wilkins.)

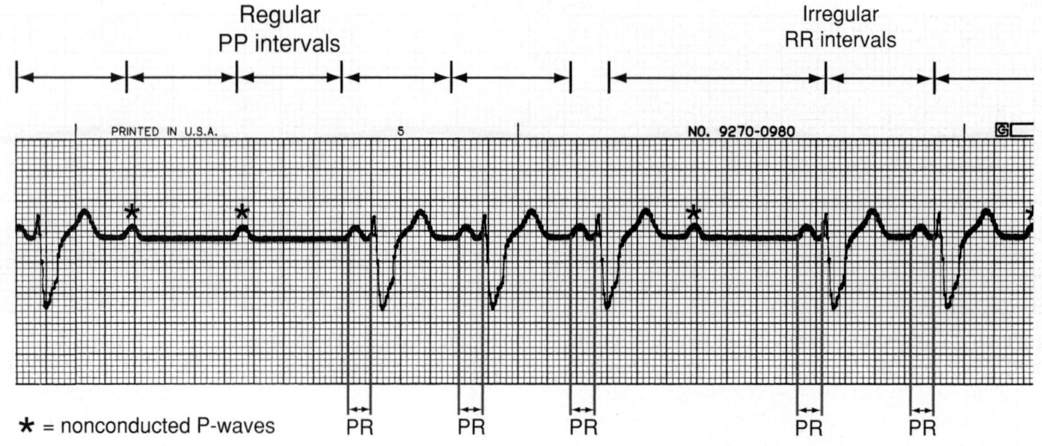

Figure 20-16. Sinus rhythm with second-degree AV block, type II in lead V_1. Note constant PR interval and presence of more P waves than QES complexes. (From Smeltzer, S. C., & Bare, B. G. [2008]. *Brunner & Suddarth's textbook of medical surgical nursing* [11th ed.]. Philadelphia: Lippincott Williams & Wilkins.)

4. Imbalanced Nutrition: Less than body requirements related to electrolyte imbalance from diuretics or other medications, nutritional imbalance
5. Risk for Injury related to adverse effects of drugs
6. Deficient Knowledge about medications, related to drug therapy

C. Planning
1. Restore normal sinus rhythm or controlled ventricular rate.
2. Maintain hemodynamic stability.
3. Relieve symptoms.
4. Promote activity tolerance.
5. Reduce anxiety.

D. Implementation: Identify and treat dysrhythmia.

E. Evaluation
1. Client's vital signs and SpO_2 are within targeted range.
2. Client affirms absence of symptoms.
3. Client exhibits conversion to NSR or controlled rate.
4. Client's laboratory values are within normal range.

CN

III. Client needs

A. Physiologic adaptation: Acute, symptomatic dysrhythmias require immediate treatment with antidysrhythmics, cardioversion, defibrillation, or temporary pacemaker. Provide appropriate fluid and electrolyte replacement and evaluate the client's response to treatment. See pharmacologic and parenteral therapies for antidysrhythmic drugs used to restore a normal cardiac rhythm and prevent life-threatening complications of dysrhythmias.

B. Management of care: Care of the client experiencing cardiac dysrhythmias requires critical thinking skills and knowledge of assessment, and teaching and evaluation methods unique

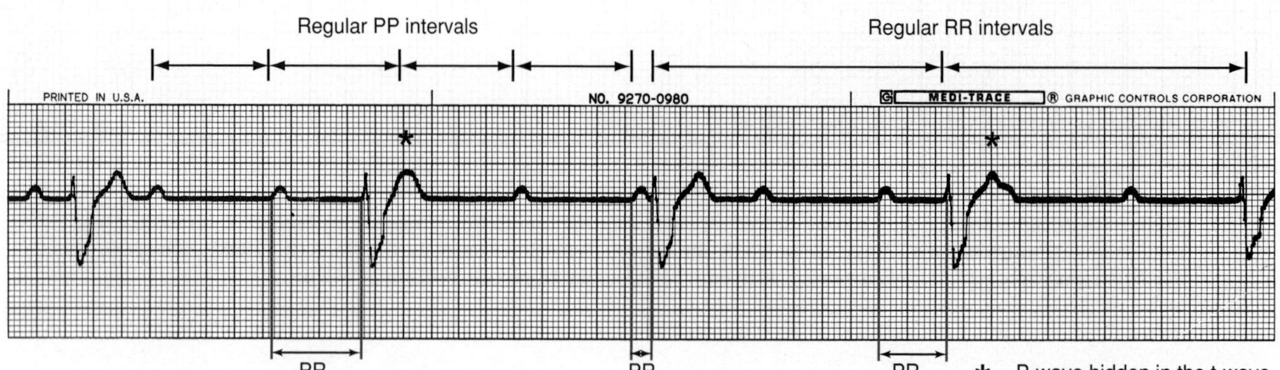

Figure 20-17. Sinus rhythm with third-degree AV block and idioventricular rhythm in lead V_1. Note irregular PR intervals. (From Smeltzer, S. C., & Bare, B. G. [2008]. *Brunner & Suddarth's textbook of medical surgical nursing* [11th ed.]. Philadelphia: Lippincott Williams & Wilkins.)

to the RN role. These skills cannot be delegated to an LPN or UAP.

1. Perform comprehensive physical assessments and provide care to the client with acute dysrhythmias and symptoms.
2. Delegate responsibly those activities that can be delegated, including basic care needs, assessment of vital signs, and measuring of intake and output for the stable client. All monitoring information is reported to the RN.
3. Assess for signs of inadequate cardiac output and tissue perfusion, including changes in BP, activity tolerance and LOC, and intervene with appropriate follow-through and treatments.
4. Provide information on changes in client status to the physician and appropriate members of the multidisciplinary team: Health care team discusses with client and family treatment options for clients with refractory dysrhythmias—includes implantable cardioverter defibrillator (ICD), permanent pacemaker, and cardiac ablation.
5. Provide client and family teaching about purpose for, dosage, timing, and side effects of medications.
6. Instruct client about pacemaker care.
   a. Take pulse and report slowing of rate; wear a medical alert bracelet or carry a medical alert card.
   b. Avoid high-magnetic fields and magnetic resonance imaging (MRI); airport or store alarms do not interfere with pacemaker at security checkpoints (e.g., airport or government buildings); request hand search.
   c. Monitor settings and report changes.
7. Facilitate follow-up outpatient care.

C. Safety and infection control
   1. Instruct client to monitor for signs and symptoms of infection after pacemaker insertion; avoid contact sports.
   2. Monitor vital signs during dosage adjustment.

D. Health promotion and maintenance: Provide teaching on promoting a healthy lifestyle, as well as routine physical assessments and follow-up care.

E. Psychologic integrity
   1. Assist client and family in coping with lifestyle changes.
   2. Assess client for social support and community resources.

F. Basic care and comfort: Maintain a calm environment.

G. Reduction of risk potential
   1. Inform client about major side effects of antidysrhythmic drugs, including hypotension, dizziness, nausea, vomiting, heart block, blood dyscrasias; toxicity includes diarrhea and central nervous system disturbances.
   2. Provide client teaching: Monitor heart rate daily; modify activity when symptomatic with dysrhythmias; avoid operating electrical appliances or have cell phones directly over the pacemaker or ICD site—if unusual sensations occur when near any electrical devices, move 5 to 10 feet away and check a pulse.
   3. Encourage certification in CPR for family members of client with history of life-threatening dysrhythmia—terminate CPR on return of pulse and spontaneous breathing, rescuer exhaustion, or arrival of professional help (e.g., paramedics).

H. Pharmacologic and parenteral therapies: Client and family will state the purpose, dosage, timing, and side effects of all antidysrhythmic drugs. Classifications of antidysrhythmic drugs and associated side effects are as follows (see reduction of risk potential for major side effects of antidysrhythmic drugs):
   1. Class I drugs—fast sodium channel blockers used to treat both atrial and ventricular dysrhythmias. Side effects include hypotension, nausea, vomiting, diarrhea, HF, increase in dysrhythmias; lupuslike syndrome with procainamide (Pronestyl); CNS changes (e.g., confusion, lethargy) with lidocaine (Xylocaine).
      a. Disopyramide (Norpace), procainamide (Pronestyl, Procanbid), quinidine (Quinidex, Cardioquin, Quinaglute)—treat symptomatic premature ventricular contractions, supraventricular tachycardia, ventricular tachycardia, and prevention of ventricular fibrillation.
      b. Lidocaine (Xylocaine), mexiletine (Mexitil), phenytoin (Dilantin), tocainide (Tonocard)—treat symptomatic premature ventricular contractions, ventricular tachycardia, and prevention of ventricular fibrillation.
      c. Propafenone (Rythmol), moricizine (Ethmozine)—treat life-threatening ventricular tachycardia or fibrillation and supraventricular tachycardia unresponsive to other drugs; has proarrhythmic effects.
   2. Class II drugs—beta-blockers used to treat supraventricular tachycardia. Side effects

include dizziness, fatigue, hypotension, HF, dysrhythmias, bronchospasms, and GI distress.
   a. Acebutolol (Sectral)
   b. Atenolol (Tenormin)
   c. Esmolol (Brevibloc)
   d. Metoprolol (Lopressor)
   e. Nadolol (Corgard)
   f. Propranolol (Inderal)
   g. Sotalol (Betapace)—also has a Class III effect
3. Class III drugs—potassium channel blockers used to treat ventricular tachycardia and ventricular fibrillation. Side effects include hypotension, nausea and vomiting, and bradycardia; amiodarone may cause hypothyroidism, pulmonary fibrosis, photosensitivity, bluish skin discoloration, corneal deposits, peripheral neuropathy, tremor.
   a. Amiodarone hydrochloride (Cordarone)
   b. Dofetilide (Tikosyn)
   c. Ibutilide (Corvert)
4. Class IV drugs—calcium channel blockers used to treat atrial fibrillation, atrial flutter, and supraventricular tachycardia. Side effects include dizziness, hypotension, edema, bradycardia, and constipation.
   a. Verapamil (Calan)
   b. Diltiazem (Cardizem)
5. Other antidysrhythmic drugs
   a. Adenosine (Adenocard) used to treat supraventricular dysrhythmias
   b. Digoxin (Lanoxin) used to treat atrial fibrillation and atrial flutter
   c. Magnesium sulfate used to treat ventricular dysrhythmias

Shock and Multiple Organ Dysfunction Syndrome

I. Definition: Shock is a clinical complex syndrome that manifests itself as a result of attempts by the body to achieve homeostasis in direct response to inadequate tissue perfusion; this results in impaired cellular metabolism. Shock often leads to systemic inflammatory response (SIRS) and multiple organ dysfunction syndrome (MODS).
   A. Shock—cellular hypoperfusion results when the cardiovascular system fails to function properly because of an alteration in blood volume, myocardial contractility, blood flow, and vascular resistance. Any disruption of components within the cardiovascular system results in the body's attempt to compensate, which manifests itself in the classic signs and symptoms of shock.
      1. Stages of shock—the generalized response to shock is very individualized, but the compensatory mechanism for all types progress on a continuum through four similar stages.
         a. Initial: Decreased cardiac output resulting in impaired tissue perfusion; aerobic to anaerobic metabolism resulting in buildup of lactic academia; changes occur at cellular level and may see no visible changes in client parameters.
         b. Compensatory: Sympathetic nervous system stimulation results in neural, hormonal, and chemical responses.
            (1) Neural—increased heart rate, increased myocardial contractility, arteriolar and venous constriction, and shunting of blood to vital organs
            (2) Hormonal—activation of renin-angiotensin system resulting in vasoconstriction, release of aldosterone and antidiuretic hormone, resulting in sodium and water retention, secretion of ACTH, resulting in increased serum glucose levels and release of epinephrine and norepinephrine
            (3) Chemical—hyperventilation as a result of lactic acidosis
         c. Progressive: Compensatory mechanisms fail and cells begin to die as a result of the hypoxic state; this leads to release of biochemical mediators. Organ systems begin to decompensate (respiratory, cardiovascular, neurologic, renal, hepatic, GI, and hematologic).
         d. Refractory (irreversible): Cellular death results in MODS.
      2. Classification of shock
         a. Hypovolemia: Involves decrease in circulating intravascular volume (greater than 15%), whether from external losses or internal fluid shifts; characterized by loss of circulating fluid volume, either blood or plasma resulting in circulatory dysfunction and inadequate tissue perfusion—most common classification; occurs with other types of shock.
         b. Cardiogenic: Pumping ability of the heart is compromised, leading to inadequate cardiac output and inadequate tissue perfusion.

c. Distributive or circulatory:
   (1) Anaphylaxis—antigen-antibody reaction evoking a life-threatening hypersensitivity response; histamine release leads to increased capillary permeability and massive vasodilation.
   (2) Neurogenic—involves loss or suppression of sympathetic (vasomotor) tone, resulting in vasodilation, decreased venous return, decreased cardiac output, and decreased tissue perfusion. Risk factors included with traumatic injury; CNS depressants and anesthesia; vital signs; skin color and temperature; urinary output; mentation. Parasympathetic nervous system dominates, and peripheral vasodilation and bradycardia occurs.
   (3) Septic—leading cause of death in intensive care units (mortality rate, 45%). Involves abnormal distribution of intravascular volume from vasodilation initiated by the body's response to overwhelming systemic infection, micro-organism byproducts, systemic inflammatory and immune response, and chemical mediator release.
      (a) Warm phase (early or hyperdynamic)—characterized by a high cardiac output with systemic vasodilation
      (b) Cold phase (late or hypodynamic)—characterized by deterioration of the client's hemodynamic status, with a fall in cardiac output and profound hypotension
   (4) Obstructive: Heart or great vessels become obstructed, resulting in decreased venous return, impairment of cardiac pumping; decreased BP; reduced tissue perfusion and cellular metabolism—most common cause is pulmonary embolus.

B. Multiple organ dysfunction syndrome—MODS results from SIRS and pertains to progressive failure of two or more body systems after a major insult to the body from infection, trauma, or severe illness with persistent hypotension and hypoxia. The four major organ systems affected by MODS are the pulmonary, renal, cardiovascular, and coagulation. MODS may be classified as primary or secondary.
   1. Primary MODS—results from a direct tissue insult; leads to impaired perfusion or ischemia.
   2. Secondary MODS—results as a complication from inadequate tissue perfusion.

II. Nursing process

A. Assessment
   1. Assess history of risk and presence of causative factors related to each type of shock.
      a. Hypovolemic—external excessive fluid losses from trauma, surgery, vomiting, diarrhea, diuresis, diabetes insipidus; fluid shifts from hemorrhage burns, ascites, peritonitis, dehydration.
      b. Cardiogenic—severe left ventricular myocardium damage as a result of anterior wall MI; noncoronary cardiogenic shock may result from conditions that stress the myocardium (e.g., severe hypoxemia, acidosis, hypoglycemia, hypocalcemia, and tension pneumothorax); ineffective myocardial function (e.g., cardiomyopathies, valvular damage, cardiac tamponade, dysrhythmias).
      c. Anaphylaxis—antigen-antibody reaction; pre-existing exposure to medication, foods associated with high allergic reactions (iodine-containing foods, coarse wheat products, various nuts), animals or insects, and other risk factors.
      d. Neurogenic—spinal cord damage or loss of vasomotor function; traumatic injury; CNS depressants and anesthesia.
      e. Septic—presence of endogenous mediators causing an overwhelming inflammatory response and massive vasodilation; immunosuppression; extreme age (less than 1 year and over 65 years); malnourishment; chronic illness; invasive procedures.
      f. Obstructive—predisposing diagnoses such as thrombophlebitis, DVT, and risk factors for DVT such as smoking and/or contraceptive use.
   2. Perform a comprehensive physical assessment.
      a. Assess vital signs, fluid status, hemodynamic status, and SpO_2.
      b. Assess clinical manifestations of shock in the respiratory, cardiovascular, neurologic, GI, renal, and integumentary systems such as LOC, vital signs, skin color and temperature, capillary refill, urinary output, client's ability to cope, cardiac rhythm, heart and lung sounds and movement, and peripheral pulses.

3. Assess for signs and symptoms of type of shock.
   a. Hypovolemia
      (1) Altered mentation
      (2) Tachypnea
      (3) Cool and clammy skin, weak and thready pulse, poor capillary refill
      (4) Tachycardia
      (5) Decreased urine output
      (6) Hypotension
      (7) Hemodynamics
         (a) Decreased cardiac output (CO), central venous pressure (CVP), pulmonary artery pressure (PAP), and pulmonary artery wedge pressure (PAWP)
         (b) Increased peripheral vascular resistance (PVR) and systemic vascular resistance (SVR)
   b. Cardiogenic
      (1) Hypotension (systolic BP less than 90 mmHg and mean arterial pressure less than 70 mmHg)
      (2) Thready, rapid pulse, narrow pulse pressure, distended neck veins, dysrhythmias, chest pain, cool, pale, moist skin, oliguria, altered mentation
      (3) Shallow, rapid respirations, dyspnea, crackles (pulmonary edema), S3 gallop, systolic murmur, diastolic murmur, heart sounds distant in cardiac tamponade
      (4) Hemodynamics
         (a) Decreased CO
         (b) Increased CVP, PAP, PAWP, PVR, and SVR
   c. Anaphylactic
      (1) Altered mental status; feeling of impending doom or fright
      (2) Hives; itching; flushed, warm skin
      (3) Increased heart rate, decreased BP
      (4) Tachypnea, stridor, wheezing
      (5) Abdominal cramping, nausea, vomiting, diarrhea
      (6) Hemodynamics: Decreased CO, CVP, PAP, PAWP, and SVR
   d. Neurogenic
      (1) Restlessness and confusion
      (2) Warm, dry skin
      (3) Bradycardia
      (4) No sweating below the level of injury; temperature-regulating center altered: Risk for overheating, chilling
      (5) Paralysis
      (6) Apnea, tachypnea, diaphragmatic breathing
      (7) Profound hypotension
      (8) Nausea, vomiting
      (9) Decreased urinary output
      (10) Hemodynamics
         (a) Decreased CO, CVP, PAP, PAWP, and SVR
         (b) Decreased heart rate (due to lost of sympathetic tone)
   e. Septic
      (1) Confusion, decreased LOC
      (2) Fever, chills, nausea, vomiting, diarrhea (early stage)
      (3) Tachycardia
      (4) Tachypnea
      (5) Cyanosis
      (6) Oliguria
      (7) Hemodynamics
         (a) Early (hyperdynamic)—increased CO; normal CVP, normal or elevated PAP, normal PAWP; and decreased SVR
         (b) Late (hypodynamic)—decreased CO; CVP, PAP; normal PAWP; and increased SVR
      (8) Clinical manifestations: Early signs of sepsis are signs of inflammation such as fever more than 38°C (100.4°F), tachypnea, hypocarbia, tachycardia, restlessness, hyperglycemia; late signs will include diminished LOC, coma, respiratory failure, HF, and oliguria.
   f. Obstructive
      (1) Change in LOC, tachycardia, hypotension, distended neck veins
      (2) Hemodynamics: Decreased CO, increased CVP, PAP, and PAWP
4. Obtain diagnostic tests: Test indicated by clinical manifestations.
   a. Radiographic tests such as chest x-ray, CT scan
   b. 12-Lead ECG—compare with earlier tracing
   c. Serum electrolytes, fasting blood glucose, BUN, creatinine, CBC, coagulation studies, serum lactate, end-tidal carbon dioxide monitoring ($ETCO_2$), and ABGs
   d. Urinalysis, blood, and wound culture and sensitivity
   e. Cardiac enzymes/markers
5. Assess for risk factors for MODS.
   a. Assess for primary and secondary risk factors.

(1) Primary: Severity of injury, shock, or SIRS
(2) Secondary: Infection, transfusion, multiple surgical procedures

b. Assess client's age (more common in older adult clients); pre-existing medical problems; presence of malnutrition, immunosuppression, and surgical or traumatic wounds.
c. Assess for signs of decreased tissue perfusion, cellular death, organ failure, microvascular coagulopathy—if hypermetabolic phase not reversed, will see jaundice, hyperbilirubinemia, oliguria, less response to vasoactive medications, fluids, and other treatments.

B. Analysis
1. Decreased Cardiac Output related to left ventricular failure, intravascular volume depletion, or vasodilation
2. Decreased Cardiac Output related to relative hypotension and bradycardia secondary to neurogenic shock
3. Decreased Cardiac Output related to alterations in heart rate, preload, contractility, and/or afterload
4. Ineffective Tissue Perfusion: Cardiopulmonary, Cerebral, Renal, GI, and Peripheral, related to decreased myocardial contractility, hypovolemia, or fluid shift from vascular spaces
5. Imbalanced Nutrition: Less Than Body Requirements related to increased metabolic demands or lack of exogenous nutrients
6. Impaired Gas Exchange related to ventilation/perfusion mismatching or intrapulmonary shunting
7. Hopelessness related to poor prognosis, decreased role performance, and quality of life
8. Anxiety related to dyspnea, activity intolerance, poor prognosis, decreased quality of life
9. Compromised Family Coping related to critically ill family member

C. Planning
1. Maintain hemodynamic stability and normovolemia.
2. Improve sensory, motor, and reflex functions.
3. Reduce anxiety and feelings of hopelessness.
4. Enhance functional capacity and quality of life.
5. Provide adequate oxygenation and tissue perfusion.
6. Prevent further alterations in body systems affected.
7. Prevent and treat infection.
8. Provide nutritional and metabolic support.

D. Implementation
1. Monitor and document hemodynamic status, vital signs, SpO_2, cardiac rhythm, lung sounds, and fluid status.
2. Assess perfusion by monitoring LOC, peripheral circulation, and urinary output.
3. Administer medications used in shock (see pharmacologic and parenteral therapies).
4. Provide nonpharmacologic interventions.
   a. Intra-aortic balloon pump
   b. Ventricular assist devices
   c. Ventilator support
   d. Hemodynamic monitoring (pulmonary artery catheter, arterial line)
5. Provide collaborative supportive measures based on type of shock and monitor effects of pharmacologic therapy and nonpharmacologic interventions.
   a. Hypovolemic—minimize fluid loss and monitor for complications.
   b. Cardiogenic—limit myocardial oxygen demand and monitor client's response to care.
   c. Anaphylactic—facilitate ventilations, administer volume replacement, emotional support, and maintain surveillance for complications.
   d. Neurogenic—provide DVT prophylaxis therapy: Calf and thigh measurement, antiembolic stockings, and/or sequential pneumatic stockings; administer prescribed anticoagulation therapy.
   e. Septic—identify clients at risk using evidence-based collaborative practice; monitor for complications and provide continual observation of process.
   f. Obstructive—limit myocardial oxygen demand and monitor client's response to care.
6. Provide interventions for MODS, including promoting early recognition, and supporting the client and monitoring organ perfusion.
7. Provide client and family teaching, including emotional and comfort measures, and anticipated course and treatment of shock.

E. Evaluation
1. Client has adequate cellular perfusion as measured by hemodynamic stability, improved LOC, and urinary output.
2. Client has effective breathing pattern and oxygenation/ventilation.

3. Client's fluid and electrolyte levels fall within reference limits.
4. Client and family verbalize understanding of plan of care and follow-up care needed.
5. Client's functional capability is optimized through tailored interventions and self-care behaviors based on individualized assessments and needs.

CN

III. Client needs
   A. Physiologic adaptation: Therapeutic management is directed toward supportive measures of vital organ systems with supplemental oxygen, mechanical ventilation, and fluid administration to maintain an adequate cardiac output. Assess for resolving symptoms of shock, improved cardiac output, perfusion, and tolerance to increasing levels of activity. Pathophysiologic sequences are as follows:
      1. Hypovolemic shock: Decreased blood volume, venous return, stroke volume, cardiac output, and tissue perfusion.
      2. Cardiogenic shock: Decreased cardiac contractility, stroke volume, cardiac output, pulmonary congestion, decreased systemic tissue perfusion, and decreased coronary artery perfusion.
      3. Anaphylactic, neurogenic, septic shock: Vasodilatation, maldistribution of blood volume, decreased venous return, decreased stroke volume, decreased cardiac output, decreased tissue perfusion.
      4. Obstructive shock: Decreased cardiac output and perfusion.
      5. MODS: If hypermetabolic state is not reversed—multiorgan failure of the GI, hepatobiliary, pulmonary, renal, cardiovascular, and coagulation systems.
   B. Management of care: Care of the client experiencing shock and MODS requires critical thinking skills and knowledge of assessment, and teaching and evaluation methods unique to the RN role. These skills cannot be delegated to an LPN or UAP.
      1. Perform frequent comprehensive assessments, assessing severity of symptoms, adequacy of cardiac output and oxygenation, perfusion, effectiveness of ventilation, and hemodynamic stability.
      2. Monitor client's hemodynamic status and report deviations to the HCP; assist in identifying and treating underlying disorder.
      3. Delegate responsibly those activities that can be delegated, including basic care needs and assessment of vital signs for the stable client. All monitoring information is reported to the RN.
      4. Facilitate client's plan of care with appropriate health care team.
      5. Help to reduce the risk of related complications from supportive technologies, therapies, decreased mobility, and compromised status.
         a. Monitor laboratory and diagnostic tests.
         b. If client is on a ventilator, position client for maximum alveolar ventilation and perfusion; maintain soft restraints to prevent accidental extubation; maintain ventilator settings; monitor ABGs, and SpO_2; administer sedation and other medications as appropriate.
         c. Perform mouth care every 2 hr and suctioning of endotracheal tube as needed, based on respiratory assessment.
         d. Monitor IV and hemodynamic monitoring device (arterial line, pulmonary artery catheter) sites every 2 hr and as needed—monitor distal pulses.
         e. Monitor nutritional status: Use antacids, histamine-2 blockers, or antipeptic agents to reduce the risk of damage to the GI system.
            (1) Enteral: Oral supplementation, tube feeding
               (a) Maintain tube placement; administer feedings and monitor client tolerance to feedings; detect and prevent complications.
               (b) Keep head of bed elevated 30 degrees, unless contraindicated.
               (c) For septic shock—maintain high protein to enhance client's overall nutritional status, immune system, and promote wound healing.
            (2) Total parenteral nutrition: Provide catheter care, administer solutions, prevent or correct complications, and evaluate client's response to feeding.
   C. Safety and infection control
      1. Use aseptic technique at all times to prevent infective processes; administer organism-specific antibiotics as ordered.
      2. Monitor all invasive sites for signs and symptoms of infection.
      3. Use appropriate restraints for client with altered mentation resulting in disruption of IV lines, catheters, endotracheal tubes, and assistive devices (IAPB, VAD).

4. Assess infusion pump function, IV site, and accurate dosage of IV fluids and medications.

D. Health promotion and maintenance
1. Monitor very young children and very old adults for hypovolemic shock; these clients are at greater risk because of dehydration or other underlying medical problems.
2. Promote self-care behaviors and compliance with diet and medication regimen in client with history of antigen-antibody reactions.
3. Instruct client and family about strategies to optimize health status and prevent further complications of shock and/or MODS.
4. Provide client and family teaching about emergency administration of medications, IV therapy, parenteral nutrition, skin care, exercise, ambulation, dietary needs, rehabilitation needs, and complications to assess for upon discharge.

E. Psychologic integrity
1. Encourage frequent and open communication about treatment modalities and options to ensure client's wishes are met regarding plan of care.
2. Promote client and family teaching by health care team regarding treatment options, living will, and advance directive to determine preferences while the client is able to participate in decisions with end-of-life care.

F. Basic care and comfort
1. Provide calm, quiet environment and encourage rest to reduce workload of the heart and promote optimal perfusion.
2. Allow family to participate in care as appropriate; encourage use of touch, relaxation, and imagery therapies, and manage physiologic symptoms as ordered.
3. Reduce fever through antipyretics and hyperthermia measures.
4. Promote end-of-life management, including assessment and adequate management of symptoms, and assessment and arrangement for palliative care needs.

G. Reduction of risk potential
1. Recognize client at risk for complications associated with decreased mobility.
2. Identify client at risk for insufficient vascular perfusion.
3. Monitor for side effects of medications.
4. Intervene to prevent aspiration: Check NG tube placement; recognize cultural differences contributing to potential complications following tests and procedures.
5. Plan and implement body system-specific interventions to prevent complications, including elastic stockings to prevent thrombus formation.
6. Assess client for abnormal neurologic status.
7. Determine client and family understanding of relevant information prior to procedure or surgery.

H. Pharmacologic and parenteral therapies: Client and family will state the purpose, dosage, timing, and side effects of all medications used to treat shock and MODS.
1. Hypovolemic shock
   a. Crystalloids (lactated Ringer solution or 0.9 % normal saline); and colloids (blood products, albumin, synthetic volume expanders such as Hespan)
      (1) Observe for and identify symptoms of fluid overload, coagulation disorders, and hypersensitivity reactions.
      (2) Observe blood precautions when administering blood products.
   b. Vasopressors after established blood-volume replacement
2. Cardiogenic shock
   a. Narcotic analgesics and sedatives: Morphine sulfate can minimize the SNS response to increase venous capacitance, decrease resistance to ejection, and relieve chest pain.
   b. Sympathomimetics (vasoconstrictors)
      (1) Norepinephrine (Levophed) and epinephrine (Adrenalin): Enhance cardiac output by increasing contractility, heart rate, or SVR—these drugs are used cautiously because of peripheral vascular dilation that robs vital organs of blood.
      (2) Dopamine (Intropin): Dose-dependent, and at high rates can cause tachycardiac and dysrhythmias.
   c. Positive inotropic agents
      (1) Dobutamine (Dobutrex): Increases strength of myocardial activity and improves cardiac output. Stimulates myocardial alpha-adrenergic receptors, resulting in decreased PAP and SVR. Improves stoke volume and ejection.
      (2) Milrinone (Primacor) used short term to improve myocardial contractility in HF.
   d. Venous and arterial vasodilators: Decrease preload and afterload, includes nitroprusside (Nipride),

nitroglycerin (Tridil). (See also pharmacologic and parenteral therapies in section on heart failure and cardiomyopathy for treatment of chronic HF.)
   e. Diuretics: Furosemide (Lasix)—decrease preload and achieve "optimal filling pressures" if client has pulmonary edema resulting in less workload of the heart. Monitor for signs of hypokalemia and dysrhythmias.
   f. Other medications: Thrombolytics/fibrinolytics, anticoagulants, antiplatelet agents, heparin, aspirin, GPIIb/IIA inhibitors (acute non-STEMI or STEMI MI).
3. Anaphylactic shock
   a. Oxygen
   b. Antihistamine (subcutaneous or IV diphenhydramine [Benadryl])
   c. Epinephrine (reverse vasodilatation and bronchoconstriction)
   d. Corticosteroids
   e. Bronchodilators
   f. Vasopressors
   g. Norepinephrine (Levophed) and dopamine (Intropin) if hypotensive
4. Neurogenic shock
   a. Fluids (isotonic) if BP is low
   b. Methylprednisolone (Solu-Medrol)
   c. Vasopressor (dopamine [Intropin] or norepinephrine [Levophed]) if BP does not respond to fluids
5. Septic shock
   a. Fluid (crystalloids or colloids)
   b. Broad-spectrum antibiotics
   c. Inotropics
   d. Other medications (drotrecogin alfa [Xigris]): Activated protein C—helps to decrease mortality in clients with severe sepsis and modulate inflammatory process; limits abnormal coagulation and fibrinolytics processes. Side effect is bleeding.
6. Obstructive shock
   a. Vasopressors (norepinephrine [Levophed])
   b. Thoracostomy tube, if tension pneumothorax
   c. Pericardiocentesis to relieve cardiac tamponade
7. MODS: Antibiotics (broad-spectrum antibiotics)
8. All types of shock
   a. Protein pump inhibitors
   b. Prophylaxis for deep vein thrombosis (DVT; heparin or low-molecular-weight heparin)

Bibliography

Abrams, A. C. (2004). *Clinical drug therapy: Rationales for nursing practice* (7th ed.). Philadelphia: Lippincott Williams & Wilkins.

American College of Cardiology/American Heart Association Task Force (2002). *ACC/AHA 2002 guideline update for the management of patients with chronic stable angina—summary article.* Retrieved May 15, 2008 from http://www.acc.org/qualityandscience/clinical/guidelines/stable/update_index.htm.

American College of Cardiology/American Heart Association Task Force (2002). *ACC/AHA guideline update for the management of patients with unstable angina and non–ST-segment elevation myocardial infarction.* Retrieved May 15, 2008 from http://www.acc.org/qualityandscience/clinical/guidelines/unstable/update_index.htm.

American College of Cardiology/American Heart Association Task Force (2005). *ACC/AHA 2005 guideline update for the diagnosis and management of chronic heart failure in the adult.* Retrieved May 15, 2008 from http://circ.ahajournals.org/cgi/content/full/112/12/e154.

Heart Failure Society of America (2006). *HFSA 2006 comprehensive heart failure practice guideline.* Retrieved May 15, 2008 from http://www.heartfailureguideline.com/index.cfm?id=130.

Hogan, M. A. (2005). *Pharmacology: Review & rationales.* Upper Saddle River, NJ: Pearson Prentice Hall.

Ignatavicius, D. D., & Workman, M. L. (2006). *Medical-surgical nursing* (5th ed.). Philadelphia: Saunders.

Lewis, S., Heitkemper, M., Dirksen, S., O'Brien, P., & Bucher, L. (2007). *Medical-surgical nursing: Assessment and management of clinical problems* (7th ed.). St. Louis: Mosby.

Morton, P. G., Fontaine, D. K., Hudak, C. M., & Gallo, B. M. (2005). *Critical care nursing: A holistic approach* (8th ed.). Philadelphia: Lippincott Williams & Wilkins.

Smeltzer, S. C., & Bare, B. G. (2004). *Brunner & Suddarth's textbook of medical-surgical nursing* (10th ed.). Philadelphia: Lippincott Williams & Wilkins.

Smeltzer, S. C., Bare, B. G., Hinkle, J. L., & Cheever, K. H. (2008). *Brunner & Suddarth's textbook of medical-surgical nursing* (11th ed.). Philadelphia: Lippincott Williams & Wilkins.

Urden, L. D., Stacy, K. M., & Lough, M. E. (2006). *Thelan's critical care nursing: Diagnosis and management* (5th ed.). St. Louis: Mosby.

U.S. Department of Health and Human Services. (2004). *The seventh report of the Joint National Committee on Prevention, Detection, Evaluation, and Treatment of High Blood Pressure.* Retrieved May 15, 2008 from http://www.nhlbi.nih.gov/guidelines/hypertension/jnc7full.pdf.

CHAPTER 20

Practice Test

Acute Coronary Syndrome

1. A client with acute MI receives alteplase, recombinant t-PA. The nurse should report which of the following to the physician as being an untoward effect of the medication?
   - □ 1. Absent pedal pulses
   - □ 2. Vomiting
   - □ 3. Epistaxis
   - □ 4. ST-segment elevation of ECG

2. AF A middle-aged client is hospitalized for a cholecystectomy and has an acute onset of chest pain. In which order should the nurse perform the following interventions? Place in order from first to last.
   - _____ 1. Administer sublingual nitroglycerin.
   - _____ 2. Check vital signs.
   - _____ 3. Draw serum CK- MB and troponin levels.
   - _____ 4. Obtain 12-lead ECG.

3. A client with a diagnosis of unstable angina is going to have a cardiac catheterization. Prior to the procedure the nurse should:
   - □ 1. Administer a dose of nitroglycerin.
   - □ 2. Assess and record peripheral pulses.
   - □ 3. Verify the client had an echocardiogram.
   - □ 4. Insert a central line.

Coronary Artery Disease

4. The client diagnosed with hypertension and chronic angina is receiving metoprolol (Lopressor). The current vital signs are: BP 132/80 and apical heart rate of 62. The nurse should:
   - □ 1. Administer the medication as ordered.
   - □ 2. Hold the drug until the vital signs are reported to the physician.
   - □ 3. Wait 1 hr and recheck vital signs, then decide whether to administer the drug.
   - □ 4. Withhold the drug because the vital signs are normal.

5. A client with CAD is taking atorvastatin (Lipitor). The nurse should instruct the client to:
   - □ 1. Be admitted to the hospital to regulate the dose.
   - □ 2. Increase exercise if muscle cramps occur.
   - □ 3. Have periodic laboratory tests for liver function.
   - □ 4. Monitor BP daily.

Heart Failure and Cardiomyopathy

6. AF When assessing a client with HF, which of the following findings does the nurse report to the HCP? Select all that apply.
   - □ 1. Bibasilar crackles.
   - □ 2. BP 108/62, heart rate 88.
   - □ 3. O_2 saturation 94%.
   - □ 4. 2-pound weight gain in 5 days.
   - □ 5. Urine output 20 ml/hr.
   - □ 6. Confusion.

7. The nurse is planning care for a client with hypertropic cardiomyopathy. The physician orders a dopamine (Intropin) IV infusion to start at 3 mcg/kg per minute and titrate to keep the BP more than 100 systolic. The nurse should:
   - □ 1. Question the order and call the physician.
   - □ 2. Initiate the dopamine drip to increase cardiac output.
   - □ 3. Start the dopamine at 1 mcg/kg per minute and titrate to the ordered dose.
   - □ 4. Weigh the client prior to starting the infusion.

8. A client with acute HF is receiving IV antibiotics mixed in 100-ml bags of fluid every 4 hr. The nurse should monitor the client for signs and symptoms of:
   - □ 1. Decrease in afterload.
   - □ 2 Reduction in preload.
   - □ 3. Increase in cardiac workload.
   - □ 4. Improvement in pulmonary gas exchange.

9. A client with symptoms of fluid volume overload is hospitalized for acute exacerbation of HF and is to start on an IV infusion of nesiritide (Natrecor). The nurse should:
   - □ 1. Assess urine output.
   - □ 2. Check BP.
   - □ 3. Insert an arterial line.
   - □ 4. Instruct client to report swelling of the feet.

Hypertension

10. A client's BP has continued to be greater than 150/95 after 4 months of a low-sodium diet and daily exercise of walking for 30 min. The nurse should instruct the client to:
    - □ 1. Contact the HCP.
    - □ 2. Decrease calorie count by 10%.

□ 3. Increase exercise by jogging.
□ 4. Continue current treatment plan.

11. A female client who is 32 years of age has been diagnosed with stage 1 hypertension. The client's height is 5 feet 5 inches, and her weight is recorded as 125 pounds; she reports that she frequently eats at "fast food" restaurants and enjoys a glass of wine to relax on weekends. In developing a teaching plan for this client, the nurse should first address which of the following topics?
□ 1. Use of nitroprusside (Nipride).
□ 2. Adverse effects of alcohol.
□ 3. Decreasing dietary caloric intake.
□ 4. Low-sodium food choices.

12. During a home visit, the nurse assesses a client who is taking hydrochlorothiazide (HydroDIURILl) and lisinopril (Prinivil) for the treatment of hypertension. Which symptom would indicate a need to inform the physician of a need to change medication therapy?
□ 1. BP is 132/80.
□ 2. Persistent cough.
□ 3. Potassium level is 4.1 mEq/L.
□ 4. Waking up at night to void.

Inflammatory and Valvular Diseases

13. A nurse is evaluating a client for cardiac tamponade immediately following a pericardiocentesis. The nurse should report which of the following to the HCP?
□ 1. Rising CVP.
□ 2. Increase in BP.
□ 3. Client expression of relief.
□ 4. Audible heart sounds.

Valvular and Cardiac Surgery

14. The nurse is providing care for a client after a mechanical aortic valve replacement. The nurse determines the need for further discharge teaching when the client tells the nurse:
□ 1. "I will avoid alcohol now that I am taking my daily warfarin (Coumadin)."
□ 2. "I will limit my physical activity to avoid stress on my new valve."
□ 3. "I will need prophylactic antibiotic therapy prior to any surgery."
□ 4. "I will start a cardiac rehabilitation program on discharge."

15. Following open heart surgery, a nurse is administering sodium nitroprusside (Nipride) to a client by IV drip. The nurse should assess the client for which of the following?
□ 1. LOC.
□ 2. BP.
□ 3. Pulse oximetry.
□ 4. Breath sounds.

Cardiac Dysrhythmias

16. AF The nurse is assessing a client diagnosed with an MI. The nurse identifies the following rhythm on the monitor as:

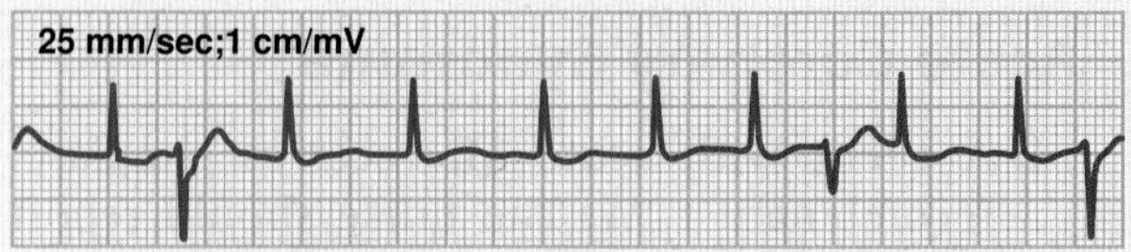

□ 1. Atrial flutter.
□ 2. Premature ventricular contractions.
□ 3. Third-degree heart block.
□ 4. Ventricular tachycardia.

17. A nurse is caring for a client following implantation of an automatic internal cardioverter-defibrillator (AICD). The nurse should first determine:
□ 1. Activation status of the device.
□ 2. Client's anxiety level.
□ 3. Provision of a medic-alert card.
□ 4. Postdischarge physical activity order.

Shock and Multiple Organ Dysfunction Syndrome

18. A client is admitted to the ICU with a MI. Which assessment indicates to the nurse the development of cardiogenic shock?
□ 1. Bradycardia.
□ 2. Increased BP.
□ 3. Oliguria.
□ 4. Warm, flushed skin.

19. A client is started on digoxin (Lanoxin). The physician prescribes IV doses of 0.5 mg now, 0.25 mg in 8 hr, and another 0.25 mg in another 8 hr. The client has a 1,000-ml bag of NS infusing at 25 ml/hr. The nurse should next:
□ 1. Add the medication to the fluid remaining in the IV bag of solution.
□ 2. Infuse each dose over 30 min using an IV piggyback set-up.
□ 3. Question the physician over the dosing and frequency of the medication.
□ 4. Administer each dose of medication over 5 min via IV push.

20. A client who is in cardiogenic shock following a MI is receiving IV nitroglycerin. The nurse documents which of the following to indicate nitroglycerin is achieving the desired therapeutic effect?
□ 1. The client's chest pain is relieved.
□ 2. There is a decrease in the client's edema.
□ 3. The client has fewer bleeding episodes.
□ 4. The client's skin is no longer diaphoretic.

Answers and Rationales

1. 3 t-PA promotes thrombolysis and is used to restore blood flow to the occluded coronary artery. Bleeding is a major side effect. Absence of pedal pulses suggests arterial occlusion or a decrease in cardiac output. Vomiting is not an adverse affect of the medication. ST elevation represents myocardial injury associated with the MI. (D)

2. 2, 1, 4, 3 With the onset of acute chest pain, the nurse first assesses vital signs to determine the client's hemodynamic stability and guide further interventions. Prior to administration of nitroglycerin, BP is assessed because of increased risk of hypotension. NTG is a vasodilator that reduces myocardial oxygen requirements, improves coronary artery perfusion, and can be administered if systolic BP is above 90 mmHg to relieve chest pain. The nurse can then obtain a 12-lead ECG to identify ischemia or injury to the heart; it may show changes during symptoms and in response to treatment. Cardiac markers are drawn last to assist in establishing the diagnosis of MI because ST elevation by ECG may not be evident. (M)

3. 2 Prior to a cardiac catheterization, baseline vital signs and peripheral pulses are assessed and recorded. Catheter access to the left side of the heart is through arterial insertion. A decrease or absence of peripheral pulse warrants investigation. Nitroglycerin and an echocardiogram may have been provided in client care, but are not prerequisites for a cardiac catheterization. A central line is not required, but peripheral IV access is needed for the procedure. (R)

4. 1 Metoprolol is a cardioselective beta blocker that decreases BP and heart workload through blocking beta 1 receptors, which decreases heart rate and force of contraction. Client's BP is high normal range and heart rate is greater than 60; the drug can safely be given by the nurse. The client requires treatment to maintain a normal BP and prevent angina. (D)

5. 3 "Statin" drugs are used to treat hyperlipidemia. Serious side effects of atorvastatin (Lipitor) are liver toxicity and myopathy. The client requires baseline and periodic assessment of liver function. Advise client to report muscle pain or weakness immediately and to discontinue use of the drug until evaluated by a HCP. BP monitoring is not required for this medication. Lipid profiles are used to assess the drug's effectiveness. (D)

6. 4, 5 The nurse reports signs of decreased tissue perfusion to the HCP; these include a decrease in urine output and confusion. Crackles, edema, and weight gain are monitored closely, but are not as high a priority as decreasing tissue perfusion. Vital signs and oxygen saturation are within normal limits. (M)

7. 1 Dopamine is a positive inotrope, which is contraindicated in the treatment for hypertrophic cardiomyopathy. The left ventricular outflow tract will be further obstructed by increasing the myocardial contraction of the hypertrophic ventricle. Dopamine less than 3 mcg/kg per minute has a dopaminergic effect, which increases urine output. Weighing the client is needed for dosing. (S)

8. 3 The amount of IV fluids may increase rather than decrease preload and thus increase the workload of the heart in a client with HF. Pulmonary congestion may interfere with gas exchange. A decrease in afterload results from vasodilation of the arterioles. (R)

9. 2 Nesiritide is not administered for a systolic BP less than 90 mmHg. Nesiritide causes a balanced vasodilation of arterioles and veins. Hypotension is a side effect. An arterial line is not required, but should be considered in an unstable client for close monitoring of BP. Nesiritide causes a diuresis, not edema and swelling of the feet. (D)

10. 1 The goal of therapy in the management of hypertension is a BP less than 140/90. Lifestyle modifications such as a low-sodium diet and physical activity may reduce BP, but often are not sufficient. The nurse refers the client to the HCP, who will likely prescribe antihypertensive drugs along with lifestyle management as the BP is above the recommendation. Increasing the exercise and decreasing calorie count may be helpful, but likely will not bring the BP into the desired range. The client should not continue with the current plan of care as the BP is not in the desired range. (M)

11. 4 Lifestyle modification to lower BP includes weight reduction in clients who are overweight, reducing the intake of dietary sodium, and an increase in physical activity. Client teaching involves instruction on low-sodium diet and foods because of the propensity for high-sodium foods at fast food restaurants. The client is of a normal weight and alcohol intake is in moderation. Nipride is a treatment for hypertensive crisis. (H)

12. 2 A persistent cough is a side effect of the ACE inhibitor that may warrant a change to another antihypertensive medication. BP and potassium are within normal limits. The nurse assesses when the drug is taken and changes to an earlier time of administration. (D)

13. 1 Following pericardiocentesis, a rise in BP and a fall in CVP are expected; the nurse reports increased CVP as a sign of increasing fluid. The client expresses immediate relief of the symptoms such as dyspnea. Heart sounds are no longer muffled or distant. (R)

14. 2 Physical activity is gradually increased and encouraged. Alcohol potentiates warfarin (Coumadin) and alters PT/INR levels. Antibiotics are used prophylactically prior to any invasive medical or dental procedures. Cardiac rehabilitation is started once the client is stable. (H)

15. 2 Sodium nitroprusside causes the release of intravascular nitric oxide and is considered a potent vasodilator of arteries and veins. Frequent monitoring of BP is needed to achieve optimal effect and prevent unwanted hypotension. Changes in LOC may result, but typically secondary to severe hypotension. Monitoring pulse oximetry and breath sounds are unrelated to sodium nitroprusside therapy. (D)

16. 2 The rhythm strip displays multifocal PVCs. The abnormal complexes are wide and bizarre in appearance. (A)

17. 1 After insertion of an AICD, the nurse assesses device settings. The nurse needs to know whether the device is activated, the heart rate cutoff above which it will fire, and the number of shocks it is programmed to deliver. Anxiety level, medic alert card or bracelet, and postdischarge activity order are important considerations, but not the highest priority directly after insertion of the AICD. (R)

18. 3 Cardiogenic shock occurs with severe damage (greater than 40%) to the left ventricle. Classic signs include hypotension, rapid pulse that becomes weaker, decreased urine output, and cool, clammy skin. (A)

19. 4 Digoxin (Lanoxin) is a potent cardiovascular drug that both slows conduction and increases contractility of the heart. Digoxin is administered slowly via IV push. Although each 1 ml can be diluted in 4 ml of SW, NS, D5W, or LR for injection, it is not added to the IV bag of solution or given over a 30-min duration. There is no need to question the physician at this time. Because digoxin (Lanoxin) is a new medication for this client and because it takes this type of dosing to reach a therapeutic level, dosing such as the one described is typical when the medication is first initiated. It is a type of loading dose protocol and for digoxin, sometimes referred to as *digitalization*. (D)

20. 1 Cardiac ischemia associated with MI causes the client to experience pain. Nitroglycerin helps improve coronary blood flow to ischemic regions, which then decreases pain. Nitroglycerin does not directly affect fluid volume status to decrease edema, and does not have an effect on blood clotting or any bleeding episodes. Diaphoresis associated with MI is related to sympathetic system stimulation and is not treated with nitroglycerin. (D)

chapter 21

The Client With Vascular Disease

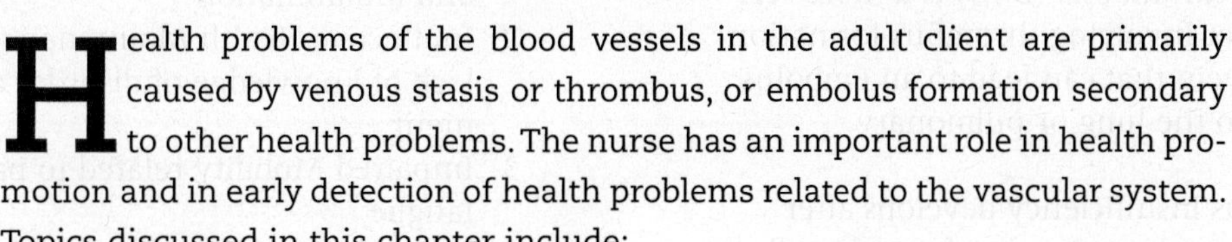

Health problems of the blood vessels in the adult client are primarily caused by venous stasis or thrombus, or embolus formation secondary to other health problems. The nurse has an important role in health promotion and in early detection of health problems related to the vascular system. Topics discussed in this chapter include:

- Venous Disorders: Venous Thrombosis, Chronic Venous Insufficiency, and Varicose Veins
- Arterial Diseases: Peripheral Arterial Disease, Thromboangiitis Obliterans, and Raynaud Disease
- Aortic Aneurysm

Venous Disorders: Venous Thrombosis, Chronic Venous Insufficiency, and Varicose Veins

I. Definition: Diseases of the vein include inflammation, clotting, and distention. The legs are particularly affected because of the effect of gravity on venous circulation.
   A. Venous thrombosis is the formation of a thrombus (clot) in a vein and is associated with inflammation. The disorder results from at least one component of Virchow triad: Venous stasis, damage to the endothelial lining of the vein, and hypercoagulopathy. Associated disease processes include the following:
      1. Superficial thrombophlebitis is thrombosis of a superficial vein and is usually treated at home. Thrombophlebitis refers to inflammation caused by a clot in a vein and occurs more commonly in the lower extremities.
      2. Deep vein thrombosis (DVT) is a more serious disorder involving thrombus formation in a deep vein that can lead to an embolus traveling to the lung or pulmonary embolism.
   B. Chronic venous insufficiency develops after prolonged venous hypertension from thrombus obstruction or incompetent valves. Increase in hydrostatic pressure stretches vein walls and prevents valves from closing fully, causing a backward flow of venous blood. Prolonged venous stasis results in lower extremity edema, discoloration of the skin, and venous stasis ulceration.
   C. Varicose veins or varicosities are distended, tortuous, palpable subcutaneous veins resulting from pooled blood.

II. Nursing process
   A. Assessment
      1. Assess risk factors for venous disorders.
         a. Modifiable: Immobility, obesity, use of oral contraceptives.
         b. Nonmodifiable: Vein trauma, pregnancy, surgery, cancer, blood dyscrasias, and heart failure.
      2. Obtain a detailed health history, including past medical and surgical history and family history; and perform a detailed physical assessment.
      3. Assess for signs and symptoms.
         a. Venous thrombosis: Superficial thrombophlebitis can be palpated as a linear hardened cord with associated tenderness, pain, warmth, and erythema. Deep vein thrombosis may be asymptomatic or may manifest as tenderness, pain, warmth over the involved area with swelling of the extremity, skin discoloration, and prominent superficial veins; fever may be present; Homans sign is not a reliable assessment.
         b. Chronic venous insufficiency causes edema, stasis dermatitis with a brown discoloration extending from the ankle to the calf; venous stasis ulcers and cellulitis may develop.
         c. Varicose veins appear as darkened, protruding, tortuous veins that cause swelling, heaviness, aching after standing, and nocturnal cramping.
      4. Obtain diagnostic tests.
         a. CBC, platelet count, PT/INR, APTT, bleeding time, D-dimer
         b. Duplex ultrasound, plethysmography, venography
   B. Analysis
      1. Acute Pain related to venous congestion and inflammation
      2. Ineffective Health Maintenance related to lack of knowledge of disorder and treatment
      3. Impaired Mobility related to pain and leg fatigue
      4. Disturbed Body Image related to skin discoloration and disfigured, protruding veins
      5. Risk for Impaired Skin Integrity related to edema, venous stasis, decreased nutrition
      6. Risk for Bleeding related to anticoagulation therapy
      7. Risk for Pulmonary Embolism related to venous thrombus formation
   C. Planning
      1. Relieve pain.
      2. Decrease edema.
      3. Maintain skin integrity.
      4. Prevent complications such as pulmonary embolism.
   D. Implementation
      1. Provide anticoagulation therapy.
      2. Elevate extremity.
      3. Provide wound care.
      4. Obtain elastic compression stockings.
      5. Provide client and family teaching (see management of care).
      6. Restrict physical activity to prevent release of emboli; when client is able to resume activity, encourage to promote venous return.
   E. Evaluation
      1. Client experiences absence of pain and edema.

2. Client exhibits intact skin or restoration of skin integrity.
3. Client has no signs of respiratory and bleeding complications.

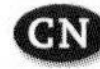

III. Client needs

A. Physiologic adaptation: The primary goal of treatment of venous disorders is to prevent release of emboli. Venous disorders can be treated with anticoagulants, thrombolytic therapy, and with bed rest and use of heat. Surgically placed filters can be inserted into the inferior vena cava to trap emboli. For varicose veins, sclerotherapy or laser treatment can be performed for cosmetic purpose. Surgical ligation and dissection may be performed for venous insufficiency uncontrolled by conservative therapy or recurrent thrombophlebitis in varicose veins.

B. Management of care: Care of the client with a venous disorder requires critical thinking skills and knowledge of assessment, and teaching and evaluation methods unique to the RN role. These skills cannot be delegated to an LPN or UAP.

1. Monitor vital signs, peripheral pulses, extremity circumference, edema, skin breakdown, wound healing, fluid status to maintain adequate hydration, and for signs of pulmonary embolism (dyspnea, tachypnea, chest pain, and decrease in SpO_2).
2. Delegate responsibly those activities that can be delegated, including basic hygiene needs to clients on bed rest with limited mobility, recording of vital signs, and measurement of intake and output. All monitoring information is reported to the RN.
3. Manage DVT.
   a. Provide DVT prophylaxis for clients on bed rest.
      (1) Unfractionated heparin or low-molecular-weight heparin (LMWH) subcutaneous injections
      (2) Sequential compression device (SCD)
      (3) Leg exercises
   b. Promote bed rest; elevate the extremity 10 to 20 degrees above the heart.
   c. Administer IV or subcutaneous heparin, LMWH, or hirudin derivatives (for clients with heparin-induced thrombocytopenia) until warfarin (Coumadin) at therapeutic level.
   d. Start warfarin (Coumadin) PO and continue for 3 to 6 months.
   e. Surgeon can insert vena cava filter for clients at high risk for pulmonary embolism.
   f. Promote thrombolytic therapy or surgical thrombectomy to dissolve clot.
   g. Apply elastic compression stockings or 4-inch elastic bandages once client begins ambulation.
   h. Obtain customized elastic compression stockings, such as Jobst stockings, or sleeve for upper extremity once edema has resolved.
4. Manage chronic venous insufficiency and venous stasis ulcers.
   a. Elevate extremity frequently; elevate foot of bed when sleeping.
   b. Apply elastic compression stockings, wraps, or bandages.
   c. Provide wound assessment and moist environment dressing for wound care.
   d. Promote wound debridement.
   e. Administer antibiotics for wound infection or cellulitis.
   f. Provide care for complicated ulceration: Unna paste boot or bed rest with elevation and compression dressing.
5. Manage varicose veins.
   a. Promote rest with limb elevated; promote walking, and compression stockings.
   b. Prepare client for sclerotherapy or laser treatment (used for cosmetic purpose) of surgical ligation and dissection.
6. Provide information on changes in client status to the physician and appropriate members of the multidisciplinary team.
7. Instruct client regarding medications and associated side effects; nutritious diet; management of risk factors, including signs of a pulmonary embolism and when to seek medical attention; reasons for compression or antiembolism stockings, activity, and leg elevation; methods for skin and wound care; avoidance of restrictive clothing; and need for regular follow-up care.
8. Assess need for home health assistance and social support.

C. Safety and infection control

1. Avoid heating pads, hot water bottles, and hot baths.
2. Observe bleeding and fall precautions if client receiving anticoagulation therapy.

D. Health promotion and maintenance: Promote nutritious diet and smoking cessation.

E. Psychologic integrity: Encourage client to adjust lifestyle to use devices such as support hose, and to increase activity.

F. Basic care and comfort

1. Reposition client on bed rest every 2 hr; use therapeutic bed or mattress.

2. Avoid tape application to skin.
3. Apply moisturizing lotion to skin.
4. Provide pain management.
5. Brush teeth with soft toothbrush—no vigorous flossing for clients on anticoagulation.

G. Reduction of risk potential
1. Inspect IV sites every hour.
2. Monitor for signs of bleeding. Monitor laboratory results: PT, INR, APTT, Hgb, Hct, platelets.
3. Avoid IM injections for clients on anticoagulation therapy and review medications that may interfere with anticoagulation.
4. Eliminate modifiable risk factors for DVT (see assessment for risk factors).
5. Avoid alcohol with anticoagulation therapy.
6. Avoid sitting or stationery standing for long periods.
7. Promote proper use of elastic compression stockings without restriction of circulation.
8. Discontinue estrogen once DVT has occurred.
9. Administer stool softeners for clients on anticoagulation therapy to avoid straining and bleeding.

H. Pharmacologic and parenteral therapies: Client will state the purpose, dosage, timing, and side effects of medications to treat venous disorders. The following drugs are used to manage venous thrombosis.
1. Heparin (IV, SC): Heparin IV 3 to 5 days until warfarin (Coumadin) is at therapeutic level, INR 2.0 to 3.0 for DVT
   a. Expected outcome: Prevents emboli formation.
   b. Reduction of risk potential: Monitor APTT for therapeutic level with IV infusion; protamine sulfate or fresh-frozen plasma (FFP) to reverse effects.
   c. Management of care: Monitor platelet count for heparin-induced thrombocytopenia (HIT) requiring discontinuation and no further use of any heparin product.
2. Hirudin derivatives (IV): Lepirudin (Refludan), bivalirudin (Angiomax), argatroban (Acova)
   a. Expected outcome: Used in clients with HIT when anticoagulation is still required.
   b. Reduction of risk potential: Monitor APTT for therapeutic levels; no known antidote.
   c. Management of care: Monitor platelet level.
3. Low-molecular-weight heparin (SC): Enoxaparin (Lovenox), dalteparin (Fragmin), ardeparin (Normiflo)
   a. Expected outcome: Anticoagulation; more predictable dose response than heparin.
   b. Reduction of risk potential: Protamine sulfate or FFP reverses effects.
   c. Management of care: Monitor platelet level for HIT.
4. Warfarin (Coumadin), PO
   a. Expected outcome: Anticoagulation (requires a few days to obtain therapeutic dose).
   b. Management of care: Provide steady diet of vitamin K (green, leafy vegetables) to maintain stable drug levels.
   c. Reduction of risk potential: Monitor PT/INR for therapeutic level.

Arterial Diseases: Peripheral Arterial Disease, Thromboangiitis Obliterans, and Raynaud Disease

I. Definition: Arterial diseases involve degeneration or inflammation of the arteries. Common arterial diseases include peripheral arterial disease, thromobangiitis obliterans and Raynaud disease.

A. Peripheral arterial disease (PAD) is a progressive narrowing and degeneration of the arteries occurring most commonly as a result of atherosclerosis, which involves diminishing of arterial blood supply beyond the area of narrowing. The most common sites of atherosclerosis are peripheral areas of artery bifurcation, iliac arteries, femoral arteries, and popliteal arteries. Diabetics tend to develop the disease in the distal popliteal, anterior and posterior tibial, and peroneal arteries. The classic symptom of PAD is intermittent claudication.

B. Thromboangiitis obliterans (Buerger disease) is a segmental inflammatory disorder characterized by a combination of acute inflammation and thrombosis of the arteries and veins in the hands and feet. The disease is not caused by atherosclerosis. Obstruction of blood flow can lead to skin ulcerations and gangrene of fingers and toes. The disorder occurs predominately in men age 20 to 40 years and is strongly associated with heavy cigarette smoking.

C. Raynaud disease is an episodic disorder with vasospasm of the small cutaneous arteries and reduced blood supply most commonly in the fingers and toes, but may occur in the nose and ears. Skin color changes are, first, white (pallor) as the blood supply is reduced; second, blue (cyanosis) as oxygen supply to the area is depleted; and lastly, bright red (rubor) as blood returns to the area. As blood returns, it is often accompanied by a throbbing or burning sensation, cold, and numbness. Episodes can be triggered by exposure to cold, emotions, stress, and anxiety. Attacks typically last a few minutes.

1. Primary Raynaud disease has the typical symptoms of pain or numbness and skin color changes with no other causative medical problem.
2. Secondary Raynaud disease, or Raynaud phenomenon, occurs when the vasospasm are secondary to another medical condition, such as connective tissue diseases, scleroderma, rheumatoid arthritis, lupus; vibration white finger, occlusive arterial disease, thoracic outlet syndrome, or carpel tunnel syndrome. Raynaud phenomenon can be associated with migraine headaches, variant angina, and pulmonary hypertension.

II. Nursing process

A. Assessment

1. Assess for risk factors for atherosclerosis (see Chapter 20).
2. Obtain a detailed heath history, including past medical and surgical history, as well as psychosocial history.
3. Perform a comprehensive physical assessment: Assess vital signs; peripheral pulses; capillary refill; color, temperature, sensation, and movement of the extremity; edema; activity tolerance; and presence and location of claudication pain.
4. Assess signs and symptoms of acute arterial occlusion, such as:
   a. Sudden onset of severe pain, pallor, coldness, numbness, and absence of pulses distal to the occlusion.
   b. Sensory and motor loss occur.
5. Assess for signs and symptoms of PAD, including:
   a. Presence of pain, ache, cramp, or tired feeling with walking—can occur in the calf, foot, thigh, hip, or buttocks. Pain location correlates with the level of occlusion. Similar symptoms related to exertion can occur with involvement of the arm.
   b. Diminished or absent pulses distal to the occlusion, decreased capillary refill, and sensations of coldness and numbness.
   c. Pallor on elevation of extremity; rubor with dependent positioning of extremity.
   d. Skin observed as thin and shiny, with loss of hair on extremity; presence of skin breakdown with ulceration. Nails thickened or brittle.
6. Assess for signs and symptoms of Buerger disease.
   a. Claudication or pain occurs when the hands or feet are at rest (not following exercise).
   b. Pain typically begins in the distal extremity but may radiate to more central area of the body.
   c. Presence of numb or tingling sensation.
   d. Skin color changes similar to those seen in Raynaud phenomenon.
   e. Skin ulceration and gangrene of the fingers and toes accompanied by intense pain.
7. Assess for signs and symptoms of Raynaud disease: Color changes (pallor, cyanosis, and rubor as discussed in definition) in fingers and toes (less common in nose, ears, or lips) in response to exposure to cold or emotional stress. May also experience numb, cold, or painful sensation in affected area.
8. Obtain diagnostic tests.
   a. Ankle/brachial index (ABI)
      (1) Normal ABI more than 90 mm Hg
      (2) Mild arterial insufficiency, ABI 70–90 mm Hg
      (3) Moderate arterial insufficiency, ABI 50–70 mm Hg
      (4) Severe arterial insufficiency, ABI less than 50 mm Hg
   b. Doppler ultrasound, Duplex ultrasound imaging
   c. Angiography
   d. Magnetic resonance angiography
   e. Cold stimulation test for Raynaud disease

B. Analysis

1. Ineffective Tissue Perfusion: Arterial, related to decreased arterial blood flow
2. Chronic Pain related to tissue ischemia
3. Activity Intolerance related to ischemic pain, oxygen demand greater than supply
4. Impaired Skin Integrity related to impaired perfusion, decreased sensation, and vulnerability to infection
5. Ineffective Therapeutic Regimen Management related to lack of knowledge of disease, treatment, and self-care measures

C. Planning

1. Maintain tissue perfusion.
2. Relieve pain.
3. Improve exercise tolerance.
4. Maintain skin integrity.

D. Implementation

1. Manage risk factors.
2. Administer medications to reduce claudication and vasospasm.

3. Promote walking exercise therapy.
4. Perform ischemic leg and wound care.
5. Surgeon may initiate percutaneous endovascular therapy or surgical procedures for incapacitating pain or threatened viability of the limb.
6. Provide teaching on control of modifiable risk factors, medications and associated side effects, diet, exercise, and self-care behaviors.

E. Evaluation
1. Client's peripheral pulses are palpable; ABI more than 90.
2. Client exhibits activity tolerance without pain.
3. Client exhibits intact skin or restoration of skin integrity.
4. Client has normal lipid levels and BP.

CN

III. Client needs

A. Physiologic adaptation: Management of arterial disease is directed at increasing blood flow to the affected part. Arterial disease may improve by reducing risk factors by losing weight, increasing exercise, stopping smoking, and managing hypertension and/or diabetes. Blood flow can be improved with antiplatelet or anticoagulants. Surgical approaches include endarterectomy and revascularization procedures.

B. Management of care: Care of the client with an arterial disease requires critical thinking skills and knowledge of assessment, and teaching and evaluation methods unique to the RN role. These skills cannot be delegated to an LPN or UAP.
1. Delegate responsibly those activities that can be delegated, including basic hygiene needs to clients on bed rest with limited mobility, recording of vital signs, and measurement of intake and output. All monitoring information must be reported to the RN.
2. Provide interventions to manage PAD.
   a. Administer medications (see pharmacologic and parenteral therapies).
   b. Promote exercise therapy: Instruct client to walk 30 to 60 min/day to improve circulation; rest on experience of pain, then resume walking.
   c. Encourage appropriate diet.
      (1) Low fat, 2-g sodium, weight reduction based on individual risk factors
      (2) Vitamin B_6, B_{12}, and folic acid supplements for elevated homocysteine levels
   d. Assure that the client has had daily foot care and inspection, especially in diabetics.
   e. Relieve pain when client at rest: Elevate head of bed to improve arterial flow to lower extremities.
   f. Provide care following interventional procedures: Percutaneous transluminal angioplasty (PTA) and stent placement.
   g. Provide interventions for surgical procedures.
      (1) Peripheral arterial bypass graft surgery: Uses a substitute vessel (saphenous vein) or synthetic graft.
         (a) Aortofemoral bypass graft
         (b) Femoropopliteal bypass graft
         (c) Femorotibial bypass graft
      (2) Endarterectomy to remove plaque from the artery.
      (3) Embolectomy for acute arterial occlusion.
      (4) Amputation for an ischemic or gangrenous extremity that is not viable.
   h. Provide interventions for postprocedural or postoperative care.
      (1) Monitor vital signs frequently and SpO_2 per protocol starting with every 15 min and progressing to every hour to 4 hr when client is stable.
      (2) Assess peripheral pulses and neurovascular status with vital signs—ABI measurements may be ordered after peripheral bypass surgery.
      (3) Notify physician immediately for loss of a palpable pulse, decreasing ABI, increase in pain, or presence of cold sensation, numbness, or tingling in extremity.
      (4) Monitor sheath site of PTA or surgical dressing for signs of bleeding or hematoma.
      (5) Promote bed rest with immobilization of extremity for PTA; turn and position postsurgery clients every 2 hr; avoid knee flexed position.
      (6) Monitor intake and output closely, and hourly urine output.
      (7) Use incentive spirometry or deep-breathing exercises every 1 to 2 hr while awake postoperatively.
      (8) For amputation, support stump on pillow and maintain compression bandage. Periods of extension may be needed with splint or positioning to prevent flexion contractures.

(9) Monitor CBC, PT/INR, APTT, platelets, electrolytes, BUN, creatinine, glucose.
(10) Provide wound care and incisional care; monitor for signs of infection.
(11) Provide pain management.

3. Provide interventions to manage Buerger disease: Provide client with teaching and resources to quit smoking and abstain from all tobacco products.
4. Provide interventions to manage Raynaud disease.
   a. Teach client to protect extremities from cold; teach relaxation techniques to reduce emotional stress; instruct avoidance of vibrating tools, and smoking cessation.
   b. Administer medications to reduce vasospasm.
      (1) Calcium channel blockers
      (2) Alpha blockers
      (3) Vasodilators such as nitroglycerin cream

C. Safety and infection control
   1. Instruct client to keep extremity warm (wear nonrestrictive socks) but do not apply direct heat.
   2. Avoid thermal injury or mechanical trauma to the extremities.

D. Health promotion and maintenance
   1. Assist client in identifying personal risk factors for CAD.
   2. Provide teaching on health behaviors that promote a healthy lifestyle.
      a. Eliminate all forms of tobacco.
      b. Maintain ideal weight, or encourage weight loss, if indicated.
      c. Maintain regular physical exercise.
      d. Promote stress management.
   3. Teach client about self-care behaviors for monitoring at home, such as monitoring BP, assessing peripheral pulses, foot care, and blood sugar, if client is diabetic.

E. Psychologic integrity: Atherosclerosis is more common in older adults and occurs earlier in clients with diabetes mellitus. Older adults may have deconditioning with less endurance for exercise and resilience with postoperative recovery.
   1. Assist client and family in coping with lifestyle changes.
   2. Identify stress factors and anxiety that may interfere with recovery.
   3. Introduce counseling and support groups to assist the client with smoking cessation.
   4. Assess client's ability to independently manage social support and home health care needs.

F. Basic care and comfort
   1. Inspect and care for skin to prevent severe dryness, cracking, and breakdown.
   2. Keep feet dry and clean.
   3. Provide adequate pain management.

G. Reduction of risk potential
   1. Teach client to avoid extremity exposure to cold, sitting with legs crossed, restrictive clothing, and walking barefoot.
   2. Instruct client to notify HCP of decrease in pulses or changes in color, sensation, movement, and temperature of extremities.
   3. Instruct client to wear proper-fitting shoes.
   4. Provide postoperative discharge teaching after peripheral bypass surgery.
      a. Client should refrain from driving until he or she is able to perform an emergency stop—usually 4 weeks.
      b. Client should avoid heavy lifting or straining for 6 weeks after the operation.
      c. Client should call HCP on experience of fever; productive cough; shortness of breath; chest pain; redness, swelling, hotness, or discharge from incision site; nausea or vomiting; difficulty, pain, burning, frequency, urgency, or bleeding with urination; pain or swelling in feet, calves, or legs.

H. Pharmacologic and parenteral therapies: Client will state the purpose, dosage, timing, and side effects of medications to treat arterial diseases.
   1. Antiplatelets: Aspirin, ticlopidine (Ticlid), or clopidogrel (Plavix)
   2. Pentoxifylline (Trental): Increases erythrocyte flexibility and reduces blood viscosity, improving blood supply to the muscle.
   3. Cilostazol (Pletal): Inhibits platelet aggregation and increases vasodilation.

Aortic Aneurysm

I. Definition: An aortic aneurysm is an area of dilation or outpouching from an underlying weakness in the wall of the aorta caused by atherosclerosis and degeneration of elastin and collagen. An aortic aneurysm can be asymptomatic and life-threatening, as rupture of an aneurysm results in extravasation of blood into the thoracic or abdominal region. An aneurysm may be true or false (pseudoaneurysm), and one of several types.

A. A true aneurysm involves all three layers of the artery wall. A false or pseudoaneurysm occurs from disruption of the intimal layer or intimal

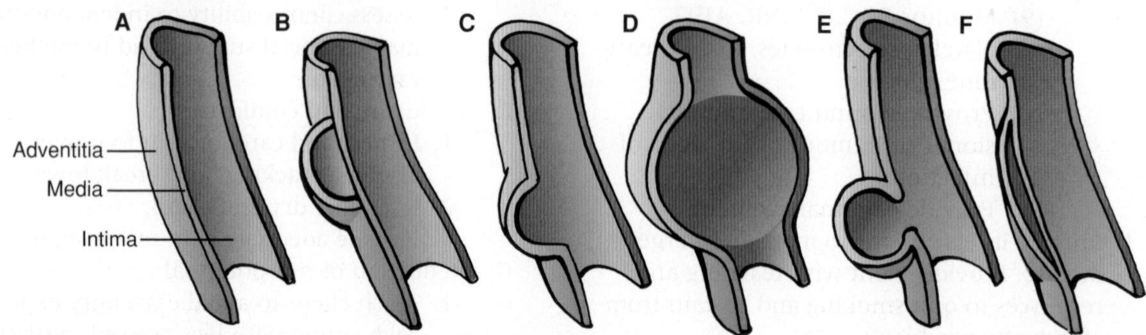

Figure 21-1. Characteristics of arterial aneurysm. **A.** Normal artery. **B.** False aneurysm—actually a pulsating hematoma. The clot and connective tissue are outside the arterial wall. **C.** True aneurysm—one, two, or all three layers of the artery may be involved. **D.** Fusiform aneurysm—symmetric, spindle-shaped expansion of entire circumference of involved vessel. **E.** Saccular aneurysm—a bulbous protrusion of one side of the arterial wall. **F.** Dissecting aneurysm—this usually is a hematoma that splits the layers of the arterial wall. (From Smeltzer, S. C., Bare, B. G., Hinkle, J. L., & Cheever, K. H. [2008]. *Brunner & Suddarth's textbook of medical-surgical nursing* [11th ed.]. Philadelphia: Lippincott Williams & Wilkins.)

and medial layers, is caused by trauma or infection, and results in containment of blood.

B. Aortic aneurysms are classified by the area of the aorta (thoracic or abdominal) and shape (fusiform, saccular, dissecting). An aortic dissection is a longitudinal tear in the intimal layer of the aorta forming a false lumen. Dissections may involve the ascending aorta, the descending thoracic and abdominal aorta, or the entire aorta (Fig. 21-1).

II. Nursing process

A. Assessment

1. Assess for risk factors: Atherosclerosis, hypertension, male gender, age 50 to 70 years, family history, congenital defect, infection, inflammation, smoking, and blunt chest or abdominal trauma.
2. Obtain a detailed health history, including medical and surgical history, and a comprehensive physical assessment.
3. Assess for signs and symptoms (most clients are asymptomatic).
   a. Abdominal aortic aneurysm: Diminished femoral pulses, lower back and abdominal pain, pulsatile abdominal mass, bruit over site, BP differences between extremities, peripheral ischemia.
   b. Thoracic aortic aneurysm: Chest pain, dysphagia, dyspnea, hoarseness, pericardial friction rub, increased intensity of heart murmur.
   c. Rupture or dissection: Sudden intense, severe, stabbing, tearing pain in chest, abdomen, or back; pain radiates to back and extremities; pallor; tachycardia; fleeting peripheral pulses; ischemia; cyanosis; possible neurologic deficits (mental status changes and paralysis of lower extremities); hypovolemic shock.
4. Obtain diagnostic tests.
   a. Chest x-ray
   b. Echocardiogram
   c. Ultrasound
   d. MRI, CT scan
   e. Angiography
   f. CBC, PT/INR, APTT, platelets, basic metabolic panel (Chem 7), calcium

B. Analysis

1. Ineffective Tissue Perfusion: Peripheral, related to impaired arterial blood flow
2. Chronic Pain related to tissue ischemia
3. Activity Intolerance related to claudication, dyspnea
4. Fear related to life-threatening diagnosis

C. Planning

1. Control hypertension and maintain adequate tissue perfusion.
2. Improve client symptoms and comfort.
3. Reduce anxiety and fear.
4. Prevent aneurysm rupture and complications.
5. Promote adherence to the therapeutic regimen.
6. Prepare client for surgical repair, if indicated.

D. Implementation

1. Monitor vital signs with close attention to BP, SpO_2, pulses, heart sounds, and lung sounds.
2. Monitor urine output.
3. Provide client teaching regarding control of modifiable risk factors, medications and associated side effects, monitoring of BP, and signs and symptoms that require immediate medical attention.

E. Evaluation
   1. Client's vital signs, SpO_2, and urine output are within targeted range.
   2. Client's peripheral pulses are palpable.
   3. Client has intact neurologic and motor function.
   4. Client affirms absence of symptoms.
   5. Client's laboratory results are within normal range.

CN

III. Client needs
A. Physiologic adaptation: Treatment is based on client symptoms, and size progression of the aortic aneurysm, which varies among clients. Assess client's need for and response to administration of antihypertensive and analgesic medications.
   1. Open surgical or endovascular stent graft repair considered for aneurysm size greater than 5 cm, impending rupture, symptoms from cerebral or coronary ischemia, pericardial tamponade, uncontrollable pain, severe aortic insufficiency.
      a. Assess for increase in pain intensity, pulse deficits, ischemic changes, increase in dyspnea or heart murmur, abnormal vital signs, neurologic changes, or palpable mass.
      b. Monitor for sudden onset of severe, tearing chest or abdominal pain unrelieved by position change, indicating aortic rupture or dissection.
      c. Assess need for and response to blood transfusions, if indicated.
   2. Surgical emergency indicated by aortic aneurysm rupture, symptomatic expansion or leak.
   3. Surgical emergency for aortic aneurysm dissection: Risk of death is highest for dissection of the ascending aorta; dissection of the descending thoracic aorta may be treated with antihypertensive medications and aggressive control of BP and heart rate while the aorta heals.
B. Management of care: Care of the client with an aortic aneurysm requires critical thinking skills and knowledge of assessment, and teaching and evaluation methods unique to the RN role. These skills cannot be delegated to an LPN or UAP.
   1. Delegate responsibly those activities that can be delegated, including basic care needs, and measurement of intake and output. All monitoring information must be reported to the RN. RN assesses and documents vital signs when rapid changes are occurring.
   2. Perform comprehensive physical assessments and provide care to the client with acute symptoms of an aortic aneurysm.
   3. Provide information on changes in client status to the physician and appropriate members of the multidisciplinary team.
   4. Provide teaching to the client and family.
      a. Administer antihypertensive and analgesic medications.
      b. Observe self-care behaviors for client monitoring BP, pulse, and symptoms requiring immediate attention.
      c. Manage pre- and postoperative care.
   5. Provide nursing interventions after aortic surgical or endovascular graft repair.
      a. Monitor vital signs and peripheral pulses every hour.
      b. Provide continuous monitoring of ECG, arterial line BP, and SpO_2.
      c. Monitor heart sounds and lung sounds.
      d. Provide neurologic and neurovascular checks.
      e. Monitor fluid and electrolytes, hemoglobin, hematocrit, renal function, and coagulation studies.
      f. Assess for hypovolemia; monitor urine output and intake and output every hour.
      g. Manage hypertension.
         (1) Beta blockers
         (2) $Alpha_1$ blockers
         (3) Vasodilators, such as sodium nitroprusside (Nipride)
      h. Manage pain with morphine or other prescribed medication.
      i. Assess wounds and provide incision care per protocol.
      j. Promote deep-breathing exercises or incentive spirometry after extubation.
      k. Instruct initial bed rest and gradual increase in activity.
   6. Facilitate outpatient follow-up care.
   7. Assess client social support and home health care needs prior to discharge.
C. Safety and infection control: Monitor BP closely and maintain systolic BP in the targeted range.
D. Health promotion and maintenance
   1. Assess ability of client and family to adapt to control of risk factors, monitor symptoms, and perform necessary interventions for an aortic aneurysm.
   2. Provide client teaching on health behaviors that decrease the risk for atherosclerosis and promote a healthy lifestyle.
   3. Reinforce regular follow-up care.

E. Psychologic integrity: Assess level of understanding of the client and family; provide emotional support and teaching on the postoperative course.
   1. Assist client and family in coping with lifestyle changes.
   2. Identify factors such as anxiety that may interfere with recovery.
   3. Introduce counseling and support groups to assist the client with smoking cessation and medication management, if indicated.

F. Basic care and comfort
   1. Provide adequate pain management.
   2. Promote turning and position changes every 2 hr while on bed rest.
   3. Provide skin care.

G. Reduction of risk potential
   1. Assess for and treat hypovolemia.
   2. Monitor for decreasing hemoglobin and hematocrit and risk for bleeding (increased PT/INR, APTT, and decreased platelets).
   3. Provide teaching on smoking cessation and BP control.

H. Pharmacologic and parenteral therapies: Client will state the purpose, dosage, timing, and side effects of medications prescribed to treat chronic hypertension (see Tables 20-3 and 20-4).

Bibliography

Altman, G. (2004). *Delmar's fundamental and advanced nursing skills.* (2nd ed.) Albany, NY: Delmar.

Ellis, J., & Hartley, C. (2005). *Managing and coordinating nursing care.* Philadelphia: Lippincott Williams & Wilkins.

Karch, A. (2006). *Lippincott's nursing drug guide.* Philadelphia: Lippincott Williams & Wilkins.

Nursing 2008 drug handbook. Ambler, PA: Springhouse.

Purnell, L., & Paulanka, B. (Eds.). (2003). *Transcultural healthcare: A culturally competent approach.* Philadelphia: Davis.

Smeltzer, S. C., Bare, B. G., Cheever, K. H., & Hinkle, J. L. (2008). *Brunner & Suddarth's textbook of medical-surgical nursing* (11th ed.). Philadelphia: Lippincott Williams & Wilkins.

Taylor, C., Lillis, C., LeMone, P., & Lynn, P. (2006). *Fundamentals of nursing.* Philadelphia: Lippincott Williams & Wilkins.

Weber, J. R. & Kelley, J. (2007). *Nurses handbook of health assessment.* Philadelphia: Lippincott Williams & Wilkins.

CHAPTER 21 Practice Test

Venous Disease: Venous Thrombosis, Chronic Venous Insufficiency, and Varicose Veins

1. A client diagnosed with deep vein thrombosis (DVT) of the left lower left extremity is on bed rest. The nurse should instruct the UAP providing routine morning care for the client to:
- ☐ 1. Check that the legs are in a low, dependent position.
- ☐ 2. Ensure that the lower extremity is elevated.
- ☐ 3. Massage the leg and foot with lotion.
- ☐ 4. Place one or two pillows under the client's left knee.

2. The nurse is assessing a client with superficial thrombophlebitis in the greater saphenous vein of the left leg. Which of the following indicate the nurse should contact the physician to request an order to improve the client's comfort?
- ☐ 1. Brown discoloration of the skin with edema.
- ☐ 2. Dark, protruding veins that ache.
- ☐ 3. IV infusion in an arm with prominent superficial veins.
- ☐ 4. Red, painful, palpable linear cord along the vein.

3. A client with a recent diagnosis of DVT has sudden onset of shortness of breath and chest pain that increases with a deep breath. The nurse should first:
- ☐ 1. Assess the oxygen saturation.
- ☐ 2. Call the physician.
- ☐ 3. Administer morphine sulfate, 2 mg IV.
- ☐ 4. Perform range of motion exercises in the involved leg.

4. A client with DVT is on bed rest and receiving a heparin IV infusion. The physician orders warfarin (Coumadin) to start today. The nurse should do which of the following?
- ☐ 1. Monitor partial thromboplastin time (APTT) to assure the effectiveness of Coumadin and heparin combination.

- □ 2. Contact physician to verify the order.
- □ 3. Administer Coumadin and monitor INR level to assure a therapeutic level prior to stopping the IV heparin.
- □ 4. Discontinue heparin when the client receives the first dose of Coumadin.

5. The nurse is planning care for a client with venous stasis ulcers. Which of the following interventions is a priority?

- □ 1. Apply heat to the extremity.
- □ 2. Elevate leg above heart level.
- □ 3. Restrict fluids.
- □ 4. Encourage client to walk.

6. A client is talking with the nurse about her unsightly varicose veins and their discomfort. What information should the nurse provide to the client?

- □ 1. Avoid walking to reduce the discomfort.
- □ 2. Keep your legs elevated when sitting or lying down.
- □ 3. Sclerotherapy can be used for cosmetic improvement.
- □ 4. Contact a surgeon for a femoral-popliteal bypass graft.

Arterial Disease: Peripheral Arterial Disease, Thromboangiitis Obliterans, and Raynaud Disease

7. AF The nurse is assessing a client with peripheral arterial insufficiency. Where should the nurse palpate the client's pulse to identify tibioperoneal artery involvement?

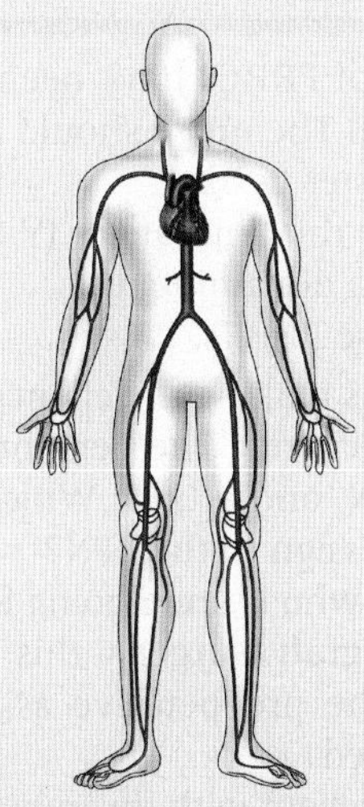

8. The nurse is assessing a client with peripheral arterial disease who had a femoral-popliteal bypass. Which of the following indicates improved arterial blood supply to the lower extremity?

- □ 1. Decrease in muscle pain when walking.
- □ 2. Dependent rubor.
- □ 3. Absence of pulse using a Doppler Ultrasound.
- □ 4. Reduction in pitting edema.

9. A nurse is assessing a client who had femoral-popliteal bypass graft surgery 24 hr ago. The nurse is unable to palpate the dorsalis pedis and posterior tibial arterial pulses that were palpable and strong 2 hr ago. Vital signs are stable with a urine output of 40 to 60 ml/hr. The pedal pulses are now present using a Doppler Ultrasound. The nurse should do which of the following first?

- □ 1. Increase IV fluid rate to improve perfusion to lower extremities.
- □ 2. Notify the surgeon immediately of the change.
- □ 3. Place a warm pack on the lower leg to improve circulation and restore the pulse.
- □ 4. Reassess pulses in 4 hr with the next set of vital signs.

10. The nurse is conducting a health assessment of a client who is 70 years of age. The client tells the nurse about cramping leg pain that occurs when walking 15 min; the pain is relieved with rest. The lower extremities are slightly cool to touch and pedal pulses are palpable +1. The nurse should instruct the client to:

- □ 1. Increase the length of time for walking.
- □ 2. Include more potassium in the diet.
- □ 3. Perform leg circles and ankle pumps.
- □ 4. Seek consultation from the HCP.

11. A client with peripheral arterial disease has had surgery for placement of an aortobifemoral bypass graft. Immediately following surgery, which of the following is a nursing priority?

- □ 1. Elevate lower extremities.
- □ 2. Assist client to use incentive spirometry.
- □ 3. Start client on a liquid diet.
- □ 4. Assess peripheral pulses every 4 hr.

12. The nurse is teaching a client with Buerger disease about health management. Which of the following topics should the nurse include in the teaching plan?

- □ 1. Exercise.
- □ 2. Low-fat diet.
- □ 3. Smoking cessation.
- □ 4. Use of warfarin (Coumadin).

13. A client is experiencing more severe and frequent symptoms of Raynaud phenomenon. Which intervention would be appropriate for the nurse to discuss with the client?

- □ 1. Adding a beta blocker to the client's treatment plan.
- □ 2. Elevating the affected extremities during an attack.

□ 3. Educating the client on the effects of a calcium channel blocker.
□ 4. Describing an angioplasty procedure for the affected extremities.

14. AF The nurse is teaching a client with Raynaud phenomenon to prevent having vasospasms. The nurse should discuss which of the following lifestyle changes with this client? Select all that apply.
□ 1. Stop smoking.
□ 2. Exercise fingers by using the keyboard or playing the piano.
□ 3. Wear mittens when taking food out of the freezer.
□ 4. Warm up the car before driving in cold weather.
□ 5. Stop vasospasm by putting the affected part in ice water.

Aortic Aneurysm

15. The nurse is planning care for a client with an abdominal aneurysm; the client has unstable vital signs, and is experiencing increasing pain. Which of the following tasks should the nurse delegate to the UAP?
□ 1. Assess peripheral pulses of the lower extremities.
□ 2. Explain the use of the morphine PCA pump.
□ 3. Reposition the client every 2 hr.
□ 4. Obtain vital signs every hour.

16. The nurse is assessing the vital signs for a client who had a repair of an abdominal aortic aneurysm 1 hr ago. The client is in pain; respirations are 22; heart rate is 88; and BP is 210/108. The heart rhythm on the cardiac monitor shows normal sinus rhythm. The nurse should do which of the following first?
□ 1. Elevate the head of the bed to 90 degrees.
□ 2. Administer morphine.
□ 3. Administer nitroprusside (Nipride).
□ 4. Anchor a nasogastric tube.

17. The nurse is assessing a client in the emergency department who has dysphagia, chest pain, and shortness of breath. The nurse auscultates an aortic heart murmur. The client complains of a sudden tearing pain sensation in the chest radiating to the upper back, and appears very pale and diaphoretic. The ECG reveals sinus tachycardia at a rate of 142. Systolic BP has decreased to 78. Peripheral pulses in the upper and lower extremities are not palpable and the patient is more somnolent. The nurse should first:
□ 1. Place an IV line.
□ 2. Assess the client's temperature.
□ 3. Begin CPR.
□ 4. Start a nitroglycerin infusion.

18. A client who is 78 years of age is admitted to the ICU with an abdominal aortic dissection. The client is refusing surgery. The nurse should collaborate with the HCP to:
□ 1. Consult social services for a referral to hospice or nursing home care.
□ 2. Tell the client and family that the client will have to remain in the hospital indefinitely if surgery is not performed now.
□ 3. Support the client's decision, and inform the client and family about the option of medical management with antihypertensive drugs to control BP and heart rate.
□ 4. Ask family members to persuade the client to have surgery as this is the only likelihood for survival.

19. AF The nurse is planning care for a client who had an abdominal aortic aneurysm repair 3 days ago. The nurse is reviewing the progress notes below.

PROGRESS NOTES

Date	Time	Progress Notes
2/20/09	0900	Temperature is 36.8 °C; Pulse is 138; BP is 86/44; CVP is 2 mm Hg ~Robin Brown, RN
2/20/09	1100	Urine output is 20 ml/hr for the last 2 hours; Hgb is 7.8 gm/dl. IV of D_5 1/2 normal saline is infusing at 75 cc/hr. ~Robin Brown, RN

Two units of PRBCs have been prescribed for transfusion. The nurse should first:
□ 1. Administer Lasix.
□ 2. Increase the drip rate of IV fluids.
□ 3. Initiate a dopamine drip.
□ 4. Transfuse PRBCs.

20. The nurse is making the client assignment for a group of clients. The personnel include the RN, an LPN, and a UAP. Which client would the nurse assign to the LPN?
□ 1. A client who is undergoing femoropopliteal bypass graft surgery this morning and needs the preoperative assessment sheet completed.
□ 2. A stable client with thrombophlebitis of the lower left extremity with limited mobility and requiring a complete bed bath.
□ 3. A client with a palpable abdominal mass, painful lower extremities, and a decreasing BP.
□ 4. A client with intermittent claudication who needs frequent assistance with getting out of bed and ambulating.

Answers and Rationales

1. 2 DVT causes edema; therefore, the UAP should elevate the extremity to promote venous return. Dependent positioning is appropriate for a client with arterial insufficiency. Placing a pillow under the knee would position the foot in a low position and pressure behind the knee may obstruct venous flow. Massaging the extremity could dislodge the thrombus. (M)

2. 4 Superficial thrombophlebitis is associated with pain, warmth, and erythema that can be palpated. The nurse can request an order for warm packs to relieve the pain. Venous insufficiency causes edema and a brown discoloration of the lower leg. Varicose veins are dark, protruding veins, and symptoms of discomfort increase with standing. There are no indicators for concern with the IV infusion in the arm. (C)

3. 1 A client with DVT is at high risk for a pulmonary embolism from an embolus traveling to the lung. Sudden onset of symptoms and worsening of chest pain with a deep breath suggest a pulmonary embolism. The nurse assesses the client and obtains oxygen saturation levels prior to calling the physician and administering morphine. Range of motion is a preventive measure for DVT and is not appropriate that this time. (A)

4. 3 The nurse administers Coumadin as ordered. Heparin is used to prevent further thrombus formation and therapeutic levels are acquired quickly with the IV infusion. Coumadin is an oral anticoagulant that requires a few days to obtain a therapeutic dose. When the INR reaches 2 to 3 times the control (therapeutic level of Coumadin), the physician will discontinue the heparin. The APTT measures the therapeutic level of IV heparin. (D)

5. 2 Venous stasis ulcers result from venous insufficiency. Elevating the leg above heart level promotes venous return. Adequate hydration is important to prevent dehydration and increased blood viscosity. Heat is not applied to the extremity. Pain with waking or claudication is associated with arterial disease. Wound care may require bed rest and continuous extremity elevation for healing. The nurse encourages walking after wound healing. (M)

6. 2 The nurse instructs the client to elevate the legs to improve venous return and alleviate discomfort. Walking is encouraged to increase venous return. Sclerotherapy or laser treatment is done for cosmetic reasons, but it does not improve circulation. Surgery may be performed for severe venous insufficiency or recurrent thrombophlebitis in the varicosities. Femoral-popliteal bypass graft is a surgical intervention for arterial disease. (H)

7. The nurse palpates the dorsalis pedis; if the pulse is obtained in that artery, the tibioperoneal artery is patent. (A)

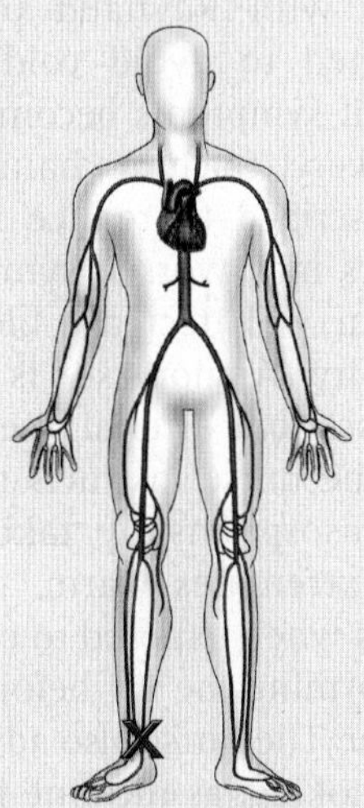

8. 1 Claudication (cramping pain in leg with walking) should decrease or be absent with improved arterial blood supply. Pulses should be palpable with improved blood supply. Edema is associated with venous disease. Pallor with elevation and dependent rubor are symptoms of peripheral arterial disease. (A)

9. 2 The loss of a palpable pulse is a significant finding after bypass surgery; the nurse notifies the surgeon of impaired perfusion. Hydration is important, but client data do not suggest dehydration. Warm packs are avoided as sensation may be decreased, leading to burns and impaired skin integrity. (R)

10. 4 This client has indications of PAD and needs additional follow-up. Increasing walking or exercising the legs and feet likely will not be sufficient to improve peripheral circulation. Muscle cramping is a result of inadequate arterial circulation. Increasing potassium will not decrease the cramping. (H)

11. 2 The nurse assists the client to use incentive spirometry every 1 to 2 hr postoperatively to prevent atelectasis and pneumonia. Starting a liquid diet is not the highest priority as the client will have an IV infusion and might have an NG tube; adequate fluid status can be maintained until intestinal function returns. The client's extremities are kept flat or lowered to promote circulation. Elevation of extremities is used to promote venous blood flow. The nurse assesses pulses and vital signs hourly in the early postoperative course. (R)

12. 3 Smoking cessation is the only treatment known to be effective with Buerger disease. Exercise and a low-fat diet are measures to reduce the risk of atherosclerosis, which is not associated with Buerger disease. Anticoagulation is not an effective treatment. (H)

13. 3 Clients with Raynaud phenomenon are instructed to avoid cold and emotional stress; if symptoms become more frequent and severe, calcium channel blockers may be prescribed to reduce vasospasm. Beta blockers may worsen symptoms. Elevating the arm will decrease blood flow to the extremity. Angioplasty is a treatment for atherosclerotic arterial disease. (D)

14. 1, 3, 4 The nurse instructs the client to prevent vasospasms by taking measures to keep extremities warm, such as wearing mittens when exposed to cold temperatures and warming the car before driving in cold weather. The nurse also advises the client to stop smoking, as nicotine is a vasoconstrictor. Repetitive motions with a keyboard can induce symptoms. The client can stop the vasospasm by putting the hands or feet in warm water. (R)

15. 3 The UAP performs basic care needs, including repositioning the client every 2 hr. The nurse assesses the client frequently, including vital signs, level of pain, and peripheral pulses, because of the frequency with which the vital signs are changing. The nurse also provides client teaching for how to use the PCA pump. (M)

16. 3 The nurse must maintain client BP within normal limits after surgery in order to prevent pressure on the graft and reduce the potential for rupture. Nipride is a potent vasodilator used to lower BP. The nurse titrates the drug while closely monitoring BP via arterial line. Once BP is stable, the nurse manages pain. The nurse elevates the head of the bed at 45 degrees to prevent tension on the suture site. An NG tube is used to manage ileus until bowel sounds return; there are no data to support that this client is experiencing ileus. (D)

17. 1 Although symptoms of an aortic dissection are similar to a heart attack, the sudden tearing sensation in the chest to the back, dysphagia, and aortic murmur are more closely associated with an ascending aortic dissection. The client has symptoms of hypotensive shock, which occur suddenly. An IV line is needed to increase blood volume. Nitroglycerin will decrease the already low BP. CPR is not indicated as the client is still breathing. Taking the temperature is not the highest priority at this time. (A)

18. 3 Because client decisions about care are respected, the nurse collaborates with the HCP to inform the client and family about various treatment options. Abdominal dissections in a stable client are managed with strict compliance with antihypertensive medications and BP and heart rate control. Once BP is under control during hospitalization, the client can be managed on an outpatient basis with good follow-up care and adherence to plan of care. (P)

19. 4 A blood transfusion is required postoperatively with significant blood loss from surgery or bleeding. Data from the progress notes indicate the client is hypovolemic and has a low hemoglobin level, which warrants transfusion at this time rather than IV fluids. The nurse continues to assess the client for signs of bleeding. Correction of hypovolemia precedes a dopamine infusion. The transfusion should improve the hemodynamics, and the hemoglobin and hematocrit are reassessed post transfusion. The client has fluid volume deficit, so Lasix is not needed at this time. (R)

20. 1 The LPN can complete the assessment sheet and care for the client before surgery. Clients who are stable and requiring complete care or frequent assistance with basic care needs along with vital signs and intake and output recordings can be assigned to a UAP. An unstable client requiring critical assessments receives care from the RN. (M)

chapter

22

The Client With Hematologic Health Problems

Hematologic health problems are relatively uncommon in adult clients, and may be chronic forms of health problems that originated in childhood or occur secondary to other health problems. The nurse has an important role in identifying health problems, health promotion, and health maintenance. Topics discussed in this chapter include:

- Anemias
- Sickle Cell Anemia
- Polycythemia Vera
- Leukemia
- Lymphomas
- Bleeding Disorders
- Disseminated Intravascular Coagulation

Anemias

I. Definition: Anemia is not a specific disease state, but an indicator of an underlying condition. Types of anemia are classified by the way in which RBCs are deficient, and include sickle cell anemia (see section on sickle cell anemia within this chapter), G6PD deficiency anemia, immune hemolytic anemia, iron deficiency anemia, folic acid deficiency anemia, vitamin B_{12} deficiency anemia, pernicious anemia, and aplastic anemia. Table 22-1 presents greater detail on each type of anemia.

II. Nursing process

A. Assessment

1. Obtain a detailed health history and perform a comprehensive physical examination.
2. Assess for signs and symptoms specific to type of anemia (see Table 22-1); general signs and symptoms include pallor, jaundice, dizziness, weakness, general malaise, dyspnea, hepatosplenomegaly, petechiae, and/or ecchymotic areas.
3. Obtain diagnostic tests (see also Table 22-1).
   a. Initial laboratory tests: Hemoglobin, hematocrit, reticulocyte, and MCV values; iron studies, vitamin B_{12}, and folic acid levels
   b. CBC—helps determine if anemia is the result of underlying hemolytic cause
   c. Bone marrow aspiration, if indicated

B. Analysis

1. Activity Intolerance related to weakness and general malaise
2. Decreased Cardiac Output related to increased cardiac workload
3. Imbalanced Nutrition: Less Than Body Requirements related to inadequate intake of essential nutrients
4. Knowledge Deficit related to disease process and treatment plan

Table 22-1 Types of Anemia

Type of Anemia	Overview	Incidence/ Prevalence	Signs and Symptoms	Diagnostic Characteristics
Sickle Cell Anemia (See also Chapter 13)	Autosomal recessive genetic disorder resulting in abnormal shape of RBCs (sickle cells). Because of the complexity of this disease, a separate section has been dedicated to it.	Can occur in all ethnicities and races, but is less prevalent in whites.	Symptoms vary depending on the severity; may include low hemoglobin levels; anorexia, joint pain, abdominal pain; frequent infections; jaundice; tachycardia; cardiac murmurs, and often an enlarged heart.	Hemoglobin electrophoresis distinguishes between sickle cell trait and sickle cell disease. Additional diagnostic tests include sickle cell prep and Sickledex.
G6PD Deficiency Anemia	Congenital hemolytic anemia resulting from deficiency of enzyme (G6PD) within RBCs. Inherited through X-linked recessive gene. Condition presents itself when susceptible patients are in certain situations where RBCs are overwhelmed, such as with a fever or with certain medications.	Occurs in African Americans, Asians, and people of Greek and Italian descent. Incidence is greater in men than in women.	Client is asymptomatic; involves normal hemoglobin levels. Client develops pallor, jaundice, and hemoglobin is excreted in the urine, then symptoms of hemolysis develop several days after they are exposed to affecting medications.	Diagnosed via screening test for G6PD.
Immune Hemolytic Anemia	Increased RBC destruction through hemolysis; the body's own immune system "attacks" RBCs; no known cause.	Equally affects all ages, genders, and races.	Symptoms vary depending on the severity of the anemia; hemolysis can be mild enough for the patient to be asymptomatic or severe enough to be life-threatening. Fatigue and dizziness, splenomegaly, hepatomegaly, lymphadenopathy, and jaundice are common.	Labs: Low hemoglobin and low hematocrit levels. Also, increase in reticulocyte count. Positive Coombs test.

Type of Anemia	Overview	Incidence/ Prevalence	Signs and Symptoms	Diagnostic Characteristics
Iron Deficiency Anemia	Most common type of anemia; can result from blood loss (GI, menstruation, malignancy), increased energy demands, GI malabsorption, and dietary inadequacy. Iron stores are depleted, including hemoglobin stores, resulting in small (microcytic) RBCs.	Most common form of anemia; seen frequently in underdeveloped countries.	Symptoms include weakness; fatigue; general malaise; pallor; smooth, red tongue; angular cheilosis (corners of mouth ulcerated); brittle, ridged, or concave nail beds; tachycardia; exertional dyspnea; and, occasionally, pica is seen.	Labs: Low ferritin and low hemoglobulin. Also elevated TIBC, decreased MCV, decreased RBC, and decreased hematocrit.
Folic Acid Deficiency Anemia	Deficiency of folic acid interferes with DNA synthesis of RBC, resulting in large RBCs (macrocytic) and fewer RBCs being released from bone marrow related to size. Most common causes are poor nutrition, malabsorption, drugs, and pregnancy. Chronic alcohol use and Crohn disease can also result in folic acid deficiency.	Increases susceptibility in chronic EtOH abusers, and patients with malabsorption diseases. Equally affects all ages, genders, and races.	Symptoms include pallor, jaundice, weight loss, and smooth, beefy, red tongue.	Labs: Serum folic acid level.
Vitamin B_{12} Deficiency Anemia	Vitamin B_{12} is associated with transport of folic acid into cells; B_{12} deficiency indirectly causes anemia. Can result from dietary deficiency or from conditions such as small bowel resection, diverticula, or tapeworm.	Equally affects all ages, genders, and races.	Symptoms include pallor, jaundice, fatigue, weight loss, smooth, beefy, red tongue, positive Romberg sign (assessed by loss of balance with eyes closed), confusion, and paresthesias of extremities.	Labs: Serum B_{12} level. Positive Schilling test (without intrinsic factor added).
Pernicious Anemia	Inability to absorb vitamin B_{12}; can result from a deficiency of intrinsic factor (necessary for absorption of B_{12} from the intestines).	Involves genetic component; increases risk of contracting gastric cancer. Equally affects all ages, genders, and races.	Symptoms include pallor; jaundice; fatigue; weight loss; sore mouth; beefy, red tongue; positive Romberg sign (assessed by loss of balance with eyes closed); confusion; and paresthesias of extremities.	Labs: Intrinsic factor antibody test (not specific for pernicious anemia). Positive Schilling test with intrinsic factor.
Aplastic Anemia	Deficiency of circulating erythrocytes as a result of the halted development of RBCs within the bone marrow. Relatively rare, can be associated with chronic exposure to toxic agents or may occur after a viral infection; mostly, cause is unknown. Usually accompanied by agranulocytopenia and thrombocytopenia. Pancytopenia is also common.	Equally affects all ages, genders, and races.	First indicators are bone marrow failure complications; otherwise, infection, fatigue, pallor, and dyspnea. Occasionally lymphadenopathy and/or splenomegaly seen.	Bone marrow aspirate. Disease usually accompanied by agranulocytosis and thrombocytopenia.

5. Risk for Infection related to impaired immune response (aplastic anemia)
6. Risk for Bleeding: Secondary to Thrombocytopenia related to bone marrow depression (aplastic anemia)
7. Impaired Physical Mobility related to altered neurologic function (B_{12} deficiency and pernicious anemias)
8. Impaired Oral Mucous Membranes related to potential glossitis and angular cheilosis

C. Planning
1. Determine underlying cause (if indicated).
2. Correct decreased RBCs via nutrition and/or medication as indicated.

D. Implementation (see management of care)

E. Evaluation
1. Client's activity level returns to baseline.
2. Client's cardiac function returns to baseline.
3. Client's diet is well balanced.
4. Client shows understanding of disease process and treatment.
5. Client remains free of infection.
6. Client is free from injury.
7. Client maintains clean, moist mucous membranes that are free of ulcerations.

CN

III. Client needs

A. Physiologic adaptation: Anemia is treated by managing the underlying cause, which may include blood transfusion or infusion of platelets for bleeding; use of oral or parenteral iron therapy for iron deficiency anemia; or administration of cyanocobalamin (B_{12}) for pernicious anemia.
1. Monitor for complications such as heart failure, paresthesias, and confusion.
2. Monitor for complications of blood transfusion, if indicated.
3. Monitor client's vital signs due to cardiac overload.
4. Monitor client with excessive alcohol intake for withdrawal.

B. Management of care: Care of the client with anemia requires critical thinking skills and knowledge of assessment, and teaching and evaluation methods unique to the RN role. These skills cannot be delegated to an LPN or UAP.
1. Delegate responsibly those activities that can be delegated, including basic hygiene needs, measurement of intake and output, and recording of vital signs for the stable client. All monitoring information is reported to the RN.
2. Review results of laboratory studies to assess effectiveness of treatment as indicated.
3. Provide nutrition and physical therapy consults as indicated. Promote rest periods throughout the day as needed.
4. Encourage ambulation and activity as tolerated as not to further decompensate; monitor client's ability to tolerate activity, and obtain assistive devices as indicated.
5. Provide oxygen therapy, if necessary (related to dyspnea).
6. Assess for signs and symptoms of fluid retention related to increased cardiac workload.
7. Monitor laboratory values, especially iron, albumin, and protein levels to ensure adequate nutrition.
8. Monitor CBC periodic levels.
9. Provide frequent neurologic assessments, including position sense and balance as indicated.
10. Assess mucous membranes frequently and provide adequate hydration.

C. Safety and infection control
1. Initiate pneumococcal vaccine for client requiring a splenectomy.
2. Instruct client receiving splenectomy about increased risk of infection for remainder of life.
3. Monitor client receiving steroid therapy for infection and glucose control.
4. Implement fall precautions, when appropriate, because of extreme weakness and fatigue.
5. Ensure prompt attention is given to wounds, ulcerations, and abrasions.

D. Health promotion and maintenance: Provide client teaching regarding nutritious diet, as indicated, and avoidance of excessive alcohol intake.

E. Psychologic integrity: Identify support groups for client and family within the community; monitor clients with excessive alcohol intake for depression, and initiate therapy as indicated.

F. Basic care and comfort
1. Manage fatigue.
2. Promote physical activity as tolerated with adequate rest periods.
3. Provide adequate hydration and nutrition.
4. Administer dietary supplements as indicated.
5. Ensure frequent oral hygiene.

G. Reduction of risk potential: Provide client and family teaching:
1. Avoid or limit any activities that cause dyspnea, palpitations, dizziness, or tachycardia.
2. Avoid razors and hard-bristled toothbrushes to prevent bleeding; recognize signs and symptoms of bleeding.

3. Avoid alcohol use or advise to limit intake, if indicated (alcohol can inhibit certain nutrients from being used).
4 Avoid using aspirin.

H. Pharmacologic and parenteral therapies: Client will state the purpose, dosage, timing, and side effects of medications to manage specific type of anemia.
   1. Sickle cell anemia (see section on sickle cell anemia)
   2. Glucose-6-phosphate dehydrogenase (G6PD) deficiency anemia: Blood transfusions (in severe circumstances)
   3. Immune hemolytic anemia: Corticosteroids
   4. Iron deficiency anemia: Iron supplements and dietary modification
   5. Folic acid deficiency anemia: Folic acid supplements/dietary modification
   6. Pernicious anemia (vitamin B_{12} deficiency anemia): Vitamin B_{12} replacement and dietary modification
   7. Aplastic anemia: Bone marrow transplant or immunosuppressive therapy and blood and/or platelet transfusions

Sickle Cell Anemia

I. Definition: Sickle cell anemia is a hemolytic anemia resulting from a defect in the synthesis of hemoglobin. The disorder occurs from an autosomal recessive trait causing abnormally shaped erythrocytes (sickle cells). See Table 22-1 for prevalence and incidence. See also Chapter 13 for discussion of sickle cell anemia in pediatric clients.

II. Nursing process
   A. Assessment
      1. Obtain a detailed health history and perform a comprehensive physical examination; assess for signs and symptoms (see Table 22-1).
      2. Assess for sickle cell crises.
         a. Fever
         b. Severe abdominal pain
         c. Joint pain
         d. Pallor
         e. Jaundice
         f. Diagnostic measures
         g. Hemoglobin electrophoresis can distinguish between the sickle cell trait and sickle cell disease.
      3. Obtain diagnostic tests (see Table 22-1).
   B. Analysis
      1. Altered Tissue Perfusion related to sickle cell crisis
      2. Acute Pain related to tissue hypoxia and joint pain
      3. Activity Intolerance related to the "sickling" of the RBCs, which decreases oxygen carried within the blood
      4. Risk for Infection related to decreased immune function
   C. Planning
      1. Relieve pain.
      2. Restore fluid and electrolyte balance.
      3. Prevent infection.
      4. Prevent hypoxia.
   D. Implementation
      1. Provide interventions to manage anemia (see basic care and comfort).
      2. Provide interventions during a sickle cell crisis.
         a. Encourage bed rest to decrease oxygen needs.
         b. Provide oxygen.
         c. Assess pain on routine basis via pain scale.
         d. Administer pain medication as indicated.
         e. Promote hydration as necessary (either PO or IV, if indicated).
         f. Initiate blood transfusions, if indicated (for severe crisis).
   E. Evaluation
      1. Client has as few sickle cell crises as possible.
      2. Client is pain-free or pain is controlled.
      3. Client is able to tolerate appropriate levels of activity.
      4. Client is free of infection.

CN

III. Client needs
   A. Physiologic adaptation: Management goals for sickle cell anemia are to restore fluid balance and prevent hemoconcentration, and to promote adequate oxygenation.
   B. Management of care: Care of the client with sickle cell anemia requires critical thinking skills and knowledge of assessment, and teaching and evaluation methods unique to the RN role. These skills cannot be delegated to an LPN or UAP.
      1. Delegate responsibly those activities that can be delegated, including basic hygiene needs, measurement of intake and output, and recording of vital signs for the stable client. All monitoring information is reported to the RN.
      2. Perform periodic complete assessments on the client having a sickle cell crisis, and provide interventions as indicated or as ordered.
      3. Report any changes in the client's condition to the physician.
      4. Provide client and family teaching (see safety and infection control).

C. Safety and infection control: Reduce frequency of sickle cell crisis (see reduction of risk potential).
D. Health promotion and maintenance: Ensure client has up-to-date immunizations because of increased susceptibility to infections.
E. Psychologic integrity
   1. Assist client and family to adapt to lifestyle changes.
   2. Identify client and family stressors and teach tools to effectively alleviate anxieties associated with condition.
   3. Identify support groups for the client and the family within the community.
F. Basic care and comfort
   1. Treat joint pain.
   2. Provide heat therapy to affected area.
   3. Obtain cushioning to support affected areas during sleep.
   4. Manage fatigue.
   5. Promote physical activity as tolerated, with adequate rest periods.
   6. Provide adequate hydration and nutrition.
G. Reduction of risk potential: Provide client and family teaching to reduce frequency of sickle cell crisis.
   1. Return to the hospital for oxygenation, hydration, and analgesic relief on experience of signs and symptoms associated with a sickle cell crisis.
   2. Avoid strenuous physical activity as increased oxygen demand may precipitate a sickle cell crisis.
   3. Avoid contact with others who are sick because of increased susceptibility to infection.
   4. Avoid high altitudes where there is low oxygen content.
   5. Ensure adequate hydration and recognize signs of dehydration.
H. Pharmacologic and parenteral therapies: Client will state the purpose, dosage, timing, and side effects of medications to manage sickle cell anemia.
   1. Analgesics as indicated
   2. Antibiotics, if infection present
   3. Oxygenation as needed
   4. Blood transfusion as needed
   5. Parenteral fluids may be administered up to twice fluid maintenance needs.

Polycythemia Vera

I. Definition: Polycythemia vera is a cancer of the RBCs characterized by a hypercellular bone marrow, resulting in elevated levels of RBCs. Frequently there is a rise of WBCs and platelets seen in the blood as well. The hematocrit is dramatically elevated (to above 50% in males, 55% in females). Males are 2 times more likely to develop this condition than women; people over 40 years of age are at an increased risk; and white individuals are more susceptible than nonwhites. Over time, polycythemia vera can evolve into myeloid metaplasia or acute myeloid leukemia; if untreated, few clients will survive longer than 2 years.

II. Nursing process
A. Assessment
   1. Obtain a detailed health history and perform a comprehensive physical examination.
   2. Assess client for signs and symptoms.
      a. Persistently elevated hematocrit level
      b. Hypertension
      c. Splenomegaly; hepatomegaly
      d. Ruddy complexion of hands and face
      e. Weight loss
      f. Fatigue
      g. Generalized pruritus
      h. Swollen joints
      i. Increased blood viscosity indicated by angina, claudication, dyspnea and thrombophlebitis
   3. Obtain diagnostic tests, including CBC, bone marrow biopsy, and uric acid.
B. Analysis
   1. Activity Intolerance related to fatigue
   2. Risk for Injury related to bleeding while on anticoagulants and splenomegaly
   3. Risk for Acute Pain related to swollen joints
   4. Risk for Ineffective Tissue Perfusion: Peripheral, related to potential clot formation
   5. Risk for Impaired Skin Integrity related to generalized pruritus
C. Planning
   1. Promote periodic phlebotomies (removal of blood from body to decrease total proportion of RBCs in body).
   2. Maintain adequate hydration (at least 3 L of fluid per day).
   3. Promote venous return.
   4. Suppress bone marrow activity (with disease progression).
D. Implementation
   1. Encourage client to exercise only as tolerated and to take frequent rest breaks.
   2. Assess client for signs and symptoms of activity intolerance (decreased O_2 saturation, postural hypotension, shortness of breath).
   3. Assess client for signs and symptoms of bleeding.
   4. Administer pain medication as indicated.
   5. Assess client for chest pain, palpitations, and dyspnea.

6. Monitor vital signs frequently.
7. Provide client teaching about signs and symptoms of a thrombus.
8. Assist client in finding ways to relieve itching (gentle soaps, cool water baths, colloidal oatmeal).

E. Evaluation
1. Client's RBCs return to normal range.
2. Client's hematocrit returns to normal range.
3. Client does not develop thrombus.
4. Client's activity level returns to baseline.
5. Client's pain is relieved or well controlled.

CN

III. Client needs

A. Physiologic adaptation: Management of polycythemia vera is directed at decreasing the proliferation of RBC mass. Phlebotomy may be used to reduce hyperviscosity. Myelosuppressive therapy with hydroxyurea (Hydrea) or radioactive phosphorus may be used to reduce marrow hyperplasia.
1. Recognize risk for decreased tissue perfusion—indicated by chest pain, severe headache, and cyanotic areas on hands and face.
2. Recognize risk for generalized pruritus and hypertension as a result of vasodilatation.
3. Monitor for signs and symptoms of thrombi.

B. Management of care: Care of the client with polycythemia vera requires critical thinking skills and knowledge of assessment, and teaching and evaluation methods unique to the RN role. These skills cannot be delegated to an LPN or UAP.
1. Delegate responsibly those activities that can be delegated, including basic hygiene needs, measurement of intake and output, and recording of vital signs for the stable client. All monitoring information is reported to the RN.
2. Perform frequent physical assessments and provide appropriate care to the client.
3. Inform the physician of any changes in client's status.
4. Provide client and family teaching (see reduction of risk potential).

C. Safety and infection control
1. Teach client signs and symptoms of a thrombus.
2. Instruct client on use of anticoagulation therapy, if indicated.

D. Health promotion and maintenance (see reduction of risk potential)

E. Psychologic integrity: Offer support while client verbalizes concerns and negative feelings.

F. Basic care and comfort: Teach client techniques to alternate massage, pressure, and vibration instead of scratching when itching is severe.

G. Reduction of risk potential: Provide client teaching about the following:
1. Exercise only as tolerated, taking rest breaks as needed.
2. Identify and avoid potential irritants that may exacerbate pruritus, including mild laundry detergents.
3. Maintain adequate hydration (at least 3 L of liquids per day).
4. Elevate lower extremities when sitting to promote venous return.
5. Wear support stockings during waking hours.
6. If client on anticoagulation therapy:
   a. Use electric razor and soft-bristled toothbrush.
   b. Consult physician before taking any new medications.

H. Pharmacologic and parenteral therapies: Client will state the purpose, dosage, timing, and side effects of medications to manage polycythemia vera. Treatment is based on a symptomatic approach:
1. Ischemic symptoms: Dipyridamole sometimes used
2. Thrombotic complications: Anticoagulation therapy
3. Disease progression: Therapies focus on suppression of bone marrow activity such as the use of hydroxyurea (Hydrea) or radioactive phosphorus.

Leukemia

I. Definition: Leukemia refers to a group of malignant conditions that involve the overproduction of WBCs in the bone marrow. (See also Chapter 13 for discussion of leukemia in pediatric clients.) Types of leukemia are classified by the specific pathway from which the abnormal cells develop and whether the condition is acute (occurring suddenly) or chronic (taking months or years to develop). The four main types of leukemia are as follows:

A. Acute myeloid leukemia (AML): AML is more prevalent in whites and has a higher incidence in males. AML is a disease of older adults, but prognosis is poorer in adult clients than in pediatric clients, and is more often curable in pediatric clients.

B. Chronic myeloid leukemia (CML): CML occurs more often in adults over 50 years of age. Prognosis is poor.

C. Acute lymphocytic leukemia (ALL): ALL is most common in children. Favorable prognosis with chemotherapy in children; less successful (30% to 40% cure rate) with chemotherapy in adults.

D. Chronic lymphocytic leukemia (CLL): CLL is more prevalent in whites and has a higher incidence in males. The condition occurs mostly in adults over 50 years of age, and is the most common form of leukemia in adults.

II. Nursing process

A. Assessment

1. Obtain a detailed health history and perform a comprehensive physical assessment.
2. Assess each body system for signs and symptoms.
   a. Integumentary system—petechiae; ecchymotic areas; open infected lesions; pallor, particularly of face, mouth, and nail beds (related to anemia)
   b. Neurologic system—weakness and fatigue (occurs not only from leukemia itself but also from the resulting anemia); headache
   c. Cardiovascular system (usually related to anemia)—tachycardia; palpitations; murmurs; bruits
   d. Respiratory system—tachypnea (related to anemia); infectious process complications (sepsis, cough, pneumonia, URI, SOB)
   e. GI system—weight loss; nausea; anorexia; hepatosplenomegaly
   f. Miscellaneous—infection; bone/joint pain; lymphadenopathy
3. Assess for signs and symptoms of bleeding (from potential for decreased platelet functioning).
   a. Tendency to easily bruise
   b. Nosebleeds
   c. Gum bleeding
   d. Rectal bleeding
   e. Hematuria
   f. Excessive or prolonged bleeding from otherwise minor wounds
   g. Petechiae
4. Obtain diagnostic tests: Classification of each type of leukemia occurs via tests such as immunophenotyping and karyotyping. The results of these tests will help guide treatment plan and determine probable diagnosis.
   a. AML: CBC with decreased erythrocytes and platelets; presence of anemia. Leukocyte count may or may not be low, but percentage of normal cells is markedly decreased. Bone marrow aspiration will show excessive immature blast cells.
   b. CML: CBC with increased WBC count; bone marrow aspiration; presence of Philadelphia chromosome via bone marrow biopsy of blood test.
   c. ALL: CBC with elevated WBC count, low platelets, and anemia. Lymphocyte count may be low or high, but always high proportion of immature cells; bone marrow aspiration—increased number of cells and lymphoblasts.
   d. CLL: CBC with elevated WBC count; increased lymphocyte count is always present; bone marrow aspiration.

B. Analysis

1. Risk for Infection and Bleeding related to decreased leukocytes and/or chemotherapy side effects
2. Risk for Impaired Skin Integrity related to chemotherapy side effects and nutritional deficits
3. Risk for Impaired Gas Exchange related to possible pneumonia
4. Risk for Impaired Mucous Membranes related to chemotherapy or prolonged use of antibiotics
5. Risk for Imbalanced Nutrition: Less Than Body Requirements, related to anorexia, nausea, medication side effects
6. Risk for Acute Pain related to cancer and infection
7. Risk for Impaired Mobility related to fatigue and weakness
8. Risk for Diarrhea related to medication side effects
9. Risk for Self-Care Deficit: Bathing and Hygiene, related to fatigue and weakness
10. Risk for Anxiety related to knowledge deficit
11. Risk for Spiritual Distress related to death and dying
12. Risk for Knowledge Deficit related to disease process treatment, and medication side effects

C. Planning

1. Treat complications associated with disease process and medication side effects.
2. Decrease pain.
3. Maintain adequate nutrition and hydration.
4. Promote self-care rituals.
5. Increase knowledge of disease process, treatments, and potential complications and outcomes.

D. Implementation

1. Prevent infection by placing client in isolation with the initiation of therapy and when lymphocyte levels are low.

2. Assess client's skin and oral mucosa as indicated to check for signs of an infection and bleeding.
3. Initiate blood transfusions to treat anemia and low platelet counts as indicated.
4. Avoid administration of aspirin.
5. Provide client with meals that he or she can tolerate, and administer nutritional supplements as indicated.
6. Provide analgesics as indicated.
7. Help client to create a balance between activity and rest.
8. Monitor intake and output status closely, especially in clients with vomiting and diarrhea.

E. Evaluation
1. Client is free of infection.
2. Client exhibits no signs of bleeding.
3. Client has intact oral mucosa.
4. Client experiences well-controlled pain levels.
5. Client maintains adequate weight with increased nutritional intake.
6. Client experiences increased energy and decrease in fatigue.
7. Client discusses concerns and fears, and uses strategies learned to cope with anxiety effectively.

CN

III. Client needs

A. Physiologic adaptation: The goal of management of leukemia is to eradicate leukemic cells. The client with leukemia is treated with chemotherapy and is monitored for associated complications. Leukapheresis, radiation, and bone marrow transplant may also be used.
1. Recognize risk for client to become very ill with infections, and experience bleeding complications and severe mucositis during induction of chemotherapy.
2. Recognize complications such as severe infection, uncontrolled bleeding, disseminated intravascular coagulation (DIC), idiopathic thrombocytopenic purpura (ITP), and autoimmune hemolytic anemia.
3. Recognize risk for complication of tumor lysis syndrome, which can lead to acute renal failure, cardiac dysrhythmias, hypotension, muscle cramping, tetany, confusion, and seizure. Promote high fluid intake and alkalization of urine.
4. Recognize risk for GI side effects—including anorexia, nausea, vomiting, and mucositis.
5. Initiate bone marrow transplant as indicated; monitor client for infections and graft-versus-host disease.

B. Management of care: Care of the client with leukemia requires critical thinking skills and knowledge of assessment, and teaching and evaluation methods unique to the RN role. These skills cannot be delegated to an LPN or UAP.
1. Delegate responsibly those activities that can be delegated, including basic hygiene needs, measurement of intake and output, and recording of vital signs for the stable client. All monitoring information is reported to the RN.
2. Assess client frequently, including assessment of vital signs; immediately report any changes to the physician.
3. Place client on cardiac telemetry, if indicated; monitor closely.
4. Assess laboratory values daily, especially CBC, platelet level, and coagulation panel, to look for neutropenia and signs of bleeding.
5. Provide frequent skin inspection, especially IV sites, for signs of infection.
6. Monitor petechiae and ecchymotic areas that indicate bleeding.
7. Assess client frequently for dehydration and fluid overload, and monitor electrolytes (especially in clients with vomiting and diarrhea).

C. Safety and infection control
1. Prevent infection: When hospitalized, place client in private room; when at home, avoid exposure to people with infection; avoid crowded areas such as theaters and malls. Teach client to observe for signs of infection such as fever, urinary tract infection, or upper respiratory infections.
2. Prevent bleeding by using soft-bristled toothbrush, electric razor, stool softeners as needed.
3. Provide low-microbial diet to decrease risk of infection.
4. Promote use of medicinal mouthwashes for clients with mucositis to decrease risk of developing yeast or fungal oral infections.

D. Health promotion and maintenance: Instruct client to perform frequent mouth care, and to maintain adequate nutrition.

E. Psychologic integrity
1. Encourage client and family to join a cancer support group through their local community.
2. Offer social services or psychiatry consult to client and family while in hospital.
3. Instruct client to cope with anxiety; encourage discussion with health care team related to concerns and fears.

F. Basic care and comfort
  1. Administer analgesics before meals to promote client eating.
  2. Provide client with small, frequent meals that are soft in texture and at a moderate temperature.
  3. Provide nutritional supplements as indicated.
  4. Instruct client to take adequate rest periods throughout day.

G. Reduction of risk potential
  1. Assess laboratory results and skin integrity frequently for clients with vomiting and diarrhea to decrease risk of dehydration.
  2. Provide client teaching regarding disease process and potential complications, and how to help prevent them.

H. Pharmacologic and parenteral therapies: Client will state the purpose for and side effects of medications and therapies to manage leukemia.
  1. Chemotherapy (involves three phases)
     a. Induction therapy—high-dose chemotherapy to eliminate leukemic cells
     b. Consolidation therapy—lower dose chemotherapy
     c. Maintenance therapy—to prevent recurrence
  2. Bone marrow (stem cell) transplantation to remove leukemic cells and replace with healthy bone marrow or stem cells.
  3. Antibiotics to treat infection
  4. Platelet transfusion to control bleeding
  5. Analgesics
  6. Radiation therapy to destroy leukemic cells in ALL
  7. Imatinib (Gleevec) is an effective oral treatment for CML. This drug is a protein-tyrosine kinase inhibitor and inhibits proliferation of abnormal cells. Side effects include edema, nausea and vomiting, musculoskeletal pain, and diarrhea.
  8. Antineoplastic drugs such as chlorambucil (Leukeran) or cyclophosphamide (Cytoxan) may be used with CLL to suppress lymphocyte proliferation.

Lymphomas

I. Definition: Lymphomas arise from the lymphatic system of the body, usually from the lymph nodes themselves, and can be classified into two different categories: Hodgkin's lymphoma (also known as Hodgkin's disease), and non-Hodgkin lymphoma (NHL). For Hodgkin disease, long-term survival is common; the prognosis varies more in NHLs, depending on the type of NHL.

A. Hodgkin disease—begins in a single lymph node and then spreads through the lymphatic system, involving primarily lymph nodes. Cause is unknown; however, viral infections may be linked and there is a familial pattern noted among first-degree relatives. Hodgkin disease is slightly more common in men than in women; highest incidences are among clients near 20 years of age and clients older than 50 years of age.

B. Non-Hodgkin lymphomas (NHLs)—consist of a group of cancers originating within the lymph nodes. Unlike Hodgkin disease, NHL malignant cells usually spread throughout all lymphatic tissues. Cause for NHLs is unknown. Incidence increases with age, and is higher in individuals with autoimmune disorders, immunodeficiencies, or viral infections. The disease is more prevalent among men.

II. Nursing process

A. Assessment
  1. Perform complete assessment of health history and detailed physical assessment.
  2. Assess for signs and symptoms.
     a. Hodgkin disease: Lymphadenopathy (painless)
     b. NHL: Painless enlargement of lymph nodes, pain in bones or chest; fever, chills, weight loss
  3. Obtain diagnostic tests:
     a. Hodgkin disease: Lymph node biopsy, checking for presence of Reed-Sternberg cells
     b. NHL: Lymph node biopsy; CBC, bone marrow aspiration; liver function studies and liver scan; lumbar puncture
  4. Assess stage of cancer following diagnosis.
     a. Stage I—one lymph node involved
     b. Stage II—two lymph nodes involved on same side of diaphragm
     c. Stage III—lymph node involvement on both sides of diaphragm
     d. Stage IV—spread of cancer outside lymph nodes

B. Analysis
  1. Knowledge Deficit about Hodgkin disease related to medication administration and side effects of radiation therapy and chemotherapy
  2. Impaired Skin Integrity related to side effect of radiation therapy
  3. Risk for Infection related to decreased immune system
  4. Risk for Injury related to thrombocytopenia and/or anemia
  5. Risk for Fluid Volume Deficit related to nausea, vomiting, and poor nutritional intake

6. Imbalanced Nutrition: Less Than Body Requirements related to nausea, vomiting, and poor nutritional intake
7. Risk for Bleeding related to chemotherapy (resulting in low blood counts)

C. Planning
1. Relieve pain.
2. Prevent infection.
3. Maintain nutrition.
4. Instruct about use of therapeutic interventions (surgery, radiation, chemotherapy, bone marrow or stem cell transplant).

D. Implementation (see implementation for leukemia)

E. Evaluation
1. Client understands treatment protocol.
2. Client's skin is intact.
3. Client is free of infection.
4. Client is free from signs of injury.
5. Client exhibits adequate fluid and food intake.
6. Client does not have any bleeding complications.

CN

III. Client needs

A. Physiologic adaptation: Hodgkin disease is treated based on the stage of the disease; NHLs are treated based on the actual classification of the disease, as well as the stage of the disease. Cancer is eradicated via radiation therapy or chemotherapy, or a combination of both, depending on staging. Enlarged lymph nodes are surgically removed. Treatment occurs on an outpatient basis unless complications occur (see physiologic adaptation for leukemia for complications).

B. Management of care: Care of the client with Hodgkin disease and NHL who is undergoing chemotherapy requires critical thinking skills and knowledge of assessment, and teaching and evaluation methods unique to the RN role. These skills cannot be delegated to an LPN or UAP. (See management of care for the client with leukemia.)

C. Safety and infection control
1. Teach client to decrease risk of infection and minimize bleeding complications.
2. Instruct client to notify the health care team of any changes in his or her condition.

D. Health promotion and maintenance
1. Monitor and screen client for other malignances as the incidence increases among lymphoma-surviving clients to develop another malignancy.
2. Initiate nutritional consult to help client find palatable foods while undergoing treatment.
3. Provide frequent assessments for bleeding, anemia, and thrombocytopenia during therapy.
4. Provide skin assessments during radiation therapy to detect and treat skin breakdown.

E. Psychologic integrity
1. Introduce client and family to a local cancer support group.
2. Assess client for signs and symptoms of depression.
3. Promote a social services consult or mental health treatment for client and family in conjunction with therapy.

F. Basic care and comfort (see basic care and comfort for client with leukemia)

G. Reduction of risk potential: Provide client teaching regarding disease process and potential complications, and how to help prevent them.

H. Pharmacologic and parenteral therapies (see pharmacologic and parenteral therapies for leukemia)

Bleeding Disorders

I. Definition: Bleeding disorders are characterized by a group of conditions that affect the blood-clotting system, in which the bleeding following an injury is prolonged and severe. The main disorders in this group are idiopathic thrombocytopenic purpura (ITP), hemophilia, and von Willebrand disease.

A. ITP—caused by too few platelets in the blood, which are destroyed by the immune system. ITP is still referred to as idiopathic because the exact mechanism of the autoimmune component is not completely understood; it can be induced by viral infections, sulfa drugs, systemic lupus erythematosus, and pregnancy. The disorder can affect individuals of all ages, but is most commonly seen among children and young women.

B. Hemophilia—inherited bleeding disorder that disrupts the blood's clotting time and results in abnormal bleeding. There are two types of hemophilia: Hemophilia A and hemophilia B; while clinically indistinguishable the two types can be identified by laboratory tests, and may occur in varying degrees of severity. Because it is an X-linked trait, hemophilia affects mostly males. The disorder is usually diagnosed in children and affects all racial groups. (See also Chapter 13 for information about hemophilia in pediatric clients.)

C. von Willebrand disease—genetic disorder caused by a deficiency of the von Willebrand factor (which is necessary for factor VIII activity), and usually passed on as a dominant trait, equally affecting both men and women. The disorder is the most common of bleeding disorders and is usually discovered during surgery or a dental procedure. Most cases of von Willebrand disease are mild.

II. Nursing process
   A. Assessment
      1. Obtain a detailed health history and perform a comprehensive physical assessment.
      2. Assess for signs and symptoms, including bruising, nosebleed, petechiae, abnormal menstrual bleeding, bleeding of the gums, pain and swelling in joints as a result of bleeding into joint (hemophilia), hemorrhaging, even after minimal trauma (hemophilia), and spontaneous hemorrhaging (severe hemophilia).
      3. Obtain diagnostic criteria.
         a. ITP: CBC with low platelet count; normal bone marrow biopsy; normal PT and PTT
         b. Hemophilia: Decreased plasma concentration of factor VIII (hemophilia A) or factor IX (hemophilia B); normal PT and PTT
         c. von Willebrand disease: Normal platelet count; prolonged PT and PTT; low von Willebrand factor level
   B. Analysis
      1. Risk for Injury related to bleeding disorder
      2. Acute Pain related to hemophilia and bleeding into joints
      3. Impaired Physical Mobility related to discomfort from hemophilia
   C. Planning
      1. Control bleeding.
      2. Replete client with blood products or factor concentrates as indicated.
   D. Implementation: Assess pain before and after administration of blood products or factor concentrates.
   E. Evaluation
      1. Client is free from injury.
      2. Client's pain is eliminated or is well managed.
      3. Client is able to perform self-care activities and ambulate at baseline.

CN

III. Client needs
   A. Physiologic adaptation
      1. Recognize increased risk of bleeding after a surgical or traumatic event.
      2. Perform frequent neurologic assessments for client suffering from a head injury.
   B. Management of care: Care of the client with a bleeding disorder requires critical thinking skills and knowledge of assessment, and teaching and evaluation methods unique to the RN role. These skills cannot be delegated to an LPN or UAP.
      1. Delegate responsibly those activities that can be delegated, including basic hygiene needs, measurement of intake and output, and recording of vital signs for the stable client. All monitoring information is reported to the RN.
      2. After a procedure or traumatic event, closely assess client for signs of bleeding and monitor vital signs frequently.
   C. Safety and infection control: Teach client how to minimize safety risks at home (use electric razor and soft-bristled toothbrush) and at work, and to notify their HCP and seek medical attention if bleeding occurs without a reason or is uncontrolled.
   D. Health promotion and maintenance: Encourage client to exercise to maintain joint function; assist client in range of motion exercises, as tolerated, to promote joint health.
   E. Psychologic integrity: Instruct client on ways to cope with chronic illness and the restrictions it puts on daily activities (hemophilia).
   F. Basic care and comfort
      1. Encourage client to restrict certain activities to decrease risk of bleeding.
      2. Promote warm baths or analgesics help to relieve joint pain (warm baths not indicated during bleeding event).
      3. Administer analgesics for the client with hemophilia to relieve joint discomfort.
   G. Reduction of risk potential
      1. Avoid administering any medication that interferes with platelet function and clotting time; this includes aspirin, ibuprofen, and warfarin, even some over-the-counter medications.
      2. Inform client with a splenectomy that he or she is at increased risk for infection, and to ensure that all vaccinations are up to date.
      3. Instruct client with von Willebrand disease to begin desmopressin acetate (DDAVP) before surgery.
      4. Encourage the client with hemophilia to wear a medical bracelet indicating his or her condition.
   H. Pharmacologic and parenteral therapies: Client will state the purpose, dosage, timing, and side effects of medications and therapies to manage bleeding disorders.
      1. ITP: Steroid therapy; splenectomy
      2. Hemophilia: Factor VIII or factor IX blood concentrates; aminocaproic acid—fibrinolytic enzyme inhibitor (used before

surgical procedures); DDAVP (very useful in mild form of hemophilia A)
3. von Willebrand disease: Cryoprecipitate or fresh-frozen plasma replacement therapy; DDAVP to raise levels of von Willebrand factor

Disseminated Intravascular Coagulation

I. Definition: Disseminated intravascular coagulation (DIC) results in increased clotting throughout the body. It is not a disease itself, but rather a sign of an underlying condition. DIC usually causes severe bleeding and can be stimulated by septicemia, severe tissue injury (as seen in burns and head injuries), cancer, blood transfusion reactions, and obstetric emergencies. Mortality rate of those who develop DIC can exceed 80%.

II. Nursing process

A. Assessment

1. Assess client for risk factors, including recent sepsis, severe hypotension, a recent trauma or surgery, complications of labor and delivery, cancer, and severe liver disease.
2. Assess for signs and symptoms.
    a. Abnormal bleeding, usually sudden and severe, involving more than one system (bleeding most notable at sites of invasive procedures such as an IV or chest tube)
    b. Sudden bruising
    c. Clot formation (in clients with cancer, DIC develops more slowly, resulting in clot formation rather than bleeding)
3. Obtain diagnostic tests.
    a. Blood studies
    b. Elevated (prolonged) PT and PTT; decreased PT and PTT in cancer client with slowly forming DIC
    c. Decreased platelets
    d. High fibrinogen-degradation products
    e. Low-serum fibrinogen

B. Analysis

1. Ineffective Tissue Perfusion: Peripheral, related to interruption of flow to organs
2. Acute Pain related to tissue trauma
3. Anxiety related to emergent situation and threat of death

C. Planning

1. Identify underlying cause and control bleeding.
2. Monitor vital signs.
3. Replace clotting factors.
4. Provide anticoagulation therapy.

D. Implementation

1. Ensure IV access.
2. Administer fresh-frozen plasma as ordered.
3. Administer IV heparin, if indicated and as ordered.
4. Observe for signs of increased bleeding (especially at sites of invasive procedures) and apply pressure as necessary.
5. Closely monitor vital signs (BP, temperature, pulse, respiratory rate) as ordered.
6. Assess neurologic status as indicated.
7. Assess arterial blood gases.
8. Administer pain medications as indicated.

E. Evaluation

1. Client's bleeding has stopped or is controlled.
2. Client does not experience new sources of bleeding.
3. Client is pain-free.
4. Client and family experience relief of anxiety.

CN

III. Client needs

A. Physiologic adaptation. Physiologic adaptation in DIC is complex and requires frequent assessment and evaluation of interventions. Management involves simultaneously treating the underlying disorder while treating bleeding with fresh-frozen plasma to replace clotting factors, platelet transfusions, and cryoprecipitate to replace clotting factors and fibrinogen. Fluid balance and replacement is critical; client may be at risk for hypovolemic shock. Oxygen is used to maintain cellular oxygenation, particularly to vital organs.

B. Management of care: Care of the client with DIC requires critical thinking skills and knowledge of assessment, and teaching and evaluation methods unique to the RN role. These skills cannot be delegated to an LPN or UAP.

1. Delegate responsibly those activities that can be delegated, including basic hygiene needs and measurement of intake and output. All monitoring information is reported to the RN.
2. Provide client with frequent assessments, including vital signs, neurologic assessments, and ECGs as indicated.
3. Inform the physician of any changes noted during each assessment.

C. Safety and infection control

1. Ensure aseptic technique throughout emergent event.
2. Ensure sites of bleeding are cleaned properly, once controlled, and appropriate wound care is provided.

D. Health promotion and maintenance
  1. Provide client and family with information regarding DIC and treatment in easy-to-understand language.
  2. Be attentive to client's nonverbal cues.

E. Psychologic integrity
  1. Identify client and family stressors associated with situation and help provide tools to alleviate them.
  2. Provide client and family with clergy, social worker, as indicated.
  3. Reassure client throughout emergent event; maintain calm environment.

F. Basic care and comfort
  1. Provide pain relief as appropriate.
  2. Ensure client is comfortable; reposition in bed, if necessary, and provide clean, dry clothes.

G. Reduction of risk potential
  1. Assess client for signs and symptoms of bleeding, particularly when risk factors are present.
  2. Monitor client's laboratory values as indicated; note slow changes in coagulation for clients with cancer.

H. Pharmacologic and parenteral therapies: Client will state the purpose for and side effects of medications and therapies to manage DIC.
  1. Fresh-frozen plasma to replace clotting factors
  2. IV heparin, if indicated, to prevent thrombosis
  3. Other blood products, if needed
  4. Analgesics for pain relief
  5. Oxygen therapy, if indicated

Bibliography

Altman, G. (2004). *Delmar's fundamental and advanced nursing skills* (2nd ed.). Albany, NY: Delmar.

Ellis, J., & Hartley, C. (2005). *Managing and coordinating nursing care.* Philadelphia: Lippincott Williams & Wilkins.

Karch, A. (2006). *Lippincott's nursing drug guide.* Philadelphia: Lippincott Williams & Wilkins.

Nursing 2008 drug handbook. Ambler, PA: Springhouse.

Purnell, L., & Paulanka, B. (Eds.). (2003). *Transcultural healthcare: A culturally competent approach.* Philadelphia: Davis.

Smeltzer, S. C., Bare, B. G., Cheever, K. H., & Hinkle, J. L. (2008). *Brunner & Suddarth's textbook of medical-surgical nursing* (11th ed.). Philadelphia: Lippincott Williams & Wilkins.

Taylor, C., Lillis, C., LeMone, P., & Lynn, P. (2006). *Fundamentals of nursing.* Philadelphia: Lippincott Williams & Wilkins.

Weber, J. R., & Kelley, J. (2007). *Nurses handbook of health assessment.* Philadelphia: Lippincott Williams & Wilkins

Yarbro, C. H., Frogge, M., & Goodman, M. (2004). *Cancer symptom management* (3rd ed.). Sudbury, MA: Jones and Bartlett.

CHAPTER 22

Practice Test

Anemias

1. A client with pernicious anemia is receiving vitamin B_{12}. The nurse should assess the client for which of the following expected outcomes of vitamin B_{12}?
- ☐ 1. Increased energy.
- ☐ 2. Healed tongue and lips.
- ☐ 3. Absence of paresthesias.
- ☐ 4. Improved clotting time.

2. The nurse is administering parenteral iron replacement for a client with iron deficiency anemia. The nurse should use which of the following injection techniques?
- ☐ 1. Administer in the subcutaneous tissue around the umbilicus.
- ☐ 2. Use a rotational pattern in the arms and legs.
- ☐ 3. Place the needle bevel up and inject intradermally.
- ☐ 4. Retract skin over the gluteus maximus using "Z-track" technique.

3. AF The nurse is giving instructions to a client with anemia who is going to have a Hematest®. The nurse should instruct the client to avoid ingesting which of the following for 7 days? Select all that apply.
- ☐ 1. Aspirin.
- ☐ 2. Penicillin drugs.
- ☐ 3. Iron preparation.
- ☐ 4. Vitamin C.
- ☐ 5. Red meat.
- ☐ 6. Corticosteroids.

4. The nurse is reviewing laboratory results of an older adult with iron deficiency anemia

who is taking ferrous sulphate and following an iron-rich diet. Which of the following indicates the diet and drug therapy is having desired effects?
- □ 1. Erythrocytes are 3,000,000 mm^3 blood.
- □ 2. Thrombocytes are 200,000 mm^3 blood.
- □ 3. Leukocytes are 7,000 mm^3 blood.
- □ 4. Hemoglobin is 14 g per 100 mL of blood.

Sickle Cell Anemia

5. The nurse is planning care for an adult client in sickle cell crisis. Which of the following indicates successful nursing management?
- □ 1. Client's fever is reduced.
- □ 2. Client's coughing and sputum production is decreased.
- □ 3. Client states decrease in pain.
- □ 4. Client exhibits no further evidence of bruising.

6. A middle-aged adult client is admitted to the hospital with a vasoocclusive sickle cell crisis. The nurse should do which of the following first?
- □ 1. Administer oxygen.
- □ 2. Obtain a nursing history.
- □ 3. Start an IV infusion.
- □ 4. Give pain medication.

Polycythemia Vera

7. The nurse is assessing a client with polycythemia vera. The nurse should conduct a focused assessment because this client is at risk for which of the following?
- □ 1. Hair loss.
- □ 2. Thrombus formation.
- □ 3. Clotting.
- □ 4. Iron deficiency.

Leukemia

8. AF A client who is having a bone marrow biopsy is worried about the pain. The nurse can explain that which of the following will be used to minimize pain and discomfort of the procedure? Select all that apply.
- □ 1. Conscious sedation at the time of the procedure.
- □ 2. Regional nerve block during the procedure.
- □ 3. Tranquilizer 30 min prior to the procedure.
- □ 4. Local anesthetic prior to the incision.
- □ 5. General anesthesia prior to beginning the procedure.

9. A client with chronic myelogenous leukemia is experiencing leukopenia secondary to chemotherapy. The nurse should plan with the client to do which of the following?
- □ 1. Cover the mouth when coughing.
- □ 2. Avoid use of aspirin.
- □ 3. Stay out of public areas.
- □ 4. Alternate activity with periods of rest.

10. A client receiving a blood transfusion begins complaining of lower back pain and dyspnea. The nurse should first:
- □ 1. Slow the transfusion until the dyspnea is relieved.
- □ 2. Obtain the client's vital signs.
- □ 3. Clear the infusion with normal saline.
- □ 4. Stop the transfusion.

11. A client with chronic myelogenous leukemia is taking imatinib (Gleevec). The nurse should instruct the client to report which of the following adverse effects of this drug?
- □ 1. Edema.
- □ 2. Numbness and tingling in extremities.
- □ 3. Bloody stools.
- □ 4. Persistent cough.

12. A client with acute lymphocytic leukemia is receiving vincristine (Oncovin). Prior to infusing the drug, the nurse administers diphenhydramine (Benadryl). The nurse should inform the client that the expected outcome of using diphenhydramine (Benadryl) is which of the following?
- □ 1. Promotes sleep, while the vincristine (Oncovin) is infusing.
- □ 2. Decreases incidence of a reaction to the vincristine (Oncovin).
- □ 3. Potentiates the action of the vincristine (Oncovin).
- □ 4. Reduces any anxiety associated with the vincristine (Oncovin) infusion.

13. A female client is receiving chemotherapy and is experiencing pancytopenia. Which laboratory result most warrants that the nurse immediately contact the physician?
- □ 1. Platelet count of 12,000/mm^3.
- □ 2. WBC count of 4,000/mm^3.
- □ 3. Absolute neutrophil count of 1,500/mm^3.
- □ 4. Hemoglobin of 12 g/100 mL.

14. A nurse is administering an IV antineoplastic agent when the client says, "My arm is burning by the IV site." What should the nurse do first?
- □ 1. Slow the infusion rate and check the IV site.
- □ 2. Call the physician to report the incident.
- □ 3. Stop infusing the medication.
- □ 4. Place a warm, moist pack on the IV site area.

15. AF A client who is receiving a blood transfusion suddenly experiences chills and a temperature of 101°F. The client also has a headache and appears flushed. In what order should the nurse perform the following? Place in order from first to last.

_____ 1. Obtain a blood culture from the client.
_____ 2. Send the blood bag and administration set to the blood bank.
_____ 3. Stop the blood infusion.
_____ 4. Infuse normal saline to keep the vein open.

16. A client being treated with IV antineoplastic drugs develops stomatitis. What should the nurse teach this client?
- ☐ 1. Eat small, frequent meals with cold foods.
- ☐ 2. Apply antibiotic ointment to the skin erosions prior to bedtime.
- ☐ 3. Use a hot water bottle on the abdomen as needed for comfort.
- ☐ 4. Sit in a semi-Fowler position after meals.

17. A client undergoing antineoplastic therapy is prescribed subcutaneous epoetin (Procrit). The nurse evaluates that the drug is effective when:
- ☐ 1. Biopsies no longer show malignancy.
- ☐ 2. Hemoglobin levels rise.
- ☐ 3. Nausea and vomiting stop.
- ☐ 4. A scan shows tumor shrinkage.

Lymphomas

18. The nurse is developing a care plan for a client who has had radiation therapy for Hodgkin's lymphoma. Which of the following is the primary goal of care for this client?
- ☐ 1. Maintain fluid balance.
- ☐ 2. Obtain sufficient exercise.
- ☐ 3. Prevent infection.
- ☐ 4. Avoid depression.

Bleeding Disorders

19. Following an automobile accident, an adolescent with a medic-alert bracelet indicating hemophilia A is admitted to the emergency department. Which of the following orders should the nurse implement first?
- ☐ 1. Transport to radiology for C-spine x-rays.
- ☐ 2. Type and cross-match for three units PRBCs.
- ☐ 3. Infuse normal saline at 200 ml/hr.
- ☐ 4. Transfuse factor VIII concentrate.

Disseminated Intravascular Coagulation

20. Which of the following findings is the most significant for a client who has DIC?
- ☐ 1. Bloody stools.
- ☐ 2. Difficulty swallowing.
- ☐ 3. Fruity-smelling breath.
- ☐ 4. Peripheral edema.

Answers and Rationales

1. 3 Pernicious anemia is caused by a lack of vitamin B_{12}. Primary symptoms include neuropathy with paresthesia of hands and feet. The nurse assesses the client to determine the effectiveness of the monthly dose of vitamin B_{12}, which is to reverse the deficiency and the related symptoms. Improved energy is associated with treatment for iron deficiency anemia. Healing of cracked lips and tongue are outcomes of taking folic acid for folic acid deficiency. Delayed clotting time is associated with hemophilia; the clotting time is not affected by vitamin B_{12}. (D)

2. 4 Iron administered parenterally can stain the tissues; therefore, the nurse uses a Z-track technique by retracting the skin over the muscle, injecting the medication, and allowing the skin to return to the muscle to prevent leakage. Heparin is administered subcutaneously, insulin is administered in a rotational pattern, and tuberculin testing uses an intradermal approach. (D)

3. 1, 5, 6 Drugs that cause GI irritation (aspirin, corticosteroids, indomethacin, anticoagulants) can cause a false-positive Hematest®, as can red meat (as well as liver, salmon, sardines, broccoli, and melons). Vitamin C can cause a false-negative test. Iron and penicillin will have no effect on the test. (A)

4. 4 The expected outcome of supplemental iron in diet and medication is to improve the RBC count and the hemoglobin. A hemoglobin of 14 g/100 ml of blood is within normal limits; normal erythrocyte count is 5 million erythrocytes mm^3 of blood. The thrombocytes and leukocytes are within normal range. (A)

5. 3 The primary symptom associated with the sickling of cells is severe pain; therefore, the nursing care plan must include measures to manage pain. Clients with sickle cell crisis generally do not present with fever, coughing, or bruising, although jaundice may be present because of hemolysis. (A)

6. 3 Vaso-oclusive sickle cell crisis is a medical emergency. Because dehydration increases sickling of cells, the nurse's first priority is to start an IV to maintain fluid balance. Next, the nurse starts oxygen, and then administers morphine for pain. The nurse can obtain a nursing history once emergent needs are met. (A)

7. 2 Polycythemia vera is a chronic disorder in which all of the bone marrow elements proliferate. There is an increase in the RBC mass and the blood is viscous, putting the client at risk for forming thrombi, which may present as MI, stroke, or DVT. The nurse instructs the client to report signs of thrombus formation. Hair loss is associated with chemotherapy. The client with polycythemia vera is more prone to bleeding from abnormal platelet functioning than to clotting disorders. Iron deficiency is associated with iron deficiency anemia. (H)

8. 3, 4 Typically, the client who is having a bone marrow biopsy can have an oral tranquilizer 30 min prior to the procedure to relieve anxiety. Prior to making an incision, the HCP will administer a local anesthetic. It is not necessary to use conscious sedation, regional nerve block, or general anesthesia for this procedure. (C)

9. 3 Leucopenia is an abnormal low number of leukocytes or WBCs. The client is at increased risk for infection because WBCs help prevent infection; therefore, the nursing goal is to assist the client to avoid large, closely crowded areas that may increase the chance of exposure to infected persons. Instructing the client to cover his or her mouth when coughing may protect others from the possible spread of pathogens, but not the client. Aspirin products are avoided with chemotherapy because of a low number of platelets rather than leukocytes. Alternating activity and rest may help relieve fatigue associated with chemotherapy-induced anemia, but will not prevent infection. (R)

10. 4 The client is exhibiting signs of a hemolytic blood transfusion reaction. The nurse stops the blood transfusion to prevent further reactions and notifies the physician before further therapy can be initiated. Once the infusion is discontinued, the nurse removes and changes the tubing (because blood remains in the tubing) and infuses normal saline in order to keep the IV line open. The transfusion must be stopped, not slowed. The first step is to stop the transfusion; the nurse can take vital signs after (or while, if assistance is available) notifying the physician. (R)

11. 1 Imatinib (Gleevec) works by inhibiting the proliferation of abnormal cells. Adverse effects include edema and GI irritation. Typical side effects of this drug do not include edema, numbness and tingling, bloody stools, or persistent cough. If the client has these symptoms, they may relate to disease occurrence or recurrence. (D)

12. 2 Diphenhydramine (Benadryl) is an antihistamine. This drug helps reduce the incidence of allergic response by blocking the release of histamine. Diphenhydramine also possesses anticholinergic effects and can reduce the incidence of nausea and vomiting for clients receiving chemotherapy. Although diphenhydramine may promote sleep, it is not the primary reason for its administration in this instance. Diphenhydramine will not reduce anxiety or potentiate the action of the vincristine (Oncovin). (D)

13. 1 Pancytopenia means a decrease in all blood components. Because a platelet count of less than 15,000/mm^3 can result in spontaneous bleeding, the nurse notifies the HCP of this laboratory result. Neutrophils are a type of WBC. An absolute neutrophil count between 1,000 and 1,800/mm^3 suggests mild neutropenia and represents a low risk of infection. Although references vary, normal range for WBC counts are 5,000 to 11,000/mm^3, and a female's normal hemoglobin (Hgb) value is roughly 12 to 16 g/100 ml. Therefore, the WBC count and Hgb levels are a bit low, but not critical. (R)

14. 3 Antineoplastic agents can cause severe tissue damage if they extravasate; therefore, the nurse immediately stops the infusion and then notifies the physician. If extravasation has occurred, it may be appropriate to apply ice packs to the site. Ice packs cause desired vasoconstriction; warm, moist packs cause vasodilation. Ice packs should not remain in place for more than 15 to 20 min because rebound vasodilation can occur; the ice packs are removed for a short time and then reapplied as needed. (D)

15. 3, 4, 1, 2 The client is experiencing a septic reaction to the blood transfusion. The nurse first stops the infusion and notifies the HCP and blood bank; then the nurse uses an infusion of normal saline to keep the vein open, and follows by obtaining a sample of the client's blood for a blood culture. Lastly, the nurse sends the blood bag and the administration set to the blood bank for culture. (M)

16. 1 Stomatitis is inflammation of the mouth, lips, tongue, and mucous membranes caused by a variety of situations, including antineoplastic drug therapy. Teaching the client to eat small, frequent meals with cold foods will reduce discomfort and help ensure that the client consumes needed nutrients. Open skin erosions are not associated with stomatitis, and antibiotic ointments are not needed unless there is an infection. A hot water bottle does not address oral inflammation, and sitting upright after meals is primarily intended for those with gastric reflux. (D)

17. 2 Epoetin (Procrit) stimulates erythropoiesis and the production of RBCs. This is important for clients taking antineoplastics because they often suffer bone marrow depression as a side effect of antineoplastic therapy. Epoetin does not affect tissue malignancy or tumor size. Nausea and vomiting are commonly associated with antineoplastics, but these are treated with antiemetics. (D)

18. 3 The client with Hodgkin's lymphoma who has had radiation therapy is prone to infection; therefore, the primary goal is to prevent infection. The nurse instructs the client to perform frequent hand hygiene, avoid crowded areas, and report a temperature over 100°F. Maintaining fluid balance, exercising, and maintaining mental health are also important, but not the primary goal at this time. (H)

19. 4 When a hemophiliac client is at high risk for bleeding (e.g., after a trauma or accident), the priority intervention is to maximize the availability of clotting factors. The other orders also should be implemented rapidly, but are not as high a priority. (M)

20. 1 In disseminated intravascular coagulation, clotting factors are rapidly consumed, which causes generalized bleeding. Difficulty swallowing is most commonly associated with throat cancers or stroke. Fruity-smelling breath is associated with ketoacidosis. Peripheral edema is associated with fluid volume excesses, not clotting disorders. (A)

chapter

23

The Client With Respiratory Health Problems

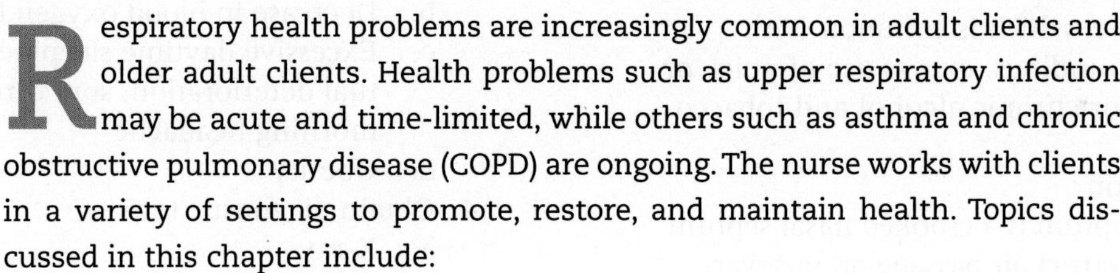

Respiratory health problems are increasingly common in adult clients and older adult clients. Health problems such as upper respiratory infection may be acute and time-limited, while others such as asthma and chronic obstructive pulmonary disease (COPD) are ongoing. The nurse works with clients in a variety of settings to promote, restore, and maintain health. Topics discussed in this chapter include:

- Upper Respiratory Disorders
- Cancer of the Larynx
- Lung Cancer
- Asthma
- Chronic Obstructive Pulmonary Disease
- Pneumonia
- Pulmonary Tuberculosis
- Acute Respiratory Distress Syndrome
- Chest Trauma

Upper Respiratory Disorders

I. Definition: Upper respiratory disorders are health problems of the nose, sinuses, throat, and trachea. These health problems are primarily caused by infection, trauma, or tumors.
   A. Upper respiratory infections (URIs)
      1. Rhinitis is an inflammation of the mucous membranes of the nose, caused by allergies (allergic rhinitis) or a virus (viral rhinitis or common cold), and rarely by bacteria (bacterial rhinitis) or a fungal infection.
      2. Sinusitis occurs from narrowing or blocking of the ostia or exit from the sinuses from inflammation or hypertrophy of the mucosa. The secretions that collect provide a medium for bacterial, viral, or fungal growth. Acute sinusitis is resolving. Chronic sinusitis is a persistent infection associated with allergies, nasal polyps, and recurrent episodes of acute sinusitis.
      3. Pharyngitis is an inflammation of the pharyngeal wall, which may include the tonsils, palate, and uvula, with an acute presentation of a sore throat. Chronic pharyngitis is a persistent inflammation of the pharynx, which is common with dusty surroundings, excess use of voice or coughing, or chronic alcohol and tobacco use.
   B. Nasal obstruction
      1. Deviated septum is a crooked nasal septum that can obstruct air passage or, in severe cases, block drainage from the sinuses.
      2. Nasal fracture is caused by traumatic force to the middle of the face that can cause airway obstruction, epistaxis (see later discussion), cosmetic deformity, and meningeal tear. Nasal fractures are classified as unilateral, bilateral, or complex.
      3. Nasal polyps are benign, grapelike swellings of the mucous membrane of the sinuses that form from repeated inflammation of the sinus or nasal mucosa.
   C. Epistaxis is hemorrhage from the nose caused from trauma, inhalation of drugs, infection, blood dyscrasias, low humidity, foreign body, anatomic malformation, and tumors. Anterior septal bleeding is more common and easier to self-treat. Posterior bleeding usually requires medical intervention with packing.
   D. Obstructive sleep apnea (OSA) is a condition characterized by partial or complete obstruction of the airway during sleep, causing apnea and hypoxia.

II. Nursing process
   A. Assessment
      1. Obtain a detailed health history, psychosocial history, and perform a comprehensive physical examination focusing on the head and neck, nose, ears, mouth sinuses, pharynx and chest, breathing patterns, and adequacy of oxygenation.
      2. Assess for signs and symptoms.
         a. Nasal drainage, congestion, purulent discharge, or bleeding
         b. Obstructed or diminished air flow from the nose
         c. Headache
         d. Sneezing, sore throat
         e. Fever
         f. Inflamed, reddened membranes, sore throat, difficulty swallowing
         g. Facial pain or pressure over the sinus area, facial edema
         h. Decreased sense of smell
         i. Decreased SpO_2
         j. Fatigue
         k. Intellectual deterioration
      3. Assess for signs and symptoms of OSA.
         a. Loud snoring and breathing cessation for at least 10 s for five or more episodes per hour, followed by abrupt awakening
         b. Decrease in blood oxygen levels
         c. Excessive daytime sleepiness, intellectual deterioration, sore throat, and morning headache
         d. Obesity
      4. Obtain diagnostic tests.
         a. X-ray
         b. CT scan
         c. MRI
         d. Nasal endoscopy
         e. Sleep study
         f. CBC, PT, INR, aPTT or PTT, platelets
   B. Analysis
      1. Ineffective Airway Clearance related to increased mucus production
      2. Acute Pain related to upper airway inflammation and irritation
      3. Altered Breathing Pattern related to airflow obstruction and ineffective airway clearance
      4. Ineffective Therapeutic Regimen Management related to knowledge deficit
   C. Planning
      1. Maintain a patent airway.
      2. Relieve pain and associated symptoms.
      3. Control secretions, bleeding, or infection.
      4. Prevent complications.
   D. Implementation
      1. Monitor vital signs, SpO_2, patency of airway, and extent of airflow obstruction.

2. Monitor amount, color, and consistency of secretions or drainage.
3. Provide client and family teaching about risk factors, interventions, promoting a healthy lifestyle, self-care behaviors, and signs and symptoms that require medical attention.

E. Evaluation
1. Client exhibits a patent airway and adequate oxygenation.
2. Client has absence of bleeding or minimal secretions.
3. Client acknowledges absence of pain and reduction of symptoms.
4. Client is free from infection.

CN

III. Client needs

A. Physiologic adaptation: A tracheostomy is indicated for an upper airway obstruction to facilitate removal of copious secretions, and for clients who require long-term mechanical ventilation. Treatments for individual upper respiratory disorders are as follows:
1. URIs—for viral URIs, interventions include rest, fluids, antipyretics, and analgesics; antibiotics may be indicated for bacterial infections.
2. Nasal obstructions
   a. Deviated septum—submucous resection to remove obstructions or straighten the septum.
   b. Nasal fractures—rhinoplasty, septoplasty, or nasal fracture reduction surgery may be performed.
   c. Nasal polyps—removed by endoscopic or laser surgery, but recurrence is common.
3. Epistaxis—first aid: Keep client upright and leaning forward to prevent swallowing blood; if bleeding is in anterior part of the nose, apply pressure by compressing the nose between finger and thumb for 5 to 10 min. For uncontrolled epistaxis, treatment may include nasal packing to the area of the bleeding, treating abnormal coagulation factors, and controlling hypertension. Cauterization or application of a vasoconstricting agent on a cotton pledget may also be used.
4. OSA—an oral appliance may be prescribed for a client with mild OSA; for more severe OSA, nasal continuous positive airway pressure or bi level positive airway pressure (BiPAP) is applied for sleeping.

B. Management of care: Care of the client with an upper respiratory disorder requires critical thinking skills and knowledge of assessment, and teaching and evaluation methods unique to the RN role. These skills cannot be delegated to an LPN or UAP.
1. Delegate responsibly those activities that can be delegated, such as taking vital signs and performing dressing changes. All monitoring information is reported to the RN.
2. Perform physical assessments and monitor vital signs, SpO_2, patency of airway, quality of respirations, lung sounds, quantity and characteristics of secretions or drainage, and symptoms.
3. Provide teaching and interventions for symptom and pain management, positioning for improving ventilation and reducing inflammation and edema, and reduction of anxiety.
4. Provide interventions to manage epistaxis.
   a. Keep client calm and place in a sitting position or with head and shoulders elevated.
   b. Apply pressure by pinching the nares together for 10 to 15 min.
   c. Apply ice compress to the nose.
   d. If bleeding continues, identify the site and notify the health care provider (HCP), who will apply a vasoconstrictive agent, or perform cauterization or anterior packing.
   e. Tape a drip pad or nasal sling below the nares to absorb and monitor drainage.
5. Provide interventions to manage tracheostomy.
   a. Assess respirations, lung sounds, and SpO_2.
   b. Encourage deep breathing and coughing.
   c. Maintain semi-Fowler to high Fowler positions.
   d. Assess secretions and provide tracheal suctioning to maintain airway patency.
      (1) Keep suction equipment, suction supplies, and Ambu bag at bedside.
      (2) Preoxygenate prior to suctioning.
      (3) Suction for maximum of 5 to 10 s during removal of catheter.
   e. Assess cuff pressure.
   f. Assess stoma and clean tracheostomy site and inner cannula per agency protocol.
      (1) Remove disposable inner cannula and replace with a new one or clean nondisposable cannula with half-strength hydrogen peroxide; rinse with saline, reinsert, and lock into place using sterile technique.

(2) Change tracheostomy securing tape.
(3) Place tracheostomy dressing below stoma to absorb expelled secretions.

g. Suction secretions from mouth with a separate catheter.
h. Instruct client and family on tracheostomy care and suctioning for clients returning to home setting with a tracheostomy.

6. Assess for home health care needs such as managing tracheostomy or dressing changes.
7. Introduce client to community resources for smoking cessation therapy, weight-loss program (if indicated), and support groups.

C. Safety and infection control: Instruct client in good hand hygiene techniques and avoidance of people with respiratory infections, colds, or flu.

D. Health promotion and maintenance
1. Encourage smoking cessation.
2. Instruct client to moderate or eliminate alcohol intake.
3. Promote influenza vaccine.
4. Refer client with OSA to a weight-loss program, if indicated.

E. Psychologic integrity: Assess impact of disease on quality of life and coping strategies.

F. Basic care and comfort: Manage symptoms to maintain client comfort.

G. Reduction of risk potential
1. Instruct client to avoid vigorous nose blowing with epistaxis.
2. Facilitate treatment of hypertension to assist in controlling epistaxis.
3. Instruct client to avoid exposure to allergens.

H. Pharmacologic and parenteral therapies: Client will state the purpose, usage, and associated side effects of medications used to treat upper respiratory disorders.
1. Antihistamines
2. Decongestants
3. Corticosteroids (for severe inflammation)
4. Antipyretics
5. Analgesics

Cancer of the Larynx

I. Definition: Laryngeal cancer is a malignant tumor of the larynx, occurring in the glottic area (vocal cords), supraglottic area, or subglottic area. Squamous cell carcinoma accounts for the majority of cases. The tumor is staged by the TNM classification system, which facilitates identification of treatment modalities. Although uncommon, cancer of the larynx is significant because of the potential loss of voice, disfigurement, and social isolation; the cancer is curable if identified early.

II. Nursing process

A. Assessment
1. Obtain a detailed health history, psychosocial history, and physical examination of head and neck.
2. Assess for presence of risk factors, including prolonged use of tobacco and alcohol.
3. Assess for signs and symptoms.
   a. Hoarseness, lump in neck, sore throat
   b. Pain, dysphagia, dyspnea, and foul breath are later symptoms.
4. Obtain diagnostic tests.
   a. Indirect laryngoscopy
   b. Direct laryngoscopy with multiple biopsy specimens
   c. CT scan
   d. MRI
   e. Chest x-ray

B. Analysis
1. Ineffective Breathing Pattern related to secretions, inability to cough, or surgical creation of artificial airway
2. Impaired Verbal Communication related to laryngectomy
3. Altered Nutrition: Less Than Body Requirements related to impaired swallowing, use of chemotherapy, or radiation therapy
4. Ineffective Tissue Perfusion: Peripheral, related to laryngectomy
5. Disturbed Body Image related to creation of artificial airway.
6. Anxiety related to progress and prognosis
7. Acute Pain related to disease and surgical procedures

C. Planning
1. Maintain a patent airway.
2. Maintain stable vital signs and SpO_2.
3. Maintain adequate nutrition.
4. Decrease pain.
5. Maintain ability of client to communicate.
6. Reduce anxiety and promote positive body image.
7. Prevent complications and spread of cancer.

D. Implementation
1. Monitor vital signs, SpO_2, patency of airway, secretions, lung sounds.
2. Provide client and family teaching on risk factors, effects of interventions, alternate methods of communication, stoma care, and suctioning after total laryngectomy.
3. Provide good oral care.

E. Evaluation
1. Client's vital signs and SpO_2 are within targeted range with normal breathing pattern.
2. Client's respiratory secretions are minimal and controlled with suctioning.
3. Client affirms satisfactory pain management.
4. Client exhibits intact swallow, adequate oral intake, maintenance of weight, and healing of incision after surgery.
5. Client demonstrates effective communication.
6. Client shows a decrease in anxiety.
7. Client participates in self-care.
8. Client receives adequate oral care.

CN

III. Client needs

A. Physiologic adaptation: After staging is determined, treatment of laryngeal cancer is selected based on health history, location, size, extent of disease and cervical lymph node involvement, cosmetic concerns, urgency, and client preference. Treatment options include the following:
1. For early lesions and voice preservation—radiation, chemotherapy, or partial laryngectomy (quality of voice is affected).
2. For advanced lesions—total laryngectomy with or without chemotherapy or radiation therapy: A stoma is created in the neck for breathing with a surgical tie-off of the airway above the stoma; a modified or radical neck dissection may be performed to decrease the risk of tumor spread. Separation of the airway from the oral cavity with a total laryngectomy affects breathing, swallowing, ability to smell, and taste functions.

B. Management of care: Care of the client with laryngeal cancer requires critical thinking skills and knowledge of assessment, and teaching and evaluation methods unique to the RN role. These skills cannot be delegated to an LPN or UAP.
1. Delegate responsibly those activities that can be delegated, such as taking vital signs, providing comfort measures, and assisting with bathing and hygiene. All monitoring information is reported to the RN.
2. Promote evaluation by speech-language pathologist prior to surgery to facilitate planning of postsurgical treatment.
3. Provide postoperative care.
   a. Monitor vital signs frequently.
   b. Monitor continuous SpO_2 and ECG.
   c. Promote frequent suctioning of stoma to maintain airway patency.
   d. Titrate humidified oxygen to maintain target SpO_2.
   e. Elevate head of bed in semi-Fowler position to decrease edema to surgical site.
   f. Monitor dressing, incision site, and drainage tubes for wound management.
   g. Monitor for potential complications, including respiratory distress, hemorrhage, infection, and wound breakdown.
   h. Promote tube feedings as indicated to allow healing of the surgical sites.
   i. Facilitate postoperative diet—client may undergo a radiographic swallow study about 1 week postoperatively; if incisions are intact, client begins an oral diet, typically advancing to a soft diet by the time of discharge.
   j. Promote initial postoperative communication through a communication board or writing.
4. Promote interventions with speech-language pathologist, who instructs client on a new sound source for speech:
   a. Esophageal speech
   b. Artificial larynx
   c. Tracheoesophageal puncture
5. Enhance self-care strategies through client and family teaching:
   a. Teach care for the stoma and incision to promote ability of client to handle and monitor secretions.
   b. Teach signs and symptoms of a wound infection and to monitor temperature.
   c. Reinforce a nutritious diet and monitoring of weekly weights.
   d. Encourage a gradual return to normal activity.
   e. Teach importance of outpatient follow-up care with the HCP and speech therapist.
6. Assess for home health care needs such as laryngectomy care, dressing changes, nutritional assessment and management.
7. Promote follow-up care with home care nurse, including assessment of client's surgical incision, respiratory status, nutrition, pain management, ability to care for stoma, and adequacy of humidification.
8. Link client with community resources for smoking cessation therapy and support groups.

C. Safety and infection control: Provide client teaching to promote safety and infection control.
1. Prevent water from entering stoma while showering by turning back away from water spray of shower head.

2. Wear a loose-fitting bib over stoma to filter dust and particulate matter, and maintain humidity.
3. Avoid swimming to prevent water in the lungs.

D. Health promotion and maintenance: Introduce client to smoking cessation program; promote abstinence from alcohol; instruct a nutritious, high-protein and -calorie diet to promote healing and maintain target weight.

E. Psychologic integrity
1. Assess impact of disease on quality of life and coping strategies.
2. Assess client's social and family support and adequacy of communication to prevent social isolation.
3. For client with advanced-stage cancer, promote teaching from health care team regarding goals of treatment, living will, and an advance directive to determine client preferences while client is able to participate in decisions for end-of-life care.

F. Basic care and comfort
1. Provide frequent oral care.
2. Promote adequate pain management and control of symptoms to maintain client comfort and quality of life.

G. Reduction of risk potential
1. Monitor client for signs of infection to avoid wound breakdown.
2. Maintain adequate humidification of stoma.
3. Maintain patent airway and control of secretions.
4. Instruct client on symptoms that require medical attention.

H. Pharmacologic and parenteral therapies: Client will state the purpose, usage, and associated side effects of medications used to treat laryngeal cancer.
1. Narcotics or analgesics for pain management, if needed following surgery.
2. IV fluids and nutritional replacement for as long as necessary to promote wound healing and prevent dehydration.

Lung Cancer

I. Definition: Lung cancer is the leading cause of cancer death among men and women in the United States. There are two major types of lung cancer, small cell and non-small cell.

A. Small cell or oat cell lung cancer accounts for 15% to 20% of all lung cancers, occurring mostly in smokers. Small cell lung cancer is staged according to tumor tissue type, node involvement, and extent of metastasis (TPN). Although more responsive to chemotherapy and radiation therapy than other types of lung cancer, small cell lung cancer is aggressive and has usually metastasized by the time of diagnosis; this results in a low survival rate. This type of cancer is associated with paraneoplastic syndrome, which causes symptoms from a hormone or enzyme produced by the tumor cells.

B. Non-small cell lung cancer accounts for approximately 80% of all lung cancers. It spreads more slowly than small cell cancer and is staged by the TNM classification (size of tumor, node involvement, and metastasis). The tumor is surgically resectable if found in the early stages. There are three major forms of non-small cell lung cancer:
1. Squamous cell carcinoma (about 30% of all lung cancers) is directly linked to smoking and tends to grow near the bronchus.
2. Adenocarcinoma, the most prevalent carcinoma of the lung, is usually found in the peripheral area of the lung.
3. Large cell carcinoma (10% of all lung cancers) tends to arise peripherally and grows and spreads quickly.

II. Nursing process

A. Assessment
1. Obtain a detailed health history, psychosocial history, and perform a comprehensive physical examination.
2. Assess for risk factors.
   a. Smoking of cigarettes or inhalation of second-hand smoke
   b. Exposure to radon or asbestos
   c. Exposure to air pollution
3. Assess for signs and symptoms.
   a. Persistent cough
   b. Shortness of breath
   c. Chest pain that persists or worsens with a deep breath
   d. Wheezing
   e. Hemoptysis
   f. Recurring respiratory infections (bronchitis or pneumonia)
   g. Hoarseness
   h. Fatigue, loss of appetite, and weight loss
4. Obtain diagnostic tests.
   a. Chest x-ray
   b. Contrast-enhanced chest CT scan
   c. MRI
   d. Positron emission tomography (PET) scan
   e. Bronchoscopy with biopsy
   f. Sputum cytology
   g. Percutaneous transthoracic needle biopsy for peripheral lesions

B. Analysis
   1. Ineffective Airway Clearance related to increased secretions, obstruction, and fatigue
   2. Altered Breathing Pattern related to shortness of breath and decreased lung capacity
   3. Anxiety related to diagnosis, unknown prognosis, and necessary tests and treatments
   4. Imbalanced Nutrition: Less Than Body Requirements related to increased metabolic demands, shortness of breath, anorexia
   5. Acute Pain related to pressure of tumor on surrounding tissue
   6. Ineffective Health Maintenance related to lack of knowledge of disease and therapeutic regimen

C. Planning
   1. Promote adequate oxygenation of tissues.
   2. Relieve symptoms and pain.
   3. Promote smoking cessation.
   4. Provide adequate nutrition.
   5. Maintain effective airway clearance.
   6. Reduce anxiety.
   7. Prepare for diagnostic tests and interventions.
   8. Prevent or minimize complications.

D. Implementation
   1. Monitor vital signs, SpO_2, arterial blood gas, lung sounds, respiratory secretions, nutritional status, and exercise tolerance.
   2. Diagnose and stage lung cancer.
   3. Provide client and family teaching on risk factors, disease processes, diagnostics and treatments, medications, activity, smoking cessation, and realistic goals based on prognosis.

E. Evaluation
   1. Client's vital signs and SpO_2 are stable.
   2. Client verbalizes control of pain using pain rating scale.
   3. Client experiences reduction of dyspnea and fatigue.
   4. Client maintains target weight.
   5. Client shows no signs of infection.

CN

III. Client needs

A. Physiologic adaptation: Definitive diagnosis of cancer is made by biopsy. Tumor type and staging determines treatment options for client, which may include:
   1. Surgical treatment—performed for localized non-small cell cancer without evidence of metastasis; cure rate depends on type and stage of cancer.
      a. Lobectomy—removal of single lobe of lung
      b. Pneumonectomy—removal of entire lung
   2. Radiation—may be used for tumors that cannot be surgically resected as an adjunct to surgery, or for palliative therapy to shrink tumor to provide pain and symptom relief.
   3. Chemotherapy—used for metastatic cancer and as an adjunct to surgery or radiation therapy.

B. Management of care: Care of the client with lung cancer requires critical thinking skills and knowledge of assessment, and teaching and evaluation methods unique to the RN role. These skills cannot be delegated to an LPN or UAP.
   1. Delegate responsibly those activities that can be delegated, such as taking vital signs and assisting with bathing, hygiene, and comfort measures. All monitoring information is reported to the RN.
   2. Monitor vital signs, SpO_2, quality of respirations, lung sounds, sputum quantity and characteristics, and symptoms of pain and shortness of breath.
   3. Promote coughing and deep breathing; high-protein and -calorie diet with supplements; positioning for greater lung expansion; and reduction of anxiety.
   4. Provide surgical interventions (see physiologic adaptation for descriptions of types of surgeries); surgical interventions for the two most common surgeries are as follows:
      a. For lobectomy, maintain pleural chest tube to re-establish lung expansion
         (1) Monitor and record drainage appearance and amount.
         (2) Check for air leak and fluctuation (tidaling).
         (3) Promote patency of tube and drainage; prevent kinking of tube. Do not strip or milk chest tube.
         (4) Maintain chest tube drainage system below waist level.
         (5) Review results of daily chest x-ray.
      b. For pneumonectomy, position client on operative side or on back to allow adequate expansion of remaining lung. Assess trachea position for complication of mediastinal shift.
      c. Promote pain management with patient-controlled analgesia (PCA) pump.
      d. Provide close monitoring of vital signs, SpO_2, and ECG.
      e. Administer and titrate oxygen via nasal cannula or face mask to maintain targeted SpO_2.

f. Use incentive spirometry every 1 to 2 hr.
g. Promote tolerance of activity (e.g., out of bed to chair).

5. Assess for home health care needs such as a visiting nurse or home health care aide, home oxygen and delivery, and meal provision. For end-stage lung cancer, assess client and family desire for home care, hospice, or palliative care.
6. Link client with community resources for smoking cessation therapy, support groups, and pulmonary rehabilitation.

C. Safety and infection control: Teach good hand hygiene techniques and avoidance of people with respiratory infections, colds, or flu.

D. Health promotion and maintenance: Provide client and family teaching about self-care strategies.
1. Smoking cessation
2. Adequate nutrition with high-protein diet to maintain target weight
3. Activity tolerance and strategies to conserve energy
4. Nutritious diet
5. Importance of outpatient follow-up care

E. Psychologic integrity
1. Assess impact of disease on quality of life and coping strategies.
2. Assess client's social and family support and prevent social isolation.
3. For the client with advanced stage, promote client and family teaching from health care team regarding goals of treatment, living will, and advance directive to determine preferences while the client is able to participate in decisions for end-of-life care.

F. Basic care and comfort: Relieve pain and control symptoms to maintain client comfort and quality of life.

G. Reduction of risk potential: Counsel client to avoid irritants that may aggravate symptoms.

H. Pharmacologic and parenteral therapies: Client will state the purpose, usage, and associated side effects of medications used to treat underlying disorders or complications of lung cancer, including bronchodilators, corticosteroids, and antibiotics.

Asthma

I. Definition: Asthma is defined as a chronic inflammatory disorder of the airways causing recurrent episodes of wheezing, breathlessness, chest tightness, and coughing, particularly at night or early morning. Inflammation contributes to airway hyperresponsiveness and airflow limitation. Acute bronchoconstriction, airway edema, mucus plug formation, and airway wall remodeling lead to bronchial obstruction.

A. Classification of severity of asthma is based on clinical features before treatment allows for a stepwise approach for managing asthma.
1. Step 1, mild intermittent
   a. Symptoms occur less than 2 times a week; client has normal peak expiratory flow (PEF) rate between exacerbations; exacerbations are brief, lasting from a few hours to a few days, with varying intensity.
   b. Nighttime symptoms occur less than 2 times a month.
   c. Forced expiratory volume in 1 second (FEV_1) or PEF 80% or more predicted; PEF variability less than 20%.
2. Step 2, mild persistent
   a. Symptoms occur more than 2 times a week, but less than one time a day; exacerbations may affect activity.
   b. Nighttime symptoms occur less than 2 times a month.
   c. FEV_1 or PEF 80% or more predicted; PEF variability 20% to 30%.
3. Step 3, moderate persistent
   a. Client experiences daily symptoms and uses short-acting beta-2 agonist daily; exacerbations affect activity; exacerbation occurs more than 2 times a week and may last days.
   b. Nighttime symptoms occur more than one time per week.
   c. FEV_1 or PEF more than 60% to more than 80% predicted; PEF variability more than 30%.
4. Step 4, severe persistent
   a. Client's symptoms are persistent and exacerbations frequent; physical activity is limited.
   b. Nighttime symptoms are frequent.
   c. FEV_1 or PEF 60% or less predicted; PEF variability more than 30%.

B. Status asthmaticus is a severe, life-threatening asthma attack that is unresponsive to the usual intervention with adrenergic drugs and places the client at risk for respiratory failure. The combination of hypoxia, hypercapnia, and acidosis along with the mechanical effects of increased lung volumes may result in cardiovascular depression or arrest.

II. Nursing process

A. Assessment
1. Obtain a detailed health history, family history, and psychosocial history.

2. Perform a comprehensive physical examination.
   a. Vital signs, SpO_2, lung sounds, and heart sounds
   b. Upper respiratory tract, chest, and skin are the focus of the physical exam for asthma—including hyperexpansion of the chest, use of accessory muscles, hunched shoulders, chest deformity, wheezing during normal breathing, increased nasal secretion, mucosal swelling, nasal polyps, and allergic skin condition.
3. Assess for presence of signs and symptoms, including coughing, wheezing, shortness of breath, chest tightness, and sputum production; assess for symptom's patterns:
   a. Perennial, seasonal, or both
   b. Continual, episodic, or both
   c. Onset, duration, frequency
   d. Diurnal variations, especially at night and on awakening early morning
4. Assess for precipitating or aggravating factors, including exercise, viral infection, indoor or outdoor environmental allergens, occupational chemicals or allergens, irritants (smoke, odors, dust, air pollutants, aerosols), strong emotion, drugs (aspirin, beta blockers, NSAIDs), food or food additives or preservatives, changes in weather, exposure to cold air, or endocrine factors (menses, pregnancy, thyroid disease), presence of GERD.
5. Obtain diagnostic tests.
   a. Spirometry measurements
      (1) FEV_1
      (2) Forced vital capacity (FVC)
      (3) FEV_1/FVC
   b. Chest x-ray
   c. Allergy testing
   d. Evaluation of the nose for nasal polyps and sinuses
   e. Evaluation for gastroesophageal reflux
   f. Bronchoprovocation with methacholine, histamine, or exercise challenge with suspected asthma and near-normal spirometry
   g. CBC with differential, electrolytes, arterial blood gas, serum IgE, sputum (eosinophils, C&S, Gram stain)

B. Analysis
1. Ineffective Breathing Pattern related to airway narrowing and secretions
2. Impaired Gas Exchange related to decreased expiratory volume, secretions, atelectasis, or infection
3. Ineffective Airway Clearance related to thick tenacious secretions and weak cough force
4. Activity Intolerance related to shortness of breath, impaired gas exchange, work of breathing, and fatigue
5. Anxiety related to shortness of breath and symptoms
6. Risk for Infection related to respiratory secretions and ineffective airway clearance
7. Ineffective Therapeutic Regimen Management related to knowledge deficit

C. Planning
1. Control and eliminate precipitating cause.
2. Maintain personal best pulmonary function.
3. Prevent or control symptoms.
4. Maintain normal activity levels.
5. Enhance quality of life.
6. Prevent recurrent exacerbations.
7. Provide optimal pharmacotherapy with minimal side effects.
8. Reduce anxiety.

D. Implementation
1. Monitor vital signs, lung sounds, SpO_2, laboratory values, response to respiratory medications, symptoms and clinical signs of asthma.
2. Provide client with a written action plan of medications to treat signs and symptoms and PEF measurements.
3. Provide client and family teaching on triggers of asthma, long-term control medications that are taken regularly, and quick-relief medications to rapidly treat bronchoconstriction, peak flow monitoring, signs and symptoms that indicate inadequate asthma control, when to seek medical attention, and importance of follow-up care.

E. Evaluation
1. Client's vital signs, SpO_2, spirometry, and PEF are within targeted range.
2. Client affirms absence of daytime symptoms and nocturnal awakening with symptoms.
3. Client affirms absence of wheezing.
4. Client exhibits tolerance to normal activity without symptoms.
5. Client states the purpose, dosage, timing, and side effects of medications.
6. Client's functional capability is optimized through medications and self-care behaviors.

CN

III. Client needs
A. Physiologic adaptation: Asthma is controlled by inhaled and oral medication with dose

adjustments on a routine, outpatient basis, unless symptoms are severe and warrant hospitalization. Persistent asthma is most effectively controlled with daily anti-inflammatory medications.

B. Management of care: Care of the client with acute exacerbation of asthma and status asthmaticus requiring hospitalization requires critical thinking skills and knowledge of assessment, and teaching and evaluation methods unique to the RN role. These skills cannot be delegated to an LPN or UAP.
   1. Delegate responsibly those activities that can be delegated, including basic care needs and monitoring of vital signs for the stable client. All monitoring information is reported to the RN.
   2. Perform comprehensive physical assessments and provide care to the hospitalized, symptomatic client with acute exacerbation.
   3. Provide respiratory interventions (may be performed by the nurse or respiratory therapist):
      a. Promote first-line therapy for severe bronchoconstriction—bronchodilator treatment with a beta-2 agonist; typically albuterol via nebulizer administered either continuously or frequent dosing.
      b. Administer corticosteroid PO or IV for moderate-to-severe exacerbations.
      c. Monitor response to therapy with PEF and spirometry.
   4. Place client on bed rest in high Fowler position, as tolerated.
   5. Promote continuous ECG and pulse oximetry monitoring and frequent monitoring of vital signs.
   6. Administer titrate oxygen to maintain SpO_2 in targeted range; oxygen, 2 to 6 L via nasal cannula or 40% to 100% via face mask.
      a. Arterial blood gas
      b. Endotracheal intubation with mechanical ventilation may be required for severe hypoxia and hypercapnia
   7. Auscultate heart and lung sounds frequently.
   8. Promote IV fluid replacement.
   9. Provide information on changes in client status to the physician and appropriate members of the multidisciplinary team.
   10. Administer medications used to manage asthma (see pharmacologic and parenteral therapies).
      a. Amount and frequency of long-term control medications are based on severity of asthma and suppressing airway inflammation.
      b. Medication is initiated at a higher level at the onset of asthma to establish prompt control and then a cautious stepdown approach is used once control is sustained.
      c. Stepdown therapy is necessary to identify the minimum medication needed to maintain control.
      d. Continual monitoring is essential to ensure that asthma control is attained.
   11. Provide client and family teaching (see health promotion and maintenance).
   12. Teach client, or assist respiratory therapist in teaching client, to perform PEF monitoring in the morning, and more frequent monitoring if the reading is less than 80% of personal best PEF rate.
   13. Facilitate and reinforce the need for outpatient follow-up care at 1- to 6-month intervals (see health promotion and maintenance).
   14. Assess for home health care needs and community resources for support groups, smoking cessation, and pulmonary rehabilitation, based on client needs.

C. Safety and infection control: Assess characteristics of home, including age, location, and heating and cooling system; presence of wood-burning stove, humidifier, carpeting, mold or mildew, potential dust mites; and condition of bedding, floor coverings, and furniture (e.g., stuffed).
   1. Reduce house mites.
      a. Encase mattress and pillow in allergen-impermeable cover.
      b. Wash sheets and blankets weekly in hot water at 130°F.
      c. Vacuum with high-efficiency particulate air (HEPA) filter.
   2. Reduce indoor humidity to less than 50% and eliminate water sources to decrease mold.
   3. Use poison baits or traps to control cockroaches.

D. Health promotion and maintenance
   1. Provide client and family teaching about the following:
      a. Correct use of long-term control medications and quick-relief medications (see pharmacologic and parenteral therapy).
      b. Proper technique and use of nebulizer, dry powder inhaler (DPI), or metered dose inhalers (MDI) with spacer and peak flow meter.

c. Symptom patterns that indicate inadequate control and need for additional therapy.
d. Need to follow action plan stating interventions based on signs and symptoms and PEF measurements (green zone, yellow zone, and red zone).

2. Monitor client on a periodic outpatient basis to confirm that goals of therapy are being met; perform the following evaluations:
   a. Signs and symptoms of asthma within the last 2 to 4 weeks
   b. Daytime symptoms, nocturnal awakening from symptoms, and symptoms early in the morning not relieved 15 min after inhaling a short-acting beta-2 agonist
   c. Pulmonary function (spirometry)
   d. Functional status, quality of life
   e. Exacerbations
   f. Medications and side effects
   g. General satisfaction of client and family
3. Encourage smoking cessation and avoidance of second-hand smoke.
4. Introduce methods to manage stress.
5. Promote annual influenza vaccine for clients with persistent asthma.

E. Psychologic integrity: Assess ability of client and family to cope with asthma; level of family support; and client's ability to recognize severity of an exacerbation.

F. Basic care and comfort
1. Provide a quiet, calm environment.
2. Instruct client on positioning to optimize breathing, such as arms outstretched over bedside table.

G. Reduction of risk potential
1. Promote skin or in vitro testing to assess sensitivity to allergens.
2. Teach client to avoid nonselective beta blocker drugs and side effects of bronchoconstriction.
3. Treat client for rhinitis, sinusitis, and GERD.

H. Pharmacologic and parenteral therapies: Client will state the purpose, usage, and associated side effects of medications used to manage asthma.
1. Long-term control medications (see Table 23-1).
2. Quick-relief medications (see Table 23-2).
3. Bronchodilators
   a. Beta-2 agonists
   b. Anticholinergics
   c. Methylxanthines
4. Anti-inflammatory medications
   a. Corticosteroids
   b. Cromolyn and nedocromil
   c. Leukotriene modifiers
5. Monoclonal antibody to IgE—omalizumab (Xolair) subcutaneous injection
   a. Blocks the allergic immune response by removing and deactivating IgE, preventing allergic mediated early- and late-phase hyperresponsiveness of asthma.
   b. Treats moderate-to-severe allergy-related asthma inadequately controlled with inhaled steroid treatment.
   c. Dose based on body weight and pretreatment serum IgE levels.
   d. Side effects include injection site reaction, viral infection, URI, sinusitis, headache, and pharyngitis.

Chronic Obstructive Pulmonary Disease

I. Definition: Chronic obstructive pulmonary disease (COPD) is characterized by airflow limitation that is progressive and largely irreversible. The disorder is associated with an abnormal inflammatory response of the lungs to noxious particles or gases. Onset occurs in midlife and symptoms slowly progress; severity is classified in stages based on spirometry measurement and symptoms. COPD involves chronic bronchitis, emphysema, or a combination of both disorders.

A. Chronic bronchitis—a chronic, productive cough for 3 consecutive months for at least 2 successive years.

B. Emphysema—results from abnormal enlargement of the alveoli and alveolar ducts with destruction of the alveolar walls.

II. Nursing process

A. Assessment
1. Obtain a detailed health history and psychosocial history, and perform a comprehensive physical examination.
2. Assess for risk factors.
   a. Tobacco smoke
   b. Occupational chemicals and dust
   c. Outdoor and indoor air pollution
   d. History of severe childhood respiratory infections
   e. Alpha-1 antitrypsin deficiency
   f. Airway hyperresponsiveness and asthma
3. Assess for signs and symptoms.
   a. Chronic cough
   b. Chronic sputum production

Table 23-1 Long-Term Control Medications for Asthma

Classification	Generic/Trade Name	Expected Outcomes	Reduction of Risk Potential	Management of Care
Corticosteroids	**Inhaled drugs:** Beclomethasone (Vanceril, Beclovent); budesonide (Pulmicort); flunisolide (AeroBid); fluticasone (Flovent); triamcinolone acetonide (Azmacort) **Systemic drugs:** Prednisone; prednisolone; methylprednisolone	**Inhaled drugs:** Decrease and control inflammation and prevent symptoms. **Systemic drugs:** Gain prompt control when initiating long-term therapy; prevent symptoms in severe persistent asthma, and reverse and control inflammation.	**Inhaled drugs:** Monitor client for oral candidiasis. **PO and IV systemic drugs:** Monitor for hyperglycemia, fluid retention, weight gain, hypertension, and mood alterations. Prophylactic antiulcer agents to prevent peptic ulcer.	**Inhaled drugs:** Teach proper use of spacer for aerosol inhalants; rinse mouth after inhalation. **Systemic drugs:** Perform Accu-Chek, assess daily weight and BP; prophylactic proton pump inhibitor or H_2 antagonist.
Long-Acting Beta-2 Agonists	Salmeterol (Serevent); formoterol (Foradil); albuterol sustained-release	Promotes bronchodilation; prevents long-term symptoms, especially nocturnal; prevents exercise-induced bronchospasm.	Not used for acute symptoms. Monitor for tachycardia, tremor, hypokalemia.	Added to anti-inflammatory treatments. Monitor pulse, check potassium, and ECG for prolonged QT.
Mast Cell Stabilizers	Cromolyn sodium (Intal); nedocromil (Tilade)	Decreases inflammation; prevents bronchospasm and acute response to exercise and cold and dry air.	Prophylactic use prior to exercise. Monitor for coughing, skin rash, headache, sore throat, unpleasant taste, nausea, and abdominal pain.	Teach proper use of spacer with MDI.
Leukotriene Modifiers	Montelukast (Singulair); zafirlukast (Accolate); zileuton (Zyflo)	Promotes long-term control of symptoms, bronchodilation, and anti-inflammatory effects.	Monitor LFTs.	Administer with meals; monitor for interference with warfarin (Coumadin) and theophylline.
Methylxanthines	Theophylline sustained release	Promotes bronchodilation; prevents symptoms, especially nocturnal.	Monitor serum levels; monitor for tachycardia, nausea and vomiting, headache, insomnia, GI distress, and seizures.	Assess theophylline level and pulse; assess for hyperglycemia and hypokalemia with high levels.

c. Dyspnea that worsens over time, present every day, worsens with exercise, and during respiratory infections; described as air hunger or gasping
d. Decrease in FEV_1 and FVC
e. Increase in anteroposterior chest wall diameter
f. Longer expiratory time I-to-E ratio 1:3-4

4. Assess for complications of COPD.
   a. Acute exacerbation
   b. Pneumonia
   c. Acute respiratory failure
   d. Pulmonary hypertension
   e. Cor pulmonale
   f. Peptic ulcer disease
   g. Gastroesophageal reflux disease
5. Obtain diagnostic tests.
   a. Spirometry—FEV_1, FVC, FEV_1/ FVC
   b. Chest x-ray
   c. Bronchodilator reversibility testing to rule out asthma
   d. Alpha-1 antitrypsin deficiency screening
   e. SpO_2, arterial blood gas
   f. CBC with differential, basic metabolic panel (Chem 7), sputum culture and sensitivity (C&S)

Table 23-2 Quick-Relief Medications for Asthma

Classification	Generic/Trade Name	Expected Outcomes	Reduction of Risk Potential	Management of Care
Short-acting Inhaled Beta-2 Agonists	Albuterol (Proventil, Ventolin); levalbuterol (Xopenex); bitolterol (Tornalate); pirbuterol (Maxair); terbutaline (Brethine, Brethaire);	Promotes bronchodilation; relieves acute symptoms; prevents exercise-induced bronchospasm.	Monitor for tachycardia, tremor, and hypokalemia.	Use cautiously in clients with cardiovascular disease. Monitor vital signs prior to, during, and after administration.
Anticholinergics	Ipratropium (Atrovent)	Promotes bronchodilation.	Monitor for drying of mouth and respiratory secretions.	Can be used as an additive or alternative to beta-2 agonists; treatment of choice for bronchospasm due to beta blocker medication.
Systemic Corticosteroids	Prednisone; prednisolone; methylprednisolone	Reverses inflammation and prevents progression of exacerbation; reduces rate of relapse.	Monitor for hyperglycemia, fluid retention, weight gain, hypertension, and mood alterations. Administer prophylactic antiulcer agents to prevent peptic ulcer.	Promote short-term therapy until client achieves 80% PEF; perform Accu-Chek, assess daily weight and BP; prophylactic use of proton pump inhibitors or H_2 antagonist.

B. Analysis
1. Ineffective Airway Clearance related to weak cough force, airflow limitation, and thick tenacious secretions
2. Impaired Gas Exchange related to pulmonary secretions, alveolar hypoventilation, and altered breathing pattern
3. Altered Nutrition: Less Than Body Requirements related to dyspnea, fatigue and anorexia
4. Disturbed Sleep Pattern related to dyspnea, anxiety, hypoxemia, and hypercapnia
5. Activity Intolerance related to dyspnea, fatigue, and hypoxia
6. Anxiety related to dyspnea, activity intolerance, reduced socialization, and prognosis
7. Ineffective Therapeutic Regimen Management related to lack of knowledge of disease process, medications, and self-care behaviors

C. Planning
1. Optimize gas exchange and spirometry volumes.
2. Promote effective airway clearance.
3. Improve client symptoms and comfort.
4. Encourage smoking cessation.
5. Reduce anxiety.
6. Enhance functional capacity and quality of life.
7. Promote adherence to therapeutic regimen.
8. Prevent complications.
9. Reduce hospitalizations.

D. Implementation
1. Monitor vital signs, SpO_2, arterial blood gas, lung sounds, respiratory secretions, fluid status, and exercise tolerance.
2. Administer bronchodilator and anti-inflammatory medications based on severity of symptoms.
3. Provide client and family teaching (see safety and infection control).

E. Evaluation
1. Client's vital signs, SpO_2, and arterial blood gas are within targeted range.
2. Client affirms improvement or absence of symptoms.
3. Client is able to eat and sleep without frequent awakening by dyspnea.
4. Client exhibits tolerance to increasing levels of activity.
5. Client states the purpose, dosage, timing, and side effects of medications.
6. Client demonstrates proper use of inhalers and spacer, and delivery device.
7. Client's functional capability is optimized through pulmonary rehabilitation and self-care behaviors.
8. Client stops smoking and avoids second-hand smoke.

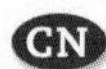

III. Client needs

A. Physiologic adaptation: Management of COPD involves a stepwise increase in medications based on severity of symptoms to decrease and control symptoms and prevent complications. Bronchodilator medications are fundamental to symptomatic management of COPD, given on a regular or as needed basis.
   1. Presence of postbronchodilator FEV_1 less than 80% of predicted along with FEV_1/FVC less than 70% confirms airflow limitation is not fully reversible.
   2. Noninvasive mechanical ventilation (noninvasive intermittent positive pressure ventilation) or intubation and mechanical ventilation may be required.
   3. Surgical treatment for COPD is performed in carefully selected clients; surgery may involve:
      a. Bullectomy
      b. Lung volume-reduction surgery
      c. Lung transplantation

B. Management of care: Care of the client with COPD exacerbation requiring hospitalization requires critical thinking skills and knowledge of assessment, and teaching and evaluation methods unique to the RN role. These skills cannot be delegated to an LPN or UAP.
   1. Delegate responsibly those activities that can be delegated, including basic care needs and monitoring of vital signs for the stable client. All monitoring information is reported to the RN.
   2. Perform comprehensive physical assessments, including assessment of severity of symptoms, adequacy of oxygenation, effectiveness of ventilation, and hemodynamic stability.
   3. Perform frequent vital signs and neurologic checks.
   4. Control oxygen therapy and repeat arterial blood gas 30 min after a change in oxygen level delivered or ventilator change.
   5. Review results of continuous SpO_2 and ECG monitoring.
   6. Administer medications for COPD exacerbation (see pharmacologic and parenteral therapies).
   7. Monitor noninvasive mechanical ventilation or intubation and mechanical ventilation, if indicated.
      a. Assess client first and then the ventilator (vital sings, lung sounds, respiratory and breathing patterns, bilateral chest expansion); monitor skin color.
      b. Note ventilator settings and assess for correct functioning.
         (1) If a cause for an alarm is not found, ventilate the client with an Ambu bag until problem is corrected.
         (2) High-pressure alarms may be due to increased secretions, displaced endotracheal tube and client coughing or biting of tubing, client anxiousness or fighting of the ventilator.
         (3) Low-pressure alarms may be due to disconnection or leak in the ventilator or the client's airway cuff.
   8. Provide postsurgical interventions, if indicated.
   9. Assess for home health care needs such as a visiting nurse or home health care aide, home oxygen and delivery, and meal provision.
   10. Assess along with the HCP ability of client to meet discharge criteria.
      a. Inhaled beta-2 agonist required no more frequently than every 4 hr.
      b. Client is able to walk across room if previously ambulatory.
      c. Client's eating and sleeping patterns are not deterred by dyspnea.
      d. Hemodynamics and arterial blood gases are stable.
      e. Client has been assessed for long-term home oxygen need.
      f. Client and family fully understand correct medication administration.
      g. Home care arrangements are established.

C. Safety and infection control
   1. Provide along with the respiratory therapist client and family teaching.
      a. Medications and correct inhaler technique and care.
      b. Pursed-lip breathing to prevent collapse of the small airways with expiration.
   2. Teach client to enhance self-care strategies, including gradually increasing exercise activity and strategies to conserve energy; always exercising with a buddy; monitoring of symptoms; avoidance of temperature extremes; and have a place to rest, if needed.
   3. Promote safe management of home oxygen therapy (keep away from flame, sources of heat, and inflammable oil-based products).

D. Health promotion and maintenance
   1. Introduce programs to encourage smoking cessation.

2. Introduce client to exercise training program to improve exercise tolerance and symptoms of dyspnea and fatigue.
3. Promote long-term administration of oxygen (more than 15 hr/day) to clients with stage 4: very severe COPD with PaO_2 less than 55 and SaO_2 88% to increase survival rate.
4. Maintain target weight; prevent weight loss.
5. Promote influenza and pneumococcal vaccinations.

E. Psychologic integrity
1. Assess impact of disease on quality of life and coping strategies.
2. Assess client's social and family support and prevent social isolation.
3. For client with advanced-stage COPD, instruct client and family along with other members of health care team regarding goals of treatment, living will, and advance directive to determine preferences while the client is able to participate in decisions for end-of-life care.

F. Basic care and comfort
1. Promote adequate periods of rest between activities.
2. Provide a calm, quiet environment; teach relaxation techniques.
3. Promote management of symptoms to maintain client comfort and quality of life.

G. Reduction of risk potential
1. Treat peptic ulcer disease (PUD), if indicated.
2. Counsel client to avoid irritants that may aggravate symptoms.
3. Promote good hand hygiene and avoidance of people with respiratory infections, colds, or flu.
4. Instruct client that COPD causes vulnerability to high altitudes, beta blockers, and narcotics.

H. Pharmacologic and parenteral therapies: Client will state the purpose, usage, and associated side effects of medications used to manage COPD.
1. Inhaled bronchodilators (beta-2 agonists and/or anticholinergics, theophylline, and systemic corticosteroids).
2. Antibiotics with clinical signs of airway infection such as increased volume and change in color of sputum, and fever.
3. Inhaled corticosteroids for clients with FEV_1 less than 50% predicted and repeated exacerbations.

Pneumonia

I. Definition: Pneumonia is an acute inflammation of the lung parenchyma, including the interstitial spaces of the alveoli and the bronchioles. Infection is caused by a microbial agent such as bacteria, viruses, fungi, parasites, mycoplasma, and chemicals. The inflammation that occurs in pneumonia results in edema causing the lungs to become very "stiff"; this is followed by a decrease in lung compliance and vital capacity, which interferes with the ventilation process and results in severe hypoxemia.

A. Pneumonia is described as bacterial, or atypical and nonbacterial:
1. Bacterial
   a. Lobar—occurs abruptly from an infection and affects a large portion of a lobe; causes pleuritic pain and large amount of sputum.
   b. Bronchopneumonia—general patchy infiltration in lungs; more common than lobar pneumonia.
   c. Alveolar
2. Atypical
   a. *Mycoplasma pneumoniae* or *Legionella pneumophila*—infection that can result in serious complications (e.g., multisystem failure from ARDS, DIC, and renal failure, inflammation of heart, neurologic disorders, and death).
   b. *Pneumocystis carinii*—seen in immunocompromised clients with AIDS.
3. Aspiration
   a. Noninfectious materials introduced into the airway (e.g., gastric secretions, foods, liquids, enteral feedings).
   b. Bacterial aspiration pneumonia may be related to poor cough reflex due to anesthesia, coma.
   c. Clients receiving mechanical ventilation.
4. Hematogenous pneumonia bacterial infections—spread of infection from the bloodstream into the lungs.

B. Pneumonia may also be classified as:
1. Community-acquired pneumonia (CAP)—involves lower respiratory tract infection of the lung parenchyma with onset in the community or during the first 2 days of hospitalization; occurs more frequently in winter months.
2. Hospital-acquired pneumonia (HAP)—occurs 48 hr or longer after hospital admission and not incubating at the time of hospitalization; involves highest morbidity and mortality rate of any nosocomial infection.

3. Immunocompromised (opportunistic)—*Pneumocystis carinii* in persons with AIDS.
4. Aspiration—results from the entry of endogenous or exogenous substances in the lower respiratory tract.
5. Ventilated-associated pneumonia (VAP)—involves critically ill, vulnerable clients who are mechanically ventilated.

II. Nursing process

A. Assessment

1. Obtain a detailed health history, including history of allergies, prior hospitalizations, family medical history, and psychosocial history.
2. Perform a comprehensive physical examination; assess for signs and symptoms (signs and symptoms will vary based on type of pneumonia).
   a. Viral pneumonia usually presents with low-grade fever, nonproductive cough, and normal to low elevation WBC, minimal chest x-ray changes, and clinical course less severe than bacterial.
   b. Bacterial pneumonia usually presents with high fever, productive cough, elevated WBC; chest x-ray reveals wide area infiltrates; and clinical course is more severe than viral.
   c. Other general symptoms include:
      (1) Fever, chills, chest pain, weakness with generalized malaise.
      (2) Cough with greenish to rust-colored sputum production; rust (blood) or yellowish sputum (greenish with atypical pneumonia).
      (3) Rapid, shallow respirations with an expiratory grunt, nasal flaring, intercostal rib retraction, use of respiratory accessory muscles.
      (4) Dullness to flatness on percussion, possible pleural friction rub, high-pitched bronchial breath sounds (rales or crackles progressing to coarse).
      (5) Tachycardia, circumoral cyanosis, profuse perspiration.
      (6) Sudden onset of fever, chills, cough productive of purulent sputum, and pleuritic chest pain for clients with CAP.
      (7) Headache, fatigue, sore throat, nausea, vomiting, diarrhea, and abdominal distention.
      (8) Facial herpes simplex (fever blisters).
      (9) Confusion or stupor (related to hypoxia) for older adult client who is debilitated.
3. Assess for risk factors such as:
   a. Age: Older adults are at higher risk.
   b. Presence of altered conscious state because of alcoholism, head injury, seizures, anesthesia, drug overdose, or stroke.
   c. Exposure to air pollution, smoking, inhalation or aspiration of noxious substances.
   d. Chronic and debilitating illnesses and diseases such as COPD, heart failure, diabetes mellitus, cancer, end-stage renal disease, or immunosuppressive clients (e.g., client who is HIV-positive).
   e. Prolonged immobility.
   f. History of immunosuppressive drugs (corticosteroids, cancer chemotherapy, immunosuppressive therapy after organ transplant).
   g. Malnutrition.
4. Obtain diagnostic tests.
   a. Chest x-ray—displays consolidation over affected areas
   b. Gram stain of sputum and blood cultures—identifies causative organism
      (1) CAP—typical pneumonia syndrome; most common pathogens are *Streptococcus pneumoniae, Haemophilus influenzae*
      (2) VAP—protected-specimen brush culture with at least 10^3 cfu/ml, a positive result of a bronchoalveolar lavage fluid smear or a bronchoalveolar lavage fluid culture is considered; most common organism is *pseudomonas aeruginosa*
   c. Sputum culture and sensitivity test
   d. Bronchoscopy, if sputum cultures inconclusive
   e. ABGs and pulse SpO_2
   f. CBC with differential

B. Analysis

1. Impaired Gas Exchange related to pulmonary secretions, alveolar hypoventilation, and altered breathing pattern
2. Ineffective Airway Clearance related to copious tracheobronchial secretions
3. Activity Intolerance related to impaired respiratory function
4. Risk for Deficient Fluid Volume related to fever and dyspnea
5 Altered Nutrition: Less Than Body Requirements related to dyspnea, fatigue, and anorexia
6. Ineffective Therapeutic Regimen Management related to lack of knowledge of disease process, medications, and self-care behaviors

C. Planning
1. Facilitate adequate ventilation and removal of secretions.
2 Provide adequate rest and relief or control of pain.
3. Control and eliminate the precipitating cause.
4. Maintain adequate nutritional status.
5. Prevent potential complications.
6. Reduce anxiety and fear.

D. Implementation
1. Monitor vital signs with close attention to BP, SpO_2, pulses, heart sounds, and lung sounds.
2. Administer oxygen therapy as appropriate.
3. Monitor arterial blood gas, respiratory secretions, fluid status, and exercise tolerance.
4. Administer antibiotics, bronchodilator, anti-inflammatory, and other medications based on severity of symptoms.
5. Provide client and family teaching about risk factors, medications, and associated side effects, activity tolerance, breathing techniques, promoting a healthy lifestyle, self-care behaviors, signs and symptoms that require medical attention, and setting of realistic goals for pulmonary function and symptom relief.

E. Evaluation
1. Client's vital signs, SpO_2, and arterial blood gas are within targeted range.
2. Client exhibits improved gas exchange demonstrated by improved pulmonary function, acid-base and fluid balance within normal range for client.
3. Client tolerates increasing levels of activity.
4. Client's sputum production is decreased and is of normal color; client's cultures are negative.
5. Client verbalizes relief of pain and associated symptoms.
6. Client states understanding of medications, diet, and treatments.

CN

III. Client needs

A. Physiologic adaptation: Pneumonia often effects both ventilation and diffusion; it is treated by rest, fluids, and prevention (see management of care), including good hand hygiene by HCPs. Noninvasive mechanical ventilation (noninvasive intermittent positive pressure ventilation) or intubation and mechanical ventilation may be required. Associated complications of pneumonia may include the following:
1. Atelectasis, pleurisy, pleural effusion, lung abscess, empyema
2. Superinfection
3. Respiratory failure
4. Shock

B. Management of care: Care of the client hospitalized with pneumonia requires critical thinking skills and knowledge of assessment, and teaching and evaluation methods unique to the RN role. These skills cannot be delegated to an LPN or UAP.
1. Delegate responsibly those activities that can be delegated, such as assisting with bathing, and hygiene comfort measures. All monitoring information is reported to the RN.
2. Perform physical assessments and monitor vital signs, SpO_2, patency of airway, quality of respirations, lung sounds, quantity and characteristics of secretions or drainage, and symptoms.
   a. Observe color and characteristics of sputum and report any changes; encourage client to perform good oral hygiene after expectoration.
   b. Administer antibiotics as ordered; monitor for side effects and possible toxicity.
   c. Control fever and chills; monitor temperature and administer antipyretics as ordered; maintain increased fluid intake and provide frequent clothing and linen change.
3. Prevent transmission (respiratory isolation may be required with clients with staphylococcal pneumonia/MRSA).
4. Provide care to client receiving mechanical ventilation (see management of care for COPD for care of client receiving mechanical ventilation).
5. Monitor temperature and administer antipyretics as ordered.
6. Provide client and family teaching and interventions for symptom and pain management (see basic care and comfort); provide teaching and discharge planning concerning prevention of recurrence.
   a. Maintain adequate rest and proper nutrition and fluids (high-calorie, high-protein diet with small, frequent meals; fluids up to 3 L/day unless contraindicated).
   b. Avoid individuals with respiratory infections or viruses.
   c. Use medications and inhalants as prescribed.
   d. Receive immunizations (pneumococcal pneumonia and influenza), especially for elderly clients and other high-risk clients.

7. Assess for home health care needs, including community resources and support groups.

C. Safety and infection control: Reinforce appropriate universal precautions and use of hand hygiene, isolation, and aseptic technique in care of client with infectious disease.

D. Health promotion and maintenance: Instruct client to report signs and symptoms of respiratory infection (persistent or recurrent fever; changes in characteristics or color of sputum; chills; increased pain; increased shortness of breath; weight loss; and increased fatigue). High-risk groups including health care professionals should receive vaccines for pneumonia (Pneumovax) and influenza.

E. Psychologic integrity: Assess impact of illness on quality of life and coping strategies.

F. Basic care and comfort: Provide client and family teaching and interventions for symptom and pain management, including positioning for improving ventilation and reducing inflammation and edema.

1. Place client in semi-Fowler position.
2. Turn and reposition immobilized client every 2 hr.
3. Plan uninterrupted rest periods, and space nursing care to ensure periods of rest.

G. Reduction of risk potential: Assess client for confusion and changes in cognitive status resulting from pneumonia; provide appropriate interventions to promote client's safety (see also management of care).

H. Pharmacologic and parenteral therapies: Client will state the purpose, usage, and associated side effects of medications used to treat pneumonia.

1. Antipyretics
2. Antibiotics
3. Bronchodilators
4. Analgesics for pain
5. Decongestants
6. Corticosteroids may be considered for severe inflammation

Pulmonary Tuberculosis

I. Definition: Pulmonary tuberculosis (TB) is an infection of the lungs caused by *Mycobacterium tuberculosis,* an acid-fast bacterium, commonly transmitted by inhalation of droplets from infected persons. Once the droplets are inhaled, the organisms implant in the lungs and begin dividing, causing inflammation, development of the primary tubercle, and eventual caseation necrosis and fibrosis. TB may also be transmitted to other parts of the body through the lymph and circulatory systems, including the lymph nodes, meninges, bones, and kidneys.

A. Chronic progressive, reinfection phase is frequently encountered in adults and involves progression or reactivation of primary lesions after months or years of latency.

B. The emergence of drug-resistant TB has complicated disease management.

1. Primary drug resistance—disease resistant to one of the first-line antituberculosis agents.
2. Secondary or acquired drug resistance—disease resistant to one or more antituberculosis agents in a client undergoing therapy.
3. Multidrug resistance—disease caused by TB bacilli resistant to at least isoniazid and rifampicin, the two most powerful anti-TB drugs.

II. Nursing process

A. Assessment

1. Obtain a detailed health history (related to exposure, travel, or bacille Calmette-Guerin [BCG] inoculation) and psychosocial history.
2. Assess for risk factors.
   a. Migration from a country with a high incidence of TB
   b. Socially and economically disadvantaged, malnourished, and alcoholic individuals
   c. Persons over 65 years of age; high incidence among Native Americans, nonwhites, and men more affected than women
   d. History of TB, personally or others with close personal contact
   e. Compromised immunity because of illness (e.g., HIV infection and chemotherapy)
3. Perform a comprehensive physical examination; assess for signs and symptoms.
   a. Low-grade fever, anorexia, malaise, weight loss, pallor, pain, fatigue, and night sweats
   b. Cough (yellow mucoid sputum), dyspnea, chest tightness, hemoptysis, or crackles
4. Obtain diagnostic tests.
   a. Tuberculin skin test (Mantoux)—most reliable determent of TB infection; positive if induration of 10 mm or more in diameter after 48 hr (purified protein derivative [PPD] or intradermal skin test)
   b. Sputum cultures for acid-fast bacillus (AFB)—three positive samples is diagnostic for TB
   c. Chest x-ray
   d. Laboratory values
      (1) Increased WBC and ESR
      (2) Decreased RBC

B. Analysis
   1. Ineffective Airway Clearance related to increased tracheobronchial secretions and fatigue
   2. Ineffective Health Maintenance related to lack of knowledge of disease and therapeutic regimen
   3. Activity Intolerance related to fatigue, altered nutritional status, and fever
   4. Disturbed Body Image related to feelings about tuberculosis diagnosis and social stigma
   5. Social Isolation related to fear of spreading infection

C. Planning
   1. Maintain patent airway.
   2. Increase knowledge about the disease and treatment regimen.
   3. Promote adherence to the therapeutic regimen.
   4. Increase activity tolerance.
   5. Prevent complications.
   6. Improve client symptoms and comfort.
   7. Reduce anxiety.

D. Implementation
   1. Monitor client's signs and symptoms in relationship to diagnostic studies (e.g., sputum cultures).
   2. Provide client and family teaching regarding risk factors, disease process, diagnostics and treatments, medications and associated side effects, activity tolerance, and goals of individualized care.
   3. Initiate follow-up care with client.

E. Evaluation
   1. Client complies with medication regimen and is able to list desired effects and side effects of medications.
   2. Client maintains target weight and diet high in protein and carbohydrates.
   3. Client's sputum culture is negative.
   4. Client and family roles are intact.
   5. Client is free from complications (e.g., no bacillus spread to others or no hemorrhage).
   6. Client's vital signs and labs are within normal range.

CN

III. Client needs

A. Physiologic adaptation: Definitive diagnosis of TB is made by positive sputum acid fast (smear and culture); positive equals greater than 10 AFB per field.
   1. For clients treated on an outpatient basis, observe closely to ensure compliance of the long-term medication regimen.
   2. For clients who have drug-resistant TB, assess for compliance and follow-through with therapy (strict adherence to the prescribed drug regimen is crucial to suppressing the disease).

B. Management of care: Care of the client hospitalized with acute TB symptoms requires critical thinking skills and knowledge of assessment, and teaching and evaluation methods unique to the RN role. These skills cannot be delegated to an LPN or UAP.
   1. Delegate responsibly those activities that can be delegated, including basic care needs and monitoring of vital signs for the stable client. All monitoring information is reported to the RN.
   2. Monitor vital signs, SpO_2, quality of respirations, lung sounds, sputum quantity and characteristics, and symptoms of pain and shortness of breath.
   3. Monitor side effects of antitubercular medications (hepatitis, neurologic changes [hearing loss, neuritis], rash). Monitor liver enzymes, blood urea nitrogen, and serum creatinine levels. Initiate sputum cultures for acid-fast bacillus to evaluate effectiveness of medications.
   4. Provide teaching to client and family about the following:
      a. Airborne and droplet precautions to reduce spread of disease:
         (1) Use good hand hygiene technique.
         (2) Cover mouth and nose when coughing, sneezing, and using disposable tissues.
         (3) Maintain good ventilation of fresh air.
         (4) Use mask when in contact with other people.
      b. Signs and symptoms to report (may indicate complications), including persistent cough, fever, or hemoptysis. Stress the need for follow-up care, including physical exam, sputum cultures, and chest x-ray.
      c. Medications, medication regimen, and associated side effects (see also pharmacologic and parenteral therapies):
         (1) Consult with pharmacist, nurse, or physician prior to taking OTC drugs to avoid drug interactions.
         (2) Follow instructions for taking medications (including labs being drawn).
         (3) For INH, instruct client to take on empty stomach or 1 hr prior to meals; avoid foods with tyramine and histamine (tuna, aged cheese, red wine, soy sauce, yeast extract)

to avoid headache, flushing, hypotension, light-headedness, palpitations, and diaphoresis.

(4) For rifampin, instruct client drug may discolor contact lenses, so may need to wear glasses; may discolor secretions, especially urine.

d. Diet management:

(1) Maintain high-carbohydrate, high-protein, high-vitamin diet with supplemental vitamin B_6 if receiving isoniazid (INH).

(2) Consume small, frequent meals with nutritional supplements to assist in meeting basic caloric requirements.

5. Provide information on changes in client status to the physician and appropriate members of the multidisciplinary team.

C. Safety and infection control: Reduce spread of TB.

1. Protect immunocompromised clients and those at risk (young and elderly).
2. Place client in a well-ventilated, private room with the door kept closed at all times while in hospital. (Strict isolation not required if client adheres to special respiratory precautions for TB.)
3. Use standard precautions and airborne precautions with high-efficiency particulate air (HEPA) filter; teach the proper techniques to prevent spread of infection: Frequent hand hygiene; covering the mouth when coughing; use of disposable tissues; cleaning of eating utensils and disposal of food wastes.
4. Avoid direct contact with sputum.

D. Health promotion and maintenance

1. Provide teaching on self-care behaviors.
2. Monitor daily weights; promote maintenance of ideal weight.
3. Encourage wholesome diet specific to level of disease and complications.
4. Encourage client to maintain role in family while home treatment is ongoing and to return to work and social contacts as soon as it is determined safe for progress of treatment goal.

E. Psychologic integrity

1. Assist client and family in coping with lifestyle changes; encourage client to express feelings about disease and the many implications related to stigma, isolation, and fear of prognosis.
2. Support groups for client and family members when risks factors are present (homeless, drug or alcohol history).

F. Basic care and comfort: For client with advanced stage, promote client and family teaching from health care team regarding goals of treatment, living will, and advance directive to determine preferences while the client is able to participate in decisions for end-of-life care.

G. Reduction of risk potential: Refer client to a clinic for daily medication administration if client is not compliant with medical regimen for directly observed therapy (DOT).

H. Pharmacologic and parenteral therapies: Client will state the purpose, usage, and associated side effects of medications used to treat TB.

1. First line

a. Isoniazid (INH)

(1) Individuals with positive skin test reactors may be prescribed 300 mg INH daily for 1 year as prophylactic measures (e.g., persons immunosuppressed, diabetic, or who have had a gastrectomy).

(2) Side effects include pyridoxine (vitamin B_6 deficiency), hypersensitivity, peripheral neuritis, neurotoxicity, hepatotoxicity, dry mouth, hyperglycemia, vision changes, hepatitis, nausea, and vomiting.

b. Rifampin (Rifadin, Rimactane, Rofact)—side effects include ototoxicity, nephrotoxicity, and red-colored secretions; can increase metabolism of other medications, such as beta blockers, oral anticoagulants, digoxin, quinidine, corticosteroids, and oral hypoglycemic agents.

c. Pyrazinamide (Pyrazinamide, Tebrazid)—side effects include hyperuricemia, hepatotoxicity, skin rash, arthralgias, and GI distress.

d. Ethambutol (Myambutol)—side effects include optic neuritis (may lead to blindness).

e. Streptomycin—side effects include nephrotoxicity, neurotoxicity, and ototoxicity.

2. Second line

a. Capreomycin (Capastat)—side effects include hepatoxicity and pruritus.

b. Cycloserine (Seromycin)—side effects include drowsiness, dizziness.

c. Ethionamide (Trecator)—side effects include nausea, vomiting, dizziness.

d. Kanamycin (Kantrex)—side effects include ototoxicity and nephrotoxicity.

3. Other drugs used to treat TB
   a. Aminosalicylate sodium (Tubasal)—used in the treatment of pulmonary and extrapulmonary TB in combination with other antituberculosis drugs.
   b. Rifabutin (Mycobutin)—antimycobacterial used in persons with immunodeficiency virus infections as prophylaxis for disseminated *Mycobacterium avium.*
   c. Rifampin and isoniazid (Rifamate)—used in combination therapy after separate medications have been tried.

Acute Respiratory Distress Syndrome

I. Definition: Acute respiratory distress syndrome (ARDS) is a clinical syndrome characterized by a sudden and progressive noncardiogenic pulmonary edema unrelated to left-sided heart failure, increasing bilateral infiltrates on chest x-ray, hypoxemia refractory to oxygen supplementation, and reduced lung compliance. Damage to alveolar capillary membrane results in noncardiogenic pulmonary edema and impaired gas exchange. Decreased surfactant production leads to atelectasis and severe hypoxia. Refractory hypoxemia is a landmark finding. Mortality can be as high as 60%, but is less if recognized and treated at the inception; thus, it is very important that the nurse be knowledgeable about risk factors, assessment tools, protocols, and preventive strategies throughout the different phases of ARDS the client may exhibit. Phases of ARDS include the following:

A. Exudative phase—occurs 24 hr after onset and involves increased capillary membrane permeability; protein-rich fluid leaks into pulmonary interstitium, which overwhelms pulmonary lymphatics and forces fluid into alveoli. The end result is alveolar edema.

B. Proliferative phase—occurs 7 to 10 days prior to healing.
   1. There is an increase in type II pneumocytes.
   2. The specialized cells synthesize new pulmonary surfactant and differentiate into type I pneumocytes.
   3. Hypoxemia from intrapulmonary shunting and ventilation and perfusion mismatching second to compression; collapse and flooding of the alveoli and small airway.
   4. Increased work of breathing from increased airway resistance and decreased functional residual capacity (FRC); lung compliance second to atelectasis and compression of small airway.
   5. Hypoxemia and work of breathing leads to client fatigue and alveolar hypoventilation.
   6. Pulmonary hypertension results from damage to capillaries and microthrombi; hypoxic vasoconstriction results in increased dead space and right ventricular hypertrophy.
   7. Increased right ventricular afterload leads to right ventricular dysfunction and a decrease in cardiac output.

II. Nursing process

A. Assessment
   1. Obtain a detailed health history and perform a comprehensive physical examination.
   2. Assess for risk factors; clients at risk include the very young, elderly, and immunosuppressed clients.
      a. Direct, primary—shock, sepsis, multiple trauma, disseminated intravascular coagulation (DIC), multiple blood transfusions, burns, pancreatitis, emboli, drug overdose, and eclampsia.
      b. Indirect, secondary—oxygen toxicity, aspiration (e.g., gastric fluids, near-drowning), pneumonitis, and pulmonary infections.
   3. Assess for signs and symptoms.
      a. Restlessness, anxiety, dyspnea, tachycardia, grunting respirations, intercostal retractions, cyanosis, crackles, and hypotension
      b. $PaCO_2$ initially decreases and later increases
      c. Progressively decreasing PaO_2 arterial blood gas (ratio less than 200)
      d. Chest x-ray examination reveals pulmonary edema; bilateral infiltrates
      e. Changes in orientation and level of consciousness
      f. Pulmonary capillary wedge pressure less than 18 mmHg
   4. Obtain diagnostic tests (clinical manifestations indicate performance of diagnostic studies).
      a. ABGs—$PaCO_2$ increased and PaO_2 decreased, hypoxemia (initially may see respiratory alkalosis, but deteriorates to respiratory and metabolic acidosis with refractory hypoxemia)
      b. Chest x-ray, intrapulmonary shunt measurement, lung compliance, airway resistance, and pressure
      c. Serum electrolytes, fasting blood glucose, BUN, creatinine, CBC, coagulation studies, serum lactate, and end tidal carbon dioxide monitoring ($ETCO_2$)

  d. Urinalysis, blood and wound culture and sensitivity
  e. 12-lead ECG compared with earlier tracing

B. Analysis
  1. Impaired Gas Exchange related to ventilation and perfusion mismatching or intrapulmonary shunting and refractory hypoxemia
  2. Decreased Cardiac Output related to left ventricular failure, intravascular volume depletion, or vasodilatation
  3. Ineffective Breathing Patterns related to inadequate gas exchange, increased secretions, decreased ability to oxygenate adequately, and fear and exhaustion
  4. Risk for Infection related to invasive monitoring devices and endotracheal tube
  5. Anxiety related to dyspnea, severity of illness, fear of death, role changes, or permanent disability
  6. Compromised Family Coping related to critically ill family member

C. Planning
  1. Restore oxygen delivery, uptake, and utilization.
  2. Decrease oxygen consumption.
  3. Maintain hemodynamic stability and normovolemia.
  4. Optimize cardiac function; improve cardiac output.
  5. Improve sensory, motor, and reflex functions.
  6. Reduce anxiety and feelings of hopelessness.
  7. Enhance functional capacity and quality of life.
  8. Maintain adequate oxygenation and tissue perfusion.
  9. Prevent further alterations in body systems affected.
  10. Identify and treat the underlying cause(s).

D. Implementation: Provide collaborative supportive measures based on severity of ARDS and monitor effects of pharmacologic therapy and nonpharmacologic interventions.
  1. Minimize fluid loss and monitor for complications.
  2. Limit myocardial oxygen demand and monitor client's response to care.
  3. Facilitate ventilations and administer volume replacement.
  4. Initiate immobility, DVT prophylaxis therapy—calf and thigh measurement for antiembolic stockings and/or sequential pneumatic stockings; administer prescribed anticoagulation therapy.
  5. Identify clients at risk using evidence-based collaborative practice monitoring for complications, and providing continual observation of process.
  6. Promote early recognition of client for multiple organ dysfunction syndrome (MODS) so supportive therapies can be initiated as soon as possible—prevent and treat infection; maintain tissue oxygenation and nutritional and metabolic support, and support of individual organs.

E. Evaluation
  1. Client maintains adequate gas exchange.
  2. Client maintains patent airway.
  3. Client's hemodynamic stability (BP, cardiac output, central venous pressure [CVP]) and pulmonary artery wedge pressures remain stable as a result of mechanical ventilation and therapy.
  4. Client shows no evidence of complications related to bed rest and immobility.
  5. Client maintains adequate calorie and nutritional intake to meet metabolic needs.
  6. Client is comfortable as evidenced by stable vital signs and cooperation with therapy.
  7. Client demonstrates decreased anxiety.
  8. Client and family understand and verbalize plan of care.
  9. Client achieves successful weaning from mechanical ventilation.

CN

III. Client needs

A. Physiologic adaptation: Care for the client with ARDS is typically provided in an intensive care setting. The underlying cause of ARDS is treated while assuring ventilatory support with positive end-expiratory pressure (PEEP). Fluid management is essential as the client may be hypovolemic because of fluid shifts into interstitial tissue of the lung.
  1. Recognize risk for complications of ARDS, such as systemic inflammatory response syndrome (SIRS) and MODS.
  2. Recognize risk for complications related to mechanical ventilation with high levels of PEEP, immobility because of bed rest, sedation, or pharmacologically induced paralysis.

B. Management of care: Care of the client with ARDS and hemodynamic instability requires critical thinking skills and knowledge of assessment, and teaching and evaluation methods unique to the RN role. These skills cannot be delegated to an LPN or UAP.
  1. Delegate responsibly those activities that can be delegated, including assisting with positioning the client and measurement and recording of vital signs, daily weights, and intake and output for the stable client.

All monitoring information is reported to the RN.

2. Optimizing oxygenation and ventilation—monitor mechanical ventilation (high PEEP increases the risk for pneumothorax) to increase PaO_2 without raising FiO_2, thereby reducing risk of O_2 toxicity, and provide suction, as necessary, to aid removal of secretions.
   a. Promote oxygen therapy.
      (1) Lowest level possible to maintain saturation more than 90%
      (2) FIO_2 preferably less than 65% (0.65)
      (3) Positive end-expiratory pressure (PEEP) to open alveoli and decrease FIO_2 levels; generally PEEP less than 10-15 cm H_2O
         (a) If PEEP too high, can overdistend alveoli.
         (b) If PEEP too low alveoli, collapse during expiration.
   b. Promote ventilation.
      (1) Assist control or synchronized intermittent mandatory ventilation (SIMV; traditional methods).
      (2) Permissive hypercapnia—smaller tidal volumes (5–8 ml/kg)
      (3) Pressure control ventilation (PCV)
         (a) Maintain plateau pressure less than 30 to 40 cm H_2O.
         (b) Inverse ratio ventilation to reverse inspiratory to expiratory (I:E) ratio.
   c. Monitor ABGs, SpO_2 saturation, and report.
   d. Assess respiratory, cardiovascular, and neurologic status to detect evidence of hypoxemia, such as tachycardia, tachypnea, and irritability.
3. Monitor hemodynamic changes for improvement of cardiac output and perfusion.
4. Optimize hemodynamic stability by decreasing preload and afterload, increasing contractility, and attaining a normal cardiac rhythm and fluid status.
   a. Monitor pulmonary artery and capillary wedge pressure (PAWP/PAOP) and central venous pressure (CVP); monitor arterial line for BP; keep within acceptable range.
   b. Keep vital signs in targeted range.
   c. Assess skin (should be pink and warm without pallor); peripheral pulses (palpable or present with Doppler).
   d. Resolve or control dysrhythmias.
   e. Monitor intake and output.
   f. Promote mental alertness, and activity tolerance.
5. Provide information on changes in client status to the physician and appropriate members of the multidisciplinary team.

C. Safety and infection control
   1. Prevent infection through proper hand hygiene, appropriate suctioning techniques, and wearing protective clothing, when appropriate.
   2. Provide mouth care every 2 hr and as needed.
   3. Elevate head of bed at 30 degrees.

D. Health promotion and maintenance: Maintain adequate nutrition (enteral or parenteral feedings as prescribed) and monitor daily weight.
   1. Promote early nutritional support with a balanced calorie, protein, carbohydrate, and fat intake calculated based on the client's metabolic needs.
   2. Avoid high-carbohydrate intake to prevent excess carbon dioxide production.

E. Psychologic integrity
   1. Promote client and family teaching from health care team regarding treatment options, living will, and advance directive to determine preferences while client is able to participate in decisions with end-of-life care.
   2. Briefly explain procedures as they are happening (emergency situation can be very frightening); support client during recovery phase and while weaning from mechanical ventilator as client may have become dependent on it (use prone positioning or special rotating beds).
   3. Determine client and family understanding of relevant information prior to procedure or surgery.
   4. Encourage client to express feelings about fear of suffocation to reduce anxiety and, therefore, O_2 demands.

F. Basic care and comfort
   1. Provide a calm, quiet environment and encourage rest to reduce workload of the heart and promote optimal perfusion.
   2. Keep client comfortable and begin attempts to reduce fever, such as use of antipyretics and hyperthermia measures.
   3. Promote rest by spacing activities and treatments.

G. Reduction of risk potential
   1. Promote early identification of clients at risk for development of ARDS.
   2. Monitor for side effects of medications.

3. Intervene to prevent aspiration—check NG tube placement; recognize cultural differences contributing to potential complications following tests and procedures.
4. Plan and implement body system-specific interventions to prevent complications; use elastic stockings to prevent thrombus formation.
5. Assess client for abnormal neurologic status.

H. Pharmacologic and parenteral therapies: Client will state the purpose, usage, and associated side effects of medications used to manage ARDS.
1. Antibiotics—infecting organism determines which drug is used
2. Bronchodilators and mucolytics—maintains airway patency and reduces inflammatory reaction and secretions in the airways
3. Corticosteroids—decreases inflammatory response in late stages of ARDS; may be useful in stabilizing alveolar-capillary membrane to prevent further deterioration. Includes hydrocortisone (Solu-Cortef) and methylprednisolone sodium succinate (Solu-Medrol).
4. Analgesics—morphine, fentanyl citrate (Sublimaze)
5. Sedatives—benzodiazepines; propofol (Diprivan)
6. Neuro-blocking agents—vecuronium bromide (Norcuron); cisatracurium (Nimbex); and Pancuronium (Pavulon)

Chest Trauma

I. Definition: Chest trauma depends on the type and extent of injury, which may be described as blunt or penetrating. Trauma to the chest and lungs may interfere with ventilation, oxygenation, and perfusion. There are several types of problems that may result:

A. Pulmonary contusion—bruising of the lung parenchyma.
B. Rib fractures—most common injury; may lacerate lung.
C. Flail chest—blunt chest trauma associated with accident. Instability of the chest wall also caused by fractures of the ribs or sternum; may result in hemothorax and rib fractures; asymmetrical chest expansion (paradoxical movement).
D. Pneumothorax—presence of air within the pleural cavity as result of trauma, or can occur spontaneously via accumulation of atmospheric air in the pleural space, which results in a rise in intrathoracic pressure and reduced vital capacity.
1. Closed or spontaneous—rupture of bulla, pulmonary infarction, and severe coughing attack.
2. Open or traumatic—communication between atmosphere and pleural space because of sucking chest wound.
3. Tension—air enters the pleural space with each inspiration but cannot escape; results in increased intrathoracic pressure and shifting of the mediastinal contents to the unaffected side (mediastinal shift).

E. Hemothorax—presence of blood in pleural cavity.
F. Cardiac contusion—bruising of the myocardium.
G. Cardiac tamponade—blood in pericardium and compressing the heart, resulting in decreased cardiac filling and leading to reduced cardiac output and potential shock and death.

II. Nursing process

A. Assessment
1. If related to trauma, obtain a primary survey of injury followed by a secondary survey.
2. Perform a comprehensive physical assessment; complaint varies with type of injury.
3. Assess for signs and symptoms.
   a. Pulmonary contusion—restlessness, dyspnea, decreased breath sounds, crackles, wheezes, hypoxemia, increased bronchial secretions, and hemoptysis.
   b. Rib fractures—pain at injury site that increases with inspiration, shallow respirations, client splints chest, and fractures noted on chest x-ray.
   c. Flail chest—paradoxical respirations, severe chest pain, tachypnea, shallow respirations, dyspnea, hypoxemia, tachycardia, hypotension, and diminished breath sounds.
   d. Pneumothorax—absent breath sounds on affected side; decreased chest expansion (unilaterally or bilaterally); cyanosis; dyspnea; hypoxemia; hypotension; sharp chest pain; subcutaneous emphysema as evidence by crepitus on palpation; sucking sound with open chest wound; tachycardia, tachypnea, tracheal deviation to the unaffected side with tension pneumothorax.
   e. Hemothorax—blood in the pleural space; may be hidden blood loss and client may be asymptomatic;

if symptomatic the client will be dyspneic or in shock.

f. Cardiac contusion—signs and symptoms of congestive heart failure may be present; dysrhythmias.
g. Cardiac tamponade—hypotension, muffled heart sounds, and increased central venous pressure manifested by distended neck veins (Beck triad).
h. Additional signs and symptoms include increased work of breathing (use of accessory muscles, intercostal retraction) and dullness to percussion with hemothorax, hemopneumothorax, or parenchymal hemorrhage.

4. Obtain diagnostic tests (based on signs and symptoms of trauma).
   a. Chest x-ray
   b. Pericardiocentesis for suspected cardiac tamponade
   c. ABGs
   d. 12-lead ECG, echocardiography, or multigated angiography (MUGA) if cardiac trauma
   e. Creatine kinase (CK-MB), troponin I, hemoglobin, hematocrit, type and cross-match

B. Analysis
1. Ineffective Airway Clearance related to shallow respirations and pain
2. Impaired Gas Exchange related to asymmetrical chest expansion, collapsed lung, and abnormal chest movement
3. Acute Pain related to chest injury, chest tubes
4. Decreased Cardiac Output and Perfusion related to injury
5. Anxiety related to serious physical condition
6. Risk for Trauma related to fractured ribs
7. Risk for Infection related to open chest wound
8. Activity Intolerance related to decreased cardiac output and imbalance between oxygen supply and demand

C. Planning
1. Maintain patent airway.
2. Stabilize vital signs and hemodynamic status.
3. Restore ABGs and pulmonary parameters and maintain within client's normal range.
4. Maintain chest wall stability and integrity.

D. Implementation
1. Implement mechanical ventilation, if indicated; prepare for intubation with mechanical ventilation, with PEEP for severe flail chest associated with respiratory failure and shock.
2. Position client in high Fowler position.
3. Administer humidified oxygen as prescribed.
4. Monitor for increased respiratory distress.
5. Encourage coughing and deep breathing.
6. Administer pain medication as prescribed.
7. Maintain bed rest and limit activity to reduce oxygen demands.

E. Evaluation
1. Client has patent airway with adequate oxygenation and ventilation.
2. Client's ABGs and vital signs are appropriate.
3. Client indicates pain relief and ease of breathing.

III. Client needs

A. Physiologic adaptation: Chest injuries are treated to restore pulmonary function. For pneumothorax and hemothorax this will involve inserting a chest tube to remove air or fluid intubation, and mechanical ventilation may be required, depending on the extent and duration of the injury. For rib fractures, management involves splinting or taping the ribs and providing analgesics. Complications and risks can include cardiovascular collapse, acute respiratory failure, and infection.

B. Management of care: Care of the client with chest trauma requires critical thinking skills and knowledge of assessment, and teaching and evaluation methods unique to the RN role. These skills cannot be delegated to an LPN or UAP.
1. Delegate responsibly those activities that can be delegated, such as taking vital signs, assisting with hygiene, and comfort measures. All monitoring information is reported to the RN.
2. Perform comprehensive physical assessments and provide care to the client with acute heart failure and hemodynamic instability.
   a. Administer pain medication as prescribed to maintain adequate ventilatory status.
   b. Monitor for increased respiratory distress.
   c. Instruct client to self-splint with hands and arms.
   d. Prepare client for an intercostal nerve block as prescribed, if the pain is severe.

3. Prepare to assist physician with chest tube placement, pericardiocentesis, intubation, and placement on mechanical ventilator.
4. Position client for optimal ventilation and prevent aspiration; provide symptomatic treatment for uncomplicated chest trauma to ensure the ability to cough and deep breathe.
5. Keep skin clean, reinforce dressings, and provide wound care around chest tubes and other invasive devices.
6. Provide adequate nutrition to promote healing; maintain adequate intake and output; measure daily weights.
7. Provide discharge planning and evaluate need for rehabilitation and home care needs if client using equipment such as incentive spirometry, or follow up with medications or nutrition management.

C. Safety and infection control
1. Monitor chest tube site and drainage closely for signs of complications.
2. Promote frequent skin inspection and care to prevent infection.
3. Maintain sterile technique.
4. Practice fall precautions when chest tube in place.
5. Provide teaching on ways to decrease risk factors (e.g., risky behaviors while driving, alcohol, drug use).

D. Health promotion and maintenance: Promote nutritious diet to promote wound healing.

E. Psychologic integrity
1. Assist client and family in coping with unexpected trauma.
2. Explain procedures to client during emergency situations to help decrease anxiety.

F. Basic care and comfort
1. Provide adequate pain management.
2. Teach client to splint chest when moving or coughing.

G. Reduction of risk potential
1. Instruct client about chest tubes and appropriate management.
2. Pad around chest tube when turning on operative site to maintain tube patency and promote comfort.
3. For open pneumothorax, place a dressing that is taped on only three sides to prevent a tension pneumothorax.

H. Pharmacologic and parenteral therapies: Client will state the purpose, usage, and associated side effects of medications used to treat chest trauma.
1. Antibiotics
2. Analgesics
3. Sedatives

Bibliography

Abrams, A. C. (2004). *Clinical drug therapy: Rationales for nursing practice* (7th ed.). Philadelphia: Lippincott Williams & Wilkins.

Global Initiative for Chronic Obstructive Lung Disease Executive Committee. (2006). *Global strategy for the diagnosis, management, and prevention of COPD.* Retrieved May 19, 2008 from, http://www.goldcopd.com/Guidelineitem.asp?l1=2&l2=1&intId=996

Hogan, M. A., & Silvestri, L. (2005). *Pharmacology:Review & rationales.* Upper Saddle River, NJ: Prentice Hall.

Ignataviciuc, D. D., & Workman, M. L. (2006). *Medical-surgical nursing* (5th ed.). Philadelphia: Saunders.

Lewis, S., Heitkemper, M., Dirksen, S., O'Brien, P., & Bucher, L. (2007). *Medical-surgical nursing: Assessment and management of clinical problems.* (7th ed.). St. Louis: Mosby.

Morton, P. G., Fontaine, D. K., Hudak, C. M., & Gallo, B. M. (2005). *Critical care nursing: A holistic approach* (8th ed.). Philadelphia: Lippincott Williams & Wilkins.

National Heart, Lung, and Blood Institute. (2002). *National Asthma Education and Prevention Program, NAEPP Expert Panel Report: Guidelines for the diagnosis and management of asthma. Update on selected topics.* Retrieved May 19, 2008 from, http://www.nhlbi.nih.gov/guidelines/asthma/execsumm.pdf

Porth, C. M. (2007). *Essentials of pathophysiology.* Philadelphia: Lippincott Williams & Wilkins.

Smeltzer, S. C., Bare, B. G., Cheever, K. H., & Hinkle, J. L. (2008). *Brunner & Suddarth's textbook of medical-surgical nursing* (11th ed.). Philadelphia: Lippincott Williams & Wilkins.

Urden, L. D., Stacy, K. M., & Lough, M. E. (2006). *Thelan's critical care nursing: Diagnosis and management* (5th ed.). St. Louis: Mosby.

CHAPTER 23

Practice Test

Upper Respiratory Disorders

1. The nurse is planning care with a client who has adult-onset diabetes and is experiencing frequent URIs. The nurse should instruct the client that which of the following is the most effective strategy to decrease the risk of infection?
   - □ 1. Assure adequate oral intake.
   - □ 2. Control blood sugar.
   - □ 3. Obtain daily exercise.
   - □ 4. Perform frequent hand hygiene.

Cancer of the Larynx

2. The nurse is caring for a client who had a radical neck dissection for laryngeal cancer 28 hr ago. Which of the following is the priority in the nursing care plan for this client?
   - □ 1. Start a clear liquid diet within 48 hr.
   - □ 2. Keep client on bed rest in supine position.
   - □ 3. Suction laryngeal tube frequently.
   - □ 4. Take vital signs every 8 hr.
3. The nurse is teaching a client who had a total laryngectomy about home care. Which of the following statements indicates the client needs additional teaching?
   - □ 1. "I will face away from the water when showering."
   - □ 2. "I will gradually return to my previous activities."
   - □ 3. "I will no longer be able to communicate through speech."
   - □ 4. "I will periodically check the batteries in my smoke detector."

Lung Cancer

4. Following a thoracotomy, a client has a pleural chest tube connected to water seal drainage. The client suddenly has labored breathing with an increase in heart rate and respiratory rate. Which of the following actions does the nurse first perform?
   - □ 1. Assess tubing for impaired drainage.
   - □ 2. Clamp the chest tube.
   - □ 3. Increase the suction chamber to −30 cm of water pressure.
   - □ 4. Lower the head of the bed.
5. A client had a right lobectomy for cancer of the lung 2 days ago. Today, the nurse auscultates crackles in both lung bases. The nurse should:
   - □ 1. Decrease fluid intake.
   - □ 2. Encourage deep-breathing exercises.
   - □ 3. Administer antitussive medications.
   - □ 4. Keep the client on bed rest.

Asthma

6. A client is experiencing an acute asthmatic attack. Prior to treatment with levalbuterol (Xopenex), respirations were 40, pulse 132, oxygen saturation 86%, and wheezing was audible. Which of the following indicates that the desired outcome of asthma treatment is achieved?
   - □ 1. Decreased PEF rate.
   - □ 2. Wheezing inaudible with diminished breath sounds.
   - □ 3. Pulse 96 and SpO_2 92% on room air.
   - □ 4. Inspiratory cycle twice as long as the expiratory cycle.
7. For a client with asthma, the physician prescribes albuterol (Proventil), two puffs twice a day via MDI, and beclomethasone (Vanceril, Beclovent) two puffs twice a day via MDI. Which of the following instructions should the nurse provide the client?
   - □ 1. Administer medications 1 hr apart, 2 times a day.
   - □ 2. Administer albuterol first and follow with beclomethasone, 2 times a day.
   - □ 3. Administer albuterol on awakening, and alternate the medications every 4 hr.
   - □ 4. Administer beclomethasone inhaler first and follow with albuterol.
8. The nurse is teaching a client with asthma how to take fluticasone (Flonase) via MDI. Which client statement indicates teaching is successful?
   - □ 1. "I will monitor my heart rate before using this inhaler."
   - □ 2. "I will rinse my mouth after I use this inhaler."
   - □ 3. "I will use this inhaler before I administer my bronchodilator."
   - □ 4. "I will use this inhaler with meals since nausea and vomiting are common side-effects."

9. The nursing is giving discharge instructions to a client with persistent asthma. The nurse should be sure the client understands to do which of the following?
- ☐ 1. Use inhalers only when wheezing.
- ☐ 2. Avoid exposure to known triggers.
- ☐ 3. Reduce fluid intake.
- ☐ 4. Limit activity level.

Chronic Obstructive Pulmonary Disease

10. AF The nurse is assessing a client with COPD. Which of the following indicates that the client is experiencing an exacerbation of COPD? Select all that apply.
- ☐ 1. Dyspnea.
- ☐ 2. Increased FEV_1.
- ☐ 3. Improved SpO_2 with activity.
- ☐ 4. Low carbon dioxide level.
- ☐ 5. Productive cough.
- ☐ 6. Pain on taking a deep breath.

11. The nurse is instructing a client with COPD how to perform pursed-lip breathing. The nurse should tell the client that pursed-lip breathing will:
- ☐ 1. Slow the respiratory rate and increase the inhaled air.
- ☐ 2. Loosen secretions so that they may be coughed up more easily.
- ☐ 3. Prevent airway collapse to assist with more effective expiration.
- ☐ 4. Promote maximal inhalation for better oxygenation of the lungs.

12. A client with COPD tends to stay at home rather than going out to dinner with friends because of shortness of breath while eating. The nurse should teach the client to:
- ☐ 1. Eat five to six small meals per day.
- ☐ 2. Consume warm rather than cold foods.
- ☐ 3. Decrease activity level.
- ☐ 4. Follow a high-carbohydrate diet.

13. The client with emphysema is receiving ipratropium (Atrovent) via MDI. The nurse should assess the client for which one of the following side effects?
- ☐ 1. Lethargy.
- ☐ 2. Dry mouth.
- ☐ 3. Diarrhea.
- ☐ 4. Flushing.

Pneumonia

14. The nurse is caring for a client with bacterial pneumonia. The effectiveness of the client's oxygen therapy can be best determined by the:
- ☐ 1. Absence of cyanosis.
- ☐ 2. Client's respiratory rate.
- ☐ 3. Analysis of ABG levels.
- ☐ 4. Client's level of consciousness.

15. The HCP has prescribed amoxicillin (Amoxil) for a client with streptococcal pneumonia. Before administering the drug, which of the following actions should the nurse perform first?
- ☐ 1. Take the client's temperature.
- ☐ 2. Review culture reports for resistant organisms.
- ☐ 3. Order an IV pump and additional tubing.
- ☐ 4. Check the client's allergies.

Pulmonary Tuberculosis

16. Which one of the following clients is at greatest risk for acquiring TB?
- ☐ 1. Female client who is 16 years of age and smokes cigarettes.
- ☐ 2. Male client who is 40 years of age and an alcoholic.
- ☐ 3. Male client who is 55 years of age with heart failure.
- ☐ 4. Female client who is 70 years of age and lives alone.

17. The nurse is reading a client's tuberculin skin test. The nurse should interpret which of the following reactions at the injection site as positive?
- ☐ 1. Erythema and itching, no induration.
- ☐ 2. Induration of 15 mm with erythema.
- ☐ 3. Blistering around injection site.
- ☐ 4. Painful induration of 3 mm.

Acute Respiratory Distress Syndrome

18. AF The nurse is assessing a client with ARDS. The client is on a ventilator with positive end-expiratory pressure and receiving oxygen via endotracheal tube. The nurse evaluates the client's blood gas report below.

LABORATORY RESULTS

Test	Result
PaO_2	50 mmHg
$PaCO_2$	35 mmHg
HCO_3^-	24 mEq/L
pH	7.40

Which of the following indicates the client is not receiving sufficient oxygenation?
□ 1. PaO_2.
□ 2. $PaCO_2$.
□ 3. HCO_3.
□ 4. pH.

Chest Trauma

19. AF During a motor vehicle accident, a client is ejected from her vehicle. While in the emergency department, the nurse notes the client is short of breath, has a significant decrease in respiratory excursion on the right side of her chest, and is tachycardic. The nurse should do which of the following in order of priority?
_____ 1. Prepare for a chest tube insertion.
_____ 2. Obtain vital signs.
_____ 3. Start an IV line.
_____ 4. Call a technician to obtain an ECG.

20. At 9 a.m. the nurse administers morphine as ordered for pain for a client who has six fractured ribs. At 10 a.m., considering the following changes within 1 hr, which outcome indicates that the morphine is achieving the desired effect?
□ 1. Client's respiratory rate decreases from 20 to 14.
□ 2. Client's pain on a scale of 1 to 10 decreases from 9 to 4.
□ 3. Client's urinary output increases from 200 to 210 ml.
□ 4. Client's oxygen saturation changes from 95% to 98%.

Answers and Rationales

1. 4 Hand hygiene is the best way to control the spread of infection. A nutritious diet, exercise, and control of blood sugar in diabetics are important in health-promotion strategies, but hand washing is the most effective method for reducing the incidence of upper respiratory infections. (H)

2. 3 The postoperative client requires frequent suctioning of secretions from the laryngeal tube. The nurse positions the client and elevates the head of bed to decrease edema and promote lung expansion. Frequent monitoring of vital signs is required in early postoperative course; the nurse should obtain and document vital signs every 2 to 4 hr, depending on the client's status. A swallow study is performed after 1 week to ensure intact suture lines before any oral diet is initiated. (A)

3. 3 The speech pathologist provides teaching on alternative forms of speech, such as esophageal speech, transesophageal puncture, or mechanical larynx. Clients need to avoid getting foreign material or water into the stoma; a cover can be worn. Clients gradually return to normal activities. Smell is altered as the client no longer breathes through the nose and mouth. (H)

4. 1 The nurse's first action is to assess chest tube patency, checking for kinks or blockage, which would cause increased pressure on the lung and potential collapse. Clamping the chest tube may cause air to become trapped in the pleural space and result in a tension pneumothorax. When a chest tube is first inserted, the water seal drainage is usually set at a negative pressure of −20 cm of water pressure to assist with drainage. When the chest tube is placed to water seal, the suction source is detached from the suction control chamber, which has been done. An order is needed to change the suction on the water seal drainage. The client is placed with head of bed elevated to assist with lung expansion and breathing. (R)

5. 2 Atelectasis is a common postoperative complication causing crackles in the lung bases. Because of incisional discomfort, the client may have shallow respirations and inability to achieve full lung expansion. The nurse encourages the client to perform deep-breathing exercises and get out of bed to promote lung expansion. There is no indication of fluid volume overload causing interstitial edema and crackles in the lung to require a decrease in fluid intake; the nurse routinely assesses for any intake and output imbalance. There is no indication for an antitussive medication. Coughing is encouraged, not suppressed, if there are secretions to expectorate, and a deep breath should follow. (R)

6. 3 Quick-acting bronchodilators are used in acute asthma to improve airflow and relieve symptoms; following treatment, tachycardia resolves as gas exchange and work of breathing are improved. SpO_2 and PEF rates improve and wheezing from a constricted airway resolves. The normal inspiratory to expiratory ratio is 1:2. (A)

7. 2 The nurse instructs the client to administer the bronchodilator first (the beta-2 agonist always leads) in order to open the airway and allow for improved delivery of the corticosteroid to the lung tissue, which follows after 1 min between puffs. Using a spacer device with an MDI provides the best delivery of medication to the lungs. (D)

8. 2 Client teaching is effective when the client states the need to rinse the mouth after using a corticosteroid inhaler; this prevents candidiasis from the drug's interference with natural defenses in the mouth and the throat. Tachycardia is a side effect of beta-2 agonists, not corticosteroids. The bronchodilator is given first and then followed with the corticosteroid. Candidiasis, sore throat, and hoarse voice are the more common side effects of inhaled corticosteroids. (D)

9. 2 The nurse ensures that the client understands to avoid exposure to known triggers and allergens. Self-care management requires adherence to the medication regimen to prevent and control symptoms with daily inhaled medication, or prior to exercise or unavoidable exposure to a known allergen, not only when wheezing occurs. Fluids are encouraged to liquefy secretions so that the client can easily expectorate and reduce mucus plugs. A goal of care is for the client's tolerance to normal activity without symptoms. (H)

10. 1, 5 Major signs and symptoms of COPD are shortness of breath, productive cough, chronic sputum production, and carbon dioxide retention. Expiratory volumes are decreased. Activity uses more oxygen, causing the SpO_2 to decrease. Pain with a deep breath may be a symptom of pleurisy. (A)

11. 3 Pursed-lip breathing increases pressure and prevents collapse of the bronchi during expiration. Pursed-lip breathing prolongs expiratory phase, and there is less resistance with expiring air. The client is encouraged to increase fluid intake to loosen secretions. (A)

12. 1 Adequate food intake can be disrupted by shortness of breath; therefore, the nurse teaches the client to eat smaller meals more frequently. Eating warm food does not improve shortness of breath. Clients with COPD benefit from exercise. Carbohydrates increase production of carbon dioxide and should be eaten in moderation. (P)

13. 2 The major side effects of ipratropium (Atrovent) are dry mouth and drying of secretions. Lethargy, diarrhea, and flushing are not side effects of Atrovent. (D)

14. 3 The client's ABG levels are the most sensitive indicator of the effectiveness of the client's oxygen therapy. Cyanosis is a late sign of decreased oxygenation and is not a reliable indicator. The client's respiratory rate and level of consciousness may be altered because of other problems not related to the client's oxygenation. (M)

15. 4 Antibiotics commonly cause allergy responses in a variety of clients. No antibiotic should be given without first confirming the client's history of allergies. The client's temperature is important but does not need to be obtained before antibiotic administration. Culture reports may not be available prior to the initiation of antimicrobial therapy. Many antibiotics are given orally and do not require IV equipment. (D)

16. 2 A male client who is 40 years of age and an alcoholic has a compromised immune system from the alcoholism and is at highest risk for acquiring TB. The other clients are at risk, but not as high at risk as the alcoholic. (R)

17. 2 The nurse reads the tuberculin skin test within 48 to 72 hr. Induration (hardening) of 10 mm with erythema is considered a positive reaction. An induration of 5 mm is considered positive for clients with HIV or clients who have had recent contact with active TB. Induration of 10 mm is positive for clients diagnosed with TB in the past 2 years who have chronic illnesses such as diabetes mellitus. An induration of 15 mm is considered positive for all clients. Erythema and itching are common reactions, but in the absence of induration they are not diagnostic. Painful induration of 3 mm is usually due to injection technique. Blisters around the injection area are not common and do not indicate a positive reaction. (M)

18. 1 The PaO_2 is below the normal value of 80 to 100 mmHg. This client is experiencing hypoxia; the nurse notifies the HCP or respiratory therapist for changes in the ventilator settings or oxygen levels. The $PaCO_2$ is on the low end of normal (35 to 45 mmHg); the HCO_3^- (22 to 26 mEq/L) and pH (7.35 to 7.45) are within normal limits. (A)

19. 1, 3, 2, 4 This client is experiencing signs of a pneumothorax. The nurse's first priority is to prepare for a chest tube insertion to inflate the affected lung. Next, the nurse establishes an IV infusion, obtains vital signs, and then calls for an ECG technician to obtain the ECG. (M)

20. 2 Morphine is administered to relieve pain, and the client reports on the pain scale an improvement in pain. Morphine also slows respirations, but slowing of respirations is a secondary benefit for this client; the respirations are not too slow and the client may breathe easier as a result of pain relief. Morphine does not increase urinary output; this change is not significant. The change in the client's oxygen saturation is not significant and is within the desired range. (D)

chapter

24 The Client With Upper Gastrointestinal Tract Health Problems

Health problems of the upper gastrointestinal (GI) tract range from minor discomforts, such as an oral ulceration, to severe and potentially debilitating conditions such as cancer. Given the close interrelationship between nutritional intake and the body's overall health, the nurse is involved in planning with the client and health care team to prevent upper GI problems as well as to promote and maintain health. Topics discussed in this chapter include:

- Oral Infections and Inflammations
- Oral Cancer
- Gastroesophageal Reflux Disease
- Peptic Ulcer Disease
- Cancer of the Stomach

Oral Infections and Inflammations

I. Definition: Oral infections and inflammations may be specific mouth diseases or they may occur in the presence of some systemic diseases, such as leukemia or vitamin deficiency. A client who is immunosuppressed is most susceptible to development of oral infections and inflammations. When oral infections and inflammations are present, they can severely impair ingestion of food and fluids. They may also predispose clients to infections in other body organs. The oral cavity can be considered a potential reservoir for respiratory pathogens. Oral pathogens have also been associated with heart disease.
   A. Gingivitis—involves inflamed gingivae and interdental papillae; results in bleeding during toothbrushing, development of pus, and the formation of an abscess with loosening of teeth (periodontitis). Primary causes include inadequate oral hygiene, malocclusion, missing or irregular teeth, faulty dentistry, the eating of soft rather than fibrous foods, and side effects of some medications.
   B. Oral candidiasis (moniliasis or thrush)—a fungal infection of the mouth, oral candidiasis involves soreness within the mouth and white lesions on the mucosa of the mouth and larynx. Primary causes include *Candida albicans,* debilitation, prolonged high-dose antibiotics, or corticosteroid therapy.
   C. Herpes simplex-HSV1 (cold sore, fever blister)—involves lip lesions, mouth lesions, vesicle formation (single or clustered), and shallow, painful ulcers. Primary cause is the herpes simplex virus. Predisposing factors include upper respiratory infections, excessive exposure to sunlight, food allergies, emotional tension, and the onset of menstruation in females.
   D. Parotitis (inflammation of parotid gland)—involves pain or discomfort in the area of the gland and ear, absence of salivation, purulent exudates from the gland, erythema, and ulcerations. Primary cause is usually staphylococcus bacterium, although the streptococcus species occasionally is the etiologic agent. Parotitis may occur when there is debilitation and dehydration with poor oral hygiene, or when a client may have nothing by mouth for an extended period of time.
   E. Stomatitis (inflammation of the mouth)—involves excessive salivation, halitosis, and a sore mouth. Primary causes may include trauma; pathogens; irritants such as alcohol or tobacco; renal, liver, and hematologic diseases; and side effects of numerous cancer chemotherapeutic drugs and radiation.

II. Nursing process
   A. Assessment
      1. Perform a detailed physical assessment.
         a. Presence of lesions in oral cavity
         b. Presence of pain
         c. Restriction of movement
         d. Alteration in speech (tongue restriction)
         e. Presence of enlarged cervical lymph nodes
      2. Assess educational and cultural limitations to instruction and therapy.
      3. Obtain a detailed health and dental history.
         a. Treatment of cancer with chemotherapy and/or radiation therapy
         b. Chronic diseases (e.g., diabetes mellitus, asthma)
         c. Irritants (e.g., alcohol, tobacco, spicy or acidic foods)
         d. Denture fit
         e. Presence of tooth malocclusion
         f. Professional dental care
         g. Self-care dental practices
         h. Regular use of inhalers
         i. Malnutrition or vitamin deficiency
      4. Obtain diagnostic tests.
         a. X-ray of skull
         b. Computed tomography scan
         c. Biopsy of oral tissue
         d. Endoscopy
            (1) Bronchoscopy
            (2) Esophagoscopy
            (3) Laryngoscopy
   B. Analysis
      1. Impaired Oral Mucous Membrane related to pathologic condition, infection, or chemical/mechanical trauma
      2. Imbalanced Nutrition: Less Than Body Requirements related to oral/dental disease condition
      3. Disturbed Body Image related to physical change in appearance subsequent to oral disease condition or surgical/medical treatment
      4. Impaired Verbal Communication related to mouth disease condition, tenderness, or ill-fitting dentures
      5. Acute Pain related to altered oral mucous membrane
      6. Impaired Swallowing related to altered integrity of oral mucous membrane or edema
      7. Anxiety related to fear of the unknown
      8. Risk for Ineffective Coping related to oral disease condition

C. Planning
1. Perform regular oral hygiene.
2. Improve oral mucous integrity.
3. Increase moistness of oral mucous membrane, tongue, and lips.
4. Relieve pain and discomfort.
5. Provide teaching about cause, preventive measures, and treatment of oral infections and inflammations.
6. Provide teaching about nutrition to promote healing of oral infections and inflammations.
7. Prevent progressive weight loss and/or dehydration.
8. Provide for social interaction with family and friends.
9. Aid in identification of coping strategies.
10. Reduce anxiety via therapeutic communication.
11. Prevent aspiration of liquids.

D. Implementation
1. Lubricate lips with lip balm on regular basis.
2. Support efforts to decrease or eliminate usage of tobacco (including smokeless tobacco) and alcohol.
3. Teach client and family how to inspect oral cavity.
4. Provide for increased humidification; instruct client to avoid temperature extremes.
5. Instruct client to avoid irritating foods; provide soft or pureed diet as required.
6. Promote adequate, nonirritating fluids to prevent dehydration.
7. Administer antibiotics or antifungal agents as ordered (see pharmacologic and parenteral therapies).
8. Provide oral care using soft-bristled toothbrush or sponge applicators.
9. Encourage use of chewing gum and hard candy to stimulate saliva.

E. Evaluation
1. Client demonstrates oral hygiene interventions and complies with therapeutic regimen.
2. Client's oral mucosal condition improves as evidenced by intact mucous membrane, moist and intact tongue and lips, and absence of pain and lesions.
3. Client verbalizes knowledge about cause, preventive measures, and treatment of oral infections and inflammations and factors that potentiate oral bleeding.
4. Client describes relief of pain and discomfort.
5. Client describes optimal nutrition to promote healing of oral infections and inflammations.
6. Client describes measures to prevent dehydration.
7. Client demonstrates interaction with others.
8. Client uses coping strategies.
9. Client describes little or no anxiety.
10. Client's breath sounds are free of crackles on auscultation.

CN

III. Client needs

A. Physiologic adaptation: Oral inflammations and infections are managed with specific anti-infective drugs and symptomatically to relieve pain and discomfort.
1. Promote use of liquid, soft, or blenderized foods; nutritional supplements such as commercial liquids or milkshakes are available.
   a. Decrease irritation or discomfort from painful lesions with appropriate oral care.
   b. Maintain adequate nutrition; prevent weight loss and dehydration.
2. Recognize possibility for short-term nasogastric (NG) feeding.

B. Management of care: Care of the client with oral infections and inflammations requires critical thinking skills and knowledge of assessment, and teaching and evaluation methods unique to the RN role. These skills cannot be delegated to an LPN or UAP.
1. Delegate responsibly those activities that can be delegated, including basic care needs, recording of vital signs, and provision of oral hygiene after each meal and as often as needed. The UAP may also assist in selecting soft, bland, nonacidic and nonspicy foods from the menu. All monitoring information is reported to the RN.
2. Apply topical analgesics or anesthetics as ordered and monitor effectiveness.
3. Perform physical assessments of oral cavity and provide needed care.
4. Inform physician of changes in oral lesions, presence of fever, effectiveness of analgesics, presence of oral bleeding and drainage, and difficulty in chewing and/or swallowing food or fluids.
5. Assess the need for home health care.
6. Evaluate resources to aid in cessation of smoking or alcohol practices.

C. Safety and infection control
1. Instruct client about precautions to prevent aspiration of liquids.
2. Instruct client to notify physician if any of the following recurs/worsens: Oral pain, fever, drainage, continuous bleeding, inability to eat/drink.

D. Health promotion and maintenance: Teach client about self-care behaviors to maintain healthy oral cavity.
   1. Perform self-examination of mouth at least monthly; report any unusual findings to physician or dentist.
   2. Eat a balanced diet.
   3. Brush and floss teeth every day.
   4. Avoid stress as much as possible; learn how to maintain emotional health.
   5. Avoid contact with agents that may cause inflammation of the oral cavity, such as mouthwashes that contain alcohol.
   6. Be aware of changes in occlusion of teeth, mouth pain, or swelling; seek medical attention promptly.
   7. See dentist regularly; have problems addressed promptly.
   8. If wearing dentures, make sure they are in good repair and fit properly.

E. Psychologic integrity
   1. Encourage client to verbalize perceived change in body appearance; realistically discuss actual changes and losses.
   2. Offer support while client verbalizes fears and negative feelings.
   3. Individualize plan of care by listening attentively and determining if client needs are primarily psychosocial or cognitive-perceptual.
   4. Determine major anxieties concerning interpersonal relations in home or work environment.
   5. Be alert to signs of grieving.

F. Basic care and comfort
   1. Promote mouth care—monitor intake of irritating substances. Evaluate offensive agents.
   2. Promote nutritional intake—record weight, age, and level of activity to adequate daily caloric intake. Recommend changes in consistency of foods, frequency of eating based on disease condition, and client preference. Encourage nonirritating and nonacidic foods and fluids.
   3. Dentures—assure dentures fit properly and are in good repair.

G. Reduction of risk potential
   1. Review current oral hygiene patterns and encourage proper oral hygiene practices.
   2. Provide information as required or desired to correct deficiencies in oral hygiene.
   3. Discuss special mouth care required during/after treatment for other illnesses/trauma.
   4. Review information regarding medications that make high risk for oral infections/inflammations.
   5. Monitor for superinfection such as fungal infection of the mouth, lungs, or vagina.
   6. Promote general health; provide nutritional information to correct deficiencies, reduce irritation or gum disease, and prevent dental caries.
   7. Identify community resources (low-cost dental clinics, Meals on Wheels/food stamps, home-care aide).

H. Pharmacologic and parenteral therapies: Client will state the purpose, dosage, timing, and side effects of medications to manage oral infections and inflammations.
   1. Anti-infectives—broad-spectrum: Amoxicillin (Amoxil); erythromycin (Erythrocin)
      a. Monitor for superinfection.
      b. Monitor GI upset; take with food if GI upset present.
   2. Analgesics—opioid and nonopioid
      a. Opioid: Hydrocodone (Vicodin); codeine (Paveral)
         (1) Monitor respiratory rate; hold if respirations less than 12 per minute.
         (2) Instruct client to avoid taking with alcohol as alcohol augments central nervous system depressant effects.
      b. Nonopioid: Acetaminophen (Tylenol)

Oral Cancer

I. Definition: Oral (oropharyngeal) cancer may occur on the lips or anywhere within the mouth, including the tongue, floor of the mouth, buccal mucosa, hard palate, soft palate, pharyngeal walls, and tonsils. While curable if discovered early (before spreads to lymph nodes), mortality rates have been decreasing; the 10-year survival rate is 43%. Oral cancer is more common after 40 years of age, with 60 years of age being the average age of onset. The cancer occurs in all ethnic groups and is more common in men, with a male-to-female ratio of 2:1, although incidence in women is increasing.

A. Types of oral cancer
   1. Basal cell carcinoma of the lip has the most favorable prognosis; lip lesions are more apparent and are usually diagnosed earlier.
   2. Squamous cell carcinoma is the most common oral malignant tumor (more than 90%); most occur on the lower lip or palate.

B. Etiology—although the definitive cause is unknown, the most significant etiologic factors influencing the development of oral cancer include a past or current use of tobacco (cigar, cigarette, pipe, and snuff) and excessive alcohol intake. Additional causes may include chronic irritation from factors such as a jagged tooth, poor-fitting dentures, or poor dental care.

C. Clinical manifestations
   1. Leukoplakia—whitish patch on mucosa of mouth or tongue from chronic irritation, especially from smoking.
   2. Erythroplasia—red velvety patch on mouth or tongue that is considered precancerous (90% chance of malignancy).
   3. Ulcerations, rough, or thickened areas, or sores that bleed easily and do not heal—may occur on the lip or tongue. The ulcer or area of thickening on the tongue may involve soreness or pain (primarily the proximal half), increased salivation, slurred speech, dysphagia (difficulty swallowing), toothache, and earache.
   4. Later symptoms—difficulty in moving jaw (chewing, speaking).

II. Nursing process

A. Assessment
   1. Perform a detailed physical assessment.
      a. Assess for mucosal erythroplasia:
         (1) Smooth
         (2) Granular
         (3) Minimally elevated
         (4) May present with or without leukoplakia
         (5) Persists longer than 10 to 14 days
      b. Assess lip for lesion that fails to heal.
      c. Assess tongue for edema, ulceration, areas of tenderness or bleeding, abnormal texture, and limited movement.
      d. Assess floor of mouth for red, slightly elevated, mucosal lesions with ill-defined borders; leukoplakia; induration; ulceration; and wartlike growths.
      e. Assess for neck mass, throat edema, painful swallowing, dysphagia, ear pain, difficulty opening mouth, epistaxis, and palsies of cranial nerves II, III, IV, VI, IX-XII.
   2. Perform assessment for advanced oral cancer, involving ulceration, bleeding, pain, induration, cervical lymphadenopathy, and weight loss.
   3. Perform a detailed health history for influencing factors such as tobacco use (cigarette smoking, smokeless tobacco, pipe smoking), heavy alcohol intake (especially in combination with smoking), marijuana use, and chronic sun exposure.
   4. Obtain diagnostic tests.
      a. Flexible/rigid nasopharyngoscopy
      b. Staining of oral lesions with toluidine blue distinguishes abnormal from normal tissue
      c. Biopsy of suspected lesions or mass
      d. Chest x-ray
      e. Computed tomography
      f. Magnetic resonance imaging (detects local invasiveness/metastasis)

B. Analysis
   1. Acute Pain related to disease process
   2. Disturbed Body Image related to alteration in appearance
   3. Fear related to threat to/change in health
   4. Imbalanced Nutrition: Less Than Body Requirements related to decreased taste, dysphagia, and pain
   5. Ineffective Coping related to unidentified coping strategies to meet ongoing treatment needs
   6. Risk for Infection related to impaired tissue integrity
   7. Risk for Injury related to fatigue and disease process
   8. Ineffective Airway Clearance related to ineffective cough
   9. Impaired Oral Mucous Membranes related to oral lesions

C. Planning
   1. Maintain patent airway.
   2. Maintain fluid, electrolyte, and nutritional balance.
   3. Relieve dryness of mouth.
   4. Manage pain.
   5. Manage decreased excessive salivation and mouth odors.
   6. Provide assistance with personal appearance.
   7. Prevent infection.
   8. Prevent injury.
   9. Promote healing of impaired oral mucous membrane.

D. Implementation
   1. Keep a tracheostomy set at bedside.
   2. Administer total parenteral nutrition as ordered.
   3. Provide saline mouthwashes and ample fluid if client is receiving radiation therapy.
   4. Use time and distance protocol when providing care if receiving radiation therapy.
   5. Provide prescribed analgesics as ordered (see pharmacologic and parenteral therapies) and diversion to alleviate pain intensity.
   6. Acknowledge pain experience; convey acceptance of response to pain.
   7. Provide for individualized exercise program.
   8. Instruct about signs and symptoms, and changes requiring attention.

E. Evaluation
   1. Client maintains airway patency.
   2. Client maintains nutritional status.

3. Client experiences little or no pain or discomfort.
4. Client's excessive oral secretions are managed.
5. Client participates in diversional activities.
6. Client's fear and anxiety are lessened.
7. Client directs attention to self-care that enhances personal appearance.
8. Client's oral mucous membrane in process of healing with no further breakdown.
9. Client is free from injury.
10. Client demonstrates no signs or symptoms of infection.

III. Client needs

A. Physiologic adaptation: Management of oral cancer depends on the type of cancer, size of the lesion, and tissue involvement. Lesions that are small and detected early may be excised and treated with radiation therapy. Larger lesions may require extensive surgical resection, reconstructive surgery, radical neck dissection, and use of radiation and chemotherapy.
   1. Evaluate maintenance of food, fluids, and electrolyte balance.
   2. Recognize risk for aspiration of fluid—indicated by dyspnea, elevated pulse and respirations, lung crackles, and presence of coughing and choking.
   3. Assess ability of client to swallow.
   4. Evaluate effectiveness of placing client in upright position while eating and drinking.
   5. Check for retention of food inside mouth, indicative of poor tongue movement.

B. Management of care: Care of the client with cancer requires critical thinking skills and knowledge of assessment, and teaching and evaluation methods unique to the RN role. These skills cannot be delegated to an LPN or UAP.
   1. Delegate responsibly those activities that can be delegated, including basic care needs such as mouth care following surgery and recording of vital signs. All monitoring information is reported to the RN.
   2. Perform ongoing physical and psychosocial assessment.
   3. Keep physician informed of changes in client's status.
   4. Consult with occupational and speech therapist when swallowing difficulty exists.
   5. Collaborate with discharge planner to make needed arrangements for outpatient follow-up care.
   6. Evaluate home health care needs for use of suctioning equipment or dressing changes.

C. Safety and infection control: Minimize opportunity for development of infection, such as thorough hand hygiene and use of sterile technique with dressing changes. Provide client and family teaching (see reduction of risk potential).

D. Health promotion and maintenance
   1. Provide client with accurate information about disease process of oral cancer.
   2. Inform client of immediate and long-term implications for needed health care when chemotherapy, radiation therapy, or surgery is selected for treatment.
   3. Optimize health through modifications in self-care behaviors.
   4. Emphasize need for continued follow-up care from physicians, dentists, dietitians, and/or occupational or speech therapists.
   5. Encourage adequate rest to prevent fatigue.

E. Psychologic integrity
   1. Assist client in coping with lifestyle modifications.
   2. Identify stressors for both client and family.
   3. Correct distorted perceptions with provision of accurate information.
   4. Acknowledge fears related to pain, isolation, altered lifestyle, and loss of control.
   5. Support adaptive behaviors, encourage expression of emotions, emphasize client's strengths and abilities, and foster positive self-esteem.
   6. Encourage counseling and psychologic support from clinical psychologist, member of clergy, counselor, social worker, and cancer support group.

F. Basic care and comfort
   1. Use alternative means to enhance effective communication, such as communication board.
   2. Maintain environment conducive for rest.

G. Reduction of risk potential: Provide client and family teaching.
   1. Evaluate integrity of oral mucous membranes and skin intactness on regular basis and inform physician/dentist of alterations.
   2. Maintain healthy oral cavity by regular oral hygiene, regular dental and medical visits, and avoidance of irritants such as alcohol, smoking, and sun overexposure.
   3. Apply lip moisturizers/balm as needed.
   4. Modify food texture and consistency to decrease likelihood of aspiration.
   5. Assure intake of noncaffeinated, nonirritating fluids.

H. Pharmacology and parenteral therapies: Client will state the purpose, dosage, timing, and side effects of medications to manage oral cancer.

1. Local mucosal anesthetics—benzocaine (Orajel); tetracaine hydrochloride (Pontocaine); and dyclonine (Dyclone, Sucrets): Side effects include allergic reactions; monitor for skin lesions, urticaria, and edema.
2. Analgesics
   a. Opioid—meperidine (Demerol), oxycodone (OxyContin):
      (1) Monitor client's response closely for light-headedness, vertigo, sedation, or fainting.
      (2) Instruct client to check with physician before taking over-the-counter drugs for colds, stomach distress, allergies, insomnia, or pain.
   b. Nonopioid—nonsteroidal anti-inflammatory drugs—ibuprofen (Motrin), aspirin (Ecotrin):
      (1) Monitor for GI tract distress, and signs and symptoms of GI bleeding and vertigo.
      (2) Instruct client to avoid alcohol and to avoid taking aspirin with other nonsteroidal anti-inflammatory drugs.
3. Antifungal antibiotics—nystatin (Mycostatin); fluconazole (Diflucan); and ketoconazole (Nizoral)
   a. Give reconstituted powder for oral suspension immediately after mixing.
   b. Inform client to remove dentures before each rinse with oral suspension and before use of troche; avoid food and drink during period of dissolving troche.
   c. Monitor for allergic response; lab results, blood urea nitrogen, creatinine, liver function; signs and symptoms of hepatotoxicity and loss of glycemic control.
4. Broad-spectrum antibiotics—cefazolin (Kefzol); cephalexin (Keflex); and cefepime (Maxipime)
   a. Instruct client to report promptly any signs and symptoms of superinfection, and signs of hemostatic defects (ecchymoses, petechiae, and/or nosebleeds).
   b. Monitor for changes in blood urea nitrogen and creatinine.
   c. Determine history of hypersensitivity to cephalosporins and penicillins before therapy is initiated.
   d. Instruct client to promptly report onset of diarrhea, which may indicate pseudomembranous colitis (potentially life-threatening condition).
5. Parenteral therapies
   a. Isotonic solutions: Replace deficits of total body water; expand intravascular volume.
      (1) Normal saline (0.9% NaCl)
      (2) Dextrose 5%/water (D5W); becomes hypotonic
      (3) Lactated Ringer (LR)
   b. Hypotonic solutions: For cellular dehydration
      (1) One-half normal saline (0.45% NaCl)
      (2) One-fourth normal saline (0.225% NaCl)
6. For chemotherapy with squamous cell carcinoma:
   a. General pharmacologic therapy includes methotrexate (Trexall); bleomycin (Blenoxane); cisplatin (Platinol); cyclophosphamide (Cytoxan); doxorubicin (Adriamycin); vincristine (Oncovin); 5-fluorouracil (Adrucil); and hydroxyurea (Hydrea)
   b. Foam brushes soaked in nystatin (Mycostatin) is effective in reducing bacteria and controlling candidiasis.
   c. Topical solution containing diphenhydramine (Benadryl), 2% viscous lidocaine, kaolin with pectin, and nystatin (Mycostatin) decreases pain and helps prevent secondary oral infections and inflammations such as stomatitis. (See also Chapter 32.)
7. Vitamins
   a. Vitamin C—strengthens connective tissue in gums.
   b. Niacin, riboflavin— promotes efficient cellular growth.

Gastroesophageal Reflux Disease

I. Definition: Gastroesophageal reflux disease (GERD) is a condition in which there is a backflow of gastric or duodenal contents, or both, into the esophagus and past the lower esophageal sphincter without associated belching or vomiting. Excessive reflux may result from impaired or partial gastric outlet obstruction or motility disorders such as achalasia, scleroderma, or esophageal spasm.

II. Nursing process
   A. Assessment
      1. Perform detailed physical assessment, including assessment for positive signs and symptoms of GERD (one third of clients experience minimal to no symptoms).

a. Presence of reflux pain and heartburn (pyrosis):
(1) Typically occurs 1½ to 2 hr after eating.
(2) Pain worsens with vigorous exercise, bending, lying down, wearing tight clothing, coughing, and during constipation.
(3) Relief experienced on use of antacids or sitting upright.
b. Reported regurgitation without associated nausea or belching
c. Feeling of fluid accumulation in throat without sour or bitter taste
d. Chronic pain radiating to neck, jaws, and arms that may mimic angina pectoris
e. Odynophagia (sharp substernal pain on swallowing), possibly followed by dull substernal ache
f. Bright red or dark brown blood in emesis
g. Other symptoms may include nocturnal hypersalivation or wheezing, laryngitis or morning hoarseness, and chronic cough.
2. Obtain a detailed health history. GERD may be aggravated by fatty foods, acidic foods (coffee, citrus juices, tomatoes), and obesity.
3. Obtain diagnostic tests.
a. Barium swallow with fluoroscopy—reveals evidence of recurrent reflux
b. Esophageal acidity test—reveals degree of gastroesophageal reflux
c. Gastroesophageal scintillation test—reveals reflux
d. Esophageal manometry—reveals abnormal lower esophageal sphincter pressure and sphincter incompetence
e. Acid perfusion (Bernstein) test—confirms esophagitis
f. Esophagoscopy/biopsy—confirms pathologic changes in mucosa
g. 24-hr pH monitoring to determine amount of gastroesophageal acid reflux

B. Analysis
1. Acute or Chronic pain related to tissue trauma resulting from reflux
2. Imbalanced Nutrition: More Than Body Requirements related to excess intake
3. Deficient Knowledge: Disease Process, related to management of GERD

C. Planning
1. Monitor for signs of aspiration.
2. Prevent complications such as esophagitis and aspiration.
3. Manage or relieve pain.
4. Promote diet modification.

D. Implementation (see management of care)

E. Evaluation
1. Client reports incidence of reflux pain is greatly reduced.
2. Client maintains desirable body weight.
3. Client reports understanding of GERD and its management.
4. Client shows no signs of aspiration.

III. Client needs

A. Physiologic adaptation: GERD is managed with diet therapy and medications (see pharmacologic and parenteral therapies). Surgical correction (Nissen fundoplication) may be indicated when client does not respond to other approaches—upper portion of stomach wrapped around distal esophagus and sutured, creating a tight lower esophageal sphincter.
1. Permit dressings to remain in place until removed by surgeon in 1 week; Steri-Strips fall off in 7 to 10 days.
2. Monitor wounds for redness, edema, and drainage.
3. Prevent fluid volume overload if receiving IV fluid therapy.

B. Management of care: Care of the client with GERD requires critical thinking skills and knowledge of assessment, and teaching and evaluation methods unique to the RN role. These skills cannot be delegated to an LPN or UAP.
1. Delegate responsibly those activities that can be delegated, including basic hygienic care and recording of vital signs. All monitoring information must be reported to the RN.
2. Monitor for complications of GERD, including:
a. Stricture (may require series of mechanical dilation)
b. Ulceration and possible fistula formation
c. Aspiration pneumonia
d. Barrett esophagus (presence of columnar epithelium above gastroesophageal junction), which increases risk of adenocarcinoma
3. Perform postoperative assessment and nursing care, if surgery is indicated.
4. Consult with dietitian and encourage diet modification to maintain pressure in lower esophageal sphincter pressure, which predisposes client to reflux.
a. Promote low-fat, high-fiber diet; avoid caffeine and carbonated beverages.
b. Promote avoidance of eating and drinking 2 hr before bedtime.

c. Instruct client to avoid drinking fluids with meals to reduce gastric distention.
d. Encourage frequent small meals to prevent gastric dilation; discourage overeating.

5. Instruct lifestyle modification such as avoiding wearing tight clothes, tobacco and alcohol cessation, and avoidance of situations and activities that increase intra-abdominal pressure.
6. Administer antacids, histamine-receptor antagonists, and gastric acid pump inhibitors as indicated.

C. Safety and infection control (see physiologic adaptation)

D. Health promotion and maintenance: Encourage client to use dietary plan and lifestyle modification.

E. Psychologic integrity: Promote client adaptation to changes in lifestyle.

F. Basic care and comfort
1. Elevate head of bed 6 to 8 inches.
2. Encourage client to remain upright for at least 3 hr after eating.

G. Reduction of risk potential
1. Advise client to sit or stand when taking pills/capsules; emphasize need to follow with at least 90 ml of liquid.
2. Advise client that many prescriptions and over-the-counter medications may exacerbate symptoms: Anticholinergics (further impair functioning of lower esophageal sphincter), antihistamines, antidepressants, antihypertensives, antispasmodics, and some neuroleptics and anti-Parkinson medications, which decrease saliva production (may decrease acid clearance from esophagus).

H. Pharmacologic and parenteral therapies: Client will state the purpose, dosage, timing, and side effects of medications to manage oral infections and inflammations.
1. Antacids—although antacids may provide symptomatic relief from reflux, they do not heal esophageal lesions.
2. Histamine-receptor antagonists
   a. Decrease gastric acid secretions
   b. Indirectly reduce pepsin secretion
3. Proton-pump inhibitors
   a. Suppress gastric acid production
   b. Helpful in healing esophagitis

Peptic Ulcer Disease

I. Definition: Peptic ulcer disease (PUD) is a condition characterized by erosion of the GI mucosa as a result of digestive action of hydrochloric acid and pepsin. Any portion of the GI tract that comes into contact with gastric secretions is susceptible to ulcer development, including the lower esophagus, stomach, duodenum, and margin of gastrojejunal anastomosis following surgical procedures. PUD occurs in approximately 10% of the population; it is estimated that approximately 10% of men and 4% of women in the United States will have ulcers during their lifetimes.

A. Types of peptic ulcers
1. Gastric ulcers—more likely to occur during the fifth and sixth decades of life.
2. Duodenal ulcers—located in the duodenum (most common type); more likely to occur during the fourth and fifth decades for men, and the occurrence for women is about 10 years later in life.

B. Etiology and pathophysiology
1. Peptic ulcers develop only in presence of an acid environment, but an excess of gastric acid may not be necessary for ulcer development. Pepsinogen (precursor of pepsin) is activated to pepsin in the presence of hydrochloric acid and a pH of 2 to 3. The stomach is normally protected from autodigestion by the gastric mucosal barrier; the surface mucosa of the stomach is renewed about every 3 days. When the barrier is broken, hydrochloric acid freely enters the mucosa and injury to tissue occurs; histamine is released from damaged mucosa, which stimulates further secretion of acid and pepsin. By generating ammonia in the mucosal layer, *Helicobacter pylori* bacteria may create a condition of chronic inflammation, rendering the mucosa vulnerable to other noxious substances.
2. There are two mechanisms that protect against damage:
   a. Mucus is secreted by superficial mucous cells.
   b. Bicarbonate is secreted by gastric and duodenal mucosa, which helps neutralize hydrochloric acid in lumen of GI tract.

C. Clinical manifestations: Client may experience no pain (sensory pain fibers minimal). When present, pain is burning epigastric pain, and occurs 1.5 to 3 hr after eating. Pain in duodenal ulcers is more "cramplike" while pain in gastric ulcers is more "gaseous."

D. Complications: All complications are considered emergency situations and are initially treated conservatively. Surgery may become necessary at any time during course of therapy. (See management of care for signs and symptoms of complications.)

1. Hemorrhage is the most common complication; develops from erosion of granulation tissue found at base of ulcer during healing or from erosion of ulcer through major blood vessel. Duodenal ulcers account for greater percentage of upper GI bleeding.
2. Perforation is considered the most lethal complication. Duodenal ulcers perforate more frequently; mortality rates associated with perforation of gastric ulcers are higher.
3. Pyloric obstruction involves ulcers located in antrum, pre pyloric and pyloric areas of the stomach and duodenum. Active ulcer formation is associated with edema, inflammation, and pylorospasm that contributes to narrowing of pylorus.

II. Nursing process

A. Assessment

1. Perform a detailed physical assessment, including assessment for signs and symptoms of PUD.
   a. Assess for pain, including characteristics of pain.
      (1) Determine relationship of pain to types of food ingested, time food is consumed, and whether gnawing sensation is relieved by food.
      (2) Recognize ulcer perforation may be indicated by sudden, intense, midepigastric pain radiating to right shoulder.
   b. Assess abdomen for epigastric tenderness, guarding, and hyperactive bowel sounds.
   c. Note presence of nausea, anorexia, early satiety (common with gastric ulcers), and belching.
   d. Assess for vertigo, syncope, hematemesis, and melena with GI hemorrhage.
      (1) Positive fecal occult blood
      (2) Decreased hemoglobin, hematocrit indicative of anemia
      (3) Orthostatic hypotension, pulse changes
2. Obtain a detailed health history, including history of dietary patterns, chronic alcohol abuse, smoking, caffeine use, and family history of PUD.
3. Obtain diagnostic tests.
   a. Upper GI series—outlines ulcer, area of inflammation
   b. Endoscopy (esophagogastroduodenoscopy)—visualizes duodenal mucosa; helps identify inflammatory changes, lesions, bleeding sites, and malignancy (through biopsy/cytology)
   c. Gastric secretory studies—gastric acid secretion test, serum gastrin level test (elevated in Zollinger-Ellison syndrome)
   d. *Helicobacter pylori* antibody titer—urea breath test: Determines presence of active infection; urea is by-product of metabolism of *H. pylori* bacteria
   e. CBC: May have decreased RBC count, decreased hemoglobin, and decreased hematocrit
   f. Liver enzymes (alanine aminotransferase, aspartate aminotransferase): May be elevated, possibly from inflammation

B. Analysis

1. Acute Pain related to increased gastric secretions, decreased mucosal protection, and ingestion of gastric irritants
2. Ineffective Therapeutic Regimen Management related to lack of knowledge of long-term management of PUD, consequences of not following treatment plan, and unwillingness to modify lifestyle
3. Acute Pain related to exacerbation of disease process and inadequate comfort measures
4. Nausea related to acute exacerbation of disease process
5. Chronic Pain related to gastric secretion
6. Deficient Fluid Volume related to hemorrhage and/or dumping syndrome
7. Imbalanced Nutrition: Less Than Body Requirements related to abdominal distress

C. Planning

1. Relieve pain.
2. Promote reduction of anxiety.
3. Promote proper nutrition.
4. Facilitate attainment of adequate rest.
5. Promote acquisition of knowledge about prevention and management of PUD.
6. Teach about the need for compliance with prescribed therapeutic regimen.
7. Enable client to exhibit no signs of GI complications related to ulcerative process.
8. Facilitate attainment of complete healing of peptic ulcer.

D. Implementation

1. Provide therapeutic interventions.
   a. Promote diet therapy, including well-balanced meals at regular intervals, and avoiding dietary irritants. Reinforce importance of adherence to bland diet high in vitamin K (asparagus, broccoli, cabbage, spinach, tomatoes).
   b. Encourage elimination of caffeine, alcohol, smoking, and any other known irritants.

c. Eliminate nonsteroidal anti-inflammatory drug usage.
d. Encourage client to reduce or eliminate alcohol intake.

2. Promote pharmacologic interventions and administer parenteral therapy (see pharmacologic and parenteral therapies).
3. Provide postoperative care if surgery indicated.
4. Monitor for signs of bleeding through fecal occult blood, vomiting, persistent diarrhea, change in vital signs, and intake and output.
5. Monitor hemoglobin, hematocrit, and electrolyte levels.
6. Maintain NG tube and monitor drainage.

E. Evaluation
1. Client experiences relief of pain.
2. Client verbalizes plan to modify lifestyle and incorporate therapeutic regimen.
3. Client adheres to nutritionally balanced meal plan.
4. Client takes medications as prescribed.
5. Client verbalizes increase in energy level.
6. Client identifies anxiety-producing situations.
7. Client understands what symptoms require immediate attention from health care provider (HCP).

III. Client needs

A. Physiologic adaptation: PUD is managed with medications (see pharmacologic and parenteral therapies), lifestyle modifications, and surgical intervention, which may include gastroduodenostomy (Billroth I), gastrojejunostomy (Billroth II), antrectomy, total gastrectomy, pyloroplasty, or vagotomy (severed vagus nerve).

B. Management of care: Care of the client with PUD requires critical thinking skills and knowledge of assessment, and teaching and evaluation methods unique to the RN role. These skills cannot be delegated to an LPN or UAP.

1. Delegate responsibly those activities that can be delegated, including basic hygienic care and recording of vital signs. All monitoring information is reported to the RN.
2. Monitor for signs and symptoms of complications.
   a. Hemorrhage—cool skin; confusion; elevated pulse, labored breathing; blood in stool.
   b. Perforation
      (1) Sudden, severe upper abdominal pain spreads throughout the abdomen
      (2) Shoulder pain (irritation to phrenic nerve)
      (3) Abdominal muscles contract appearing rigid and boardlike
      (4) Respirations become rapid and shallow
      (5) Bowel sounds are absent
      (6) Vomiting
      (7) Elevated temperature and elevated pulse
   c. Pyloric obstruction—nausea, vomiting; distended abdomen; and abdominal pain.
      (1) Initially, gastric emptying is normal or near normal.
      (2) Increased contractile force is needed to empty stomach; results in hypertrophy of stomach wall.
      (3) With chronic long-standing ulcers, stomach enters decompensated phase that results in dilation, atony.
3. Contact physician to report changes in client's status.
4. Suggest consult with dietitian for nutritional counseling.
5. Emphasize to client that follow-up supervision is necessary for about 1 year, unless informed otherwise by the physician.

C. Safety and infection control: Teach client to avoid use of aspirin and bicarbonate of soda (Alka-Seltzer).

D. Health promotion and maintenance
1. Encourage good perianal care.
2. Encourage frequent rest periods and to avoid, or learn to cope with, stressful situations.
3. Instruct client to immediately report evidence of bleeding, tarry stools, or vertigo, which may indicate an acute bleeding episode.
4. Encourage follow-up to determine adequate healing.

E. Psychologic integrity
1. Encourage to express concerns and fears, and ask questions as needed.
2. Explain reasons for adhering to planned treatment schedule.
3. Help identify anxiety-producing situations.
4. Teach stress-reducing exercises such as meditation, distraction, and imagery.

F. Basic care and comfort
1. Involve family members in care, if desired and feasible.
2. Schedule rest periods that coincide with treatment regimen.
3. Provide small, frequent meals; snacks at regular times. Make environment conducive for relaxing meal.

G. Reduction of risk potential
1. Administer prescribed IV fluids and blood replacement if acute bleeding is present.

2. Encourage bed rest to reduce stimulation that may enhance gastric secretion.
3. Teach client to substitute acetaminophen (Tylenol) for aspirin.
4. Instruct client to avoid over-the-counter drugs that contain acetylsalicylic acid such as Alka-Seltzer.
5. Instruct client to monitor use of drugs that are irritating to gastric mucosa:
   a. Ulcerogenic drugs, aspirin, and nonsteroidal anti-inflammatory drugs inhibit synthesis of prostaglandins and cause abnormal permeability.
   b. Corticosteroids have ability to decrease rate of mucosal cell renewal.
   c. Lipid-soluble cytotoxic drugs can pass through barrier and destroy it.

H. Pharmacologic and parenteral therapies: Client will state the purpose, dosage, timing, and side effects of medications to treat PUD.

1. Pharmacologic therapies to treat PUD:
   a. Antacids
   b. Anticholinergics
   c. Histamine–receptor antagonists
   d. Antisecretory, proton-pump inhibitors
   e. Mucosal protective agents
   f. Antibiotics
   g. Cytoprotective drugs
2. Pharmacologic therapies to treat ulcers caused by *H. pylori* bacteria (when administered together, these medications eradicate *H. pylori* bacteria in the gastric mucosa):
   a. Bismuth subsalicylate (Pepto-Bismol)
   b. Metronidazole (Flagyl)
   c. Tetracycline (Achromycin)
3. Parenteral therapies:
   a. Normal saline (0.9%) NaCl—isotonic
   b. One half normal saline (0.45% NaCl)—hypotonic
   c. 5% dextrose/water (D5/W)—isotonic/hypotonic
   d. Lactated Ringer (LR)—isotonic
   e. Colloids, as volume expanders, require dedicated infusion line—monitor for signs of hypervolemia (hypertension, dyspnea, bounding pulse); assess for adequate tissue perfusion:
      (1) Albumin (5%; 25%)
      (2) Dextran 40; Dextran 70
      (3) Hetastarch (Hespan, Hextend)
4. Parenteral therapies to use with presence of GI bleeding:
   a. Lactated Ringer with 5% dextrose (D5/LR)—hypertonic
   b. Dextrose 5% in 0.9% NaCl (D5/NS)—hypertonic
   c. Dextrose 10% in water (D10/W)—hypertonic

Cancer of the Stomach

I. Definition: Cancer of the stomach (gastric cancer) is a malignant growth in the stomach that is usually an adenocarcinoma. The growth spreads rapidly to the lungs, lymph nodes, and liver; the client may not present with clinical manifestations until metastases are present or local invasion becomes advanced (see assessment for signs and symptoms). The etiology and risk factors include a diet high in smoked foods, lack of fruits and vegetables, chronic stomach inflammation, pernicious anemia, achlorhydria (absence of hydrochloric acid), gastric ulcers, and *H. pylori* bacteria. Alcohol and tobacco use are two additional risk factors. This cancer is most common in African Americans, Hispanic Americans, Asian/Pacific islanders, and in men older than 40 years of age; incidence increases with age.

II. Nursing process

A. Assessment

1. Perform a detailed physical assessment, including assessment for signs and symptoms of gastric cancer. Early signs may present as indigestion; later signs may include the following:
   a. Fatigue
   b. Anorexia, weight loss (loss of appetite)
   c. Nausea, vomiting (possibly with coffee-ground appearance)
   d. Indigestion, epigastric discomfort
   e. Sensation of pressure in stomach
   f. Dysphagia
   g. Anemia
   h. Dyspepsia
   i. Constipation
   j. Ascites
   k. Gastric fullness (early satiety)
   l. Stool samples positive for occult blood
   m. Pain in back
   n. Palpable mass—initially, client may present with same symptoms as gastric ulcer; later, evaluation shows lesion to be malignant.
2. Obtain a detailed health history, including family history of gastric cancer.
3. Obtain diagnostic tests.
   a. Upper GI x-ray with contrast media—may initially slow suspicious ulceration that requires further evaluation
   b. Endoscopy with biopsy, cytology—confirms malignant disease

c. Imaging studies—help determine metastasis
   (1) Bone scan
   (2) Liver scan
   (3) Computed tomography scan
d. CBC—may indicate anemia from blood loss

B. Analysis
1. Acute Pain related to disease process
2. Imbalanced Nutrition: Less Than Body Requirements related to loss of appetite (anorexia)
3. Risk for Infection related to weakened state
4. Risk for Injury related to muscle weakness and fatigue
5. Anticipatory Grieving related to diagnosis of cancer

C. Planning
1. Reduce anxiety.
2. Facilitate attainment of optimum nutrition.
3. Relieve pain.
4. Facilitate adjustment to diagnosis and to anticipated lifestyle changes.
5. Provide palliative care if metastasis to other vital organs such as liver.

D. Implementation (see management of care)

CN

III. Client needs

A. Physiologic adaptation: The only successful treatment of gastric cancer is gastric resection (surgical removal of part of stomach with involved lymph nodes). Postoperative staging is done, and further treatment may be necessary; surgery may be combined with chemotherapy to provide palliation and prolong life.
1. Complications of gastric surgery may include shock; wound evisceration; hemorrhage; pulmonary problems; thrombosis, embolism; dumping syndrome; leakage from duodenal stump; pancreatitis; and paralytic ileus. (See also management of care.)
2. Surgical options include the following:
   a. Proximal/distal subtotal gastric resection
   b. Total gastrectomy (includes adjacent organs such as tail of pancreas, portion of liver, and duodenum)
   c. Palliative surgery—subtotal gastrectomy with gastroenterostomy to maintain continuity of GI tract

B. Management of care: Care of the client with gastric cancer requires critical thinking skills and knowledge of assessment, and teaching and evaluation methods unique to the RN role. These skills cannot be delegated to an LPN or UAP.
1. Provide postoperative nursing care.
   a. Position in modified Fowler position.
   b. Monitor for complications (see physiologic adaptation).
      (1) Avoid pulmonary complications by administering analgesia before deep breathing and coughing, and providing frequent turning.
      (2) Assess for signs of pancreatitis including abdominal pain, rapid pulse, and temperature elevation.
   c. Check NG tube drainage for blood first 12 hr postoperatively; assist surgeon to readjust NG tube and for irrigation and removal.
   d. Attend to fluid needs parenterally until return of peristalsis and removal of NG tube; avoid cold fluids (which cause distress).
   e. Provide nutritional intake by adding bland foods until able to eat six small meals per day.
   f. Provide wound care; report excessive drainage on dressings.
   g. Monitor hemoglobin, hematocrit; administer blood transfusions, as prescribed.
2. Delegate responsibly those activities that can be delegated for the stable client. All monitoring information is reported to the RN.
   a. Take vital signs.
   b. Provide basic hygienic care.
   c. Assist in resumption of activities according to client's abilities.
   d. Assist in provision and ingestion of small, frequent meals.
   e. Report need for analgesics to RN.
   f. Promote frequent turning.
3. Prepare client for chemotherapy or radiation therapy as indicated.
4. Keep physician informed of client's status and significant changes.
5. Consult with dietitian to promote optimum nutrition.
6. Collaborate with discharge planner and case manager to address home health care needs such as need for equipment or dressing changes.
7. Encourage follow-up visits with physician and routine blood studies; other testing to detect complications and prevent recurrence.

C. Safety and infection control
1. Position client to prevent aspiration.
2. Provide nose and mouth care using cool water and oral sponge to prevent inflammation and potential for infection.

3. Use sterile technique when performing dressing changes.
4. Prevent thrombus formation and emboli by encouraging ambulation wearing support hose, or using commercial ThromboGuard devices.

D. Health promotion and maintenance
1. Provide parenteral nutrition as long as necessary; there may be significant protein deficiency as the result of food intolerance.
2. Provide soft diet when dysphagia is present, or if client had truncal vagotomy causing trauma to the lower esophagus.
3. Provide teaching to prevent weight loss for long-term management.
4. Supplement vitamin B_{12} and iron because there is malabsorption of organic iron and vitamin B_{12}; stress to client the importance of long-term vitamin B_{12} injections after gastrectomy to prevent surgically induced pernicious anemia.
5. Teach client to prevent phytobezoar formulation (mass of compact vegetable matter that does not pass into intestine) by avoiding fibrous foods and chewing food thoroughly.

E. Psychologic integrity
1. Request consult with clergy, psychologist, psychiatric clinical nurse specialist, and/or home health care worker to help client cope.
2. Provide relaxed, nonthreatening atmosphere so client can express fears, concerns, and possibly anger.

F. Basic care and comfort: Provide pain relief (see pharmacologic and parenteral therapies).

G. Reduction of risk potential: Prevent complications (see management of care).

H. Pharmacologic and parenteral therapies: Client will state the purpose, dosage, timing, and side effects of medications to manage gastric cancer.
1. Crystalloids: To prevent/manage hypovolemia and shock.
   a. 5% dextrose/water (D5/W)—isotonic, hypotonic
   b. Normal saline (0.9% NaCl)—isotonic
   c. Lactated Ringer (LR)—isotonic: Used to expand intravascular volume and replace extracellular fluid losses
   d. 5% dextrose in normal saline (D5/NS)—hypertonic
   e. 5% dextrose in half-normal saline (D5/0.45NS)—hypertonic
   f. 3% normal saline (3% NS)—hypertonic: Ideal fluids for hydration; must be administered slowly and with extreme caution (may cause intravascular volume overload and pulmonary edema)
2. Analgesics: For pain relief
   a. Narcotic analgesics—includes morphine (Duramorph) and hydromorphone (Dilaudid)
   b. Oral analgesics
      (1) Narcotic—hydrocodone (Vicodin) and codeine (Paveral)
      (2) Nonnarcotic—ibuprofen (Motrin) and naproxen (Naprosyn)
3. Broad-spectrum antibiotics: For infection—includes amoxicillin (Amoxil) and erythromycin (Erythrocin)

Bibliography

Altman, G. (2004). *Delmar's fundamental and advanced nursing skills* (2nd ed.). Albany, NY: Delmar.

Doenges, M., Moorhouse, M., & Murr, A. (2006). *Nurse's pocket guide: Diagnosis, prioritized interventions, and rationales* (10th ed.). Philadelphia: Davis.

Ellis, J., & Hartley, C. (2005). *Managing and coordinating nursing care.* Philadelphia: Lippincott Williams & Wilkins.

Hogan, M., & Wane, D. (2003). *Fluids, electrolytes, and acid-base balance: Review & rationales.* Upper Saddle River, NJ: Prentice Hall.

Joint Commission Universal Protocol (2003). Retrieved July 6, 2006, from http://www.jcaho.org/accredited+organizations/patient+safety/universal+protocol.htm

Karch, A. (2006). *Lippincott's nursing drug guide.* Philadelphia: Lippincott Williams & Wilkins.

Nursing 2008 drug handbook. Ambler, PA: Springhouse.

Pagana, K., & Pagana, T. (2002). *Mosby's manual of diagnostic and laboratory tests* (2nd ed.). St. Louis: Mosby.

Purnell, L., & Paulanka, B. (Eds.). (2003). *Transcultural healthcare: A culturally competent approach.* Philadelphia: Davis.

Smeltzer, S. C., Bare, B. G., Cheever, K. H., & Hinkle, J. L. (2008). *Brunner & Suddarth's textbook of medical-surgical nursing* (11th ed.). Philadelphia: Lippincott Williams & Wilkins.

Taylor, C., Lillis, C., LeMone, P., & Lynn, P. (2006). *Fundamentals of nursing.* Philadelphia: Lippincott Williams & Wilkins.

Weber, J. R., & Kelley, J. (2007). *Nurses handbook of health assessment.* Philadelphia: Lippincott Williams & Wilkins.

Yarbro, C. H., Frogge, M., & Goodman, M. (2004). *Cancer symptom management* (3rd ed.). Sudbury, MA: Jones and Bartlett.

CHAPTER 24

Practice Test

Oral Infections and Inflammations

1. A client is receiving nystatin (Mycostatin) suspension for stomatitis. Which of the following statements is an indication that the nurse's teaching about taking this drug is effective?

- □ 1. "I will not eat any dairy products for at least 1 hour before, or 2 hours after the medication."
- □ 2. "To decrease nausea, I will take the medicine with crackers."
- □ 3. "I will crush the tablet and mix it with water."
- □ 4. "I will hold the liquid in my mouth for 2 minutes, swish, and then swallow."

Oral Cancer

2. Which of the following individuals is at greatest risk for oral cancer?

- □ 1. Female client who uses scented lip balm daily.
- □ 2. Male client who chews gum regularly.
- □ 3. Teenage client who drinks four cans of carbonated beverages each day.
- □ 4. Male client who smokes three filtered cigarettes daily.

3. AF An elderly client has oral cancer. To conduct a focused assessment, the nurse should do which of the following? Select all that apply.

- □ 1. Inspect the mouth and surrounding tissues for infection and inflammation.
- □ 2. Inquire about loss of sense of taste.
- □ 3. Determine presence of dysphagia.
- □ 4. Monitor the client's height and weight.
- □ 5. Ask if the client is urinating regularly.
- □ 6. Monitor for frequent usage of narcotics.

4. A client has had an excision of an early-stage tumor of the mouth and is experiencing mild pain and a dry mouth. The nurse is instructing the client about mouth care. Which of the following is most effective in promoting oral health for this client following surgery?

- □ 1. Use a firm-bristled toothbrush to remove plaque and crusts.
- □ 2. Rinse the mouth with an alcohol-based mouth wash to dislodge food particles.
- □ 3. Restrict fluids to avoid releasing sutures.
- □ 4. Suck on lemon lozenges to stimulate salivation.

Gastroesophageal Reflux Disease

5. The nurse is developing a care plan for a male client with GERD who is average height and weight, and currently obtains about 2,000 calories in his current diet. Which of the following dietary changes should the nurse suggest?

- □ 1. Increase the fat content of the diet.
- □ 2. Avoid overeating.
- □ 3. Lie down after eating.
- □ 4. Reduce calorie intake to 1,500 calories.

6. A client with GERD has difficulty sleeping. The nurse should suggest which of the following?

- □ 1. Take a combination antacid such as aluminum hydroxide and magnesium hydroxide (Mylanta).
- □ 2. Drink a large glass of warm milk before bedtime.
- □ 3. Increase the amount of complex carbohydrates in the diet.
- □ 4. Elevate the head and upper torso by sleeping on an incline.

7. AF The nurse is developing a care management plan with a client who has been diagnosed with GERD. The nurse should instruct the client to do which of the following? Select all that apply.

- □ 1. Consume a high-protein, low-fat diet.
- □ 2. Avoid beverages that contain caffeine.
- □ 3. Eat three meals a day, with the largest meal being at dinner in the evening.
- □ 4. Avoid all alcoholic beverages.
- □ 5. Lie down after consuming each meal for 30 min.
- □ 6. Use over-the-counter (OTC) antisecretory agents rather than prescriptions.

8. AF A client with GERD is scheduled for a barium swallow test. Prior to the test, the nurse should do which of the following? Select all that apply.

- □ 1. Ensure that the barium swallow is done after a cholangiography and barium enema.
- □ 2. Inform the client that the x-rays provide a view of the entire GI tract.
- □ 3. Determine the client's known allergens, such as latex, iodine, seafood, contrast medium, and dyes.
- □ 4. Explain to the client that there will be the need to swallow contrast medium.

- □ 5. Remind the client to fast and restrict fluids for 8 hr prior to the test.
- □ 6. Inform the client that only the wristwatch needs to be removed prior to the procedure.

9. A client with GERD had antireflux surgery via an abdominal incision. Following surgery, the primary goal of nursing care is to prevent?

- □ 1. Respiratory complications.
- □ 2. Fluid and electrolyte imbalance.
- □ 3. Dumping syndrome.
- □ 4. Pain.

10. A client just returned from having an esophagogastroduodenoscopy (EGD). The nurse should first?

- □ 1. Assess swallowing.
- □ 2. Encourage fluids.
- □ 3. Offer throat lozenges.
- □ 4. Offer an analgesic.

Peptic Ulcer Disease

11. AF When administering tetracycline (Achromycin) to a client with PUD, the nurse should do which of the following? Select all that apply.

- □ 1. Give with full glass of water on an empty stomach.
- □ 2. Give at least 1 hr before a meal.
- □ 3. Keep in a dry place.
- □ 4. Administer with milk or milk products.
- □ 5. Protect from light.

12. The nurse is preparing to insert an NG tube into a client with PUD. When the tube reaches the nasopharynx, the nurse should instruct the client to do which of the following?

- □ 1. Take slow, deep breaths.
- □ 2. Hold the breath.
- □ 3. Swallow several times.
- □ 4. Tilt the head back.

13. A client diagnosed with PUD has an *H. pylori* infection. The client is following a 2-week drug regimen that includes clarithromycin (Biaxin) along with omeprazole (Prilosec) and amoxicillin (Amoxil). The nurse should instruct the client to:

- □ 1. Alternate the use of the drugs.
- □ 2. Take the drugs at different times during the day.
- □ 3. Discontinue all drugs if nausea occurs.
- □ 4. Take the drugs for the entire 2-week period.

14. A client has had an antrectomy for PUD. To minimize the effects of dumping syndrome, the nurse advises the client to:

- □ 1. Drink plenty of fluids with meals.
- □ 2. Eat three meals at regularly scheduled intervals.
- □ 3. Lie down for a half an hour after meals.
- □ 4. Minimize the intake of high-protein foods.

15. The nurse is teaching a client with a gastric ulcer about dietary management for the disease. Teaching is successful when the client states:

- □ 1. "I should eat a low-fiber diet to delay gastric emptying."
- □ 2. "I cannot eat fruits or vegetables because they cause too much gas."
- □ 3. "As long as they don't bother my stomach, I can eat most foods."
- □ 4. "I can eat bland foods to help my stomach heal."

16. A client with an open-crater-peptic ulcer is taking omeprazole (Prilosec) 20 mg PO twice a day and cimetidine (Tagamet) 300 mg PO 4 times a day. The nurse instructs the client to:

- □ 1. Ingest frequent small meals.
- □ 2. Test for occult blood weekly.
- □ 3. Take medications as prescribed.
- □ 4. Expect signs of gastroesophageal pain.

17. A client with PUD is admitted to the hospital for a gastric resection. The client reports a sudden sharp pain in the midepigastric area that radiates to the shoulder. The nurse should first:

- □ 1. Establish an IV line.
- □ 2. Administer pain medication.
- □ 3. Notify the surgeon.
- □ 4. Call for a stat ECG.

Cancer of the Stomach

18. A client with cancer of the stomach had a total gastrectomy 2 days earlier. Which of the following indicate the client is ready to try a liquid diet?

- □ 1. The client tells the nurse he is hungry.
- □ 2. The client has not requested pain medication for 8 hr.
- □ 3. Bowel sounds are present.
- □ 4. The client has had a bowel movement.

19. A client had a subtotal gastrectomy. The nurse is instructing the client about preventing dumping syndrome. The nurse should instruct the client to do which of the following?

- □ 1. Drink 8 to 16 ml of fluid with meals.
- □ 2. Avoid food with high sugar content.
- □ 3. Remain standing for 30 min after meals.
- □ 4. Concentrate daily intake of food into three meals.

20. Within 6 hr following a subtotal gastrectomy, the drainage from the client's NG tube is bright red. The nurse's first responsibility is to:

- □ 1. Clamp the NG tube.
- □ 2. Remove the existing NG tube.
- □ 3. Irrigate the NG tube with iced saline.
- □ 4. Chart the finding.

Answers and Rationales

1. 4 Nystatin (Mycostatin) suspension is prescribed to treat an oral fungal infection. Effective teaching is indicated by the client's statement about holding the medication in the mouth for 2 min, swishing, and then swallowing the medication. Avoiding dairy products would be appropriate when tetracycline (Achromycin) is prescribed. Nystatin (Mycostatin) suspension is not taken with food. The medication is in a suspension to be swished in the mouth; it is not in tablet form. (D)

2. 4 Oral (oropharyngeal) cancer may occur on the lips or anywhere within the mouth. Factors that influence the development of oral cancer include tobacco use, excessive alcohol intake, and chronic irritation, such as from a jagged tooth or poor dental care. There is no indication that use of scented lip balm, sugar-free chewing gum, or drinking carbonated beverages puts one at a greater risk to develop oral cancer. (H)

3. 1, 3, 4 The nurse is conducting a focused assessment of the client's mouth and ability to obtain nutrition. Therefore, the nurse focuses on inspecting the mouth, determining if the client has difficulty swallowing, and assuring nutrition by weighing the client and noting weight loss or gain. Urinary output, while important, is not focused toward this client's health problem. The client may have pain, and for a more general assessment, the nurse can inquire about use of pain medications. (A)

4. 4 Following oral surgery for cancer of the mouth, the nurse instructs the client to promote hygiene; because the client has decreased salivation, using lozenges will stimulate saliva production. The nurse instructs the client to use a soft toothbrush, if tolerated; some clients will require oral lavage. Alcohol-based mouth washes irritate the gums and mucosa. The client should have an adequate or increased fluid intake to keep the oral cavity moist and prevent dryness. (H)

5. 2 The client with GERD should avoid overeating by consuming several small meals a day. The nurse instructs the client to follow a bland diet and to avoid coffee, cola drinks, and acid juices such as citrus or tomato juice. Increasing the fat content of the diet will not alter the reflux. The client should not lie down for 3 to 4 hr after eating. The client should maintain an ideal weight; a 2,000 calorie diet for an adult male of average height is not excessive. (H)

6. 4 Sleeping on pillows or elevating the head of the bed on blocks raises the upper torso and minimizes reflux of gastric contents. The effect of a combination antacid is not long-lasting enough to promote sleeping through the night. Increasing the stomach's contents before lying down would aggravate the symptoms associated with GERD. Milk products should be avoided, especially at bedtime, because milk increases gastric acid secretion. Complex carbohydrates have no effect on the reflux of gastric contents. (C)

7. 1, 2, 4 No specific diet is necessary, but foods that cause reflux are avoided, including fatty foods (which decrease the rate of gastric emptying) and foods that decrease lower esophageal sphincter (LES) pressure such as chocolate, peppermint, coffee, and tea. The client should also avoid alcohol. The client should not lie down for 3 to 4 hr after eating. Antisecretory agents decrease the secretion of hydrochloric acid (HCI) by the stomach; some are available in both OTC and prescription formulations, but the OTC preparations have lower drug dosages compared with prescription drugs. Cimetidine (Tagamet), ranitidine (Zantac), famotidine (Pepcid), and nizatidine (Axid) are available in both formulations. (M)

8. 1, 3, 4, 5 The barium swallow is a radiologic examination of the esophagus that evaluates motion and anatomic structures of the esophageal lumen by recording images of the lumen while the client swallows a barium solution. In clients with esophageal reflux, the radiologist may identify reflux of the barium from the stomach back into the esophagus. Prior to a barium swallow, the nurse obtains the client's history of allergies or sensitivities to latex, iodine, seafood, contrast media, and dyes, as iodine may be an element of the contrast medium. The client does have to fast and restrict fluids for 8 hr prior to the procedure. All jewelry or other metallic objects are removed. (M)

9. 1 When an abdominal incision is used, respiratory complications can occur because of the high abdominal incision; therefore, the primary goal of the nurse is to prevent respiratory complications by assessing respiratory rate, rhythm, and signs of pneumothorax (i.e., dyspnea, chest pain, and cyanosis). Deep breathing is essential to fully expand the lungs. The client receives IV fluids and electrolytes until the return of peristalsis; the nurse maintains an accurate recording of intake and output and observes for fluid and electrolyte imbalances. Dumping syndrome occurs as a result of surgical removal of a large portion of the stomach and the pyloric sphincter; antireflux surgery reduces reflux of gastric contents by enhancing the integrity of the LES. The client will have incisional pain and although the pain cannot be prevented, the nurse can offer pain medication as needed to control the pain. (S)

10. 1 For an EGD, a fiberoptic scope is inserted into the esophagus and advanced to the duodenum for visualization. Because the client's throat is anesthetized to facilitate passage of the fiberoptic scope, the first priority of the nurse is to assess swallowing and to maintain NPO status until the gag reflex and safe swallowing return. Once the gag reflex returns, the nurse can offer fluids, lozenges, and analgesia. (R)

11. 1, 2, 3, 5 Oral tetracycline (Achromycin) is administered with a full glass of water on an empty stomach at least 1 hr before or 2 hr after meals (food, milk, and milk products can reduce absorption by 50% or more). The nurse does not administer the drug immediately before bed, or with foods high in calcium such as milk or milk products. Tetracycline (Achromycin) decomposes with age, exposure to light, and when stored incorrectly. Correct storage involves a tightly sealed container stored in a dry place protected from light, with a temperature of 59° to 86°F. (D)

12. 3 The nurse instructs the client to swallow several times to aid in guiding the tube from the oral pharynx to the esophagus. Tilting the head forward helps, but tilting the head back makes it more likely the tube will descend the trachea. Taking slow, deep breaths is avoided because this opens the glottis to the trachea; the client is instructed to mouth-breathe or pant. (R)

13. 4 The use of the triple therapy approach to the *H. pylori* infection has proved effective; therefore, the nurse advises the client to take the drugs as ordered for the duration of the prescription. The nurse instructs the client to avoid alternating the use of the drugs and to take all medication at the same time, 3 times a day unless otherwise noted by the physician. Drugs have very few side effects; however, the nurse instructs the client to continue taking medications and contact the HCP if adverse effects occur. (D)

14. 3 Dumping syndrome, which can follow gastric surgery or vagotomy, includes signs and symptoms such as faintness, diaphoresis, palpitations, and diarrhea that occur soon after or up to 90 min after eating. Symptoms are due to rapid jejunal distention and hypertonic intestinal contents drawing extracellular fluid in. Management includes limiting fluids with meals, eating small but frequent meals, lying down after meals, and minimizing high-fat foods. (H)

15. 3 The antiulcer diet is not severely restricted; it is ideal to have small, frequent feedings, but the client can eat foods as long as they do not cause upset. The nurse instructs the client to avoid foods known to increase gastric acidity such as coffee, alcohol, seasonings, and milk. A low-fiber diet is used with acute diverticulitis and ulcerative colitis. Fruits and vegetables are restricted only if they bother the stomach. A bland diet is used for severe inflammation. (H)

16. 3 Because clients become symptom-free in a few days to a week, they often discontinue medications before the ulcer heals. The nurse instructs the client to take the medication as prescribed to reduce the risk of hemorrhage. Frequent small meals reduce the exposure of an impaired gastric wall to acid, but do not contribute to the healing at the same level as the drugs. Testing for occult blood provides evidence of bleeding, which provides evidence of the effectiveness of the drugs. Pain is not an expected side effect of omeprazole (Prilosec) and cimetidine (Tagamet). (D)

17. 3 The sharp, sudden midepigastric pain indicates the client may have a perforated ulcer. The nurse notifies the surgeon and may then obtain orders for pain medication and IV fluids. It is not necessary to first obtain an ECG because the pain from ulcer perforation is different from that of chest pain that may indicate coronary artery syndrome (crushing pain radiating to the jaw). (A)

18. 3 The client can begin eating with a liquid diet when bowel sounds return, usually in 2 to 3 days. The client may be hungry but cannot have oral fluids or foods until intestinal motility has been established. The client may continue to have postoperative pain for several days; because receiving a liquid diet does not depend on the client being pain-free, the nurse can continue to offer pain medication. The client does not have to experience a bowel movement to receive fluids and food. (S)

19. 2 When high-osmotic fluid passes quickly into the small intestine, it causes hypovolemia, which leads to dumping syndrome; a sympathetic response with tachycardia, diaphoresis, and vertigo result. The symptoms are also due to a rise and fall in blood glucose, and thus the client should avoid eating concentrated sugars. The nurse instructs the client to eat small, frequent meals, rather than three large meals, and to limit fluids while eating, but take them between meals. The client does not need to stand after meals, and can rest following eating. (A)

20. 4 NG drainage is expected to be bright red during the first 12 hr after surgery and then darken within 24 hr. The nurse notes the color of the drainage on the chart and then monitors the change of color of the drainage throughout the immediate postoperative period. To prevent stress on the suture line, NG suction is applied and patency of the tube maintained. Removal of the NG tube may traumatize the surgical site. The NG tube is irrigated only if the physician orders irrigation because there is danger of injury to the suture line; saline at room temperature is usually ordered. (A)

chapter

25

The Client With Lower Gastrointestinal Tract Health Problems

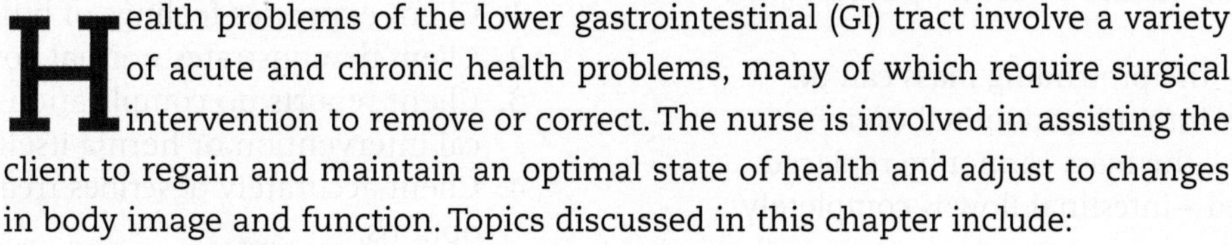

Health problems of the lower gastrointestinal (GI) tract involve a variety of acute and chronic health problems, many of which require surgical intervention to remove or correct. The nurse is involved in assisting the client to regain and maintain an optimal state of health and adjust to changes in body image and function. Topics discussed in this chapter include:

- Inguinal Hernia
- Inflammatory Bowel Disease
- Diverticular Disease
- Intestinal Obstruction
- Appendicitis
- Hemorrhoids
- Cancer of the Colon

Inguinal Hernia

I. Definition: A hernia, often called a *rupture*, is a protrusion of an organ, tissue, or structure through the wall of the cavity in which it is normally contained.
   A. Types of hernias are classified by site.
      1. Inguinal hernia—the most common type of hernia; involves protrusion of viscera into the inguinal canal at a point where the spermatic cord emerges in the male, and the round ligament in the female. A hernia may be indirect or direct.
         a. An indirect inguinal hernia extends down the inguinal canal and even into the scrotum or labia. The indirect hernia is more common, and 3 times more common for males. It may develop at any age and is especially prevalent in infants.
         b. A direct inguinal hernia protrudes through the posterior inguinal wall. The direct hernia occurs more commonly in middle-aged and elderly people.
      2. Femoral—involves protrusion into the femoral canal.
      3. Ventral—involves protrusion through a weakness in the abdominal wall.
      4. Umbilical—involves a protrusion through the umbilicus.
      5. Incisional—involves a protrusion through an incision, usually during the healing process.
   B. Classifications of hernias by severity include the following:
      1. Reducible—the protruding mass can be placed back into the abdominal cavity.
      2. Irreducible—the mass cannot be replaced.
      3. Incarcerated—intestinal flow is completely obstructed.
      4. Strangulated—part of the herniated intestine becomes twisted or edematous, interfering with normal blood flow and peristalsis, and possibly leading to obstruction and necrosis.
   C. Complications of inguinal hernia include bowel obstruction and recurrence of hernia.

II. Nursing process
   A. Assessment
      1. Obtain a detailed health history and comprehensive physical examination.
      2. Assess for signs and symptoms.
         a. Hernia bulges when client stands or strains (Valsalva maneuver) and disappears when client is supine.
         b. Client verbalizes discomfort or pulling sensation.
         c. For strangulation, client experiences severe pain, vomiting, swelling of hernial sac, rebound tenderness, and fever.
      3. Assess for risk factors.
         a. Obesity
         b. Postsurgical recovery from abdominal surgery
         c. Pregnancy
         d. Heavy lifting
      4. Obtain diagnostic tests.
         a. Abdominal x-ray—shows abnormally high level of gas in bowel, or a bowel obstruction.
         b. CBC and serum electrolytes—shows hemoconcentration elevated hematocrit, increased WBCs, and electrolyte imbalance if strangulation occurs.
   B. Analysis
      1. Acute Pain related to ischemic bowel
      2. Deficient Knowledge related to treatment options
      3. Risk for Constipation related to intestinal obstruction
      4. Risk for Infection related to break in skin integrity (incisions)
   C. Planning
      1. Promote relief of symptoms.
      2. Promote normal bowel function.
      3. Prevent complications.
      4. Increase client knowledge of treatment options.
      5. Prevent infection.
   D. Implementation (see management of care)
   E. Evaluation
      1. Client expresses feelings of little or no pain.
      2. Client demonstrates normal bowel function.
      3. Client reports no complications from surgical intervention or hernia itself.
      4. Client accurately describes treatment options.
      5. Client shows no signs of infection.

CN

III. Client needs
   A. Physiologic adaptation: Reducible hernias can be managed conservatively with risk management (avoid lifting, straining) and mechanical measures such as a truss or belt. Surgical approaches (herniorrhaphy to remove hernial sac; hernioplasty to suture area with mesh) used if hernia presents risk for strangulation or cannot be reduced.
      1. Truss positioned snugly over area—to prevent viscera from entering hernial sac when hernia is reducible; client poor surgical candidate.
      2. Protect site from increased intra-abdominal pressure.

3. Check scrotum/labia for edema after inguinal hernia repair.
4. Avoid heavy lifting for 4 to 6 weeks after surgery.

B. Management of care: Care of the client with an inguinal hernia requires critical thinking skills and knowledge of assessment, and teaching and evaluation methods unique to the RN role. These skills cannot be delegated to an LPN or UAP.
   1. Delegate responsibly those activities that can be delegated such as comfort measures and reapplying truss. All monitoring information is reported to the RN.
   2. Apply truss after hernia has been reduced.
   3. Following surgery (herniorrhaphy/hernioplasty):
      a. Insert NG tube to reduce intra-abdominal pressure above obstruction and relieve pressure on herniated sac.
      b. Administer analgesics as ordered.
      c. Encourage coughing and deep breathing while splinting incision with pillow.
      d. Monitor vital signs.
      e. Observe for signs of strangulation and incarceration.
      f. Provide wound care.
      g. Check incision for redness, edema; report signs of infection (fever, chills, malaise, diaphoresis).

C. Safety and infection control
   1. Use sterile technique during dressing changes.
   2. Administer antibiotics as ordered.
   3. Encourage fluids and monitor diet to promote healing.

D. Health promotion and maintenance: Provide client and family teaching.
   1. Wear truss under clothing; apply truss before getting out of bed in morning when hernia is reduced.
   2. Avoid standing for prolonged periods of time.
   3. Prevent constipation to avoid straining.

E. Psychologic integrity
   1. Provide information regarding preoperative and postoperative care.
   2. Provide emotional support throughout healing process.

F. Basic care and comfort
   1. Encourage ambulation as soon as permitted.
   2. Check scrotum or labia for edema after repair, and apply ice and other comfort measures.
   3. Administer analgesics as ordered.
   4. Instruct client to splint incision site with hand or pillow when coughing to lessen pain and protect site from increased intra-abdominal pressure.
   5. Position client in semi-Fowler position to reduce pressure on hernia.

G. Reduction of risk potential: Provide client and family teaching.
   1. Monitor for signs of infection, including fever, chills, malaise, and diaphoresis.
   2. Monitor for and report difficulty in voiding.
   3. Avoid extremes of exertion for 8 to 12 weeks postsurgical intervention; avoid heaving lifting for 4 to 6 weeks.

H. Pharmacologic and parenteral therapies: Client will state the purpose, usage, and associated side effects of medications used to treat an inguinal hernia.
   1. IV fluids containing electrolytes, if needed.
      a. Normal saline (NS; 0.9% NaCl)—isotonic: Includes sodium, chloride
      b. Lactated Ringer (LR)—isotonic: Includes sodium, potassium, calcium, chloride, lactate
      c. 5% dextrose with Lactated Ringer (D5/LR)—hypertonic: Includes same electrolytes as Lactated Ringer and dextrose
      d. 5% dextrose and normal saline (D5/0.9%NaCl)—hypertonic: Includes sodium, chloride, and dextrose
      e. 5% dextrose and one-half normal saline (D5/0.45% NaCl)—hypertonic: Includes sodium, chloride, and dextrose
      f. 5% dextrose and one-fourth normal saline (D5/0.2% NaCl)—hypertonic Includes sodium, chloride, and dextrose
   2. Broad-spectrum antibiotics as directed—kills both gram-positive and gram-negative micro-organisms (ciprofloxacin [Cipro]; trimethoprim sulfamethoxazole [Bactrim]).
   3. Analgesics as ordered—propoxyphene (Darvon); hydromorphone (Dilaudid).

Inflammatory Bowel Disease

I. Definition: Inflammatory bowel disease refers to two chronic inflammatory GI disorders, including regional enteritis (Crohn disease) and ulcerative colitis. Regional enteritis and ulcerative colitis are separate entities with similar causes; both are characterized by exacerbations and remissions. Exacerbations may be triggered by stress, other short-term illnesses, pesticides, food additives, tobacco, radiation exposure, and immunologic influence. A hereditary predisposition exists.

A. Regional enteritis is a subacute, chronic inflammation extending through all layers of the bowel wall, usually affecting the ileum and ascending colon. Fistulas, fissures, and abscesses extend into the peritoneum, and inflammation occurs next to segments of normal intestinal tissue.

B. Ulcerative colitis is an inflammatory disease of submucosal layer of colon and rectum usually occurring in the descending colon and rectum. The condition is characterized by recurring ulcerations and shredding of intestinal epithelium. Fat deposits and muscular hypertrophy result in a narrow, short, and thickened bowel. Ulcerative colitis is more common than regional enteritis.

II. Nursing process
  A. Assessment
    1. Complete a detailed health history and comprehensive physical examination.
    2. Assess for signs and symptoms.
      a. Regional enteritis
        (1) Abdominal tenderness and pain, typically colicky; increased after meals
        (2) Diarrhea, flatulence, steatorrhea (fatty stools)
        (3) Fever, malaise, anorexia
        (4) Signs of nutritional deficits
        (5) Perianal fistulas, abscesses
      b. Ulcerative colitis
        (1) Severe diarrhea containing pus, blood, and mucosa
        (2) Anorexia, weight loss
        (3) Abdominal cramping, tenderness, fever
    3. Obtain diagnostic tests.
      a. Regional enteritis
        (1) Barium study of upper GI tract (most conclusive diagnostic test)—reveals classic "string sign" on x-ray study of terminal ileum, indicating constriction of segment of intestine.
        (2) Barium enema—shows ulceration and "cobblestone" appearance because of fissures surrounded by submucosal edema.
        (3) Colonoscopy—visualizes distinct ulcerations separated by relatively normal mucosa in ileum and ascending colon.
        (4) Computed tomography scan—shows bowel wall thickening and fistula tracts.
      b. Ulcerative colitis
        (1) Barium enema—shows mucosal irregularities, shortening of bowel, and dilation of bowel loops.
        (2) Colonoscopy—shows friable mucosa with pseudopolyps, and ulcers in descending colon and sigmoid colon.
        (3) Stool analysis—determines presence of blood in stool; entamoeba histolytica, which causes dysentery, must be ruled out.
  B. Analysis
    1. Imbalanced Nutrition: Less Than Body Requirements related to hypermotility and malabsorption
    2. Diarrhea related to hypermotility
    3. Deficient Fluid Volume related to diarrhea
    4. Risk for Impaired Skin Integrity related to chemical constituents of excretions
  C. Planning
    1. Assist in maintaining or regaining weight.
    2. Promote adherence to prescribed dietary regimen.
    3. Promote adequate bowel movements.
    4. Provide instruction for ostomy care.
    5. Aid in development of strategies to reduce emotional stress.
    6. Reduce or eliminate pain.
    7. Maintain fluid and electrolyte balance.
  D. Implementation
    1. Regional enteritis
      a. Monitor frequency and consistency of stools; monitor for rectal bleeding.
      b. Monitor dietary therapy.
      c. Monitor electrolytes, especially potassium.
      d. Monitor for signs of obstruction, including distention, fever, hypotension.
      e. Observe and record changes in client pain status.
    2. Ulcerative colitis
      a. Monitor intake and output.
      b. Monitor glucose if client is receiving corticosteroids or hyperalimentation, or if client has glucose intolerance or diabetes mellitus.
      c. Measure daily weights.
      d. Observe for complications (perforation, toxic megacolon) including sudden abdominal distention, pain, and fever.
      e. Observe for signs of dehydration including decreased skin turgor; dry skin; oliguria; weakness; and increased hematocrit, blood urea nitrogen, and an elevated urine specific gravity.
  E. Evaluation
    1. Regional enteritis
      a. Client reports a reduction in pain.
      b. Client reports a decreased number of bowel movements.

c. Client maintains nutritional status.
d. Client maintains fluid and electrolyte balance.
e. Client implements strategies to reduce emotional stress.

2. Ulcerative colitis
a. Client maintains or regains weight.
b. Client adheres to dietary regimen.
c. Client establishes an acceptable pattern of soft, formed bowel movements.
d. Client demonstrates ability to perform ostomy care.
e. Client implements strategies to reduce emotional stress.

CN

III. Client needs

A. Physiologic adaptation: Treatment for inflammatory bowel disease involves dietary management, medications (see pharmacologic and parenteral therapies), and surgical interventions when medical management is unsuccessful.

1. Dietary management
a. Unrestricted fluid intake, if tolerated
b. High-protein, high-calorie diet
c. Avoidance of food allergens, especially milk
2. Replacement of fluids and electrolytes lost because of diarrhea.
3. Surgical intervention involves the creation of an ostomy; the ostomy can be created within the ileum or at various sites within the large bowel. An ileostomy is the surgical creation of an opening into the ileum or small intestine that allows for drainage of fecal matter from the ileum to outside the body. A colostomy is the surgical creation of an opening into the colon that allows for drainage of fecal matter from colon to outside of body.
a. Segmental/partial colectomy with anastomosis
b. Total colectomy with ileostomy
c. Total colectomy with continent ileostomy (Koch pouch)
d. Total colectomy with ileoanal anastomosis (creation of an ileal pouch that maintains anal sphincter function)
4. Replace iron, calcium, and zinc losses with supplements.
5. For ileal involvement, injections of vitamin B_{12}, IM, for each month to reduce anemia.
6. Maintain NPO status to rest bowel, and provide total parenteral nutrition (TPN) when inflammatory episodes are severe, as prescribed. Complications may develop quickly and may include infection (insertion site or bacteremia), catheter occlusion, leakage or catheter puncture, and pneumothorax.

B. Management of care: Care of the client with an inflammatory bowel disease requires critical thinking skills and knowledge of assessment, and teaching and evaluation methods unique to the RN role. These skills cannot be delegated to an LPN or UAP.

1. Delegate responsibly those activities that can be delegated, such as care and comfort measures, providing oral fluids and nutrition. All monitoring and intake/output information is reported to the RN.
2. Monitor vital signs and laboratory results.
a. Monitor daily weight, vital signs, and intake and output.
b. Observe feces for color and consistency.
c. Measure fingerstick blood glucose.
d. Assist client in dietary selection.
e. Assist with small, frequent feedings of high-protein, high-calorie foods.
f. Encourage client to avoid irritating foods.
g. Provide nutrition supplements, if ordered.
3. Request enterostomal therapy nurse assist in preoperative stoma assessment and marking.
4. Request dietitian consult to provide instruction regarding:
a. Initial low-residue diet to promote healing
b. Avoidance of kernels or seeds that can cause obstruction
c. Increased fluid intake to compensate for losses
5. Monitor for hyperglycemia:
a. Nondiabetic: Every 6 hr for 24 to 48 hr, then discontinue
b. Glucose-intolerant: Every 4 hr, with sliding scale regular insulin as prescribed
c. Diabetic: Every 4 hr, with sliding scale regular insulin as prescribed; consult with endocrinologist
6. Promote diet low in residue, fiber, fat, and high in calories, protein, and carbohydrates, with vitamin supplements (especially vitamin K).
7. During exacerbation, administer hyperalimentation to maintain nutrition while allowing bowel to rest.
8. During remission, promote regular balanced diet to maintain reasonable body weight.
9. Monitor frequency/consistency of stools to evaluate volume losses/effectiveness of therapy.

10. Monitor acid-base balance because diarrhea can lead to metabolic acidosis.
11. Monitor for distention, increased temperature, hypotension, and rectal bleeding.
12. Observe and record changes in pain frequency, location, characteristics, precipitating events, and duration.
13. Instruct client on prescribed medications to encourage compliance and understanding of management.
14. Instruct postoperative client about wound care or ostomy care, if applicable.

C. Safety and infection control
1. Observe for fever and dehydration.
2. Monitor for skin excoriation around stoma.
3. Assess for signs of peritonitis.
4. If receiving TPN via central venous catheter or peripheral venous catheter, monitor for infection or bacteria at insertion site.
   a. Change all dressings using sterile technique.
   b. When drainage appears at insertion site, change dressing promptly and culture drainage.
   c. If prescribed, obtain blood cultures.
   d. Change intravenous caps on each lumen per hospital policy.
5. Before physician inserts central venous catheter, obtain chest x-ray and listen for breath sounds.

D. Health promotion and maintenance: Encourage participation in Crohn's and Colitis Foundation of America.

E. Psychologic integrity
1. Encourage verbalization of feelings. Offer understanding, concern, and encouragement; client may be embarrassed about frequent, malodorous stools, and fearful of eating.
2. Refer to local ostomy organizations.
3. Use stress management strategies as stress can precipitate peristalsis.
4. Encourage support person/s to be involved in management of disease.

F. Basic care and comfort: Clean rectal area and apply ointments as necessary to decrease discomfort from skin breakdown.

G. Reduction of risk potential: Explain to client and family signs and symptoms of postoperative complications to report, including elevated temperature, nausea and vomiting, abdominal distention, changes in bowel function or stool consistency, and hemorrhage.

H. Pharmacologic and parenteral therapies: Client will state the purpose, usage, and associated side effects of medications used to treat inflammatory bowel disease.
1. Pharmacologic interventions include the following:
   a. Salicylate compounds such as oral mesalamine (Asacol), an anti-inflammatory agent, may be prescribed during the acute phase of illness. 5-aminosalicylic acid releases mesalamine (Asacol) to have topical, rather than systemic, anti-inflammatory effect within intestines.
   b. Sulfasalazine (Azulfidine) inhibits inflammatory process; effective only for colonic disease.
   c. Corticosteroids (controversial) reduces inflammation by various routes, depending on severity of disease.
   d. Antibiotics such as metronidazole (Flagyl) treat infection and may induce remission.
   e. Immunomodulators such as 6-mercaptopurine (Purinethol), cyclosporine (Neoral), and tacrolimus (Prograf) are used in severe cases to improve healing of fistulas.
   f. Infliximab (Remicade) is a new monoclonal antibody given by injection to block action of tumor necrosis factor. It is indicated in moderate-to-severe disease not responsive to other treatments or those with draining fistulae.
   g. Antispasmodics (dicyclomine [Antispas]) and bulking agents (psyllium [Metamucil]) help reduce abdominal pain.
   h. Antidiarrheal agents such as loperamide (Imodium) control diarrhea related malabsorption of bile salts.
   i. Fish oil may be used to maintain remission; adverse effects include diarrhea, flatulence, halitosis, and heartburn.
   j. Anticholinergics to reduce intestinal muscle spasms.
   k. Opioid analgesics to manage pain.
2. Intravenous fluids containing electrolytes include Lactated Ringer (LR)—isotonic; and normal saline (NS; 0.9% NaCl)—isotonic.
3. Customized combinations of dextrose (carbohydrate), amino acids (protein), intralipids (fat), electrolytes, vitamins, and trace metals.
   a. Dextrose provides bulk of calories, energy needs with concentrations ranging from 5% to 70%. (All solutions that use greater than 12.5% dextrose solution must be administered via central venous catheter). The more carbohydrate delivered, the greater potential

for complications, which may include fatty liver syndrome, increased carbon dioxide production, and hyperglycemia.
b. Protein—synthetic essential/nonessential amino acid formulations are available in concentrations of 3% to 10%. The amount delivered depends on client's renal/hepatic function.
c. Fat—intralipid (10%, 20%, 30%) is isotonic solution providing essential fatty acids and source of concentrated calories. Need to determine if client has egg allergy because long-chain triglycerides in lipids may originate from phospholipids in egg yolks.

Diverticular Disease

I. Definition: Diverticular disease most often occurs in the sigmoid colon, but diverticula (bulging pouches) may develop anywhere from the proximal end of the pharynx to the anus. Other typical sites include the duodenum, near the pancreatic border or the ampulla of Vater, and the jejunum. Diverticular disease of the ileum (Meckel diverticulum) is the most common congenital anomaly of the GI tract. Complications include hemorrhage, peritonitis, perforation, bowel obstruction, fistula formation, and septicemia. The cause of diverticular disease is unclear, but a low-residue diet is a contributing factor. Diverticular disease has three clinical forms including prediverticular disease, diverticulosis, and diverticulitis.
   A. Prediverticular disease: Involves weakening and degeneration of the colonic musculature and narrowing of the bowel lumen.
   B. Diverticulosis: Involves multiple diverticula or saccular dilatations at weak points of the colonic wall where nutrient blood vessels penetrate; occurs more often in persons older than 60 years of age.
   C. Diverticulitis: Involves inflammation of one or more of the pouches; inflammation may perforate the thin diverticular wall as a result of a fecalith plug and accumulating bacteria. If the diverticulum perforates, local abscess or peritonitis may occur. Minimally inflamed diverticula may erode adjacent arterial branches, causing acute massive rectal bleeding.

II. Nursing process
   A. Assessment
      1. Complete a detailed health history and comprehensive physical assessment.
      2. Assess for signs and symptoms. (Client may be asymptomatic.)
         a. Complaints of moderate dull or steady pain in left lower abdominal quadrant aggravated by straining, lifting, or coughing; tenderness in the area; palpable mass.
         b. Mild nausea, gas, diarrhea, or intermittent bouts of constipation, sometimes accompanied by rectal bleeding.
         c. For diverticulitis, low-grade fever; frequent constipation; and guarding and rebound tenderness (signs of peritoneal irritation, if acute).
      3. Obtain diagnostic tests.
         a. CBC reveals leukocytosis.
         b. Erythrocyte sedimentation rate is elevated (diverticulitis).
         c. Stool test of occult blood is positive (in 25% of clients with diverticulitis).
         d. Barium studies reveal barium-filled diverticula and outlines; does not fill diverticula blocked by impacted stool (barium studies not performed for acute diverticulitis because of risk of rupture).
         e. Radiography may show colonic spasm if irritable bowel syndrome accompanies diverticular disease.
         f. Abdominal x-rays rule out perforation.
         g. Colonoscopy/flexible sigmoidoscopy reveals diverticula and inflamed mucosa (not usually performed in acute phase).
         h. Biopsy rules out cancer.
         i. Computed tomography scan of abdomen
   B. Analysis
      1. Acute Pain related to gas and stool accumulation
      2. Constipation related to low-residue diet
      3. Diarrhea related to disease process
      4. Risk for Deficient Fluid Volume related to diarrhea
      5. Risk for Infection related to accumulation of bacteria in diverticulum
   C. Planning
      1. Promote comfort.
      2. Maintain normal fluid volume.
      3. Promote normal bowel movements.
      4. Promote understanding of disease process and treatment regimen.
   D. Implementation (see management of care)
   E. Evaluation
      1. Client expresses feelings of increased comfort.
      2. Client maintains normal fluid volume.
      3. Client reports normal bowel movements.
      4. Client verbalizes understanding of disease process, treatment regimen.

5. Client is free from signs and symptoms of infection.

III. Client needs

A. Physiologic adaptation: Diverticular disease is treated on an outpatient basis with diet and medication and management of symptoms (e.g., rest, analgesics, and antispasmodics when symptoms occur).
   1. For acute cases of diverticulitis—rest bowel with IV therapy, instituting NG tube and maintaining NPO status.
   2. Complications indicate need for surgical intervention; involves one-stage resection or multiple-stage procedures (obstruction or perforation). For abscesses, possible temporary colostomy.

B. Management of care: Care of the client with diverticular disease requires critical thinking skills and knowledge of assessment, and teaching and evaluation methods unique to the RN role. These skills cannot be delegated to an LPN or UAP.
   1. Delegate responsibly those activities that can be delegated. All monitoring information must be reported to the RN.
      a. Provide routine hygienic care.
      b. Monitor vital signs, daily weight, and intake and output.
      c. Promote activity, if appropriate.
      d. Assist with nutritional intake.
   2. Monitor for complications.
      a. Signs of peritonitis include increased pain, nausea and vomiting, guarding, distention, and rebound tenderness.
      b. Signs of shock caused by hemorrhage include tachycardia, thready pulse, and hypotension.
   3. Monitor dietary intake, fiber content, bowel sounds, and stool consistency to determine bowel status.
   4. If surgery is scheduled, provide routine preoperative care.
   5. Provide colostomy care, if appropriate.
   6. Assess stools for color, consistency, and frequency.

C. Safety and infection control
   1. Administer antibiotics, if ordered.
   2. Provide meticulous wound care.
   3. Encourage coughing and deep breathing.
   4. Monitor for signs and symptoms of infection.

D. Health promotion and maintenance: Provide client and family teaching.
   1. Use bran products to add bulk to stool; can be taken with milk or sprinkled over cereal.
   2. Add fiber gradually, as tolerated, and avoid foods that aggravate symptoms.
   3. Continue periodic medical supervision and repeat CBC to follow up for anemia; report problems and untoward symptoms.

E. Psychologic integrity: If surgical intervention is needed:
   1. Provide emotional support while caring for temporary colostomy.
   2. Involve support persons in client's care, as desired.
   3. Enlist support from enterostomal nurse therapist, social worker, clergy, another ostomate, ostomy support group.

F. Basic care and comfort:
   1. Provide analgesics and complementary therapies to relieve pain.
   2. If client has a colostomy, provide skin care and hygiene.

G. Reduction of risk potential: Inform client when to contact physician.
   1. Increasing abdominal pain and rigidity
   2. Abdominal tenderness
   3. Abdominal distention
   4. Nausea and vomiting
   5. Fever, decreased BP

H. Pharmacologic and parenteral therapies: Client will state the purpose, usage, and associated side effects used to treat diverticular disease.
   1. Broad-spectrum antibiotics—to control infection with diverticulitis: Amoxicillin (Amoxil); erythromycin (Erythrocin); and tetracycline (Achromycin).
   2. Analgesics—to control pain in diverticulitis: Propoxyphene (Darvon); hydrocodone (Vicodin); and codeine (Paveral).
   3. Anticholinergics—to control spasms in diverticulitis: Propantheline (Pro-Banthine); glycopyrrolate (Robinul); and atropine (Atropair).
   4. Vasopressin (Pitressin) and blood replacement—for massive bleeding.
   5. IV fluids—to prevent dehydration (when administering hypertonic solutions, administer cautiously and monitor for signs of extracellular fluid volume overload such as hypertension, headache, dyspnea).
      a. 5% dextrose in water (D5/W)—isotonic/hypotonic
      b. Normal saline (NS; 0.9% NaCl)—isotonic
      c. Lactated Ringer (LR)—isotonic
      d. Lactated Ringer with 5% dextrose (D5/LR)—hypertonic
      e. 5% dextrose and normal saline (D5/0.9% NaCl)—hypertonic
      f. 5% dextrose and 0.45% normal saline (D5/0.45% NaCl)—hypertonic

g. 5% dextrose and 0.225% normal saline (NS; D5/0.2% NaCl)—hypertonic

Intestinal Obstruction

I. Definition: Intestinal obstruction is an interruption in the normal flow of intestinal contents along the intestinal tract. Severity depends on the degree of obstruction, the area affected (small or large intestine), and the degree to which circulation in the bowel wall is disrupted. The block may be complete or incomplete, may be mechanical or functional (paralytic), and may or may not compromise the vascular supply. Strangulation, vascular obstruction caused by prolonged mechanical obstruction is a risk for gangrene. Obstruction most frequently occurs in the very young and the very old.
  A. Mechanical obstruction is a physical blockage to the passage of intestinal contents and may result from postsurgical adhesions, hernia (most common nonsurgical cause), volvulus, hematoma, tumor, intussusception (telescoping of intestinal wall into itself), stricture, stenosis, foreign body, fecal or barium impaction, or polyp.
  B. Functional obstruction (paralytic ileus), in contrast, involves no physical obstruction. Peristalsis is ineffective, blood supply is not interrupted, and the condition usually disappears spontaneously after 2 to 3 days. Causes of functional obstruction include spinal cord injuries, vertebral fractures, peritonitis, pneumonia, GI or abdominal surgery, and wound dehiscence (opening).

II. Nursing process
  A. Assessment
    1. Complete a detailed health history and comprehensive physical assessment.
    2. Assess for signs and symptoms, including recent change in bowel habits, and hiccoughs.
      a. Signs and symptoms specific to mechanical obstruction:
        (1) Colicky pain
        (2) Nausea and vomiting
        (3) Constipation
        (4) Distended abdomen
        (5) Borborygmi (gurgling, splashing sounds); occasionally loud enough to be heard without a stethoscope
        (6) Abdominal tenderness
        (7) Rebound tenderness
      b. Signs and symptoms specific to functional obstruction:
        (1) Diffuse abdominal discomfort
        (2) Frequent vomiting
        (3) Severe abdominal pain (if obstruction results from vascular insufficiency or infarction)
        (4) Abdominal distention
        (5) Decreased bowel sounds (early), then absent bowel sounds
    3. Obtain diagnostic tests.
      a. Serum sodium, chloride, and potassium levels decreased
      b. WBC count elevated
      c. Serum amylase level increased if pancreas is irritated by bowel loop
      d. Blood urea nitrogen increased with dehydration
      e. Abdominal x-rays reveal presence, location of intestinal gas or fluid. (In small-bowel obstruction, a typical "stepladder" pattern emerges with alternating fluid and gas levels apparent in 3 to 4 hr.)
      f. Barium enema reveals a distended, air-filled colon or a closed loop of sigmoid with extreme distention (in sigmoid volvulus).
      g. ABG analysis may indicate metabolic acidosis or alkalosis.
      h. Flexible sigmoidoscopy or colonoscopy may be performed to identify cause.
  B. Analysis
    1. Acute Pain related to obstructive process
    2. Anxiety related to outcomes of obstructive processes
    3. Constipation related to mechanical or functional obstruction
    4. Deficient Fluid Volume related to excessive loss secondary to obstructive process and subsequent vomiting or gastric decompression and decreased intake
    5. Ineffective Breathing Pattern related to abdominal distention
    6. Risk for Injury related to alteration in fluid and electrolyte balance
  C. Planning
    1. Promote comfort.
    2. Maintain normal fluid volume.
    3. Promote normal bowel function.
    4. Maintain caloric requirement.
    5. Maintain stable vital signs.
    6. Maintain fluid and electrolyte balance.
    7. Prevent infection.
    8. Maintain clean surgical wound and stoma.
  D. Implementation
    1. Check client's level of responsiveness frequently.
    2. Monitor vital signs closely for tachycardia and drop in BP.
    3. Monitor intake and output.

4. Be alert for signs of worsening obstruction that may require surgery (report promptly):
   a. Worsening pain
   b. Increasing distention
   c. Increasing NG output
5. Assist with ostomy care.
6. Record amount and consistency of stools.
7. Keep client in high Fowler position, if tolerated.

E. Evaluation
1. Client expresses feelings of increased comfort.
2. Client maintains normal fluid and electrolyte balance.
3. Client returns to normal bowel function.
4. Client maintains caloric and fluid requirements.
5. Client maintains stable vital signs.
6. Client is free from signs and symptoms of infection.
7. Client describes procedures for self-care behaviors.
8. Client adequately provides stoma and wound care.

CN

III. Client needs

A. Physiologic adaptation: Surgery is usually treatment of choice (exception is paralytic ileus in which nonoperative therapy is usually attempted first). Type of surgery depends on cause of blockage; ileostomy or colostomy may be necessary. If untreated, intraluminal pressure increases from accumulating secretions and gas; bacteria and toxins pass across the intestinal wall and lead to peritonitis. Eventually, intestinal wall ischemia and necrosis may occur, leading to shock and death.

B. Management of care: Care of the client with diverticular disease requires critical thinking skills and knowledge of assessment, and teaching and evaluation methods unique to the RN role. These skills cannot be delegated to an LPN or UAP.
1. Delegate responsibly those activities that can be delegated. All monitoring information must be reported to the RN.
   a. Monitor vital signs and daily weight.
   b. Assist with ambulation.
   c. Provide basic hygienic care.
   d. Measure intake and output.
   e. Promote turning, coughing, deep breathing at least every 2 hr.
2. Assess IV fluids, hyperalimentation, blood products, and urine measurements.
3. Maintain NG suction and monitor drainage.
4. Following ostomy procedure, empty drainage bag frequently or connect tubing to drainage bottle at side of bed; expect considerable amount of fecal drainage during first 12 to 15 hr (500 to 1,000 ml).
   a. Observe drainage equipment frequently for patency.
   b. Protect skin around ostomy with skin barrier such as a karaya preparation.
5. Provide parenteral nutrition until bowel is functioning.
6. Promote structured bowel regimen, especially if client had mechanical obstruction from fecal impaction.
7. Consult dietitian and enterostomal therapy nurse specialist as appropriate.
8. Evaluate need for continued follow-up care on outpatient basis.

C. Safety and infection control
1. Provide antibiotics as prescribed.
2. Provide instructions on wound and ostomy care.
3. Administer oral hygiene frequently.
4. Use special care for intestinal tubes.

D. Health promotion and maintenance (see reduction of risk potential)

E. Psychologic integrity
1. Allow client to verbalize concerns and fears freely.
2. Identify coping measures to deal with stress.
3. Contact support persons (clergy, social worker, enterostomal nurse therapist, another ostomate).

F. Basic care and comfort
1. Position client in Fowler position to promote ventilation and relief from abdominal distention.
2. Prevent irritation around stoma with use of skin barrier such as karaya preparation.
3. Provide gentle cleansing of perianal area and use skin barrier.

G. Reduction of risk potential: Provide client and family teaching.
1. Maintain adequate diet, fluid intake, and activity to prevent constipation and recurrence of partial obstruction.
2. Avoid lifting and contact sports postoperatively.
3. Recognize and promptly report recurrent symptoms and complications such as bleeding, abdominal distention, diarrhea dehydration, shock, and dumping syndrome, indicated by weakness, diaphoresis, cramping pains, pallor, headache, dizziness, drowsiness.
4. Teach ileostomy or colostomy care after bowel resection or temporary colostomy to

prevent complications of surgical interventions. Instruct client to examine stoma for:
   a. Edema—slight edema due to surgical manipulation is normal.
   b. Color—should be pink.
   c. Discharge—small amount of oozing is normal.
   d. Bleeding—abnormal sign.

H. Pharmacologic and parenteral therapies: Client will state the purpose, usage, and associated side effects of medications used to treat intestinal obstruction.
   1. To correct fluid/electrolyte imbalances:
      a. Sodium, potassium, blood component therapy
      b. Normal saline (NS; 0.9% NaCl)—isotonic
      c. Lactated Ringer (LR)—isotonic
   2. To treat shock and peritonitis:
      a. Dextrose 10%/water (D10/W—hypertonic
      b. 3% saline (3% NaCl)—hypertonic
      c. Dextrose 5% in one-half normal saline (D5/0.45% NaCl)—hypertonic
      d. Dextrose 5% in saline (D5/0.9% NaCl)—hypertonic
         (1) Administer cautiously because of fluid shift into the vascular compartment.
         (2) Monitor for hypertension, headache, and pulmonary edema.
   3. Prescribed intestinal anti-infectives: Kanamycin (Kantrex); erythromycin (Erythrocin); neomycin (Mycifradin)
   4. Stool softeners: Docusate sodium (Colace); docusate calcium (Surfak)

Appendicitis

I. Definition: Appendicitis is inflammation of the vermiform appendix caused by an obstruction attributable to infection, stricture, fecal mass, foreign body, or tumor. Appendicitis is the most common disease requiring surgery; if left untreated, complications may include abscess, perforation, subsequent peritonitis, and death. Appendicitis can affect either gender at any age, but is most common in males between 10 and 30 years of age.

II. Nursing process

A. Assessment
   1. Complete a detailed health history and comprehensive physical assessment.
   2. Assess for signs and symptoms.
      a. Initially, generalized, localized abdominal pain occurs in epigastric/periumbilical areas and in upper right abdomen.
      b. Within 2 to 12 hr, pain localizes in right lower quadrant (McBurney point) and intensity increases.
      c. Guarding, rebound tenderness in right lower quadrant, and referred rebound pain when palpating left lower quadrant.
      d. Additional symptoms may include anorexia, fever, nausea, vomiting, and constipation. Bowel sounds may be diminished.
   3. Obtain diagnostic tests.
      a. WBC count shows moderate leukocytosis.
      b. Urinalysis rules out urinary disorders.
      c. Abdominal x-ray visualizes shadow consistent with fecalith in appendix.
      d. Pelvic sonogram rules out ovarian cyst or ectopic pregnancy.

B. Analysis
   1. Acute Pain related to inflammatory process
   2. Constipation related to stricture
   3. Risk for Deficient Fluid Volume related to vomiting
   4. Risk for Infection related to inadequate primary defenses (danger or rupture, peritonitis, abscess formation) secondary to inflammatory process

C. Planning
   1. Prevent infection.
   2. Relieve pain.
   3. Maintain fluid volume balance.
   4. Restore normal bowel movements.

D. Implementation (see management of care)

E. Evaluation
   1. Client verbalizes decrease in pain.
   2. Client is free from signs and symptoms of infection.
   3. Client maintains fluid volume balance.
   4. Client demonstrates normal bowel movement.

CN

III. Client needs

A. Physiologic adaptation: Appendicitis is treated by removal of the appendix with immediate laparoscopic appendectomy or abdominal laparotomy (less desirable). See also pharmacologic and parenteral therapies. Signs and symptoms of postoperative complications include elevated temperature, nausea or vomiting, and abdominal distention.

B. Management of care: Care of the client with appendicitis requires critical thinking skills and knowledge of assessment, and teaching and evaluation methods unique to the RN role. These skills cannot be delegated to an LPN or UAP.

1. Delegate responsibly those activities that can be delegated, including basic hygienic care, monitoring of vital signs, assisting with menu selection, and assisting with ambulation as ordered. All monitoring information is reported to the RN.
2. Monitor frequently for signs and symptoms of worsening condition.
3. Notify physician promptly if pain or discomfort suddenly ceases.
4. Apply ice bag to abdomen.
5. Avoid indiscriminate palpation of abdomen.
6. Prepare client for surgery once diagnosis is established.
7. Ensure arrangements are made with discharge planner for follow-up visit to surgeon.

C. Safety and infection control
1. Use sterile technique with dressing changes; if laparotomy is done, allow Steri-Strips to fall off in 7 to 10 days.
2. Administer antibiotics as prescribed.
3. Monitor for signs and symptoms of infection.

D. Health promotion and maintenance: Provide client and family teaching about well-balanced diet and maintaining regular aerobic activity.

E. Psychologic integrity: Provide client and family comfort preoperatively.

F. Basic care and comfort
1. Position client in semi-Fowler position with knees flexed.
2. Apply ice bag to abdomen for comfort, if ordered.

G. Reduction of risk potential: Provide client and family teaching for recovery period.
1. Promote steady increase of ambulation.
2. Use frequent turning, coughing, and deep breathing; use incentive spirometer.
3. Use stool softeners and increase fluids to prevent constipation; avoid enemas and harsh laxatives.
4. Avoid heavy lifting or driving (until cleared by surgeon).

H. Pharmacologic and parenteral therapies: Client will state the purpose, usage, and associated side effects for medications used for appendicitis.
1. Broad-spectrum antibiotics, as directed—ampicillin (Amcill); erythromycin (Erythrocin)
2. Analgesia, as ordered—propoxyphene (Darvon); hydrocodone (Vicodin)
3. Intravenous fluids
a. Normal saline (0.9% NaCl)—isotonic
b. Lactated Ringer (LR)—isotonic
c. Dextrose 5%/water (D5/W)—isotonic/hypotonic

Hemorrhoids

I. Definition: Hemorrhoids are vascular masses that protrude into the lumen of the lower rectum or perianal area, and are the most common variety of anorectal disorders.

A. Hemorrhoids may be internal, external, or prolapsed.
1. Internal—occur above anal sphincter and cannot be seen on inspection of perianal area.
2. External—occur below anal sphincter and can be seen on inspection.
3. Prolapsed—can become thrombosed or inflamed.

B. Hemorrhoids occur when increased intra-abdominal pressure causes engorgement in vascular tissue lining the anal canal. Loosening of vessels from surrounding connective tissue occurs with protrusion and prolapse into the anal canal.

II. Nursing process

A. Assessment
1. Complete a detailed health history and comprehensive physical assessment.
2. Assess for signs and symptoms.
a. Pain (more so with external hemorrhoids)
b. Sensation of incomplete fecal evacuation
c. Constipation
d. Anal itching
e. If external hemorrhoids thrombosed, sudden rectal pain may occur
f. Bleeding may occur during defecation—bright red blood on stool caused by injury of mucosa covering hemorrhoid
g. Visible/palpable masses at anal area
3. Assess for risk factors.
a. Pregnancy
b. Prolonged sitting or standing
c. Straining during bowel movement
d. Chronic constipation or diarrhea
e. Anal infection
f. Rectal surgery or episiotomy
g. Genetic predisposition
h. Alcoholism
i. Portal hypertension (as in cirrhosis)
j. Loss of muscle tone attributable to old age
k. Anal intercourse
4. Obtain diagnostic tests.
a. External examination with anoscope/proctoscope—determines single or multiple hemorrhoids.
b. Barium enema/colonoscopy—rules out more serious colonic lesions causing rectal bleeding, such as polyps.

B. Analysis
   1. Constipation related to fear of pain on defecation
   2. Acute Pain related to inflammation
   3. Deficient Knowledge related to lack of information about hemorrhoids
C. Planning
   1. Relieve pain.
   2. Manage diet.
   3. Promote client and family teaching.
   4. Provide postoperative care, if indicated.
D. Implementation (see management of care)
E. Evaluation
   1. Client reports increased comfort, particularly on defecation.
   2. Client adheres to treatment regimen.
   3. Client establishes a pattern of regular bowel movements.
   4. Client describes what hemorrhoids are, their causes, and how they are treated and managed.

CN

III. Client needs
A. Physiologic adaptation: Hemorrhoids are treated through diet, prevention, and management. Surgery is required when prolapsed hemorrhoids can no longer be reduced spontaneously or manually.
   1. Diet:
      a. Low-roughage diet (elimination of raw fruits/vegetables) during acute exacerbations.
      b. High-fiber diet during remissions to prevent constipation.
   2. Laxatives and stool softeners to regulate bowel function; bulking agent may also be used (see pharmacologic and parenteral therapies).
   3. Surgical intervention:
      a. Ligation (internal hemorrhoids may be ligated with rubber bands)
      b. Cryosurgery
      c. Laser
      d. Sclerotherapy
      e. Hemorrhoidectomy
B. Management of care: Care of the client being treated for hemorrhoids requires critical thinking skills and knowledge of assessment, and teaching and evaluation methods unique to the RN role. These skills cannot be delegated to an LPN or UAP.
   1. Delegate responsibly those activities that can be delegated. All monitoring information is reported to the RN.
      a. Relieve pain by providing sitz baths and ice compresses; apply witch hazel soaks and topical anesthetics as prescribed.
      b. Take vital signs.
      c. Administer cleansing enemas preoperatively, if ordered.
      d. Administer stool softeners as prescribed.
      e. Provide perineal care.
   2. Reduce prolapsed external hemorrhoids manually.
   3. Provide postoperative care if surgery is indicated.
      a. Observe for rectal hemorrhage and urinary retention; report if excessive—explain to client that some bleeding with bowel movements is expected.
      b. Administer stool softener or laxative soon after surgery (assists with bowel movements and reduces risk of stricture).
      c. Teach anal hygiene, measures to control moisture to prevent itching.
      d. Discourage regular use of laxatives—firm, soft stools dilate anal canal and decrease stricture formation after surgery.
   4. Determine client's normal bowel habits; identify predisposing factors.
   5. Provide client teaching (see health promotion and maintenance).
C. Safety and infection control: Test temperature of sitz bath water.
D. Health promotion and maintenance: Provide client teaching.
   1. Prevent constipation by responding quickly to urge to defecate.
   2. Modify diet to include fluids (8 to 10 glasses per day) and fiber.
   3. Obtain regular ambulation; prevent standing or sitting for prolonged periods of time.
   4. Keep perianal area clean and dry.
   5. Avoid regular use of laxatives.
E. Psychologic integrity: Provide privacy and sufficient time for defecation, especially after meals.
F. Basic care and comfort
   1. Provide perianal care, keeping area as dry and clean as possible; apply witch-hazel dressing to perianal area or anal creams or suppositories, if ordered, to relieve discomfort.
   2. Provide analgesics, warm sitz baths, or warm compresses to reduce pain, inflammation.
G. Reduction of risk potential: Provide postoperative care and teaching (see management of care).
H. Pharmacologic and parenteral therapies: Client will state the purpose, usage, and associated side effects of all medications used to treat hemorrhoids. Client will understand that overuse of laxatives can cause laxative

dependence; it is not necessary to have a bowel movement every day.

1. Stool softeners—maintain soft stools; relieve symptoms: Docusate sodium (Colace); docusate calcium (Surfak).
2. Bulk laxatives: Psyllium (Metamucil). Administer with fluid; administer immediately before it congeals.
3. Stimulant laxatives: Bisacodyl (Dulcolax); Senna; Senokot.
4. Saline (osmotic) laxatives: Magnesium citrate (Citrate of Magnesia); magnesium hydroxide (Milk of Magnesia).
5. Nonopioid analgesics—promotes normal bowel elimination without pain, aspirin (Ecotrin); acetaminophen (Tylenol). If client does not have a bowel movement within 1 week, the client should contact the health care provider (HCP).

Cancer of the Colon

I. Definition: Cancer of the colon involves tumors in the sigmoid, descending, and ascending colon. Malignant tumors of the colon are almost always adenocarcinomas. One-half are sessile lesions of rectosigmoid area; others are polypoid lesions. Tumors in the sigmoid and descending colon undergo circumferential growth and constrict intestinal lumen. Tumors in ascending colon are large at diagnosis and are palpable on physical examination.

II. Nursing process

A. Assessment

1. Complete a detailed health history and comprehensive physical assessment.
2. Assess for signs and symptoms.
   a. Change in bowel habits
   b. Passage of blood in stools
   c. Changes in shape of stool (narrowing)
   d. Unexplained anemia, anorexia, weight loss, fatigue
   e. Right-sided tumors: Abdominal pain, melena
   f. Left-sided tumors: Abdominal pain, cramping, narrowing stools, constipation, distention
3. Assess for risk factors.
   a. Familial history
   b. Chronic inflammatory bowel disease
   c. Polyps
   d. Low-fiber, high-fat diet
   e. Older than 40 years of age
   f. Male gender
4. Obtain diagnostic tests.
   a. Fecal occult blood testing—reveals evidence of carcinoma when client is otherwise asymptomatic.
   b. Barium enema—useful in detecting smaller tumors (not to precede colonoscopy).
   c. Colonoscopy with biopsy—procedure of choice.
   d. Pelvic magnetic resonance imaging, endorectal ultrasonography—provides information about penetration and lymph node involvement.
   e. Computed tomography scan of liver, lung, brain—determines presence of metastatic disease.
   f. Carcinoembryonic antigen—monitors metastasis or tumor recurrence.
   g. Proctoscopy and sigmoidoscopy—permit visualization of lower GI tract.

B. Analysis

1. Acute Pain related to tissue compression due to obstruction
2. Anxiety related to treatments and prognosis
3. Constipation related to disease process
4. Diarrhea related to disease process
5. Fatigue related to anemia from chronic blood loss
6. Imbalanced Nutrition: Less Than Body requirements related to malabsorption
7. Risk for Deficient Fluid Volume related to anorexia, diarrhea, and vomiting
8. Disturbed Body Image related to alteration in GI structure, function
9. Risk for Infection related to possible contamination of abdominal cavity during surgical procedure
10. Deficient Knowledge related to lack of information about diagnosis, surgical procedure, and self-care
11. Impaired Skin Integrity related to surgical incisions and formation of stoma

C. Planning

1. Reduce anxiety.
2. Relieve or reduce pain.
3. Maintain optimal level of nutrition.
4. Maintain fluid and electrolyte balance.
5. Prevent infection.
6. Promote acquisition of information about diagnosis, surgical procedure, and self-care after discharge.
7. Promote optimal tissue healing.
8. Promote positive body image.
9. Maintain skin integrity.

D. Implementation

1. Observe vital signs, increasing abdominal pain, nausea, and vomiting.
2. Monitor patency of gastric and intestinal tubes.
3. Administer chemotherapeutic drugs, if ordered.

4. Administer electrolyte and parenteral fluid replacement as ordered.
5. Administer progressive diet as ordered.

E. Evaluation
1. Client maintains adequate fluid and electrolyte balance.
2. Client resumes regular pattern of bowel elimination.
3. Client demonstrates ability to perform ostomy care.
4. Client discusses feelings concerning diagnosis, prognosis, and ostomy.
5. Client maintains nutritional status.
6. Client reports relief from pain.
7. Client reports decrease in anxiety and fatigue.
8. Client demonstrates ability to cope with altered body function.
9. Client is free from signs and symptoms of infection.
10. Client's skin is intact, with exception of stoma.

CN

III. Client needs

A. Physiologic adaptation: Cancer of the colon is treated with radiation therapy, chemotherapy, and surgical intervention (may or may not involve colostomy).
1. Recognize risk for side effects of chemotherapeutic drugs, such as stomatitis, dehydration, nausea and vomiting, diarrhea, and leukopenia.
2. Recognize risk for side effects of chemotherapy, such as stomatitis, dehydration, nausea and vomiting, diarrhea, and leukopenia.

B. Management of care: Care of the client with cancer of the colon requires critical thinking skills and knowledge of assessment, and teaching and evaluation methods unique to the RN role. These skills cannot be delegated to an LPN or UAP.
1. Delegate responsibly those activities that can be delegated, including basic hygienic care, checking vital signs, assisting with ambulation, and assisting with food and fluid ingestion. All monitoring information must be reported to the RN.
2. Provide preoperative and postoperative care for colon surgery.
   a. Preoperatively: Administer enemas and drugs for intestinal antisepsis as ordered.
   b. Postoperatively: Assess reaction to colostomy; provide colostomy care—periodically dilate stoma to prevent strictures. Observe vital signs, increasing abdominal pain or discomfort to detect signs of complications.
3. Teach client how to care for colostomy; colostomy drainage begins in 3 to 4 days. Request consult with wound/ostomy nurse specialist. (See also reduction of risk potential.)
4. Promote diet management (see health promotion and maintenance). Request consult with dietitian.
5. Request consult with psychiatric nurse specialist or psychiatrist, as appropriate.
6. Determine home health care needs for ostomy care, wound care, pain management, diet management, or managing effects of chemotherapy or radiation therapy.
7. Evaluate community resources for cancer support and continued education; arrange for follow-up care with community agencies, as desired.

C. Safety and infection control
1. Provide preoperative intestinal asepsis.
2. Use sterile technique for postoperative dressing changes.
3. Support body's natural defenses through adequate fluid intake and foods high in nutrients—includes dense foods from fruit, vegetable, cereal, grain, and legume groups with some lean meat, fish, and poultry.
4. Increase immunity through vitamin and mineral supplements.

D. Health promotion and maintenance
1. Teach about self-care behaviors for colostomy care.
2. Teach measures to facilitate resumption of activities (including sexual) and need for regular medical supervision.
3. Assess ongoing functioning of ostomy.

E. Psychologic integrity
1. Identify level of anxiety (mild, moderate, severe) and coping mechanisms.
2. Recognize client is sensitive to gestures, odors, and facial expressions; teach measures to facilitate acceptance and adjustment.

F. Basic care and comfort
1. Monitor pouch system for proper fit and signs of leakage.
2. Do not allow fecal matter to remain on skin.
3. Empty pouch when one-third full.
4. Implement measures to aid in management of undesirable odors (air/room fresheners, regular hygienic care of body).

G. Reduction of risk potential: Provide client and family teaching.
1. Avoid heavy lifting.
2. Monitor for signs of complications, including increasing abdominal pain, and nausea and vomiting.
3. Monitor stoma for size, unusual bleeding, and necrotic tissue; monitor skin

around stoma for signs of redness and irritation.

4. Monitor for color changes in stoma:
   a. Normal stoma color is red or pink.
   b. Pale pink stoma indicates low hemoglobin/hematocrit levels.
   c. Purple-black stoma indicates compromised circulation, requiring physician notification.
5. Expect stool to be:
   a. Liquid stool for ascending colon colostomy.
   b. Loose or semiformed stool for transverse colon colostomy.
   c. Stool is close to normal for descending colon colostomy.

H. Pharmacologic and parenteral therapies: Client will state purpose, usage, and associated side effects of medications used to treat cancer of the colon.

1. Intravenous fluids containing electrolytes, as ordered in situations of bleeding, vomiting, and/or obstruction.
   a. Lactated Ringer (LR)—isotonic: Contains sodium, potassium, calcium, chloride, and lactate
   b. Normal saline (NS; 0.9% NaCl)—isotonic: Contains sodium and chloride
   c. Lactated Ringer solution with 5% dextrose (D5/LR)—hypertonic: Contains dextrose and all electrolytes as in Lactated Ringer
   d. 5% dextrose and normal saline (D5/0.9NS)—hypertonic: Contains dextrose, sodium, and chloride
2. Broad-spectrum antibiotics such as tobramycin (Nebcin); gentamicin (Garamycin); and neomycin (Mycifradin): Used for preoperative intestinal antisepsis because active against wide variety of gram-negative bacteria; also effective against certain gram-positive organisms.

Bibliography

Altman, G. (2004). *Delmar's fundamental and advanced nursing skills* (2nd ed.). Albany, NY: Delmar.

Doenges, M., Moorhouse, M., & Murr, A. (2006). *Nurse's pocket guide: Diagnosis, prioritized interventions, and rationales* (10th ed.). Philadelphia: Davis.

Ellis, J., & Hartley, C. (2005). *Managing and coordinating nursing care.* Philadelphia: Lippincott Williams & Wilkins.

Hogan, M., & Wane, D. (2003). *Fluids, electrolytes, and acid-base balance: Review & rationales.* Upper Saddle River, NJ: Prentice Hall.

Joint Commission Universal Protocol (2003). Retrieved July 6, 2006, from http://www.jcaho.org/accredited+organizations/patient+safety/universal+protocol.htm

Karch, A. (2006). *Lippincott's nursing drug guide.* Philadelphia: Lippincott Williams & Wilkins.

Nursing 2008 drug handbook. Ambler, PA: Springhouse.

Pagana, K., & Pagana, T. (2002). *Mosby's manual of diagnostic and laboratory tests* (2nd ed.). St. Louis: Mosby.

Purnell, L., & Paulanka, B. (Eds.). (2003). *Transcultural healthcare: A culturally competent approach.* Philadelphia: Davis.

Smeltzer, S. C., Bare, B. G., Cheever, K. H., & Hinkle, J. L. (2008). *Brunner & Suddarth's textbook of medical-surgical nursing* (11th ed.). Philadelphia: Lippincott Williams & Wilkins.

Taylor, C., Lillis, C., LeMone, P., & Lynn, P. (2006). *Fundamentals of nursing.* Philadelphia: Lippincott Williams & Wilkins.

Weber, J. R., & Kelley, J. (2007). *Nurses handbook of health assessment.* Philadelphia: Lippincott Williams & Wilkins.

Yarbro, C. H., Frogge, M., & Goodman, M. (2004). *Cancer symptom management* (3rd ed.). Sudbury, MA: Jones and Bartlett.

CHAPTER 25

Practice Test

Inguinal Hernia

1. The nurse is teaching a male client with an uncomplicated inguinal hernia. The nurse should instruct the client to use which of the following?

- ☐ 1. Scrotal support.
- ☐ 2. Cold pack.
- ☐ 3. T-binder.
- ☐ 4. Truss.

2. The nurse is providing discharge instructions for a client who had an inguinal herniorrhaphy. The nurse should teach the client to do which of the following?

- ☐ 1. Cough and deep breathe every 2 hr.
- ☐ 2. Apply warm, moist heat to the groin.
- ☐ 3. Sneeze with mouth closed.
- ☐ 4. Avoid lifting items weighing more than 5 pounds.

Inflammatory Bowel Disease

3. AF The nurse has identified four nursing diagnoses for a client who is 45 years of age and has ulcerative colitis. The nursing care plan is designed to assist the client with these diagnoses in which order of priority?

_____ 1. Acute pain.
_____ 2. Activity intolerance.
_____ 3. Imbalanced nutrition.
_____ 4. Risk for deficient fluid volume.

4. A client has Crohn disease. Which one of the following medications is most effective in the treatment of Crohn disease involving the large intestine?

- ☐ 1. Sulfasalazine (Azulfidine).
- ☐ 2. Propantheline (Pro-Banthine).
- ☐ 3. Metronidazole (Flagyl).
- ☐ 4. Hydrocortisone enema (Cortenema).

5. A client has anemia resulting from bleeding from ulcerative colitis and is to receive two units of packed red blood cells (PRBCs). The client is receiving an infusion of TPN. In preparing to administer the PRBCs, the nurse should do which of the following to ensure client comfort and safety?

- ☐ 1. Discontinue the TPN infusion.
- ☐ 2. Start an IV infusion of normal saline.
- ☐ 3. Administer PRBCs in the same IV as the TPN.
- ☐ 4. Wait until the TPN infusion is completed and use the same IV line to infuse the PRBCs.

6. AF A client with ulcerative colitis is receiving TPN. To prevent metabolic complications, the nurse assesses the client for which of the following? Select all that apply.

- ☐ 1. Thrombosis.
- ☐ 2. Fungus.
- ☐ 3. Hyperosmolar state.
- ☐ 4. Magnesium deficiency.
- ☐ 5. Hyperglycemia.

7. A client had a bowel resection and creation of an ileostomy. The nurse is assessing the client on the first postoperative day. Which of the following are expected?

- ☐ 1. Stool is loose to semisoft.
- ☐ 2. Stoma is dark blue.
- ☐ 3. Ileostomy drainage is dark green.
- ☐ 4. Dry dressing on stoma.

8. AF A client with an ileostomy has a serum potassium level of 3.0 mEq/L. The surgeon has ordered IV potassium. The nurse should do which of the following? Select all that apply.

- ☐ 1. Assess heart rate and rhythm.
- ☐ 2. Evaluate electrocardiogram (ECG) changes.
- ☐ 3. Restrict foods high in potassium.
- ☐ 4. Administer potassium chloride IV push.
- ☐ 5. Monitor client's cognitive abilities.

9. The nurse is discussing home care instructions with a client who has an ileostomy. Which of the following symptoms does the nurse instruct the client to report to the HCP?

- ☐ 1. Temperature of 101°F.
- ☐ 2. Liquid stool in the ileostomy pouch.
- ☐ 3. Undigested food in ileostomy pouch.
- ☐ 4. Continuous drainage from the ileostomy.

10. A client who has an ileostomy has a red rash with pustules around the stoma. The client reports that the stoma itches continuously. What is first action the nurse should take?

- ☐ 1. Clean the area with normal saline before reapplying the pouch.
- ☐ 2. Apply a dry dressing between the skin and pouch until the rash clears.
- ☐ 3. Change the pouch more frequently.
- ☐ 4. Contact the HCP for an order for an antifungal powder.

Diverticular Disease

11. When a client has an acute attack of diverticulitis, the nurse should first?

- ☐ 1. Prepare the client for a colonoscopy.
- ☐ 2. Encourage the client to eat a high-fiber diet.
- ☐ 3. Assess the client for signs of peritonitis.
- ☐ 4. Encourage the client to drink a glass of water every 2 hr.

12. Which of the following instructions does the nurse provide to the client with diverticulitis to prevent an exacerbation of the disease?

- ☐ 1. Avoid eating whole-grain breads and cereals.
- ☐ 2. Follow a high-fiber diet to increase fecal volume.
- ☐ 3. Have an annual colonoscopy to detect changes in polyps.
- ☐ 4. Use stool softeners to prevent bowel spasms.

Intestinal Obstruction

13. A client has a bowel obstruction from a paralytic ileus following abdominal surgery. The client has a distended abdomen and is in severe pain. The nurse should do which of the following first?

- ☐ 1. Request an order for opiate pain medication.
- ☐ 2. Assist the client to ambulate.
- ☐ 3. Encourage the client to drink carbonated beverages.
- ☐ 4. Place the client in a supine position.

Appendicitis

14. An adult admitted to the hospital with appendicitis has severe abdominal pain. Which of the following interventions is most effective

to assist the client to manage pain prior to surgery?
- ☐ 1. Position the client in semi-Fowler with knees up.
- ☐ 2. Apply moist heat to the abdomen.
- ☐ 3. Teach client to massage the painful area.
- ☐ 4. Provide distraction with music.

Hemorrhoids

15. A client has had a hemorrhoidectomy. To reduce discomfort of the first bowel movement, the nurse administers which of the following?
- ☐ 1. Docusate sodium (Colace).
- ☐ 2. Psyllium hydrophilic mucilloid (Metamucil).
- ☐ 3. Alprazolam (Xanax).
- ☐ 4. Propoxyphene (Darvon).

16. AF A client with internal hemorrhoids and a history of prolonged constipation is following a high-fiber diet. The nurse should instruct the client to eat which of the following? Select all that apply.
- ☐ 1. Whole-wheat bread.
- ☐ 2. Oatmeal.
- ☐ 3. Brown rice.
- ☐ 4. Smooth peanut butter.
- ☐ 5. Cottage cheese.
- ☐ 6. Cream of wheat cereal.

Cancer of the Colon

17. Three days after a colon resection, a client has abdominal pain. The nurse auscultates bowel sounds in all four quadrants. The orders are "up ad lib." Which of the following nursing measures would assist the client in alleviating the cause of pain?
- ☐ 1. Provide a sitz bath.
- ☐ 2. Apply warm abdominal compresses.
- ☐ 3. Increase walking activity as tolerated.
- ☐ 4. Administer analgesics as prescribed.

18. The nurse is assessing a client who has had a sigmoid colostomy for cancer of the colon. Which of the following can be expected by the fourth postoperative day?
- ☐ 1. Bowel sounds are less than two per minute.
- ☐ 2. The client has pain of 1 on scale of 1 to 10 without pain medication.
- ☐ 3. Fecal drainage includes soft stool.
- ☐ 4. The stoma is flush with the skin.

19. The nurse is preparing for discharge a client who received a colectomy 4 days earlier. Which of the following nursing care goals has the highest priority prior to discharge?
- ☐ 1. Lungs are clear per auscultation.
- ☐ 2. Incision is healed without redness or drainage.
- ☐ 3. Bowel sounds present; client expels flatus.
- ☐ 4. Vital sign within normal limits.

20. AF Neomycin sulfate (Mycifradin) is ordered preoperatively for a client with colon cancer. The physician orders are to: "Administer 1 gram every 1 hour times 4 doses, then 1 gram every 4 hours times 5 doses." The client receives his first dose of 1 g at 9:00 a.m. When will the client receive the 1-g dose that must be given every 4 hr? ______________ p.m.

Answers and Rationales

1. 4 The nurse instructs the client to wear a truss, a pad placed over the hernia and held in place with a belt; the truss is worn to keep the hernia from protruding. The nurse checks for skin irritation caused by the continual rubbing of the truss. Scrotal edema is a painful complication after an inguinal hernia repair. A scrotal support with application of an ice bag may help relieve pain and edema. Cloth T-binders are rarely used because commercial elastic perineal belts and disposable protective underwear are available. (C)

2. 4 The client is instructed to avoid lifting items heavier than 5 pounds for 4 to 6 weeks following hernia repair. The client continues to take deep breaths and expand the lungs, but is instructed to avoid coughing. Ice, rather than heat, is used to reduce scrotal swelling. The client is instructed to sneeze with the mouth open to avoid sudden stress on the sutures. (H)

3. 1, 4, 3, 2 Planning to relieve acute pain is performed first in order to promote management of other diagnoses. While experiencing pain, a client is less likely to eat, drink, or move about. The immediacy of the effects of a fluid volume deficit takes priority over malnutrition. Although long-term inactivity or immobility can result in several irreversible outcomes, it lacks the immediacy associated with malnutrition. (M)

4. 1 Sulfasalazine (Azulfidine) is effective when Crohn disease involves the large intestine; it is much less effective when only the small intestine is involved. Corticosteroid therapy is effective in reducing inflammation and suppressing the disease; the dosage and route of administration depend on the severity of the illness and the area involved. Metronidazole (Flagyl) is useful in treating Crohn disease of the perianal area; marked exacerbations have been reported when the drug is stopped. Propantheline (Pro-Banthine) decreases motility (smooth muscle tone) in the GI, biliary, and urinary tracts, and results in antispasmodic action. (D)

5. 2 The nurse administers the PRBCs using a separate infusion line and appropriate tubing, with normal saline as the priming solution. It is not necessary to discontinue the TPN infusion or wait until the TPN infusion is completed. (S)

6. 3, 4, 5 TPN base solutions contain dextrose and protein in the form of amino acids. The pharmacy department adds the prescribed electrolytes (i.e., sodium, potassium, chloride, calcium, magnesium, and phosphate), vitamins, and trace elements (i.e., zinc, copper, chromium, and manganese) to customize the solution for the client. Parenteral nutrition solutions are hyperosmolar (osmotic pressure is greater than normal plasma pressure). Hyperglycemia is a metabolic complication of parenteral nutrition. The pancreas attempts to adapt to the increased amount of glucose in the circulation by producing more insulin. Blood glucose levels are checked bedside every 4 to 6 hr with a glucose-testing meter. Some increase in blood glucose level is expected during the first few days after TPN is started; a sliding scale dose of insulin may be ordered. Thrombosis in the great vein is a mechanical complication of TPN; fungus is an infection. (R)

7. 3 Immediately after surgery the ileostomy drainage is dark green and progresses to yellow as the client begins to eat. Postoperatively, a healthy stoma is red. The nurse reports to the surgeon a color change to dark blue or black. Stool is liquid with an ileostomy. A petroleum jelly gauze is placed over a colostomy stoma to keep it moist, followed later by a dry sterile dressing if a pouching system is not in place. (A)

8. 1, 2, 5 The client with an ileostomy is at high risk for fluid and electrolyte imbalances. This client has hypokalemia; normal serum potassium levels are 3.5 to 5.0 mEq/L. With hypokalemia, there are ECG changes: ST segment depression, flattened T wave, appearance of U wave, ventricular dysrhythmias (especially premature ventricular contractions [PVCs]), and heart block. There is a variable pulse rate, a weak thready pulse, and the pedal pulses are difficult to palpitate when hypokalemia is present. Because the serum potassium level is low in hypokalemia, dietary interventions are used to promote normal potassium levels. Good food sources of potassium include vegetables, such as spinach, broccoli, carrots, green beans, acorn squash, and potatoes; fruits, such as bananas, cantaloupe, watermelon, grapefruit, and strawberries; milk, milk products, yogurt; meat; legumes, nuts, seeds, and whole grains. The nurse monitors the client's mental status for confusion, a common symptom of hypokalemia that can progress to coma. Potassium chloride is never administered IV push or IM routes as this can lead to development of fatal arrhythmias. Potassium is diluted in a solution that provides no more than 1 mEq/10 ml. The IV site is monitored closely as potassium chloride (KCl) is irritating to vessels and can lead to infiltration, phlebitis, and tissue necrosis. (M)

9. 1 The client is instructed to report an elevated temperature to the HCP, as this is a sign of infection and requires follow-up. The stool in the pouch is liquid and drains continuously. Occasionally, there is undigested food in the pouch. (H)

10. 4 The client likely has candidiasis, which can develop easily around moist surfaces. The nurse's first action is to contact the HCP and obtain an order for an antifungal powder. Cleaning with saline, using a dry dressing, and/or changing the pouch more frequently are not sufficient ways to manage the rash. (S)

11. 3 Complications of diverticulitis include perforation with peritonitis, abscess, and fistula formation, bowel obstruction, ureteral obstruction, and bleeding. A computed tomography (CT) scan with oral contrast is the test of choice for diverticulitis. A client with acute diverticulitis does not receive a barium enema or colonoscopy because of the possibility of peritonitis and perforation. With acute diverticulitis, the goal of treatment is to allow the colon to rest and inflammation to subside. The client is kept on NPO status; parenteral fluid therapy is provided. (A)

12. 2 Uncomplicated diverticular disease is treated with a high-fiber diet and bulk laxatives, such as psyllium hydrophilic mucilloid (Metamucil). A colonoscopy may be performed to rule out possible hidden polyps or lesions, but does not prevent an exacerbation. Stool softeners do not prevent bowel spasms; instead, their detergent action lowers surface tension, permitting water and fats to penetrate and soften stools for easier passage. (H)

13. 2 Paralytic ileus is a cause of intestinal obstruction and can occur following abdominal surgery. The nurse assists the client to ambulate to stimulate peristalsis; obstruction is usually relieved within 2 to 3 days. Opiate pain medications are not used because they slow peristalsis. Carbonated beverages increase gas accumulation and pain. The nurse instructs the client to turn frequently while in bed. (H)

14. 1 Appendicitis typically begins with periumbilical pain followed by anorexia, nausea, and vomiting. The pain is persistent and continuous, eventually shifting to the right lower quadrant and localizing at McBurney point (located halfway between the umbilicus and the right iliac crest). To relieve pain prior to surgery, the nurse assists the client to a comfortable position with the knees drawn to the chest and the head of the bed slightly elevated. The nurse also administers analgesics and ice packs, if ordered. Warm heat is avoided as heat may precipitate rupture. The abdomen is not palpated or massaged more than necessary to avoid increasing the pain. Distraction with music may be helpful, but positioning, using ice packs, and analgesics are most effective. (C)

15. 4 Propoxyphene (Darvon) is an analgesic with potency about one-half to two-thirds that of codeine, and is used to relieve mild-to-moderate pain. Unlike codeine, propoxyphene has little or no antitussive effect. Docusate sodium (Colace) is a stool softener, usually ordered within the first few postoperative days. If the client does not have a bowel movement within 2 to 3 days, an oil-retention enema is given. Psyllium hydrophilic mucilloid (Metamucil) is a bulk-producing laxative that promotes peristalsis and natural elimination; it is used for chronic atonic/spastic constipation and constipation associated with rectal disorders. Alprazolam (Xanax) is a CNS depressant; it contains antidepressant as well as antianxiety actions and is used for management of anxiety disorders or for short-term relief of anxiety symptoms; it is also used as an adjunct in management of anxiety associated with depression and agitation, and for panic disorders, such as agoraphobia. (D)

16. 1, 2, 3 Breads and cereals with adequate fiber provide 2 to 5 g of fiber per serving. High-fiber cereals provide 7 to 11 g of fiber per serving. The best choices are whole-wheat bread, bran cereals, oatmeal, oat bran, brown rice, wheat germ, and whole-wheat pasta. A high-fiber diet is rich in both soluble and insoluble fiber even though only insoluble fiber has been credited with increasing stool bulk and stimulating peristalsis; diet is achieved by substituting high-fiber foods for refined, low-fiber foods. Exactly how much fiber is needed to prevent or alleviate constipation varies among individuals. The nurse instructs the client to gradually increase fiber intake to avoid symptoms of intolerance, such as increased intestinal gas production, cramping, and diarrhea; if these side effects do occur, they are usually temporary and subside within several days. (H)

17. 3 Pain following a colon resection is partly caused by flatulence. The nurse promotes an increase in walking activity to stimulate peristalsis and thereby relieve the "gas pains." Warm compresses and analgesics are useful in relieving pain, but do not alleviate the cause. A sitz bath is not helpful. (C)

18. 3 By the forth postoperative day, the client with a sigmoid colostomy is expected to pass soft stool in the stoma. Bowel sounds are expected to return within 24 to 48 hr (5 to 25 per minute). The nurse continues to assess the client for pain and provides analgesia as indicated. The stoma appears bright red and shiny; there is some edema and the stoma has not yet shrunk to the size it will be later. (A)

19. 3 Because a colectomy involves the GI tract, the return of normal GI function is most important; the nurse assures the client is expelling gas prior to discharge. While the wound is not completely healed at this time and drainage is present, there are no signs of infection at the incision site. The client has clear lungs and normal vital signs prior to discharge, but these are not the priority for this client. (M)

20. The first 4 doses are given at 9 a.m., 10 a.m., 11 a.m., and 12 noon. The next dose is due 4 hr later at 4 p.m. (D)

chapter

26

The Client With Biliary Tract Disorders

Health problems of the biliary tract include diseases that affect the gallbladder, liver, and pancreas. The nurse must have an understanding of the structure and function of the biliary tract and pancreas, and understand how biliary tract disorders are closely linked with liver disease. The nurse plans care with the client and family to manage acute and chronic diseases that can affect these organs. The following topics are discussed in this chapter:

- Disorders of the Gallbladder: Cholelithiasis, Cholecystitis
- Disorders of the Liver: Hepatitis, Cirrhosis, Cancer of the Liver
- Disorders of the Pancreas: Pancreatitis and Pancreatic Cancer

Disorders of the Gallbladder: Cholelithiasis, Cholecystitis

I. Definition: Common health problems of the gallbladder include gallstone formation (cholelithiasis) and inflammation (cholecystitis).
  A. Cholelithiasis, or gallstone formation, is the most common biliary disorder. The gallbladder stores and concentrates bile produced by the liver and releases bile into the duodenum via the biliary ducts; this process assists in emulsifying fat. Gallstones form in the gallbladder from the solid components of bile (cholesterol, calcium, and bile salts).
  B. Cholecystitis is inflammation of the gallbladder and may present as an acute or chronic disease. The major cause of cholecystitis is cholelithiasis. Gallstones obstructing the cystic duct cause an inflamed gallbladder that may be associated with infection. Gallstones can migrate to the common bile duct (choledocholithiasis). Cholangitis and pancreatitis are complications of cholelithiasis.

II. Nursing process
  A. Assessment
    1. Obtain a detailed health history, including past medical, surgical, and psychosocial history, as well as a comprehensive physical assessment.
    2. Assess for risk factors.
      a. Female gender
      b. Obesity
      c. Older age
      d. White, Native American, Hispanic
      e. Rapid weight loss or frequent changes in weight
      f. Pregnancy, multiparity, estrogen therapy
      g. High cholesterol
      h. Familial tendency
    3. Assess for signs and symptoms.
      a. Epigastric discomfort or pain after eating fatty foods
      b. Severe, steady RUQ pain near the rib cage that radiates to right shoulder and scapula
      c. Biliary colic
      d. Nausea, vomiting, indigestion, belching, or flatulence
      e. Leukocytosis and fever with acute cholecystitis
      f. Positive Murphy sign
      g. Abdominal guarding or rigidity
      h. Common bile duct obstruction
        (1) Jaundice
        (2) Clay-colored stools
        (3) Dark, foamy urine
        (4) Steatorrhea
    4. Obtain diagnostic tests.
      a. Abdominal ultrasound
      b. CT scan, MRI
      c. Gallbladder radionuclide imaging
      d. Oral cholecystography or IV cholangiography
      e. Endoscopic retrograde cholangiopancreatography (ERCP)
      f. CBC, electrolytes including calcium and phosphorus, BUN, creatinine, glucose, alkaline phosphatase, ALT, AST, LDH, gamma GT, bilirubin (total, direct, indirect), total protein, cholesterol, amylase, lipase
  B. Analysis
    1. Acute Pain related to fat ingestion, gallstones, and invasive interventions
    2. Imbalanced Nutrition: Less Than Body Requirements related to pain or discomfort with eating, obstructed bile flow, and decreased absorption of vitamins A, D, E, and K
    3. Ineffective Therapeutic Regimen Management related to lack of knowledge of diet and treatment
    4. Anxiety related to symptoms, lack of knowledge of the disorder, and treatments
    5. Risk for Impaired Gas Exchange related to pain and altered breathing pattern
    6. Risk for Infection related to biliary obstruction or procedure complication
    7. Risk for Bleeding related to malabsorption of vitamin K or procedure complication
  C. Planning
    1. Relieve pain, nausea, vomiting, and discomfort.
    2. Resolve underlying cause.
    3. Prevent complications.
    4. Maintain adequate nutritional status.
  D. Implementation
    1. Provide analgesics, antiemetics, antispasmodics, antipyretics, antibiotics, as needed.
    2. Monitor for relief of symptoms.
    3. Promote treatment with low-fat diet, nonsurgical interventions for eliminating gallstones, or cholecystectomy.
    4. Provide client and family teaching about disease process, diagnostic tests, diet, medications, and interventional or surgical therapy.
  E. Evaluation
    1. Client is afebrile, and vital signs and laboratory results are within normal range.
    2. Client confirms relief of pain and associated symptoms.

3. Client states understanding of diet, medications, treatments, and any activity restrictions.

III. Client needs

A. Physiologic adaptation: Acute pain from gallbladder disorders is treated in the hospital setting. An expectant management (wait-and-see) approach may be used for clients having gallstones with no symptoms or at low risk. Surgical interventions may be indicated (see following discussion). Complications include infection, bile duct obstruction, respiratory compromise, bleeding, pancreatitis, and liver dysfunction.
   1. Nonsurgical interventions for cholelithiasis:
      a. ERCP with endoscopic sphincterotomy (ES) is the most frequently used procedure for detecting and managing common bile duct stones.
      b. Dissolution therapy
         (1) Oral dissolution therapy for clients with small, cholesterol gallstones—ursodeoxycholic acid (ursodiol) Actigall or chenodiol (Chenix).
         (2) Contact dissolution therapy—injection of organic solute, MTBE, into the gallbladder.
      c. Extracorporeal shock wave lithotripsy.
   2. Surgical intervention: Cholecystectomy—usually indicated for clients with acute cholecystitis. Clients with pain and presence of gallstones without inflammation may electively choose a cholecystectomy.
      a. Laparoscopic cholecystectomy is performed in the majority of cases for acute cholecystitis not accompanied by infection or perforation.
      b. Open, incision cholecystectomy may be used for clients with extensive previous abdominal surgery, technical difficulty, or with complications such as empyema, gangrene, or perforation.

B. Management of care: Care of the client with a disorder of the gallbladder requires critical thinking skills and knowledge of assessment, and teaching and evaluation methods unique to the RN role. These skills cannot be delegated to an LPN or UAP.
   1. Delegate responsibly those activities that can be delegated, including basic care needs and checking of vital signs for the stable client. All monitoring information must be reported to the RN.
   2. Perform comprehensive physical assessments and provide care to the symptomatic client with acute cholecystitis.
   3. Provide information on changes in client status to the physician and appropriate members of the multidisciplinary team.
   4. Provide teaching to the client and family regarding medications, maintaining a low-fat diet, and information to prepare the client for diagnostic tests and nonsurgical or surgical interventions.
   5. Provide interventions for ERCP procedure for diagnosis and gallstone removal.
      a. Explain procedure to client and obtain informed consent.
      b. Maintain NPO status after midnight or 8 hr prior to procedure.
      c. Assure IV placement.
      d. Administer sedation medication; monitor client and perform safety precautions.
      e. Spray pharynx with local anesthetic to minimize the gag reflex and discomfort from passage of endoscope.
      f. Monitor for signs of respiratory depression—keep naloxone (Narcan) available for narcotic reversal; keep resuscitation equipment readily available.
      g. Maintain NPO status postprocedure until return of gag and swallow reflex.
      h. Monitor client for development of abdominal pain, nausea, vomiting, fever, signs of bleeding and infection, and pancreatitis.
      i. Inform client of possible sore, hoarse throat for several days following procedure.
   6. Provide pre- and postoperative interventions for laparoscopic cholecystectomy.
      a. Explain procedure to client (four small incision are made for laparoscope and instrument insertion) and obtain informed consent.
      b. Administer general anesthesia.
      c. Maintain NPO status after midnight prior to surgery.
      d. Manage pain with oral narcotic medications—less postoperative pain with laparoscopic rather than the open procedure; client may complain of referred pain to shoulder from CO_2 not absorbed.
      e. Monitor for signs of respiratory complications from CO_2 including irritation of phrenic nerve and diaphragm, bleeding, and infection.
      f. Provide discharge teaching (see health promotion and maintenance).
   7. Provide pre- and postoperative care for open, incisional cholecystectomy.

a. Explain procedure to client (gallbladder is removed from a right subcostal incision) and obtain informed consent.
b. Administer general anesthesia.
c. Maintain NPO status after midnight prior to surgery.
d. Assess vital signs, SpO_2, pain level, incision, and signs of infection or bleeding.
e. Maintain NPO status, NG tube to low continuous suction until return of bowel sounds.
   (1) Monitor amount and appearance of drainage and for return of bowel sounds.
   (2) Manage diet following discontinuation of NG tube and return of bowel sounds; begin with clear liquids and advance diet as tolerated.
f. Instruct and reinforce deep-breathing exercises or incentive spirometry every hour while awake; encourage ambulation (see also basic care and comfort).
g. Provide discharge teaching (see health promotion and maintenance).

C. Safety and infection control: Promote interventional treatment for client with gallstones larger than 3 cm—client at risk for gallbladder cancer, and Pima Native Americans are considered at high risk for complications.

D. Health promotion and maintenance: Provide client and family discharge teaching.
1. For client with laparoscopic cholecystectomy, discharge occurs on day of surgery or next day.
   a. Resume previously tolerated diet and gradually add fat back into diet as tolerated.
   b. Remove dressings from incision the day after surgery; Steri-Strips remain until they fall off. Inspect incisions daily for redness, swelling, bile or pus drainage, and wash sites with mild soap and water.
   c. Resume bathing or showering 1 to 2 days after surgery.
   d. Resume driving a car after 3 to 4 days, unless taking narcotics for pain.
   e. Monitor temperature daily for a week after returning home; report signs of infection at incision sites, severe abdominal pain, nausea, vomiting, chills, fever, or jaundice.
   f. Begin ambulating immediately after surgery and gradually resume full activity and return to work in 1 week.
2. For open, incisional cholecystectomy, discharge occurs within 2 to 4 days.
   a. Resume previously tolerated diet and gradually add fat back into diet as tolerated.
   b. Inspect incision daily for redness, swelling, bile or pus drainage, and wash with mild soap and water.
   c. Monitor temperature daily for 1 week after returning home; report signs of infection at incision site, severe abdominal pain, nausea, vomiting, chills, fever, or jaundice.
   d. Resume activity as tolerated; avoid heavy lifting for 4 to 6 weeks.
   e. Resume driving a car in 2 to 4 weeks.
   f. Return to work in 4 to 6 weeks.
   g. If client has a T-tube, provide instructions on care until it is removed—position to maintain drainage flow; measure drainage; and perform dressing changes and skin care.
   h. Follow up with health care provider (HCP).

E. Psychologic integrity
1. Recognize older clients have higher risk of complications and less endurance for exercise and resilience during postoperative recovery.
2. Identify stress factors and anxiety that may interfere with recovery.
3. Assess client's social support and home health care needs, especially with shorter length of stay after gallbladder surgery.

F. Basic care and comfort
1. Teach pain management to promote postoperative activities following surgery, such as deep breathing and increased activity.
2. Administer pain medication prior to postoperative activities.
3. Teach client to splint incision, if indicated.

G. Reduction of risk potential: Monitor for complications of ERCP and surgery, including infection, bleeding, pancreatitis, and injury of common bile duct.

H. Pharmacology and parenteral therapies: Client will state the purpose, usage, and associated side effects for all medications used to treat disorders of the gallbladder. Some HCPs avoid use of morphine sulfate for pain control because of concern for potential sphincter of Oddi spasms.
1. Meperidine (Demerol) IV is suggested in most reference books, but concerns exist with effectiveness in control of pain and neurologic side effects.
2. Hydromorphone (Dilaudid) IV is an appropriate alternative used in the clinical setting.

Disorders of the Liver: Hepatitis, Cirrhosis, Cancer of the Liver

I. Definition: Common disorders of the liver include inflammation (hepatitis), fibrosis (cirrhosis), and tumors (liver cancer).
   A. Hepatitis is an inflammation of the liver. There are several types of hepatitis, including viral (most common), toxic, autoimmune, and nonalcoholic steatohepatitis (NASH). Hepatitis involves inflammatory infiltration of hepatic tissue, causing swelling, hepatic cell degeneration, and localized areas of necrosis. This process distorts the normal lobular pattern, increasing portal vein pressure and obstructing bile channels. Systemic effects are caused by circulating immune complexes and a major inflammatory response. Liver cell regeneration can occur with return of normal hepatic function if no complications result and the causative factor is resolved.
      1. Viral hepatitis
         a. Hepatitis A virus (HAV) is transmitted though the fecal-oral route, is usually self-limiting, has an acute onset, and mild symptoms.
         b. Hepatitis B virus (HBV) is transmitted percutaneously through contact with blood and body secretions or by blood transfusions, as well as sexual contact and perinatal transmission. HBV can develop into a chronic state with risk of hepatocellular carcinoma and cirrhosis.
         c. Hepatitis C virus (HCV) is primarily transmitted percutaneously or through blood or blood products. High-risk sexual behavior and perinatal transmission are also means of transmission. HCV is usually mild in presentation and the patient may be asymptomatic. Seventy-five percent to 85% of clients develop chronic infection; 20% of clients develop cirrhosis. HCV is the leading indication for liver transplantation in the United States. Clients are at risk for hepatocellular carcinoma.
         d. Hepatitis D virus (HDV) is a defective RNA virus causing infection only in the presence of HBV as a coexistent infection with HBV or suprainfection in an HBV carrier. HDV can accelerate chronic active hepatitis and has a higher rate of causing fulminant hepatitis than HBV alone. HDV is transmitted parenterally.
         e. Hepatitis E virus (HEV) is transmitted via the fecal-oral route and contaminated water primarily in developing countries. Clinical symptoms are similar to HAV, usually mild, and resolve on their own.
      2. Toxic hepatitis involves liver injury and necrosis as a result of exposure to a toxic substance or drug. Pathophysiologic changes are similar to those of viral hepatitis. Timely removal of the toxic substance may curtail damage to the liver. Complications include fulminant hepatic failure and cirrhosis.
      3. Autoimmune hepatitis is caused by the body's own immune system attacking the liver. Immunosuppressive drugs are used to deter progression. Progressive necrosis and inflammation lead to cirrhosis.
      4. Nonalcoholic steatohepatitis (NASH) involves fatty accumulation in the liver, along with inflammation occurring in clients who drink little or no alcohol. NASH can progress to cirrhosis.
   B. Cirrhosis is a chronic, progressive liver condition with extensive degeneration and destruction of liver cells and lobules with fibrotic tissue replacement. Fibrotic changes are irreversible, resulting in chronic liver dysfunction and eventual end-stage liver disease. Types of cirrhosis are as follow:
      1. Alcoholic or Laënnec cirrhosis involves fibrosis around portal areas; due to alcohol toxicity and related malnutrition.
      2. Postnecrotic cirrhosis involves scar tissue; can be caused by acute viral hepatitis.
      3. Biliary cirrhosis involves scaring around the bile ducts; can be caused by infection of the gallbladder (cholangitis).
      4. Cardiac cirrhosis is due to right-sided heart failure, which causes congestion in the liver.
   C. Cancer of the liver may be primary (rare) or secondary, involving metastases.
      1. Primary liver cancer arises directly from the liver. It is uncommon and usually associated with chronic liver disease, HBV, HCV, and cirrhosis. Hepatocellular carcinoma is the most common primary liver cancer.
      2. Secondary or metastatic cancer of the liver originates from another organ and spreads to the liver via the blood, lymphatic channels, or direct extension of the tumor. The liver is a common site for metastases from cancer originating in the colon, rectum, stomach, breast, and lung.

II. Nursing process
A. Assessment
1. Obtain a detailed health and psychosocial history.
a. Recent travel
b. Diet, alcohol consumption
c. Alteration in sleep patterns or bowel habits
d. Recent flulike symptoms
e. Cultural and sexual practices
f. Exposure to viral hepatitis or hepatotoxic drugs or agents
g. History of IV drug abuse, tattoos, and body piercing
h. History of blood transfusions, dental procedures, and surgery
2. Perform a comprehensive physical examination to assess for signs and symptoms of liver dysfunction.
a. General malaise and fatigue
b. GI symptoms
(1) Anorexia; nausea and vomiting; weight loss or malnutrition; change in bowel habits
(2) Ascites, abdominal pain, hepatomegaly, splenomegaly, and clay-colored stools
(3) Esophageal, gastric, and rectal varices
c. Integumentary symptoms, including fever, jaundice, pruritus, spider angiomas, caput medusae, palmar erythema, edema ecchymosis, and bleeding tendency
d. Neurologic symptoms, including personality changes; peripheral neuropathy; asterixis; and hepatic encephalopathy, the most advanced stage of which is hepatic coma
(1) Stage 1—mild confusion, irritability, disturbed sleep, slowing of mental tasks
(2) Stage 2—drowsiness, marked slowing of mentation, confusion, and disorientation
(3) Stage 3—somnolence, but arousable; marked confusion; incomprehensible speech; unable to perform mental tasks; may be disruptive or violent
(4) Stage 4—coma
e. Cardiovascular, pulmonary, and renal symptoms
(1) Activity intolerance, dysrhythmias
(2) Diminished lung expansion and breath sounds, dyspnea, decreased SpO_2
(3) Dark urine, decreased urine output
f. Reproductive symptoms, including gynecomastia, testicular atrophy, impotence, and erratic menses
3. Assess for complications of liver failure.
a. Jaundice
b. Portal hypertension
c. Ascites
d. Esophageal, gastric, and rectal varices
e. Coagulopathy
f. Hepatic encephalopathy
g. Infection
h. Hepatorenal syndrome
i. Cerebral edema
4. Obtain diagnostic tests.
a. Abdominal x-ray
b. Abdominal ultrasound
c. CT scan
d. MRI
e. Arteriography
f. Hepatobiliary scintography
g. Endoscopy
h. Liver biopsy
i. Diagnostic paracentesis
j. Laboratory results
(1) CBC, basic metabolic panel (Chem 7), calcium, magnesium, phosphorus
(2) Prothrombin time (PT)/international normalized ratio (INR), partial thromboplastin time (aPTT), platelet count, fibrinogen level
(3) Hepatitis serologic testing
(4) Aspartate aminotransferase (AST), alanine aminotransferase (ALT), alkaline phosphatase, gamma-glutamyl transpeptidase (GGT or GGTP), lactate dehydrogenase (LDH)
(5) Total, direct, and indirect serum bilirubin; urine bilirubin and urobilinogen
(6) Serum albumin, prealbumin, total protein
(7) Serum ammonia
(8) ABGs

B. Analysis
1. Acute Pain: Abdominal, related to enlarged liver, ascites, and abdominal distention
2. Altered Breathing Pattern related to pressure of ascites on diaphragm, atelectasis, and pleural effusion
3. Activity Intolerance related to fatigue, discomfort, and muscle wasting
4. Imbalanced Nutrition: Less than Body Requirements related to anorexia, nausea, vomiting, and decreased GI motility

5. Impaired Skin Integrity related to jaundice, edema, and impaired immune response
6. Disturbed Body Image related to jaundice, skin alterations, and ascites
7. Risk for Bleeding related to altered clotting factors and esophageal varices
8. Risk for Infection related to decrease in Kupffer cells and filtering of blood in liver, reduced hepatocellular synthesis of immune-related proteins, malnourishment, and invasive procedures
9. Risk for Disturbed Thought Processes related to hepatic encephalopathy, impaired filtering of neurotoxins from blood, electrolyte imbalances, and increased serum ammonia levels
10. Risk for Imbalanced Fluids and Electrolytes related to sodium and water retention, decreased serum albumin, and increased aldosterone

C. Planning
1. Promote liver regeneration.
2. Maintain hemodynamic stability, fluid and electrolyte balance.
3. Relieve abdominal pain and discomfort.
4. Promote nutritional support.
5. Prevent infection.
6. Prevent or resolve complications related to liver dysfunction.
7. Maintain skin integrity.

D. Implementation
1. Monitor physical assessment data, vital signs, SpO_2, and laboratory results.
2. Monitor for relief of symptoms.
3. Provide nutritional diet based on caloric need, presence of edema and ascites, presence of encephalopathy, chronic hepatic disease, infection, and nutritional status prior to hospitalization.
4. Provide client and family teaching about disease process, diagnostic tests, diet, medications, and interventional or surgical therapy.
5. Provide skin care.

E. Evaluation
1. Client is afebrile, and vital signs, SpO_2, and laboratory results are within normal range.
2. Client confirms relief of pain and associated symptoms.
3. Client's neurocognitive function returns to baseline.
4. Client tolerates increasing levels of activity.
5. Client states understanding of diet, medications, and treatments.
6. Client's skin integrity is maintained.

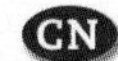

III. Client needs

A. Physiologic adaptation: Stable clients with hepatitis or chronic liver disease are managed on an outpatient basis to promote rest and relieve symptoms of nausea and vomiting, and promote nutrition with high-calorie, low-fat diets and correction of nutritional deficits. The client with severe fluid and electrolyte imbalance may be hospitalized; abdominal paracentesis may be performed to remove fluids. Transjugular intrahepatic portosystemic shunt (TIPS) may be performed for the client with cirrhosis to relieve portal hypertension.
1. Recognize risk for chronic hepatitis from viral, toxic, or autoimmune hepatitis—indicated when symptoms and abnormal laboratory findings persist for greater than 6 months. Liver function tests and serum viral antigens remain elevated. Clients with chronic HBV or HCV are carriers of the virus and remain contagious. Necrosis, active inflammation, and fibrosis may lead to liver failure, cirrhosis, end-stage liver disease, and death.
2. Recognize risk for hepatic failure—initial signs are vague; approximately 75% of liver cell function loss occurs before symptoms of liver failure may be seen. Nonspecific signs and symptoms of malaise are followed by jaundice and onset of altered mental status.
3. Administer medication carefully to older adult client with liver dysfunction because of a decline in blood flow and reduced drug metabolism and drug clearance ability.

B. Management of care: Care of the client with a disorder of the liver requires critical thinking skills and knowledge of assessment, and teaching and evaluation methods unique to the RN role. These skills cannot be delegated to an LPN or UAP.
1. Delegate responsibly those activities that can be delegated. All monitoring information must be reported to the RN.
2. Provide comprehensive physical assessments and monitor the client with acute symptoms of liver dysfunction.
   a. Provide frequent monitoring of vital signs and neurologic signs.
   b. Elevate head of bed at least 30 degrees.
   c. Assess for hepatic encephalopathy; monitor for asterixis, reflexes, ammonia levels (see assessment).
   d. Maintain strict intake and output; measure daily weight and monitor diuretic

response—close monitoring of sodium, potassium, BUN, and creatinine.
e. Assess edema and ascites, abdominal girth, and serum albumin.
f. Monitor SpO_2, respiratory rate, and pattern; auscultate lungs every 4 hr.
g. Encourage deep-breathing exercises or incentive spirometry.
h. Assess for respiratory complications; obtain ABGs and administer oxygen as prescribed.
i. Monitor for signs of bleeding; assess gastric sample and stool for occult blood.
j. Monitor serum glucose levels and Accu-Cheks.
k. Monitor CBC, LFTs, and coagulation factors.

3. Provide information on changes in client status to the physician and appropriate members of the multidisciplinary team.
4. Assist HCP in performing liver biopsy—involves a needle inserted into the eighth or ninth intercostal space midaxillary line to obtain a liver specimen.
   a. Maintain NPO status for 8 hr prior to procedure.
   b. Ensure HCP explains procedure to client and obtains consent for procedure and possible transfusion. Ensure HCP orders PT/INR, aPTT, platelet count, CBC, and type and cross-match prior to procedure.
   c. Instruct client to remain still during procedure—coach client to exhale and stop breathing while needle is inserted during biopsy, or manually ventilate intubated client to prevent lung inflation during puncture.
   d. Assure sterile technique is used throughout procedure.
   e. Provide postprocedure care.
      (1) Position client on right side for 2 hr to tamponade puncture site.
      (2) Auscultate breath sounds and respiratory rate immediately after procedure and every 1 to 2 hr for 8 hr after the procedure for pneumothorax.
      (3) Provide frequent assessment of vital signs and puncture site per agency protocol; monitor for signs of bleeding and infection.
      (4) Instruct bed rest for 8 hr after biopsy to minimize risk of hemorrhage.
      (5) Send biopsy specimen to lab.
      (6) Instruct client to avoid heavy lifting for 1 week.
5. Assist HCP in performing paracentesis—involves a trocar inserted below umbilicus to drain and collect fluid.
   a. Ensure HCP explains procedure to client and consent is obtained.
   b. Assess PT/INR, aPTT, platelet count, CBC.
   c. Instruct client to void.
   d. Place client in an upright position on side of bed, in a chair, or in Fowler position, if on bed rest; place BP cuff.
   e. Assure sterile technique is used throughout procedure.
   f. Monitor BP and heart rate frequently, assessing for signs of hemodynamic instability.
   g. Provide postprocedure care.
      (1) Return client to bed or to comfortable sitting position.
      (2) Measure and assess fluid collected; send samples to lab.
      (3) Provide frequent assessment of vital signs per agency protocol; monitor for hypovolemia and infection.
      (4) Assess puncture site with vital signs.
      (5) Instruct client to avoid heavy lifting.
6. Provide client and family teaching (see health promotion and maintenance, and reduction of risk potential).
7. Facilitate and reinforce need for outpatient follow-up care.
8. Assess for home health care needs such as use of IV fluids, dressing changes, dietary management.
9. Evaluate community resources for support and rehabilitation needs.

C. Safety and infection control
1. For a client with hepatic encephalopathy, ensure a safe environment and use safety and seizure precautions.
2. For a client with a history of alcoholism, monitor and treat for delirium tremens.
3. For a client with HBV, monitor closely for liver dysfunction once treatment for chronic HBV is complete—severe, acute exacerbations of HBV have been reported with discontinuation of antihepatitis B therapy.

D. Health promotion and maintenance: Provide client and family teaching.
1. Decrease metabolic needs of liver with rest and a nutritious diet to help liver tissue

(without fibrotic changes) to regenerate—diet is specific to level of disease and complications:
   a. For client with severe ascites and edema—restrict sodium to 500 mg/day.
   b. For client with hepatic encephalopathy—restrict protein; primarily vegetable sources, or no protein may be indicated for severe encephalopathy.
   c. For client with stable liver disease without evidence of encephalopathy—intake of 0.8 g of protein per kilogram per day.
   d. For client with alcoholism—daily thiamine and folate replacement.
2. Consult with pharmacist, nurse, or physician prior to taking over-the-counter drugs to avoid hepatotoxic drugs.
3. Provide teaching on self-care behaviors, including eliminating alcohol, monitoring daily weights, and maintenance of ideal weight.

E. Psychologic integrity
1. Assess client's adequacy of social support.
2. Assist client and family in coping with lifestyle changes.
3. Introduce support groups for client and family members when hepatic failure is associated with alcohol ingestion, including Alcoholics Anonymous and Al-Anon.

F. Basic care and comfort
1. Monitor and treat pain, nausea, and vomiting.
2. Turn and position client every 2 hr while on bed rest.
3. Provide skin care and protect and monitor skin for areas of bruising, bleeding, and lesions.
4. Provide frequent mouth care.
5. Assist client in maintaining circadian rhythm.

G. Reduction of risk potential
1. Provide client and family teaching.
   a. For clients with chronic viral hepatitis—prevent spread of virus as they are carriers and remain contagious; risk of transmission begins prior to onset of symptoms.
   b. For clients traveling to areas with increased rates of HAV; for known drug users, male homosexuals; and clients with clotting disorders or chronic liver disease—recommend HAV vaccine; immune globulin provides short-term protection within 2 weeks before and after contact with HAV.
   c. For clients with chronic HCV—recommend vaccination against HAV and HBV; HBV vaccine given in the deltoid muscle is available and recommended for all age groups to prevent HBV.
   d. For clients with hepatitis—prevent spread of disease: Use latex condoms correctly; do not share personal care items that may have blood on them (razor, toothbrush, nail clippers, earrings); assure sterile needles used for piercing, tattoos, acupuncture; avoid illegal drugs.
2. Use cautious administration with all medications metabolized by the liver and toxic to the kidneys.
3. Provide close monitoring of drug levels; reduced dosages may be needed to prevent medication toxicity, especially in older adults with liver failure.
4. Provide close monitoring of client having a paracentesis for acute hypovolemia—can occur after the procedure from a fluid shift out of the intravascular space.
5. Keep scissors at bedside for a client with a balloon tamponade tube to allow prompt cutting of balloon to remove tube if sudden acute respiratory distress occurs from a displaced tube blocking the airway.

H. Pharmacology and parenteral therapies: Client will state the purpose, usage, and associated side effects of all medications used to treat disorders of the liver.
1. Diuretics: See Table 20-3
2. Reduction of ammonia level
   a. Lactulose (Cephulac) PO, NGT, or retention enema—dosing adjusted to produce two to three semiformed stools per day; side effects include diarrhea.
   b. Metronidazole (Flagyl)—side effects include nausea, GI disturbance, headache, dizziness, and peripheral neuropathy.
   c. Neomycin sulfate PO, NGT—side effects include nausea, vomiting, diarrhea, renal toxicity, and ototoxicity.
3. Treatment of chronic HBV: Monitor for acute exacerbation of HBV on discontinuation of antihepatitis B therapy.
   a. Interferon alfa-2b (Intron A) IM; peginterferon alfa-2a (Pegasys)—side effects include flu-like symptoms, depression, nausea, vomiting, and diarrhea; following each injection treat with acetaminophen (Tylenol) and diphenhydramine (Benadryl).

b. Lamivudine (Epivir, 3TC) PO—side effects include nausea, vomiting, headaches, peripheral neuropathy, lactic acidosis, pancreatitis, and myopathy.
c. Adefovir dipivoxil (Hepsera) PO—side effects include headache, fatigue, dizziness, fever, increased cough, nausea, vomiting, diarrhea, and lactic acidosis.
d. Entecavir (Baraclude) PO—side effects include headache, fatigue, dizziness, and nausea.
e. Pegylated interferon alfa-2a (Pegasys) SC.

4. Treatment of chronic HCV
   a. Combination therapy:
      (1) Ribavirin (Rebetron) PO—side effects include flu-like symptoms, fatigue, dizziness, nausea, vomiting, musculoskeletal pain, depression, insomnia, black, tarry stools, bleeding gums, blood in urine or stools, chest pain, dyspnea, and hemolytic anemia
      (2) Pegylated interferon alfa-2b (Peg Intron) or pegylated interferon alfa-2a (Pegasys) SC—side effects include flu-like symptoms following each injection, depression, nausea, vomiting, and diarrhea
   b. Interferon alfa-2a (Roferon-A) or interferon alfa-2b (Intron A)—side effects include flu-like symptoms, depression, nausea, vomiting, and diarrhea.

5. Treatment of complications
   a. Ascites and edema not controlled by low-sodium diet:
      (1) Diuretics: Administer with caution because of intravascular volume depletion—includes spironolactone (Aldactone) and furosemide (Lasix).
      (2) IV 25% albumin: Corrects hypoalbuminemia.
      (3) Paracentesis: Temporary measure for refractory ascites with severe respiratory impairment or uncontrolled abdominal pain.
      (4) Peritoneal-venous shunt: For chronic, unresolved ascites—includes LeVeen shunt, Denver shunt.
   b. Antiulcer agents: Histamine 2 antagonists, proton pump inhibitors, or sucralfate (Carafate).
   c. Hepatic encephalopathy/high ammonia levels: Lactulose (Cephulac), metronidazole (Flagyl), or neomycin sulfate.
   d. Coagulopathy/bleeding: Vitamin K, fresh-frozen plasma, platelets, and PRBCs.
   e. Esophageal varices and portal hypertension: Beta blockers, propranolol (Inderal), nadolol (Corgard); and nitrates.
   f. Bleeding esophageal varices:
      (1) Pharmacologic therapy: Octreotide (Sandostatin), more commonly used; and vasopressin (Pitressin), administered with nitroglycerin.
      (2) Endoscopic sclerotherapy or endoscopic ligation (banding).
      (3) Balloon tamponade (Sengstaken-Blakemore tube most common) may be considered if sclerotherapy and vasoconstrictor therapy fail to control variceal bleeding or are contraindicated.
      (4) Shunts to reduce portal hypertension, decompress varices, and control recurrent variceal bleeding:
         (a) Transjugular intrahepatic portosystemic shunt (TIPS procedure).
         (b) Portosystemic shunt surgery—portocaval shunt or distal splenorenal shunt.
   g. Acetaminophen toxicity: *N*-acetylcysteine (Mucomyst).

Disorders of the Pancreas: Pancreatitis and Pancreatic Cancer

I. Definition: Common disorders of the pancreas include inflammation (pancreatitis) and tumors (pancreatic cancer).
   A. Pancreatitis involves acute or chronic inflammation of the pancreas. Major causes include alcoholism and biliary disease.
      1. Acute pancreatitis occurs suddenly and usually resolves; however, the disorder can be severe and life-threatening. Acute pancreatitis results from the premature activation of the digestive enzymes within the pancreas, causing inflammation, necrosis, and autodigestion of the pancreas, which can spread to surrounding organs.
         a. Mild, edematous pancreatitis is more common and has a lower mortality rate. Parenchymal edema and fat necrosis develop.

b. Severe, necrotizing pancreatitis is accompanied by tissue necrosis with associated hemorrhage and infection. Acute necrotizing pancreatitis has a high mortality rate because of serious blood volume depletion and systemic complications.

2. Chronic pancreatitis develops from acute pancreatitis, or in the absence of any acute history. Progressive damage and fibrosis lead to permanent functional loss. Fibrotic changes, strictures, and calcifications damage the exocrine tissue and ductal system, impairing digestion and nutrient absorption. Injury can also occur to endocrine function, leading to diabetes.

B. Pancreatic cancer is rarely detected in its early stage as symptoms of pain, weight loss, jaundice, and digestive problems do not usually appear until the cancer is advanced. Adenocarcinoma is the most common type of pancreatic cancer. Malignant cells often shed into the peritoneum, increasing chances of metastasis. Major risk factors include smoking, long-standing diabetes, chronic pancreatitis, and family history. Prognosis is poor.

II. Nursing process

A. Assessment

1. Obtain a detailed health history and medical, surgical, and psychosocial history.
2. Assess for risk factors for pancreatitis.
   a. Excessive alcohol consumption
   b. Gallstones
   c. Abdominal or surgical trauma to the pancreas
   d. ERCP
   e. Drugs: Thiazide diuretics, furosemide, corticosteroids, estrogen, azathioprine
   f. Hyperlipidemia, high triglycerides
   g. Hypercalcemia, hyperparathyroidism
3. Perform a comprehensive physical examination; assess for signs and symptoms of pancreatitis.
   a. GI symptoms
      (1) Severe abdominal or midepigastric pain (may radiate to the back or flank)
      (2) Nausea, vomiting, and weight loss
      (3) Abdominal tenderness, guarding, distention
      (4) Diminished bowel sounds
      (5) Mild-to-moderate ascites
      (6) Clay-colored stools with biliary obstruction
      (7) Steatorrhea
   b. Cardiovascular, pulmonary, and renal symptoms
      (1) Tachycardia, hypotension, diminished peripheral pulses
      (2) Dyspnea, hypoxia, crackles, diminished breath sounds
      (3) Decreased urine output
   c. Integumentary symptoms
      (1) Fever
      (2) Jaundice with biliary tract disease
      (3) Grey Turner sign and Cullen sign
   d. Neurologic symptoms
      (1) Numbness or tingling in the extremities, tetany
      (2) Chvostek sign, Trousseau sign
4. Assess Ranson's criteria or acute physiology and chronic health evaluation (APACHE) grading system for prediction of severity and mortality.
5. Assess for complications of pancreatitis.
   a. Hypovolemic shock, myocardial depression
   b. Respiratory distress, hypoxia, atelectasis, pleural effusion, ARDS
   c. Pseudocyst, abscess formation
   d. Hypocalcemia
   e. Hyperglycemia
   f. Peritonitis
6. Obtain diagnostic tests.
   a. Abdominal x-ray
   b. Contrast-enhanced computed tomography (CT) of the abdomen
   c. MRI
   d. Ultrasound
   e. ERCP
   f. Biopsy for pancreatic cancer
   g. Laboratory results: Serum and urine amylase, serum lipase, trypsin, electrolytes including calcium, ionized calcium, magnesium, glucose, BUN, creatinine, albumin, CBC, lipid profile, triglycerides, liver function tests, bilirubin, PT/INR, aPTT, platelets, arterial blood gas, stool sample for fat

B. Analysis

1. Acute Pain related to pancreatic inflammation, obstruction, and decreased blood supply
2. Impaired Nutrition: Less Than Body Requirements related to decreased digestive enzymes, malabsorption of nutrients, decreased intake, and alcoholism
3. Risk for Imbalanced Fluids and Electrolytes related to vomiting, inflammation, fluid sequestration, and fat necrosis
4. Impaired Gas Exchange related to altered breathing pattern, inflammatory process extending through diaphragm, atelectasis, and pleural effusion

5. Impaired Skin Integrity related to impaired nutritional status and bed rest
6. Anxiety related to unrelenting pain, lack of knowledge of disease process, and symptoms
7. Risk for Infection related to pseudocyst or abscess formation, and peritonitis

C. Planning
1. Maintain hemodynamic stability, fluid and electrolyte balance.
2. Relieve pain.
3. Promote normal breathing pattern and oxygenation.
4. Maintain normal amylase and lipase levels.
5. Provide adequate nutritional support.
6. Decrease anxiety.
7. Include client and family in care and decision-making.
8. Achieve optimal level of functioning.
9. Prevent or resolve complications.

D. Implementation
1. Monitor physical assessment data, vital signs, SpO_2, and laboratory results; treat abnormalities.
2. Monitor for relief of symptoms.
3. Maintain NPO status initially; assess nutritional status and initiate appropriate nutrition.
4. Provide client and family teaching about disease process, diagnostic tests, diet, medications, and interventional or surgical therapy.

E. Evaluation
1. Client is afebrile, and vital signs, SpO_2, and laboratory results are within normal range.
2. Client verbalizes relief of pain and associated symptoms.
3. Client tolerates PO diet with maintenance of weight.
4. Client exhibits normal patterns of elimination.
5. Client tolerates increasing levels of activity.
6. Client states understanding of diet, medications, and treatments.

CN

III. Client needs

A. Physiologic adaptation: The client with acute pancreatitis is monitored in the intensive care unit until hemodynamically stable (see management of care). The stable client with chronic pancreatitis is managed on an outpatient basis and hospitalized for acute symptoms; surgery may be indicated. Cancer of the pancreas is treated with surgery, radiation therapy, or chemotherapy.
1. Surgical intervention for chronic pancreatitis:
   a. Pancreaticojejunostomy (Puestow procedure) for chronic daily unrelenting pain with narcotic dependence—improves drainage of pancreatic secretions into the jejunum
   b. Drain pseudocyst or debridement of pancreatic necrosis
2. Surgical intervention for pancreatic cancer
   a. Pancreaticoduodenectomy (Whipple procedure)
   b. Total or distal pancreatectomy

B. Management of care: Care of the client with acute pancreatitis occurs within the intensive care unit and requires critical thinking skills and knowledge of assessment, and teaching and evaluation methods unique to the RN role. These skills cannot be delegated to an LPN or UAP.
1. Delegate responsibly those activities that can be delegated. All monitoring information is reported to the RN.
2. Perform comprehensive assessments, and monitor client while in intensive care unit until client is hemodynamically stable.
   a. Perform frequent monitoring of vital signs and neurologic signs.
      (1) Volume replacement for hypovolemia
      (2) Bleeding into the peritoneum: Cullen sign or Turner sign (Grey-Turner's sign)
   b. Monitor peripheral pulses, capillary refill, and skin for pallor and cool extremities.
   c. Assess need for inotropic support with medications such as dopamine or dobutamine.
   d. Monitor amylase, lipase, electrolytes, and CBC.
   e. Monitor calcium levels closely and provide replacement if indicated—monitor for numbness or tingling in the extremities, tetany, Chvostek sign, or Trousseau sign.
   f. Monitor serum glucose levels and Accu-Cheks with insulin sliding scale.
   g. Monitor for signs of infection and sepsis, and systemic complications.
   h. Provide continuous ECG and SpO_2 monitoring.
   i. Monitor respiratory rate and pattern, auscultate lungs; administer oxygen.
   j. Promote deep-breathing exercises or incentive spirometry.
   k. Encourage bed rest; elevate head of bed at 30 degrees.
   l. Initiate Foley catheter insertion.

m. Monitor fluid status; maintain strict intake and output; measure daily weights.
n. Monitor bowel sounds, assess for ascites.
o. Initiate nasogastric tube for severe vomiting, abdominal distention, or ileus—administer medications to treat nausea and vomiting.
p. Perform pain assessment at least every 4 hr, beginning 30 min after pain intervention.
   (1) Provide individualized pain medication scheduling, IV, patient-controlled analgesic (PCA) pump.
   (2) Discuss appropriate opioid use with health care team.
   (3) Monitor hemodynamics, respiratory status, and sedation level.
   (4) Provide nonpharmacologic therapies.
q. Anticipate treatments and procedures and provide explanations and reassurance to client and family.

3. Initiate NPO status to rest the pancreas (stomach or duodenal route of feeding will stimulate pancreas and may induce further inflammation of the pancreas); initiate nutrition once client is hemodynamically stable through a nasoenteric feeding beyond the ligament of Treitz into the jejunum, or with TPN if the client remains NPO.
   a. Bland, low-fat, high-carbohydrate, high-protein diet when PO diet resumes
   b. Pancreatic enzyme replacement prescribed for client with chronic pancreatitis (see pharmacologic and parenteral therapies)
   c. Vitamin replacement for patients with alcoholism; includes multivitamin, thiamin, and folate
4. Provide information on changes in client status to the physician and appropriate members of the multidisciplinary team.
5. Provide client and family teaching (see health promotion and maintenance).
6. Facilitate and reinforce need for continued outpatient follow-up care.
7. Assess for home health care needs such as teaching about dietary management and to assure client is taking medications.
8. Evaluate community resources for support and rehabilitation needs.

C. Safety and infection control: Ensure a safe environment; use safety and seizure precautions when indicated.

D. Health promotion and maintenance: Provide client and family teaching on medications and associated side effects; interventions; low-fat, nonirritating diet; abstinence from alcohol; smoking cessation; monitoring of daily weight; importance of continued follow-up care; need for consultation with physician, nurse, or pharmacist regarding over-the-counter medications; and diabetes management, if needed.

E. Psychologic integrity
   1. Assess client's anxiety level; encourage client and family to verbalize fears and concerns.
   2. Introduce support groups for patient and family members when pancreatitis is associated with alcohol ingestion, including Alcoholics Anonymous and Al-Anon.
   3. Promote client teaching from multidisciplinary team regarding end-of-life considerations for clients with pancreatic cancer; discuss and arrange palliative or hospice care.

F. Basic care and comfort
   1. Monitor and treat pain, nausea, and vomiting.
   2. Consider liberal use of opioid medication and patient-controlled analgesia for the client with advanced pancreatic cancer with severe, escalating pain.
   3. Turn and position client every 2 hr while on bed rest.
   4. Protect and monitor skin for areas of bruising and breakdown.
   5. Provide frequent mouth care; client may be intubated, NPO, susceptible to oral *Candida* with antibiotic administration.
   6. Structure environment to promote rest; limit stimuli and assist in maintaining normal circadian rhythm.

G. Reduction of risk potential: Avoid lipid supplementation with TPN resulting from risk for hyperlipidemia and exacerbation of pancreatitis.

H. Pharmacology and parenteral therapies: Client will state the purpose, usage, and associated side effects used to treat disorders of the pancreas.
   1. Pancreatic enzymes: Pancrelipase (Cotazym, Pancrease, Ultrase, Viokase, Zymase); and pancreatin (Donnazyme, Creon)—promotes weight gain, fewer daily bowel movements, less steatorrhea, and improved feeling of general well-being.
      a. Administer with meals and snacks; do not chew or crush tablets.
      b. Side effects include nausea, vomiting, and diarrhea.

2. For treatment of complications:
   a. Hypovolemia
      (1) Fluid resuscitation with IV normal saline.
      (2) PRBCs, albumin, or fresh-frozen plasma—treats abnormal laboratory findings and complication of hemorrhage.
   b. Pain—hydromorphone (Dilaudid).
   c. Hypocalcemia resulting from fat necrosis—IV calcium replacement for low calcium levels.
   d. Prophylactic antiulcer agents—histamine 2 antagonists, proton pump inhibitors, or sucralfate (Carafate).
   e. Antibiotics for the treatment of identified infections or for necrotizing pancreatitis to reduce the incidence of sepsis.
   f. Hyperglycemia and clients on TPN:
      (1) Perform Accu-Cheks every 4 hr and sliding scale insulin during acute phase.
      (2) Insulin SC or oral hypoglycemic medications to control diabetes.
   g. Antiemetics and anticholinergics to treat symptoms.

Bibliography

Abrams, A. C. (2004). *Clinical drug therapy: Rationales for nursing practice* (7th ed.). Philadelphia: Lippincott Williams & Wilkins.

Cole, L. (1999). Early enteral feeding after surgery. *Critical Care Nursing Clinics of North America, 11*(2), 227–231.

Hogan, M. A. (2005). *Pharmacology: Review & rationales.* Upper Saddle River, NJ: Pearson Prentice Hall.

Ignataviciuc, D. D., & Workman, M. L. (2006). *Medical-surgical nursing* (5th ed.). Philadelphia: Saunders.

Lewis, S., Heitkemper, M., Dirksen, S., O'Brien, P., & Bucher, L. (2007). *Medical-surgical nursing: Assessment and management of clinical problems* (7th ed.). St. Louis: Mosby.

Morton, P. G., Fontaine, D. K., Hudak, C. M., & Gallo, B. M. (2005). *Critical care nursing: A holistic approach* (8th ed.). Philadelphia: Lippincott Williams & Williams.

Porth, C. M. (2007). *Essentials of pathophysiology.* Philadelphia: Lippincott Williams & Wilkins.

Smeltzer, S. C., Bare, B. G., Cheever, K. H., & Hinkle, J. L. (2008). *Brunner & Suddarth's textbook of medical-surgical nursing* (11th ed.). Philadelphia: Lippincott Williams & Wilkins.

Society of American Gastrointestinal and Endoscopic Surgeons. (2004). Patient information for laparoscopic gallbladder removal (cholecystectomy). Retrieved May 20, 2008, from http://www.sages.org/sagespublication.php?doc=PI11

Urden, L. D., Stacy, K. M., & Lough, M. E. (2006). *Thelan's critical care nursing: Diagnosis and management* (5th ed.). St. Louis: Mosby.

CHAPTER 26
Practice Test

Disorders of the Gallbladder: Cholelithiasis, Cholecystitis

1. A client with an incisional cholecystectomy has a nursing diagnosis of ineffective breathing pattern related to splinted, shallow respirations secondary to a high abdominal incision. The client is refusing to get out of bed. The nurse should first:

☐ 1. Administer pain medication.
☐ 2. Assess lung sounds during physical assessment for each shift, particularly the right side.
☐ 3. Instruct client on coughing and deep-breathing every hour.
☐ 4. Lower the head of the bed and position the client on the right side to splint the incision.

2. A client who had a laparoscopic cholecystectomy is receiving discharge teaching on postoperative day 1. What statement by the client shows a need for further teaching?

☐ 1. "I will start with the activity I was doing in the hospital my first day home."
☐ 2. "I will probably have some discomfort for a few days after I go home."
☐ 3. "I will not be able to return to work for 4 to 6 weeks."
☐ 4. "I will monitor my body's response as I gradually add fat back into the regular diet."

3. Which of the following interventions does the nurse place as highest priority when planning care for a client who had an ERCP for cholelithiasis?

- ☐ 1. Assess for return of the gag reflex.
- ☐ 2. Provide saline gargles for an irritated throat.
- ☐ 3. Inform the physician immediately if the client has a hoarse voice.
- ☐ 4. Monitor for bowel sounds.

4. Which diet choice by a client with chronic cholecystitis who is slightly malnourished suggests to the nurse to reinforce diet teaching?

- ☐ 1. Baked, skinless chicken for dinner.
- ☐ 2. Fruit plate for lunch.
- ☐ 3. Oatmeal with bananas for breakfast.
- ☐ 4. Regular milk with meals.

Disorders of the Liver: Hepatitis, Cirrhosis, Cancer of the Liver

5. The nurse is providing discharge information to a client with hepatitis B. The nurse instructs the client to prevent transmission via:

- ☐ 1. Airborne pathogens.
- ☐ 2. Blood and body secretions.
- ☐ 3. Skin contact.
- ☐ 4. Fecal and oral routes.

6. The nurse is assessing a client with chronic hepatitis C who has received interferon alfa-2a (Roferon-A) injections for the last month. The nurse informs the HCP about which of the following?

- ☐ 1. Frequent episodes of nausea, vomiting, and diarrhea.
- ☐ 2. Temperature of 99°F orally and a headache.
- ☐ 3. Fatigue and muscle aches.
- ☐ 4. Daily record indicates a 4-pound weight loss over the last month.

7. A homeless client with jaundice and a history of alcoholism is diagnosed with viral hepatitis. Which client outcome receives lowest priority in the plan of care?

- ☐ 1. Client abstains from alcohol.
- ☐ 2. Client adapts to temporary changes in skin appearance.
- ☐ 3. Client follows good hygiene practices.
- ☐ 4. Client obtains adequate rest and nutrition.

8. A client with cirrhosis is admitted to the hospital with fatigue, shortness of breath, ascites, and 3+ pedal edema. The client has bruises on the hands and arms, is afebrile, with heart rate of 114, respirations 28, and BP at 110/85. Hemoglobin is 8 g/dl. Which of the following nursing goals is a priority for this client?

- ☐ 1. Protect skin integrity.
- ☐ 2. Reduce ascites.
- ☐ 3. Correct nutritional imbalance.
- ☐ 4. Prevent bleeding.

9. A client had a liver biopsy 1 hr ago. The nurse's first action is to:

- ☐ 1. Auscultate lung sounds.
- ☐ 2. Check for fever.
- ☐ 3. Obtain a CBC.
- ☐ 4. Apply packing to the biopsy site.

10. A client is admitted to the hospital with hepatic failure. The nurse assesses the client and finds marked ascites, shortness of breath, pulse 110, and BP of 102/60. What is the first measure taken by the nurse to improve the client's comfort level?

- ☐ 1. Administer 250 ml of 5% albumin IV.
- ☐ 2. Promote diet restriction of protein and fluids.
- ☐ 3. Elevate the head of the bed.
- ☐ 4. Start oxygen at 2 L via nasal cannula.

11. AF The nurse is assessing a client for ascites. Where does the nurse place hands to percuss for the presence of fluid?

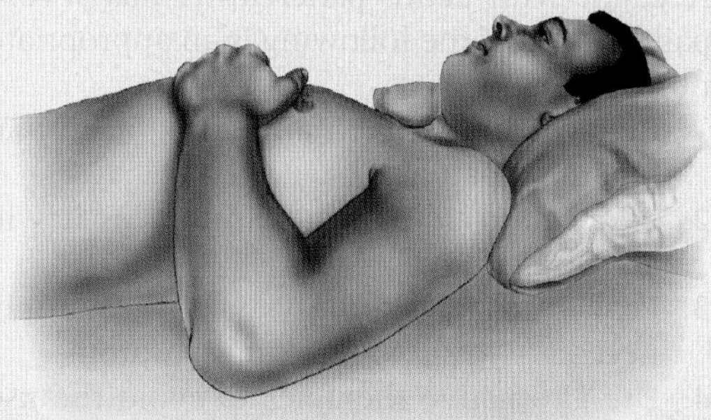

12. AF A client with postnecrotic cirrhosis is receiving lactulose (Cephulac). Which of the following indicate that the drug is having intended outcomes? Select all that apply.

- ☐ 1. Decreased ammonia levels.
- ☐ 2. Reduction in ascites.
- ☐ 3. Improved osmotic pressure.
- ☐ 4. Client alert and oriented.
- ☐ 5. Decreased potassium levels.

13. A client who is 30 years of age with fulminant hepatic failure is not responding to medications. The client has provided clear directives to the family and health care team to use all possible interventions. In collaborating with the surgeon to discuss the next steps in the plan of care, the nurse prepares to teach the family about which of the following interventions?

- ☐ 1. Distal splenorenal shunt.
- ☐ 2. Liver transplantation.
- ☐ 3. Paracentesis.
- ☐ 4. Sengstaken-Blakemore tube placement.

14. The nurse is caring for a client with esophageal varices. The nurse should discuss which of the following laboratory report findings with the HCP?

- ☐ 1. Normal serum albumin.
- ☐ 2. Decreased ammonia.
- ☐ 3. Slightly decreased levels of calcium.
- ☐ 4. Elevated PT/INR.

Disorders of the Pancreas: Pancreatitis and Pancreatic Cancer

15. The nurse is preparing a teaching plan for a client with chronic pancreatitis. Which of the following health behaviors is a priority concern?
- ☐ 1. Client uses low-dose aspirin daily to prevent myocardial infarction.
- ☐ 2. Client drinks four to six alcoholic beverages after work.
- ☐ 3. Client follows high-carbohydrate diet.
- ☐ 4. Client has a prior history of smoking.

16. A client with acute pancreatitis has severe pain. Which of the following is an appropriate nursing goal?
- ☐ 1. Relieve pain while maintaining a normal breathing pattern.
- ☐ 2. Avoid narcotic pain medication as it will accelerate the disorder.
- ☐ 3. Provide analgesics only when absolutely necessary to avoid masking symptoms.
- ☐ 4. Use alternative therapies to avoid the use of narcotics.

17. Which of the following measures should the nurse include in the plan of care for a client with acute pancreatitis?
- ☐ 1. Promote deep-breathing exercises every 2 hr.
- ☐ 2. Restrict IV and PO fluids.
- ☐ 3. Promote frequent ambulation.
- ☐ 4. Prepare client for biopsy.

18. The client is taking pancrelipase (Viokase). The nurse should instruct the client to:
- ☐ 1. Chew pills thoroughly before swallowing.
- ☐ 2. Swallow medication with minimal fluid on an empty stomach.
- ☐ 3. Take medication with meals and snacks.
- ☐ 4. Decrease dose if steatorrhea is present.

19. A client is hospitalized with acute pancreatitis. The client is vomiting, and the serum amylase and lipase levels are elevated. Which of the following will be most effective in initially restoring fluid and electrolyte balance for this client?
- ☐ 1. Offer high-carbohydrate, low-fat diet.
- ☐ 2. Give feedings through a gastrostomy tube.
- ☐ 3. Provide IV fluids and electrolyte replacement.
- ☐ 4. Administer TPN.

20. AF On 1/16/09 at 0800 the nurse is caring for a client with acute pancreatitis and reviewing progress notes as listed below:

PROGRESS NOTES

Date	Time	Progress Notes
1/15/09	0800	*Vital signs are: temperature 37.4 °C; heart rate, 138; BP is 80/48; pain is 9 on a 10-point scale; client is restless.* —Robin Brown, RN
1/15/09	1000	*Discussed following lab values with A. Smith, MD; hematocrit is 27.6%, hemoglobin is 7.6 g/dl, platelet count is 245,000 mm³, and INR is 0.8.* —Robin Brown, RN
1/15/09	1100	*PRBCs infused; no adverse reactions.* —Robin Brown, RN

Which of the following indicates that the desired outcome of the transfusion is obtained at this time?
- ☐ 1. BP is 110/80.
- ☐ 2. Pain is 4 on a 10-point scale.
- ☐ 3. Hemoglobin is 12 g/dl.
- ☐ 4. Platelet count is $144,000/mm^3$.

Answers and Rationales

1. 1 Abdominal incisions are painful. The nurse's first action is to administer pain medication to promote deep breathing and to assist the client in getting out of bed, which decreases the risk of postoperative complications such as atelectasis and pneumonia. The nurse assesses lung sounds more frequently in the postoperative period. Clients with abdominal pain will find it difficult to take deep breaths and cough. The first step is to relieve the pain so the client can get out of bed and then do deep-breathing and coughing exercises. The head of bed is elevated to promote lung expansion. (R)

2. 3 A client can gradually increase to normal activity, and return to work within 1 week of surgery. The client may need oral pain medication for a few days; the nurse instructs the client to contact the HCP if pain persists. The client can return to a regular diet, but should gradually increase fat as tolerated because bile is no longer concentrated and directly flows from the liver. (H)

3. 1 After an endoscopic procedure, the nurse's highest priority is assessing gag and swallow reflex before the client takes anything by mouth. The client may have a sore or hoarse voice for a few days. Bowel sounds should be monitored but are not the top priority. (R)

4. 4 A low-fat diet is prescribed for clients with chronic cholecystitis; fat stimulates gallbladder and symptoms. Nonfat milk is substituted for regular milk. (H)

5. 2 Hepatitis B is transmitted via blood and body secretions. The nurse instructs the client to prevent transmission through correct usage of latex condoms, and by not sharing personal care items that may have blood on them. Diseases such as pneumonia are spread by airborne pathogens; hepatitis A is spread by fecal and oral routes. Hepatitis B is not transmitted by skin contact. (S)

6. 1 The nurse reports to the HCP side effects of interferon alfa-2 such as nausea, vomiting and diarrhea, as they can lead to complications such as fluid and electrolyte imbalances and malnutrition. Fatigue and muscle aches are symptoms of hepatitis and are expected at this time. The mild elevation of temperature and weight loss are monitored closely, but are not as significant as the persistent nausea, vomiting, and diarrhea. (D)

7. 2 Abstinence from alcohol, prevention of infection with good hygiene, rest, and nutrition are essential for recovery from hepatitis. Once the client recovers from hepatitis, the jaundice will resolve. (A)

8. 2 This client has many needs, but the nurse's priority is to reduce ascites; the nurse keeps the client on bed rest to aid diuresis, administers diuretics as ordered, and restricts fluid intake if indicated. The client has impaired skin integrity from ascites and poor nutritional state. The client is anemic; therefore, the nurse promotes high-calorie, moderate-protein foods and supplementary feedings. Because the client is at risk for bleeding (as indicated by the bruising), the nurse assesses for signs of external and internal bleeding. (A)

9. 1 Because the biopsy needle insertion site is close to the lung, there is a risk of lung puncture and pneumothorax; therefore, the nurse's first measure immediately after the procedure is to determine diminished or absent lung sounds in the right lung. Although fever indicates infection, a rise in temperature is not seen immediately. A CBC is warranted if the vital signs and client symptoms indicate potential hemorrhage. The needle insertion site is covered with a pressure dressing; there is no need for a dressing requiring packing. (R)

10. 3 The nurse reduces pressure of ascites on the diaphragm and lungs by raising the head of the bed. Additional fluid and sodium (5% albumin in normal saline) will increase ascites. Ascites is treated with a low-sodium diet and diuretics. No data support using oxygen. (A)

11. The nurse places the client in supine position and percusses each flank for shifting dullness. If fluid is present, dullness is noted. (A)

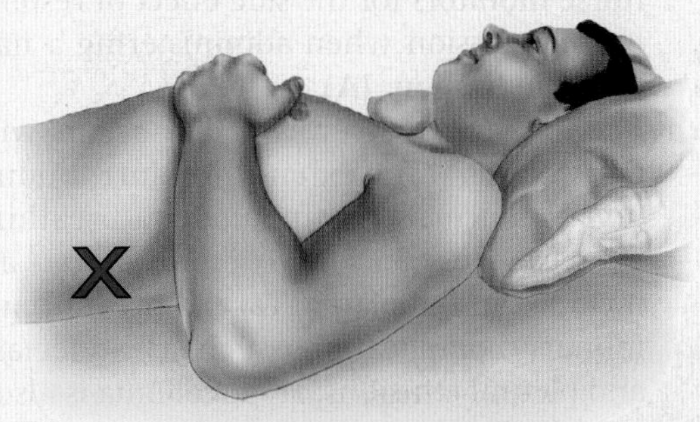

12. 1, 4 Lactulose (Cephulac) is a medication used to lower ammonia levels and decrease hepatic encephalopathy; therefore, the client has lower ammonia levels and improved mentation. Albumin is used to increase colloid osmotic pressure to pull fluid back into the vascular space. A paracentesis is a treatment for severe, symptomatic ascites. Diuretics are also used to reduce ascites; the nurse assesses the client for decreased potassium levels as a potential side effect of diuretic use. (D)

13. 2 A client with an acutely failing liver who is unresponsive to therapy requires transplantation for survival. Distal splenorenal shunt, paracentesis, and Sengstaken-Blakemore tube placement are treatments for liver failure complications from chronic liver disease. (P)

14. 4 The client with esophageal varices is at even higher risk for bleeding with elevated PT/INR. The nurse and HCP collaborate to prevent bleeding. The other laboratory findings are not as life-threatening. A decreased serum albumin can cause fluid to move into the interstitial tissues. Increased ammonia levels are toxic to the brain. Calcium loss is more common to pancreatitis. (R)

15. 2 Because alcoholism and gallstones are the leading causes of pancreatitis, the nurse assists the client to stop drinking. A bland, low-fat, high-carbohydrate, high-protein diet is indicated for pancreatitis. Smoking increases the risk of pancreatitis, especially in association with consumption of alcohol, but the client has stopped smoking. Although aspirin is not a drug that induces pancreatitis, the nurse considers the side effect of risk of bleeding. (H)

16. 1 The most common symptom of pancreatitis is severe pain; therefore, the nurse develops a nursing care plan to manage pain. Narcotics are usually required to achieve pain relief; analgesics or alternative therapies are not sufficient to manage severe pain. The nurse monitors for the side effect of respiratory depression when administering a narcotic medication. (A)

17. 1 The inflammatory process that occurs with pancreatitis can extend to surrounding organs, such as the lung. Deep-breathing exercises or incentive spirometry are included in the plan of care to prevent pulmonary complications such as atelectasis and pleural effusions. Hypovolemia is also a complication, requiring an increased fluid volume. During the initial stages of acute pancreatitis, clients are NPO. Hemodynamic instability with acute pancreatitis requires bed rest. A biopsy is not a normal diagnostic procedure for acute pancreatitis; the client may have enzyme studies, CT scans, and x-rays. (R)

18. 3 Pancreatic enzymes are swallowed to prevent activation while in the mouth. The medication is taken with meals to assist with digestion. Steatorrhea indicates a need to increase the dose. (D)

19. 3 The client with acute pancreatitis does not receive oral food or fluids in order to rest the GI tract and decrease pancreatic secretions. The nurse first administers IV fluids to replace lost fluids and electrolytes. Once the client is stable, the nurse considers nasoenteric feedings into the jejunum. TPN is not used as long as nutrition can be otherwise managed. The client will not have oral fluids until the acute inflammation has been managed. (A)

20. 3 PRBCs are ordered to improve the low hemoglobin level; therefore, the nurse assesses for an increase in hemoglobin. The PRBCs do not increase BP; colloid solutions are needed to increase the circulating blood volume and raise the BP. The client has acute pain and requires the use of analgesia to minimize the pain. The platelet count is within normal limits and is not affected by the infusion of PRBCs. (R)

chapter

27 The Client With Endocrine Health Problems

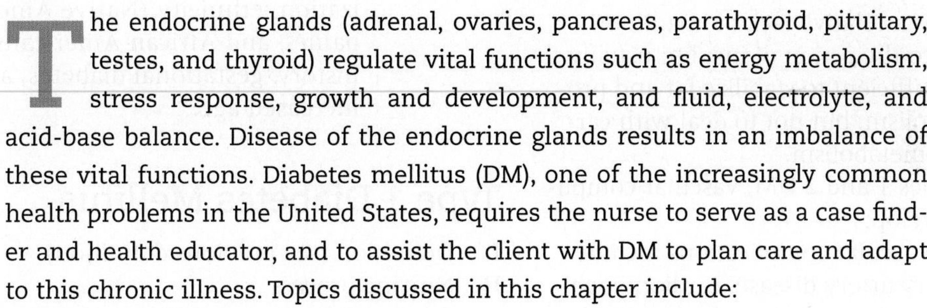

The endocrine glands (adrenal, ovaries, pancreas, parathyroid, pituitary, testes, and thyroid) regulate vital functions such as energy metabolism, stress response, growth and development, and fluid, electrolyte, and acid-base balance. Disease of the endocrine glands results in an imbalance of these vital functions. Diabetes mellitus (DM), one of the increasingly common health problems in the United States, requires the nurse to serve as a case finder and health educator, and to assist the client with DM to plan care and adapt to this chronic illness. Topics discussed in this chapter include:

- Diabetes Mellitus
- Thyroid Disease: Hypothyroidism and Hyperthyroidism
- Disorders of the Anterior Pituitary: Hypopituitarism and Hyperpituitarism
- Disorders of the Posterior Pituitary: Diabetes Insipidus and Syndrome of Inappropriate Antidiuretic Hormone
- Adrenal Disease: Addison Disease and Cushing Disease (Cushing Syndrome)
- Pheochromocytoma

Diabetes Mellitus

I. Definition: Diabetes mellitus (DM) is a chronic, multisystem disease affecting about 20% of the total United States population. DM results from dysfunctional glucose transport into the body.
   A. Pathophysiology
      1. Insulin facilitates glucose transport into cells for oxidation and energy production. Food intake, glycogen breakdown, and gluconeogenesis increase the serum glucose level, which stimulates the beta cells in the islets of Langerhans in the pancreas to release the required insulin for transport of glucose from the bloodstream into cells.
      2. In DM, there is impaired glucose transport because of decreased or absent insulin secretion and/or ineffective insulin action. Metabolism of carbohydrates, protein, and fat is altered. The client is unable to store glucose in liver and muscle as glycogen, store fatty acids and triglycerides in adipose tissue, and transport amino acids into cells.
   B. Type 1 and type 2 DM
      1. *Type 1 DM* is a nearly absolute deficiency of insulin; if insulin is not given exogenously, fats are metabolized, resulting in ketonemia (metabolic acidosis).
      2. *Type 2 DM* is a relative lack of insulin or resistance to the action of insulin; usually insulin is sufficient to stabilize fat and protein metabolism, but not to deal with carbohydrate metabolism.
      3. In both types 1 and 2 DM, vascular complications develop:
         a. Macrovascular complications include coronary artery disease, cardiomyopathy, hypertension, cerebrovascular disease, peripheral vascular disease, and infection.
         b. Microvascular complications include nephropathy (kidney), neuropathy (nerves), and retinopathy (eyes).
   C. Additional types and variations of DM
      1. *Gestational DM* is detected during 24 to 28 weeks' gestation; glucose levels are generally normal 6 weeks' postpartum. The client with gestational DM is more likely to develop type 2 DM 5 to 10 years after delivery. The neonate exhibits macrosomia, hypoglycemia, hypocalcemia, and hyperbilirubinemia. (See also Chapter 5.)
      2. *Secondary DM* is associated with other conditions or syndromes such as Cushing syndrome and pancreatic disease. Treatment with glucocorticoid medication (prednisone [Deltasone]) or the use of TPN may also produce secondary DM. Once the underlying condition is treated, secondary DM is usually resolved.
      3. Although not an official classification category by the American Diabetes Association, *prediabetes,* or *impaired glucose tolerance,* refers to mild alteration in beta cell function; blood glucose level is higher than normal, but not high enough for a diagnosis of diabetes. Most clients with impaired glucose tolerance are at increased risk for developing type 2 DM within 10 years. Overweight clients with impaired glucose tolerance can prevent or delay the onset of type 2 DM through a program of weight loss and regular physical activity.
      4. *Insulin resistance syndrome* (metabolic syndrome) is a cluster of abnormalities acting synergistically to greatly increase the risk for cardiovascular disease. The syndrome is characterized by elevated insulin levels, high levels of triglycerides, decreased levels of high-density lipoproteins, increased levels of low-density lipoproteins, and hypertension. Risk factors include central obesity, sedentary lifestyle, polycystic ovary syndrome, urbanization/Westernization, ethnicity (Native Americans, Hispanics, and African Americans), family history, gestational diabetes, and increased age.

Type 1 Diabetes Mellitus

I. Definition (see previous definition)
II. Nursing process
   A. Assessment
      1. Assess onset—occurs rapidly (usually over a few weeks).
      2. Assess for signs and symptoms.
         a. Major symptoms: Increased thirst and appetite, frequent urination, enuresis (involuntary discharge of urine), weight loss, and fatigue
         b. Minor symptoms: Dry skin, skin infections, poor wound healing, and candidal vaginitis (in females)
      3. Assess for manifestations of diabetic ketoacidosis.
         a. Early manifestations include:
            (1) Polydipsia
            (2) Polyuria
            (3) Fatigue
            (4) Malaise
            (5) Drowsiness

(6) Anorexia
(7) Nausea, vomiting
(8) Abdominal pain
(9) Muscle cramps

b. Later signs include:
(1) Kussmaul (deep, rapid) respirations
(2) Acetone breath (fruity, sweet odor)
(3) Hypotension
(4) Weak pulse
(5) Stupor, coma

4. Obtain diagnostic tests.
   a. Random blood glucose 200 mg/dl or greater
   b. Fasting blood glucose 126 mg/dl or greater

B. Analysis
1. Deficient Knowledge related to diabetes self-management
2. Fear related to unknown outcomes
3. Imbalanced Nutrition: Less Than Body Requirements related to altered utilization of ingested food
4. Ineffective Family Therapeutic Regimen Management related to ongoing time demands
5. Risk for Deficient Fluid Volume related to polyuria
6. Risk for Infection related to impaired wound healing

C. Planning
1. Maintain optimal body weight.
2. Remain free from infection.
3. Avoid complications.
4. Increase understanding of disorder and treatment.
5. Promote adaptive coping behaviors.

D. Implementation (see basic care and comfort)

E. Evaluation
1. Client maintains optimal body weight.
2. Client has no signs or symptoms of infection.
3. Client is free from evidence of complications.
4. Client verbalizes knowledge of DM and its treatment.
5. Client demonstrates adaptive coping behaviors.

CN

III. Client needs

A. Physiologic adaptation: The goal of management of type 1 DM is to maintain normal blood glucose levels with diet, exercise, and insulin therapy.
1. Insulin therapy, including diabetic ketoacidosis treatment (low-dose continuous IV infusion of regular insulin only). *Note: Lispro (Humalog) insulin is not approved for IV administration.*
   a. Reduces hyperglycemia and inhibits lipolysis and ketogenesis.
   b. Dosages adjusted through daily monitoring of blood glucose levels.
2. Balanced diet with controlled carbohydrate and adequate protein and fat to meet energy and growth requirements.

B. Management of care: Care of the client with type I DM requires critical thinking skills and knowledge of assessment, and teaching and evaluation methods unique to the RN role. These skills cannot be delegated to an LPN or UAP. (See Chapter 15 for management of care of the child with type 1 DM.)
1. Provide client and family teaching about managing diet, exercise, and insulin therapy (see safety and infection control).
2. Instruct client about maintaining overall health.
3. Collaborate with interdisciplinary team (health care provider [HCP], dietician, and others as needed).

C. Safety and infection control: Provide client and family teaching about factors that influence insulin therapy, especially exercise and preventing infection.
1. Exercise lowers blood glucose level—encourage normal activity, regulated in amount and time.
2. Infection and illness increase insulin requirement (insulin still administered during illness)—alert client to signs of infection and dehydration; instruct about prevention of infection:
   a. Perform regular body hygiene with special attention to foot care.
   b. Report breaks in skin; treat promptly.
   c. Wear properly fitted shoes; do not wear vinyl or plastic, which lack ventilation. Take measures to prevent calluses and blisters.
   d. Dress appropriately for weather.
   e. Promote regular dental checkups (maintenance every 6 months).
   f. Follow routine immunizations according to recommended schedule.

D. Health promotion and maintenance: Provide client and family teaching.
1. Observe activity tolerance, emotional stress, and other illnesses as influences on both insulin and nutritional needs.
2. Recognize causes, signs and symptoms, and treatment for hypoglycemia.
   a. Watch for pattern of activity and time of day that precedes hypoglycemic reactions, and work with client to alter behavior to prevent.

b. Use glucagon in emergency (include family member in teaching).
3. Teach home blood glucose monitoring.
a. Determine blood glucose at least 4 times per day—before meals and before bedtime snack (may be more frequently).
b. Manage DM by testing blood glucose, recording results, and reporting results to physician, certified diabetes educator, and caretaker.
4. Carry medical identification; when traveling, carry insulin because baggage may be subjected to extreme temperatures and pressures incompatible with insulin's stability.

E. Psychologic integrity
1. Encourage verbalization of feelings.
2. Offer emotional support.
3. Help to develop effective coping strategies.
4. Encourage client to seek counseling; aid in consult with clinical psychologist, as needed.
5. Encourage client to obtain diabetes self-management training.

F. Basic care and comfort
1. Administer prescribed medications.
2. Provide meticulous skin care, especially to feet and legs.
3. Encourage adequate fluid intake.
4. Assess renal and cardiovascular status.
5. Watch for signs and symptoms of hypoglycemia, hyperglycemia; treat as needed.
6. Promote regular aerobic exercise.
7. Reinforce nutrition instruction provide by dietitian.

G. Reduction of risk potential
1. Develop systematic plan for giving insulin injections, emphasizing spacing sites about 1 inch apart:
a. Rotate sites, but stay in same area of body for 1 week: Arms, thighs, abdomen, buttocks, while maintaining the rotation schedule.
b. Never inject into scar, bruised area, reddened area, or areas of lipodystrophy (hypertrophy, atrophy of subcutaneous tissue).
2. Cold insulin is irritating to tissues; instruct client to bring insulin to room temperature.
3. Teach sick-day guidelines: Continue treatment for diabetes, during times of illness because counterregulatory mechanisms increase blood glucose levels dramatically.
a. Continue with regular meal plan, if possible, and continue to increase intake of noncaloric fluids (broth, water, other decaffeinated beverages).
b. Continue taking oral agents and/or insulin as prescribed.
c. Check blood glucose at least every 4 hr.
d. If BG is greater than 240 mg/dl, test urine for ketones every 3 to 4 hr.
(1) Report moderate-to-large ketone levels to physician.
(2) Administer additional insulin as prescribed.
e. When unable to eat, or eating less than normal, continue to take oral antidiabetic medications and/or insulin as prescribed while supplementing food intake with carbohydrate-containing fluids (soups, juices, regular decaffeinated soft drinks).
f. Notify physician promptly if unable to keep any food or fluids down.
4. When surgical intervention needed:
a. Administer IV fluids; administer insulin immediately before, during, after surgery.
b. If client used oral agents, discontinue 48 hr before surgery.
(1) Depending on client's needs, an insulin infusion may be ordered.
(2) Instruct client that discontinuation of oral agents is temporary.
c. When caring for unconscious surgical client receiving insulin, be alert for hypoglycemic signs (sweating; cool, moist skin; tremors, elevated pulse).
5. Teach client and family signs and symptoms of, and differences between, hyperglycemia and hypoglycemia; teach family members how to administer glucagon if severe hypoglycemic reaction occurs (see Table 27-1).

H. Pharmacologic and parenteral therapies: Client will state the purpose for and associated side effects of all medications used to treat type 1 DM.
1. For risk for impending hypoglycemia (blood glucose less than 70 mg/dl) with all insulins, treatment includes:
a. 10 to 15 g of concentrated carbohydrate (five hard candies, 1 tablespoon honey, 1 tablespoon jelly, one very small box of raisins)
b. Glucagon must be available (0.5 to 1 mg) to be administered by family member—IM or SC—if client unresponsive
2. For dehydration or diabetic ketoacidosis—replace fluid losses from osmotic diuresis and vomiting:
a. Infuse IV fluids at slow rate; too rapid infusion in cases of severe dehydration can cause cerebral edema and death.

Table 27-1 Comparison of Hyperglycemia and Hypoglycemia

Manifestations		Treatment	
• Blood glucose greater than 180 mg/dl • Increase in urination • Increase in appetite followed by lack of appetite • Weakness, fatigue • Blurred vision • Headache • Glucosuria • Nausea and vomiting • Abdominal cramps • Progression to diabetic ketoacidosis or hyperglycemic hyperosmolar nonketotic syndrome	• Blood glucose less than 70 mg/dl • Cool, clammy skin • Numbness in fingers, toes, mouth • Rapid pulse • Emotional changes • Headache • Nervousness, tremors • Faintness, dizziness • Unsteady gait • Slurred speech • Hunger • Changes in vision • Seizures, coma	• Contact physician. • Continue diabetes medication as ordered. • Perform frequent checking of blood glucose. • Check urine for ketones. • Drink noncaloric fluids hourly.	• Immediately ingest 10 to 15 g of simple carbohydrates such as hard candy, juice; ingest another 10 to 15 g of simple carbohydrates in 15 min if no relief is obtained. • Administer 0.5 to 1 mg glucagon IM or SC if unable to swallow; assess response. • Call 911 for emergency assistance if unresponsive. • Contact physician. Discuss with physician about medication dosage.
Causes		**Preventive Measures**	
• Too much food • Too little or no diabetes medication • Inactivity • Emotional, physical stress • Poor absorption of insulin	• Alcohol intake without food • Too little food—delayed, omitted, inadequate intake • Too much diabetic medication • Too much exercise without compensation • Diabetes medication or food taken at wrong time • Loss of weight • Use of β-adrenergic blockers interfering with recognition of symptoms of hypoglycemia	• Take prescribed dose of medication at proper time. • Accurate administration of insulin/oral agents. • Maintain diet. • Maintain good personal hygiene. • Adhere to sick-day rules when ill. • Check blood glucose as ordered. • Contact physician regarding ketonuria. • Wear medical identification.	• Take prescribed dose of medication at proper time. • Provide accurate administration of insulin/oral agents. • Ingest all ordered food at proper time. • Provide compensation for exercise. • Recognize and know symptoms of hypoglycemia and treat them immediately. • Carry simple carbohydrates at all times. • Instruct friends, family, fellow employees about symptoms and treatment. • Check blood glucose as ordered. • Wear medical identification.

b. Administer short-acting IV regular insulin drip to increase glucose utilization and decrease lipolysis; treat hyperkalemia by promoting return of potassium back into cells.

3. Replace electrolytes.
   a. Administer sodium chloride and phosphate, as required.
   b. Begin potassium chloride as soon as urine output and renal function are established.
   c. Administer bicarbonate for severe or refractory acidosis.
   d. Start with 0.9% normal saline—isotonic.
   e. Change to 5% dextrose in 0.45% normal saline—hypertonic when glucose falls below 250 mg/dl.
4. Administer insulins.
   a. Classification: Rapid-acting—Lispro (Humalog), aspart (NovoLog), and glulisine (Apidra)
   b. Classification: Short-acting—Regular (R) and inhaled regular (Exubera)
   c. Classification: Intermediate-acting—Lente (L) and NPH (N)
   d. Classification: Long-acting—Ultralente (U), glargine (Lantus), and detemir (Levemir)
   e. Classification: Combination insulins—70/30; 50/50; and 75/25 and 50/50 Humalog mix
5. Administer injectable noninsulin (may be used with insulin)—classification: Analogue of amylin—Pramlintide (Symlin).

6. Administer regular (R) insulin drip through peripheral or central IV site.
   a. Flush entire IV infusion site with solution containing insulin; discard first 50 ml because plastic IV bag and tubing may absorb some insulin, thereby reducing insulin concentration of initial solution.
   b. Glucose normalizes before metabolic acidosis resolves—continue IV insulin until bicarbonate levels normalize, subcutaneous insulin takes effect, and the client starts eating.

Type 2 Diabetes Mellitus

I. Definition (See previous definition)

II. Nursing process

A. Assessment
   1. Assess onset—usually insidious.
   2. Assess for symptoms of hyperglycemia.
      a. Polyuria (excessive urination)
      b. Polydipsia (excessive thirst)
      c. Polyphagia (excessive hunger)
      d. Weight loss
      e. Fatigue
      f. Blurred vision
   3. Assess for signs of altered tissue response, including poor wound healing and recurrent infections, especially of skin.
   4. Obtain diagnostic tests.
      a. Elevated serum glucose levels:
         (1) Fasting blood glucose greater than or equal to 126 mg/dl on two occasions: Confirms DM.
         (2) Random blood glucose greater than or equal to 200 mg/dl in presence of classic symptoms (polyuria, polydipsia, polyphagia, and weight loss): Confirms DM.
         (3) 2-hr postprandial blood sample: Evaluates glucose metabolism and assists with control.
      b. Glucose tolerance test may be indicated:
         (1) Fasting blood sugar is obtained before ingestion of 50 to 200 g glucose load, and blood samples are taken at 30 min, 1, 2, 3, and possibly, 4 and 5 hr.
         (2) Diagnostic for DM if 2-hr result is 200 mg/dl or greater.
      c. Glycosylated hemoglobin (A1c): Measures glycemic control over 60- to 120-day period; fructosamine assay measures control over 20 days and is more accurate in clients with hemoglobin variants.

B. Analysis
   1. Activity Intolerance related to fatigue
   2. Anxiety related to potential complications
   3. Deficient Knowledge related to diabetes self-management
   4. Imbalanced Nutrition: More Than Body Requirements related to increased caloric consumption
   5. Risk for Impaired Skin Integrity related to compromised circulation
   6. Risk for Injury related to blurred vision, fatigue

C. Planning
   1. Maintain optimal body weight.
   2. Remain free from infection.
   3. Avoid complications.
   4. Increase understanding of disorder and treatment.
   5. Promote adaptive coping behaviors.

D. Implementation (see basic care and comfort)

E. Evaluation
   1. Client maintains optimal body weight.
   2. Client has no signs or symptoms of infection.
   3. Client is free from evidence of complications.
   4. Client verbalizes knowledge of DM and its treatment.
   5. Client demonstrates adaptive coping behaviors.

CN

III. Client needs

A. Physiologic adaptation: The goal of management of type 2 DM is to maintain normal blood glucose levels with diet, exercise, and insulin therapy.
   1. Promote tight glycemic control for prevention of complications.
   2. Provide modest calorie restriction for weight loss and maintenance for improved sensitivity of cells to insulin; decreases insulin resistance.
   3. Aim toward reaching target glucose, glycosylated hemoglobin, lipid, and BP levels according to American Diabetes Association.
   4. Instruct regular aerobic exercise to promote utilization of carbohydrates, assist with weight control, enhance action of insulin, and improve cardiovascular fitness.

B. Management of care: Care of the client with type 2 DM requires critical thinking skills and knowledge of assessment, and teaching and evaluation methods unique to the RN role. These skills cannot be delegated to an LPN or UAP.
   1. Keep endocrinologist and diabetologist informed of client's status and significant changes.

2. Reinforce information provided by dietitian and certified diabetes educator that assists in teaching ways to gain control.
3. Encourage client to see a podiatrist for foot care.
4. Encourage client to see an ophthalmologist annually.
5. Refer adult clients who are planning families for preconception counseling.
6. Encourage client to participate in diabetes support groups.

C. Safety and infection control
1. For hyperglycemic crisis, administer IV fluids with insulin drip and insulin replacement.
2. Treat all injuries, cuts, and blisters promptly.
3. Watch for signs and symptoms of urinary tract infections and vaginal infections; treat promptly.
4. Assess for cognitive and sensory impairment, which may interfere with ability to accurately administer insulin.
5. After treatment of hypoglycemia, provide protein source to prolong effect of concentrated carbohydrate if full meal cannot be eaten.
6. Advise client to inject insulin into abdominal site on days when arms and legs are aggressively exercised.
7. Use safety precautions to prevent injury: Encourage client to always wear supportive shoes on feet; do not walk with bare feet.

D. Health promotion and maintenance
1. For newly diagnosed clients or those undergoing stressful circumstances that preclude more in-depth teaching, focus on skills management related to insulin and oral agents, hypoglycemia treatment, blood glucose monitoring, and basic dietary information.
2. For ongoing teaching, include advanced skills and rationale for treatment and management. Focus on lifestyle management issues such as sick-day management exercise adjustments, travel preparations, foot care guidelines, intensive insulin management, and dietary concerns when dining out.

E. Psychologic integrity: Provide access to support from American Diabetes Association, American Association of Diabetes Educators, and/or Juvenile Diabetes Research Foundation (see also psychologic integrity for type 1 DM).

F. Basic care and comfort
1. Administer prescribed medications.
2. Provide meticulous skin care especially to feet and legs.
3. Encourage adequate fluid intake.
4. Assess renal and cardiovascular status.
5. Watch for signs and symptoms of hypoglycemia, hyperglycemia; treat as needed.
6. Avoid constricting hose, slippers, and bed linens.
7. Check vital signs, intake and output, and daily weight.
8. Monitor laboratory values, especially serum glucose and urine acetone.
9. Use bedside fingerstick to determine blood glucose.
10. Encourage ambulation.

G. Reduction of risk potential
1. Demonstrate and explain thoroughly procedure for insulin self-injection (achievement of mastered understanding very important).
2. Stress importance of accuracy in insulin preparation and meal timing to avoid hypoglycemia.
3. Advise client that prolonged strenuous exercise may require increased food at bedtime to avoid nocturnal hypoglycemia.
4. Watch for signs and symptoms of acute complications from therapy including altered thinking; dizziness, weakness; pallor, tachycardia, diaphoresis; and seizures, coma.
   a. If client is conscious, give 10 to 15 g of carbohydrate in form of fruit juice, hard candy, honey.
   b. If unconscious, give glucagon (SC or IM) and dextrose (IV).
5. Instruct client to avoid strenuous exercise whenever blood glucose levels exceed 240 mg/dl and urine ketones are present to prevent progressive hyperglycemia and metabolic acidosis.
6. Assess feet and legs daily for:
   a. Skin temperature
   b. Sensation
   c. Soft tissue injuries
   d. Corns, calluses, dryness
   e. Hammertoe or bunion deformation
   f. Hair distribution
   g. Pulses and deep tendon reflexes
7. Maintain skin integrity by protecting feet from breakdown.
   a. When client on bed rest, use special mattresses or foot cradles.
   b. Avoid drying agents to skin (alcohol).
   c. Apply skin moisturizers to maintain suppleness; prevent cracking and fissures.
8. If client smokes, promote smoking cessation program to decrease vasoconstriction and enhance peripheral blood flow.
9. Inform client regarding need to contact physician.

Table 27-2 Drug Table of Oral Antidiabetic Medications

Classifications	Generic/Trade Name	Expected Outcomes	Reduction of Risk Potential	Management of Care
Sulfonylureas	Chlorpropamide (Diabinese) first generation	Stimulates pancreas to decrease blood glucose.	Use with caution in the elderly. May cause hypoglycemia.	Administer with meals. Have available fast-acting carbohydrate source if needed. Review signs/ symptoms of hypoglycemia.
	Tolazamide (Tolinase) first generation	Lowers blood glucose; stimulates pancreas.	May cause hypo-glycemia; stimulates pancreas to produce more insulin.	Administer with meals. In case of hypoglycemia, have available 10 to 15 g of carbohydrate.
	Glyburide (Micronase, DiaBeta, Glynase) second generation	Lowers blood glucose; stimulates pancreas to produce more insulin.	May cause hypo-glycemia; have avail-able 10 to 15 g of fast-acting carbohy-drate such as juice, hard candy.	Administer with meals to decrease likelihood of hypoglycemia.
	Glipizide (Glucotrol, Glucotrol XL–extended release) second generation	Lowers blood glucose.	Take 2 times per day or once with (XL) – extended release. May cause hypoglycemia.	Administer 30 min before meals. Have available 10 to 15 g of fast-acting carbohydrate.
	Glimepiride (Amaryl) third generation	Lowers blood glucose.	Take once daily. May cause hypoglycemia.	Administer with meals. Have available 10 to 15 g of fast-acting CHO.
Biguanides	Metformin (Glucophage, Glucophage XR—extended release)	Lowers blood glucose.	Do not use with heart failure, renal, or liver problems. Check creatinine clearance if client over 65 years of age. Monitor liver enzymes. Do not take with alcohol; may lead to lactic acidosis. Do not take 48 hr before or 48 hr after a diagnostic test containing contrast medium.	Administer with meals. Adjust dose gradually as may cause severe diarrhea, GI distress.
Alpha-glucosidase Inhibitors	Acarbose (Precose); miglitol (Glyset)	Slows absorption of carbohydrate in the intestine; slowly lowers blood glucose.	May have GI side effects—flatulence, diarrhea, nausea, vomiting, and abdominal distention.	Administer with first bite of food to lessen GI side effects and enhance effect. Treat hypoglycemia with dextrose, not sucrose (table sugar).
Thiazolidinediones (TZDs)	Rosiglitazone (Avandia); pioglitazone (Actos)	Lowers blood glucose by increasing cell's sensitivity to insulin.	May reduce effectiveness of birth control pills. Need to check liver enzymes, as directed.	Take at relatively same time each day. Monitor for edema.

Classifications	Generic/Trade Name	Expected Outcomes	Reduction of Risk Potential	Management of Care
Meglitinides	Repaglinide (Prandin); nateglinide (Starlix)	Lowers postprandial blood glucose by causing pancreas to release burst of insulin.	May cause hypoglycemia if not enough food consumed at mealtime.	Take before each meal. Have available fast-acting carbohydrate. (10 to 15 g) such as fruit juice, sugar, hard candy.
DPP-4 Inhibitors	Sitagliptin (Januvia)	Deactivates glucagonlike peptide1; stimulates pancreas.	Do not use with heart failure, renal, or liver problems. Monitor creatinine clearance; liver enzymes.	Administer twice daily with meals. Adjust dose gradually.

H. Pharmacologic and parenteral therapies: Client will state the purpose for and associated side effects of all medications used to manage type 2 DM.
   1. Oral antidiabetic agents (see Table 27-2)
   2. Insulins
      a. Classification: Rapid-acting— Lispro (Humalog), aspart (NovoLog), and glulisine (Apidra)
      b. Classification: Short-acting—Regular (R) and inhaled regular (Exubera)
      c. Classification: Intermediate-acting—Lente (L) and NPH (N)
      d. Classification: Long-acting—Ultralente (U), glargine (Lantus), and detemir (Levemir)
      e. Classification: Combination insulins—70/30; 50/50; and 75/25 and 50/50 Humalog mix
   3. Injectable: Classification: Incretin mimetic—exenatide (Byetta)
   4. Injectable noninsulin (may be used with insulin)—Classification: Analogue of amylin—pramlintide (Symlin)

Thyroid Disease: Hypothyroidism and Hyperthyroidism

I. Definition: Thyroid disease involves the thyroid gland, which overlies thyroid cartilage below the larynx. Thyroid hormones accelerate cellular reactions in body cells. (See following definitions of hypothyroidism and hyperthyroidism.)
   A. Thyroxine (T_4)—stimulates metabolic rate and is essential for normal physical, mental development.
   B. Triiodothyronine (T_3)—inhibits anterior pituitary secretion of thyroid-stimulating hormone (TSH).
   C. Calcitonin (thyrocalcitonin)—decreases loss of calcium from bone and decreases the serum calcium level. Its action is opposite that of parathormone (PTH) from the parathyroid glands.

Hypothyroidism

I. Definition: Hypothyroidism (myxedema) is characterized by a decreased metabolic rate resulting from hyposecretion of thyroid hormones T_3 and T_4. Congenital hypothyroidism is also known as *cretinism,* and involves a deficiency of thyroid hormones at birth.

II. Nursing process
   A. Assessment
      1. Obtain a detailed health history and perform a comprehensive physical examination; assess for the following signs and symptoms:
         a. Fatigue, lethargy
         b. Muscle aches, weakness
         c. Intolerance to cold
         d. Weight gain
         e. Dry skin, hair
         f. Loss of body hair
         g. Bradycardia
         h. Constipation
         i. Loss of memory, forgetfulness
         j. Menstrual disturbances
         k. Myxedema coma—a severe manifestation of hypothyroidism resulting in:
            (1) Hypotension
            (2) Hypoventilation
            (3) Hypothermia
            (4) Stupor, progressing to coma

2. Obtain diagnostic tests.
   a. Decreased T_3 and T_4 levels
   b. Increased thyroid-stimulating hormone (TSH), primary
   c. Antithyroid antibodies (autoimmune)
   d. Increased cholesterol
   e. Increased creatine phosphokinase

B. Analysis
   1. Risk for Injury related to muscle weakness
   2. Activity Intolerance related to decreased metabolic rate
   3. Ineffective Coping related to loss of memory
   4. Hypothermia related to decreased metabolic rate
   5. Imbalanced Nutrition: More Than Body Requirements related to decreased metabolic rate

C. Planning
   1. Decrease risk for injury.
   2. Increase activity tolerance.
   3. Promote effective coping.
   4. Maintain normal body temperature.
   5. Facilitate understanding of disease process and treatments.
   6. Improve nutritional status.

D. Implementation (see management of care)

E. Evaluation
   1. Client is free from injury.
   2. Client has increased ability to tolerate activity.
   3. Client demonstrates ability to cope effectively.
   4. Client describes disease process and treatments.
   5. Client maintains normal body temperature.
   6. Client exhibits improved nutritional status.

CN

III. Client needs

A. Physiologic adaptation: Hypothyroidism is treated through thyroid hormone replacement and diet management. Recognize risk for severe hypothyroidism with myxedema coma, which can lead to increased myocardial oxygen requirements and cardiovascular collapse (see management of care for preventing complications).

B. Management of care: Care of the client with hypothyroidism requires critical thinking skills and knowledge of assessment, and teaching and evaluation methods unique to the RN role. These skills cannot be delegated to an LPN or UAP.
   1. Delegate responsibly those activities that can be delegated, including basic hygienic care, checking of vital signs, measuring of daily weights and intake and output, and keeping client warm, as needed. All monitoring information is reported to the RN.
   2. Monitor client for successful response to treatments.
      a. Diuresis, decreased puffiness
      b. Improved reflexes, muscle tone
      c. Accelerated pulse rate
      d. Slightly higher T_4 level, decreased TSH level
   3. Support vital body functions in severe hypothyroidism with myxedema coma; avoid rapid rewarming techniques to prevent increased oxygen requirements, possible cardiovascular collapse.
   4. Keep physician or endocrinologist informed of client's status, including any significant changes.
   5. Provide client and family teaching (see health promotion and maintenance, and reduction of risk potential).

C. Safety and infection control
   1. Provide meticulous skin care.
   2. Assess cardiovascular and pulmonary status.
   3. Monitor mental and neurologic status.

D. Health promotion and maintenance: Provide client and family teaching.
   1. Monitor for signs and symptoms of myxedema (decrease in heart rate, BP, level of consciousness, convulsions).
   2. Adhere to lifelong hormone replacement therapy; undergo periodic blood evaluations to determine thyroid hormone levels.
   3. Adhere to well-balanced, low-fat, low-cholesterol, high-fiber, low-sodium diet.
   4. Make provisions for energy conservation; increase activity gradually.
   5. Recognize signs and symptoms of insufficient and excessive medication:
      a. Underdosage—fatigue, slow pulse, constipation.
      b. Overdosage—feeling jittery, insomnia, increased pulse, palpitations.

E. Psychologic integrity: Stress importance of avoiding physical and emotional stress, and ways to maximize coping mechanisms. Advise client to obtain further information through American Thyroid Association, www.thyroid.org.

F. Basic care and comfort
   1. Provide adequate rest periods.
   2. Encourage coughing and deep-breathing exercises.
   3. Keep client warm, as needed.
   4. Assess for presence of edema.
   5. Record and evaluate intake and output.

G. Reduction of risk potential
   1. Administer IV fluids with caution if hyponatremia is present to prevent water intoxication.

2. As thyroid hormone levels gradually return to normal, monitor for arrhythmias, chest pain, and signs of heart failure.
3. Prevent chilling to avoid increasing metabolic rate, which places strain on heart.
4. Administer all prescribed medications with caution before and after thyroid replacement begins: After thyroid replacement is initiated, thyroid hormones may increase the effects of digoxin (Lanoxin)—monitor pulse and anticoagulants—watch for signs of bleeding.

H. Pharmacologic and parenteral therapies: Client will state the purpose for and associated side effects of all medications used to manage hypothyroidism: Levothyroxine (T_4; Synthroid) and liothyronine (T_3; Cytomel):
1. Administer T_3 by nasogastric tube if client is unconscious (T_3 acts more quickly than T_4).
2. Steroid therapy may be initiated: With rapid administration of thyroid hormone, plasma thyroxine levels may initiate adrenal insufficiency.
3. Use caution when administering medication to the elderly; avoid coronary ischemia caused by increased oxygen demands of heart.

Hyperthyroidism

I. Definition: Hyperthyroidism is characterized by an increased metabolic rate resulting from hypersecretion of thyroid hormones T_3 and T_4. The most common type of hyperthyroidism is Graves disease (toxic diffuse goiter), which is caused by an autoimmune response. Thyrotoxicosis, or "thyroid storm"/"thyroid crisis," occurs when the metabolic rate increases dramatically.

II. Nursing process

A. Assessment
1. Obtain a detailed health history and perform a comprehensive physical examination; assess for the following signs and symptoms:
   a. Enlarged thyroid gland (goiter)
   b. Hypertension
   c. Palpitations, cardiac dysrhythmias (tachycardia, atrial fibrillation)
   d. Nervousness, irritability, hyperactivity, emotional lability, decreased attention span
   e. Weight loss, increased appetite
   f. Insomnia, interrupted sleep
   g. Frequent stools, diarrhea
   h. Menstrual irregularities
   i. Warm, flushed skin
   j. Exophthalmos and staring gaze
   k. Hair loss
   l. Thyrotoxicosis/thyroid storm
      (1) Hyperthermia
      (2) Hypertension
      (3) Delirium
      (4) Abdominal pain, vomiting
      (5) Tachyarrhythmias
2. Obtain diagnostic tests.
   a. Increased T_3 and T_4 levels
   b. Radioactive iodine uptake—increased uptake
   c. TSH assay—nondetectable TSH level
   d. Thyroid scan—increased function (hot areas) in thyroid gland

B. Analysis
1. Imbalanced Nutrition: Less Than Body Requirements related to hypermetabolism
2. Risk for Injury related to disease process
3. Disturbed Body Image related to exophthalmos and weight loss
4. Ineffective Coping related to nervousness
5. Hyperthermia related to increased metabolic rate

C. Planning
1. Improve nutritional status.
2. Decrease risk for injury.
3. Increase activity tolerance.
4. Improve body image.
5. Augment ability to cope.
6. Maintain normal body temperature.

D. Implementation
1. Assist in exploring treatment options.
2. Promote adequate rest.
3. Promote adequate nutrition.
4. Prevent injury.
5. Maintain normothermia.
6. Provide teaching.
7. Provide postoperative care, if appropriate.
8. Provide referrals.

E. Evaluation
1. Client exhibits improved nutritional status.
2. Client demonstrates decreased risk for injury.
3. Client demonstrates increased activity tolerance.
4. Client verbalizes positive statements about body image.
5. Client demonstrates ability to cope.
6. Client maintains normal body temperature.

CN

III. Client needs

A. Physiologic adaptation: Medical and surgical management for hyperthyroidism is as follows (see also pharmacologic and parenteral therapy).
1. Restore and maintain basal metabolic rate: Radioactive iodine therapy—limits thyroid hormone secretion by destroying thyroid tissue.

2. Manage thyrotoxicosis/thyroid storm.
   a. Treat hyperthermia with cooling blanket and acetaminophen (Tylenol).
   b. Reverse dehydration with IV fluids and electrolytes.
3. Administer thyroid hormone antagonists.
4. Prepare client for surgical interventions, if indicated; includes subtotal thyroidectomy—preferred for nodular toxic goiter and thyroid carcinoma.

B. Management of care: Care of the client with hyperthyroidism requires critical thinking skills and knowledge of assessment, and teaching and evaluation methods unique to the RN role. These skills cannot be delegated to an LPN or UAP.
1. Delegate responsibly those activities that can be delegated. All monitoring information is reported to the RN.
   a. Take vital signs.
   b. Bathe client with cool to warm (not hot) water (avoid soap to prevent drying skin) to counteract diaphoresis; change linens when damp.
   c. Use lubricant skin lotions to protect pressure points.
   d. Dispose of urine or feces promptly if receiving radioactive iodine (as small levels of radiation will be eliminated through these sources).
   e. Promote sleep, relaxation through use of massage, relaxation exercises, and clustering nursing care activities.
   f. Assess for fatigue and prevent overactivity.
2. Reinforce information provided by dietitian—high-calorie foods and fluids; restrict stimulants (tea, coffee, chocolate) and alcohol.
3. Keep physician and endocrinologist informed of client's status, significant changes.
4. Reinforce measures taught by physical therapist to aid in muscle strengthening.
5. Provide client and family teaching (see reduction of risk potential).

C. Safety and infection control
1. Employ safety measures to reduce risk of trauma, falls if client is agitated.
2. Teach client to recognize and immediately report signs and symptoms of thyroid storm, including tachycardia, elevated temperature, and extreme agitation.

D. Health promotion and maintenance (see reduction of risk potential)

E. Psychologic integrity
1. Monitor nervousness, emotional lability, irritability, and apprehension.
2. Promote positive body image (may be effected by enlarged thyroid gland [goiter]).
3. Acknowledge that diminished attention span may impair relationships with others.

F. Basic care and comfort
1. Promote sleep and relaxation through use of massage, relaxation exercises, and clustering nursing care activities.
2. Provide quiet, calm environment; reduce environmental stressors (light, television, radio, visitors) as necessary.

G. Reduction of risk potential: Provide client and family teaching.
1. Recognize signs of hypothyroidism due to overtreatment (see assessment in section on hypothyroidism).
2. Recognize predisposing factors of thyroid storm, including infection, surgery, stress, and abrupt withdrawal of antithyroid medications and adrenergic blockers.
3. Undergo periodic blood evaluations to monitor CBC and thyroid hormone levels.
4. Observe possible adverse effects of medications.
5. Recognize and immediately report signs and symptoms of thyroid storm.
6. Seek continued follow-up care with physician or endocrinologist.

H. Pharmacologic and parenteral therapies
1. Thyroid hormone antagonists: Thionamide drugs such as propylthiouracil (Propyl-Thyracil) and methimazole (Tapazole) inhibit thyroid hormone formation.
   a. Duration depends on reduction of thyroid gland and normalization of T_4 and T_3 uptake.
   b. Withdraw gradually to prevent exacerbation.
   c. Radiation or surgery recommended if drugs do not result in euthyroid state.
   d. Observe for evidence of iodine toxicity.
      (1) Swelling of buccal mucosa
      (2) Excessive salivation
      (3) Coryza
      (4) Skin eruptions
2. Beta-adrenergic blocker: Propranolol (Inderal)—controls tachycardia, tremor, excess sweating, and nervousness until antithyroid drugs or radioiodine takes effect; inhibits peripheral conversion of T_4 to T_3.
3. Glucocorticoids—suppress peripheral conversion of T_4 to T_3.
4. Lugol iodine solution—inhibits hormone release in thyroid storm.
5. Diuretics—for ophthalmopathy with lubricating eyedrops; in severe cases, corticosteroids or orbital radiation may be necessary.

6. IV fluids:
   a. Normal saline (NS; 0.9% NaCl)—isotonic
   b. Lactated Ringer (LR)—isotonic
   c. 5% dextrose in water (D5/W)—isotonic, hypotonic

Disorders of the Anterior Pituitary: Hypopituitarism and Hyperpituitarism

I. Definition: The pituitary gland is considered to be the "master gland" of the human body; it is located at the base of the brain, and is influenced by the hypothalamus. Not only does the pituitary gland affect the function of the other endocrine glands, but it also promotes growth of body tissue, influences water absorption by the kidney, and controls sexual development and function. The anterior lobe produces adrenocorticotropic hormone (ACTH), follicle-stimulating hormone (FSH), growth hormone (GH), luteinizing hormone (LH), melanocyte-stimulating hormone (MSH), prolactin (PRL), somatotropic growth-stimulating hormone, and thyroid-stimulating hormone (TSH).

Hypopituitarism

I. Definition: Hypopituitarism is undersecretion of anterior pituitary hormones ACTH, TSH, GH, LH, and PRL. Thyroid, adrenal, and gonadal function is affected.

II. Nursing process

A. Assessment
   1. Obtain a detailed health history and perform a comprehensive physical examination; assess for the following signs and symptoms:
      a. Extreme weight loss
      b. Atrophy of all endocrine glands and organs
      c. Hair loss
      d. Impotence
      e. Amenorrhea
      f. Hypoglycemia
   2. Obtain diagnostic tests.
      a. Computed tomography scan (CTS) and magnetic resonance imaging (MRI) show presence, extent of pituitary tumors.
      b. Levels of pituitary hormones—decreased

B. Analysis
   1. Imbalanced Nutrition: Less Than Body Requirements related to dysfunction
   2. Activity Intolerance related to extreme weight loss
   3. Disturbed Body Image related to hair loss
   4. Sexual Dysfunction related to atrophy of endocrine glands
   5. Ineffective Coping related to inadequate ACTH hormones
   6. Hypothermia related to decreased thyroid function
   7. Deficient Knowledge related to options available for treatment of altered pituitary function

C. Planning
   1. Improve fluid and nutritional status.
   2. Increase activity tolerance.
   3. Enhance body image.
   4. Improve sexual function.
   5. Improve coping effectiveness.
   6. Facilitate attainment of normal body temperature.
   7. Promote understanding of options available for treatment of altered pituitary function.

D. Implementation (see management of care)

E. Evaluation
   1. Client shows improved fluid and nutritional status.
   2. Client exhibits increased activity tolerance.
   3. Client verbalizes positive body image.
   4. Client verbalizes improved sexual function.
   5. Client exhibits ability to cope.
   6. Client has normal body temperature.
   7. Client verbalizes options available for treatment of altered pituitary function.

CN

III. Client needs

A. Physiologic adaptation: Prognosis for hypopituitarism is good with adequate replacement therapy and correction of underlying causes (see pharmacologic and parenteral therapies).
   1. Recognize risk for medical emergency of pituitary apoplexy (copious effusion of blood into an organ)—indicated by sudden, severe headache; vomiting; and visual changes.
   2. Recognize risk for hypoglycemia—indicated by increasingly lower blood glucose levels.

B. Management of care: Care of the client with hypopituitarism requires critical thinking skills and knowledge of assessment, and teaching and evaluation methods unique to the RN role. These skills cannot be delegated to an LPN or UAP.
   1. Administer prescribed medications.
   2. Monitor postsurgical client for signs of complications.
   3. Promote fluid and nutritional balance.
   4. Protect client from injury and infection.
   5. Enhance activity tolerance.
   6. Enhance client's body image, sexual functioning, and coping.

7. Maintain normothermia.
8. Provide client and family teaching (see reduction of risk potential).

C. Safety and infection control: Provide continuous monitoring of hormone levels during hormone-replacement therapy.

D. Health promotion and maintenance: Emphasize need for long-term hormonal-replacement therapy and adverse reactions.

E. Psychologic integrity: Provide emotional support; encourage verbalization of feelings indicative of a positive self-esteem.

F. Basic care and comfort
1. Administer small, frequent meals; encourage maintenance of adequate caloric intake.
2. Keep client warm.
3. Measure daily weight.
4. Monitor vital signs.

G. Reduction of risk potential: Provide client and family teaching.
1. Know when to contact physician.
2. Keep regular follow-up appointments.
3. Obtain adequate rest.
4. Consume balanced diet.

H. Pharmacologic and parenteral therapies: Client will state the purpose for and associated side effects of all medications used to manage hypopituitarism. Replacement therapy with hormonal supplements involves the following:
1. Thyroxine-based medications
2. Cortisone (Cortone)
3. Sex hormones—estrogen, progesterone
4. Growth hormones—somatrem (Protropin) or somatropin (Nutropin)

Hyperpituitarism

I. Definition: Hyperpituitarism is oversecretion of anterior pituitary hormones ACTH, TSH, GH, LH, and PRL. The oversecretion commonly results from a secretory adenoma, which stimulates the target gland (adrenal or thyroid) or tissue (acromegaly from increased production of growth hormone).

A. Assessment
1. Obtain a detailed health history and perform a comprehensive physical examination; assess for the following signs and symptoms:
   a. Effects of excessive GH secretion (acromegaly in adults; gigantism in children):
      (1) Coarse features, including broad skull; protruding jaw; and broadening of hands and feet
      (2) Thickened heel pads
      (3) Thick tongue
      (4) Change in ring or shoe size
   b. Effects of excessive PRL secretion:
      (1) Decreased libido
      (2) Amenorrhea
      (3) Erectile dysfunction
   c. Effects of excessive ACTH secretion (Cushing syndrome):
      (1) Central obesity with round (moon) face and buffalo hump
      (2) Muscle weakness and fatigue
      (3) Frequent infections
      (4) Hirsutism
      (5) Edema
2. Obtain diagnostic tests.
   a. Visual field examination—diminished visual fields
   b. CTS, MRI—may detect a tumor
   c. Serum pituitary hormone levels may be elevated

B. Analysis
1. Imbalanced Nutrition: Less Than Body Requirements related to excessive growth
2. Risk for Injury related to diminished visual fields and muscle weakness
3. Excess Fluid Volume related to Cushing syndrome
4. Risk for Infection related to Cushing syndrome
5. Activity Intolerance related to fatigue
6. Disturbed Body Image related to coarse features; hirsutism
7. Sexual Dysfunction related to decreased libido, erectile dysfunction, and mood swings
8. Hyperthermia related to increased metabolic rate
9. Ineffective Coping related to mood swings and mental status changes
10. Deficient Knowledge related to effects of excessive treatments for hyperpituitarism

C. Planning
1. Improve fluid and nutritional status.
2. Decrease risk for injury.
3. Decrease risk for infection.
4. Increase activity tolerance.
5. Promote positive body image.
6. Improve sexual functioning.
7. Improve ability to cope effectively.
8. Enhance understanding of disease process and treatments.
9. Maintain normal body temperature.

D. Implementation (see management of care)

E. Evaluation
1. Client demonstrates balanced nutrition with adequate foods and fluids.
2. Client is free from signs of injury, edema, and infection.

3. Client tolerates daily activity.
4. Client verbalizes positive body image.
5. Client verbalizes improved sexual functioning.
6. Client maintains normal body temperature.
7. Client describes ability to cope effectively with stressors.
8. Client demonstrates ability to describe effects of excessive treatment options for hyperpituitarism.

CN

II. Client needs

A. Physiologic adaptation: The goal of therapy is to reduce the overproduction of hormones. Surgical removal (hypophysectomy), radiation therapy, or specific medications may be used.

B. Management of care: Care of the client with hyperpituitarism requires critical thinking skills and knowledge of assessment, and teaching and evaluation methods unique to the RN role. These skills cannot be delegated to an LPN or UAP.

1. Delegate responsibly those activities that can be delegated. All monitoring information must be reported to the RN.
2. Administer prescribed medications.
3. Prepare for indicated procedures or surgery.
4. Monitor postsurgical client for signs of complications.
5. Promote fluid and nutritional balance.
6. Protect from injury and infection.
7. Enhance activity tolerance.
8. Enhance client's body image, sexual functioning, and coping.
9. Maintain normothermia.
10. Provide teaching about effects of excessive hormones and treatments.
11. Provide consultations with endocrinologist, dietitian, and physical therapist as indicated.

C. Safety and infection control: Same as those for acromegaly (excess growth hormone), Cushing syndrome (excess adrenocortical hormones and mineralocorticoids), and Graves disease (excess thyroid hormone).

D. Health promotion and maintenance: Same as those for excessive hormones from other endocrine glands (thyroid, adrenal).

E. Psychologic integrity: Refer to measures for excess of other hormones (thyroid, ACTH).

F. Basic care and comfort: See measures for other excess hormones.

G. Reduction of risk potential: Refer to measures used for excess of other hormones (thyroid, ACTH).

H. Pharmacologic and parenteral therapies: Client will state the purpose for and associated side effects of all medications used to manage hyperpituitarism. Treatment depends on:

1. Hormone alterations
2. Gender, age of client
3. Surgical interventions performed
4. Radiation therapy provided
5. Availability of replacement hormone modalities

Disorders of the Posterior Pituitary: Diabetes Insipidus and Syndrome of Inappropriate Antidiuretic Hormone

I. Definition: The pituitary gland is considered to be the "master gland" of the human body; it is located at the base of the brain, and is influenced by the hypothalamus. Not only does the pituitary gland affect the function of the other endocrine glands, but it also promotes growth of body tissue, influences water absorption by the kidney, and controls sexual development and function. The posterior lobe produces oxytocin, antidiuretic hormone (ADH or vasopressin). Posterior pituitary dysfunction includes specific disorders involving oversecretion or undersecretion of ADH.

Diabetes Insipidus

I. Definition: Diabetes insipidus (DI) is a disorder involving undersecretion of ADH.

A. Results in excessive dilute urine production

B. Etiology may include:

1. Posterior pituitary destruction from tumors
2. Vascular accidents
3. Surgery, hypothalamic damage
4. Certain drugs that can interfere with antidiuretic hormone secretion/action: Phenytoin (Dilantin), alcohol, and lithium carbonate (Eskalith)
5. Nephrogenic diabetes insipidus, familial or arising from various renal disorders

II. Nursing process

A. Assessment

1. Obtain a detailed health history and perform a comprehensive physical assessment; assess for the following signs and symptoms.
   a. Profoundly increased urine output (5 to 20 L per day of dilute urine)
   b. Nocturia
   c. Extreme thirst
   d. Weight loss
   e. Possible tachycardia, hypotension, weakness

2. Obtain diagnostic tests.
   a. Plasma osmolality, serum sodium levels are elevated.
   b. Water (fluid) deprivation test: Shows inability of kidneys to concentrate urine despite increased plasma osmolality, low plasma vasopressin level.
   c. Vasopressin test: Kidneys can concentrate urine after administration of antidiuretic hormone—differentiates central (pituitary) or (hypothalamic) from nephrogenic (kidney) diabetes insipidus.

B. Analysis
1. Deficient Fluid Volume related to excessive urine output
2. Activity Intolerance related to hypotension
3. Risk for Injury related to weakness
4. Deficient Knowledge related to lack of information about disease process, treatment options

C. Planning
1. Improve fluid status.
2. Decrease risk for injury.
3. Increase activity tolerance.
4. Provide information about disease process and possible treatments available.

D. Implementation
1. Promote fluid balance; monitor signs of dehydration (thirst, headache); poor skin turgor, and dry mucous membranes.
2. Protect from injury.
3. Enhance activity tolerance.
4. Provide teaching about diabetes insipidus, treatment options.
5. Monitor vital signs—tendency for hypotension, tachycardia.

E. Evaluation
1. Client demonstrates improved fluid status.
2. Client is free from injury.
3. Client experiences increase in activity tolerance.
4. Client accurately describes diabetes insipidus and treatment options.

CN

III. Client needs

A. Physiologic adaptation: DI is treated by administration of antidiuretic hormone (ADH) or vasopressin.

B. Management of care: Care of the client with DI requires critical thinking skills and knowledge of assessment, and teaching and evaluation methods unique to the RN role. These skills cannot be delegated to an LPN or UAP.
1. Keep physician and endocrinologist informed of client's status and significant changes.
2. Reinforce information provided by dietitian for low-sodium diet with nephrogenic diabetes insipidus.
3. Reinforce measures taught by physical therapist to help strengthen muscles.
4. Provide client and family teaching (see health promotion and maintenance, and reduction of risk potential).

C. Safety and infection control
1. Provide meticulous skin and mouth care.
2. Watch for signs and symptoms of hypovolemic shock.
3. Monitor cardiac rhythm; telemetry may be required.

D. Health promotion and maintenance: Provide client and family teaching about the following measures:
1. Weigh self daily (teach importance).
2. Measure intake and output daily.
3. Wear medical identification.
4. Seek ongoing medical care.
5. Prevent dehydration.

E. Psychologic integrity
1. Encourage verbalization of feelings.
2. Offer encouragement while providing realistic assessment of situation.
3. Help client develop effective coping strategies.
4. Assess for changes in mental or neurologic status.
5. Refer to mental health professional for additional counseling, if indicated.

F. Basic care and comfort
1. Check vital signs, intake and output, and daily weight.
2. Provide fluids.
3. Assist with care when weakness and fatigue are present.
4. Promote measures to prevent constipation.
5. Encourage ambulation.

G. Reduction of risk potential
1. Provide client and family teaching regarding the following measures:
   a. Medications and potential adverse effects
   b. When to notify physician
   c. Signs and symptoms of dehydration
   d. Signs/symptoms of hypovolemic shock
2. Monitor urine specific gravity, serum electrolytes, BUN.

H. Pharmacologic and parenteral therapies: Client will state the purpose for and associated side effects of all medications used to manage DI.
1. Central diabetes insipidus: Promote daily replacement of vasopressin (Pitressin) using desmopressin acetate (DDAVP), a synthetic analogue.

2. Nephrogenic diabetes insipidus: Use thiazide diuretics to reduce serum osmolality.
   a. Monitor intake, output, and urine specific gravity to adjust medication dosage.
   b. Monitor for signs of water intoxication while on desmopressin acetate (DDAVP) therapy, including drowsiness, listlessness, headache, confusion, anuria, and weight gain.

Syndrome of Inappropriate Antidiuretic Hormone

I. Definition: The syndrome of inappropriate antidiuretic hormone (SIADH) involves oversecretion of ADH.
   A. Results in excessive water conservation
   B. Etiology may include:
      1. Central nervous system disorders and traumatic brain injury
      2. Stimulation from hypoxia or decreased left atrial filling pressure
      3. Pharmacologic agents: Chemotherapy, chlorpropamide (Diabinese)
      4. Overuse of vasopressin (Pitressin) therapy
      5. Ectopic antidiuretic hormone production associated with some cancers
      6. Nausea, opioid use, which can stimulate antidiuretic hormone secretion

II. Nursing process
   A. Assessment
      1. Obtain a detailed health history and perform a comprehensive physical examination; assess for the following signs and symptoms.
         a. Decreased urine output
         b. Weight gain
         c. Altered mental status, including headache, confusion, lethargy, seizures, and coma
         d. Delayed deep tendon reflexes
      2. Obtain diagnostic tests.
         a. Plasma osmolality, sodium levels: Decreased
         b. Urinalysis: Increased urine sodium, decreased urine osmolality
         c. Serum antidiuretic hormone level: Elevated
   B. Analysis
      1. Excess Fluid Volume related to decreased urine output
      2. Activity Intolerance related to fluid retention
      3. Risk for Injury related to fluid retention and edema
      4. Deficient Knowledge related to lack of information about disease process and treatment options
   C. Planning
      1. Improve fluid status.
      2. Decrease risk for injury.
      3. Increase activity tolerance.
      4. Provide information about disease process and available treatment options.
   D. Implementation
      1. Provide nursing care for SIADH.
      2. Promote fluid balance.
      3. Protect from injury.
      4. Provide client and family teaching.
   E. Evaluation
      1. Client's fluid status improves without signs of edema and with ease in breathing.
      2. Client is free from injury.
      3. Client's tolerance for activity is improved.
      4. Client describes SIADH and possible treatments.

CN

III. Client needs
   A. Physiologic adaptation: The goal of therapy is to correct overproduction of ADH and establish a normal fluid and electrolyte balance.
      1. Monitor serum electrolytes, including sodium and potassium.
      2. Restrict fluid intake, as indicated.
      3. With severe hyponatremia, monitor altered mental status (see assessment).
      4. Note delayed deep tendon reflexes.
   B. Management of care: Care of the client with SIADH requires critical thinking skills and knowledge of assessment, and teaching and evaluation methods unique to the RN role. These skills cannot be delegated to an LPN or UAP.
      1. Keep physician and endocrinologist informed of client's status and significant changes.
      2. Reinforce information provided by dietitian—high-salt, high-protein diet or urea supplements to enhance water excretion.
      3. Delegate responsibly those activities that can be delegated. All monitoring information is reported to the RN.
         a. Provide client orientation, as needed.
         b. Restrict fluids (500 to 1,000 ml/day).
         c. Reduce unnecessary environmental stimuli.
         d. Monitor intake and output.
         e. Monitor vital signs.
         f. Measure daily weight.
      4. Provide client and family teaching (see reduction of risk potential).
   C. Safety and infection control
      1. Provide safe environment.
      2. Institute seizure precautions, as needed.
      3. Monitor breath and heart sounds.
      4. Perform neurologic checks; monitor changes in level of consciousness.

D. Health promotion and maintenance
   1. Restrict fluids.
   2. Provide client and family teaching regarding self-monitoring techniques for fluid retention (e.g., measuring daily weight).
   3. Administer prescribed medications.
E. Psychologic integrity: Provide emotional support to client and family as needed.
F. Basic care and comfort
   1. Promote methods to decrease discomfort from thirst.
   2. Monitor vital signs.
   3. Measure daily weight.
   4. Monitor intake and output.
   5. Maintain fluid restriction as ordered by HCP.
   6. Encourage activity as tolerated.
G. Reduction of risk potential: Provide client and family teaching.
   1. Watch closely for signs and symptoms of heart failure, which may occur because of fluid retention.
   2. Recognize signs and symptoms requiring immediate medical intervention.
   3. Perform self-monitoring techniques for fluid retention.
   4. Understand medications and possible adverse effects.
   5. Take measures to prevent complications such as cerebral edema, water intoxication, severe hyponatremia, and coma.
H. Pharmacologic and parenteral therapies: Client will state the purpose for and associated side effects of all medications used to manage SIADH.
   1. Demeclocycline (Declomycin)
   2. Lithium (Eskalith)—for long-term treatment
   3. Loop diuretics for:
      a. Fluid overload
      b. History of heart failure
      c. Resistance to treatment
   4. IV fluid: 3% sodium chloride (3% NS)—hypertonic if serum sodium level is less than 120 mEq/L or if client is seizing.

Adrenal Disease: Addison Disease and Cushing Disease

I. Definition: Adrenal disease results in over- or undersecretion of hormones produced by the adrenal gland: Epinephrine/norepinephrine; glucocorticoids, cortisone, and hydrocortisone; mineralocorticoids, aldosterone, and desoxycorticosterone; and adrenosterones, adrenal androgens. Addison disease and Cushing disease are the two most common health problems.

Addison Disease

I. Definition: Addison disease is a deficiency of adrenocortical hormones following destruction of the adrenal cortex. The disorder most commonly occurs gradually, but can occur suddenly as a result of such stressors as trauma, infection, or surgery. Primary Addison disease is a pathologic condition of the adrenal glands themselves, whereas secondary Addison disease is often caused by prior treatment with glucocorticoids or other diseases of the pituitary gland that inhibit primary adrenocorticotropic hormone release. Extreme adrenal cortical insufficiency produces an addisonian (adrenal) crisis that can result in death.

II. Nursing process
A. Assessment
   1. Obtain a detailed health history, including history of previous trauma or surgery.
   2. Perform a comprehensive physical examination; assess for the following signs and symptoms:
      a. Lethargy, fatigue, muscle weakness, arthralgias
      b. GI complaints, including anorexia; nausea, vomiting, and diarrhea; and abdominal pain
      c. Decreased alertness, confusion
      d. Weight loss
      e. Dry skin, decreased body hair, increased pigmentation with excessive adrenocorticotropic hormone stimulation
   3. Addisonian (adrenal) crisis:
      a. Hypotension
      b. Rapid, weak pulse
      c. Rapid respiratory rate
      d. Pallor, extreme weakness
      e. Hyperthermia
   4. Obtain diagnostic tests.
      a. *Suggestive* findings:
         (1) Blood glucose: Decreased
         (2) Serum sodium: Decreased
         (3) Serum potassium: Increased
         (4) White blood cell count: Increased
      b. *Definitive* findings:
         (1) Serum cortisol levels: Decreased
         (2) Adrenocorticotropic hormone stimulation test: Shows low-to-normal cortisol response
B. Analysis
   1. Deficient Fluid Volume related to disease process
   2. Imbalanced Nutrition: Less Than Body Requirements related to anorexia

3. Risk for Injury related to muscle weakness
4. Risk for Infection related to diminished stress response
5. Activity Intolerance related to muscle weakness and fatigue
6. Disturbed Body Image related to dry skin, decreased body hair
7. Ineffective Coping related to diminished cortisol levels
8. Hyperthermia related to disease process
9. Deficient Knowledge related to lack of information about Addison disease and its management

C. Planning
1. Improve food and nutrition status.
2. Decrease risk for injury and infection.
3. Increase activity tolerance.
4. Enhance body image.
5. Promote effective coping.
6. Maintain normal body temperature.
7. Increase knowledge about Addison disease and its management.

D. Implementation
1. Administer prescribed medications.
2. Provide immediate treatment for addisonian crisis.
3. Help prevent adrenal crisis.
4. Provide client and family teaching.
5. Promote fluid and nutrition balance.
6. Protect client from injury and infection.
7. Enhance activity tolerance.
8. Enhance body image and coping.
9. Maintain normothermia.

E. Evaluation
1. Client attains and maintains normal fluid and electrolyte balance.
2. Client maintains nutritionally balanced diet and verbalizes appropriate dietary modifications.
3. Client remains injury-free and is free from signs and symptoms of infection.
4. Client verbalizes adequate energy to perform activities of daily living.
5. Client openly discusses feelings about the effects of Addison disease on body image.
6. Client demonstrates appropriate coping mechanisms.
7. Client has stable vital signs.
8. Client verbalizes importance of complying with prescribed medication regimen and plans for follow-up care.

CN

III. Client needs

A. Physiologic adaptation
1. Provide cardiovascular support, if indicated:
   a. Cardiac and hemodynamic monitoring
   b. Oxygen therapy
2. Monitor for impending addisonian crisis indicated by decrease in BP and increase in temperature.
3. Evaluate effectiveness of prescribed medications, including glucocorticoids and mineralocorticoids (see also pharmacologic and parenteral therapies).
4. Promote lifelong therapy and follow-up.
   a. Variable doses of hydrocortisone (Hydrocortone) when under stress
   b. Be aware of adverse effects of corticosteroids with long-term use

B. Management of care: Care of the client with Addison's disease requires critical thinking skills and knowledge of assessment, and teaching and evaluation methods unique to the RN role. These skills cannot be delegated to an LPN or UAP.
1. Delegate responsibly those activities that can be delegated, including basic care needs and vital signs. All monitoring information is reported to the RN.
2. Reinforce information provided by dietitian to provide high-sodium, low-potassium diet; fluids to restore and maintain fluid and electrolyte balance.
3. Reinforce measures taught by physical therapist to increase muscle strength.
4. Consult with discharge planner to aid in making arrangements (e.g., transportation) for needed follow-up care.

C. Safety and infection control: Protect infection with good hand hygiene technique and avoiding contact with staff or visitors who may be carriers.

D. Health promotion and maintenance
1. Instruct client about need for lifelong therapy (required) with mineralocorticoid and glucocorticoid therapy; and follow-up:
   a. Do not miss a medication dose.
   b. Take more hormones when under stress.
      (1) Dose may be doubled for minor illness; tripled for an illness keeping client home from school or work.
      (2) Injection hydrocortisone may be needed for:
         (a) Trauma
         (b) Surgery
         (c) Severe fatigue
         (d) Other highly stressful situations
   c. Wear medical identification.
2. Identify factors that may precipitate addisonian crisis, including infection, extremes of temperature, and trauma.

E. Psychologic integrity
1. Client with long-term use of corticosteroids may experience psychosis.

2. Client receiving steroid replacement therapy may experience adverse effects such as Cushingoid-type appearance, weight gain, hirsutism, and mood swings.

F. Basic care and comfort: Administer prescribed glucocorticoids and mineralocorticoids.

G. Reduction of risk potential
   1. Monitor vital signs frequently to detect impending addisonian crisis.
   2. Minimize stressful situations to avoid risk of adrenal crisis.
   3. Maintain constant room temperature and avoid drafts, dampness, and extremes in temperature to prevent addisonian crisis.

H. Pharmacologic and parenteral therapies: Client will state the purpose for and associated side effects of all medications used to treat Addison disease.
   1. IV fluids—sodium chloride solutions:
      a. Normal saline (NS) (0.9% NaCl)—isotonic
      b. Lactated Ringer (LR)—isotonic
      c. 5% dextrose, normal saline (D5/0.9NS)—hypertonic
      d. 3% normal saline (3% NS)—hypertonic
      e. 10% normal saline (10% NS)—hypertonic
      f. 5% dextrose and 0.45% normal saline (D5/ 1/2 NS)—hypertonic
      g. 5% dextrose and 0.225% normal saline (D5/ 1/4 NS)—hypertonic
   2. Corticosteroids to treat glucocorticoid deficiency—hydrocortisone (Hydrocortone) and prednisone (Deltasone). Adverse effects include:
      a. Fluid overload
      b. Osteoporosis
      c. Pathologic fractures
      d. Hyperglycemia
      e. Masking of signs of infection
      f. Poor tissue regeneration, growth
      g. Peptic ulcer formation
      h. Psychosis
   3. Mineralocorticoid to treat mineralocorticoid deficiency—fludrocortisone (Florinef). Adverse effects include:
      a. Hypertension
      b. Edema from sodium, water retention
      c. Weakness caused by potassium loss
   4. Injection of circulatory stimulants if addisonian crisis or circulatory collapse is imminent:
      a. Atropine (Atropair)
      b. Calcium chloride (Calciject)
      c. Epinephrine (Epifrin)

Cushing Disease

I. Definition: Cushing disease (Cushing syndrome or hypercortisolism) is a spectrum of symptoms associated with prolonged elevated plasma concentration of adrenal glucocorticoids (cortisol). Cushing disease is caused by autonomous adrenal tumors (adenomas or carcinomas), adrenocorticotropic hormone-secreting tumors outside the pituitary, or iatrogenic causes such as long-term administration of corticotropin (adrenocorticotropic hormone) or cortisol (steroids).

II. Nursing process

A. Assessment
   1. Obtain a detailed health history, including history of synthetic steroid use.
   2. Perform a comprehensive physical examination; assess for signs and symptoms.
      a. Complaints of fatigue, muscle weakness, sleep disturbances
      b. Polyuria, thirst, other symptoms of hyperglycemia
      c. Frequent infections
      d. Water retention
      e. Amenorrhea
      f. Decreased libido; erectile dysfunction
      g. Irritability; emotional instability
      h. Headache
      i. Alopecia of scalp hair in women, and hirsutism of face
      j. Moon-shaped face
      k. Buffalo humplike back
      l. Central obesity
      m. Thin extremities, muscle wasting, and weakness
      n. Petechiae, ecchymosis, and purplish striae
      o. Delayed wound healing
      p. Acne
      q. Hypertension
      r. Edematous ankles
   3. Obtain diagnostic tests.
      a. Serum cortisol—elevated
      b. Elevated sodium, elevated glucose, decreased potassium, decreased calcium
      c. Free cortisol level—elevated
      d. Glucosuria
      e. CTS, MRI, ultrasonography—shows presence of tumor

B. Analysis
   1. Activity Intolerance related to fatigue
   2. Disturbed Body Image related to hirsutism and acne
   3. Excess Fluid Volume related to water retention
   4. Risk for Impaired Skin Integrity related to thin extremities, delayed wound healing
   5. Risk for Injury related to muscle weakness

C. Planning
  1. Maintain skin integrity.
  2. Prevent infection.
  3. Provide client teaching about Cushing disease.
D. Implementation
  1. Administer prescribed medications.
  2. Reinforce nutrition instruction provided by the dietitian.
  3. Use protective measures to reduce risk of infection; perform meticulous hand hygiene.
  4. Schedule adequate rest periods.
  5. Institute safety precautions; prevent falls.
  6. Provide meticulous skin care.
  7. Help to develop effective coping strategies.
E. Evaluation
  1. Client is free from breaks in skin integrity.
  2. Client is free from infection.
  3. Client verbalizes positive feelings about self.
  4. Client verbalizes knowledge about Cushing disease.

III. Client needs
A. Physiologic adaptation
  1. Provide high-protein, high-potassium, low-calorie, low-sodium diet.
  2. Promote postoperative hormone-replacement therapy.
    a. Adrenalectomy—glucocorticoids, mineralocorticoids
    b. Pituitary irradiation, hypophysectomy—adrenal replacement plus thyroid, posterior pituitary, gonadal hormone replacement
    c. Transsphenoidal adenomectomy—hydrocortisone replacement therapy for 12 to 18 months, and additional hormones if excessive loss of pituitary function has occurred
    d. Protein anabolic steroids may be given to facilitate protein replacement; potassium replacement usually required
  3. After hypophysectomy, monitor for diabetes insipidus, hypothyroidism, and other endocrine changes.
  4. After adrenalectomy, monitor for adrenal crisis.
B. Management of care: Care of the client with Cushing disease requires critical thinking skills and knowledge of assessment, and teaching and evaluation methods unique to the RN role. These skills cannot be delegated to an LPN or UAP.
  1. Delegate responsibly those activities that can be delegated. All monitoring information is reported to the RN.
    a. Monitor intake and output.
    b. Measure daily weights.
    c. Perform bedside fingerstick glucose determination.
    d. Monitor vital signs, especially temperature.
    e. Monitor skin to detect reddened areas, skin breakdown or tearing.
    f. Encourage client to turn in bed frequently or ambulate to reduce pressure on bony prominences, areas of edema.
  2. Consult with dietitian:
    a. Provide foods low in sodium to minimize edema.
    b. Provide foods high in potassium (bananas, orange juice, tomatoes).
    c. Provide foods high in calcium (dairy products, broccoli) to prevent osteoporosis caused by glucocorticoid replacement.
  3. Consult with physical therapist:
    a. Instruct on weight-bearing activity to prevent osteoporosis.
    b. Instruct on use of correct body mechanics to avoid pain or injury during activities.
    c. Teach how to use assistive devices during ambulation to prevent falls and fractures.
  4. Provide client and family teaching (see health promotion and maintenance).
  5. Refer client for counseling, if indicated.
C. Safety and infection control
  1. Monitor for signs of infection and stress prompt reporting of infection.
  2. Teach client to recognize signs and symptoms of excessive exertion.
  3. Teach client to prevent injury during activities with use of assistive devices, proper body mechanics, and provision of scheduled exercise and rest periods.
D. Health promotion and maintenance: Provide client and family teaching.
  1. Comply with lifelong hormone-replacement therapy; seek regular follow-up visits to determine if dosage is appropriate or to detect adverse effects.
  2. Perform proper skin care and stress prompt reporting of trauma and infection.
  3. Monitor blood glucose; report results as directed.
  4. Prevent hyperglycemia through low-calorie, low-concentrated carbohydrate, low-fat diet, and increase activity as tolerated.
E. Psychologic integrity
  1. Encourage client to verbalize concerns about illness, changes in appearance, and altered role functions.

2. Observe for evidence of depression, which may progress to suicide.
   a. Mood changes
   b. Sleep disturbances
   c. Change in activity level
   d. Change in appetite
   e. Loss of interest in others and experiences

F. Basic care and comfort
   1. Handle skin and extremities gently.
   2. Assist with ambulation and hygiene when client is weak and fatigued.

G. Reduction of risk potential
   1. Provide information about medications and potential adverse effects.
   2. Discuss with client when to notify physician of changes in health status.
   3. Instruct client about need for lifelong steroid replacement and adverse effects.
   4. Teach signs and symptoms of adrenal crisis.
   5. Instruct client on stress reduction strategies.

H. Pharmacologic and parenteral therapies: Client will state the purpose for and associated side effects of all medications used to manage Cushing disease.
   1. Aminoglutethimide (Cytadren)—hormone antagonist
   2. Antifungal agents
   3. Antihypertensives
   4. Diuretics
   5. Glucocorticoids—administered morning of surgery to help prevent acute adrenal insufficiency during surgery. Cortisol therapy essential during, after surgery to tolerate physiologic stress caused by removal of pituitary or adrenal glands.
   6. Potassium supplements
   7. IV fluid: 5% dextrose in water (D5/W)—isotonic, hypotonic

Pheochromocytoma

I. Definition: Pheochromocytoma is a rare condition characterized by a tumor of the adrenal medulla, which produces excessive catecholamines (epinephrine, norepinephrine). Pheochromocytoma can occur at any age and in either gender, but is found most commonly in young to middle-aged adults. In most cases, the tumor is benign, encapsulated, unilateral, and solitary; occasionally, bilateral tumors are found. The secretion of excessive catecholamines results in severe hypertension. If undiagnosed and untreated, pheochromocytoma may be fatal.

II. Nursing process

A. Assessment
   1. Assess for hypermetabolic and hyperglycemic effects.
      a. Excessive perspiration
      b. Tremor
      c. Pallor or facial flushing
      d. Nervousness
      e. Elevated blood glucose
      f. Polyuria
      g. Nausea, vomiting, diarrhea
      h. Abdominal pain
      i. Paresthesias
   2. Assess for hypertension.
      a. May be paroxysmal (intermittent) or persistent (chronic); chronic form of hypertension mimics essential hypertension, but does not respond to antihypertensives.
      b. Headache, vision disturbances (common)
   3. Assess for changes in emotional status; psychosis may occur.
   4. Assess for predisposing factors that trigger symptoms, including physical exertion, emotional upset, and allergic reactions.
   5. Obtain diagnostic tests.
      a. 24-hr urine: Elevated vanillylmandelic acid (VAMA); metanephrine (metabolites of epinephrine and norepinephrine)
      b. If symptomatic, elevated epinephrine, norepinephrine in blood, urine
      c. Clonidine (Catapres) suppression test: No significant decrease in catecholamines
      d. Computed tomography scan, magnetic resonance imaging exam of adrenal glands or entire abdomen: Identifies tumor

B. Analysis
   1. Anxiety related to disease process
   2. Ineffective Tissue Perfusion: Peripheral, related to vasoconstriction of blood vessels
   3. Risk for Injury related to elevated BP

C. Planning
   1. Encourage expression of feelings of less anxiety.
   2. Prevent injury.
   3. Promote oxygenation of tissues.

D. Implementation
   1. Monitor BP frequently while client is symptomatic.
   2. Remain with client during acute episodes of hypertension.
   3. Ensure bed rest and elevate head of bed 45 degrees during severe hypertension.
   4. Instruct client about use of relaxation exercises.
   5. Monitor vital signs.

E. Evaluation
   1. Client describes decreased perception of anxiety.
   2. Client is free from signs and symptoms of injury.
   3. Client's tissues are pink, warm, and dry.

CN

III. Client needs
A. Physiologic adaptation: Pheochromocytoma is managed medically by alpha-adrenergic blocking agents, and surgically by removal of one or both adrenal glands.
   1. Reduce events that bring about episodes of hypertension, including palpation of tumor, physical exertion, and emotional upset.
   2. Eliminate stimulants (coffee, tea, cola) from diet.
   3. Use relaxation exercises.
   4. Prepare client for surgery, if needed.
B. Management of care: Care of the client with pheochromocytoma requires critical thinking skills and knowledge of assessment, and teaching and evaluation methods unique to the RN role. These skills cannot be delegated to an LPN or UAP.
   1. Keep physician and endocrinologist informed of client's status and significant changes.
   2. Prepare client for surgery, if required.
      a. Unilateral/bilateral adrenalectomy
      b. Removal of nonadrenal tumor
   3. Provide client and family teaching (see health promotion and maintenance).
C. Safety and infection control
   1. Recognize risk for infection following corticosteroid replacement postsurgical intervention.
   2. Use sterile technique when doing dressing changes.
   3. If metyrosine (Demser) used for medical management of effects of pheochromocytoma, may cause sedation; avoid activities that require alertness.
D. Health promotion and maintenance
   1. Instruct client how to take metyrosine (Demser) and potential side effects:
      a. Avoid taking other central nervous system depressants.
      b. Observe for signs of sedation.
      c. Promote fluid intake of at least 2,000 ml/day to prevent kidney stones.
   2. Inform client regarding need for continued follow-up for:
      a. Recurrence of pheochromocytoma
      b. Assessment of any residual renal and cardiovascular injury related to preoperative hypertension
      c. Documentation that catecholamine levels are normal 1 to 3 months after surgery (by 24-hr urine)
   3. Teach about corticosteroid replacement:
      a. Comply with therapy for rest of life when have bilateral adrenalectomy.
      b. Replacement therapy may be used for 2 to 3 weeks—if 1 adrenal gland is removed, until stress of surgery is over; the remaining adrenal gland can compensate.
E. Psychologic integrity
   1. Instruct client about use of relaxation exercises.
   2. Encourage client to reduce environmental stressors by providing a calm and quiet environment.
F. Basic care and comfort
   1. Reduce environmental stressors by providing calm, quiet environment; restrict visitors.
   2. Provide good skin care if symptomatic with diarrhea, diaphoresis.
   3. Encourage oral fluids.
G. Reduction of risk potential
   1. Maintain adequate hydration with IV fluid postoperatively to prevent hypotension.
   2. Maintain IV infusion preoperatively to ensure adequate volume expansion going into surgery.
   3. Administer sedatives to promote relaxation and rest.
   4. Because reduction of catecholamines postoperatively causes vasodilation, hypotension may occur; caution client to rise slowly.
H. Pharmacologic and parenteral therapies: Client will state the purpose for and associated side effects of all medications used to manage pheochromocytoma.
   1. Alpha-adrenergic blocker such as phentolamine (Regitine) administered preoperatively—to inhibit effects of catecholamines on BP.
   2. Catecholamine synthesis inhibitors such as metyrosine (Demser) administered preoperatively or for long-term management of inoperable tumors. Adverse effects include sedation, crystalluria leading to kidney stones.

Bibliography

Altman, G. (2004). *Delmar's fundamental and advanced nursing skills* (2nd ed.). Albany, NY: Delmar.

Ellis, J., & Hartley, C. (2005). *Managing and coordinating nursing care.* Philadelphia: Lippincott Williams & Wilkins.

Karch, A. (2006). *Lippincott's nursing drug guide.* Philadelphia: Lippincott Williams & Wilkins.

Nursing 2008 drug handbook. Ambler, PA: Springhouse.
Purnell, L., & Paulanka, B. (Eds.). (2003). *Transcultural healthcare: A culturally competent approach.* Philadelphia: Davis.
Smeltzer, S. C., Bare, B. G., Cheever, K. H., & Hinkle, J. L. (2008). *Brunner & Suddarth's textbook of medical-surgical nursing* (11th ed.). Philadelphia: Lippincott Williams & Wilkins.
Taylor, C., Lillis, C., LeMone, P., & Lynn, P. (2006). *Fundamentals of nursing.* Philadelphia: Lippincott Williams & Wilkins.
Weber, J. R., & Kelley, J. (2007). *Nurses handbook of health assessment.* Philadelphia: Lippincott Williams & Wilkins.
Yarbro, C. H., Frogge, M., & Goodman, M. (2004). *Cancer symptom management* (3rd ed.). Sudbury, MA: Jones and Bartlett.

CHAPTER 27

Practice Test

Diabetes Mellitus

1. An adult client with type 1 diabetes is scheduled for cataract surgery in the Same-Day Surgery Department. On arrival, the client's fingerstick blood glucose is 210 mg/dl. The nurse should:
- ☐ 1. Add an insulin drip to the IV therapy.
- ☐ 2. Reschedule the surgery for another date.
- ☐ 3. Instruct the client to ambulate.
- ☐ 4. Contact the client's HCP.

2. An adult client who has type 2 diabetes and requires insulin tells the nurse about feeling trembly, weak, and anxious before supper. The nurse should:
- ☐ 1. Tell the client to lie down for 30 min.
- ☐ 2. Have the client drink a glass of milk or orange juice.
- ☐ 3. Contact the client's physician to decrease the insulin dose.
- ☐ 4. Administer the next dose of insulin.

3. The HCP has prescribed detemir (Levemir) for a client with type 2 diabetes requiring insulin. The nurse should tell the client:
- ☐ 1. "You may mix your sliding scale aspart (NovoLog) insulin with this insulin."
- ☐ 2. "You do not need to rotate injection sites with this insulin."
- ☐ 3. "You do not need to mix detemir (Levemir) insulin; the solution is clear."
- ☐ 4. "You may refill the detemir (Levemir) FlexPen."

4. The nurse is instructing a client with DM about a diet plan comprised of 45 g of carbohydrate at each meal. Which selections does the nurse encourage?
- ☐ 1. 1 cup of skim milk, 1/2 cut unsweetened applesauce with cinnamon, 2 ounces of pork chop, 1/2 cup mashed potatoes, 1 cup coffee with cream.
- ☐ 2. 1 cup sugar-free hot chocolate, 3/4 cup unsweetened cold cereal, 1 slice bacon, 1/2 cup scrambled egg, 1 cup skim milk, 1 slice whole wheat toast.
- ☐ 3. 1 cup yogurt (100 calorie, lite), 1/3 cup pasta, 1/2 cup peas, 1 cup canned pineapple in its own juice.
- ☐ 4. 2 ounces chicken breast, 1 cup cooked carrots, 1 cup ice cream, 5 radishes, 1 can diet soda.

5. When evaluating teaching to a client on how to administer insulin, which of the following indicates that additional teaching is necessary?
- ☐ 1. Client draws up the regular insulin first and then the NPH.
- ☐ 2. Client rotates sites from legs to arms.
- ☐ 3. Client identifies that the syringe is U-100.
- ☐ 4. Client waits 30 min to eat breakfast after injecting rapid-acting insulin.

6. A client with newly diagnosed DM is scheduled to receive regular insulin 10 units and NPH insulin 20 units every morning. When should the nurse schedule the administration of these medications?
- ☐ 1. Regular insulin with breakfast; NPH after breakfast.
- ☐ 2. Both insulins 0.5 hr before breakfast.
- ☐ 3. In two separate syringes with breakfast.
- ☐ 4. NPH 1 hr before and regular 0.5 hr before breakfast.

7. A client receives NPH insulin at 0800. Given the peak time of NPH insulin, when should the nurse anticipate a hypoglycemic reaction?
- ☐ 1. 0900.
- ☐ 2. 1600.
- ☐ 3. 2200.
- ☐ 4. Midnight.

8. A client is to receive NPH and regular insulin. How should the nurse prepare these medications?
- □ 1. Draw up the NPH insulin first, then the regular insulin into the syringe.
- □ 2. Roll the NPH insulin between the palms of the hands for 1 min.
- □ 3. Prepare the insulins in one syringe at least 5 to 10 min before administration.
- □ 4. Use two different syringes because these two insulins are not compatible.

9. An insulin-dependent client complains of feeling shaky, weak, and cold. What does the nurse do first?
- □ 1. Administer orange juice with two packages of sugar.
- □ 2. Determine if the client has been eating between hospital meals.
- □ 3. Check the client's blood glucose with a bedside glucometer.
- □ 4. Start an IV and prepare to administer fluids.

10. The nurse is instructing a client with DM who takes insulin about the causes of hypoglycemia. The client understands the underlying cause of hypoglycemia when telling the nurse hypoglycemia is caused by:
- □ 1. Drinking too much water.
- □ 2. Getting too little exercise.
- □ 3. Eating too much food.
- □ 4. Taking too much insulin.

Thyroid Disease: Hypothyroidism and Hyperthyroidism

11. A client with hyperthyroidism is taking potassium iodide (SSKI) prior to having a thyroidectomy. The nurse instructs the client to do which of the following?
- □ 1. Discontinue all other medications.
- □ 2. Take on an empty stomach.
- □ 3. Take with water.
- □ 4. Take with milk.

12. A client with hyperthyroidism is hospitalized to have a thyroidectomy. The physician has prescribed propranolol (Inderal). In reviewing the client's history, the nurse notes that the client has asthma. The nurse should next:
- □ 1. Take the client's pulse and hold the propranolol (Inderal) if the pulse is less than 100 beats per minute.
- □ 2. Count the client's respirations and hold the propranolol (Inderal) if the respirations are less than 20 breaths per minute.
- □ 3. Contact the physician; question the order for propranolol (Inderal) with the client's asthma history.
- □ 4. Instruct the client to make position changes slowly.

13. A client who takes levothyroxine (Synthroid) had a cholecystectomy yesterday. Laboratory results indicate a normal T_4 level and a decreased thyroid-stimulating hormone (TSH) level. The nurse should:
- □ 1. Hold the medication and notify the physician of the lab results.
- □ 2. Explain to the client that the medication is not needed after surgery.
- □ 3. Schedule the medication for early each morning to mimic normal thyroid release.
- □ 4. Teach the client about the manifestations of hyperparathyroidism following surgery.

Disorders of the Anterior Pituitary: Hypopituitarism and Hyperpituitarism

14. A client with a pituitary tumor had a transsphenoidal hypophysectomy. Following surgery, the nurse places the head of the bed in which of the following positions?
- □ 1. Flat.
- □ 2. Lowered 20 degrees.
- □ 3. Elevated 90 degrees.
- □ 4. Elevated 30 degrees.

Disorders of the Posterior Pituitary: Diabetes Insipidus and Syndrome of Inappropriate Antidiuretic Hormone

15. A client with DI is taking desmopressin acetate (DDAVP). The nurse should assess which of the following to determine that the expected outcome of this drug is being achieved?
- □ 1. Intake is equal to output.
- □ 2. Serum glucose is in normal range.
- □ 3. Weight is within normal range for height.
- □ 4. BP is stable.

Adrenal Disease: Addison Disease and Cushing Disease

16. A client with Addison disease is hospitalized for an acute crisis. During the crisis, which of the following nursing diagnoses is a priority?
- □ 1. Deficit fluid volume.
- □ 2. Activity intolerance.
- □ 3. Anxiety.
- □ 4. Risk for injury.

17. AF A client with Addison disease is taking corticosteroid replacement therapy. The nurse should instruct the client about which of the following side effects of corticosteroids? Select all that apply.

- □ 1. Hyperkalemia.
- □ 2. Skeletal muscle weakness.
- □ 3. Mood changes.
- □ 4. Hypocalcemia.
- □ 5. Increased susceptibility to infection.
- □ 6. Hypotension.

18. A client with Cushing disease had a bilateral adrenalectomy 24 hr ago. The nurse should monitor the client closely for which of the following?

- □ 1. Neurogenic shock.
- □ 2. Hypovolemic shock.
- □ 3. Cardiogenic shock.
- □ 4. Anaphylactic shock.

19. A client with Cushing disease has an order to receive IV solution of 3% sodium chloride (NaCl). The nurse contacts the physician to verify the order because:

- □ 1. 3% sodium chloride (NaCl) is a hypertonic solution that will increase the extracellular fluid (ECF) volume.
- □ 2. 3% sodium chloride (NaCl) is a hypotonic solution that will cause extracellular fluid (ECF) volume depletion.
- □ 3. 3% sodium chloride (NaCl) is like normal saline.
- □ 4. 3% sodium chloride (NaCl) is an isotonic solution with no net effect on cellular dynamics.

Pheochromocytoma

20. When sympathetic blocking agents are used to decrease the BP prior to removal of an adrenal tumor, the nurse should instruct the client to:

- □ 1. Continue current prescriptions.
- □ 2. Change position cautiously.
- □ 3. Walk 30 min daily.
- □ 4. Place furniture for support.

Answers and Rationales

1. 4 Blood glucose over 180 mg/dl is considered to be hyperglycemia. Both emotional and physical stress can elevate the blood glucose level and result in hyperglycemia. Acute illness, injury, and surgery are situations that may evoke a counterregulatory hormone response resulting in hyperglycemia. If the glucose is greater than 240 mg/dl, urine is tested for ketones every 3 to 4 hr. With surgery, the client is given IV fluids and insulin immediately before, during, and after surgery when there is no oral intake. Frequent monitoring of blood glucose prevents episodes of severe hypoglycemia in this client. The nurse does not initiate an insulin drip without orders from a physician. There is no reason to have to reschedule the cataract surgery to another date; the stress of surgery elevates the blood glucose level. Walking exercise increases insulin sensitivity and can have a direct effect on lowering the blood glucose levels. Clients who use insulin are at increased risk for hypoglycemia when there is an increase in physical activity; this is undesirable during surgery as the effects of exercise can last up to 48 hr after the activity. (M)

2. 2 Hypoglycemia is a blood glucose level below 70 mg/dl. The signs and symptoms of hypoglycemia include confusion, irritability, diaphoresis, tremors, hunger, weakness, and visual disturbances. Untreated hypoglycemia can progress to loss of consciousness, seizures, coma, and death. With effective treatment, hypoglycemia can usually be quickly reversed. If the client has manifestations of hypoglycemia and monitoring equipment is not available, hypoglycemia is assumed, and treatment is initiated. Hypoglycemia is treated by ingesting 10 to 15 g of simple (fast-acting) carbohydrate, such as 4 to 8 ounces of fruit juice or regular (nondiet) soft drink or 8 ounces of low-fat milk. The client is then advised to eat the regularly scheduled meal or a snack that has protein, such as cheese or peanut butter, to prevent hypoglycemia from recurring. Without treating the possible hypoglycemia, the blood glucose level will go down even lower and the client may lose consciousness, develop seizures, or go into a coma. Contacting the physician would delay treating the possible hypoglycemia. Decreasing the insulin dose or increasing the meal plan may prevent episodes of hypoglycemia in the future. Administering insulin would cause the blood sugar to go even lower. (A)

3. 3 Detemir (Levemir) is used only if the solution appears clear and colorless with no visible particles. Detemir (Levemir) is not diluted or mixed with any other insulin preparations. As with any insulin therapy, lipodystrophy may occur at the injection site and delay insulin absorption. Continuous rotation of the injection site within a given area may help to reduce or prevent this reaction. Levemir is available in the Levemir FlexPen, a prefilled insulin pen. When the FlexPen is empty, it may not be refilled; instead the FlexPen is discarded. (D)

4. 1 Carbohydrate "carb" counting is a meal-planning method especially useful for those on rapid-acting insulin, such as lispro (Humalog), aspart (NovoLog), or on an insulin pump. Carbohydrate is the primary nutrient that affects the after-meal (postprandial) blood glucose level because carbohydrates turn into glucose within the first 1 to 2 hr after being eaten. Counting carbs correctly helps in calculating a more accurate dose of rapid-acting insulin. Carbohydrate groups include fruit, starch, milk, and other carbohydrates. One serving = 15 g = 1 carbohydrate. One cup skim milk = 1 carbohydrate; 1/2 cup unsweetened applesauce = 1 carbohydrate; cinnamon is free; 2 ounces pork chop = 0 carbohydrate, it is protein; 1/2 cup mashed potatoes = 1 carbohydrate; 1 cup coffee is free; cream = 0 carbohydrate, it is fat. Total = 3 carbohydrates = 45 g carbohydrate. Options 2 and 4 contain 4 carbohydrates = 60 g carbohydrate. Option 3 contains 5 carbohydrates = 75 g carbohydrate. (H)

5. 4 The nurse instructs the client to not wait any longer than 5 to 15 min to eat after injecting rapid-acting insulin, which has an onset action of 5 min and duration of 1 hr. The client is using proper technique for mixing the insulins, rotating sites, and using the U-100 syringe. (H)

6. 2 Regular and NPH insulins are scheduled together one-half hour before breakfast. They do not need to be given separately or in different syringes. (D)

7. 2 NPH insulin has an onset in 3 to 4 hr and peaks in 6 to 12 hr. Morning NPH insulin, given at 0800, is most likely to cause a hypoglycemic reaction between 1400 and 2000. (D)

8. 2 NPH insulin is supplied as a suspension containing protamine particles, which help to delay onset and peak times. The NPH vial is rolled between the palms of the hands, not shaken, to assure a uniform solution. NPH and regular insulin can be drawn into the same syringe, starting with the regular; this keeps the regular bottle from contamination by NPH. Insulins mixed together into one syringe are given very soon after they are drawn up to avoid interactions. (D)

9. 3 Although the symptoms suggest hypoglycemia, the nurse checks the blood glucose to be certain before intervening further. Administering orange juice with two packages of sugar generally exceeds the amount of sugar needed to treat simple hypoglycemia and should not be done without knowing the blood glucose value. Knowing the client's between-meal snacks is helpful, but not the first thing the nurse should do. And unless ordered, an IV is not needed as a first step in this situation. (D)

10. 4 Insulin assists glucose transport into the cells and causes the blood glucose levels to drop. Taking too much insulin could significantly drop blood levels and cause symptoms of hypoglycemia. Drinking excessive water does not directly drop blood glucose levels. Decreasing exercise or eating excessively causes elevations in blood glucose levels. (D)

11. 4 Potassium iodide (SSKI) is used in the immediate preoperative period prior to a thyroidectomy to decrease the vascularity, fragility, and size of the thyroid gland. The client is instructed to take the solution with meals in a full glass of water or juice. SSKI is not taken with milk; absorption of the drug may be decreased by diary products. The client can take other medications along with the SSKI. (D)

12. 3 Propranolol hydrochloride (Inderal) is a nonselective beta blocker of both cardiac and bronchial adrenoreceptors, which competes with epinephrine and norepinephrine for available beta-receptor sites. Propranolol (Inderal) blocks cardiac effects of beta-adrenergic stimulation; as a result, it reduces heart rate; a hypertensive effect is associated with decreased cardiac output. A contraindication of propranolol (Inderal) is bronchial asthma; propranolol (Inderal) can cause bronchiolar constriction even in normal clients. The nurse takes the apical pulse and BP before administering propranolol (Inderal). The medication is held if the heart rate is less than 60 beats per minute or the systolic BP is less than 90 mmHg. (D)

13. 3 Levothyroxine (Synthroid) is synthetic T_4. The normal T_4 levels indicate that the client's current dosing regimen is therapeutic and should be continued. Holding the medication is unnecessary; once started, supplemental thyroid hormone therapy is typically continued for the client's lifetime. Hyperparathyroidism is associated with elevated calcium levels and is unrelated to thyroid therapy. (D)

14. 4 After surgery in which a transsphenoidal approach has been used, the head of the client's bed is elevated at a 30-degree angle at all times. This elevation avoids pressure on the sella turcica and decreases headaches, a frequent postoperative problem. The nurse monitors neurologic status, including pupillary response, in order to detect neurologic complications. None of the other head-of-bed positions avoids pressure on the sella turcica or prevents increased intracranial pressure. (R)

15. 1 DI is a disorder of water metabolism. Desmopressin is a vasopressin derivative and has antidiuretic effects; the client should attain a urinary output equal to intake. Desmopressin does not affect serum glucose; insulin is used to regulate glucose levels. Desmopressin does not affect weight or BP. (D)

16. 1 When the client with Addison disease is experiencing a crisis, restoration of fluid and electrolyte imbalance is the priority for care. The client may be at risk for injury from ineffective stress response, will likely have anxiety because of the crisis situation, and may have activity intolerance related to decreased cortisol production. However, these diagnoses have lower priority and can be addressed once the fluid and electrolyte levels are stabilized. (A)

17. 2, 3, 4, 5 The long-term administration of corticosteroids in therapeutic doses often leads to serious complications or side effects. Corticosteroid therapy is not recommended for minor chronic conditions; the potential benefits of treatment must always be weighed against the risks. Hypokalemia may develop; corticosteroids act on the renal tubules to increase sodium reabsorption and enhance potassium and hydrogen excretion. Corticosteroids stimulate the breakdown of protein for gluconeogenesis, which can lead to skeletal muscle wasting. CNS adverse effects are euphoria, headache, insomnia, confusion, and psychosis. The nurse watches for changes in mood and behavior, emotional stability, sleep pattern, and psychomotor activity, especially with long-term therapy. Hypocalcemia related to anti-vitamin D effect may occur. Corticosteroids cause atrophy of the lymphoid tissue, suppress the cell-mediated immune responses, and decrease the production of antibodies. The nurse must be alert to the possibility of masked infection and delayed healing (anti-inflammatory and immunosuppressive actions). Retention of sodium (and subsequently water) increases blood volume and, therefore, BP. (D)

18. 2 Treatment for Cushing disease may involve surgical removal of a pituitary, adenoma, an adrenal tumor, or one/both adrenal glands. Surgery on glands poses risks beyond those of other types of operations. Because glands are highly vascular, the risk of hemorrhage is increased. Manipulation of glandular tissue during surgery may release large amounts of hormone into the circulation, producing marked fluctuations in the metabolic processes affected by these hormones. Postoperatively, BP, fluid balance, and electrolyte levels tend to be unstable. Neurogenic shock is a hemodynamic phenomenon that occurs after a spinal cord injury at the fifth thoracic (T5) vertebra or above. Cardiogenic shock occurs when either systolic or diastolic dysfunction of the myocardium results in compromised cardiac output. Anaphylactic shock is an acute and life-threatening hypersensitivity (allergic) reaction to a sensitizing substance (i.e., drug, chemical, vaccine, food, or insect venom). (R)

19. 1 In Cushing disease, there is marked sodium and water retention and a tendency toward edema. There is also hypertension and hypervolemia. The nurse questions the physician's order to give a 3% sodium chloride (NaCl) solution because it is hypertonic and would increase the extracellular fluid (ECF) volume even further. With sodium and water retention and hypertension and hypervolemia already in Cushing disease, the additional extracellular fluid (ECF) volume would increase even further an elevated BP and contribute to ECF volume overload. Hypotonic solutions cause fluids to shift out of blood vessels and into the intestinal space, causing ECF volume depletion. Normal saline is an isotonic solution that expands the ECF volume, but has no net effect on cellular dynamics. (D)

20. 2 The primary treatment for pheochromocytoma is surgical removal of the tumor. Preoperatively, sympathetic blocking agents such as prazosin (Minipress), doxazosin (Cardura), or terazosin (Hytrin) are used to reduce the BP and alleviate other symptoms of catecholamine excess. The use of these drugs may result in orthostatic hypotension; the nurse instructs the client to make postural changes slowly and cautiously. The current prescriptions may not include the most therapeutic antihypertensive agents. Walking daily promotes circulation, but it may also increase the BP. Placement of furniture for support may become obstacles for safe ambulation. When a client experiences orthostatic hypotension or an abnormally low BP occurs when assuming a standing position, vertigo may be present also. (S)

chapter 28

The Client With Urinary Tract Health Problems

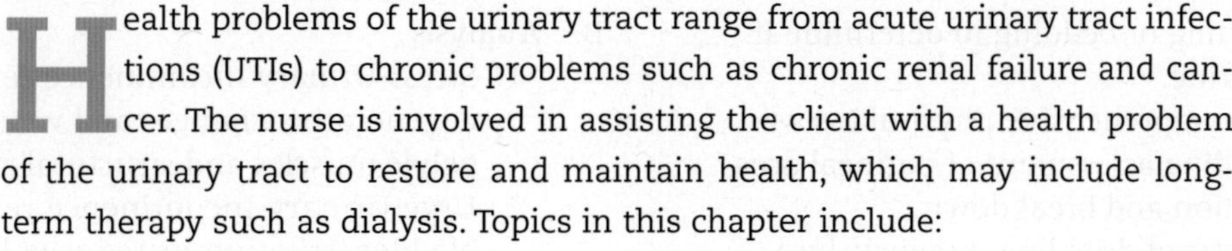

Health problems of the urinary tract range from acute urinary tract infections (UTIs) to chronic problems such as chronic renal failure and cancer. The nurse is involved in assisting the client with a health problem of the urinary tract to restore and maintain health, which may include long-term therapy such as dialysis. Topics in this chapter include:

- Urinary Incontinence
- Urinary Tract Infections
- Pyelonephritis
- Renal Calculi
- Acute Renal Failure
- Chronic Renal Failure
- Dialysis
- Bladder Cancer

Urinary Incontinence

I. Definition: Urinary incontinence is the inability of the urinary sphincter to control the release of urine. Incidence increases with age. There are several forms of incontinence, including the following:

A. Nocturnal enuresis (bedwetting) occurs primarily in children and hospitalized adult clients.

B. Stress incontinence involves dribbling resulting from any kind of physical stress (coughing, sneezing, or laughing), and most commonly affects women.

C. Urgency incontinence involves inability to hold back urine flow when feeling the urge to void.

D. Overflow incontinence involves frequent, sometimes almost constant, loss of urine from the bladder; the bladder cannot empty normally and becomes overdistended.

E. Continuous incontinence is completely uninhibited micturition reflex with an unpredictable voiding pattern.

F. Functional incontinence occurs when the function of the lower urinary tract is intact, but other factors (physical or mental impairments) make it difficult to identify need to void.

II. Nursing process

A. Assessment

1. Assess clothing or bedding to determine if wet with urine.
2. Perform a comprehensive physical assessment including assessment of perineal area for excoriation and breakdown.
3. Assess reports of dribbling, urgency, hesitancy, or inability to get to the bathroom before voiding starts.
4. Assess whether cause of incontinence is anatomic or psychosocial.
   a. Anatomic—may include weak abdominal and perineal muscle tone because of obesity and a sedentary lifestyle; sphincter weakness or damage from obstetric trauma, surgery, or congenital conditions; and urethral deformity.
   b. Psychosocial—may be an exhibition or expression of anxiety or frustration; may involve factors such as rebellion, dependence, regression, or attention-getting behavior.
5. Assess whether episodes are persistent/permanent or temporary.
   a. Temporary episodes may result from inflammation, stress, certain medications (opioids, tranquilizers, diuretics, antihistamines, antihypertensives).
   b. Persistent/permanent incontinence may result from neuromuscular dysfunction associated with disorders such as spinal cord injury, multiple sclerosis, bladder lesions, or large bowel disease.
6. Obtain diagnostic tests.
   a. Urinalysis—cloudy/hazy appearance, foul odor, pH of 7.8, and presence of RBCs, WBCs, and WBC casts.
   b. Urine culture—detects type of bacteria present.
   c. Urodynamic studies—evaluates cause and extent of incontinence.
   d. Uroflowmetry—provides information about bladder strength and opening ability of urethral sphincter.
   e. Cystometry—provides ability of bladder to accommodate fluid, sense bladder-filling, and presence of appropriate detrusor muscle contraction.
   f. Electromyography (EMG)—evaluates function of striated pelvic floor.
   g. Postvoid residual—measures amount of urine in bladder after normal voiding.
   h. Blood urea nitrogen, creatinine—increases as renal-urinary function declines.

B. Analysis

1. Stress Urinary Incontinence related to degenerative changes and weakness in pelvic muscles and structural supports
2. Urge Urinary Incontinence related to bladder irritation or reduced bladder capacity
3. Functional Urinary Incontinence related to sensory, cognitive, or mobility deficits related to environmental changes
4. Risk for Impaired Skin Integrity related to incontinence of urine
5. Disturbed Body Image related to odor, discomfort, and embarrassment

C. Planning

1. Implement bladder training program.
2. Implement bowel and bladder toileting program.
3. Promote maintenance of skin integrity.
4. Encourage verbalization of feelings, frustrations without self-deprecating statements.

D. Implementation

1. Administer prescribed medications.
2. Promote measures to decrease physiologic or psychologic complications.
3. Provide bladder training.
4. Assess medication regimen.

5. Discuss, prepare for surgical correction for stress incontinence.
6. Provide health teaching.

E. Evaluation
1. Client experiences urine continence as a result of bladder training program.
2. Client experiences stool and urine continence as a result of toileting program.
3. Client exhibits intact perineal skin.
4. Client verbalizes feelings and frustrations without self-deprecating statements.

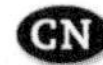

III. Client needs

A. Physiologic adaptation: Urinary incontinence may be treated through performance of Kegel exercises and bladder training (see management of care), electrical stimulation, and use of inserts/pessaries and medications. Surgical correction may be indicated for stress incontinence (vaginal repair, abdominal suspension of bladder).

B. Management of care: Care of the client experiencing urinary incontinence requires critical thinking skills and knowledge of assessment, and teaching and evaluation methods unique to the RN role. These skills cannot be delegated to an LPN or UAP.
1. Teach client to perform Kegel exercises—encourage client to contract perineal muscles as though stopping urination; sustain contraction for 5 to 10 s and release; perform 10 to 15 sets of 10 repetitions daily.
2. Teach client to time intake of fluids to avoid incontinence.
3. Teach client bladder training: To increase the time between when feels the urge to void until the time of voiding, gradually increasing voiding control. Provide client with information about surgery and pre- and postoperative care.

C. Safety and infection control
1. Provide client teaching regarding care of catheters and drains in the home setting, if indicated.
2. Stress importance of maintaining fluid intake of at least 2,000 ml per day; avoid caffeine, and alcohol.
3. Provide client teaching regarding care of incision postsurgical intervention.

D. Health promotion and maintenance
1. Administer prescribed medication, which may include antibiotics for treatment of infection.
2. Promote measures to ensure adequate nutrition.
3. Promote measures to maintain fluid and electrolyte balance.

E. Psychologic integrity
1. Refer client for psychological evaluation as appropriate.
2. Promote effective coping strategies.

F. Basic care and comfort
1. Supply bedpan and urinal within easy reach.
2. Change clothing and bed linens as necessary.
3. Advise client to select clothing that is easy to remove when using toilet.
4. Promote easy access to bathroom.
5. Provide adequate food and fluids.
6. Promote skin integrity by keeping perineal area dry.
7. Encourage client to use protective pads and undergarments.
8. Provide pain relief.

G. Reduction of risk potential
1. Provide health teaching about maintaining skin integrity and preventing skin excoriation.
2. Provide health teaching on measures to prevent UTIs.
3. Assess medication regimen for any drugs that could cause or contribute to incontinence.

H. Pharmacologic and parenteral therapies: Client will state the purpose for and associated side effects of all medications used to treat urinary incontinence.
1. Antibiotics: Ciprofloxacin (Cipro), nitrofurantoin (Nitrofan), sulfisoxazole (Gantrisin), and trimethoprim-sulfamethoxazole (Bactrim)—prevent or treat bacterial growth in kidneys or bladder.
   a. Assess for allergies before first dose; determine whether culture has been obtained.
   b. Assess for superinfection (thrush, yeast infection, diarrhea) after multiple doses; notify physician on observation.
   c. Assess insertion site for phlebitis if antibiotics being administered intravenously.
   d. Assess effectiveness of antibiotic therapy by monitoring urinalysis.
2. Cholinergics: Bethanechol chloride (Urecholine)—stimulates bladder contraction.
3. Antispasmodics: Tolterodine (Detrol) to reduce bladder spasms.
4. IV fluids—for hydration of acutely ill.
   a. Normal saline (NS—0.9% NaCl)—isotonic

b. Lactated Ringer (LR)—isotonic
c. Dextrose 5% in water (D5/W)—isotonic, hypotonic

Urinary Tract Infections

I. Definition: Urinary tract infections (UTIs) occur in the bladder, ureter, or in the urethra as a result of pathogenic micro-organisms in the urinary tract such as *Escherichia coli, Proteus, Klebsiella,* or *Enterobacter* (see assessment for predisposing factors). Women develop UTIs more frequently than men because of the shorter urethra. Incidence among women increases with aging, and incidence among men peaks after 50 years of age. Inflammation and infection of urinary tract structures are classified as being either upper UTIs or lower UTIs.
  A. Upper UTIs are known as *pyelonephritis,* which involves inflammation of the kidney.
  B. Lower UTIs include the following:
    1. Cystitis—involves inflammation of the bladder wall, and is the most common type of UTI.
    2. Ureteritis—involves inflammation of the ureter.
    3. Urethritis—involves inflammation of the urethra.

II. Nursing process
  A. Assessment
    1. Perform a comprehensive physical assessment, including assessment for signs and symptoms. The only sign of UTI in elderly clients may be mental status change.
      a. Upper UTI: Flank pain; costovertebral angle tenderness; fever, chills; dysuria; frequency, urgency; malaise; possibly bloody/cloudy urine
      b. Lower UTI: Frequency, urgency; burning on urination; nocturia; inflamed, edematous meatus in urethritis
    2. Assess client for predisposing factors.
      a. Loss of resistance to invading micro-organisms
      b. Sexual intercourse
      c. Indwelling catheterization
      d. Urine stasis
      e. Urinary tract instrumentation
      f Residual urine
      g. Urinary reflux
      h. Bladder overdistention
      i. Loss of intact mucosal lining
      j. Metabolic disorders
      k. Improper hygienic practices
    3. Obtain diagnostic tests.
      a. Upper UTI: Urinalysis—elevates WBC count; white cell casts, bacteria.
      b. Lower UTI:
        (1) Urinalysis—bacteriuria, RBCs in urine
        (2) Urine culture—identifies causative organism: 100,000 bacterial colonies per milliliter of urine or greater, tends to indicate infection.
      c. Urologic workup with renal ultrasound, IV pyelogram, and voiding cystourethrogram—evaluates cause of recurrent infections.
  B. Analysis
    1. Acute Pain related to disease process
    2. Anxiety related to diagnostic test results and treatment options available
    3. Deficient Knowledge related to cause of UTI
    4. Impaired Urinary Elimination related to urethral inflammation
  C. Planning
    1. Administer prescribed medications.
    2. Relieve pain.
    3. Eliminate infection.
    4. Maintain fluid and electrolyte balance.
    5. Provide teaching to prevent additional UTIs.
    6. Promote client, family coping with current alteration in health.
  D. Implementation (see management of care)
  E. Evaluation
    1. Client verbalizes decrease in pain.
    2. Client demonstrates ability to describe tests, significance of the results, and treatment options available.
    3. Client verbalizes risk factors of UTI.
    4. Client demonstrates adequate urine output of at least 2,000 ml/day.

CN

III. Client needs
  A. Physiologic adaptation: UTIs are treated with antibiotics and/or antispasmodics, increased fluid to flush bacteria from urinary tract, and surgery to correct underlying obstruction or congenital anomaly (defect), if indicated.
  B. Management of care: Care of the client with a UTI requires critical thinking skills and knowledge of assessment, and teaching and evaluation methods unique to the RN role. These skills cannot be delegated to an LPN or UAP.
    1. Administer/teach self-administration of prescribed antibiotic and/or antispasmodic.
    2. Encourage fluids to promote urinary output; encourage voiding every 2 to 3 hr.
    3. Monitor fluid and electrolyte balance.
    4. Provide client teaching (see safety and infection control).
    5. Refer client to urologist, if indicated.

C. Safety and infection control—provide client teaching about the following:
 1. Promote frequent voiding to prevent reinfection.
 2. Minimize spread of bacteria from anal/vaginal areas to urethra by cleansing from front to back.
 3. Decrease entry of micro-organisms into bladder by voiding immediately after sexual intercourse.
 4. Make sure bladder is completely emptied when voiding.
 5. Avoid urinary irritants such as alcohol, caffeinated coffee, tea, and soft drinks.
 6. Wear cotton underwear.
 7. Take a shower rather than a bath.
 8. Avoid external irritants such as bubble baths, perfumed vaginal cleaners, and deodorants.
 9. Consume a high-fiber diet to avoid constipation.
 10. Drink liberal amounts water to lower bacterial concentration in urine.

D. Health promotion and maintenance: Encourage follow-up care for recurrent or severe infections.

E. Psychologic integrity: Support client efforts to prevent infections.

F. Basic care and comfort
 1. Administer antipyretics, analgesics, antibiotics, or antiemetics as ordered.
 2. Provide liberal fluids (nonstimulant) and encourage frequent voiding (every 2 to 3 hr).
 3. Encourage ambulation.

G. Reduction of risk potential: Teach client to prevent recurrent UTIs by taking medication exactly as prescribed; do not save any pills.

H. Pharmacologic and parenteral therapies: Client will state the purpose for and associated side effects of all medications used to treat UTIs. Follow-up culture is recommended to establish effectiveness of treatment.
 1. Antibiotics—indwelling catheters are changed at start of antibiotic therapy; long-term antibiotic therapy may be needed for recurrent UTIs.
  a. For uncomplicated UTIs—treat with 3-day course of antibiotics: Amoxicillin (Amoxil), trimethoprim-sulfamethoxazole (Bactrim), or ciprofloxacin (Cipro).
  b. For UTI with associated complications—treat with a 7- to 10-day course of nitrofurantoin (Macrobid). Complications may include obstruction, resistant pathogens, upper UTI, or urologic dysfunction, as well as clients who are pregnant, and in most cases involving men and children.
 2. Analgesics—Propoxyphene (Darvon) or antispasmodic—propantheline (Pro-Banthine) if pain is severe.

Pyelonephritis

I. Definition: Pyelonephritis is an acute inflammation and infection of the renal pelvis, tubules, and interstitial tissue. Infection typically spreads as a result of vesicoureteral reflux, moving from the bladder, to the ureters, and then the kidneys; one or both kidneys may be affected. After multiple bouts of acute pyelonephritis, chronic pyelonephritis can occur and lead to permanent kidney damage.

II. Nursing process

A. Assessment
 1. Perform a comprehensive physical assessment—assess for signs and symptoms of pyelonephritis; observe older adult clients for signs of confusion and GI or pulmonary symptoms as they may not show usual febrile response.
  a. Burning during urination
  b. Dysuria, nocturia, hematuria
  c. Anorexia, vomiting, diarrhea
  d. Fatigue
  e. Flank pain
  f. Cloudy urine
  g. Ammonialike or fishy odor to urine
  h. Fever of 102°F or higher, shaking chills
 2. Obtain a detailed health history, including a history of urinary urgency and frequency.
 3. Assess for predisposing factors.
  a. Urinary obstruction
  b. Recurrent infection
  c. Trauma
  d. Blood-borne infection
  e. Pregnancy
  f. Metabolic disorders
 4. Obtain diagnostic tests.
  a. Urinalysis and culture/sensitivity—reveals pyuria, significant bacteriuria, low specific gravity, osmolality, slightly alkaline urine, proteinuria, glycosuria, gross or microscopic hematuria.
  b. CBC: Elevated WBCs; elevated erythrocyte sedimentation rate.
  c. Radiography of the kidneys, ureters, or bladder—shows calculi, tumors, or cysts in urinary tract.
  d. Excretory urography—reveals asymmetrical kidneys, possibly indicating a high frequency of infection.

B. Analysis
 1. Acute Pain related to inflammatory process
 2. Hyperthermia related to infection

3. Readiness for Enhanced Knowledge related to cause of and means to prevent pyelonephritis

C. Planning
1. Maintain fluid balance.
2. Maintain urine specific gravity within normal range.
3. Identify risk factors that exacerbate decreased tissue perfusion.
4. Promote increased comfort.

D. Implementation
1. Assess vital signs frequently.
2. Monitor intake and output.
3. Monitor renal function.
4. Administer prescribed antibiotics, analgesics, antiemetics, and antipyretics.
5. Correct dehydration.

E. Evaluation
1. Client reports decreased perception of pain.
2. Client demonstrates body temperature below 100° F.
3. Client describes cause of and means to treat pyelonephritis.

CN

III. Client needs

A. Physiologic adaptation. The goal of management is to treat infection, reduce inflammation, and treat or prevent complications.
1. Assist with percutaneous drainage as needed; prolonged antibiotic therapy needed to treat renal/perinephric abscess.
2. Administer antibiotic therapy for chronic or recurring infections to preserve renal function.
3. Follow-up care required for acute infection (may be for 2 years after infection) to ensure eradication of infection and stabilization of kidney function.
4. Complications include renal insufficiency, bacteremia with sepsis, chronic renal failure, hypertension, and renal abscess.

B. Management of care: Care of the client with pyelonephritis requires critical thinking skills and knowledge of assessment, and teaching and evaluation methods unique to the RN role. These skills cannot be delegated to an LPN or UAP.
1. Delegate responsibly those activities that can be delegated. All monitoring information is reported to the RN.
   a. Check routine vital signs.
   b. Measure and record intake and output.
   c. Assist with adequate hydration.
2. Consult with urologist and or nephrologist as indicated.
3. Provide client and family teaching (see health promotion and maintenance).

C. Safety and infection control
1. Assess vital signs often for impending sepsis.
2. Take measures to decrease body temperature, if indicated (cooling blanket).
3. Review signs and symptoms of lower UTI.
4. Avoid bacterial contamination.

D. Health promotion and maintenance: Provide client and family teaching.
1. Always use hygienic toileting practices.
2. Follow through with routine checkups when history of UTIs is present.
3. Promptly report to physician signs and symptoms of UTI.
4. Consume generous amount of fluids; avoid caffeinated beverages (e.g., coffee, tea, and colas); want intake of at least 2,000 ml/day unless contraindicated (heart failure, renal failure).

E. Psychologic integrity: Elderly may become confused; orient to time, place, and person.

F. Basic care and comfort
1. Make available ample noncaffeinated fluids.
2. Measure intake and output.
3. Use comfort measures, such as positioning and heat to relieve local flank pain.
4. Provide analgesics, antiemetics as ordered.

G. Reduction of risk potential
1. Explain preventive measures including:
   a. Adequate fluid intake (2,000 ml/day)
   b. Healthy personal hygienic measures
   c. Voiding habits
2. Encourage follow-up visits with regular physician or urologist.
3. Review antibiotic therapy; stress importance of taking all prescribed antibiotics and having follow-up urine cultures.

H. Pharmacologic and parenteral therapies: Client will state the purpose for and associated side effects of all medications used to treat pyelonephritis.
1. Organism-specific antimicrobial therapy:
   a. Begin promptly to cover prevalent gram-positive and gram-negative pathogens; then adjust according to urine culture results.
      (1) Obtain urine specimen for culture/sensitivity before antibiotic therapy is begun.
      (2) Obtain midstream urine specimen or urine specimen via straight catheterization.
   b. Provide treatment for at least 2 weeks.
   c. Follow up with urine culture after completion of therapy.
2. Parenteral antimicrobial therapy—used if client cannot tolerate oral intake, is dehydrated, or acutely ill.

3. Maintenance antimicrobial therapy may be used for chronic/recurring infections to preserve renal function.
4. IV fluids (may be ordered):
   a. Normal saline (NS; 0.9% NaCl)—isotonic
   b. Dextrose 5% in water (D5/W)—isotonic, hypotonic
   c. Lactated Ringer (LR)—isotonic

Renal Calculi

I. Definition: Urolithiasis refers to the presence of stones (calculi) in the urinary system; nephrolithiasis refers to the presence of stones in the renal pelvis. Calculi are formed by crystallization of urinary solutes (calcium, oxalate, uric acid, calcium phosphate, struvite, and cystine), and vary in size; stones vary from granular (gravel, sand) deposits to bladder stones, which can be as large as an orange. Gravel stones, which are most common, generally pass on their own. Incidence peaks between 30 and 50 years of age; men are affected more frequently than women.

II. Nursing process

A. Assessment

1. Perform a comprehensive physical assessment, including assessment for signs and symptoms. (Signs and symptoms vary with location, size, and cause of calculi.)
   a. Acute, sharp, intermittent pain (ureteral colic)
   b. Dull, tender ache in flank (renal colic)
   c. Nausea, vomiting accompanying severe pain
   d. Fever, chills
   e. Hematuria, dysuria, frequency
   f. Abdominal distention
   g. Pyuria
   h. Rarely, oliguria and anuria
2. Assess for predisposing factors in calculi formation.
   a. Immobility
   b. Hypercalcemia and hypercalciuria
   c. UTI
   d. Urine stasis
   e. High urine specific gravity
   f. Genetic predisposition (cystinuria)
   g. Multiple myeloma
   h. Excessive intake of vitamin D, milk, alkali
   i. Chronic dehydration, poor fluid intake
   j. Abnormal purine metabolism (hyperuricemia, gout)
   k. Chronic obstruction by foreign bodies in urinary tract
   l. Excessive oxalate absorption in inflammatory bowel disease, bowel resection, or ileostomy
3. Obtain diagnostic tests.
   a. Radiograph of kidneys, ureters, and bladder—shows visible calculi.
   b. Stone analysis—shows mineral content of calculi.
   c. IV pyelography—shows size and location of calculi.
   d. Renal ultrasound—shows obstructive changes such as hydronephrosis.
   e. Spiral computed tomography technique—shows stone in ureter; faster than IV pyelogram and no preparation needed.
   f. Urinalysis—shows hematuria, pyuria; culture, sensitivity studies identify infective organism/s.
   g. Serum renal function tests, electrolytes, calcium, phosphorus, uric acid, magnesium, and parathyroid hormone levels—evaluated.

B. Analysis

1. Acute Pain related to attempted passage of calculi
2. Impaired Urinary Elimination related to obstruction
3. Risk for Infection related to urinary stasis

C. Planning

1. Manage pain.
2. Prepare for surgical and/or nonsurgical procedures.
3. Institute measures to prevent calculi recurrence.
4. Maintain comfortable (not hot) environmental temperature.
5. Provide health-related teaching.

D. Implementation

1. Provide pharmacologic therapy.
2. Provide comfort measures.
3. Prepare for nonsurgical and/or surgical procedures.
4. Make provision for analysis of calculi.
5. Institute measures to help prevent recurrent calculi.
6. Instruct client to avoid sudden increases in environmental temperature.
7. Provide teaching on measures to prevent UTIs.

E. Evaluation

1. Client reports little or no pain.
2. Client has adequate amount of urine output in relation to intake.
3. Client is free from signs and symptoms of UTIs.

CN

III. Client needs

A. Physiologic adaptation: Calculi may pass through the urinary tract, or lodge in the urinary tract, causing obstruction, infection, and perhaps hydronephrosis (collection of urine in renal pelvis). If the calculi do not pass, extracorporeal shock wave lithotripsy or surgical intervention may be required.

1. Extracorporeal shock wave lithotripsy—treatment of choice; procedure directed at disintegrating calculi into very small particles to pass in the urine. Eliminates need for surgery; can be repeated for recurrent stones.
   a. Stones smaller than 3/4 inch in diameter
   b. Stones located in ureter above iliac crest
2. Surgical interventions:
   a. Percutaneous nephrolithotomy—calculi broken apart with hydraulic shock waves/laser beam via nephroscope; may be combined with extracorporeal shock wave lithotripsy.
      (1) Stones larger than 1 inch
      (2) Fragments removed using forceps, graspers, basket
   b. Percutaneous stone dissolution (chemolysis)—used to dissolve struvite, uric acid, cystine calculi; solvent infused into calculus via nephrostomy tube placed in kidney.
   c. Ureteroscopy—used for distal ureteral calculi; may be used for midureteral calculi.
      (1) Stones are fragmented with electrohydraulic, ultrasonic, laser equipment and removed by ureteroscope
      (2) Stent may be inserted to maintain patency of ureter

B. Management of care: Care of the client with renal calculi requires critical thinking skills and knowledge of assessment, and teaching and evaluation methods unique to the RN role. These skills cannot be delegated to an LPN or UAP.
1. Delegate responsibly those activities that can be delegated, including vital sign checks, encouraging ambulation, straining all urine, and monitoring of intake and output. All monitoring information is reported to the RN.
2. Assure adequate fluid intake (PO and IV if needed).
3. Provide pain relief—opioids are most effective. Client may require large doses; monitor for respiratory depression.
4. Manage nausea; use rectal suppository.
5. Prepare client for procedure/surgery as needed.
6. Provide postsurgical monitoring and care (see safety and infection control).
7. Provide client and family teaching (see health promotion and maintenance).
8. Consult with nephrologist, urologist as indicated.
9. Consult with dietitian to aid in food/fluid selections based on stone analysis (see reduction of risk potential).

C. Safety and infection control: Provide postsurgical monitoring and care.
1. Monitor for complications of procedures.
   a. Infection—indicated by fever, dysuria, frequency, foul-smelling urine
   b. Hemorrhage
   c. Extravasation of urine
   d. Obstruction from remaining stone fragments
2. Encourage oral fluid intake, if able, or administer intravenously if client is vomiting to ensure adequate urine output; monitor urine output, pattern of voiding; report oliguria, anuria.
3. Strain urine to harvest stones/fragments; inspect sides of urinal and/or bedpan for clinging stones/fragments.

D. Health promotion and maintenance: Provide client and family teaching.
1. Drink enough fluids (noncaffeinated) to achieve urinary volume of at least 2,000 to 3,000 ml/day to aid in prevention of calculi and, if present, to accelerate passage of stone particles.
2. Ambulate to assist in passage of stone fragments.
3. Comply with prescribed drug therapy (see pharmacologic and parenteral therapies).
4. Perform weight-bearing activity; avoid prolonged bed rest, which alters calcium metabolism.

E. Psychologic integrity: Promote relaxation techniques.

F. Basic care and comfort
1. Encourage client to assume position of comfort.
2. Encourage oral fluid intake, if able.
3. Provide analgesics, antiemetics as needed.

G. Reduction of risk potential
1. Instruct client to quickly report signs and symptoms of UTI.
2. For client with uric acid/cystine stones—monitor urine pH with test strip to maintain urine alkalinity.
3. Promote dietary requirements related to specific stone type:
   a. For calcium, oxalate stones—avoid excessive calcium, phosphorus.

b. For uric acid stones—reduce purine intake (red meat, fish, fowl).

H. Pharmacologic and parenteral therapies: Client will state the purpose for and associated side effects of all medications used to treat renal calculi.
1. Analgesics—hydrocodone (Vicodin); morphine (Duramorph)
2. Antiemetics—promethazine (Phenergan); dimenhydrinate (Dramamine); ondansetron hydrochloride (Zofran)
3. Thiazide diuretics to reduce urine calcium excretion
4. Allopurinol (Alloprim) to reduce uric acid concentration
5. D-penicillamine (Depen) to lower cystine concentration
6. Sodium bicarbonate to alkalinize urine
7. IV fluids:
a. Normal saline—NS (0.9% NaCl)—isotonic
b. Lactated Ringer (LR)—isotonic
c. Dextrose 5% in water (D5/W)—isotonic, hypotonic

Acute Renal Failure

I. Definition: Acute renal failure is a clinical syndrome characterized by a rapid loss of renal function with progressive azotemia (an accumulation of nitrogenous waste products such as blood urea nitrogen and increasing levels of serum creatinine). Most commonly, acute renal failure follows severe, prolonged hypotension, hypovolemia, or exposure to nephrotoxic agents. Acute renal failure can be reversed with medical treatment; if untreated, the health problem progresses to chronic renal failure, end-stage renal disease, and death.

A. Causes are classified as prerenal, postrenal, and intrarenal.
1. Prerenal failure results from conditions that interrupt the renal blood supply, reducing renal perfusion (e.g., hypovolemia, shock, hemorrhage, burns, impaired cardiac output or diuretic therapy).
2. Postrenal failure results from obstruction or impairment of urine flow.
a. Ureteral obstruction due to calculi, strictures, trauma, or pregnancy
b. Bladder obstruction due to tumors or prostatic hypertrophy
3. Intrarenal failure results from injury to the kidneys themselves from ischemia, toxins, immunologic processes, and systemic or vascular disorders.

B. Acute renal failure progresses through four clinical phases: Initiation, oliguric-anuric, diuretic, and recovery phase. Phases are primarily distinguished by changes in urine volume, blood urea nitrogen, and creatinine levels.
1. Initiation phase—involves sudden interruption of renal function; may last a few hours or several days.
2. Oliguric-anuric phase:
a. Urine volume less than 400 ml/day.
b. Increase in serum creatinine, urea, uric acid, organic acids, potassium, magnesium.
c. Duration is 10 to 14 days.
3. Diuretic phase:
a. Begins when urine output exceeds 500 ml/day.
b. Ends when blood urea nitrogen and creatinine levels stop rising.
c. Duration varies.
4. Recovery phase:
a. Duration is several months to 1 year.
b. Some scar tissue may remain.

II. Nursing process
A. Assessment
1. Perform a comprehensive physical assessment including assessment for general signs and symptoms.
a. Tachycardia
b. Crackles in bases of both lungs
c. Irritability, drowsiness, confusion
d. Bleeding abnormalities
e. Dry, pruritic skin
f. Nausea, vomiting, diarrhea, lethargy
2. Assess client for signs and symptoms specific to disease type.
a. Prerenal disease:
(1) Decreased tissue turgor
(2) Dryness of mucous membranes
(3) Weight loss
(4) Flat neck veins
(5) Hypotension
b. Postrenal disease:
(1) Difficulty in voiding
(2) Changes in urine flow
c. Intrarenal disease:
(1) Edema
(2) Fever
(3) Skin rash
3. Obtain diagnostic tests.
a. Blood urea nitrogen, creatinine, potassium levels—elevated
b. Hematocrit, hemoglobin, bicarbonate, blood pH—decreased
c. Urine casts, cellular debris—present

d. Proteinuria, urine osmolality—close to serum osmolality level (in glomerular disease)
e. Urine creatinine clearance—decreased
f. The following procedures reveal obstruction:
(1) Kidney ultrasonography
(2) Kidney-ureter-bladder radiography
(3) Retrograde pyelography
(4) Computed tomography scan
g. Electrocardiogram—tall, peaked T waves; widening QRS complex if hyperkalemia present

B. Analysis
1. Excess Fluid Volume related to fluid retention
2. Risk for Infection related to invasive lines, uremic toxins, and altered immune responses
3. Imbalanced Nutrition: Less Than Body Requirements related to altered metabolic state and dietary restrictions
4. Disturbed Thought Processes related to effects of uremic toxins on central nervous system
5. Fatigue related to anemia, metabolic acidosis, and uremic toxins
6. Anxiety related to disease process, therapeutic interventions, and uncertainty of prognosis
7. Ineffective Tissue Perfusion, cardiopulmonary related to electrolyte imbalances and potential for arrhythmia
8. Impaired Urinary Elimination and risk for metabolic acidosis related to inability to excrete hydrogen ions, impaired bicarbonate reabsorption, and decreased synthesis of ammonia

C. Planning
1. Promote recovery without any loss of kidney function.
2. Maintain normal fluid and electrolyte balance.
3. Decrease anxiety.
4. Promote compliance with follow-up care.
5. Provide information as to why follow-up care is needed.
6. Prevent development of complications.
7. Maintain hemodynamic stability.
8. Assist in identification of risk factors for decreased tissue perfusion with strategies to prevent further deterioration.
9. Facilitate management of urinary elimination problems.
10. Enhance understanding of diet-medication regimen and rationale.

D. Implementation
1. Ensure adequate hydration.
2. Avoid exposure to various nephrotoxins (see reduction of risk potential).
3. Avoid abuse of chronic analgesics.
4. Prevent/treat shock; prevent prolonged hypotension.
5. Monitor vital signs, urinary output.
6. Schedule diagnostic tests so client does not become dehydrated.
7. Take measures to prevent infection.
8. Ensure right client receives right blood/blood product to avoid severe transfusion reaction.
9. Monitor weight daily.
10. Monitor dialysis access site (fistula or graft) for bruit/thrill; these accesses are surgically placed and cannot be used immediately.

E. Evaluation
1. Client is free from signs and symptoms of fluid retention.
2. Client is free from signs and symptoms of infection.
3. Client attains and maintains body weight with normal body mass index.
4. Client demonstrates clear cognitive function.
5. Client is free from signs and symptoms of fatigue.
6. Client verbalizes decreased perception of anxiety.
7. Client does not exhibit signs of cardiac arrhythmia.
8. Client's serum pH is within normal range.
9. Client's dialysis access remains patent.

CN

III. Client needs
A. Physiologic adaptation: Treatment for acute renal failure may involve the following:
1. Surgical relief of obstruction—may be required to enhance urine flow
2. Correction of underlying fluid excesses or deficits
3. Correction/management of biochemical imbalances
4. Restoration/maintenance of BP via IV fluids and vasopressors
5. Maintenance of adequate nutrition: Low-protein diet with supplemental amino acids, vitamins
6. Initiation of hemodialysis, peritoneal dialysis, or continuous renal replacement therapy for clients with progressive azotemia or other life-threatening complications

B. Management of care: Care of the client with renal calculi requires critical thinking skills and knowledge of assessment, and teaching and evaluation methods unique to the RN role. These skills cannot be delegated to an LPN or UAP.

1. Delegate responsibly those activities that can be delegated. All monitoring information is reported to the RN.
   a. Vital signs
   b. Daily weight
   c. Intake, output, and documentation
   d. Bedside fingerstick blood glucose monitoring, as needed
   e. Signs of mental status changes (lethargy, fatigue, irritability, disorientation, twitching)
2. Provide client and family teaching (see health promotion and maintenance).
3. Consult with nephrologists as indicated.
4. Consult with hemodialysis nurses as indicated.
5. Consult with dietitian—regulate protein intake according to type of renal impairment: Restrict protein and potassium, and large amounts of sodium and phosphorus.
6. Consult with IV therapists as indicated.

C. Safety and infection control
1. Institute seizure precautions; provide padded side rails.
2. Provide meticulous wound care.
3. Employ intensive pulmonary hygiene because incidence of pulmonary edema and infection is high.
4. Remove bladder catheter as soon as possible.
   a. Watch for signs of UTI.
   b. Encourage noncaffeinated fluids, as permitted.
5. Treat hyperkalemia as ordered.
6. Watch for cardiac dysrhythmias, heart failure from hyperkalemia, electrolyte imbalance, or fluid overload.

D. Health promotion and maintenance: Provide client and family teaching.
1. Report for routine urinalysis and follow-up examinations.
2. Avoid any medication unless specifically prescribed.
3. Space activity with periods of rest (muscle weakness may be from excessive catabolism).
4. Consume high-carbohydrate meals (carbohydrates have greater protein-sparing power).
5. Inform physician of signs and symptoms of edema and daily weight changes (2 pound gain or loss).

E. Psychologic integrity
1. Encourage client to express feelings and provide emotional support.
2. Long-term convalescence of 3 to 12 months may cause psychosocial, financial hardships—counseling, social work, psychiatry referrals may be needed.

F. Basic care and comfort: Maintain normal homeostasis and monitor renal function.

G. Reduction of risk potential
1. Prevent health problem.
   a. Identify and monitor high-risk populations.
   b. Control nephrotoxic drugs (aminoglycoside antibiotics, nonsteroidal anti-inflammatory drugs)—most drugs and/or their metabolites are excreted by the kidneys: Adjust dosages for age and physiologic status.
   c. Prevent prolonged episodes of hypotension and hypovolemia.
2. Provide close monitoring of intake and output, and fluid and electrolyte balance.
3. Assess and record extrarenal losses of fluid (vomiting, diarrhea, hemorrhage, increased insensible losses).
4. Identify and treat streptococcal infections promptly.
   a. Comply with antibiotic regimen.
   b. Prevent acute poststreptococcal glomerulonephritis.
5. For diagnostic studies with contrast media given intravenously, adequately hydrate client before and after test.
6. Caution with chemotherapy that causes hyperuricemia—increases risk for renal injury.
7. Monitor renal function when taking potentially nephrotoxic drugs.
   a. Use sparingly in high-risk clients.
   b. Give in smallest effective dose for shortest possible period of time.
8. Caution client about overuse of over-the-counter analgesics, especially nonsteroidal anti-inflammatory drugs—may worsen renal function if client has borderline renal insufficiency.
9. Caution client with angiotensin-converting enzyme inhibitors:
   a. Decrease perfusion pressure
   b. Cause hyperkalemia
   c. Contraindicated in renal insufficiency
10. Avoid restricting fluids for prolonged periods for exams—dehydrating procedures are hazardous to clients who cannot produce concentrated urine.

H. Pharmacologic and parenteral therapies: Client will state the purpose for and associated side effects of all medications used to treat acute renal failure.
1. Hyperkalemia: Glucose and insulin to shift potassium into cells—cation exchange resin (sodium polystyrene sulfonate [Kayexalate]) to promote GI excretion of potassium.

2. Acidosis: Sodium bicarbonate—be prepared for mechanical ventilation.
3. For restoration/maintenance of BP: Vasopressin (Pitressin), desmopressin (Stimate).
4. During initiation or oliguric-anuric phase: IV fluids (dextrose 5%/water [D5/W]—isotonic, hypotonic)—give enough total fluid to equal 24-hr urine output plus 500 ml/day; monitor closely to prevent fluid volume overload.

Chronic Renal Failure

I. Definition: Chronic renal failure is a progressive deterioration of renal function that ends fatally in uremia (an excess of urea and other nitrogenous wastes in the blood) unless dialysis or kidney transplantation is performed. Before end-stage renal disease develops, a client with chronic renal failure can lead a relatively normal life managed by diet and medications; typically, there are few signs or symptoms until about 75% of renal function (glomerular filtration) is lost. According to the National Kidney Foundation's Kidney Disease Outcomes Quality Initiative, the progression of chronic renal failure is described in 5 stages and defined by the glomerular filtration rate (GFR):

Stage 1 Signs of mild kidney disease, GFR greater than 90%
Stage 2 Mild kidney disease with GFR of 60 to 89%
Stage 3 Moderate chronic renal insufficiency with GFR of 30 to 59%
Stage 4 Severe chronic renal insufficiency with GFR of 15 to 29%
Stage 5 End stage renal failure (ESRF) with GFR of less than 15%

II. Nursing process

A. Assessment

1. Obtain a detailed health history, including assessment of causes of chronic renal failure such as:
   a. Glomerulonephritis
   b. Diabetes mellitus
   c. Hypertension
   d. Polycystic kidney disease
2. Perform a comprehensive physical assessment; assess for signs and symptoms—clinical manifestations are similar because of retention of metabolic end products and accompanying fluid and electrolyte imbalances.
   a. Decreased renal reserve—client is asymptomatic unless there is exposure to severe physiologic or psychologic stress.
   b. Renal insufficiency:
      (1) Polyuria
      (2) Nocturia
      (3) Mild anemia
   c. End-stage renal disease—involves widespread systemic manifestations:
      (1) Cardiovascular—fluid overload, edema, hypertension, arrhythmias, congestive heart failure, electrolyte imbalances
      (2) GI—anorexia, nausea, vomiting, diarrhea, gastritis, bleeding, stomatitis
      (3) Hematopoietic—anemia, increased susceptibility to infection, alterations in coagulation
      (4) Integumentary—pallor, jaundice, dryness, pruritus, ecchymosis, uremic frost (rare)
      (5) Neuromuscular—drowsiness, confusion, irritability, twitching, tremors, peripheral neuropathy
      (6) Psychosocial—decreased mentation, altered perceptions
      (7) Respiratory—pulmonary edema, pneumonia, Kussmaul respirations with metabolic acidosis
      (8) Skeletal—hypocalcemia, hyperphosphatemia, osteodystrophy, metastatic calcifications
3. Obtain diagnostic tests.
   a. CBC: Anemia
   b. Elevated blood urea nitrogen, creatinine
   c. Elevated phosphorus
   d. Decreased calcium
   e. Decreased serum albumin
   f. ABGs: Low blood pH, low carbon dioxide; low bicarbonate

B. Analysis

1. Compromised Family Coping related to chronicity of disease management
2. Constipation related to hypomotility due to electrolyte imbalances and restricted fluid intake.
3. Disturbed Sleep Pattern related to altered neuromuscular function from metabolic waste buildup
4. Excessive Fluid Volume related to inability of kidneys to excrete fluid, and inadequate dialysis or excessive fluid intake
5. Imbalanced Nutrition: Less Than Body Requirements related to restricted intake of nutrients (especially protein), nausea, vomiting, anorexia, and stomatitis
6. Impaired Skin Integrity related to decrease in oil and sweat gland activity, hyperphosphatemia, capillary fragility, excess fluid, neuropathy, and pruritus

7. Risk for Injury related to alterations in calcium and phosphorus balance, and altered vitamin D metabolism
8. Activity Intolerance related to generalized weakness due to anemia and uremia

C. Planning
1. Encourage therapeutic conversation with client and family.
2. Encourage ambulation to promote peristalsis.
3. Provide environment conducive for sleep.
4. Maintain fluid control.
5. Maintain adequate nutrition.
6. Prevent skin breakdown.
7. Prevent injury.
8. Increase daily activity.

D. Implementation
1. Administer prescribed medications.
2. Provide conservative therapy with no dialysis, as needed.
3. Prepare client for peritoneal dialysis, if needed.
4. Prepare client for and assist with hemodialysis, as needed.
5. Prepare client for kidney transplantation, if indicated.
6. Provide referrals.

E. Evaluation
1. Client's family demonstrates ability to cope and complies with therapeutic regimen.
2. Client demonstrates adequate bowel elimination.
3. Client verbalizes ability to sleep majority of hours designated for sleep.
4. Client is free from signs of edema and shows no evidence of dyspnea.
5. Client maintains reasonable body weight.
6. Client exhibits intact, clean skin.
7. Client has acceptable calcium and phosphorus levels with no bone fractures.
8. Client is able to perform activities of daily living without undue fatigue.

III. Client needs

A. Physiologic adaptation: Before end-stage renal disease develops, medical management is aimed at slowing progression of chronic renal failure and avoiding complications (e.g., diabetes, hypertension volume depletion, and infection).
1. Alleviate uremic symptoms.
2. Provide dialysis (see sections on peritoneal dialysis and hemodialysis).
3. Explain kidney transplantation—surgical placement of a donor kidney into a client with irreversible renal failure. Transplant is a treatment, and not a cure. Recipient must be free of infection and cancer and healthy enough to withstand surgery. There must be a match between donor and recipient.
   a. Used synergistically with dialysis.
   b. Major advantages of transplantation over dialysis: Reversal of many of the pathophysiologic changes associated with renal failure when normal kidney function is restored; dependence on dialysis eliminated, as well as dietary and lifestyle restrictions imposed by renal failure.
   c. Rejection of the transplanted kidney is always a threat.
   d. Transplant survival rate for kidneys is approximately 10 years. Lifetime medications and medical follow-up are necessary.
4. Manage diet—sodium, potassium, and phosphorus limited; protein further restricted.
5. Maintain fluid restriction on hemodialysis—fluid weight gain limited to 3% to 4% of "dry" weight between dialysis sessions; client at risk for developing excess fluid volume.
6. Administer PRBCs—to treat severe and symptomatic anemia. *Note:* Transfusions limited because of transmittable diseases and risk of developing antibodies. Also, RBCs have shorter lifespan; therefore, results of transfusion do not last long. Epoetin alfa (Epogen) used extensively.
7. Maintain homeostasis; prevent complications by avoiding:
   a. Volume depletion
   b. Hypotension
   c. Use of contrast media
   d. Nephrotoxic substances

B. Management of care: Care of the client with chronic renal failure requires critical thinking skills and knowledge of assessment, and teaching and evaluation methods unique to the RN role. These skills cannot be delegated to an LPN or UAP.
1. Consult with nephrologist, endocrinologist, wound care specialist, and social worker as needed.
2. Consult with dietitian—diet, fluid restrictions may be altered as renal function decreases.
3. Provide referrals to the National Kidney Foundation and American Association of Kidney Patients.
4. Provide client and family teaching (see reduction of risk potential).

C. Safety and infection control
   1. Assess for local signs of infection (pain on urination, hematuria, cloudy urine; redness, edema, or drainage in areas of skin breakdown) and systemic signs of infection (chills, fever, and tachycardia).
   2. Instruct client to avoid exposure to others with infections to decrease risk of infection.
   3. Maintain aseptic technique when performing dialysis or other invasive procedures to prevent introduction of organisms.

D. Health promotion and maintenance
   1. Promote adherence to therapeutic regimen by providing client and family teaching about the following:
      a. Measure weight every morning to avoid fluid overload.
      b. Drink limited amounts only when thirsty.
      c. Measure allotted fluids and save some for ice cubes; sucking on ice is thirst-quenching.
      d. Eat food before drinking fluids to alleviate dry mouth.
      e. Use hard candy and chewing gum to moisten mouth.
      f. Teach client how to read labels and avoid foods that are high in potassium, sodium, and phosphorus.
   2. Explore alternatives that may reduce or eliminate adverse effects of treatment:
      a. Provide rest after dialysis.
      b. Provide smaller, more frequent meals to reduce nausea and facilitate the taking of medication.
   3. Promote client and family teaching regarding diet; include fact sheet listing foods to be restricted/limited.
   4. Provide care for, and observation of, dialysis access.
   5. Support need for continued medical follow-up care.

E. Psychologic integrity
   1. Contract with client for behavioral changes if client nonadherent to therapy or control of underlying condition.
   2. Support family in adjustment to chronic illness of a member.
   3. Allow client time to mourn loss of body function. Encourage verbalization of feelings and identify ways of coping with losses more effectively.
   4. Include family in discussion of client's concerns to enable them to assist the client and foster support and understanding.
   5. For client approaching end-stage renal disease, provide data concerning treatment options; support groups.

F. Basic care and comfort
   1. Weigh client daily; maintain intake and output.
   2. Monitor for edema and respiratory compromise from fluid volume excess.
   3. Monitor for signs of infection. *Note:* Renal failure clients do not always demonstrate fever, leukocytosis.
   4. Administer oral supplements as needed.
   5. Keep skin clean; relieve dryness to prevent itching. Avoid alcohol-based lotions as they are drying.
   6. Keep nails short and trimmed to prevent disruption of skin integrity with scratching.
   7. Keep hair clean and moisturized.
   8. Prevent constipation.
   9. Provide assistance with ambulation, as needed.
   10. Increase activity as tolerated; avoid immobilization because it increases bone demineralization.

G. Reduction of risk potential: Encourage strict follow-up for blood work, dialysis, and physician visits.

H. Pharmacologic and parenteral therapies: Client and family will state the purpose for and associated side effects of all medications used to manage chronic renal failure.
   1. Anemia—treated with recombinant human erythropoietin (epoetin alfa [Epogen, Procrit]), a synthetic kidney hormone that enhances RBC formation.
   2. Acidosis—treated with PO/IV sodium bicarbonate to replace bicarbonate stores.
   3. Hyperkalemia—treated with cation exchange resin (sodium polystyrene sulfonate [Kayexalate]) to promote enteric excretions of potassium.
   4. Hyperphosphatemia—treated with phosphate-binding agents (aluminum hydroxide [ALternaGEL], lanthanum carbonate [Fosrenol]) because they bind phosphorus in the intestinal tract for excretion. *Note:* ALternaGEL is usually restricted to 1 month because of body's inability to excrete aluminum. Calcium carbonate (Os-Cal, Tums) is more common.
   5. Hypocalcemia—treated with calcium supplements and vitamin D (calcitriol [Rocaltrol]) to increase calcium absorption.
   6. IV fluids that may be ordered:
      a. Lactated Ringer (LR)—isotonic
      b. Dextrose 5% in water (D5/W)—isotonic, hypotonic
      c. Normal saline (NS, 0.9% NaCl)—isotonic

Dialysis

I. Definition: Dialysis is the selective movement of water and solutes from one fluid compartment to another across a semipermeable membrane. The two fluid compartments are a client's blood and the dialysate (electrolyte, glucose solution).

A. Types of dialysis
   1. Peritoneal dialysis—client's own peritoneum serves as dialysis membrane (see following section on peritoneal dialysis for complete definition).
   2. Hemodialysis—semipermeable membrane is a synthetic one (see following section on hemodialysis for complete definition).
   3. Continuous arteriovenous hemofiltration—involves use of extracorporeal circulation through a filter; used with clients in critical care setting who have system failure such as acute renal failure, pulmonary edema, heart failure, or septic shock. Catheters are inserted in femoral artery and femoral vein.

B. Dialysis may be either temporary or permanent, depending on the kidneys' ability to resume adequate function. Indications for dialysis include the following:
   1. Acute renal failure or acute episodes of renal insufficiency that cannot be managed by diet, medications, or fluid restriction.
   2. End-stage renal disease
   3. Drug overdose
   4. Hyperkalemia
   5. Fluid overload
   6. Metabolic acidosis

Peritoneal Dialysis

I. Definition: Peritoneal dialysis uses client's own peritoneum as semipermeable membrane to remove toxins from blood. Procedure requires placement of a peritoneal catheter (Tenckhoff) by a surgeon, and does not require heparinization. Client can be trained to perform peritoneal dialysis (see physiologic adaptation for types of peritoneal dialysis).

CN

II. Client needs

A. Physiologic adaptation
   1. *Intermittent* peritoneal dialysis—performed manually or mechanically using a cycler; client dialyzed for 3 to 10 hr three to five times per week; predetermined amount dialysate (2 L) instilled for 20 to 30 min and allowed to drain by gravity.
   2. *Continuous ambulatory* peritoneal dialysis—client attaches bag of dialysate to peritoneal catheter; allows to drain out; allows new dialysate to drain in. Catheter clamped; new cap placed on tubing. Repeated every 4 to 6 hr (8 hr during night), 7 days a week.
   3. *Continuous cycling* peritoneal dialysis (combination of previous two)—cycler performs three dialysate exchanges at night; fourth exchange instilled in morning and left in peritoneal cavity throughout day. At end of day, fourth exchange drained out; process is repeated. Client is ambulatory during day; confined to bed at night. Procedure performed every night.

B. Management of care: Care of the client receiving peritoneal dialysis requires critical thinking skills and knowledge of assessment, and teaching and evaluation methods unique to the RN role. These skills cannot be delegated to an LPN or UAP.
   1. Consult nephrologists, renal dietitian, and social worker as needed.
   2. Refer client to Kidney Transplant/Dialysis Association, Inc., American Association of Kidney Patients, National Kidney Foundation.
   3. Delegate responsibly those activities that can be delegated. All monitoring information is reported to the RN.
      a. Monitor vital signs.
      b. Measure intake and output.
      c. Provide basic hygienic care, including oral hygiene.
      d. Assist with ambulation and nutritional intake.

C. Safety and infection control
   1. Assure dialysate solution is sterile.
   2. Add prophylactic antibiotics to dialysate to prevent or treat peritonitis; if peritonitis is suspected, obtain culture of outflow to determine infective organism.
   3. Monitor for signs of infection.
   4. Maintain meticulous sterile technique when connecting and disconnecting bags, and when caring for catheter insertion site.
   5. Monitor temperature closely.
   6. Observe for and report indicators of fluid overload (hypertension, dyspnea, tachycardia, distended neck veins)—fluid retention can occur because of catheter complications that prevent adequate outflow.
   7. Monitor for fever, cloudy outflow, rebound abdominal tenderness.

D. Health promotion and maintenance
   1. Promote dietary and fluid restrictions to supplement dialysis.
   2. Ensure dietary evaluation and teaching program are performed when client changes from one type of dialysis to another.

3. Provide accurate measurement and recording of outflow (critical).
4. Monitor intake and output; weigh client daily.
5. Increase intake of protein as necessary to prevent excessive tissue catabolism.
6. Provide list of restricted and encouraged foods with menus.

E. Psychologic integrity
1. Assist with development of coping strategies to manage frequent exchanges every day; assist client to identify strengths used in managing other major life stressors.
2. Promote positive body image and verbalization of feelings.
3. Provide therapeutic communication to address signs and symptoms of depression.
4. Encourage client and significant other to discuss sexuality and sexual activity.

F. Basic care and comfort
1. Monitor vital signs and intake and output.
2. Monitor for respiratory distress, pain, or discomfort.
3. Monitor for malaise, nausea, vomiting.
4. Warm dialysate before use with special dialysate warmer pad—cold temperature of dialysate aggravates discomfort.
5. Place heating pad on abdomen during inflow to relieve discomfort.

G. Reduction of risk potential
1. Add insulin to dialysate for client with diabetes mellitus.
2. Before dialysis, monitor vital signs; obtain weight; have client void, if possible; and assess electrolyte and glucose levels.
3. Monitor for signs of pulmonary edema.
4. Monitor dwell time as prescribed by physician, and initiate outflow; do not allow dwell time to extend beyond physician's order—increases the risk for hyperglycemia.
5. Maintain drainage bag below client's abdomen.

H. Pharmacologic and parenteral therapies: Client and family will state the purpose for and associated side effects of all medications used along with peritoneal dialysis. Common intraperitoneal medication additives include:
1. Antibiotics: Cefazolin (Ancef), tobramycin (Nebcin), and vancomycin (Vancocin)
   a. Monitor BP and pulse.
   b. Monitor liver and kidney function.
   c. Monitor peak/trough levels.
   d. Assess hearing.
2. Other: Heparin, insulin, and potassium
   a. Monitor potassium level.
   b. Monitor electrocardiogram results.
   c. Monitor for signs and symptoms of hyperglycemia and hypoglycemia.
   d. Monitor for easy bruising and bleeding gums.

Hemodialysis

I. Definition: Hemodialysis is a procedure to remove wastes (potassium, urea) from the client's blood; semipermeable membrane is a synthetic one. Hemodialysis is used for clients with end-stage renal failure and generally requires heparinization and specially trained staff, although partner can be trained to do home hemodialysis. Client must have adequate blood vessels for access or a centrally placed catheter.

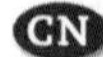

II. Client needs

A. Physiologic adaptation
1. Assure dialysate meets specific standards; water treatment systems are used to ensure safe water supply (removal of chemicals and organisms).
2. Monitor laboratory values before, during, and after dialysis.
3. Establish vascular access site—internal arteriovenous fistula used primarily for chronic dialysis clients who do not have adequate blood vessels for creation of fistula.
4. Perform hemodialysis every other day for 3 to 4 hr per session.

B. Management of care: Care of the client receiving hemodialysis requires critical thinking skills and knowledge of assessment, and teaching and evaluation methods unique to the medical-surgical nurse with specialized education in hemodialysis; the nurse performs dialysis in clinics or hemodialysis department within hospital. These skills cannot be delegated to an LPN or UAP.
1. Delegate responsibly those activities that can be delegated, including monitoring vital signs; performing basic hygienic care, including oral hygiene; measuring daily weight; monitoring intake and output; assisting with ambulation; and assisting with food and fluid intake during and after hemodialysis session.
2. Consult social worker, care coordinator, nephrologist, endocrinologist, renal dietitian, and hemodialysis nurses as needed.

C. Safety and infection control
1. Assess for fluid overload before hemodialysis.
2. Hold antihypertensives that can affect BP before hemodialysis.
3. Hold medications that could be flushed out with dialysis.

4. Monitor for hypovolemia during hemodialysis.
5. Assess access site for hematoma, bleeding, and infection.
6. Palpate/auscultate for bruit/thrill over fistula/graft.
7. Note temperature and capillary refill of extremity.
8. Provide safe environment to reduce risk of injury; explain to client the potential for fracture.

D. Health promotion and maintenance
1. Attend hemodialysis session every other day for 3 times per week.
2. Monitor intake and output, and measure daily weight as indicators of fluid status; instruct client to monitor for/report indications of fluid volume excess: Edema, hypertension, crackles, tachycardia, distended neck veins, and shortness of breath.
3. After dialysis, observe for/report indicators of fluid volume deficit: Hypotension, tachycardia, complaints of dizziness, lightheadedness.
4. Use dietary recommendations made by renal dietitian.

E. Psychologic integrity
1. Listen attentively to concerns of client to convey caring attitude and foster a relationship to ascertain how client is handling situation.
2. Allow client time to mourn loss of body function to promote identification of efficient ways to cope with losses.
3. Include family members in discussions of client's concerns to enable them to assist client and foster their support and understanding.

F. Basic care and comfort
1. Assess skin for changes in color, texture, turgor, and vascularity.
2. Provide environment conducive for rest after hemodialysis session.
3. Provide small, frequent meals to reduce nausea, vomiting.
4. Monitor intake, output, and daily weight.
5. Inspect for bruises, purpura, and signs of infection.

G. Reduction of risk potential
1. Monitor for postdialysis bleeding (needle sites, incisions), which can occur because of use of heparin during dialysis.
2. Test stool for occult blood.
3. After surgical creation of vascular access, assess for patency, auscultate for bruit, and palpate for thrill.
4. Instruct client to report severe or unrelieved pain, numbness, tingling of area of vascular access, or extremity distal to access, which is indicative of impaired tissue perfusion.
5. Notify physician if extremity distal to vascular access becomes cool, edematous, has decreased capillary refill, or is discolored because these can indicate occlusion of vascular access.
6. Follow principles of nursing care common to all types of vascular access: Prevent bleeding, clotting, and infection.
7. Do not take BP, start an IV access, or draw blood in arm with shunt, graft, or fistula.
8. Avoid restraints and constricting clothing on affected extremity.

H. Pharmacologic and parenteral therapies: Client and family will state the purpose for and associated side effects of all medications used during hemodialysis.
1. Phosphate binders: Calcium carbonate (Os-Cal), calcium acetate (PhosLo), and aluminum hydroxide (ALternaGEL)
   a. Administer with meals.
   b. Monitor calcium and phosphorus.
   c. Monitor aluminum levels.
2. Vitamin D analogue: Calcitrol (Rocaltrol) and calcitriol injection (Calcijex)—increase absorption of calcium; suppress parathyroid hormone secretion. Monitor calcium and phosphorus.
3. Vitamin B, C, folic acid—replace water-soluble vitamins lost during dialysis.
4. Mineral (iron): Ferrous sulfate (Feosol) and iron dextran (Imferon)—administer Z-track—treats anemia due to iron lost with blood during hemodialysis.
   a. Monitor monthly hemoglobin and hematocrit.
   b. Monitor for constipation, upset stomach, feces to turn black.
5. Anticoagulants: Heparin (Hepalean) and enteric-coated aspirin (Hepalean)
   a. Monitor activated partial thromboplastin time, prothrombin time levels as needed.
   b. Monitor for easy bruising, bleeding gums.
   c. Protect from injury.

Bladder Cancer

I. Definition: Bladder cancers are usually transitional cell tumors that arise from the epithelial lining of the urinary tract; others are adenocarcinomas, squamous cell carcinomas, or carcinomas. Although most are superficial and easily removed, some metastasize to the bladder wall, pelvis, para-aortic or supraclavicular nodes, liver, lungs, and bone. Bladder cancers have been linked to cigarette smoking (2 to 3 times higher risk), prolonged exposure to aromatic amines (industrial dyes), the drug cyclophosphamide (Cytoxan), pelvic radiation therapy, and to chronic bladder irritation as in long-term indwelling catheterization. Bladder cancer occurs 3 times more often in the male gender, with peak incidence between 60 and 80 years of age.

II. Nursing process

A. Assessment

1. Obtain a detailed health history and perform a comprehensive physical assessment; assess for signs and symptoms.
   a. Gross, painless, intermittent hematuria usually with clots
   b. Suprapubic pain after voiding which suggests invasive lesions
   c. Bladder irritability, urinary frequency, nocturia, and dribbling
   d. Flank pain and tenderness, which may be indicative of an obstructed ureter
   e. Pelvic or back pain may indicate distant metastases; leg edema may result from invasion of pelvic lymph nodes
2. Obtain diagnostic tests.
   a. CBC—may reveal anemia.
   b. Urinalysis—detects blood and malignant cells in urine.
   c. Excretory urography—may identify a large, early-stage tumor or an infiltrating tumor; outlines functional problems in upper urinary tract; shows hydronephrosis, rigid deformity of bladder wall.
   d. Retrograde cystography—evaluates bladder structure, integrity for functional or anatomic abnormalities; helps confirm diagnosis of bladder cancer.
   e. Bone scan—may reveal metastasis.
   f. CTS—reveals thickness of involved bladder wall, enlarged retroperitoneal lymph nodes.
   g. Ultrasonography—reveals metastases in tissues beyond bladder and distinguishes bladder cyst from bladder tumor.
   h. Cystoscopy, biopsy—confirm diagnosis.
   i. Chest x-ray, CTS, MRI bone scan—evaluate metastatic disease.

B. Analysis

1. Acute Pain related to disease process
2. Anxiety related to lack of information about diagnosis and treatment options
3. Impaired Urinary Elimination related to disease process
4. Risk for Infection related to impaired urinary tract

C. Planning

1. Maintain adequate fluid balance.
2. Express feelings of increased comfort and decreased pain.
3. Exhibit adequate coping mechanisms.
4. Express feelings about potential or actual changes in sexual activity.

D. Implementation (see basic care and comfort)

E. Evaluation

1. Client reports relief of pain.
2. Client verbalizes relief in anxiety upon being informed about disease process and treatments.
3. Client's urine output is adequate and balanced with fluid intake.
4. Client is free from signs and symptoms of infection.

CN

III. Client needs

A. Physiologic adaptation

1. Surgical interventions
   a. Transurethral resection, fulguration (destruction of tissue by means of electric sparks)—used for superficial tumors. Intravesical (within bladder) chemotherapy is used to prevent tumor recurrence.
   b. Partial cystectomy—used when tumors located in dome of bladder.
   c. Radical cystectomy—bladder removed with urinary diversion—for invasive or poorly differentiated tumors.
2. Chemotherapy within bladder allows high concentration of drug to come in contact with tumor, urothelium; minimal systemic toxicity.
3. Systemic chemotherapy—treats metastatic bladder cancer.
4. Radiation therapy—internal or external
5. Urinary diversion—ileostomy (may be necessary; includes variety of operative procedures). Potential complications include:
   a. Hemorrhage, shock
   b. Pulmonary complications—atelectasis, pneumonia, pneumothorax
   c. Thromboembolism (thrombophlebitis, pulmonary embolism)
   d. Paralytic ileus
   e. Urinary infection
   f. Obstruction of urinary drainage

B. Management of care: Care of the client with bladder cancer requires critical thinking skills and knowledge of assessment, and teaching and evaluation methods unique to the RN role. These skills cannot be delegated to an LPN or UAP.

1. Consult with enterostomal therapist—marks stoma preoperatively and assists with training in care of urinary diversion.
2. Consult with urologist and surgeon.
3. Delegate responsibly those activities that can be delegated. All monitoring information is reported to the RN.
   a. Monitor vital signs.
   b. Measure and record intake and output.
   c. Promote adequate hydration.
   d. Assist with adequate activity to prevent complications.
4. Provide client and family teaching (see reduction of risk potential).

C. Safety and infection control
1. Remove indwelling catheter as soon as possible after transurethral surgery to reduce risk of infection.
2. Monitor for complications of therapy, including hemorrhage, infection, bladder perforation, and temporary irritative voiding in transurethral resection.

D. Health promotion and maintenance
1. Advise client that irritative voiding symptoms and intermittent hematuria are possible for weeks after transurethral resection.
2. Emphasize importance of adhering to follow-up schedule: cystoscopy every 3 months for 1 year; then every 6 months to 1 year thereafter for the rest of client's life (70% of superficial tumors will reoccur).
3. Encourage participation in smoking cessation program.
4. Ensure adequate hydration, either PO or IV.

E. Psychologic integrity
1. Relieve anxiety by allowing client to verbalize fears and concerns.
2. Provide information about diagnostic studies, surgery, and treatments.
3. Be prepared to discuss concerns about sexual dysfunction, incontinence after surgery.

F. Basic care and comfort
1. Administer prescribed medications.
2. Ensure pain control.
3. Monitor urine output for clearing of hematuria.
4. Monitor intake and output, including irrigation solution.
5. Administer analgesic for pelvic discomfort.
6. Administer anticholinergic to relieve bladder spasms.

G. Reduction of risk potential: Provide client and family teaching.
1. Report signs of UTI.
2. For client with urinary stoma: Avoid lifting, performing strenuous exercise, taking long automobile rides, and contact sports.
3. Client to seek medical care if experiences fever or inability to void.
4. Provide stoma care.
5. Provide skin care and evaluation.

H. Pharmacologic and parenteral therapies: Client and family will state the purpose for and associated side effects of all medications used to treat bladder cancer.
1. Intravesical (within bladder) chemotherapy
2. Instillation of immunotherapeutic agent, bacille Calmette-Guérin to stimulate immune response to prevent recurrence of transitional cell tumors
3. Systemic chemotherapy to treat metastatic bladder cancer; combination therapy
4. Antibiotics as needed to treat UTIs—ciprofloxacin (Cipro); sulfisoxazole (Gantrisin)
5. Analgesics for pain control—hydrocodone (Vicodin); propoxyphene (Darvon)
6. Anticholinergics to relieve bladder spasms—propantheline (Pro-Banthine); trospium (Sanctura)

Bibliography

Altman, G. (2004). *Delmar's fundamental and advanced nursing skills* (2nd ed.). Albany, NY: Delmar.

Ellis, J., & Hartley, C. (2005). *Managing and coordinating nursing care.* Philadelphia: Lippincott Williams & Wilkins.

Karch, A. (2006). *Lippincott's nursing drug guide.* Philadelphia: Lippincott Williams & Wilkins.

National Kidney Foundation Definition and Classification of States of Chronic Kidney Disease retrieved on May 20, 2008 from http://www.kidney.org/professionals/KDOQI/guidelines_ckd/p4_class_g1.htm

Nursing 2008 drug handbook. Ambler, PA: Springhouse.

Purnell, L., & Paulanka, B. (Eds.). (2003). *Transcultural healthcare: A culturally competent approach.* Philadelphia: Davis.

Smeltzer, S. C., Bare, B. G., Cheever, K. H., & Hinkle, J. L. (2008). *Brunner & Suddarth's textbook of medical-surgical nursing* (11th ed.). Philadelphia: Lippincott Williams & Wilkins.

Taylor, C., Lillis, C., LeMone, P., & Lynn, P. (2006). *Fundamentals of nursing.* Philadelphia: Lippincott Williams & Wilkins.

Weber, J. R., & Kelley, J. (2007). *Nurses' handbook of health assessment.* Philadelphia: Lippincott Williams & Wilkins.

Yarbro, C. H., Frogge, M., & Goodman, M. (2004). *Cancer symptom management* (3rd ed.). Sudbury, MA: Jones and Bartlett.

CHAPTER 28

Practice Test

Urinary Incontinence

1. A client who is 70 years of age and lives alone has stress incontinence. To prevent incontinence, the nurse advises the client to:
- □ 1. Ask someone else to lift heavy objects.
- □ 2. Wear disposable protective underwear.
- □ 3. Perform perineal muscle exercises (i.e., Kegel exercises).
- □ 4. Apply estrogen vaginal cream to the urinary meatus after each intentional voiding.

2. A client is taking propantheline bromide (Pro-Banthine) for urinary bladder spasm. The nurse should teach the client to:
- □ 1. Take 30 to 60 min before meals and at bedtime.
- □ 2. Chew the tablet, and then swallow.
- □ 3. Take with an antacid.
- □ 4. Void prior to each dose.

Urinary Tract Infection

3. A client has an indwelling Foley catheter. To prevent a nosocomial UTI, the nurse should take which of the following measures?
- □ 1. Allow the emptying tube of the collection bag to hang freely.
- □ 2. Keep the collection bag at the level of the bladder.
- □ 3. Clean the urinary meatus at the catheter junction with soap and water.
- □ 4. Allow the catheter to move freely.

4. The nurse is planning care for a group of hospitalized clients. Which of the following clients is at high risk for a UTI?
- □ 1. Client with diabetes mellitus.
- □ 2. Client who had one course of antibiotic therapy.
- □ 3. Client with a family history of UTIs.
- □ 4. Client with a urinary calculus.

5. AF The nurse is providing teaching to a client who has a UTI. Which of the following instructions should the nurse include in client teaching? Select all that apply.
- □ 1. Empty the bladder regularly.
- □ 2. Prevent constipation.
- □ 3. Cleanse the perineal area with perfumed cleansing wipes.
- □ 4. Wipe the perineal area from front to back.
- □ 5. Drink 3,000 ml of cranberry juice daily.
- □ 6. Take broad-spectrum antibiotics daily.

Pyelonephritis

6. A client is at risk for acute pyelonephritis. The nurse should instruct the client about which of the following health promotion behaviors that will be most effective in preventing pyelonephritis?
- □ 1. Wash the perineum with warm water and soap, cleaning from front to back.
- □ 2. Treat fungal infections such as athlete's foot immediately.
- □ 3. Have a Pneumovax immunization to prevent streptococcal infection.
- □ 4. Treat with antibiotics and cover any open skin lesions.

7. AF A client with pyelonephritis is taking tobramycin sulfate (Nebcin). The nurse should assess the client for which of the following adverse effects? Select all that apply.
- □ 1. Depressed AST, ALT.
- □ 2. Increased LDH.
- □ 3. Anemia.
- □ 4. Increased serum creatinine.
- □ 5. Ototoxicity.

Renal Calculi

8. A client has a renal calculus in the left lower ureter. Which of the following is the priority nursing goal for this client?
- □ 1. Treat infection.
- □ 2. Relieve spasms.
- □ 3. Relieve pain.
- □ 4. Maintain client's position on the left side.

9. The nurse is teaching a client with urinary calculi about diet. Which comment by the client is an indication that the nurse needs to reinforce previous teaching?
- □ 1. "Dairy products may cause more stones to develop in the future."
- □ 2. "I should drink cranberry juice and water daily."
- □ 3. "Strenuous exercise will make bones lose their calcium, and I will have more stones."

□ 4. "I should not allow myself to get dehydrated while working in the hot sun."

10. AF A client had a lithotripsy to treat renal calculi. The client is having ureteral spasms and hematuria. The nurse should do which of the following? Select all that apply.
□ 1. Strain all urine.
□ 2. Apply a heating pad to the lower back area.
□ 3. Contact the physician to report hematuria.
□ 4. Encourage fluid intake of 1,000 ml/day.
□ 5. Assess pain level.

Acute Renal Failure

11. To prevent development of acute renal failure in a client with diabetes mellitus, the nurse should emphasize which of the following care measures?
□ 1. Conduct a urine glucose test prior to each meal and at bedtime.
□ 2. Follow a "no concentrated sweets" meal plan.
□ 3. Limit physical activity that requires lifting.
□ 4. Manage daily blood glucose.

12. A client with acute renal failure has a 24-hr urine output of 400 ml. To maintain fluid and electrolyte balance the nurse should:
□ 1. Restrict IV and PO fluids to 200 ml per 24 hr.
□ 2. Maintain IV and PO fluid intake at 3,000 ml per 24 hr.
□ 3. Replace fluid loss with 400 ml per 24 hr.
□ 4. Place the client on NPO and offer lemon lozenges.

13. AF The nurse is assessing a client with acute renal failure. Which of the following are expected findings? Select all that apply.
□ 1. Irregular apical pulse.
□ 2. Slow heart rate.
□ 3. Tall, peaked T waves on electrocardiogram (ECG) strip.
□ 4. Hypoactive bowel sounds.
□ 5. Confusion.

Chronic Renal Failure

14. AF A client with end-stage chronic renal failure is admitted to the hospital with a serum potassium level of 7 mEq/L. In what order of priority does the nurse perform the following?
_____ 1. Administer calcium gluconate.
_____ 2. Start an IV access site.
_____ 3. Administer sodium polystyrene sulfonate (Kayexalate).
_____ 4. Attach the client to a cardiac monitor.

15. A client with end-stage renal disease has had a cadaveric renal transplant, and now has secondary diabetes. The client asks, "Wasn't that kidney checked for diabetes before the surgeon transplanted it?" Which is the most helpful response by the nurse?
□ 1. "Yes, the cadaveric kidney was typed and cross-matched."
□ 2. "All kidney donors must be free of severe hypertension, long-standing diabetes mellitus, and malignancies."
□ 3. "Immunosuppressive therapy used before surgery may have caused the diabetes."
□ 4. "Your diabetes is related to the use of steroids after your surgery."

16. The most useful indicator for a nurse to assess fluid balance in a client with chronic renal failure is to:
□ 1. Measure intake and output.
□ 2. Assess skin turgor.
□ 3. Measure daily weights.
□ 4. Monitor serum sodium levels.

Dialysis

17. A nurse is performing peritoneal dialysis for a client. For two sequential exchanges, the outflow is less than the inflow. The nurse should first:
□ 1. Take the client's vital signs.
□ 2. Reposition the client.
□ 3. Irrigate the Tenckhoff dialysis catheter.
□ 4. Monitor the third exchange very closely.

18. AF A client with end-stage renal failure has an internal arteriovenous fistula created on the left arm as an access for hemodialysis. The nurse instructs the client to do which of the following? Select all that apply.
□ 1. Tell the health care providers (HCPs) to draw blood from veins on the left side.
□ 2. Avoid sleeping on the left arm.
□ 3. Wear wrist watch on the right arm.
□ 4. Assess fingers on the left arm for warmth.
□ 5. Obtain BP from the left arm.

Bladder Cancer

19. The nurse is planning care for a group of clients. Which of the following clients is at high risk for bladder cancer?
□ 1. Client with a history of aspirin use.
□ 2. Client with a history of long-term caffeine use.

□ 3. Client with a history of taking loop diuretics.
□ 4. Client with a history of chain smoking.

20. Following intravesical therapy for bladder cancer, a client tells the nurse that he "urinates blood." The nurse should tell the client:

□ 1. "You should limit the amount of fluids to 1,000 ml/day."
□ 2. "Irritation of the bladder with bleeding is normal."
□ 3. "You should contact your health care provider."
□ 4. "Be sure you are only having three servings of protein each day."

Answers and Rationales

1. 3 Perineal muscle exercises (Kegel exercises) increase the tone of the urethral sphincters; the nurse teaches the client to perform the exercises in sets of at least 10 contractions, 4 to 5 times per day. Asking someone else to lift heavy loads may not always be practical. Wearing disposable protective underwear is only a temporary measure because long-term use discourages continence, and can lead to skin problems. Applying estrogen vaginal cream to the urinary meatus after each intentional voiding can lead to UTIs. Drug therapy has a very limited role in the management of stress urinary incontinence. (H)

2. 1 Propantheline bromide (Pro-Banthine) decreases motility in the GI biliary and urinary tracts; it is useful for ureteral and urinary bladder spasms. The nurse advises the client to take the drug 30 to 60 min before meals and at bedtime. The nurse also advises the client not to chew tablets because the drug is bitter. If the client is taking antacids, the drug is taken at least 1 hr before or 1 hr after an antacid. It is not necessary to void just prior to each dose. (D)

3. 3 Principles considered by the nurse in the management of a client with a urethral catheter include the following: (a) Maintain unobstructed downhill flow of urine; (b) keep collection bag below the level of the bladder; (c) give perineal care frequently, including cleaning of the meatus-catheter junction with soap and water; and (d) keep the catheter secured to the leg to prevent movement and urethral traction. Allowing the emptying tube of the collection bag to hang freely allows germs to enter the collection bag, which could cause a UTI. (S)

4. 1 Clients who are immunosuppressed, have diabetes mellitus, or have undergone multiple courses of antibiotic therapy are prone to bacterial, fungal, and parasitic infections. Taking one course of antibiotic therapy or having a family history of UTIs does not make a client at high risk for development of a UTI. A predisposing factor for a UTI is ongoing problems of urinary calculi; one calculus would not place a client at high risk. (H)

5. 1, 2, 4 Health promotion activities can help decrease the frequency of infections and promote early detection of infection. Health promotion activities include teaching preventive measures, such as emptying the bladder regularly and completely; evacuating the bowel regularly; wiping the perineal area from front to back after urination and defecation; and drinking an adequate amount of liquid each day. The recommended daily liquid intake is about 15 ml per pound of body weight per day for the ambulatory adult. Suppressive antibiotics are not generally recommended. A daily intake of cranberry juice (consumed as pure juice, 8 oz twice daily) or cranberry essence tablets may reduce the risk of certain UTIs. The nurse instructs the client to avoid use of harsh soaps, bubble baths, powders, and sprays in the perineal area. (H)

6. 1 Acute pyelonephritis usually begins with a bacterial infection of the lower urinary tract via the ascending urethral route; most infections are due to gram-negative bacilli, such as *E. coli*, normally found in the GI tract. Thorough perineal care using soap and warm water, and cleansing from front to back, decreases the likelihood that organisms will be introduced into the urinary tract and ascend upward toward the kidneys. Although preventing and treating all infections are appropriate, fungal infections from the feet and bacterial infections in the throat or skin are less likely to be immediate sources of infection causing pyelonephritis. (H)

7. 2, 3, 4, 5 Central nervous system adverse effects include neurotoxicity (including ototoxicity), nephrotoxicity, increased liver enzymes of AST and ALT, increased LDH, and anemia. AST (aspartate aminotransferase) and ALT (alanine aminotransferase) are liver enzymes that rise when there is cellular damage to the tissues where the enzymes are found, such as in the liver. LDH (lactate dehydrogenase) is an enzyme that catalyzes the reversible conversion of lactate to pyruvate within cells. Because many tissues contain LDH, elevated total LDH is considered a nonspecific indicator of cellular damage unless other clinical data make the tissue origin obvious. Creatinine is the end product of creatine metabolism. Creatine resides almost exclusively in skeletal muscle, where it participates in energy-requiring metabolic reactions. In these processes, a small amount of creatine is irreversibly converted to creatinine, which then circulates to the kidneys and is excreted. Creatinine is the ideal substance for determining renal clearance. The creatinine clearance test reflects the kidney's glomerular filtration rate. (D)

8. 3 Managing the client's pain is the priority nursing goal. Movement of a renal stone (calculus) along the ureter produces excruciating pain, for which narcotic analgesics are usually required. Antispasmodic medications may also be administered to relax the smooth muscle of the ureter and control spasms, but this is not the priority nursing goal. Broad-spectrum antibiotics are not prescribed unless an infection is present. Having the client lay on the left side has no effect on pain relief. (A)

9. 3 More than 99% of the body's calcium is deposited in the bones, but can be mobilized from bones to keep the blood level constant when dietary intake is inadequate. Exercise promotes the deposition of calcium into bone; immobility can lead to osteomalacia and osteoporosis in adults. If calculi are primarily calcium, dairy products may promote stone formation as they are high in calcium content and reduce the urinary excretion of oxalate. Initial nutritional management includes limiting oxalate-rich foods, and thereby reducing oxalate excretion. Oxalate is a common factor in many stones. Water aids in the dilution of calcium in the urinary system, and cranberry juice promotes acidic urine that prevents calcium particles from aggregating together. When a client is dehydrated, the osmolality of serum is increased and urine is more concentrated, promoting the formation of stones (calculi). (H)

10. 1, 2, 5 Following lithotripsy, the nurse strains all urine to collect and identify stone composition. Providing heat to the flank area may be helpful to relieve muscle spasms when renal colic is present; the nurse assesses the client's pain level and administers analgesics as needed. Hematuria is common after lithotripsy and it is not necessary to notify the physician. The nurse promotes a fluid intake of at least 2,000 ml/day to flush stones and clots through the urinary tract. (A)

11. 4 Microvascular complications result from thickening of the vessel membranes in the capillaries and arterioles in response to conditions of chronic hyperglycemia. Although microangiopathy can be found throughout the body, the areas most noticeably affected are the eyes (retinopathy), kidneys (nephropathy), and the skin (dermopathy). Urine glucose testing is rarely used today; self-monitoring of blood glucose is a cornerstone of diabetes management. By providing a current blood glucose reading, self-monitoring of blood glucose enables a client to make self-management decisions regarding meal plans, activity, and medication, if required. A "no concentrated sweets" is not a recognized meal plan by the American Diabetic Association or the American Dietetic Association. Limiting physical activity that requires lifting has no effect on the prevention of the development of acute renal failure. (H)

12. 3 The client is in the oliguric phase of acute renal failure. The nurse gives only enough fluids to replace losses plus an additional 400 ml per 24 hr. It is not necessary to restrict fluids to 200 ml or place the client on NPO status. Because the fluid-regulating function of the kidney is impaired, the nurse does not increase the fluid load during the oliguric phase of acute renal failure. The nurse continues to monitor the client for other signs of fluid and electrolyte imbalance. (A)

13. 1, 2, 3 Serum potassium levels increase because the normal ability of the kidneys to excrete 80% to 90% of the body's potassium is impaired. When potassium levels exceed 6 mEq/L or arrhythmias are identified, treatment must be initiated immediately. Before clinical signs of hyperkalemia are apparent, the electrocardiogram (ECG) will show tall, peaked T waves, widening of the QRS complex (slower heart rate), and ST depression. Hypoactive bowel sounds and confusion are signs of hypokalemia. (A)

14. 2, 4, 1, 3 The nurse first assures an IV access site in case the client has respiratory or cardiac arrest. Next, the nurse monitors the client's heart rate and rhythm: Cardiovascular signs of elevated serum potassium levels are irregular, slow heart rate; decreased BP; narrow, peaked T waves; widened QRS complexes, prolonged PR intervals, flattened D waves; frequent ectopy; ventricular fibrillation; and ventricular standstill. The nurse then administers calcium gluconate, which has an immediate action to antagonize the effect of hyperkalemia on cardiac muscle. Last, the nurse administers polystyrene sulfonate (Kayexalate), which is a cation-exchange resin that removes potassium from the body by exchanging sodium ion for potassium; potassium-containing resin is then excreted; onset is in several hours to days. (M)

15. 4 Problems related to corticosteroids used posttransplant include peptic ulcer disease, glucose intolerance and diabetes, cataracts, hyperlipidemia, and an increased incidence of infections and malignancies. In the first year after transplant, corticosteroid doses are usually decreased to 5 to 10 mg/day. Secondary diabetes occurs in some clients because of another medical condition or the treatment of a medical condition that causes abnormal blood glucose levels. Medications that induce diabetes in some clients include corticosteroids, such as prednisone. When a kidney donor becomes available, the donor's HLA data, ABO type are compared with the list of potential recipients. Donors and recipients must have the same blood type. Zero antigen mismatches are given priority because statistically these grafts have much better survival rates. A donor must be free of active IV drug abuse, severe hypertension, long-standing diabetes, malignancies, sepsis, and communicable diseases including HIV, hepatitis B and C, syphilis, and tuberculosis. Although the need for immunosuppressive drugs and measures to prevent infection is reviewed preoperatively, they are actually used postoperatively to adequately suppress the immune response to prevent rejection of the transplanted kidney while maintaining sufficient immunity to prevent overwhelming infection. (A)

16. 3 Water intake depends on the daily urine output. Generally, 600 ml (from insensible loss) plus an amount equal to the previous day's urine output is allowed for the client with chronic kidney disease who is not receiving dialysis. The fluid allotment is spaced throughout the day so the client does not become thirsty. For the client with hemodialysis, fluid intake is adjusted so that weight gains are no more than 1 to 3 kg between dialysis. Skin has a yellow-gray discoloration and is dry and scaly because of a decrease in oil and sweat gland activity. Skin turgor is the resistance of the skin to deformation, especially to being grasped between the fingers. Sodium may be normal or low in renal failure. Because of impaired sodium excretion, sodium along with water is retained. If large quantities of body water are retained, dilutional hyponatremia occurs. (A)

17. 2 Peritoneal dialysis is performed using a dialysate solution and the peritoneal membrane to filter out the harmful toxins and excessive fluid. The clean dialyzing fluid passes into the peritoneal cavity through a permanent indwelling peritoneal catheter, and wastes diffuse across the peritoneal membrane into the fluid. The contaminated fluid is drained and replaced with fresh fluid. If outflow is less than inflow, the nurse changes the client's position to shift abdominal fluid and move the catheter into contact with fluid in the abdomen. Although vital signs are monitored, they are not a concern at this time. The dialysis catheter does not need to be irrigated. The nurse repositions the client before starting the third exchange. (A)

18. 2, 3, 4 The nurse instructs the client to protect the site of the fistula. The client should avoid pressure on the involved arm such as sleeping on it, wearing tight jewelry, or obtaining BP. The client is also advised to assess the area distal to the fistula for adequate circulation, such as warmth and color. When the client is hospitalized, the nurse posts a sign on the client's bed not to draw blood or obtain BP on the left side; the client is also instructed to be sure that none of the health care team members do so. (S)

19. 4 Risk factors for bladder cancer include cigarette smoking, exposure to dyes used in rubber and cable industries, and chronic abuse of phenacetin-containing analgesics. None of the other health behaviors increase a client's likelihood of developing bladder cancer. (H)

20. 2 Most clients have dysuria and hemorrhagic cystitis following installation of chemotherapy directly into the bladder by a urethral catheter. The nurse instructs the client to obtain 2,000 to 3,000 ml fluids per day. It is not necessary to limit the protein in the diet. The hematuria is expected, and it is not necessary to contact the HCP. (A)

chapter

29

The Client With Reproductive Health Problems

Reproductive health problems are common in adults. The nurse has a significant role in identifying clients at risk for acute infections, such as sexually transmitted diseases (STDs) or chronic health problems, such as cancer, as well as promoting health and assisting clients who have cancer and other chronic diseases to maintain their health. Topics discussed in this chapter include:

- Breast Disease: Fibrocystic Complex and Breast Cancer
- Health Problems of Female Reproductive Organs
- Health Problems of Male Reproductive Organs
- Sexually Transmitted Diseases

Breast Disease: Fibrocystic Complex and Breast Cancer

I. Definition: Fibrocystic complex refers to a condition resulting from exaggerated response to estrogen and is the most frequently occurring breast disorder. Cancer of the breast is the most common type of cancer in women and is second only to lung cancer as the cause of cancer death in women.

- A. Fibrocystic complex: Fibrocystic complex is a benign condition characterized by hyperplasia of breast tissue and cyst formation. The masses are often bilateral and located in the upper, outer quadrant. These lesions are round, well-delineated and mobile, and tend to increase in size and tenderness before menstruation. Occasionally, a milky, yellow, or green nipple discharge is present. Fibrocystic complex is not a premalignant lesion but can make it more difficult to assess new lesions.
- B. Breast cancer: The majority of breast cancers are infiltrating ductal carcinomas and are invasive. Although cancer of the breast occurs in many women despite absence of risk factors, those clients who do have risk factors require close monitoring (see assessment section for risk factors).

II. Nursing process

- A. Assessment
  1. Obtain a detailed health history, including family history relating to breast cancer (risk is increased if first-degree relative had breast cancer prior to menopause or had bilateral tumors) and previous history of breast, colon, endometrial, or ovarian cancer.
  2. Perform a comprehensive physical examination; assess for signs and symptoms of breast disease.
     - a. Palpable lesion(s)
       - (1) Benign lesions are round with smooth edges and move freely.
       - (2) Malignant lesions are irregular, firm, nontender, and fixed.
     - b. Tenderness
     - c. Nipple discharge
     - d. Dimpling of skin over breast
     - e. Nipple retraction
     - f. "Orange peel" skin (peau d'orange)
  3. Assess client's knowledge of and accuracy regarding performance of self-breast examination.
  4. Inspect for signs of lymphedema in mastectomy client.
  5. Assess for risk factors, including family history in a first-degree relative, increased age, personal history of cancer, early menarche, and late menopause, obesity after menopause, and possibly estrogen-replacement therapy.
  6. Obtain diagnostic tests.
     - a. Mammography
     - b. Ultrasound
     - c. Fine-needle aspiration
     - d. Open biopsy
- B. Analysis
  1. Fear related to diagnosis of cancer
  2. Acute Pain related to enlarged cysts of fibrocystic complex
  3. Disturbed Body Image related to actual or anticipated effects of treatment for breast cancer
  4. Knowledge Deficit related to self breast examination
  5. Impaired Tissue Perfusion: Cardiovascular, related to lymphedema (postmastectomy)
- C. Planning
  1. Identify coping strategies to manage fear.
  2. Relieve or manage pain and discomfort.
  3. Promote positive body image.
  4. Instruct client about correct performance of breast self-examination.
- D. Implementation
  1. Encourage client to discuss fears.
  2. Instruct client in self-help strategies such as imagery, progressive relaxation, and distraction.
  3. Administer analgesics as ordered.
  4. Assist client in identifying supportive relationships.
  5. Recommend self-help groups such as Reach to Recovery for mastectomy clients.
  6. Provide information regarding condition and treatment options.
  7. Refer client to community resources for adaptive clothing postmastectomy.
  8. Encourage client to assist in wound care postmastectomy.
  9. Encourage arm and shoulder exercise for postmastectomy clients.
  10. Instruct client in breast self-examination technique.
  11. Avoid activities that would endanger postmastectomy client such as venipuncture or injections in arm subject to lymphedema.
- E. Evaluation
  1. Client demonstrates effective coping strategies to manage fear.
  2. Client states decrease in pain.
  3. Client verbalizes positive perception of body image.
  4. Client demonstrates correct technique for breast self-examination.

5. Client states intent to perform breast self-examination monthly.
6. Client accurately lists signs of lymphedema and strategies for prevention.
7. Client expresses intent to keep affected arm elevated.

CN

III. Client needs
A. Physiologic adaptation
1. Fibrocystic complex: Administer mild analgesics for cyclic discomfort; manage tenderness and pain by suggesting avoidance of coffee and chocolate, following a low-salt diet and wearing a good support bra. Surgical management may involve needle aspiration or removal.
2. Cancer of the breast: Treatment options for breast cancer include surgery such as lumpectomy with sentinel node biopsy, partial mastectomy with breast reconstruction, or radical mastectomy followed by chemotherapy or radiation therapy. Hormonal therapy is used if the lesion tests positive for estrogen receptors.

B. Management of care: Care of the client with a breast disorder requires critical thinking skills and knowledge of assessment, and teaching and evaluation methods unique to the RN role. These skills cannot be delegated to an LPN or UAP.
1. Delegate responsibly those activities that can be delegated, including basic care needs and vital sign checks for the stable client. All monitoring information is reported to the RN.
2. Place client receiving radiation therapy in private room out of heavy traffic area.
3. Instruct client regarding signs and symptoms of recurrence of breast cancer.
   a. Firm, discrete nodules on skin at surgical site
   b. Enlarged lymph nodes
   c. Pathologic fractures
   d. Back pain
   e. Shortness of breath
   f. Headache and confusion
4. Restore arm function on affected side postmastectomy. Teach postmastectomy client preventive measures for, and signs of, lymphedema (see reduction of risk potential):
   a. Heaviness or pain in affected extremity
   b. Decreased motor function
   c. Numbness and tingling in fingers
   d. Visible edema
5. Evaluate community resources for self-help groups following mastectomy or breast cancer.
6. Provide care to the client pre- and postprocedure.
7. Teach client self-care strategies related to drains and wound management.
8. Facilitate follow-up care.

C. Safety and infection control
1. Assess postsurgical client for signs of wound infection.
2. Use hazardous material precautions for clients receiving chemotherapy.
3. Institute radiation protection measures for clients receiving radiation therapy.
4. Wear dosimeter to measure radiation exposure.
5. Limit client contact to 30 min/day.
6. Stand at foot of bed or entrance to room whenever possible.
7. Use lead shields as needed.
8. Instruct visitors to stay 6 feet away from bed.
9. Restrict visits to 3 hr per day.
10. Instruct UAP in recognition of hazardous materials used in treatment regimen.
11. Monitor immune status of client receiving chemotherapy.
12. Use protective isolation measures for clients with compromised immune system.
13. Instruct unlicensed personnel in appropriate precautions.
14. Teach postoperative client signs of infection to be reported to physician, including fever, purulent discharge, and localized redness and tenderness.

D. Health promotion and maintenance
1. Perform risk assessment related to breast cancer and fibrocystic complex.
2. Stress importance of medical evaluation of new lesions in client with fibrocystic complex.
3. Remind client with breast cancer of need for life-long medical follow-up.

E. Psychologic integrity
1. Assist client in identifying sources of support; offer information about community resources for clients with breast cancer. Facilitate visit by Reach to Recovery volunteer, if desired.
2. Encourage client to verbalize fears and concerns.
3. Suggest stress reduction techniques for client with fibrocystic complex.
4. Reassure client with fibrocystic disease that it is unrelated to breast cancer.

F. Basic care and comfort
1. Administer analgesics as indicated.
2. Provide wound and drain care postprocedure.

3. Elevate arm on operative side postmastectomy.
4. Assist with range of motion exercises on operative side.

G. Reduction of risk potential
1. Encourage breast health.
   a. Perform breast self-examination monthly after menses.
   b. Receive yearly breast examination by HCP.
   c. Receive regular mammograms based on risk level.
2. Prevent lymphedema.
   a. Avoid constriction on affected arm (no straps from purses or laptop cases).
   b. Elevate affected arm whenever possible.
   c. Use compression garment if ordered.
   d. Instruct client to avoid sunburn and other injuries to affected arm.
   e. Avoid venipuncture, injections, and BP on affected extremity.
   f. Remind client to treat minor injuries promptly and report them to her physician.

H. Pharmacologic and parenteral therapies: Client will state the purpose for and associated side effects of all medications used to treat breast disorders, including hormone therapy to remove or block estrogen (tamoxifen, anastrozole [Arimidex]). See also Chapter 32 for discussion of chemotherapy and radiation therapy.

Health Problems of Female Reproductive Organs

I. Definition: Health problems of the female reproductive organs involve uterine fibroids, cancer of the cervix, endometrial cancer, ovarian cancer, and premenstrual syndrome.

A. Uterine fibroids (leiomyomas) are benign tumors arising from the smooth muscle of the uterus. They tend to grow slowly and atrophy after menopause, but their etiology is unknown.

B. Cancer of the cervix may be invasive or noninvasive, with the noninvasive type being the most common. Repeated injuries over a number of years can cause normal cervical cells to become dysplagic and cancerous. Incidence is higher among Hispanic, African American, and Native American women. Noninvasive cervical cancer is highest in women who are in their mid-30s, whereas invasive cervical cancer is more common in women over 50 years of age.

C. Endometrial cancer is the most common cancer of the female reproductive system. Most of the tumors are adenocarcinomas, originating in the lining of the endometrium. These tumors grow slowly and metastasize late, so the disease has a low mortality rate if diagnosed in the early stages. The highest incidence occurs in women in their early 60s.

D. Ovarian cancer is the fifth leading cause of cancer death because it is usually diagnosed in the advanced stages. The cause is unknown but it is more common in women with *BRCA* gene mutations. Most of these cancers are epithelial carcinomas, which metastasize to adjacent organs.

E. Premenstrual syndrome refers to a cluster of physical and psychologic symptoms that occur during the week prior to menstruation (see assessment for symptoms). The exact cause of premenstrual syndrome is unknown. The condition may be complicated with premenstrual dysphoric disorder.

II. Nursing process

A. Assessment
1. Obtain a detailed health history, including family history relating to cancer (risk of ovarian cancer is increased if first-degree relative had breast or colon cancer) and client's previous history of breast or colon cancer.
2. Perform a comprehensive physical examination; assess for signs and symptoms.
   a. Uterine fibroids—includes heavy menstrual bleeding accompanied by abdominal pain and pelvic pressure.
   b. Cervical cancer—client may be asymptomatic in early stages; leukorrhea and midcycle bleeding are among the earlier symptoms of cervical cancer. Late symptoms include pain, weight loss, anemia, and cachexia.
   c. Endometrial cancer—client is asymptomatic in early stages, progressing to abnormal uterine bleeding (especially in postmenopausal women). Late symptoms include pain and weight loss plus symptoms related to site of metastasis.
   d. Ovarian cancer—client is asymptomatic in the early stages. Later symptoms include abdominal bloating and pressure, loss of appetite, feeling of fullness, and change in bowel habits. As the disease progresses, clients experience increased abdominal girth, bowel and bladder problems, persistent abdominal pain, ascites and abnormal vaginal bleeding.
   e. Premenstrual syndrome—symptoms vary from mild to severe; the most

common symptoms are breast tenderness, edema, bloating, food cravings, mood swings, and irritability.

3. Assess for risk factors.
   a. Cervical cancer
      (1) Sexual activity before 17 years of age
      (2) Multiple sexual partners
      (3) Infection with human papillomavirus (HPV)
      (4) Smoking
   b. Endometrial cancer
      (1) History of estrogen unopposed by progesterone
      (2) Over 55 years of age
      (3) Nulliparity
      (4) Obesity
      (5) Hypertension
      (6) Diabetes mellitus
   c. Ovarian cancer
      (1) Over 50 years of age
      (2) Nulliparity
      (3) High-fat diet
      (4) Early menarche and late menopause
      (5) Hormone-replacement therapy
      (6) Use of infertility drugs
4. Obtain diagnostic tests.
   a. Uterine fibroids—pelvic examination, ultrasound, endometrial biopsy, hysteroscopy.
   b. Cancer of the cervix—colposcopy and biopsy; routine screening with Papanicolaou (Pap) test is essential because cervical cancer is asymptomatic in early stages.
   c. Endometrial cancer—endometrial biopsy.
   d. Ovarian cancer—pelvic examination, sonography, Doppler imaging, laparotomy.
   e. Premenstrual syndrome—no specific diagnostic tests; client can keep a symptom calendar.

B. Analysis
   1. Anxiety related to possibility of cancer
   2. Acute Pain related to pressure of mass on surrounding organs
   3. Disturbed Body Image related to loss of body part
   4. Ineffective Sexuality Patterns related to physiologic limitations
   5. Ineffective coping related to inability to control symptoms

C. Planning
   1. Assist client identify strategies to cope with anxiety.
   2. Relieve or manage pain.
   3. Manage symptoms.

D. Implementation
   1. Encourage regular screening for reproductive cancers based on risk factors.
   2. Recommend lifestyle changes to reduce risk of reproductive cancers (see health promotion and maintenance).
   3. Provide information on surgical and adjuvant treatment options.
   4. Provide pre- and postoperative care for the client undergoing surgical intervention.
   5. Reduce symptoms of premenstrual syndrome.
      a. Stress management
      b. Relaxation exercises
      c. Avoidance of caffeine and alcohol
      d. Diet low in refined carbohydrates
      e. Salt limitation before menses
      f. Vitamin B_6 supplement

E. Evaluation
   1. Client lists prevention strategies based on personal risk factors.
   2. Client expresses willingness to follow prevention program.
   3. Client recognizes importance of early detection and treatment.
   4. Client actively seeks information on treatment options on diagnosis.
   5. Client expresses confidence in decisions made.
   6. Client states pain is adequately controlled.
   7. Client maintains close relationship with significant others.
   8. Client verbalizes increased satisfaction with quality of life.

CN

III. Client needs

A. Physiologic adaptation
   1. Uterine fibroids—fibroids do not require treatment unless bleeding is intensive or the tumors are large and rapidly growing; treatment includes myomectomy or hysterectomy. Embolization of the blood vessels feeding the fibroid and cryosurgery have also been used.
   2. Cancer of the cervix—treatment options include conization via cryotherapy or laser vaporization, hysterectomy, or radiation therapy for advanced cancer.
   3. Endometrial cancer—treatment includes hysterectomy sometimes followed by radiation, hormone therapy, or chemotherapy.
   4. Ovarian cancer—treatment includes complete hysterectomy with radiation or chemotherapy.

5. Premenstrual syndrome—often can be managed with diet and exercise; supplements of vitamin B_6, calcium, and magnesium; diuretics may be used to relieve fluid retention; NSAIDs for pain. Hormonal therapy with oral contraceptives may be effective for some clients.

B. Management of care: Care of the female client with health problems of the reproductive organs requires critical thinking skills and knowledge of assessment, and teaching and evaluation methods unique to the RN role. These skills cannot be delegated to an LPN or UAP.
   1. Provide rest periods for clients experiencing anemia with fatigue.
   2. Administer analgesics for pain.
   3. Provide postoperative care after hysterectomy.
      a. Use measures to prevent deep venous thrombosis, such as early ambulation, frequent position changes, leg exercises, compression hose, and sequential compression devices.
      b. Maintain urinary drainage system.
      c. Remove vaginal packing following vaginal hysterectomy 24 hr postoperatively.
      d. Restrict food and fluids until bowel sounds return.
      e. Assess for abdominal distention at regular intervals.
      f. Counsel client on effects of surgical menopause.
   4. Reduce fluid retention in clients with premenstrual syndrome.
   5. Control cramps, backache, and headache with ibuprofen.
   6. Improve mood with vitamin therapy and exercise.
   7. Refer clients with *BRCA-1* and *BRCA-2* mutations for genetic counseling.
   8. Place client receiving radiation therapy in private room out of flow of traffic.
   9. Refrain from placing client undergoing hysterectomy near nursery or postpartum unit.

C. Safety and infection control
   1 Assess postsurgical client for signs of wound infection.
   2. Use hazardous material precautions for clients receiving chemotherapy.
   3. Instruct UAP in recognition of hazardous materials used in treatment regime.
   4. Institute radiation protection measures for clients receiving radiation therapy (see safety and infection control for breast disorders).
   5. Instruct unlicensed personnel in radiation protection measures.
   6. Monitor immune status of client receiving chemotherapy.
   7. Use protective isolation measures for clients with compromised immune system.
   8. Instruct unlicensed personnel in appropriate precautions.
   9. Teach postoperative client signs of infection to be reported to physician, including fever, purulent discharge, and localized redness and tenderness.

D. Health promotion and maintenance: Perform risk assessment related to cancer of the reproductive system; recommend lifestyle changes to reduce risk of reproductive cancers.
   1. Abstinence until after adolescence
   2. Monogamous sexual relationships
   3. Condom use
   4. Prevention of HPV with safe sex and immunization
   5. Smoking cessation program
   6. Low- to moderate-fat diet

E. Psychologic integrity
   1. Encourage client to express feelings relating to hysterectomy.
   2. Provide guidelines relating to the resumption of intercourse.
   3. Assure client that symptoms of premenstrual syndrome can be managed.
   4. Counsel client's partner about nature of premenstrual syndrome.

F. Basic care and comfort
   1. Administer analgesics as indicated.
   2. Provide wound care postprocedure.

G. Reduction of risk potential
   1. Advise clients to avoid high-risk behavior (see health promotion and maintenance).
   2. Stress importance of pelvic examinations and Papanicolaou (Pap) test beginning when sexually active and following American Cancer Society guidelines.

H. Pharmacologic and parenteral therapies: Client will state the purpose for and associated side effects of all medications used to treat health problems of the reproductive organs.
   1. Chemotherapy
   2. Diuretics such as spironolactone (Aldactone) for fluid retention in premenstrual syndrome
   3. Analgesics such as ibuprofen for mild-to-moderate discomfort
   4. Antianxiety agents such as buspirone (BuSpar) for premenstrual syndrome
   5. Antidepressants such as fluoxetine (Sarafem) and amitriptyline (Elavil) for premenstrual syndrome

Health Problems of Male Reproductive Organs

I. Definition: Health problems of the male reproductive organs involve benign prostatic hypertrophy (BPH), prostate cancer, testicular cancer, and erectile dysfunction.
   A. Benign prostatic hypertrophy (BPH) is a common problem in men over 50 years of age. The tissue of the inner part of the prostate becomes enlarged and puts pressure on the urethra, causing urinary obstruction and retention. The stagnant urine is prone to infection. The cause of BPH is unknown but is believed to be related to endocrine changes. This condition is benign and does not develop into cancer. Complications include acute urinary retention, urinary tract infection (UTI), sepsis, bladder stones, and renal failure.
   B. Prostate cancer is the second leading cause of cancer death in men. Most prostate cancer occurs in older men and is slow-growing, although the cancer is often more aggressive when it occurs in younger men. Prostate cancer is fueled by testosterone.
   C. Testicular cancer is the most common type of cancer in men between 15 and 35 years of age. The cancer is asymptomatic in its early stages and is often not diagnosed until it has metastasized. The two forms of testicular cancer are seminomas, which are slow-glowing, and nonseminomas, which are aggressive tumors.
   D. Erectile dysfunction refers to the inability to attain or maintain penile erection. Most erectile dysfunction is caused by physical problems such as impaired vascular perfusion, altered nerve function, diabetes, or a side effect of medications such as antihypertensives. Psychologic causes include stress, fatigue, and depression.

II. Nursing process
   A. Assessment
      1. Assess for presence of BPH.
         a. Obtain a detailed health history, including:
            (1) Family history—risk of BPH is higher in those who have first-degree relatives with the condition.
            (2) Diet history—risk of prostate cancer is higher in those who consume a diet high in zinc, butter, and margarine.
         b. Perform a comprehensive physical assessment and determine if client has signs and symptoms of BPH.
            (1) Decreased force of urinary stream
            (2) Hesitancy
            (3) Inability to maintain steady stream
            (4) Sensation of incomplete emptying of bladder
            (5) Postvoiding dribbling
            (6) Nocturia
            (7) Incontinence
         c. Obtain diagnostic tests.
            (1) Palpate lower abdomen to detect enlarged bladder.
            (2) Perform bladder scan to measure urinary retention.
      2. Assess client for prostatic cancer.
         a. Obtain a detailed health history, including:
            (1) Family history—risk of prostatic cancer is higher in those who have first-degree relatives with the condition.
            (2) Diet history—risk of prostatic cancer is higher in those who consume a diet high in fat.
         b. Perform a comprehensive physical assessment and determine if client has symptoms of prostatic cancer (client is often asymptomatic in early stages).
            (1) Hesitancy
            (2) Postvoiding dribbling
            (3) Nocturia
            (4) Incontinence
            (5) Dysuria
            (6) Frequency and urgency
            (7) Inability to urinate
            (8) Hematuria
            (9) Back pain radiating to hips or legs (may indicate metastasis)
            (10) Fatigue
            (11) Weight loss
            (12) Pathologic fractures
         c. Obtain diagnostic tests.
            (1) Digital rectal examination
            (2) Prostate-specific antigen (PSA) levels
            (3) Biopsy
      3. Assess client for testicular cancer.
         a. Obtain a detailed health history, including:
            (1) Family history—risk of testicular cancer is higher in those who have first-degree relatives with testicular cancer or whose mothers were exposed to diethylstilbestrol (DES).
            (2) Personal history—risk of testicular cancer is higher in those who had cryptorchidism (undescended testicles), orchitis, testicular cancer in other testicle, or HIV infection.

b. Perform a comprehensive physical assessment and determine if client has symptoms of testicular cancer.
   (1) Firm, nontender scrotal mass
   (2) Scrotal heaviness
   (3) Scrotal swelling
   (4) Dull ache in lower abdomen
   (5) Signs of metastasis depend on site
   (6) Fatigue
   (7) Weight loss
   (8) Pathologic fractures
c. Obtain diagnostic tests—diagnosis begins with palpation of a tumor in the scrotal sac and is confirmed with ultrasound and blood test for alpha-fetoprotein levels.

4. Assess client for erectile dysfunction.
   a. Obtain a detailed health history, including sexual and psychosocial history.
   b. Have client complete a self-administered assessment questionnaire.
   c. Obtain diagnostic tests—physical examination, testosterone blood levels, ultrasound.

B. Analysis
1. Fear related to possible diagnosis of cancer, and sexual dysfunction
2. Acute Pain related to surgical procedure, bladder spasms
3. Decisional Conflict related to multiple treatment alternatives
4. Sexual Dysfunction related to erectile dysfunction and decreased libido
5. Deficient Knowledge related to testicular self-examination
6. Urinary Incontinence related to impaired sphincter control
7. Risk for Infection related to urinary retention
8. Low Self-Esteem related to inability to maintain a sexual relationship

C. Planning
1. Assist client to identify coping strategies to manage fear.
2. Relieve pain and discomfort.
3. Restore urinary drainage.

D. Implementation
1. Provide interventions for BPH.
   a. Promote diet limiting caffeine, artificial sweeteners, spicy or acidic foods.
   b. Advise client to avoid medications such as decongestants and anticholinergics, which exacerbate symptoms.
   c. Restrict fluids after supper time.
   d. Establish a voiding schedule.
   e. Teach client to empty bladder completely using moderate manual pressure on abdomen.
   f. Provide urinary catheter care.
   g. Irrigate bladder postprocedure to remove clots.
      (1) Intermittent irrigation via open method
      (2) Continuous irrigation via triple lumen catheter
   h. Instruct client regarding clean, intermittent, self-catheterization procedure, if indicated.
2. Provide interventions for prostatic cancer.
   a. Support client's decision-making process.
   b. Provide pre- and postsurgical care for clients undergoing prostatectomy.
   c. Administer antiandrogen medication when ordered.
   d. Provide pelvic floor muscle training for clients with incontinence.
3. Provide interventions for testicular cancer.
   a. Advise client of possibility of banking sperm, if desired.
   b. Provide pre- and postsurgical care for client undergoing orchiectomy.
   c. Implement chemotherapy or radiation therapy protocols when indicated.
4. Provide interventions for erectile dysfunction.
   a. Suggest client involve partner in treatment decision-making process.
   b. Discuss expectations of treatment with client and partner.

E. Evaluation
1. Client reports increased bladder control.
2. Client maintains satisfactory intimate relationship.
3. Client does not experience UTI.
4. Client actively participates in treatment decisions.
5. Client demonstrates correct performance of testicular self-examination.

CN

III. Client needs

A. Physiologic adaptation
1. BPH—treatment includes medications to relieve symptoms and surgery to resect or remove prostate (prostatectomy).
2. Prostate cancer—initial treatment is often watchful waiting; later treatment options include prostatectomy, radiation therapy, and hormone therapy.
3. Testicular cancer—treatment is orchiectomy followed by radiation or chemotherapy.
4. Erectile dysfunction—treatment includes removal of the cause, if possible, medication, and penile implants.

B. Management of care: Care of the male client with health problems of the reproductive organs requires critical thinking skills and knowledge of assessment, and teaching and evaluation methods unique to the RN role. These skills cannot be delegated to an LPN or UAP.
   1. Refer to continence clinic if incontinence persists.
   2. Refer for sexual counseling if erectile dysfunction persists.
   3. Identify community resources for clients with prostatic cancer.

C. Safety and infection control
   1. Assess client postprocedure for signs of UTI.
   2. Advise client to consume 2,000 to 3,000 ml of fluid daily to prevent UTI.
   3. Institute radiation protection measures for clients receiving radiation therapy.
   4. Instruct UAP in recognition of hazardous materials used in treatment regime.
   5. Instruct UAP in voiding schedule and urinary catheter care.
   6. Teach postoperative client signs to report to physician.
      a. Fever
      b. Purulent discharge
      c. Grossly bloody urine
      d. Frequency, urgency, and dysuria

D. Health promotion and maintenance
   1. Recommend yearly physical and digital rectal examination for men over 50 years of age.
   2. Encourage annual prostate-specific antigen (PSA) level beginning at 50 years of age.
   3. Suggest avoiding alcohol and caffeine to decrease bladder distention.
   4. Advise client to read labels of over-the-counter medications to determine effects on bladder emptying.
   5. Recommend client void as soon as urge is perceived.
   6. Reassure client that drinking normal amounts of fluid will prevent urinary tract infection rather than increase symptoms.
   7. Suggest smoking cessation program.
   8. Teach testicular self-examination technique.
   9. Promote stress management.

E. Psychologic integrity
   1. Warn client that retrograde ejaculation is possible after surgery on prostate.
   2. Allow client and partner to discuss concerns regarding sexual functioning.
   3. Assist client in managing incontinence so he can resume social activities without fear of embarrassment.
   4. Ensure client and partner have realistic expectations of erectile dysfunction treatment.

F. Basic care and comfort
   1. Insert urinary catheter using coude tip and lidocaine gel, when indicated, using strict aseptic technique.
   2. Encourage 2 to 3 L of fluid intake daily.
   3. Provide urinary catheter care.
   4. Prevent bladder spasms by keeping catheter free of clots and kinks in the drainage tubing.
   5. Administer analgesics as indicated.
   6. Instruct client in Kegel exercises to reduce dribbling and incontinence.
   7. Reduce intra-abdominal pressure by administering stool softeners and recommending a high-fiber diet.

G. Reduction of risk potential
   1. Suggest limiting zinc, butter and margarine, caffeine, artificial sweeteners, spicy or acidic foods in the diet to reduce risk of BPH.
   2. Avoid medications such as decongestants and anticholinergics, which cause difficulty voiding.
   3. Advise clients taking alpha-adrenergic blockers for BPH to change positions slowly to avoid postural hypotension.

H. Pharmacologic and parenteral therapies: Client will state the purpose for and side effects of all medications used to treat health problems of the reproductive system.
   1. Finasteride (Proscar)—shrinks prostatic tissue.
   2. Dutasteride (Avodart)—shrinks prostatic tissue.
   3. Tamsulosin (Flomax)—relaxes smooth muscles in the prostate.
   4. Saw palmetto—an herbal remedy for BPH used to improve urinary flow in some clients.
   5. Belladonna and opium (B&O) suppositories—used to relieve bladder spasms.
   6. Oxybutynin (Ditropan)—used to relieve bladder spasms.
   7. Sildenafil (Viagra), Tadalafil (Cialis), and vardenafil (Nuviva)—used with erectile dysfunction.

Sexually Transmitted Diseases

I. Definition: STDs are infectious diseases primarily transmitted through sexual contact; they may be viral or bacterial in nature and constitute a significant public health issue. These diseases often have a latent stage so they may be transmitted even though the infected party has no active symptoms. It is not uncommon for individuals to have more than one infection at a time. The two most common STDs in the United States are *Chlamydia* and *Gonorrhea*. Herpes simplex virus and human papillomavirus (HPV) are also common, but their exact incidence is unknown as they are not required to be reported to state boards of health.

II. Nursing process

A. Assessment

1. Obtain a detailed health history, including sexual history—risk is increased with multiple sexual partners, failure to use condoms consistently, personal history of STDs, and contact with someone infected with an STD.
2. Assess client's knowledge of need for barrier protection.
3. Perform a comprehensive physical examination and determine if client has signs and symptoms of STDs.
   a. Gonorrhea
      (1) For men—dysuria, purulent urethral drainage, painful and swollen testicles
      (2) For women—minor symptoms or vaginal discharge, dysuria, frequency, and menstrual changes
   b. Chlamydia—symptoms often minor or absent, especially in women
      (1) For men—dysuria, urethritis, and epididymitis, proctitis
      (2) For women—urethritis, cervicitis, and pelvic inflammatory disease
   c. Genital herpes (herpes simplex virus)
      (1) Painful vesicular lesions on genitals
      (2) Burning, tingling, and itching at site of lesions
      (3) Painful urination
      (4) Purulent vaginal drainage
      (5) Fever, headache, malaise with initial infection
   d. HPV
      (1) For men—itching, genital warts on penis, scrotum, anus, or urethra
      (2) For women—itching, genital warts on vulva, vagina, cervix, or perianal area
   e. Trichomonas
      (1) For men—often no symptoms as protozoa are harbored in urethra
      (2) For women—copious vaginal discharge with foul odor; pruritus; vulvar edema
   f. Syphilis
      (1) For men—primary, ulcer (chancre) on penis, non tender, indurated; secondary, rash on palms and soles; fever, lymphadenopathy
      (2) For women: Often undetected
4. Obtain diagnostic tests. Observe guidelines for reporting results to state boards of health.
   a. HPV—Pap smear; viral DNA or RNA
   b. Genital herpes—Pap smear, culture, antibody tests
   c. Chlamydia—culture, DNA test
   d. Gonorrhea—Gram stain, DNA testing
   e. Syphilis—VDRL, rapid plasma reagin blood test
   f. Trichomonas—microscopic examination

B. Analysis

1. Anxiety related to impact on personal relationships and potential complications
2. Acute Pain related to lesions and inflammatory process
3. Risk for Infection related to ignorance of mode of transmission and failure to follow safe sex guidelines
4. Ineffective Health Maintenance related to poor understanding of treatment plan and prevention strategies

C. Planning

1. Provide client teaching about disease process, treatment plan, and prevention strategies.
2. Manage pain and discomfort.

D. Implementation

1. Counsel client to abstain from sexual intercourse during treatment.
2. Advise client to avoid alcohol to reduce urethral irritation.
3. Impress on client the importance of follow-up care and notification of contacts.
4. Encourage safe sexual practices:
   a. Barrier protection such as condoms
   b. Abstinence
   c. Maintenance of monogamous sexual relationship
   d. Avoidance of high-risk sexual practices such as anal sex, drinking, or taking drugs prior to sexual activity
5. Instruct client of implications of pregnancy with an active STD.
6. Encourage use of loose-fitting cotton underwear.
7. Advise client to keep lesions clean and dry.
8. Remind female client to be screened for cervical cancer yearly as STDs increase this risk.

E. Evaluation

1. Client recognizes mode of transmission of STDs.
2. Client states intention to use condoms regularly.
3. Client verbalizes understanding of need to abstain from sexual intercourse when herpes lesions are present.

4. Client completes course of medication and returns for follow-up care.
5. Client cooperates with notification of sexual partners.

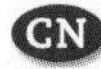

III. Client needs

A. Physiologic adaptation: STDs are treated with medications (administered by oral, topical, and IM routes) specific to the causative organism. The nurse counsels clients to avoid sexual encounters while taking the medications and to practice safe sex thereafter.

B. Management of care: Care of the male client with health problems of the reproductive organs requires critical thinking skills and knowledge of assessment, and teaching and evaluation methods unique to the RN role. These skills cannot be delegated to an LPN or UAP.
1. Screen all clients for risk of STDs.
2. Adhere to mandatory reporting requirements.
3. Facilitate follow-up care of infected clients.
4. Assist with notification of sexual partners in accordance with policy.

C. Safety and infection control
1. Instruct client to reduce risk of infection by inspecting partner's genitalia for symptoms prior to sexual activity.
2. Recommend voiding immediately after sexual encounter to help flush out organisms.
3. Advise client to wash genital and perineal area with soap and water after sexual activity to reduce micro-organisms.
4. Inform client that STDs can be spread by all sexual contact, including oral sex.

D. Health promotion and maintenance
1. Offer all clients opportunity to discuss issues related to sexuality.
2. Encourage all women to be screened for cervical cancer and have annual Pap tests.
3. Provide client teaching on disease prevention.
4. Recommend vaccination for human papillomavirus.
5. Participate in screening and case-finding programs.

E. Psychologic integrity
1. Allow client to verbalize feelings on diagnosis or notification of contact with infected individual.
2. Offer support for couples in committed relationships wherein one partner has been diagnosed or exposed to an STD.
3. Refer clients for counseling, if indicated.

F. Basic care and comfort
1. Assist client with perineal cleansing to reduce irritation from drainage.
2. Offer analgesics when needed.

G. Reduction of risk potential
1. Promote the use of barrier protection such as condoms in conjunction with other methods of birth control.
2. Provide written and verbal instruction on the proper use of condoms.
3. Advise clients to avoid sexual contact with IV drug users or individuals impaired by drugs or alcohol.
4. Prevent re-exposure by ensuring that both partners are treated simultaneously.
5. Encourage client to return for reculture after treatment.
6. Prevent development of pelvic inflammatory disease and infertility by providing all sexually active clients with information on STDs.
7. Advise regular screening for sexually active clients.

H. Pharmacologic and parenteral therapies: Client will state the purpose for and side effects of all medications used to treat STDs.
1. Gonorrhea
   a. Erythromycin or silver nitrate eye drops in newborns—prevents gonorrhea-induced blindness
   b. Ceftriaxone (Rocephin), ciprofloxacin (Cipro), or levofloxacin (Levaquin)—treats gonorrhea infections resistant to penicillin
   c. Penicillin
2. Chlamydia—doxycycline (Vibramycin) or azithromycin (Zithromax)
3. Herpes lesions: Acyclovir—treats and prevents outbreaks
4. HPV: Podofilox (Conylox), imiquimod (Aldara)
5. Trichomonas: Metronidazole (Flagyl)
6. Syphilis: Benzathine penicillin G

Bibliography

Altman, G. (2004). *Delmar's fundamental and advanced nursing skills.* (2nd ed.). Albany, NY: Delmar.

American Cancer Society. http://www.cancer.org

Ellis, J., & Hartley, C. (2005). *Managing and coordinating nursing care.* Philadelphia: Lippincott Williams & Wilkins.

Karch, A. (2006). *Lippincott's nursing drug guide.* Philadelphia: Lippincott Williams & Wilkins.

Nursing 2008 drug handbook. Ambler, PA: Springhouse.

Purnell, L., & Paulanka, B. (Eds.). (2003). *Transcultural healthcare: A culturally competent approach.* Philadelphia: Davis.

Smeltzer, S. C., Bare, B. G., Cheever, K. H., & Hinkle, J. L. (2008). *Brunner & Suddarth's textbook of medical-surgical nursing* (11th ed.). Philadelphia: Lippincott Williams & Wilkins.

Taylor, C., Lillis, C., LeMone, P., & Lynn, P. (2006). *Fundamentals of nursing.* Philadelphia: Lippincott Williams & Wilkins.

Weber, J. R., & Kelley, J. (2007). *Nurses' handbook of health assessment.* Philadelphia: Lippincott Williams & Wilkins.

Yarbro, C. H., Frogge, M., & Goodman, M. (2004). *Cancer symptom management* (3rd ed.). Sudbury, MA: Jones and Bartlett.

CHAPTER 29

Practice Test

Breast Disease: Fibrocystic Complex and Breast Cancer

1. The nurse is instructing a postmenopausal woman about breast self-examination. Which of the following points does the nurse include in the explanation?

- □ 1. It is not necessary to perform breast self-examination after menopause.
- □ 2. Having an annual mammogram is more useful than doing a self-exam.
- □ 3. It is more accurate to have the exam done by the HCP.
- □ 4. The exam should be performed on the same date each month.

2. Following a simple mastectomy, the nurse is assessing the drainage from a suction drain in the incision. The nurse notes there is 200 ml of serosanguinous drainage for the first 24 hr. The nurse should:

- □ 1. Document the findings.
- □ 2. Notify the surgeon.
- □ 3. Remove the drain.
- □ 4. Place the client's arm in a dependent position.

3. The nurse is providing discharge instructions to a client who had a modified radical mastectomy. Which of the following instructions is most effective in preventing infection?

- □ 1. Wear protective gloves when gardening.
- □ 2. Avoid crowded areas.
- □ 3. Keep cuticles cut.
- □ 4. Remove underarm hair with a sharp razor.

4. AF The nurse is instructing a client with fibrocystic complex. Which of the following instructions supports client management of the discomforts associated with the disease? Select all that apply.

- □ 1. Eliminate caffeine and chocolate.
- □ 2. Wear a supportive bra.
- □ 3. Avoid having mammograms.
- □ 4. Increasing the fat in the diet.
- □ 5. Take vitamin E.

Health Problems of Female Reproductive Organs

5. During the preoperative preparation for an abdominal hysterectomy, the client states she is worried that the surgery might have a negative impact on her marital relationship. The nurse should:

- □ 1. Complete the preoperative preparation.
- □ 2. Encourage client to focus on the immediate problem.
- □ 3. Schedule a counseling session with the psychologist for the couple.
- □ 4. Listen to the client's concerns about the impact of the surgery.

6. Following a vaginal hysterectomy, a client is having difficulty voiding. The nurse develops a care plan that includes which of the following?

- □ 1. Assist with ambulation.
- □ 2. Offer oral fluids every 2 hr.
- □ 3. Keep the bed at the lowest level.
- □ 4. Assess amount of vaginal drainage.

7. AF A client who had a hysterectomy 2 hr ago is returning to the postsurgical unit from the recovery room. The nurse is assessing the client. The vital signs are: T = 99°F; P = 98, R = 20, BP = 100/65. The urinary catheter is draining freely, and the client wants to try voiding without the catheter. The IV is infusing at 60 gtt/min. The perineal pad is saturated with bright red blood. The nurse reviews the progress notes from the recovery room below.

PROGRESS NOTES

Date	Time	Progress Notes
5/24/09	11:45	Client ready for transfer to room. Vital signs T = 99°F, P = 78; R = 14, BP = 114/70, O_2 Sat of 95% per pulse oximetry; catheter to straight drainage; IV in left cephalic vein infusing at keep open rate; client awake and oriented x3. Peri pad changed; moderately saturated. ~Bonnie Slater, RN

The nurse should do which of the following first?

- □ 1. Change the perineal pad.
- □ 2. Contact the surgeon.
- □ 3. Increase the IV fluids.
- □ 4. Remove the urinary catheter.

8. A client with cancer of the cervix is being treated with intracavitary radiation therapy. Which of the following are appropriate nursing care goals for this client?
- □ 1. Provide perineal care twice a day.
- □ 2. Maintain low-residue diet.
- □ 3. Restrict fluids to 1,000 ml/day.
- □ 4. Keep client on left side.

9. The nurse is instructing a group of women about early detection of ovarian cancer. The nurse emphasizes that the women should do which of the following?
- □ 1. Have an annual Pap smear according to age-appropriate standards of care.
- □ 2. Report any indications of abdominal pain.
- □ 3. Notify the HCP of signs of abdominal swelling.
- □ 4. Contact the HCP if experiencing indigestion, flatulence, or anorexia.

10. The nurse is instructing a client about managing premenstrual syndrome. The woman has symptoms of edema in extremities, breast swelling, and weight gain 5 to 7 days before her period. Which of the following health behaviors does the nurse instruct for this client?
- □ 1. Restrict sodium intake.
- □ 2. Take ibuprofen.
- □ 3. Use a calcium supplement.
- □ 4. Obtain additional sleep.

Health Problems of Male Reproductive Organs

11. The nurse is providing preoperative instructions to a client who is having a transurethral resection of the prostate. Which teaching point should the nurse include in this client's care?
- □ 1. "You will have a central venous access inserted just prior to the procedure."
- □ 2. "Plan on being in the hospital anywhere from 5 to 7 days following the procedure."
- □ 3. "You will be taught care of the incision and suture line prior to your discharge home."
- □ 4. "Expect some blood in urine in the first couple of days following the procedure."

12. A nurse is receiving a client to the postsurgical nursing unit with continuous bladder irrigation. To prepare the room for this client's arrival, the nurse should:
- □ 1. Obtain a urinary collection bag with incremental markings to measure hourly urine output.
- □ 2. Place a urinal at the client's bedside that will be easily within the client's reach.
- □ 3. Put a urine collection container in the bathroom toilet to catch and measure urinary output.
- □ 4. Have an IV pole with hooks to suspend the bladder irrigating solution.

13. When providing client teaching about continuous bladder irrigation following prostate surgery, the nurse instructs the client about which of the following?
- □ 1. "The catheter is disconnected from the drainage tubing one time per shift to enable manual irrigation of the bladder."
- □ 2. "The purpose of the irrigation is to keep bladder outflow clear and to prevent the formation of blood clots in the bladder."
- □ 3. "The fluid drips into the bladder at a slow rate to prevent the effects of overhydration and hyponatremia."
- □ 4. "The inflow catheter is clamped off approximately 4 hr after returning to the nursing unit."

14. The nurse is teaching a client with BPH and a family history of prostate cancer. Which of the following statements does the nurse provide about reducing the risk of cancer?
- □ 1. Surgical removal is the remedy for prostate cancer.
- □ 2. Follow a diet with limited amounts of red meat.
- □ 3. Frequent bladder infections are associated with prostate cancer.
- □ 4. An increased serum prostate antigen level is indicative of cancer.

15. A client had a TURP 24 hr ago and is complaining of bladder pressure, pain, and spasms. He has continuous bladder irrigation with a three-way catheter. Small amounts of urine are leaking around the catheter and the urine in the drainage bag is bloody. What action does the nurse take first?
- □ 1. Administer the prescribed belladonna and opium suppository.
- □ 2. Irrigate the catheter with 50 ml of sterile water.
- □ 3. Remove the catheter and insert a new one.
- □ 4. Stop the continuous irrigation until the spasms subside.

16. AF The nurse is teaching a client with erectile dysfunction about using sildenafil (Viagra). Which of the following points does the nurse emphasize? Select all that apply.
- □ 1. Do not use the drug if taking nitrates.
- □ 2. Take the drug on an empty stomach.
- □ 3. Report having erections that last longer than 4 hr.
- □ 4. Limit use of the drug to three in 24 hr.
- □ 5. Take 2 hr before having sex.

Sexually Transmitted Diseases

17. A client with a history of multiple sexual partners refuses to use protective barriers such as a condom during sexual activity. The nurse provides teaching to this client about which of the following?
- ☐ 1. Need for psychologic counseling.
- ☐ 2. Risk for STDs.
- ☐ 3. Importance of using protective barriers.
- ☐ 4. Specific types of protective barriers.

18. The nurse is providing teaching to a sexually active female client who is 20 years of age and has genital herpes. Which of the following statements is an important point for the nurse to include about using antiviral agents?
- ☐ 1. Antiviral agents, when used correctly, can cure genital herpes.
- ☐ 2. Herpes is transmitted only during the primary stage of the disease.
- ☐ 3. If pregnancy occurs, prenatal care is essential to monitor for fetal complications.
- ☐ 4. Secondary infections occur when drug therapy is initiated.

19. Client teaching is successful if the client states that she can best prevent a recurrence of pelvic inflammatory disease by:
- ☐ 1. Avoiding the use of tampons.
- ☐ 2. Using condoms with sexual intercourse.
- ☐ 3. Using good hand hygiene techniques.
- ☐ 4. Having yearly gynecologic examinations.

20. A nurse is instructing a female client who is 23 years of age who is to take metronidazole (Flagyl). Which of the following statements is included in client teaching?
- ☐ 1. "Possible temporary side effects of this medication include a greenish-yellow vaginal discharge and vaginal itching."
- ☐ 2. "Because oral contraceptives may not be effective when taking this medication, it is recommended that you use a second form of contraception."
- ☐ 3. "You can use alcohol as long as you do not have more than two drinks."
- ☐ 4. "You will need to taper off the dose of your medication slowly as you discontinue use."

Answers and Rationales

1. 4 Women of all ages are encouraged to perform monthly breast self-examinations. Prior to menopause, the woman examines her breasts just following menstrual periods; the nurse instructs the postmenopausal woman to perform the exam at the same time each month. While the client is also instructed to receive a mammogram according to standards of care, as well as an exam by a HCP, the breast self-exam is an important method of early detection. (H)

2. 1 The nurse documents serosanguinous drainage of 100 to 200 ml because this is normal during the first 24 hr after surgery. The nurse notifies the surgeon only if there is excessive or very bloody drainage. The surgeon removes the drain within 24 to 48 hr. The client is instructed to keep her arm on the affected side and supported in an adducted position. (A)

3. 1 Following a modified mastectomy in which lymph nodes have been removed, the client is at risk for lymphedema and infection. The nurse instructs the client to take precautions to avoid creating an entry site for infection in the affected arm by wearing protective gloves when gardening or using sharp instruments. Additional measures to prevent infection include using cuticle cream (not cutting cuticles), using an electric razor, using a thimble when sewing, and avoiding having injections or blood drawn from that arm. The woman does not need to avoid crowded areas as she is not at high risk for respiratory infection. (S)

4. 1, 2, 5 The discomforts of fibrocystic complex are often managed by nonsurgical approaches. The nurse instructs the client to eliminate caffeine and chocolate, wear a tight-fitting bra, and to take vitamin E. The client is encouraged to continue receiving mammograms and to monitor breast changes. Decreasing fat in the diet reduces discomfort. (H)

5. 4 Listening quietly is an appropriate technique for assisting the client experiencing anxiety. Psychosocial preparation is a part of preoperative preparation. Anxiety concerning the impact on the marriage is an immediate preoperative problem. Scheduling a counseling session is premature at this point. (P)

6. 2 It is important for the client who is having difficulty voiding to drink fluids to decrease the risk of bladder infections associated with vaginal surgery. Addressing safety issues such as assistance with ambulation and maintaining the bed in a safe position are important, but are unrelated to dysuria. The nurse also assesses vaginal drainage, but the amount of vaginal drainage is not directly related to the surgery. (S)

7. 2 The nurse's first action is to notify the surgeon as the amount of bleeding on the perineal pad is not normal. Excessive bleeding is also indicated by elevated heart rate and decreased BP. Urinary catheters are not removed until the second or third postoperative day. The surgeon may order an increase in the rate of the IV fluids. The nurse changes the perineal pad and offers comfort measures once the client is stable. (R)

8. 2 Nursing care while a client has intracavitary radiation is directed at protecting the placement of the radiation while maintaining comfort for the client. The client is on a low-residue diet to prevent gas and accumulation of fecal material. The nurse does not provide perineal care while the implant is in place. The client has a urinary catheter and it is not necessary to restrict fluid intake. The client is positioned on her back on strict bed rest and can only move slightly from side to side. (S)

9. 4 There are few distinct and early signs of ovarian cancer, but those that are associated with the disease include unexplained anorexia, indigestion, flatulence, weight gain or loss, or pelvic pressure. Pap smears are used to detect cervical cancer. Abdominal swelling and pain are late signs. (H)

10. 1 Premenstrual syndrome is a constellation of symptoms that range from fatigue and depression to fluid retention. The nurse instructs the client about a variety of nonpharmacologic approaches to manage symptoms based on the need of the individual client. For this client, restricting sodium intake before her period may minimize the swelling and weight gain. Clients with cramps and pain benefit from using ibuprofen and aerobic exercise. Calcium supplements may help irritability and mood swings. Obtaining sufficient sleep also helps relieve symptoms of irritability and fatigue. (H)

11. 4 Transurethral resection of the prostate (TURP) is a common surgical procedure used to treat male clients with benign prostate enlargement. The surgery commonly results in blood in the urine for the first few days. Central venous access is not expected for this type of surgery. Peripheral IV access can be expected. Clients are instructed to anticipate hospitalization for 1 to 3 days. Because the procedure is performed transurethrally (via the urethra), there is no outward incision. (A)

12. 4 A pole with hooks to suspend two 2-L bags of irrigating solution is needed. Because this type of bladder irrigation is continuous and the rate may be rapid, one bag is open and dripping, and the other is clamped and ready to be started when the first bag is instilled. This rate and volume prohibits the use of a traditional collection bag with an added urometer for hourly output measurement. A urinal and urine collection container are not necessary when the client has an indwelling urinary catheter. (A)

13. 2 Continuous bladder irrigation (CBI) is performed when urinary surgery (typically prostate surgery) results in hematuria. It is accomplished using an indwelling Foley catheter with three lumens. One port is for the balloon, a second port allows irrigant inflow, and a third port enables outflow. The purpose of the irrigation is to achieve and maintain clear outflow and to prevent clot formation within the bladder. Manual irrigation is used as an intermittent type of bladder irrigation and is not the same as CBI. CBI involves irrigation of the bladder; it is not an intravascular infusion. The rate is often initially fast to achieve a clear outflow. Stopping and clamping the irrigant inflow is done only under a physician's direction and is typically not expected until at least 1 day following the procedure. (A)

14. 2 Age, African American descent, socioeconomic level, and family history have the highest correlation with prostate cancer. A diet high in red meat is also closely associated with prostate cancer. Hormonal, radiation, and cryotherapy are used to treat prostate cancer, in addition to surgical removal. Frequent bladder infections are not associated with prostate cancer. PSA is produced by normal and neoplastic tissues. (H)

15. 2 The urethral catheter is obstructed, probably from clots; the catheter is irrigated to relieve the obstruction. The nurse prevents the bladder from distending; distention causes increased bleeding from stretching of blood vessels in the prostatic capsule. Drainage is initially a reddish-pink color and clear to light pink within 24 hr. The nurse reports continued bleeding to the surgeon. Belladonna and opium suppositories, while sometimes used to treat bladder spasms, will not be effective in this case and will delay treatment. Removing the catheter can be dangerous if a new one cannot be reinserted; this is performed by the surgeon, if necessary. Stopping the irrigation could allow irreversible catheter clotting. (R)

16. 1, 3 The nurse instructs the client to avoid using sildenafil (Viagra) if he is taking nitrates, and to report side effects such as painful erections, erections lasting longer than 4 hr, or vision problems. It is not necessary to take the drug on an empty stomach. The client is advised to limit use to one dose in 24 hr, and to take the drug 30 min to 1 hr before having sex. (D)

17. 2 The nurse explains to the client that he or she is at risk for acquiring STDs. Early detection and treatment of the diseases could decrease the risks to the client as well as the community. Counseling may assist the client in determining the etiology of the lifestyle, but is a long-term approach to an immediate problem. Because the client is already refusing to use protection, repeating this information likely will not change this client's behavior. (S)

18. 3 For the pregnant client with genital herpes, prenatal care is essential to prevent fetal complications such as microcephaly, encephalitis, or skin lesions; these risks are greater when the initial episode occurs during pregnancy. Delivery by cesarean section is always performed when the mother has active lesions at the time of delivery. Antiviral agents can arrest the infection if taken with a narrow window of time, but they do not cure the disease. Herpes is transmitted before lesions appear and until lesions are fully healed. Antiviral therapy does not cause secondary infection. (D)

19. 2 Pelvic inflammatory disease (PID) is most commonly caused by sexual transmission of gonorrheal or chlamydial organisms and so is best prevented by using condoms. The use of tampons, especially when accompanied by good hand hygiene, is not an important risk factor. Gynecologic examinations are important but are not preventive. (S)

20. 2 Metronidazole, like several other antimicrobial agents, can interfere with oral contraceptives; female clients are advised to use a second method of contraception. A frothy, greenish-yellow vaginal discharge with itching and possible dysuria is characteristic of *Trichomoniasis vaginalis*; these are not side effects of the drug. The client is instructed to avoid alcohol use, including products such as mouthwash and cough medicine that may include alcohol. Metronidazole adversely interacts with alcohol, resulting in effects such as severe nausea, vomiting, headache, abdominal cramps, flushing, and palpitations. The client does not need to taper the dose to discontinue the prescription. (D)

chapter

30

The Client With Neurologic Health Problems

Stroke is the third most common cause of death in the United States, and therefore neurologic health problems represent a significant proportion of admissions to health care services. The nurse must be prepared to plan care for clients who are unconscious, have changes in intracranial pressure (ICP), are experiencing pain, or have long-term and chronic health problems such as seizures or Parkinson disease. Topics discussed in this chapter include the following:

- The Unconscious Client
- Increased Intracranial Pressure
- Head Injury
- Stroke
- Seizure
- Pain
- Parkinson Disease
- Multiple Sclerosis
- Myasthenia Gravis
- Amyotrophic Lateral Sclerosis
- Guillain-Barré Syndrome

The Unconscious Client

I. Definition: Consciousness refers to awareness of self and environment, and one's ability to become oriented to new stimuli. Consciousness involves both arousal, or wakefulness, and content and cognition and awareness. A disturbance in level of consciousness (LOC) ranges from mild confusion to stupor or coma and indicates injury to either the reticular activating system (RAS) or both cerebral hemispheres concurrently (Fig. 30-1). Levels of consciousness exist on a continuum including consciousness, confusion, delirium, obtundation, stupor, and coma (Table 30-1).
   A. Altered LOC is demonstrated in a client who is not oriented, does not follow commands, or needs persistent stimuli to achieve a state of alertness.
   B. Persistent vegetative state (PSV) is characterized by loss of all cognitive functions and the unawareness of self and surroundings.
   C. Brain death is defined as the irreversible loss of function of the brain and brain stem.

II. Nursing process
   A. Assessment
      1. Perform a detailed health history, including allergies, prior hospitalizations, family medical history, psychosocial history, and history of medications.
      2. Perform a comprehensive physical assessment with a detailed neurologic examination.
         a. Evaluate mental status, cranial nerve function, cerebellar function (balance and coordination), reflexes, motor, and sensory function.
         b. Use Glasgow Coma Scale (GCS) to assess for best eye opening, verbal response, and motor response—score of 3 indicates severe neurologic impairment; score of 8 or less indicates coma.
         c. Assess vital signs, visual changes, pupillary response, breathing pattern, oxygenation status, cardiac rhythm, fluid and electrolyte balance, and signs of complications (e.g., increased ICP).
      3. Assess etiology—any structural lesions, metabolic, or toxic conditions may cause an altered LOC.

Table 30-1 Descending Levels of Consciousness

Level of Consciousness	Characteristics
Confusion	Client experiences disturbance in consciousness evidenced by inability to think clearly, and inability to perceive, respond to, or remember current stimuli.
Delirium	Client experiences an altered state of consciousness evidenced by disorientation, transient hallucinations, and disordered thinking and memory.
Obtundation	Client experiences decreased alertness and psychomotor retardation.
Stupor	Client is conscious, but demonstrates lack of reaction to environmental stimuli.
Coma	Client is unarousable and unresponsive to external stimuli.

Adapted from Bates D. (1993). The management of medical coma. *Journal of Neurology, Neurosurgery, and Psychiatry*, 56–59.

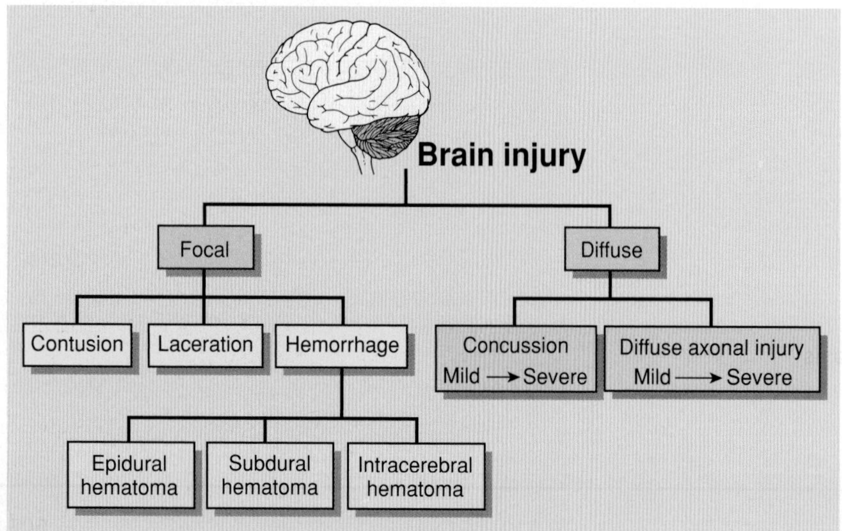

Figure 30-1. Focal and generalized brain injuries. (Adapted from Hickey, J. V. [2005]. *Neurological and neurosurgical nursing* [5th ed., p. 374]. Philadelphia: Lippincott Williams & Wilkins.)

4. Assess for factors that place client at risk for altered LOC—head injury, brain tumors, strokes, drug overdose, alcohol intoxication, hepatic or renal disease, diabetic ketoacidosis, electrolyte imbalance, sepsis, hypovolemia, myocardial infarction, respiratory arrest, hypoglycemia, and encephalopathy.
5. Obtain/monitor diagnostic tests.
   a. For altered LOC—cognitive and motor function; cranial nerve reflexes
   b. For PVS—diagnosis requires that the condition has continued for at least a month; reflex and vegetative functions remain, including sleep-wake cycles, lack of language comprehension, bowel and bladder incontinence, sufficiently preserved hypothalamic and brain stem function to maintain life, cranial nerve and spinal cord reflexes are variably preserved.

B. Analysis
1. Ineffective Airway Clearance related to altered LOC
2. Risk for Injury related to decreased LOC
3. Disturbed Sensory Perception: Visual, Kinesthetic, related to neurologic impairment
4. Impaired Oral Mucous Membranes related to mouth breathing, absence of pharyngeal reflex, and altered fluid and nutrition intake
5. Impaired Physical Mobility related to neurologic impairment

C. Planning
1. Maintain patent airway.
2. Prevent injury.
3. Maintain body temperature within normal limits.
4. Promote skin integrity.
5. Promote adequate fluid, hydration, and nutritional intake.
6. Maintain cerebral tissue perfusion.
7. Promote client and family support systems.

D. Implementation
1. Assess vital signs and perform neurologic checks at specified intervals as ordered. Report any significant changes to physician.
2. Establish and maintain adequate airway to and ensure maximum ventilation.
3. Position client to maintain optimal hemodynamic status.
4. Promote safety—pad side rails; avoid restraints; place bed in low position.
5. Maintain fluid balance and manage nutritional needs.
6. Provide mouth care, skin care, and preserve corneal integrity.
7. Achieve thermoregulation.
8. Prevent urinary retention and promote bowel function.
9. Provide sensory stimulus as needed; avoid overstimulation.
10. Provide emotional support to client and family.
11. Monitor for complications.

E. Evaluation
1. Client maintains patent airway and adequate oxygenation.
2. Client is free from injuries.
3. Client has adequate fluid and nutritional status.
4. Client maintains skin integrity.
5. Client experiences appropriate sensory stimulation.
6. Client and family cope with crisis.
7. Client is free of complications.

CN

III. Client needs

A. Physiologic adaptation: The goal of management of the unconscious client is to treat underlying causes and prevent further injury or complications.
1. Monitor temperature—hyperthermia increases metabolic needs; hypothermia can lead to dysrhythmias and metabolic compromise.
2. Monitor respiration patterns (e.g., Cheyne-Stokes, central neurogenic hyperventilation, apneustic, ataxic [Biot], and cluster breathing)—hypercapnia (increased carbon dioxide levels) or hypoxia (low oxygen levels) results in vasodilatation, increased cerebral blood volume (CBV), and increased ICP.
3. Recognize risk for seizures and intervene to avoid precipitating factors, including fever, hypoxia, and electrolyte imbalance.
4. Monitor for other complications, including aspiration, contractures, deep vein thrombosis, ICP, musculoskeletal deterioration, pneumonia, pressure ulcers, and respiratory failure.

B. Management of care: Care of the unconscious client requires critical thinking skills and knowledge of assessment, and teaching and evaluation methods unique to the RN role. These skills cannot be delegated to an LPN or UAP.
1. Delegate responsibly those activities that can be delegated, including basic care needs and vital sign checks for the stable client. All monitoring information is reported to the RN.

2. Perform comprehensive physical assessments and provide care to the symptomatic unconscious client.
3. Provide information on changes in client status to the physician and appropriate members of the multidisciplinary team.
4. Promote sensory stimulation; assist family and significant others on ways to enhance sensory stimulation, but avoid overstimulation.
   a. Explain procedures in advance.
   b. Maintain a well-lighted environment, if appropriate.
   c. Keep large calendar and clock in view.
   d. Frequently orient client to person, place, and time.
   e. Introduce self when caring for client.
   f. Provide for adequate rest periods.
5. Prevent tongue from obstructing airway—place client in a side-lying or three-quarters prone position; if tongue is obstructing, insert oral airway; prepare for insertion of a cuffed endotracheal or tracheostomy tube as the client's condition requires.
6. Provide mouth care to keep mucous membranes clear, moist, and intact.
7. Turn and reposition client every 2 hr; inspect skin for signs, symptoms of pressure or breakdown; perform passive range of motion (PROM) exercises every 4 hr; use nursing measures to prevent deformities; apply foot splints or high-topped sneakers to prevent footdrop; apply splints to prevent wrist-drop or finger contractures.
8. Provide teaching to client and family regarding rehabilitation needs; diagnostic tests, nonsurgical and surgical interventions; and medications (see also health promotion and maintenance).

C. Safety and infection control
1. Pad side rails and place bed in low position; avoiding restraints.
2. Protect client's eyes from corneal irritation.

D. Health promotion and maintenance: Provide client and family teaching.
1. Perform ROM exercises to promote muscle strength and prevent contractures.
2. Consume nutritious diet and maintain target weight.
3. Maintain progress toward recovery and prevent relapse through adequate rest periods.

E. Psychologic integrity
1. Discuss what information the family needs to make informed decisions, and inquire as to whether the client has a living will or advanced directive to guide decision-making.
2. Provide ancillary support for client and family (chaplains, social workers, and community groups).

F. Basic care and comfort
1. Speak softly and use client's name during nursing care.
2. Touch client as gently as possible.
3. Keep skin clean, dry, and pressure-free.

G. Reduction of risk potential
1. Use strict medical asepsis and adhere to universal precautions to reduce incidence of nosocomial infections.
2. Keep bed in low position and provide other protective equipment.
3. Instill artificial tears as ordered; patch eyes.

H. Pharmacology and parenteral therapies: Client or family will understand the purpose for and associated side effects of all medications.
1. Anticonvulsants
2. Sedatives
3. Stool softeners
4. Other medications based on client's specific needs

Increased Intracranial Pressure

I. Definition: Increased intracranial pressure (ICP) is also known as intracranial hypertension and is associated with altered states of consciousness. It results from disequilibrium between the volume and pressure of the three components found within the rigid cranial vault: Brain tissue, blood, and cerebral spinal fluid (CSF).

A. An increase in any one of the components necessitates a reciprocal change in one of the other components to maintain adequate cerebral pressure. This concept is referred to as the *Monro-Kellie hypothesis*. The normal ICP is 0 to 15 mmHg and normal cerebral perfusion pressure (CPP) is 60 to 100 mmHg. Cerebral edema results in an increase in tissue volume that may increase ICP. If increased ICP is untreated, displacement of brain tissue may occur in brain herniation.

B. ICP monitoring devices (see Fig. 30-2)
1. Ventriculostomy/intraventricular catheter—involves ventricular catheter placed into lateral ventricle on nondominant side level with foramen of Monro.
2. Subarachnoid bolt—involves bolt placed in subarachnoid space via burr hole.
3. Intraparenchymal space—probe placed in parenchymal space.
4. Epidural—involves probes placed into epidural space; reduces risk of infection; questionable accuracy at high ICP.

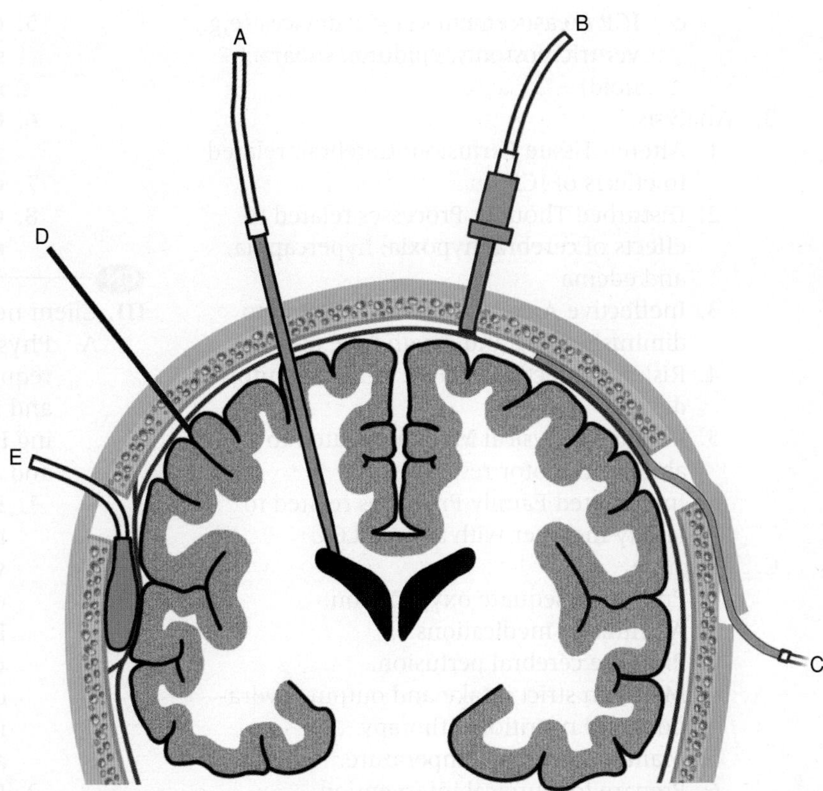

Figure 30-2. Intracranial pressure monitoring devices. **A.** Ventriculostomy/intraventricular. **B.** Subarachnoid. **C.** Subdural. **D.** Intraparenchymal. **E.** Epidural.

II. Nursing process

A. Assessment

1. Perform detailed physical assessment to assess for cause of increased ICP, including trauma, tumor, abscess, space-occupying lesion, edema, hemorrhage, hydrocephalus, head injury, infection, congenital abnormality, and encephalopathy.
2. Obtain detailed health history, and history of events leading to present illness (may need to obtain information from family, friends, or bystanders).
3. Assess and inspect client for other factors that may cause increased ICP.
   a. Increased intracranial blood volume—vasodilatation from hypoxia, hypercapnia, fluid overload
   b. Jugular venous obstruction—neck flexion, hyperextension, neck swelling, tight tracheostomy ties
   c. Increased intrathoracic pressure—positive pressure ventilation, positive end-expiratory pressure (PEEP), Valsalva maneuver
   d. Increased oxygen demand—seizures, fever, shivering, hyperactivity, pain
4. Assess for signs and symptoms—earliest signs of ICP are changes in LOC, progressing from restlessness to confusion and disorientation to lethargy and coma.
   a. Vital signs: Cushing triad—widening pulse pressure (high systolic BP rises while diastolic BP remains the same), bradycardia, bradypnea are late signs of severe complications of increased ICP
   b. Pupillary changes: Ipsilateral (same side) dilation of pupil with sluggish reaction to light from compression of cranial nerve III; pupil eventually becomes fixed and dilated
   c. Motor abnormalities
      (1) Contralateral (opposite side) hemiparesis from compression of corticospinal tracts
      (2) Decorticate or decerebrate rigidity
   d. Headache, projectile vomiting, papilledema (edema of the optic disc), visual disturbance (diplopia), and seizures
   e. Abnormal respiratory patterns (e.g., Cheyne-Stokes respirations)
5. Obtain and monitor results of diagnostic tests.
   a. Laboratory tests include ABGs and SpO_2, CBC, coagulation profile (aPTT, PT, INR), platelet count, electrolytes, BUN, Cr, liver function, and serum osmolality.
   b. CT scan (noncontrast), MRI, skull x-rays, EEG, CBF, cerebral arteriography

c. ICP measurement via ICP devices (e.g., ventriculostomy, epidural, subarachnoid)

B. Analysis
   1. Altered Tissue Perfusion: Cerebral, related to effects of ICP
   2. Disturbed Thought Processes related to effects of cerebral hypoxia, hypercapnia, and edema
   3. Ineffective Airway Clearance related to diminished gag and cough reflexes
   4. Risk for Infection related to ICP monitoring devices
   5. Impaired Physical Mobility related to abnormal motor responses
   6. Interrupted Family Processes related to family member with altered LOC

C. Planning
   1. Promote adequate oxygenation.
   2. Administer medications.
   3. Promote cerebral perfusion.
   4. Maintain strict intake and output, hydration, and nutritional therapy.
   5. Maintain normal temperature.
   6. Prepare for surgical intervention.
   7. Relieve pain.

D. Implementation
   1. Assess vital signs and perform neurologic checks (GCS) at specified intervals as ordered. Report any significant changes to physician.
   2. Maintain fluid and electrolyte balance; ensure adequate nutrition; administer IV fluids and nasogastric (NG) tube feedings as ordered; maintain accurate intake and output.
   3. Assess and maintain mechanical ventilation to limit further neurologic impairment.
   4. Monitor ABGs, SpO_2, ICP, arterial BP, and pulmonary artery pressures.
   5. Collaborate with dietician to ensure client is receiving optimal nutrition based on calorie needs and laboratory findings.
   6. Maintain client in a normovolemic state.
   7. Position client to minimize ICP and optimize CPP, and oxygenation.

E. Evaluation
   1. Client's ICP remains within normal range, and CPP, cerebral blood flow (CBF), and oxygenation remain within the desired range without interventions.
   2. Client's neurologic status improves; client regains optimal LOC.
   3. Client resumes self-care activities.
   4. Client achieves optimal level of neurologic and motor function.
   5. Client is afebrile, with vital signs and neuro signs, ABGs, SpO_2, and labs within normal range.
   6. Client affirms relief of pain and associated symptoms.
   7. Client tolerates increasing levels of activity.
   8. Client states understanding of diet, medications, and treatments.

CN

III. Client needs

A. Physiologic adaptation: Clients with ICP may require intubation and mechanical ventilation, and invasive hemodynamic monitoring including ICP monitor, pulmonary artery catheter, and arterial line.
   1. Recognize causes of increased ICP and implement measures to manage and prevent possible complications of client's condition and/or procedures. Complications of ICP include seizures, infection, hemorrhage (ICP site), coma, diabetes insipidus, syndrome of inappropriate antidiuretic hormone (SIADH), brain ischemia, herniation, and death.
   2. Recognize risk for hypoxia and hypercapnia (see management of care).
   3. Recognize risk for seizures—indicated by fever, hypoxia, hypercapnia, and electrolyte imbalance (see management of care).

B. Management of care: Care of the client with increased ICP requires critical thinking skills and knowledge of assessment, and teaching and evaluation methods unique to the RN role. These skills cannot be delegated to an LPN or UAP.
   1. Delegate responsibly those activities that can be delegated, including basic care needs and vital sign checks for the stable client. All monitoring information is reported to the RN.
   2. Perform comprehensive assessments and monitor client with potential or actual symptoms of increased ICP.
      a. Maintain and record vital signs and neuro signs, ICP, CPP, and hemodynamic pulmonary artery catheter values.
      b. Maintain patent airway, administer oxygen, and assist with turning and deep breathing.
      c. Maintain position and patency of the endotracheal tube and mechanical ventilator, arterial line, pulmonary artery catheter, indwelling Foley catheter.
      d. Maintain measures to prevent hypoxia and hypercapnia, including proper

positioning of client's head to enhance respiratory exchange and aid in optimal CPP, and decrease cerebral edema.
(1) Keep head in neutral position; prevent hip flexion to prevent blockage in outflow of cerebral venous blood flow.
(2) Before and after suctioning, hyperventilate the client with a resuscitator bag connected to 100% oxygen. Limit suctioning to 15 s.

e. Maintain measures to prevent seizures.
(1) Assess for fever, hypoxia, hypercapnia, electrolyte imbalance, drug levels.
(2) Turn client with slow, gentle movements to prevent rapid changes in ICP; close ventriculostomy ICP clamp, if present, when suctioning or turning.

f. Protect client's eyes from corneal irritation—check for corneal reflex; instill artificial tears as ordered; patch eyes.

g. Maintain patency and position of the NG tube to low suction to prevent abdominal distention.

h. Maintain fluid and electrolyte balance and ensure adequate nutrition; administer IV fluids, enteral feedings as ordered.

i. Assess client's hydration status: Skin turgor, check for dry mucous membranes.

j. Prevent further increase in ICP: Maintain quiet, comfortable environment; avoid use of restraints; prevent straining at stool, administer stool softeners and mild laxatives as ordered; prevent vomiting; administer antiemetics as ordered; prevent excessive coughing; avoid clustering nursing care activities together; prevent complications of immobility; administer medications as ordered.

3. Provide information on changes in client status to physician and appropriate members of the multidisciplinary team—late signs and symptoms of increased ICP include hypertension with widening pulse pressure, bradycardia, and bradypnea (Cushing triad).
4. Assist with insertion and maintenance of intracranial monitoring device (see safety and infection control).
5. Provide teaching on procedures and interventions, diet, medications, and importance of continuous follow-up care (see also health promotion and maintenance).
6. Evaluate community resources for support and rehabilitation needs.

C. Safety and infection control
1. Use strict aseptic technique when handling any part of monitoring system; inspect insertion site for signs of infection. Closely monitor temperature, pulse, and respirations.
2. Adjust side rails and avoid restraints.
3. Administer drugs cautiously—may cause cerebral vasodilatation (e.g., nitroprusside, nitroglycerin, halothane, nitrous oxide).

D. Health promotion and maintenance: Provide client and family teaching.
1. Enhance optimal cerebral perfusion—use stool softeners; practice proper positioning; promote relaxing environmental factors (e.g., noise, light, space activities); and avoid strenuous coughing, Valsalva maneuver, and isometric muscle exercise.
2. For client with chronic hydrocephalus requiring a ventricular peritoneal shunt (VPS)—maintain patency of, and care for, shunt; monitor for shunt malfunction; identify signs and symptoms of infection.
3. Recognize signs and symptoms requiring medical attention, including any change in LOC such as increased drowsiness or confusion.
4. Practice self-care behaviors.
5. Comply with diet, medication regimen, and exercise program.

E. Psychologic integrity: Support family in making end-of-life and palliative care decisions in client with minimal brain function or brain death. Anticipate grieving and identify community support resources.

F. Basic care and comfort
1. Speak softly and use client's name during nursing care.
2. Provide oral care to keep mucous membranes clean, moist, and intact.
3. Monitor and treat pain, nausea, and vomiting.
4. Turn and position client every 2 hr while on bed rest.
5. Provide skin care; protect and monitor skin for signs of pressure areas and breakdown.

G. Reduction of risk potential
1. Prevent complications of immobility.
2. Follow written protocols and best practice standards for care of the client with an ICP monitoring device.
3. Closely monitor drug levels and signs and symptoms of increased ICP and decreased CPP.

H. Pharmacology and parenteral therapies: Client and family will state purpose for and side effects of all medications used to treat increased ICP.
   1. Analgesic: Codeine (Paveral)—stronger opiates may be contraindicated as they may potentiate respiratory depression, altered LOC, and pupillary changes.
   2. Anticonvulsants: Phenytoin (Dilantin) and fosphenytoin (Cerebyx)—decrease risk of seizures; monitor drug level closely and assess for side effects, including bradycardia, hypotension, nystagmus/ataxia; gingival hyperplasia, agranulocytosis, rash, Stevens-Johnson syndrome; lymphadenopathy, nausea, and heart block.
   3. Osmotic diuretics: Mannitol (Osmitrol)—reduce cerebral edema.
      a. Monitor vial for crystals—shake vial and use filter needle to administer.
      b. Monitor urine output, serum electrolytes, serum osmolarity; and signs of hypotension, dehydration, tachycardiac, rebound edema.
   4. Loop diuretics: Furosemide (Lasix)—monitor side effects, including ototoxicity, polyuria, electrolyte imbalance, gastric irritation, muscle cramps, hypotension, and dehydration.
   5. Sympathomimetics (vasopressors): Dopamine (Intropin) and norepinephrine (Levophed)—maintain optimal CPP if BP is low and ICP is elevated.
   6. Corticosteroids: Dexamethasone (Decadron)—reduce cerebral edema; side effects include flushing, sweating, hypertension, tachycardia, thrombocytopenia, hyperglycemia, peptic ulcer, decreased wound healing, muscle wasting, and hypokalemia.
   7. Histamine antagonists: Ranitidine (Zantac) and famotidine (Pepcid)
   8. Mucosal barrier fortifier: Sucralfate (Carafate)
   9. Posterior pituitary hormone: Vasopressin (Pitressin) and desmopressin (DDAVP)—may be administered if client develops diabetes insipidus.
   10. Stool softeners: Docusate (Colace, Surfak) and Sennosides (Senokot)—help to prevent "straining" and therefore decrease potential for increased ICP.
   11. Antipyretics: Acetaminophen (Tylenol)
   12. Barbiturates: Pentobarbital sodium (Nembutal sodium)—induce coma artificially in the client who has not responded to conventional treatment; monitor for side effects: Hypotension, myocardial or respiratory depression (client must be intubated and mechanically ventilated), thrombocytopenia purpura.
   13. Neuromuscular blocking agents (NMBAs): Cisatracurium (Nimbex), vecuronium (Norcuron), and atracurium (Tracrium)—assist with maintaining adequate ventilation, enhancing client comfort, and decreasing work of breathing, particularly if the client is fighting the ventilator (which can compromise CPP).
      a. Administer sedatives and analgesic agents concurrently because NMBAs do not have sedative or analgesic properties.
      b. Monitor level of paralysis; protect client from environment and immobility complications.
   14. Sedatives: Propofol (Diprivan), lorazepam (Ativan), and diazepam (Valium)
   15. Antacids or H_2 antagonist—prevent stress ulcer
   16. Steroids: Dexamethasone (Decadron) for anti-inflammatory action

Head Injury

I. Definition: Head injury involves injury to the scalp, skull (cranium and facial bones), or brain; it may consist of fractures, hemorrhage, or brain trauma (concussion and/or contusion). Immediate complications include cerebral bleeding, hematomas, uncontrolled increased ICP, infections, and seizures. Effects of head injury such as changes in personality or behavior, or cranial nerve deficits depend on the area involved and extent of damage. The best approach to head injury is prevention.
   A. Primary head injury occurs with a direct impact to the head from an acceleration-deceleration or rational force and involves compression and/or shearing of vessels and nerves.
      1. Concussion involves temporary loss, or no loss of, consciousness and is reversible.
      2. Contusion involves bruising of the brain tissue, resulting in disruption of neural functioning.
      3. Laceration involves tearing of brain tissue or blood vessels because of a sharp bone fragment or object, or a tearing force.
      4. Fractures
         a. Linear—crack in skull; may result in epidural bleed.
         b. Comminuted—multiple linear fractures; depressed area at site of impact; "eggshell fracture"; may tear dura and result in leakage of CSF.

c. Depressed—broken bones may penetrate meninges or brain tissue, closed with scalp intact; compound with scalp open but dura intact; and complex with dura lacerated by bone fragments.
d. Basilar skull fracture—fracture at base of skull into either anterior, middle, or posterior fossa; usually not seen on x-ray; dural tears; spinal fluid leakage from nose and ears.

B. Secondary injury is a response to the primary injury as a result of hypoxemia, hypotension, ICP, hypocapnia, hyperthermia, and anemia, and can result in hematomas or hemorrhage (see Fig. 30-3).
1. Hematomas
a. Epidural—arterial bleed (usually tearing of middle meningeal artery), resulting in blood clot between dura mater and inner surface of skull.
b. Subdural—acute, subacute, or chronic; venous bleed resulting in blood clot between arachnoid and dura.
c. Intracerebral—within brain, causes direct damage to the brain, usually following contusion.

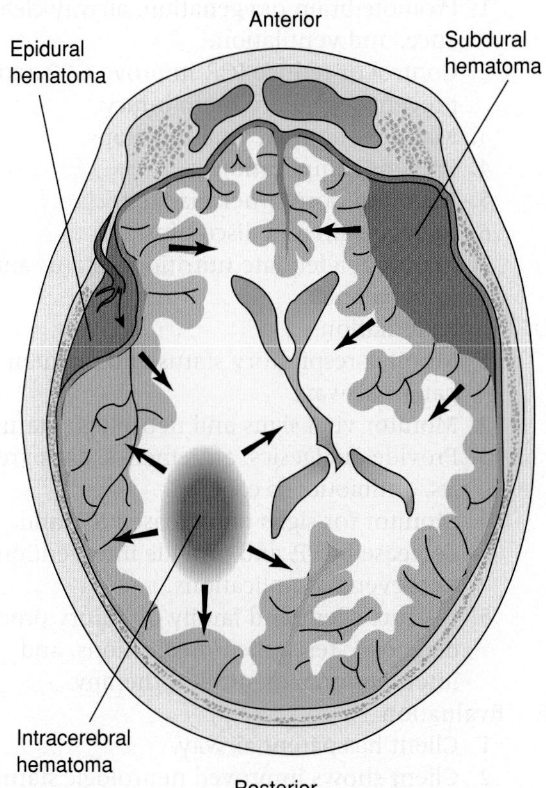

Figure 30-3. Characteristics of arterial aneurysm. (From Smeltzer, S. C., Bare, B. G., Hinkle, J. L., & Cheever, K. H. [2008]. *Brunner & Suddarth's textbook of medical-surgical nursing* [11th ed.]. Philadelphia: Lippincott Williams & Wilkins.)

2. Hemorrhage
a. Intracerebral—bleeding into the subcortical white matter of brain.
b. Subarachnoid and intraventricular—bleeding between the pia mater of the covering of the brain and spinal cord and the arachnoid membrane and ventricles.

C. Mechanisms of injury
1. Skull deformation results from a direct force to the head that alters skull contour and causing contusion, laceration, and/or hemorrhage.
2. Acceleration-deceleration is forward then backward thrusting of the head, resulting in brain movement (coup-contrecoup), causing compression, tension, and shearing of brain tissue.
3. Rotational injuries involve acceleration or deceleration injury to the brain and results in tension, stretching, and shearing of brain tissue, and diffuse axonal injury (DAI). DAI involves diffuse white matter shearing associated with severe widespread mechanical disruption of axons and neuronal pathways in the hemispheres, corpus callosum, diencephalon, and brain stem.
4. Penetrating injuries may result from gunshot wounds, stab wounds, or other types of penetrating objects.

II. Nursing process
A. Assessment
1. Assess for etiology and risk factors of traumatic brain injury (TBI).
a. Higher incidence in male clients.
b. High incidences in clients between 15 and 24 years of age, and clients over 75 years of age.
c. Major causes include blunt and penetrating trauma, motor vehicle accidents, falls, and assaults.
2. Perform a detailed health history, including neurologic history.
3. Perform a comprehensive physical assessment.
a. Vital signs and neurologic signs
b. Airway and breathing pattern changes
c. Visual disturbances, pupillary changes, papilledema, and extraocular movements
d. Weakness and paralysis
e. Posturing and seizure activity
4. Assess for signs and symptoms regarding extent, degree, and location of brain injury.
a. Concussion—temporary, or no loss of, consciousness; confusion; dizziness;

amnesia; nausea and vomiting; and headache.

b. Contusion—multiple petechial hemorrhages, bruising, swelling, ischemia, and ICP, followed by a lucid period, and then lethargy and coma. Signs and symptoms of increased ICP may develop within minutes following the lucid interval. Headache, fixed dilated pupil on affected side, hemiparesis, hemiplegia, and seizures can also develop. Tentorial herniation may occur without immediate intervention, leading to a poor prognosis.

c. Laceration—caused by extracranial trauma; presents as bleeding and tissue damage.

d. Skull fractures—may present with varying signs and symptoms depending on location. Basilar skull fractures are usually uncomplicated, but may result in classic signs.
   (1) Rhinorrhea, otorrhea, Battle sign, and raccoon eyes
   (2) Infection (meningitis) due to disruption of the sinuses and middle ear bones—signs and symptoms of meningitis include nuchal rigidity, positive Kernig sign, positive Brudzinski sign, and photophobia.

e. Subdural hematoma—confusion, drowsiness, headaches, ipsilateral pupil dilation or sluggishness, and seizures.

f. Intracerebral hematoma—varies in presentation of signs and symptoms depending on the location; may include headache, decreased LOC, hemiplegia, and ipsilateral pupil dilation as hematoma expands.

g. Epidural hematoma—client may have periods of responsiveness followed by unresponsiveness.

5. Assess for signs of increased ICP (see section on increased ICP).
6. Obtain diagnostic tests.
   a. Skull x-ray
   b. Computerized tomography (CT)
   c. Magnetic resonance imaging (MRI)
   d. Cerebral angiography
   e. Electroencephalography (EEG)
   f. Transcranial Doppler (TCD)
   g. Positron emission tomography (PET)
   h. Laboratory tests may include ABGs, CBC, electrolytes, and alcohol and drug screens
   i. Glucose test for drainage from nose or ears (indicates leakage of CSF)
   j. Lumbar puncture (contraindicated with ICP)

B. Analysis
   1. Ineffective Breathing Pattern related to increased ICP or brain stem injury
   2. Impaired Gas Exchange related to head injury
   3. Altered Tissue Perfusion: Cerebral, related to ICP and decreased CPP
   4. Risk for Injury related to impaired CNS and neuromuscular functioning
   5. Risk for Aspiration related to loss of gag reflex, or inability to cough and expectorate
   6. Self-Care Deficit: Feeding and Toileting, related to altered LOC
   7. Risk for Disuse Syndrome related to long-term immobility
   8. Ineffective Role Performance related to impaired neuromuscular and cognitive function
   9. Deficient Knowledge: Recovery and Rehabilitation Process, related to brain injury and treatment plan.
   10. Risk for Imbalanced Body Temperature: Increased, related to damaged temperature-regulating mechanism

C. Planning
   1. Promote brain oxygenation, airway clearance, and ventilation.
   2. Control or reduce ICP, improve CPP and prevent secondary brain injury.
   3. Maintain optimal vital functions.
   4. Prevent complications.
   5. Maintain normothermia.
   6. Relieve pain and discomfort.
   7. Maintain adequate nutritional status and fluid balance.

D. Implementation
   1. Monitor respiratory status and maintain patent airway.
   2. Monitor vital signs and neurologic status.
   3. Provide analgesics, antiemetics, antipyretics, antibiotics as ordered.
   4. Monitor for signs of increased ICP and decreased CPP, and provide interventions to prevent complications.
   5. Instruct client and family on injury process, diagnostic tests, diet, medications, and interventional or surgical therapy.

E. Evaluation
   1. Client has patent airway.
   2. Client shows improved neurologic status.
   3. Client remains free from complications of immobility.
   4. Client and family participate in plan of care.

5. Client verbalizes relief of pain and associated symptoms.
6. Client and family accurately state understanding of diet, medications, treatments, and any activity restrictions.

III. Client needs

A. Physiologic adaptation: Head injury may or may not require hospitalization, depending on severity of the injury (see section on increased ICP for treatment of ICP).
   1. Recognize types of surgical interventions indicated for evacuation of hematomas, debridement and elevation of depressed fractures of the skull, and suture of severe scalp lacerations.
      a. Craniotomy—surgical opening of skull to gain access to intracranial structures.
      b. Craniectomy—excision of a portion of the skull.
      c. Cranioplasty—repair of a cranial defect with a metal or plastic plate.
   2. Recognize risk for missed diagnosis of head injury for elderly clients because of previous behaviors and history of confusion. Causes of confusion and disorientation may result from decreased cardiac output, hypoxia and respiratory acidosis, neurologic, metabolic, or environmental factors.

B. Management of care: Care of the client with a head injury requires critical thinking skills and knowledge of assessment, and teaching and evaluation methods unique to the RN role. These skills cannot be delegated to an LPN or UAP.
   1. Delegate responsibly those activities that can be delegated, including basic care needs and vital sign checks for the stable client. All monitoring information is reported to the RN.
   2. Perform comprehensive physical assessment and provide care to client based on type and severity of head injury—priority objectives are to maintain a patent airway, prevent hypoxia and hypercapnia, and to identify signs and symptoms of increased ICP.
   3. Provide information on changes in client status to the physician and appropriate members of the multidisciplinary team.
   4. Provide interventions for acute care management.
      a. Promote optimal oxygenation.
         (1) Maintain patent airway, supplemental oxygen, intubation and mechanical ventilation, IV fluids, blood replacement, vasopressors, antihypertensives, vasodilator agents, and anticonvulsives.
         (2) Administer oxygen, provide pulmonary hygiene to reduce risk of pulmonary complications. Suction secretions only as needed.
      b. Control and/or reduce increased ICP with CSF drainage, osmotic diuretics, evacuation of hematomas, mild hyperventilation; provide care for client in a barbiturate coma and/or receiving paralyzing agents.
         (1) Administer and monitor barbiturate and paralytic therapy (see pharmacologic and parenteral therapies).
         (2) Monitor client's ICP, BP, pulmonary pressures, ABGs, serum barbiturates levels, level of paralysis (train of four and ECG).
         (3) Monitor closely for hyperthermia that may result in secondary to hypothalamic damage.
      c. Detect and prevent complications of head injury.
         (1) Monitor ECG for changes in rate and rhythm, ICP trends, and hemodynamic status with pulmonary artery catheter (CVP, PA pressures).
         (2) Monitor intake and output with administration of diuretics for decrease in urine specific gravity in the presence of diabetes insipidus or syndrome of inappropriate antidiuretic hormone (SIADH).
         (3) Perform frequent neurologic assessment for sudden changes in LOC, pupil changes, and respiratory patterns.
      d. Monitor for complications of skull fracture—perform neurologic assessments, provide pain management, and monitor for signs and symptoms of infection. For basilar skull fracture:
         (1) Assess for signs of periorbital ecchymosis, mastoid ecchymosis, otorrhea, rhinorrhea, or facial nerve paralysis.
         (2) Test any drainage from the ear or nose with a glucose reagent strip; clear drainage that tests positive for glucose indicates CSF fluid.
      e. Provide interventions to manage hematomas.
         (1) Epidural: Promote surgical evacuation with possible placement of ICP monitor.

(2) Subdural: Monitor LOC and perform regular and frequent neurologic assessments.

f. Prevent secondary injury by maintaining adequate CPP (more than 60 mmHg) and oxygenation, avoiding brain ischemia and preventing systemic and neurologic complications.

5. Provide client and family teaching about medications, diagnostic tests, nonsurgical and surgical interventions, and rehabilitation needs (also see health promotion and maintenance).

C. Safety and infection control
1. Use sterile technique when caring for a client with invasive devices, such as ICP monitor.
2. Perform debridement and irrigation of contaminated scalp wound prior to closure.
3. Avoid putting anything into client's nose or ears, including tissue, dressings, packing, suction catheters, NG tubes, or nasal airway.
4. Place a dry, sterile dressing loosely over the client's ear or under nose to absorb drainage.
5. Administer prophylactic antibiotics as ordered.
6. Monitor drug levels (e.g., phenytoin [Dilantin], pentobarbital [Nembutal]).

D. Health promotion and maintenance: Assess client and family understanding of consequences of illness. Provide written and verbal instructions.
1. Report signs and symptoms of changes in LOC, vision, drainage, increased sleepiness, worsening headache not responsive to medications, and upon occurrence of seizure.
2. Reduce risk factors related to head injuries (e.g., driving safety and contact sports).
3. Seek routine medical and follow-up care.

E. Psychologic integrity
1. Identify stress or anxiety-producing factors that may interfere with recovery.
   a. Prepare family for emergence of client from coma; explain process of awakening may take several weeks or months.
   b. Review potential chronic problems related to motor and sensory deficits, communication, memory, and intellectual function.
2. Collaborate with discharge planner or case manager to arrange for home health, hospice, or palliative care needs.
3. Provide end-of-life/palliative care for client with poor prognosis. Provide support system for family and significant others; involve family with option of organ donation based on client's wishes.

F. Basic care and comfort
1. Position client to provide optimal hemodynamic status and adequate cerebral perfusion and to decrease restlessness.
2. Provide frequent skin care to prevent skin breakdown due to immobility.
3. Provide plan of care to optimize balance in sensory stimulation and motor activity, and enhance functional capacity and decrease agitation.
4. Provide adequate pain management to promote postoperative activities required of clients after surgery, such as deep breathing, increased activity, and therapy sessions.
5. Manage symptoms to maintain client comfort, including lubricating eye drops, an eye patch for diplopia, antiemetics for nausea and vomiting, and aspirin or small doses of codeine for headache (if not contraindicated).

G. Reduction of risk potential
1. Monitor for signs and symptoms of neurologic changes. Immediately report acute changes.
2. Instruct client to avoid blowing nose if a basilar skull fracture was sustained.
3. Instruct client to avoid activities that increase ICP, such as Valsalva maneuver, lifting, sneezing, and neck flexion; administer stool softeners.

H. Pharmacology and parenteral therapies: Client and family will state the purpose for and side effects of all medications used to treat head injuries.
1. Blood and IV fluids—maintain normovolemia.
2. Antibiotics (prophylactic broad spectrum)—for penetrating head injuries that will cross the blood–brain barrier.
3. Analgesics: Codeine (Paveral)—stronger opiates may be contraindicated because of potential respiratory depression, altered LOC, and pupillary changes.
4. Anticonvulsants: Phenytoin (Dilantin)—monitor drug level closely; assess and monitor for side effects including bradycardia, hypotension, nystagmus/ataxia, gingival, hyperplasia, agranulocytosis; rash, Stevens-Johnson syndrome; lymphadenopathy; nauseas; heart block.
5. Osmotic diuretics: Mannitol (Osmitrol)—reduces cerebral edema.

a. Monitor urine output, serum electrolytes, serum osmolarity; signs of hypotension, dehydration, tachycardia, rebound edema.
b. Monitor vial for crystals; shake vial and use filter needle to administer.

6. Loop diuretics: Furosemide (Lasix)—monitor side effects, including ototoxicity, polyuria, electrolyte imbalance, gastric irritation, muscle cramps, hypotension, and dehydration.
7. Sympathomimetics (vasopressors): Dopamine (Intropin) and norepinephrine (Levophed)—maintain optimal CPP if BP is low and ICP is elevated.
8. Corticosteroids: Dexamethasone (Decadron)—reduces cerebral edema; controversial use because of side effects of drug, including flushing, sweating, hypertension, tachycardia, thrombocytopenia, hyperglycemia, peptic ulcer perforation, decreased wound healing, muscle wasting, and hypokalemia.
9. Histamine antagonists
10. Mucosal barrier fortifier: Sucralfate (Carafate)
11. Posterior pituitary hormone: Vasopressin (Pitressin) and desmopressin (DDAVP)—administered if client develops diabetes insipidus; indications for improvement include decreased urine output and increased specific gravity.
12. Stool softeners: Docusate (Colace, Surfak) and Sennosides (Senokot)—prevent "straining" and therefore decrease potential for increased ICP.
13. Antipyretics: Acetaminophen (Tylenol)—increased temperature can increase cerebral metabolic demand.
14. Barbiturates: Pentobarbital sodium (Nembutal sodium)—induces coma artificially in the client who has not responded to conventional treatment; monitor for side effects, including hypotension, myocardial or respiratory depression (client must be intubated and mechanically ventilated), thrombocytopenia purpura.
15. Neuromuscular blocking agents (NMBAs)
16. Sedatives: Propofol (Diprivan), lorazepam (Ativan), and diazepam (Valium)

Stroke

I. Definition: Stroke or brain attack, previously known as cerebrovascular accident (CVA), occurs when there is ischemia or hemorrhage into the brain that results in functional abnormality of the central nervous system (CNS). Stroke is the third most common cause of death and is the leading cause of serious, long-term disability in the United States. Functions such as movement, sensation, or emotions that were controlled by the affected brain area are lost or impaired. The severity of the loss of function varies according to the location and extent of the brain involved, rapidity of onset, size of lesion, and presence of collateral circulation. The progression of a stroke may take several hours or days. The progression of neurologic deterioration is referred to as *stroke in evolution*. A stroke is complete when symptoms have stabilized and the neurologic deficits are permanent.

A. Transient ischemic attacks (TIAs) involve neurologic changes resolving in less than 24 hr. TIAs are caused by temporary, complete, or relatively complete cessation of CBF to a localized area of brain, and may be considered a warning sign of impending stroke.

B. Ischemic strokes occur with decreased blood flow to the brain secondary to partial or complete occlusion of an artery.
1. Thrombotic stroke is the most common type and is associated with atherosclerosis.
2. Embolic strokes evolve rapidly over a few seconds or minutes and are associated with hypercoagulability, heart disease, atrial fibrillation, and cardiac or vascular surgery.
3. Lacunar strokes result from small vessel occlusive disease and are caused by chronic hypertension and diabetes.
4. Cryptogenic strokes are a subtype of stroke with undetermined cause.

C. Hemorrhagic stroke or intracerebral hemorrhage (ICH)
1. Cerebral aneurysm is a localized dilation of the cerebral arterial wall causing the arterial wall to weaken and become susceptible to rupture. Cerebral aneurysm occurs during the fifth and sixth decades of life. Types include:
a. Saccular—involves a saclike outpouching
b. Fusiform—elongated outpouching, without a stem
c. Berry—type of saccular aneurysm that looks like a "berry"; (has a neck or stem)
d. Other— dissecting and traumatic Charcot-Bouchard
2. Arteriovenous malformation (AVM) is shunting of arterial blood directly into the venous system without the intervening capillary bed. High pressure can result in hemorrhage and bleeding into the

subarachnoid space and parenchymal space. AVM is diagnosed after the client presents with seizures or significant signs and symptoms (e.g., headache, blurred vision). AVM is congenital, usually occurs in the second to fourth decades of life, and is more common in males.

3. Subarachnoid hemorrhage is most frequently caused by a cerebral aneurysm or AVM.

D. Neuromuscular deficits of a stroke are due to motor neuron damage of the pyramidal tract.

1. Right-brain damage involves right-sided stroke and results in hemiplegia left side, left-sided neglect, spatial perceptual deficits, rapid performance, short attention span, impulsivity, safety problems, impaired judgment, and impaired time concepts.
2. Left-brain damage involves paralysis or weakness on right side of body; right visual field deficit; aphasia (expressive, receptive, or global); altered intellectual ability; and slow, cautioned behaviors.

II. Nursing process

A. Assessment

1. Perform a comprehensive physical assessment (client complaints vary with the type of stroke). For ischemic stroke, the National Institutes of Health Stroke Scale (NIHSS) is used routinely to measure neurologic function following an acute ischemic stroke to assess overall level of consciousness, visual function, motor skills, sensation and inattention, language, and cerebellar integrity.
2. Assess for risk factors.
   a. Modifiable factors include hypertension, cardiac disease, atrial fibrillation, diabetes, obesity, stress, use of oral contraceptives, lifestyle habits such as cigarette smoking, a diet high in fat and sodium, heavy alcohol consumption, and recreational drug use (e.g., cocaine).
   b. Nonmodifiable risk factors include age, race, and family history. African Americans have the highest incidence of stroke and death; Hispanics, Native Americans, and Asian Americans have a higher incidence than whites.
3. Assess for signs and symptoms (based on anatomic location of the lesion and severity of problem); classic findings include a sudden onset of focal neurologic findings such as numbness or weakness of the face or extremities, change in LOC, visual changes, difficulty walking, dizziness or loss of balance or coordination, dysphagia, or aphasia.
   a. Ischemic stroke: Sudden onset of signs for more than 24 hr; hemiparesis, aphasia, and hemianopia; stupor, confusion, and agitation, and coma.
   b. Hemorrhagic: Abrupt onset of pain, brief loss of consciousness, nausea, vomiting, focal neurologic deficits, stiff neck and photophobia. Client may have history of headaches with dizziness or syncope.
4. Obtain diagnostic tests.
   a. CT scan without contrast—primary diagnostic study to indicate lesion size and location and differentiate between ischemic and hemorrhagic stroke
   b. MRI—to reveal ischemic stroke
   c. Electroencephalogram (EEG)
   d. CT angiography (CTA)—provides visualization of vasculature
   e. Cardiac monitoring and diagnostic cardiac tests—assesses for underlying cardiac condition
      (1) 12-lead ECG
      (2) TEE
      (3) ECHO
   f. Serum glucose, electrolytes, CBC, liver and renal functions, lipid profile, and coagulation studies—assess stroke risk factors and rule out conditions that mimic stroke
   g. Platelet count, PT, INR, APTT—assess for coagulation state
   h. Lumbar puncture—assesses for subarachnoid hemorrhage (contraindicated if client is candidate for fibrinolytics and has increased ICP)

B. Analysis

1. Ineffective Tissue Perfusion: Cerebral, related to altered cerebral blood flow, hemorrhage, and rupture of vessel
2. Impaired Physical Mobility related to hemiparesis, loss of balance and coordination, spasticity, and brain damage
3. Acute Pain related to hemiplegia and disuse
4. Self-Care Deficit: Hygiene, Toileting, Grooming, and Feeding, related to complications from stroke
5. Disturbed Sensory Perception: Visual and Kinesthetic, related to altered sensory reception, transmission, and/or integration
6. Impaired Swallowing related to complications from stoke
7. Anxiety related to pain, lifestyle change, ineffective coping, and fear
8. Impaired Urinary Elimination and Bowel Incontinence related to altered motor reception, transmission, and/or integration

9. Ineffective Health Maintenance related to lack of knowledge of stroke, risk factors, and unhealthy lifestyle
10. Ineffective Therapeutic Regimen Management related to lack of knowledge of medications and self care behaviors
11. Risk for Impaired Skin Integrity related to hemiparesis or hemiplegia, or decreased mobility

C. Planning
1. Maintain adequate CPP and blood flow.
2. Maintain stable or improve LOC.
3. Maximize physical functioning.
4. Improve client symptoms and comfort.
5. Maximize communication abilities.
6. Maximize self-care abilities and skills.
7. Maintain adequate nutrition and hydration.
8. Prevent complications of stroke.
9. Maintain effective personal and family coping.
10. Promote adherence to therapeutic regimen.
11. Maintain skin integrity.

D. Implementation
1. Monitor vital signs and neurologic status, with close attention to ICP and CPP (if appropriate); monitor BP, SpO_2, pulses, heart sounds, and lung sounds.
2. Monitor intake and output closely.
3. Instruct client and family about control of modifiable risk factors, medications, and side effects, monitoring of BP, and signs and symptoms that require immediate medical attention.

E. Evaluation
1. Client's vital signs, neurologic signs, ICP, CPP, and hemodynamic status are within normal limits.
2. Client does not experience complications (e.g., increased ICP, pneumonia, aspiration, skin breakdown).
3. Client regains functional independence and resumes self-care activities.
4. Client exhibits return of control over body functions, including bowel, bladder, speech.
5. Client accurately states the purpose, dosage, timing, and side effects of medications.
6. Client's functional capability is optimized through rehabilitation.
7. Client's labs are within normal range.
8. Client and family verbalize understanding of interventions, possible complications, and outcomes.

CN

III. Client needs

A. Physiologic adaptation: Goals of acute care include preserving life, preventing further brain damage, and reducing disability. Treatments vary according to type of stroke and as the client progresses from the acute to rehabilitation phase.

1. Provide interventions for treatments according to type of stroke.
   a. For acute ischemic stroke—treated with airway protection and ventilatory assistance to maintain adequate tissue oxygenation; pharmacologic interventions include thrombolytic therapy with IV rt-PA within 3 hr of onset to dissolve clot and reperfuse ischemic brain. Additional therapies may involve surgical decompression, carotid endarterectomy, embolectomy.
      (1) Recognize risk for side effect of bleeding, especially intracranial hemorrhage.
      (2) Monitor for signs and symptoms of cerebral edema or seizures (administer diuretics and anticonvulsives, if indicated).
   b. For hemorrhagic stroke—early diagnosis important; treatment involves airway management and ventilatory assistance, insertion of ventriculostomy to control ICP. Surgical interventions include craniotomy to expose and isolate aneurysm, and a clip or coil. AVM: Embolization.
      (1) Recognize risk for rebleeding within first 24 hr following first bleed (e.g., nitroprusside, metoprolol, or hydralazine to maintain or reduce systolic BP greater than 160 mmHg).
      (2) Recognize risk for seizures (administer prophylactic anticonvulsant therapy).
   c. For ICH—prognosis is poor; treatment involves pharmacologic therapy, intubation and mechanical ventilation, and reducing BP.
2. Recognize increased risk for stroke with chronic inflammation—indicated by elevated serum C-reactive protein and chronic periodontitis.
3. Observe cerebral angioplasty as treatment for cerebral vasospasm when pharmacologic and congenital therapy fails.
4. Recognize risk for sensory-perceptual alterations, including homonymous hemianopsia (blindness in the same half of each visual field); agnosia (disturbance in sensory information); diplopia (often treated with an eye patch); loss of corneal reflex

(involves risk for corneal abrasion); and ptosis, particularly if the stroke is in the vertebrobasilar distribution.

B. Management of care: Care of the client with acute stroke requires critical thinking skills and knowledge of assessment, and teaching and evaluation methods unique to the RN role. These skills cannot be delegated to an LPN or UAP.
   1. Delegate responsibly those activities that can be delegated, including basic care needs and vital sign checks for the stable client. All monitoring information is reported to the RN.
   2. Perform comprehensive physical assessments and provide care to the symptomatic client.
   3. For acute stroke, closely monitor ICP, hemodynamic status, laboratory values, and cardiac function.
   4. Maintain patent airway; monitor client closely for signs of increasing neurologic deficit.
   5. Monitor neurologic status to detect changes suggesting extension of stroke, ICP, and vasospasm. Administer GCS; assess mental status, pupillary responses, extremity movement, and strength.
   6. Monitor cardiovascular status—closely monitor intake and output; carefully regulate IV therapy.
   7. Manage integumentary system—keep client moving to prevent thrombophlebitis and deep vein thrombosis in the weak or paralyzed lower extremity: Teach active ROM exercises; if hemiplegic, teach passive ROM exercises to be performed several times a day.
   8. Maintain optimal function of musculoskeletal system by preventing joint contractures and muscular atrophy through ROM exercise and positioning (acute phase), and positioning of joints higher than the joint proximal to it.
   9. Prevent constipation or diarrhea.
   10. Promote normal bladder function and avoid use of indwelling catheter; long-term use of an indwelling catheter is associated with urinary tract infections and delayed bladder retraining. An intermittent catheterization program may be used for clients with urinary retention.
   11. Accommodate sensory-perceptual alterations (see basic care and comfort).
   12. Provide information on changes in client status to the physician and appropriate members of the multidisciplinary team.
   13. Provide client and family teaching (see health promotion and maintenance).

C. Safety and infection control: Avoid administration of aspirin, heparin, warfarin, ticlopidine, or any other antithrombotic or antiplatelet drugs for 24 hr for client receiving rt-PA therapy.

D. Health promotion and maintenance: Provide client and family teaching.
   1. Tailor treatment based on functional ability.
      a. Participate in rehabilitation program (e.g., physical therapy; occupational, speech, and recreational therapy).
      b. Increase self-care behaviors (e.g., compliance with diet, medications, and exercise).
   2. Identify signs and symptoms that require medical attention, including change in LOC (increased drowsiness, confusion, headache not responsive to medications), loss of feeling or sensation in any extremity, blurriness, drainage from incisions (if applicable), and seizures.

E. Psychologic integrity
   1. Assess need for home health assistance and social support.
   2. Assist client and family in coping with lifestyle changes.
   3. Distinguish with client and family short- and long-term interventions for reversible stroke versus prolonged life support in severe brain damage without expected return to optimal functional capacity.
   4. Promote client and family teaching from health care team for neurologic client with poor outcomes regarding treatment options, living will, and advanced directives.
   5. To assist the caregiver to stay healthy after the client is discharged, plan for respite or time away from caregiving activities on a regular basis. Assist caregivers in identifying resources.

F. Basic care and comfort
   1. Assist the client to ambulate using an assistive device (e.g., gait belt, lift, transfer board, crutches, walker, wheelchair, and cane).
   2. Use alterative methods to communicate with a client verbally and in writing (e.g., touch pad, sign board).
   3. Position client to minimize the effects of dependent edema and the use of elastic compression gradient stockings.
   4. For client with sensory-perceptual alterations (homonymous hemianopsia), arrange environment within the client's perceptual field—place food tray so that all

food is on the right side or the left side to accommodate for field of vision. Instruct client to consciously attend to the neglected side.

G. Reduction of risk potential
   1. Avoid administering aspirin, heparin, warfarin, ticlopidine, or any other antithrombotic or antiplatelet drugs for at least 24 hr after treatment for clients receiving thrombolytics.
   2. Observe bleeding and fall precautions if client is receiving anticoagulation therapy.
   3. Provide for client's safety by adjusting side rails and avoiding restraints. Encourage use of seatbelt in wheelchair.
   4. Prevent complications for client on bed rest.
      a. Assess for fever, hypoxia, electrolyte imbalance, and skin integrity.
      b. Turn client every 2 hr; position for optimal functional status and oxygenation.
      c. Place client in a side-lying or three-quarters prone position to prevent tongue from obstructing airway.

H. Pharmacology and parenteral therapies: Medications used for treatment of stroke will depend on the type of stroke or brain insult. Drug therapy may vary. Client will state the purpose for and side effects of all medications used to treat stroke.
   1. Anticonvulsants: Phenytoin (Dilantin) and fosphenytoin (Cerebyx)
   2. Antihypertensives: Labetalol (Normodyne), sodium nitroprusside (Nipride), and hydralazine (Apresoline)
   3. Anticoagulants and antiplatelets: Heparin, enoxaparin sodium (Lovenox, low-molecular heparin), warfarin; and aspirin, ticlopidine, and clopidogrel bisulfate (Plavix)
   4. Antipyretics: Acetaminophen (Tylenol)
   5. Barbiturates: Phenobarbital and pentobarbital
   6. Osmotic diuretics: Mannitol
   7. Loop diuretics: Furosemide (Lasix)
   8. Calcium channel blockers: Nimodipine (Nimotop)
   9. Sedatives: Propofol (Diprivan), lorazepam (Ativan), and diazepam (Valium)
   10. Thrombolytics: Tissue plasminogen (tPA) and rt-PA
   11. Vasopressors: Dopamine (Intropin) and norepinephrine (Levophed)
   12. Other
      a. Oxygen
      b. Blood and IV fluids to maintain normovolemia
      c. Corticosteroids (dexamethasone [Decadron])

Seizure

I. Definition: Seizures involve sudden, excessive discharge of electrical activity within the brain, resulting in episodes of abnormal motor, sensory, autonomic, or psychic activity, or a combination of these activities. Epilepsy is a disorder characterized by chronic seizure activity and indicates brain or central nervous system (CNS) irritation. Status epilepticus is a potential complication that can occur with any type of seizure involving a rapid succession of epileptic spasms without intervals of consciousness; it is an emergent situation and may result in brain damage. Types of seizures include partial and generalized (see Box 30-1).
   A. Partial seizures: Arise from region in motor cortex (posterior frontal lobe); most commonly begins in upper extremities, spreading to face and lower extremity (Jacksonian march); noting progression is important in identifying area of cortex involved.

Box 30-1. International Classification of Seizures

Partial Seizures (Seizures Beginning Locally)

Simple partial seizures (with elementary symptoms, generally without impairment of consciousness)

- With motor symptoms
- With special sensory or somatosensory symptoms
- With autonomic symptoms
- Compound forms

Complex partial seizures (with complex symptoms, generally with impairment of consciousness)

- With impairment of consciousness only
- With cognitive symptoms
- With affective symptoms
- With psychosensory symptoms
- With psychomotor symptoms (automatisms)
- Compound forms

Partial seizures secondarily generalized

Generalized Seizures (Convulsive or Nonconvulsive, Bilaterally Symmetric, Without Local Onset)

Tonic-clonic seizures
Tonic seizures
Clonic seizures
Absence (petit mal) seizures
Atonic seizures
Myoclonic seizures (bilaterally massive epileptic)
Unclassified seizures

From Smeltzer, S. C., Bare, B. G., Cheever, K. H., & Hinkle, J. L. (2008). *Brunner & Suddarth's textbook of medical-surgical nursing* (11th ed., p. 2190). Philadelphia: Lippincott Williams & Wilkins.

1. Simple partial—affects focal sensory or motor activities without loss of consciousness.
2. Complex partial—affects cognitive, psychosensory, psychomotor, or affective activities with brief loss of consciousness.

B. Generalized seizures usually result in a loss of consciousness; the client may or may not have a seizure.
1. Tonic-clonic—begins with aura, loss of consciousness, and rigidity and is followed by tonic-clonic movements; hyperventilation or altered respirations; and loss of bladder and bowel control. Seizure usually lasts 2 to 5 min, and full recovery may take several hours.
2. Absence—may or may not involve loss of consciousness and minor motor movements. Client has fixation of gaze; blank facial expression; flickering of eyelids; and jerking of facial, muscle, or arm. Absence seizures are more common in children (see Chapter 17).
3. Myoclonic—involves brief, transient stiffening or jerking of extremities. Client may fall to the ground from seizure.
4. Atonic or akinetic (drop attacks)—involve loss of muscle control and brief loss of consciousness.
5. Tonic—involve sudden stiffening of arms and legs; the client is usually conscious.

II. Nursing process

A. Assessment
1. Perform a detailed health history, including past medical, neurologic, surgical, family, and psychosocial history, and history of past illness, trauma, infection, alcohol or drug use. Obtain history description of seizure from client or witness, including antecedent events, precipitating factors and postictal events, and frequency and duration.
2. Perform a comprehensive neurologic and physical examination, including assessment for signs and symptoms.
   a. Seizure activity, including length and progression of jerking, time started, and involved extremity, as well as presence of oral bleeding, postictal stages, vital signs, and posturing.
   b. Signs and symptoms such as mood changes, irritability, insomnia, aura (a sensation that warns the client of the impending seizure), loss of motor activity, bowel and bladder function, or loss of consciousness during the seizure; and occurrences during the postictal state, such as headache, loss of consciousness, sleepiness, and impaired speech or thinking.
3. Assess for risk factors.
   a. Brain injury or trauma
   b. Infections (meningitis, encephalitis)
   c. Fluid and electrolyte disturbances
   d. Hypoglycemia, hypocalcemia, hyponatremia
   e. Tumors
   f. Vascular disorders (hypoxia and acidosis)
   g. Other (e.g., drug- and alcohol-induced)
   h. Toxicity of sedatives, hypnotics, heavy metals, drug interactions, "street" drugs, theophylline, and abnormal anticonvulsant drug levels
4. Obtain diagnostic tests.
   a. Serum electrolytes, glucose, BUN, Cr, ABG, CBC, drug screens
   b. Lumbar puncture (LP)
   c. CT, MRI, PET scan, EEG

B. Analysis
1. Risk for Injury related to convulsive disorder
2. Anxiety related to potential for sudden loss of consciousness
3. Situational Low Self-Esteem related to chronic illness
4. Impaired Social Interaction related to self-consciousness about having seizures
5. Powerlessness related to unpredictable nature of disease and limitations imposed on lifestyle

C. Planning
1. Prevent injury during seizure.
2. Provide postseizure care.
3. Prevent or reduce recurrences of seizure activity.
4. Provide health teaching.

D. Implementation: Provide interventions during a seizure and following a seizure (see Box 30-2). Document all details of seizure, including observations prior to and following seizure activity (see management of care).

E. Evaluation
1. Client does not experience injuries or complications during seizure activity.
2. Client's seizure activity is controlled.
3. Client displays effective individual coping.
4. Client exhibits knowledge and understanding of seizures and epilepsy.
5. Client shows no toxic effects from anticonvulsants.
6. Client follows a healthy lifestyle.

CN

III. Client needs

A. Physiologic adaptation: Seizure activity is controlled with anticonvulsants and dose adjustment on an outpatient basis. Biofeedback may

Box 30-2. Guidelines for Seizure Care

Nursing Care During a Seizure

- Provide privacy and protect the patient from curious onlookers. (The patient who has an *aura* [warning of an impending seizure] may have time to seek a safe, private place.)
- Ease the patient to the floor, if possible.
- Protect the head with a pad to prevent injury (from striking a hard surface).
- Loosen constrictive clothing.
- Push aside any furniture that may injure the patient during the seizure.
- If the patient is in bed, remove pillows and raise side rails.
- If an aura precedes the seizure, insert an oral airway to reduce the possibility of the patient's biting the tongue or cheek.
- *Do not attempt to pry open jaws that are clenched in a spasm or to insert anything.* Broken teeth and injury to the lips and tongue may result from such as action.
- No attempt should be made to restrain the patient during the seizure, because muscular contractions are strong and restraint can produce injury.
- If possible, place the patient on one side with head flexed forward, which allows the tongue to fall forward and facilitates drainage of saliva and mucus. If suction is available, use it if necessary to clear secretions.

Nursing Care After the Seizure

- Keep the patient on one side to prevent aspiration. Make sure the airway is patent.
- There is usually a period of confusion after a grand mal seizure.
- A short apneic period may occur during or immediately after a generalized seizure.
- The patient, on awakening, should be reoriented to the environment.
- If the patient becomes agitated after a seizure (postictal), use calm persuasion and gentle restraint.

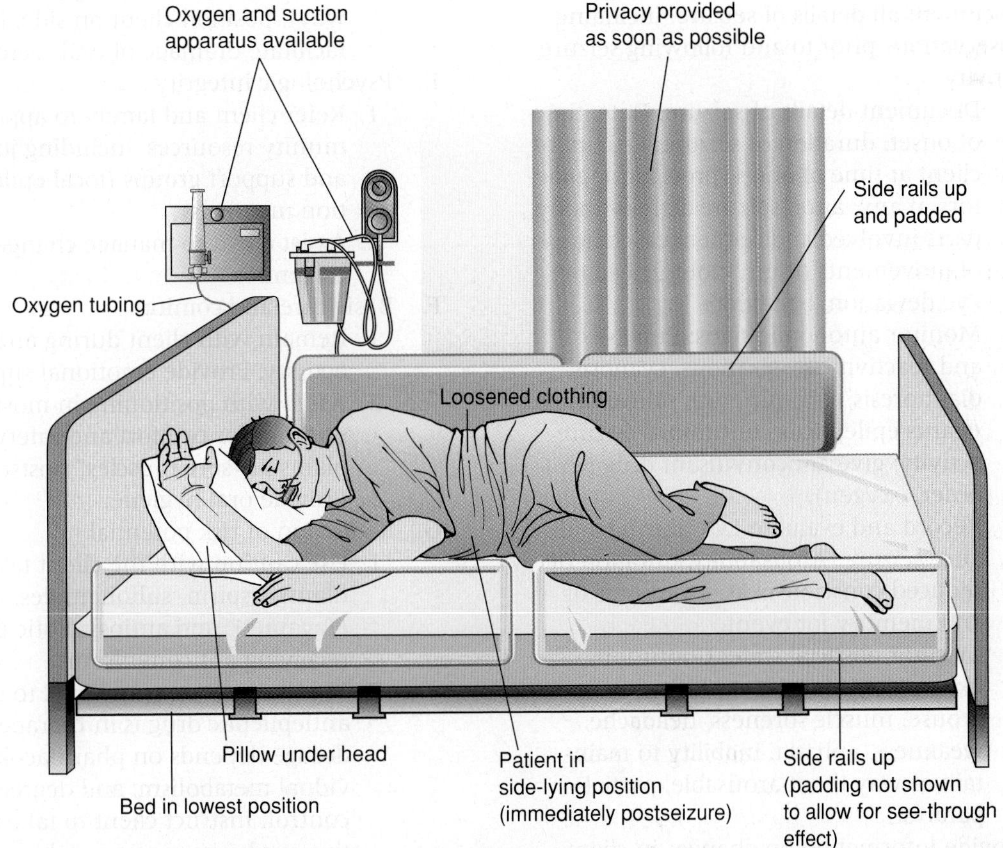

From Smeltzer, S. C., Bare, B. G., Cheever, K. H., & Hinkle, J. L. (2008). *Brunner & Suddarth's textbook of medical-surgical nursing* (11th ed., p. 2192). Philadelphia: Lippincott Williams & Wilkins.

be used with clients who can identify auras. Surgery (temporal lobectomy, hemispherectomy) may be used.

1. Recognize risk for status epilepticus—indicates emergent situation involving a rapid succession of epileptic spasms without intervals of consciousness and may result in brain damage. May be precipitated by withdrawal of anticonvulsants, fever, and concurrent infections.
2. Recognize risk for fractures in clients receiving long-term therapy—results from

bone disease (osteoporosis, osteomalacia, and hyperparathyroidism) as side effect of therapy.

3. Women with epilepsy often have an increase in seizures during menses and are considered at high risk during pregnancy.
4. Elderly have a high incidence of new-onset of epilepsy; associated with stroke, head injury, dementia, infection, alcoholism, and aging.

B. Management of care: Care of the symptomatic client with seizures requires critical thinking skills and knowledge of assessment, and teaching and evaluation methods unique to the RN role. These skills cannot be delegated to an LPN or UAP.

1. Delegate responsibly those activities that can be delegated, including basic care needs and vital sign checks for the stable client. All monitoring information is reported to the RN.
2. Document all details of seizure, including observations prior to and following seizure activity.
    a. Document details of seizure: Date, time of onset, duration of seizure; activity of client at time of onset; precipitating factors, if any; aura; seizure activity (body parts involved and sequence); character of movements (tonic, clonic, head or eye deviation, behavior).
    b. Monitor autonomic signs: Pupil size and reactivity, respirations, cyanosis, diaphoresis, incontinence, salivation (status epilepticus continuous seizure activity; give anticonvulsant drug per order, oxygen).
    c. Record and evaluate LOC during and after seizure: Arousability, duration of reduced consciousness, awareness of and memory for event.
    d. Monitor postictal state: Confusion, exhaustion, sleepiness, difficulty to arouse, muscle soreness, headache, weakness, aphasia, inability to maintain airway if not arousable, partial paralysis.
3. Provide information on changes in client status to the physician and appropriate members of the multidisciplinary team.
4. Provides client and family teaching about disease process, safety issues, diagnostic tests, diet, medications and side effects, and interventional or surgical therapy.
5. Promote home and community-based care.

C. Safety and infection control: Maintain large vein access while client is hospitalized for treatment of status epilepticus.

D. Health promotion and maintenance: Provide client and family teaching.

1. Use medications as directed; understand actions and side effects (e.g., apathy, ataxia, hyperplasia of gums with phenytoin [Dilantin]); and complications associated with sudden withdrawal.
2. Maintain normal activities, with exception of driving (return to driving depends on state law, usually until seizure-free for period of time).
3. Avoid stress, lack of sleep, emotional upset, and stimulants such as alcohol; practice relaxation and stress-management techniques.
4. Wear medic-alert band or necklace.
5. Prevent complications from seizures: Provide protection from injury during and after seizure; avoid placing anything in the mouth (may cause tongue to occlude airway); position client on side, if possible, to facilitate drainage of oral secretions.

E. Psychologic integrity

1. Refer client and family to appropriate community resources, including job counseling and support groups (local epilepsy association meetings).
2. Assist client to manage changes in self-esteem.

F. Basic care and comfort

1. Remain with client during and after seizure activity. Provide emotional support.
2. Assist with positioning in most optimal position for comfort and safety (often complains of "sore muscles" postseizure).
3. Provide oral hygiene.

G. Reduction of risk potential

1. Use caution with the client taking anticoagulants, aspirin, sulfonamides, cimetidine (Tagamet), and antipsychotic drugs when receiving anticonvulsants.
2. Monitor serum drug levels to determine if antiepileptic drug is in therapeutic range—dosage depends on pharmacokinetics, individual metabolism, and degree of seizure control. Instruct client to take drug on continuous basis; continue taking drug if adverse effects occur, and contact physician who will lower dose or prescribe a different drug.
3. Provide close monitoring of client on long-term therapy and the elderly client to prevent adverse and toxic effects of anticonvulsants and osteoporosis.

H. Pharmacology and parenteral therapies: Client will state the purpose for and side effects of all medications used to treat seizures.

1. Hydantoins: Ethotoin (Peganone), fosphenytoin (Cerebyx), mephenytoin (Mesantoin), phenytoin (Dilantin)—used for overall seizure treatment. Side effects may include gingival hyperplasia (Dilantin), blood dyscrasias, elevated serum glucose, alopecia, and hirsutism.
   a. Phenytoin (Dilantin) may decrease effectiveness of birth control pills.
   b. Normal Dilantin drug level is 10 to 20 mcg/mL.
2. Barbiturates: Amobarbital (Amytal), mephobarbital (Mebaral), phenobarbital, primidone (Mysoline)—used to treat tonic-clonic seizures and acute episodes of status epilepticus seizures. Side effects may include hypotension, respiratory depression, and drowsiness.
3. Benzodiazepines: Clonazepam (Klonopin), clorazepate (Tranxene), diazepam (Valium), lorazepam (Ativan)—used to treat absence seizures; diazepam and lorazepam are used with status epilepticus; clorazepate may be used to treat partial seizures. Side effects may include ataxia, respiratory and cardiac depression.
4. Succinimides: Ethosuximide (Zarontin), methsuximide (Celontin), phensuximide (Milontin)—used to treat absence seizures. Side effects may include blood dyscrasias.
5. Oxazolidinediones: Paramethadione (Paradione)—used to treat absence seizures. Side effects may include drowsiness and photophobia.
6. Valproates: Valproic acid (Depakene) and divalproex (Depakote)—used to treat tonic-clonic, partial, myoclonic, and psychomotor seizures. Side effects may include hepatotoxicity.
7. Iminostilbenes: Carbamazepine (Tegretol), felbamate (Felbatol), gabapentin (Neurontin), lamotrigine (Lamictal), oxcarbazepine (Trileptal), tiagabine (Gabitril), topiramate (Topamax), zonisamide (Zonegran)—used to treat seizures not responsive to other anticonvulsants. Side effects may include drowsiness, visual disturbances, dry mouth, and headache.

Pain

I. Definition: Pain is a subjective perception consisting of complex sensory, emotional, and cognitive elements. Pain may be acute or chronic, and consists of several dimensions.
   A. Types of pain (see also Chapter 32 for additional discussion of pain in clients with cancer)
      1. Acute pain involves sympathetic nervous system response; symptoms are mild to severe and last less than 6 months. Acute pain is associated with pressure on organs, nerves, skin, or bones, and often follows injury.
         a. Somatic pain arises from skin, muscle, or bone and is described as sharp, dull, aching, or cramping.
         b. Visceral pain arises from organs and is described as a sharp, stabbing, deep ache.
         c. Cutaneous pain is localized to cutaneous tissue.
         d. Referred pain has origins in the body at a location different from where it is experienced.
      2. Chronic pain is associated with the parasympathetic nervous system; symptoms are mild to severe and last longer than 6 months. Client may have behaviors associated with acute pain, such as withdrawal and depression.
   B. Dimensions of pain
      1. Physiologic
         a. Transduction is the conversion of a mechanical, thermal, or chemical stimulus.
         b. Transmission is the movement of pain impulses from the site of transduction to the brain.
         c. Perception results when pain is recognized, defined, and responded to by the individual experiencing the pain.
         d. Modulation involves the activation of descending pathways that exert inhibitory or facilitatory effects on the transmission of pain, thus decreasing intensity perception, decreasing distress perception, and modifying meaning.
      2. Sensory—intensity, location, quality
      3. Affective—distress, anxiety, depression, suffering
      4. Behavioral—behavioral responses such as crying, gritting teeth
      5. Cognitive—expectations, beliefs, attitudes, evaluations, goals
      6. Sociocultural—effect of culture on pain perception and pain management

II. Nursing process
   A. Assessment: Assess location, severity, intensity, frequency, and timing of pain (see Table 30-2).
      1. Obtain a detailed health history, including past medical and surgical history, and psychosocial history. Obtain information regarding antecedent factors if pain related to injury.

Table 30-2 Pain Assessment Tool

Parameter	Assessment
Frequency	Are you in pain now? How often do you have pain?
Intensity	How much pain are you having? Rate your pain now (use an appropriate pain rating scale).
Location and radiation	Where is your pain? (Ask client to use a diagram.) Does your pain radiate to another part of your body? Describe the quality and character of your pain.
Timing	When does your pain start? Does it improve or become worse at various times? Is there a pattern to your pain?
Factors that increase or improve pain	What makes your pain worse? What makes your pain better?
Effect of pain on quality of life	How does your pain impact your daily life (eating, sleeping, working, concentration, relaxation, interaction with others)?
Pain-management history	What do you do to manage your pain? Are you taking medication now? What medications? What is the dose and frequency? How long have you been using pain-relief strategies? What works? What does not work?
Goal for pain relief	What is your goal for relieving your pain? Do you expect your pain to be totally relieved? How will relieving pain help you manage your daily activities?

2. Perform a detailed physical examination; assess for type of pain (acute, chronic) and site and quality, as well as client behavior.
3. Assess client's cultural background and perception of and response to pain.
4. Obtain diagnostic tests.
   a. Blood work to identify organ dysfunction (e.g., liver, lung)
   b. Imaging studies to outline underlying pathology
   c. Nerve blocks to distinguish type or source of discomfort and pain
   d. Electrodiagnostic test to identify myopathies and neuropathies

B. Analysis
1. Pain: Acute or Chronic, related to specific client condition
2. Activity Intolerance related to pain and discomfort
3. Disturbed Sleep Pattern related to pain and discomfort
4. Fatigue related to state of discomfort or emotional stress
5. Ineffective Coping and Ineffective Role Performance related to chronic pain
6. Powerlessness related to feeling of loss of control

C. Planning
1. Relieve pain and discomfort.
2. Prepare client for surgical intervention of pain control, if appropriate.
3. Promote adherence to therapeutic pain regimen.

D. Implementation
1. Monitor and document client's pain and associated symptoms, including physiologic indicators of pain (e.g., increased respiratory rate, heart rate, BP, dilated or constricted pupils, pallor, diaphoresis).
   a. Assess level of pain—ask client to rate on scale of 0 to 10 (0 signifies no pain; 10 signifies worst pain).
   b. Use age-, condition-, and language-appropriate scale to assess client's pain.
2. Provide client teaching on medications and optional therapies for control of pain and discomfort (see physiologic adaptation).
3. Provide preoperative and postoperative care for clients requiring surgical intervention (e.g., rhizotomy, cordotomy, sympathectomy, dorsal column).

E. Evaluation
1. Client verbalizes or demonstrates decreased pain or adequate pain relief.
2. Client uses alternative measures for pain relief.
3. Client adequately copes with pain.

CN

III. Client needs

A. Physiologic adaptation: Pain is treated with pharmacologic and nonpharmacologic interventions (complementary and alternative therapies) to control pain and discomfort, as well as surgical procedures used to block pain-impulse transmission.
1. Alternative and complementary therapies
   a. Relaxation techniques, guided imagery, and distraction (e.g., music, TV)—relaxes and distracts the client's focus on pain; can increase circulation and lower BP
   b. External transcutaneous electric nerve stimulation (TENS) unit: Adjustable electronic simulation via surface electrodes to prevent complete

depolarization or block transmission of pain impulses

c. Heat (muscle relaxation) or cold (local anesthesia)

d. Patient-controlled anesthesia (PCA)—allows client to control the timing of the administration of the medication

e. Acupuncture—stimulates nerves and blocks transmission of pain impulses

f. Aromatherapy—induces relaxation response

g. Biofeedback—promotes muscle relaxation

h. Massage—promotes deep relaxation, increases circulation to affected part, increases energy flow

i. Meditation and faith—relaxation and external focus

j. Reflexology—induces relaxation, increases circulation, promotes energy flow, reduces anxiety

k. Therapeutic touch—decreases anxiety, improves immune response, alters pain perception

2. Procedures

a. Injection of local anesthetic into nerve (e.g., dental)

b. Cordotomy—severs anterolateral spinal cord nerve tracts

c. Electrical stimulation—transcutaneous (skin surface), percutaneous (peripheral nerve)

d. Peripheral nerve implant electrode to major sensory nerve

e. Dorsal column stimulator electrode to dorsal column

B. Management of care: Care of the client experiencing pain requires critical thinking skills and knowledge of assessment, and teaching and evaluation methods unique to the RN role. These skills cannot be delegated to an LPN or UAP. Delegate responsibly those activities that can be delegated.

1. Collaborate with health care providers (HCPs) regarding use of a continuous, multimodal, and multidisciplinary approach to manage pain.

a. Determine cause of pain and discomfort and initiate comfort measures before giving drugs (e.g., environmental factors, physiologic needs, emotional fear, anxiety, boredom, and loneliness).

b. Report sudden, severe, new pain; pain not relieved by comfort measures or medications; pain associated with casts or traction.

c. Assist with medical and surgical intervention to block pain-impulse transmission (see physiologic adaptation).

d. Monitor client to evaluate effectiveness of pain interventions.

2. Provide client and family teaching about medications, alternative pain-relief methods, and self-care behaviors (see safety and infection control, and health promotion and maintenance).

C. Safety and infection control: Provide client and family teaching.

1. Avoid cold to reduce immediate tissue reaction to trauma.

2. Use caution with application of heat to relieve ischemia.

3. Check with HCP prior to taking OTC medications.

4. Avoid driving or using heavy equipment when receiving narcotics or medications causing drowsiness.

D. Health promotion and maintenance: Instruct client and family to decrease GI side effects of narcotics by consuming a high-fiber diet, increasing fluids, and promoting activity in lifestyle routines.

E. Psychologic integrity

1. Understand that all clients are different; cultural perceptions of pain and past experiences may interfere with quality control of pain.

2. Recognize that older adults may expect pain or may fear addiction; may require lower dosages of medications related to altered metabolic, hepatic, and renal functioning.

F. Basic care and comfort

1. Minimize barriers to effective pain management; achieve "balanced analgesia"; around-the-clock administration of NSAIDs or acetaminophen, if possible; continuous infusion, PCA; and combination therapy (opioids, nonopioids, adjuvants).

2. Observe terminally ill client for increase in pain at the end of life (indicated by restlessness, grimacing, or moaning); increase doses of analgesics as appropriate.

3. Identify client's need for PRN medications for breakthrough pain if receiving scheduled pain medications.

4. Initiate nonpharmacologic techniques to manage pain (e.g., heat or cold, positioning or external support, massage, guided imagery, relaxation).

G. Reduction of risk potential
1. Do not abruptly discontinue opioids in clients who have been receiving opioids for 1 or more weeks; taper doses by 25% every other day.
2. Monitor closely for potential risk when using heat or cold for pain control.
3. Promote appropriate use of equianalgesic dose when need to change from one medication to another to manage pain more effectively with fewer side effects.

H. Pharmacology and parenteral therapies: Client will state the purpose, usage, and associated side effects of all medications used to manage pain.
1. Opioid analgesics: Meperidine (Demerol) is no longer recommended as a first-line opioid for pain management because it produces the active metabolite normeperidine. This metabolite is a central nervous system (CNS) stimulant and can cause irritability, tremors, muscle twitching, jerking, agitation, and seizures.
   a. Morphine sulfate
   b. Codeine
   c. Hydromorphone (Dilaudid)
   d. Fentanyl (Sublimaze)
   e. Methadone (Dolophine)
   f. Propoxyphene (Darvon)
   g. Hydrocodone (Vicodin)
2. Nonopioids
   a. Acetaminophen (Tylenol)
   b. Aspirin (ASA)
   c. Ketorolac (Toradol)
   d. Ibuprofen (Motrin, Advil)
   e. Naproxen (Naprosyn)
   f. Celecoxib (Celebrex)
3. Adjuvants
   a. Corticosteroids
   b. Antidepressants: Amitriptyline (Elavil), doxepin (Sinequan), imipramine (Tofranil-PM), nortriptyline (Pamelor)
   c. Antiseizure: Clonazepam (Klonopin), gabapentin (Neurontin), carbamazepine (Tegretol)
   d. Muscle relaxant: Baclofen (Lioresal)
   e. Alpha-2-adrenergic agonist: Clonidine (Duraclon)
   f. Anesthetics—systemic, oral, or local: Mexiletine (Mexitil); topical EMLA; capsaicin (Zostrix)
   g. Psychostimulants: Methylphenidate (Ritalin)
   h. Other
      (1) Sedatives
      (2) Anxiolytics (benzodiazepines, propofol)—used to complement analgesia and improve client's overall comfort
4. Nonpharmacologic pain management (see physiologic adaptation)
5. Narcotic antagonists: Nalmefene (Revex), naloxone hydrochloride (Narcan), naltrexone (ReVia)—reverses effects of narcotics; treats respiratory depression from narcotics
   a. Place client on cardiac monitor and assess rhythm, vital signs, especially respiratory rate, every 15 min until client is stable.
   b. Have resuscitation equipment available and do not leave client unattended.

Parkinson Disease

I. Definition: Parkinson disease (PD) is a chronic, neurodegenerative disease involving client inability to control or regulate movements. The disease is caused by degeneration of dopamine-producing neurons in the substantia nigra of the midbrain, resulting in an imbalance between acetylcholine and dopamine. Parkinson disease affects men more frequently than women, and usually presents after 60 years of age.

II. Nursing process

A. Assessment
1. Obtain a detailed health history, psychosocial history, physical assessment, and neurologic examination.
2. Perform a detailed physical examination, including assessment for signs and symptoms. Cardinal symptoms include tremor, muscle rigidity, and bradykinesia; other symptoms are as follows.
   a. Postural instability, shuffling of feet when walking, freezing gait
   b. Dysphagia, slow facial expressions, speech impairment
   c. Depression, sleep disturbance, personality changes, dementia
3. Obtain diagnostic tests: There are no diagnostic studies that confirm Parkinson disease; clinical diagnosis is based on health history and presence of two of three cardinal symptoms.

B. Analysis
1. Impaired Physical Mobility related to rigidity, bradykinesia, or freezing gait
2. Impaired Nutrition: Less Than Body Requirements related to dysphagia, tremor, and difficulty chewing
3. Impaired Verbal Communication related to slowing of facial muscles, and dysarthria
4. Constipation related to medications and reduced activity

5. Self-Care Deficit: Feeding and Grooming related to tremors and bradykinesia
6. Ineffective Coping related to depression and sleep disturbance
7. Risk for Falls related to postural instability
8. Risk for Aspiration related to dysphagia

C. Planning
1. Improve mobility.
2. Promote independence.
3. Promote effective communication.
4. Maintain adequate nutritional intake.
5. Maintain normal elimination pattern.
6. Prevent falls.
7. Optimize psychosocial well-being.

D. Implementation
1. Monitor vital signs, neurologic status, and progression of symptoms.
2. Encourage an exercise program to enhance muscle strength.
3. Introduce speech therapy for dysphagia and communication.
4. Provide client and family teaching about diet, medications and side effects, mobility, preventing constipation, preventing falls, and promoting a safe environment.

E. Evaluation
1. Client exhibits stable vital signs and neurologic status.
2. Client independently performs activities of daily living.
3. Client participates in an exercise program.
4. Client is free from falls.
5. Client maintains target body weight.
6. Client maintains normal daily bowel pattern.
7. Client participates in social activities.

CN

III. Client needs

A. Physiologic adaptation: Management of Parkinson disease is based on symptom control. Pharmacologic therapy is initiated to correct imbalance of neurotransmitters. Surgical intervention may be used in select clients who are unresponsive to medications and have developed severe motor complications; deep brain stimulation is more commonly performed.
1. Deep brain stimulation—involves electrical stimulation to targeted areas in the brain to assist client control movement. Fine wires are placed deep in the brain and attached to a small electrical stimulator inserted adjacent to the collar bone to deliver electronic stimulation and block abnormal nerve signals, causing tremor and other symptoms.
2. Pallidotomy—involves destruction of part of the globus pallidus of the brain responsible for stiffness, slow movements, and tremors.
3. Thalamotomy—involves surgical ablation of selected portion of the thalamus of the brain responsible for tremors.

B. Management of care: Care of the client with Parkinson disease requires critical thinking skills and knowledge of assessment, and teaching and evaluation methods unique to the RN role. These skills cannot be delegated to an LPN or UAP.
1. Delegate responsibly those activities that can be delegated, including basic care needs and vital sign checks for the stable client. All monitoring information is reported to the RN.
2. Monitor vital signs, neurologic status, symptoms, and medication adjustments. Administer all medications according to agency policy.
3. Introduce Parkinson disease nurse specialist to client as a continuing contact for support, home visits, and information on clinical and social matters of concern for clients and families.
4. Provide client and family teaching.
   a. Adhere to medication regimen: Understand action, dose, route, timely administration, and side effects.
   b. Promote mobility: Manage Freezing when walking
      (1) Do not pull person forward.
      (2) Suggest stepping over log, marching in place, attention to lines on carpet or cracks in pavement, taping sections of floor to promote walking.
   c. Prevent falls:
      (1) Maintain activity and exercise.
      (2) Avoid soft surfaces, loose carpeting, or throw rugs.
      (3) Create safe pathways in the home.
      (4) Use assistive devices.
      (5) Avoid low light (night lights).
   d. Prevent constipation:
      (1) Develop a bowel program.
      (2) Follow high-fiber diet, adequate fluid intake.
      (3) Use stool softeners, laxatives, suppositories, and enemas in moderation, as needed.
   e. Manage dysphagia:
      (1) Sit upright and position chin slightly downward to enhance swallowing.
      (2) Use thickeners for liquids.

(3) Give sip of water prior to medication and food.

(4) Promote meals when medication is working.

(5) Prepare pureed foods, or advance to moist semi-solid food.

5. Collaborate with dietician, physical therapist, occupational therapist, speech pathologist, and social service to develop a comprehensive plan of care.
6. Assess for home health care needs and support, and client and family desire for home care, hospice, or palliative care.
7. Link client with community resources for support groups and exercise programs.

C. Safety and infection control: Instruct client and family to provide a safe environment to prevent falls—discuss installation of railings where more support is needed, such as the bathtub and toilet area; keep floors and halls clear of clutter and loose rugs.

D. Health promotion and maintenance

1. Promote exercise to improve muscle strength.
2. Promote nutritious diet and maintenance of target weight.

E. Psychologic integrity

1. Assess impact of disease on quality of life and coping strategies.
2. Assess client's social and family support and prevent social isolation.
3. Provide clients and family with opportunity to make informed decisions about care and treatment, and to discuss end-of-life issues.

F. Basic care and comfort

1. Provide adequate periods of rest between activities.
2. Manage symptoms to maintain client comfort and quality of life.

G. Reduction of risk potential

1. Thicken liquids to prevent aspiration for clients with dysphagia.
2. Avoid abruptly withdrawing antiparkinson drugs to prevent neuroleptic malignant syndrome.

H. Pharmacology and parenteral therapies: Client will state the purpose for and side effects of all medications used to treat Parkinson disease (see Table 30-3).

Multiple Sclerosis

I. Definition: Multiple sclerosis (MS) is a chronic, degenerative disorder of the central nervous system (CNS), and is characterized by inflammation, demyelination, and scarring in multiple areas of the brain and spinal cord. Symptoms are produced as nerve fibers are damaged or destroyed, and nerve impulses are slowed or blocked. There are four categories for clinical courses of MS.

A. Relapsing-remitting—the most common clinical course, relapsing-remitting MS involves clearly defined relapses or exacerbations followed by partial or complete remissions.

B. Primary-progressive—involves slow, progressive worsening from disease onset with occasional plateaus and temporary minor improvements.

C. Secondary-progressive—initial period involves relapsing-remitting disease and is followed by steady worsening with or without occasional relapses, remissions, or plateaus. Secondary-progressive clinical course is found in half of clients with MS, and develops within 10 years of disease onset.

D. Progressive-relapsing—involves steady progression of disease from onset with clear acute exacerbations with or without recovery; periods between relapses are characterized by continuing disease progression.

II. Nursing process

A. Assessment

1. Obtain a detailed health history and psychosocial history.
2. Perform a comprehensive physical and neurologic examination, including assessment for signs and symptoms. Onset of MS is often insidious and gradual. Because of the scattered distribution of plaque lesions, symptoms differ between individuals and can vary over time with exacerbations and remissions. There is a continuous decline in neurologic function.
   a. Fatigue, weakness, spasticity, loss of balance, numbness, paresthesia, pain, depression
   b. Visual disturbances: Diplopia, patchy blindness, nystagmus
   c. Dizziness, vertigo
   d. Cognitive dysfunction: Memory loss, decreased concentration
   e. Spastic or flaccid bladder dysfunction: Urgency, frequency, hesitancy, nocturia, incontinence
   f. Constipation
   g. Sexual dysfunction
3. Obtain diagnostic tests.
   a. MRI
   b. Cerebral spinal fluid (CSF) analysis
   c. Evoked potential studies

B. Analysis

1. Impaired Mobility related to weakness, spasticity, fatigue, and loss of balance

Table 30-3 Drugs Used to Treat Parkinson Disease

Classification	Generic/ Trade Name	Expected Outcomes	Reduction of Risk Potential	Management of Care
Levodopa	Carbidopa, levodopa (Sinemet, Parcopa)	Improves symptoms.	Monitor for nausea and vomiting; orthostatic hypotension (occurs when first initiated but subsides); dyskinesia; "on-off" phenomenon; hallucinations, paranoia, and nightmares. Administer drug at exact time ordered (very short half-life). If GI slowing is severe, consider administering as a liquid. Effectiveness decreased in presence of dietary protein.	Initiate treatment when symptomatic relief from other drugs no longer effective; drug effects wearing off generally 5 years. Administer on an empty stomach, 1 hr prior to meals or 2 hr following meals. Promote timely administration. Parcopa dissolves on the tongue; can be administered on waking in AM when movement is limited; when difficulty swallowing; and during "off" times.
Dopamine agonists	Pramipexole (Mirapex), ropinirole (Requip), bromocriptine (Parlodel), pergolide (Permax); rotigotine skin patch; apomorphine injectable (Apokyn)	Used early in course of PD. Improves symptoms; helps to delay use of levodopa treatment. Used in combination with levodopa, lower dosages of levodopa are needed, thus delaying side effects.	Avoid sudden changes in posture. Avoid alcohol. Monitor for nausea and vomiting, orthostatic hypotension; dyskinesia; hallucinations; confusion; sleepiness; leg edema; severe irritation of the skin. Evaluate when starting apomorphine injectable to determine dosage and effect prior to starting medication because of risk for drop in BP, dyskinesia, and severe nausea.	Rotigotine skin patch: Administer for client with difficulty swallowing and decreased GI motility. Apomorphine injectable: Administer in subcutaneous tissue of abdomen.
Anticholinergics	Trihexyphenidyl (Artane), benztropine (Cogentin)	Treats tremors.	Poorly tolerated by elderly; monitor carefully if prescribed. Prevent falls from sedation effect and orthostatic hypotension. Monitor for blurred vision, drowsiness, constipation, urinary retention in men, dry mouth, and cognitive impairment (memory, hallucinations, confusion).	Provide safe environment; prevent falls.
Monoamine oxidase B inhibitors	Selegiline (Eldepryl), rasagiline (Azilect)	Used in early and advanced PD. Inhibits metabolism of dopamine; improves symptoms.	Monitor for insomnia, nausea, and exacerbation of dyskinesia. Do not administer Demerol with Eldepryl as interaction causes adverse reactions that may be fatal.	Eldepryl: Administer in AM because affects sleep. Rasagiline: Does not cause insomnia so can be administered close to bedtime.
Antivirals	Amantadine (Symmetrel)	Improves symptoms in 50% of PD clients; effects are short term.	Monitor for insomnia, confusion, hallucinations, nightmares, lower extremity edema, and purplish mottling of skin (livedo reticularis).	May regain effectiveness if stopped for short time.
Catechol-O-methyl transferase (COMT) inhibitor	Entacapone (Comtan), tolcapone (Tasmar)	Improves "on" time and decreases "off" time.	Monitor for increased side effects of levodopa, especially dyskinesia.	Always administer in combination with levodopa and at same time. Side effects are reduced by decreasing dosage of levodopa.

2. Impaired Urinary Elimination related to spastic or flaccid bladder
3. Bowel Incontinence related to constipation
4. Impaired Swallowing related to nerve involvement, fatigue, and weakness
5. Impaired Thought Process related to nerve involvement in the brain, and fatigue
6. Risk for Falls related to weakness, impaired mobility, and sensory and visual impairment
7. Ineffective Coping related to depression and uncertainty of MS progression

C. Planning
1. Promote mobility.
2. Promote independence.
3. Maintain bladder and bowel continence.
4. Maintain adequate fluid and nutritional intake.
5. Promote effective communication.
6. Prevent falls and injury.
7. Optimize psychosocial well-being.

D. Implementation
1. Monitor vital signs, neurologic status, and progression of symptoms.
2. Promote daily exercise or exercise program.
3. Introduce speech therapy for dysphagia and communication.
4. Provide client and family teaching about diet, medications and side effects, mobility, preventing constipation, preventing falls, and promoting a safe environment.

E. Evaluation
1. Client has stable vital signs and neurologic status.
2. Client performs activities of daily living.
3. Client participates in daily exercise.
4. Client is free from injury and falls.
5. Client has bladder continence.
6. Client has normal daily bowel pattern.
7. Client participates in social activities.
8. Client is free from exacerbations.
9. Client shows no signs of contractures or skin breakdown.
10. Client adheres to therapeutic regimen.

CN

III. Client needs

A. Physiologic adaptation: During exacerbations, existing symptoms worsen and new symptoms appear; exacerbations can be associated with physical or emotional stress. Interventions for MS are based on managing chronic symptoms, delaying progression, and resolving acute exacerbations.

B. Management of care: Care of the client with MS requires critical thinking skills and knowledge of assessment, and teaching and evaluation methods unique to the RN role. These skills cannot be delegated to an LPN or UAP.
1. Delegate responsibly those activities that can be delegated, including basic care needs, turning and positioning, measuring intake and output, and vital sign checks for the stable client. All monitoring information is reported to the RN.
2. Monitor vital signs, neurologic status, symptoms, and medication adjustments.
3. Promote continuing care for client in outpatient or home setting; provide contact for support, home visits, and information on clinical and social matters of concern.
4. Provide client and family teaching.
   a. Discuss medication action, dose, route, administration times, and side effects.
   b. Promote mobility and prevent falls—maintain activity and daily exercise; avoid strenuous physical activity and take short rest periods between activities; perform ROM exercises for clients with severe limitation.
   c. Inspect skin; prevent and treat pressure ulcers.
   d. Prevent constipation.
   e. Promote bladder control.
   f. Promote proper positioning for eating to reduce risk of aspiration.
   g. Provide for cognitive impairment through structured environment and daily routine; provide memory aids, lists, recorded messages, and promote calendar use.
   h. Promote relaxation techniques.
5. Consult and collaborate with dietician, physical therapist, occupational therapist, speech pathologist, counseling, and social services.
6. Assess for home health care needs and support; provide client and family with community resources for support groups and community services such as local chapter of the National MS Society, International MS Support Foundation, Multiple Sclerosis Association of America, and MS Foundation.

C. Safety and infection control: Instruct client and family to provide a safe environment to prevent falls—discuss installation of railings where more support is needed, such as the bathtub and toilet area; keep floors and halls clear of clutter and loose rugs.

D. Health promotion and maintenance
1. Promote exercise to improve muscle strength.

2. Promote nutritious diet and maintenance of target weight.

E. Psychologic integrity
1. Assess impact of disease on quality of life and coping strategies.
2. Assess client's social and family support and prevent social isolation.
3. Provide clients and family with opportunity to make informed decisions about care and treatment, and to discuss end-of-life issues.

F. Basic care and comfort
1. Provide adequate periods of rest between activities.
2. Manage symptoms to maintain client comfort and quality of life.

G. Reduction of risk potential
1. Promote skin integrity—identify areas of decreased sensation and pressure points; instruct client to avoid applying extreme heat or cold, and to test bath water.
2. Thicken liquids to prevent aspiration for clients with dysphagia.

H. Pharmacology and parenteral therapies: Client will state the purpose for and side effects of all medications used to manage MS.
1. Beta interferons: Interferon beta-1a (Avonex, Rebif); interferon beta-1b (Betaseron)
   a. Treats relapsing-remitting MS; reduces number of exacerbations and slows progression
   b. Side effects include flulike symptoms during initial weeks of treatment, depression
2. Antineoplastic with immunosuppressive effects: Mitoxantrone (Novantrone)
   a. Treats secondary-progressive MS; decreases relapse and progression
   b. Side effects to report immediately: Fever or chills, lower back or side pain; painful or difficult urination; swelling of feet and lower legs; black, tarry stools; cough, dyspnea; sores in mouth and lips; stomach pain. Common side effects include nausea, temporary hair loss, and menstrual disorders.
3. Corticosteroids: Dexamethasone (Decadron), prednisone (Deltasone), and methylprednisolone (Solu-Medrol)—treats exacerbations
4. Muscle relaxants and tranquilizers: Baclofen (Lioresal), clonazepam (Klonopin), dantrolene (Dantrium), diazepam (Valium), tizanidine (Zanaflex)—treat spasticity
5. For treatment of urinary retention (flaccid bladder): Desmopressin (DDAVP), bethanechol (Urecholine)
6. For treatment of urinary frequency and urgency (spastic bladder): Tolterodine (Detrol), oxybutynin (Ditropan, Oxytrol), propantheline (Pro-Banthine), trospium (Sanctura), and imipramine (Tofranil)

Myasthenia Gravis

I. Definition: Myasthenia gravis is a chronic progressive autoimmune disorder affecting transmission of nerve impulses at the neuromuscular junction, and is characterized by varying degrees of weakness in certain skeletal muscles.
   A. Myasthenia crisis is an acute exacerbation with severe muscle weakness and requires intubation for mechanical ventilation support or airway protection. Myasthenia crisis is usually triggered by infection, emotional stress, surgery, or insufficient anticholinesterase medication. Symptoms are treated with administration of anticholinesterase medication.
   B. Cholinergic crisis results from an overmedication of anticholinesterase drugs. Symptoms mimic myasthenia crisis. Deterioration or no improvement occurs if an anticholinesterase medication is given.

II. Nursing process
   A. Assessment
      1. Obtain a detailed health history and psychosocial history.
      2. Perform a comprehensive physical examination and neurologic examination, including assessment for signs and symptoms.
         a. Weakness of the face, jaw, neck, shoulder, and hips; weakness usually improves with rest, eventually leading to fatigue and weakness not relieved by rest.
         b. Diplopia, ptosis
         c. Impaired chewing, swallowing, and speaking; dysphonia
      3. Obtain diagnostic tests.
         a. Electromyography (EMG) studies
         b. Edrophonium chloride (Tensilon) test
            (1) Improvement of symptoms with myasthenia gravis or myasthenia crisis
            (2) No improvement or deterioration of symptoms with cholinergic crisis
         c. Acetylcholine receptor antibody titers
         d. MRI to assess thymus gland
   B. Analysis
      1. Activity Intolerance related to fatigue, weakness
      2. Ineffective Breathing Pattern related to intercostal muscle weakness

3. Impaired Verbal Communication related to fading voice, weakness of the facial and throat muscles
4. Disturbed Sensory Perception: Visual, related to diplopia, ptosis, decreased eye movement
5. Impaired Nutrition: Less Than Body Requirements related to dysphagia, difficulty chewing
6. Risk for Aspiration related to dysphagia, ineffective airway clearance, impaired gag reflex
7. Ineffective tissue perfusion cardiopulmonary related to respiratory muscle weakness
8. Anxiety related to disease process, fatigue, weakness, decreased quality of life

C. Planning
1. Improve muscle function and endurance.
2. Maintain patent airway, normal breathing pattern, and adequate oxygenation.
3. Maintain target weight.
4. Maintain quality of life.
5. Prevent complications.

D. Implementation
1. Monitor vital signs, neurologic status, respiratory status, and symptoms.
2. Treat underlying cause of myasthenia exacerbation.
3. Provide client and family teaching about medications and side effects, diet, strategies to conserve energy, symptoms of respiratory distress, and factors that exacerbate symptoms.

E. Evaluation
1. Client has stable vital signs, SpO_2, and neurologic vital signs.
2. Client performs usual activities of daily living.
3. Client is free from complications.
4. Client maintains target body weight.
5. Client confirms adequate control of symptoms.

CN

III. Client needs

A. Physiologic adaptation: Management of myasthenia gravis is guided by improving muscular function and reducing circulating antibodies with medications, plasmapheresis to treat exacerbations, and surgical removal of thymus (thymectomy).

B. Management of care: Care of the client with myasthenia gravis requires critical thinking skills and knowledge of assessment, and teaching and evaluation methods unique to the RN role. These skills cannot be delegated to an LPN or UAP.
1. Monitor vital signs, oxygen saturation, neurologic status, respiratory rate and depth, lung sounds, symptoms, medication adjustments, and for complications: Signs of respiratory distress, aspiration, myasthenia crisis, and cholinergic crisis.
2. Provide teaching to the client and family (see also health promotion and maintenance, and reduction of risk potential).
   a. Promote understanding of medication action, dose, route, timely administration, and side effects.
   b. Plan activities with periods of rest to avoid fatigue.
   c. Promote nutritious, well-balanced diet with foods that can be chewed and swallowed easily.
      (1) Place client in upright position, or encourage sitting upright while eating.
      (2) Promote meals 1 hr after medication administration and when client is experiencing good muscle strength.
   d. Discuss when to seek medical attention: Increase in weakness, signs of respiratory distress, myasthenia, or cholinergic crisis.
3. Assess for home health care needs and support; provide information on community resources such as the Myasthenia Gravis Foundation of America or a local support group.

C. Safety and infection control: Instruct client and family to provide a safe environment to prevent falls—discuss installation of railings where more support is needed, such as the bathtub and toilet area; keep floors and halls clear of clutter and loose rugs.

D. Health promotion and maintenance: Provide client and family teaching.
1. Avoid exposure to infections.
2. Avoid alcohol and sedatives.
3. Consume nutritious diet and maintain target weight.

E. Psychologic integrity
1. Assess impact of disease on quality of life and coping strategies.
2. Assess client's social and family support, and prevent social isolation.
3. Provide clients and family with opportunity to make informed decisions about care and treatment, and to discuss end-of-life issues.

F. Basic care and comfort
1. Manage symptoms to maintain client comfort and quality of life.

2. Provide adequate periods of rest between activities.
3. Promote relaxation techniques; reduction of stress.

G. Reduction of risk potential: Provide client and family teaching.
1. Wear a medic-alert bracelet.
2. Provide eye care: Artificial tears, patch over one eye with diplopia, sunglasses with bright light.
3. Avoid triggers and drugs that can exacerbate myasthenia gravis.

H. Pharmacology and parenteral therapies: Client and family will state the purpose, usage, and associated side effects of all medications used to treat myasthenia gravis.
1. Anticholinesterases: Pyridostigmine bromide (Mestinon), neostigmine bromide (Prostigmin)—enhances function at the neuromuscular junction.
   a. Individually tailor doses to prevent myasthenia or cholinergic crisis.
   b. Side effects include nausea, vomiting, abdominal cramps, diarrhea, increased bronchial and oral secretions. Overdose causes severe, generalized weakness and respiratory failure (cholinergic crisis).
2. Immunosuppressants
   a. Corticosteroids: Prednisone (Deltasone)
   b. Azathioprine (Imuran)
   c. Cyclosporine (Gengraf, Neoral, Sandimmune)
   d. Cyclophosphamide (Cytoxan)

Amyotrophic Lateral Sclerosis

I. Definition: Amyotrophic lateral sclerosis (ALS), also known as Lou Gehrig disease, is a progressive neurodegenerative disorder from a loss of motor neurons in the brain and spinal cord. As the motor neuron cells degenerate, atrophy occurs in the muscle fibers supplied and results in loss of voluntary muscle action. Total paralysis occurs in later stages of the disease and permanent mechanical ventilation is eventually needed. Intellectual function remains intact. The cause for ALS is unknown.

II. Nursing process

A. Assessment
1. Obtain a detailed health history and psychosocial history.
2. Perform a comprehensive physical and neurologic examination; assess for signs and symptoms.
   a. Progressive muscle weakness involving the arms, legs, speech, swallowing, and breathing
   b. Fasciculations (twitching) and cramping of muscles
   c. Fatigue
   d. Incoordination
   e. Dysarthria, dysphonia, dysphagia
3. Obtain diagnostic tests: There are no diagnostic studies specific to ALS. Diagnosis is based on signs and symptoms.
   a. Electromyography (EMG) studies to determine extent of muscle atrophy
   b. MRI to rule out other causes of symptoms

B. Analysis
1. Impaired Physical Mobility related to motor neuron loss
2. Impaired Verbal Communication related to impairment of bulbar muscles, difficulty in articulation and projecting the voice
3. Imbalanced Nutrition: Less Than Body Requirements related to dysphagia, weakness
4. Ineffective Breathing Pattern related to respiratory muscle loss
5. Self-Care Deficit related to motor function loss
6. Ineffective Coping related to paralysis, depression, loss of control
7. Anxiety related to disease progression, paralysis, role change, loss of function
8. Risk for Aspiration related to dysphagia, ineffective airway clearance
9. Ineffective tissue perfusion cardiopulmonary related to respiratory muscle loss
10. Risk for Impaired Skin Integrity related to immobility

C. Planning
1. Maintain adequate oxygenation.
2. Promote optimal motor function.
3. Facilitate effective communication.
4. Maintain adequate nutritional intake.
5. Relieve symptoms.
6. Prevent complications.
7. Optimize psychosocial well-being.

D. Implementation
1. Monitor vital signs, neurologic status, SpO_2, respiratory status, and progression of symptoms.
2. Assess need for enteral feedings.
3. Provide client and family teaching regarding disease progression; medications, and associated side effects; nutrition; signs of aspiration; symptoms of respiratory distress; and management of ventilatory support when needed.

E. Evaluation
1. Client has stable vital signs, SpO_2, and neurologic vital signs.
2. Client maintains best possible functioning.
3. Client is free from complications.
4. Client maintains target body weight.
5. Client confirms adequate control of symptoms.

CN

III. Client needs
A. Physiologic adaptation: Onset of ALS is insidious, beginning with muscle weakness or stiffness, progressing to muscle atrophy, paralysis in the limbs and trunk, and finally inevitable paralysis. At this point permanent ventilatory support is required to survive. Most clients are managed at home with hospitalization for acute problems.
B. Management of care: Care of the client with ALS requires critical thinking skills and knowledge of assessment, and teaching and evaluation methods unique to the RN role. These skills cannot be delegated to an LPN or UAP.
1. Delegate responsibly those activities that can be delegated, including basic care needs and vital sign checks for the stable client. All monitoring information is reported to the RN.
2. Monitor vital signs, oxygen saturation, respiratory rate and depth, lung sounds, neurologic status, progression of symptoms, responses to medications, and for complications: Respiratory failure, aspiration, pneumonia, dehydration, and malnutrition.
3. Provide client and family teaching.
a. Promote understanding of medication action, dose, route, timely administration, and side effects.
b. Encourage client's optimal participation in self-care.
c. Promote nutritious, balanced diet with foods that can be chewed and swallowed easily; promote adequate fluid intake.
(1) Keep client seated or positioned upright when eating.
(2) Observe for signs of aspiration.
d. Assist client and family to determine when a feeding tube may be required for nutritional intake.
e. Promote turning and positioning, ROM exercises, inspection of skin, prevention of skin breakdown, and treatment of pressure ulcers.
f. Instruct when to seek medical attention: Signs and symptoms of aspiration, respiratory infection, and respiratory distress.
g. Discuss choices related to life support; availability of mechanical ventilation for survival when respiratory failure occurs and need for tracheostomy.
h. Provide interventions for mechanical ventilation, suctioning, care of tracheostomy, if needed.
4. Consult and collaborate with respiratory therapist, dietician, physical therapist, speech pathologist, and social service to develop a comprehensive plan of care.
5. Provide support of cognitive and emotional functions.
6. Assess for home health care needs and support; assess client's and family's desire for home care, hospice, or palliative care.
7. Introduce client and family to community resources such as the ALS Society for local support groups.
C. Safety and infection control: Instruct client and family to provide a safe environment to prevent falls—discuss installation of railings where more support is needed, such as the bathtub and toilet area; keep floors and halls clear of clutter and loose rugs.
D. Health promotion and maintenance: Promote a nutritious diet and maintenance of target weight.
E. Psychologic integrity
1. Assess impact of disease on quality of life and coping strategies.
2. Assess client's social and family support and prevent social isolation.
3. Provide client and family with opportunity to make informed decisions about care and treatment, and to discuss end-of-life issues.
F. Basic care and comfort
1. Turn and position client every 2 hr; promote preventive skin care.
2. Provide frequent oral care.
3. Manage symptoms to maintain client comfort and quality of life.
G. Reduction of risk potential
1. HCP will insert gastrostomy tube for clients experiencing problems with swallowing and aspiration.
2. Avoid complications leading to hospitalization: Injury from falls, dehydration, malnutrition, respiratory infection, and respiratory distress.
H. Pharmacology and parenteral therapies: Client will state the purpose for and associated side effects of riluzole (Rilutek).
1. Glutamate antagonist slows the deterioration of motor neurons in the early stages and prolongs survival.

2. Side effects include asthenia, nausea, dizziness, decreased lung function, diarrhea, abdominal pain, pneumonia, vomiting, vertigo, circumoral paresthesia, anorexia, and somnolence.
3. Dose adjustment for side effects may be needed.

Guillain-Barré Syndrome

I. Definition: Guillain-Barré syndrome (GBS) is an autoimmune disorder causing a rapid, segmental demyelination and inflammation of peripheral nervous system and some cranial nerves. The disorder disables motor and sensory nerve impulses, causing weakness, numbness, or paralysis. Progressive muscle weakness usually begins and ascends from the legs, spreading to the arms and upper body. Severe cases may result in total paralysis, fluctuations in heart rate and BP from autonomic nervous system dysfunction, and respiratory failure from paralysis progressing to the thoracic area. The etiology of GBS is unknown, but it is often preceded by immune system stimulation from a viral or bacterial infection 1 to 4 weeks prior to onset of symptoms and less commonly after trauma, surgery, or immunization. Most clients recover with minimal residual symptoms.

II. Nursing process

A. Assessment
1. Obtain a detailed health history, including recent viral or bacterial illness, and psychosocial history.
2. Perform a comprehensive physical and neurologic examination, including assessment for signs and symptoms.
   a. Progressive muscle weakness, paralysis
   b. Diminished reflexes, hypotonia
   c. Paresthesia
   d. Pain
   e. Facial weakness and paresthesia
   f. Extraocular eye movement difficulty, blindness
   g. Dysphagia
   h. Difficulty breathing
   i. Bradycardia
   j. Orthostatic hypotension, hypertension
   k. Bowel and bladder dysfunction
3. Obtain diagnostic tests. Diagnosis is based on client history and signs and symptoms.
   a. Cerebrospinal fluid to determine protein level (elevated in clients with GBS)
   b. Electromyography (EMG) and nerve conduction studies to determine muscle weakness and nerve conduction
   c. ABGs to determine oxygenation status

B. Analysis
1. Impaired Physical Mobility related to motor neuron demyelination
2. Chronic Pain related to paresthesia, muscle cramps
3. Impaired Verbal Communication related to loss of function to the face and throat, intubation
4. Self-Care Deficit related to impaired mobility, paralysis
5. Impaired Breathing Patterns related to respiratory muscle paralysis
6. Risk for Aspiration related to dysphagia, loss of gag reflex
7. Anxiety related to loss of function, paralysis
8. Fear related to unknown outcome, paralysis, inability to breathe

C. Planning
1. Maintain adequate ventilation and oxygenation.
2. Relieve pain.
3. Maintain adequate nutritional intake.
4. Maintain effective communication.
5. Promote return to previous function level.
6. Avoid complications of respiratory dysfunction, autonomic dysfunction, and immobility.

D. Implementation
1. Monitor vital signs, neurologic status, ECG, SpO_2, respiratory status, reflexes, and progression of symptoms.
2. Assess need for mechanical ventilation.
3. Assess need for enteral feedings.
4. Provide client and family teaching about disease progression, medications, and associated signs and symptoms, plasmapheresis, nutrition, signs of aspiration, symptoms of respiratory distress, mechanical ventilation.

E. Evaluation
1. Client's vital signs and SpO_2 are within targeted range.
2. Client has normal spontaneous breathing pattern.
3. Client confirms adequate control of pain.
4. Client returns to previous level of physical function.
5. Client has normal reflexes.
6. Client is free from complications.

CN

III. Client needs

A. Physiologic adaptation: Most clients recover from even the most severe cases of GBS, but it can be fatal. Treatment involves pain management, supportive care, symptom management, and prevention of complications:

1. Ventilator support, mechanical ventilation.
2. Tube feeding (for severe dysphagia) and total parenteral nutrition with a paralytic ileus.
3. Plasmapheresis—used during the first 2 to 3 weeks to reduce circulating antibody levels, improve symptoms, and promote recovery.
4. Immunoglobulin therapy to reduce severity of the disease.

B. Management of care: Care of the client with GBS requires critical thinking skills and knowledge of assessment, and teaching and evaluation methods unique to the RN role. These skills cannot be delegated to an LPN or UAP.
   1. Provide interventions during acute phase.
      a. Perform comprehensive physical assessments, evaluating severity of symptoms, adequacy of oxygenation, effectiveness of ventilation, hemodynamic stability, response to interventions, and for complications: Respiratory failure, aspiration, pneumonia, urinary tract infection, dehydration, malnutrition, deep vein thrombosis, and skin breakdown.
         (1) Perform frequent vital sign assessment, and assessment of neurologic status and corneal, gag, swallow, and peripheral reflexes.
         (2) Assess rate, depth, quality of respirations, vital capacity, cough and airway clearance, ABG, signs of hypoxia, need for mechanical ventilation, suctioning.
         (3) Provide continuous monitoring of SpO_2 and ECG.
         (4) Assess for orthostatic hypotension.
         (5) Assess bowel sounds.
         (6) Assess for urinary retention and need for intermittent or indwelling catheterization.
         (7) Monitor temperature closely; sputum, urine, and blood cultures if fever develops.
         (8) Perform frequent skin assessments.
      b. Assess for adequacy of nutritional intake, severe dysphagia, and symptoms of paralytic ileus.
         (1) Promote nutritious, balanced diet with foods that can be chewed and swallowed easily. Seat client or position upright when eating.
         (2) Promote adequate fluid intake.
         (3) Assess for signs of aspiration.
         (4) Provide tube feedings with severe dysphagia—check residuals every 4 hr.
         (5) Provide total parenteral nutrition with paralytic ileus or intolerance to tube feedings—monitor electrolytes and blood glucose levels.
      c. Promote adequate hydration and renal function with immunoglobulin therapy.
      d. Facilitate communication.
      e. Prevent deep vein thrombosis (DVT)—promote ROM, turning, and positioning; prophylactic subcutaneous anticoagulation; elastic compression stockings; and sequential compression device.
   2. Provide information and teaching to the client and family regarding all procedures; mechanical ventilation, suctioning, care of tracheostomy, if needed; turning and positioning, and ROM exercises; pain management; bowel and bladder management; and signs of respiratory insufficiency, aspiration, infection, impaired skin integrity.
   3. Consult and collaborate with a respiratory therapist, dietician, physical therapist, speech therapist, and social service to develop a comprehensive plan of care.
   4. Assess for home health care needs and support; link client and family with rehabilitation and community resources, including Guillain-Barré Syndrome Foundation International.

C. Safety and infection control: Instruct client and family to provide a safe environment to prevent falls—discuss installation of railings where more support is needed, such as the bathtub and toilet area; keep floors and halls clear of clutter and loose rugs.

D. Health promotion and maintenance: Promote adequate nutritional intake and maintenance of target weight.

E. Psychologic integrity
   1. Assess impact of disease on quality of life and coping strategies.
   2. Assess client's social and family support.
   3. Provide interventions that increase sense of control and diminish sense of isolation.

F. Basic care and comfort
   1. Promote turning and positioning, ROM exercises, inspection of skin, and prevention of pressure ulcers.
   2. Perform frequent oral care.
   3. Provide effective pain management.

G. Reduction of risk potential: Implement strategies to minimize the effects of immobility.

H. Pharmacology and parenteral therapies: Client will state the purpose for and side effects of medications used to treat GBS.

1. Acetaminophen (Tylenol), NSAIDs or narcotics—for pain management
2. Immunoglobulin IV

Bibliography

Abrams, A. C. (2004). *Clinical drug therapy: Rationales for nursing practice* (7th ed.). Philadelphia: Lippincott Williams & Wilkins.

ALS Association. (2004). *Facts you should know about ALS.* Retrieved June 6, 2008 from http://www.alsa.org/als/facts.cfm?CFID=2475677&CFTOKEN=97320641

Hogan, M. A. (2004). *Pathophysiology: Review & rationales*. Upper Saddle River, NJ: Pearson-Prentice Hall.

Hogan, M. A. (2005). Hogan, M. A., Johnson, J. F., Franlensen, G. F., & Warren, L. (Eds). *Pharmacology: Review & rationales*. Upper Saddle River, NJ: Pearson-Prentice Hall.

Ignataviciuc, D. D., & Workman, M. L. (2006). *Medical-surgical nursing* (5th ed.). Philadelphia: Saunders.

Joint Commission. http://jointcommission.org

Lewis, S., Heitkemper, M., Dirksen, S., O'Brien, P., & Bucher, L. (2007). *Medical-surgical nursing: Assessment and management of clinical problems* (7th ed.). St. Louis: Mosby.

Morton, P. G., Fontaine, D. K., Hudak, C. M., & Gallo, B. M. (2005). *Critical care nursing: A holistic approach* (8th ed.). Philadelphia: Lippincott Williams & Wilkins.

National Collaborating Centre for Chronic Conditions. (2006). *Parkinson's disease: National clinical guideline for diagnosis and management in primary and secondary care.* London: Royal College of Physicians. Retrieved from http://guidance.nice.org.uk/CG35/guidance/pdf/English

National Institute of Neurological Disorders and Stroke & National Institute of Health. (2006). *Amyotrophic lateral sclerosis fact sheet.* Retrieved from http://www.ninds.nih.gov/disorders/amyotrophiclateralsclerosis/detail_amyotrophiclateralsclerosis.htm

National Institute of Neurological Disorders and Stroke & National Institute of Health. (2007). *Guillain-Barré syndrome fact sheet.* Retrieved from http://www.ninds.nih.gov/disorders/gbs/detail_gbs.htm

Smeltzer, S. C., Bare, B. G., Cheever, K. H., & Hinkle, J. L. (2008). *Brunner & Suddarth's textbook of medical-surgical nursing* (11th ed.). Philadelphia: Lippincott Williams & Wilkins.

Urden, L. D., Stacy, K. M., & Lough, M. E. (2006). *Thelan's critical care nursing: Diagnosis and management* (5th ed.). St. Louis: Mosby.

CHAPTER 30
Practice Test

Unconscious Client

1. AF One hour following abdominal surgery, a client is found unconscious and not breathing. The nurse should do which of the following in order of priority?

_____ 1. Obtain client's carotid pulse.
_____ 2. Administer oxygen.
_____ 3. Establish an airway.
_____ 4. Call for the resuscitation team.

2. A client suffered a head injury and is emerging from a coma. The client is confused and restless, and keeps trying to pull out the NG tube. The nurse should first:

☐ 1. Apply soft restraints loosely to the client's arms.
☐ 2. Contact the physician for a sedation order.
☐ 3. Place mitts on the client's hands.
☐ 4. Remove the NG tube.

Increased Intracranial Pressure and Head Injury

3. AF A client who is 23 years of age is admitted to the hospital with a head injury and possible temporal skull fracture sustained in a motorcycle accident. On admission the client was conscious, but lethargic; vital signs included: Temperature 99°F, pulse 100, respirations 18, and BP 140/70. The nurse immediately reports which of the following changes to the HCP? Select all that apply.

☐ 1. Decreasing urinary output.
☐ 2. Decreasing systolic BP.
☐ 3. Bradycardia.
☐ 4. Widening pulse pressure.
☐ 5. Tachycardia.
☐ 6. Increasing diastolic BP.

4. While assisting a client with a skull fracture into bed, the nurse notices a clear substance exuding from his nose. The nurse should first:

☐ 1. Test drainage for glucose.
☐ 2. Pack the nose with sterile gauze.
☐ 3. Gently suction the nose and mouth.
☐ 4. Instruct client to gently blow the nose.

Stroke

5. A client survives the acute phase of stroke and needs help adjusting to residual deficits resulting from her left intercerebral hemorrhagic CVA. The client is right-handed. Which of the following is not appropriate to include in the plan of care?

☐ 1. Provide passive ROM exercises, or teach joint ROM exercises, using unaffected limbs to move affected limbs.

- □ 2. Place the comb, toothbrush, and mirror on the left side of the overbed table.
- □ 3. Teach medication purpose, dose, schedule, side effects, and interactions.
- □ 4. Provide a clear liquid diet until the client indicates readiness to progress.

6. AF Which of the following outcomes indicates effective management of a conscious client who is being treated with recombinant tissue plasminogen therapy during the initial phase of an ischemic CVA? Select all that apply.
- □ 1. Headache reduced.
- □ 2. Dysphagia improved.
- □ 3. Visual disturbances improved.
- □ 4. Responds to comfort measures.
- □ 5. No signs or symptoms of bleeding.

7. Following a stroke, a client has dysphagia and left-sided facial paralysis. Which of the following feeding techniques will be most helpful at this time?
- □ 1. Encourage sipping diluted liquid meal supplements from a straw.
- □ 2. Position the client with the bed at a 30-degree angle.
- □ 3. Offer solid foods from the unaffected side of the mouth.
- □ 4. Feed the client a soft diet from a spoon into the left side of the mouth.

Seizure

8. A client newly diagnosed with epilepsy is being discharged from the hospital with a prescription for phenytoin (Dilantin). The nurse should advise the client to:
- □ 1. Brush teeth and gums, and floss regularly.
- □ 2. Check stool color with each bowel movement.
- □ 3. Have BP checked monthly.
- □ 4. Take medication with a full glass of water.

9. A client just had a seizure. During the postictal phase of the seizure, the nurse should first:
- □ 1. Make sure the client is awake.
- □ 2. Ask the client if he or she had an aura.
- □ 3. Prevent injuries.
- □ 4. Assess breathing.

Pain

10. To prevent a common adverse effect of a narcotic analgesic, the nurse takes which of the following measures?
- □ 1. Administer smaller than the ordered dosage of pain medication.
- □ 2. Administer antidiarrheal medications.
- □ 3. Obtain respiratory rate at specific intervals.
- □ 4. Immobilize the client to prevent falls.

11. AF A client who is 89 years of age is in traction for a broken hip. At 1100 on 3/26/09 the client is experiencing pain. Her orders are morphine sulfate 2 to 4 mg intravenous push every 2 to 4 hr for pain. The client rates the pain as an 8 on the visual analog scale (0–10). Prior to intervening to manage the pain, the nurse reviews the progress notes as noted below.

PROGRESS NOTES

Date	Time	Progress Notes
3/26/09	0900	Client is alert and oriented. Vital signs: pulse 80, respirations 14, BP 100/80, and oxygen saturation by pulse oximeter 92%. Received Morphine Sulfate 2 mg by intravenous push (IVP). ~Fred Lewis, RN
3/26/09	1000	Client has pain of 4 on the Visual Analog Scale (0-10). Respirations are 10. ~Fred Lewis, RN

At 1100 on 3/26/09 the nurse should do which of the following?
- □ 1. Reposition the client for comfort and administer pain medication in another 2 hr.
- □ 2. Administer 2 mg morphine sulfate IVP now and reassess in 10 to 15 min.
- □ 3. Call the physician for supplemental medication to relax the client and promote sedation.
- □ 4. Administer 2 mg morphine sulfate IVP in 2 hr if her respirations are above 12 breaths per minute.

Parkinson Disease

12. A client with Parkinson disease is having difficulty swallowing. To assist the client to eat, the nurse should take which of the following measures?
- □ 1. Give thin, soft food with broth or juice.
- □ 2. Raise the head of the bed to 45 degrees.
- □ 3. Provide dry solid foods.
- □ 4. Have client tuck chin downward to swallow.

13. Which of the following is most helpful to a client with Parkinson disease who is

experiencing a freezing gait (difficulty initiating movement)?
- □ 1. Pull client forward to initiate walking.
- □ 2. Instruct client to use a wheelchair.
- □ 3. Have client remain still.
- □ 4. Tell client to march in place.

Multiple Sclerosis

14. The nurse is reviewing the nursing diagnoses and a standardized care plan for a client with MS. The nurse validates which of the following nursing diagnoses before implementing the plan of care?
- □ 1. Impaired mobility.
- □ 2. Risk for falls.
- □ 3. Risk for seizures.
- □ 4. Self-care deficit.

15. The nurse is planning care for a client with MS. The client is concerned about weakness and the variability of the symptoms. Which of the following is the priority nursing care goal at this time?
- □ 1. Increase protein and carbohydrates.
- □ 2. Provide rest between activities.
- □ 3. Reinforce need for bed rest.
- □ 4. Administer baclofen (Lioresal).

Myasthenia Gravis

16. A client with myasthenia gravis is at highest risk for which of the following?
- □ 1. Aspiration.
- □ 2. Bladder dysfunction.
- □ 3. Hypertension.
- □ 4. Sensory loss.

17. The nurse is discussing discharge instructions to a client with myasthenia gravis. The nurse instructs the client about which of the following?
- □ 1. Administering artificial tears.
- □ 2. Avoiding contact with crowds.
- □ 3. Taking pyridostigmine (Mestinon) in the afternoon.
- □ 4. Decreasing protein in the diet.

Amyotrophic Lateral Sclerosis

18. When teaching the client with ALS about the effects of riluzole (Rilutek), the nurse explains that the expected outcome of this drug is to:
- □ 1. Cure the disease.
- □ 2. Improve movement.
- □ 3. Prevent respiratory failure.
- □ 4. Slow disease progression.

Guillain-Barré Syndrome

19. The nurse is planning care for a client with GBS. Which of the following is the highest priority?
- □ 1. Provide frequent mouth care and positioning.
- □ 2. Insert indwelling Foley catheter.
- □ 3. Promote ROM exercises.
- □ 4. Relieve pain.

20. The nurse should teach the client admitted with GBS about which of the following?
- □ 1. Need for total bed rest.
- □ 2. Potential need for mechanical ventilation.
- □ 3. Preparation for permanent paralysis.
- □ 4. Use of antibiotics to resolve the syndrome.

Answers and Rationales

1. 4, 3, 2, 1 The nurse's first priority is to obtain personnel qualified to provide advanced airway management and advanced cardiac life support. The nurse then follows the priorities of airway, breathing, and circulation (ABC), by establishing an airway, administering oxygen, and determining if the client has a pulse. If the client does not have an IV infusion, the nurse establishes a large-bore IV line to provide a route for delivery of emergency medications as needed for the client. (M)

2. 3 The nurse uses the least restrictive measure possible to maintain safety; mitts reduce the ability of the client to pull out tubes while still maintaining mobility of the upper extremities. Restraints are used only as a last resort. Sedation could mask signs of neurologic deterioration. The NG tube is not removed without a physician's order. (R)

3. 3, 4 The nurse immediately reports changes that indicate ICP; these include bradycardia, increasing systolic pressure, and widening pulse pressure. As ICP increases and the brain becomes more compressed, respirations become rapid, BP decreases, and the pulse slows further; these are very ominous signs. Decreased arterial BP and tachycardia can indicate bleeding elsewhere in the body. Decreasing urinary output indicates decreased tissue perfusion. The nurse monitors changes and notifies the HCP if trends continue. (A)

4. 1 The nurse tests drainage for glucose to indicate whether drainage is spinal fluid; CSF contains a high amount of glucose. A leakage of CSF is reported to the physician immediately. The nurse never attempts to insert anything into the nose of a client with CSF drainage. The client is instructed to avoid coughing, sneezing, or blowing the nose, as those activities can increase ICP and exacerbate CSF leakage. (R)

5. 4 A liquid diet can intensify swallowing difficulties. Soft, semisolid material placed in the unaffected side of the mouth is usually better manipulated by hemispheric stroke clients; diet is ordered by the physician after evaluation of swallowing. Passive ROM to the affected extremities is crucial to restoring function. Personal items are placed where the client can reach them (with left CVA, the client's right side is affected), and all clients should be taught about medications. (H)

6. 1, 4, 5 A headache (which is treated with analgesics) is commonly associated with an ischemic CVA. A conscious client responds to comfort measures. Bleeding is a side effect of recombinant tissue plasminogen (TPA) therapy to dissolve the clots; absence of bleeding is a desired outcome. Reduction of dysphagia and visual disturbances are unpredictable and less likely to change during this phase. (A)

7. 3 Following a stroke, it is easiest for clients with dysphagia (difficulty swallowing) to swallow solid foods; the nurse introduces foods on the unaffected side. Liquid foods are difficult to swallow, and the client with facial paralysis will have difficulty sipping using a straw. The head of the bed is elevated to 90 degrees, or the client is instructed to sit up, if possible, while eating to prevent choking and aspiration. (R)

8. 1 Dilantin causes gingival hyperplasia in about 20% of clients; this can be minimized with good oral hygiene. Dilantin does not cause GI bleeding but can cause irritation, which can be minimized by taking the drug with food. Oral phenytoin has little effect on the cardiovascular system (although IV administration can cause hypotension). (D)

9. 4 During the postictal phase of a seizure (after the seizure), the nurse assesses the client's breathing; if client is not breathing, the nurse establishes an airway and administers oxygen if needed. As the client wakes up, the nurse reorients the client to time and place and inquires about precipitating events such as an aura. The nurse prevents injuries during the seizure; after the seizure there is little risk of injury. (S)

10. 3 One of the most common adverse effects of narcotics is respiratory depression. Obtaining the respiratory rate of the client at specific intervals assures the nurse that the client will not develop any respiratory compromise from the narcotic. Administering a smaller dose of a pain medication is a medication dosage error. Constipation, not diarrhea, is an adverse effect of narcotics. Immobilizing the client is inappropriate; the nurse carefully monitors the client to prevent falls. (D)

11. 2 The nurse administers between 2 and 4 mg of morphine sulfate IVP every 2 to 4 hr according to the physician's order for pain management. Even though the client received pain medication 2 hr ago, she is still experiencing pain of the intensity of 8 on a scale of 0 to 10. Elderly clients may have slowed pain perception, but not diminished pain intensity. According to the WHO ladder recommendations, the nurse starts out conservatively, administering 2 mg of morphine sulfate IVP and reassessing in 15 min to determine the effectiveness of pain management and respiratory effort. If pain is still not relieved, the titration of morphine sulfate upward to 4 mg is optional. The single provision of nonpharmacologic interventions such as repositioning is not sufficient pain management when a client rates pain at 8 on a scale of 0 to 10. Requesting an order for sedation only causes the client to be unable to express her pain, and does not treat her pain. Although the nurse continues to monitor the client's respirations, the respirations are not dangerously depressed, and waiting another 2 hr to administer pain medication does not address the client's need for pain relief. (M)

12. 4 Clients with Parkinson disease may have difficulty swallowing. Swallowing is easier if the head is positioned downward with the chin in a slightly tucked position. The client is positioned to sit upright while eating. Thickened liquids and semisolid foods cut in small pieces assist with swallowing and prevent aspiration. (R)

13. 4 When a freezing gait occurs, having the client march in place or step over actual lines, imaginary lines, or objects on the floor can promote walking. Instructing the client to take one step backward and two steps forward may also stimulate walking. Pulling the client forward can cause imbalance. The nurse does not instruct the client to use a wheelchair. The client obtains as much exercise as possible; having the client remain still does not help the client obtain the momentum needed to walk. (A)

14. 3 Clients with multiple sclerosis have motor and sensory loss that impairs mobility and ability for self-care, and increases risk for falls. Seizures typically are not associated with MS, and the nurse should verify that this is, in fact, an accurate diagnosis for this client. (H)

15. 2 The nurse provides rest between activities to decrease symptoms of weakness and fatigue. The nurse encourages a nutritious, balanced diet, but it is not necessary to increase protein and carbohydrates. The client maintains activity and daily exercise and avoids adverse effects of complete bed rest. Baclofen is a medication for spasticity. (A)

16. 1 Loss of motor function to the face and throat can cause dysphagia and places the client at risk for aspiration. Bladder dysfunction and hypertension are not associated with myasthenia gravis. Myasthenia affects nerve impulses at the neuromuscular junction, causing loss of motor function; there is no sensory deficit. (R)

17. 1 The nurse instructs the client regarding use of artificial tears because eyelid and extraocular muscles are frequently affected by myasthenia gravis and there is a risk of corneal abrasion if the eyelids do not close completely. The client is encouraged to maintain social contacts and prevent social isolation by staying at home. Medication is taken in the morning, prior to activities, so the client is able to complete them. A nutritious diet is encouraged and there is no indication to limit protein. (H)

18. 4 There is no cure for ALS. Although the exact action of riluzole (Rilutek) is not known, in studies the drug has shown to slow the progression of the disease to the time a tracheostomy is required or death occurs, but the drug does not improve symptoms. The drug does not improve movement or prevent respiratory failure. (D)

19. 4 The client with GBS experiences paresthesia, involving muscle aches and cramps that may worsen at night. Pain is treated prior to ROM or positioning to improve client comfort with these activities. An indwelling catheter may be required for a flaccid bladder, but is not a routine need. (R)

20. 2 GBS is a rapidly progressing neurologic disorder causing demyelination of the peripheral nerves, which can result in respiratory failure as muscle weakness ascends to the thorax. Clients may require mechanical ventilation until remyelination occurs and neurologic function returns. Most clients recover without residual symptoms or permanent paralysis. Clients can be positioned out of bed to avoid the complications of total bed rest. GBS is often preceded by a viral infection. Antibiotics are not indicated unless the complication of a bacterial infection occurs, such as an upper respiratory or urinary tract infection. (A)

chapter 31

The Client With Musculoskeletal Health Problems

Adult clients are at risk for musculoskeletal health problems as a result of normal aging processes such as osteoporosis. Adults, and particularly older adults, are also at risk for falls and fractures because of problems with balance and sensorimotor disturbances. The nurse has an important role in teaching adult clients about health-promotion behaviors, as well as in assisting these clients adapt to living with chronic illness and musculoskeletal pain. The following topics are discussed in this chapter:

- Fractures
- Rheumatoid Arthritis
- Osteoarthritis
- Amputation
- Herniated Intervertebral Disk
- Spinal Cord Injury

Fractures

I. Definition: A fracture is a break in the continuity of a bone when stress placed on the bone is greater than what it can absorb. Stress may be mechanical in nature (resulting from trauma), or related to a disease process (pathologic). Osteoporosis is a major risk factor in the elderly, especially for hip and vertebral compression fractures. Hip fractures are common in clients over 65 years of age, and occur more frequently in women than in men because of osteoporosis; by 80 years of age, one in five women will fracture a hip. Because of high incidence in older adult clients, this section indicates specific information related to, and care for, fractures of the hip. Other common fractures include fractures of the pelvis, ribs, and wrist (Colles fracture).
   A. Fractures are classified according to type and extent:
      1. Closed simple, uncomplicated—no break in skin
      2. Open compound, complicated—involves trauma to surrounding tissue, and a break in the skin
      3. Incomplete—partial cross-sectional break with incomplete bone disruption
      4. Complete—complete cross-sectional break severing periosteum (bone covering)
      5. Comminuted—involves several breaks of bone, producing splinters and fragments
      6. Green stick—involves break in one side of bone and a bend in the other
      7. Spiral (torsion)—involves fracture twisting around shaft of bone
      8. Transverse—occurs straight across bone
      9. Oblique—occurs at an angle across bone (less than transverse)
   B. A fracture of the hip refers to a fracture of the proximal third of the femur that extends up to 5 cm below the lesser trochanter.
      1. Fractures that occur within the hip joint capsule are called *intracapsular fractures,* and are often associated with osteoporosis and minor trauma. Intracapsular fractures are further identified by specific locations:
         a. Capsular—fracture of the head of the femur
         b. Subcapsular—fractures just below the head of the femur
         c. Transcervical—fractures of the neck of the femur
      2. Extracapsular fractures occur outside joint capsule and are usually caused by severe direct trauma or a fall.
         a. Intertrochanteric—fracture occurs between greater and lesser trochanter
         b. Subtrochanteric—fracture occurs below lesser trochanter
   C. When a fracture occurs, other body components may sustain injury, including the muscles, blood vessels, nerves, tendons and ligaments, joints, and body organs.
   D. Complications of fractures include:
      1. Problems associated with immobility, such as muscle atrophy, joint contractures, and pressure ulcers
      2. Growth problems (occur in children; see Chapter 18)
      3. Infection
      4. Shock
      5. Venous stasis, thromboembolism
      6. Pulmonary emboli, fat emboli
      7. Bone union problems

II. Nursing process
   A. Assessment: *Note: Any client with suspected fracture is treated as though fracture is present until ruled out.*
      1. Perform a comprehensive physical examination; assess for general signs and symptoms of fracture.
         a. Pain, tenderness
         b. Edema
         c. Abnormal movement, crepitus, loss of function
         d. Ecchymosis
         e. Visible deformity, loss of normal bony/limb contour
         f. Paresthesias and other sensory abnormalities
         g. Neurovascular dysfunction, joint effusion, excessive joint laxity
      2. Assess for signs and symptoms of hip fracture.
         a. External rotation of affected extremity
         b. Muscle spasm
         c. Shortening of affected extremity
         d. Pain or tenderness in affected hip or leg involving sudden or severe onset, of insidious nature, and progressive with difficulty or inability to bear weight on leg
         e. Loss of normal bony contour
         f. Edema
         g. Ecchymosis
         h. Limited or abnormal range of motion (ROM)
         i. With open fracture, bone may be exposed
      3. For older adult clients, assess for factors that contribute to occurrence of hip fracture:
         a. Tendency to fall due to gait or balance problems, decreased vision or hearing,

decreased reflexes, orthostatic hypotension, and medication use.
   b. Inadequacy of local tissue shock absorbers (fat, muscle bulk).
   c. Decreased skeletal strength.
4. Obtain diagnostic tests.
   a. Standard anteroposterior, lateral x-ray examination—identifies fracture location
   b. Bone scan—determines integrity of bone
   c. Arthroscopy—detects joint involvement; useful in diagnosing intra-articular fracture
   d. Electromyogram—detects nerve injury
   e. Angiogram—used when blood vessels are injured
   f. Laboratory work:
      (1) CBC—hemoglobin and hematocrit may be decreased
      (2) Electrolytes—with muscle damage
   g. MRI—aids in diagnosis; useful in evaluating complicated fractures
   h. CTS—shows abnormalities in complicated fractures

B. Analysis
1. Acute Pain related to edema, movement of bone fragments, and muscle spasms, and tissue trauma
2. Self-Care Deficit: Bathing/Hygiene, related to impaired physical mobility
3. Self-Care Deficit: Dressing/Grooming, related to acute pain or impairment
4. Risk for Deficient Fluid Volume related to impaired mobility
5. Risk for Infection related to disruption of skin integrity
6. Risk for Injury related to impaired physical mobility and use of analgesics
7. Risk for Impaired Gas Exchange related to alteration in blood flow and blood/fat emboli
8. Risk for Peripheral Neurovascular Dysfunction related to vascular insufficiency and nerve compression
9. Risk for Impaired Skin Integrity related to immobility and shearing forces
10. Impaired Physical Mobility related to decreased muscle strength, pain, and presence of immobilization device

C. Planning
1. Promote physiologic healing with no associated complications.
2. Provide pain relief.
3. Facilitate achievement of maximum rehabilitation potential.
4. Prevent fluid volume deficit.
5. Prevent infection.
6. Prevent further musculoskeletal injury.
7. Promote adequate ventilation and gas exchange.
8. Identify risk factors for injury.
9. Maintain muscle strength, tone, and joint ROM.
10. Promote comfort.
11. Prevent development of a thrombus.

D. Implementation: Provide appropriate nursing interventions associated with prescribed treatment modalities.
1. Cast application
   a. Prepare client, and assist with application of cast, as needed.
   b. Provide cast care.
      (1) Support cast with palms of hands (to prevent indentations—pressure sources).
      (2) Ensure that stockinet is pulled over rough edges of cast.
      (3) Elevate casted extremity above level of heart.
      (4) Expose fresh plaster cast to circulating air, uncovered, until dry (24 to 72 hr).
      (5) Expose fresh synthetic cast until is completely set (about 20 min).
      (6) Instruct client to avoid wetting cast; if synthetic cast gets wet, instruct to dry with hair dryer on cool setting.
      (7) Do neurovascular assessments on involved extremity every 4 hr.
   c. Provide pain relief as needed.
   d. Observe for signs and symptoms of cast syndrome with clients who are immobilized in large casts.
   e. Provide nursing care for compartment syndrome.
   f. Notify physician immediately if signs and symptoms of other neurovascular complications occur.
   g. Notify physician if "hot spots" occur along cast; they may indicate infection under cast.
   h. Provide client and family teaching.
   i. Ensure proper technique and procedure in cast removal.
2. Traction application
   a. Promote measures to prevent complications of immobility.
      (1) Turn/reposition regularly within limitations of traction.
      (2) Prevent constipation by increasing fluid intake of 2,000 to 2,500 ml/day and diet high in fiber.

b. Promote skin integrity.
   (1) Keep bed linens wrinkle-free.
   (2) Provide skin care to areas of potential pressure.
   (3) Inspect for signs of skin breakdown when in skin traction.
   (4) Inspect skeletal traction sites for signs of irritation or infection.
      (a) Assess pin entrance/exit sites, areas surrounding pin sites at least 2 times per day.
      (b) Clean pin sites as prescribed.
      (c) Never remove weights with skeletal traction.

c. Provide client and family teaching (see reduction of risk potential).

d. Promote self-care within traction limitations.

3. Orthopaedic surgery
   a. Provide preoperative care (see physiologic adaptation for surgical interventions).
   b. Provide postoperative care.
      (1) Monitor blood loss at operative site.
      (2) Monitor incision site for infection.
      (3) Perform regular neurovascular assessment.
      (4) Turn, reposition, and exercise unaffected body parts every 2 hr or as prescribed.
      (5) Elevate extremity to minimize edema, unless contraindicated.
      (6) Encourage early ambulation with progressive weight bearing, as prescribed.
      (7) Instruct in proper use of assistive devices.
      (8) Apply antiembolism stockings, sequential compression device to help prevent deep vein thrombosis.
      (9) Position client with total hip replacement with abductor pillow to prevent external rotation of leg; turn as prescribed.
      (10) With total knee replacement, monitor response to continuous passive motion machine, if used, on operative leg.

E. Evaluation
   1. Client's fracture heals with no associated complications.
   2. Client verbalizes control of pain with minimal or no discomfort.
   3. Client achieves maximum mobility through active participation in prescribed rehabilitation program.
   4. Client is free from signs and symptoms of fluid volume deficit.
   5. Client is free from signs and symptoms of infection.
   6. Client reports no additional injuries.
   7. Client demonstrates adequate ventilation with normal ABG analysis results.
   8. Client's distal peripheral pulses in affected lower extremity are strong with brisk capillary refill; skin temperature is warm; skin has pink color.
   9. Client's skin is intact with no redness on bony prominences.

III. Client needs
   A. Physiologic adaptation
      1. Emergency status
         a. Splint fracture above and below site of injury.
         b. Apply cold (ice packs).
         c. Elevate limb to reduce edema and pain.
         d. Control bleeding; provide fluid replacement to prevent shock, if necessary.
      2. Traction for fractures of long bones
         a. Skin traction—force applied to skin using foam rubber and tapes (Buck's traction)
         b. Skeletal traction—force applied to bony skeleton directly using wires, pins, or tongs placed into or through bone (balanced suspension traction)
         c. External fixation—metal frame and pin system used to stabilize complex and open fracture (Kirschner wires or Steinmann pins)
      3. Surgical interventions—for some older adult clients, nonoperative treatment is preferable if unable to tolerate anesthesia, or client was nonambulatory before fracture occurred. Surgery may also be delayed for brief time until general health stabilized; skeletal traction or spica casting used.
         a. Closed reduction—bony fragments are brought into contact with each other by manipulation, and manual traction restores alignment; cast or splint applied to immobilize and maintain reduction.
         b. Open reduction and internal fixation—involves visualization, realignment of fracture fragments through surgical incision. Internal fixation performed using plates, screws, rods, or pins to maintain fragment position.
         c. Endoprosthetic replacement—replacement of fracture fragment with

implanted metal device; used when fracture disrupts nutrition of bone.
   - d. Additional surgical interventions for fractures of the hip:
     - (1) Insertion of femoral head prosthesis.
     - (2) Total hip arthroplasty—replacement of damaged hip with an artificial joint.
4. Stages of fracture healing
   - a. Fracture hematoma—occurs in initial 72 hr after surgery; bleeding and edema create hematoma that surrounds ends of bone fragments.
   - b. Granulation tissue—occurs 3 to 14 days postinjury; hematoma converts to granulation tissue consisting of new blood vessels, fibroblasts, and osteoblasts.
   - c. Callus formation—occurs by end of second week after injury; involves unorganized network of bone that forms and surrounds fracture parts.
   - d. Ossification—occurs 3 weeks to 6 months after fracture; prevents movement at fracture site even though fracture is still evident.
   - e. Consolidation—ossification continues.
   - f. Remodeling—can occur up to 1 year following injury; involves excess bone tissue reabsorbed in this final stage; union is completed.

B. Management of care: Care of the client with a fracture requires critical thinking skills and knowledge of assessment, and teaching and evaluation methods unique to the RN role. These skills cannot be delegated to an LPN or UAP.

1. Delegate responsibly those activities that can be delegated. All monitoring information is reported to the RN.
   - a. Monitor vital signs.
   - b. Monitor intake and output.
   - c. Encourage coughing and deep breathing.
   - d. Apply cold (ice packs).
   - e. Apply elastic hose.
   - f. Assist with activities of daily living, as needed.
   - g. Perform passive ROM exercises to all nonimmobilized joints; encourage client to perform active ROM exercises.
   - h. Teach relaxation techniques.
   - i. Assist nurse in use of logrolling techniques—to turn in bed.
   - j. Keep skin clean and dry; prevent skin breakdown.
2. Consult dietitian regarding the following:
   - a. Need for balanced diet—to promote bone and soft tissue healing.
   - b. Need for protein of high biologic value.
   - c. Need for adequate calcium, phosphorus, magnesium, and fluids in addition to provision of vitamin D, C, and A.
3. Consult with orthopaedic physician or surgeon, as well as physical therapist, or rehabilitation personnel.
4. Consult with orthopaedic supply firm for collars, splints, slings/swathes, walkers, canes, or other assistive devices.
5. Nurse may consult occupational therapist to provide assistive devices as needed, such as elevated toilet seat; tub or shower chair; and long-handled shoehorn or stocking-helper.
6. Refer client to support group or for psychotherapy, as needed.

C. Safety and infection control

1. Assure traction lines and weights are hanging freely and in proper position.
2. Perform wound care: Clean, debride, and irrigate open fracture wound, as prescribed, to minimize risk of infection.
3. Use sterile technique during dressing changes.
4. Evaluate for pressure from equipment (casts, traction, splints, or other appliances).
5. If femoral head prosthesis was inserted, provide client and family teaching to prevent dislocation:
   - a. Use elevated toilet seat.
   - b. Remain seated on tub or shower chair while washing.
   - c. Use pillow between legs for first 8 weeks after surgery.
   - d. Notify surgeon if severe pain, deformity, or loss of function occurs.
6. If treated by hip pinning, dislocation precautions are not necessary.
7. Assess for skin breakdown on all pressure points.
8. During transfer, provide support of affected body part.

D. Health promotion and maintenance: Provide client and family teaching.

1. Explain fracture treatment and need for participation in therapeutic regimen.
2. Encourage client to become involved in active exercises as soon as possible.
3. Teach client to recognize and report symptoms needing immediate medical attention.
4. Prevent fracture of the hip:
   - a. Provide supplementation of calcium and vitamin D.

b. Provide bone growth regulator (alendronate sodium [Fosamax]) as prescribed by physician.
c. Encourage weight-bearing exercise daily (walking).
d. Eliminate loose rugs, slippery or uneven surfaces within home.
e. Provide adequate lighting at all times.
f. Encourage client to wear supportive shoes and slippers that fit appropriately.

E. Psychologic integrity
1. Assist client to move through phases of posttraumatic stress; these include outcry, denial, intrusiveness, working through, and completion.
2. Encourage client to participate in decision-making to re-establish control and overcome feelings of helplessness.
3. Teach relaxation techniques to decrease anxiety.
4. Monitor for signs and symptoms of depression during hospitalization and period of rehabilitation. Refer to clinical psychologist, psychiatrist, if needed.

F. Basic care and comfort
1. Administer oxygen as directed.
2. Elevate injured extremity unless compartment syndrome is suspected.
3. Provide appropriate nursing interventions associated with prescribed treatment modalities (see implementation).

G. Reduction of risk potential
1. Observe for symptoms of compartment syndrome, including deep, unrelenting pain; hard, edematous muscle; and decreased tissue perfusion with impaired neurovascular assessment findings. Prescribed treatments include:
a. Fasciotomy
b. Bivalve cast
c. Release of constrictive dressings
2. Observe for symptoms of life-threatening fat emboli, which include personality changes; restlessness; dyspnea; crackles; white, frothy sputum; and petechiae over chest and buccal membranes.
3. Monitor for sudden, progressive changes in respiratory status that may indicate pulmonary embolus.
4. Monitor for development of thrombophlebitis—indicated by pain, tenderness in calf, increased size, and warmth of calf (see also pharmacologic and parenteral therapies).
5. Prevent development of thromboembolism.
a. Encourage active and passive ROM exercise.
b. Use sequential compression devices, elastic hose or bandages, as prescribed.
c. Avoid pressure on blood vessels.
d. Encourage client to move within limitations posed by traction, casts, or other orthopaedic equipment.
e. Administer anticoagulants as directed.
6. Monitor for development of infection (see also pharmacologic and parenteral therapies).
7. For older adult clients, consider coexisting chronic health problems (diabetes mellitus, hypertension, cardiac disease, pulmonary disease, arthritis, bleeding disorders) and the impact on healing and recovery.
8. For large casts (body, hip spica), observe for signs and symptoms of cast syndrome:
a. Abdominal pain and distention
b. Nausea and vomiting
c. Elevated BP
d. Rapid pulse, rapid respirations
9. If client is claustrophobic, or is at risk for psychologic cast syndrome, monitor for acute anxiety and rational behavior.
10. Provide client and family teaching about the following:
a. Prescribed activity restrictions and necessary lifestyle modifications (because of impaired mobility)
b. Methods of safe ambulation with assistive devices (cane, walker, or crutches)
c. Prescribed medications
(1) Use of less potent drugs as severity of discomfort decreases
(2) Nonpharmacologic measures for pain reduction:
(a) Cutaneous stimulation
(b) Distraction
(c) Guided imagery
(d) Transcutaneous electrical nerve stimulation and biofeedback
d. Importance of following instructions concerning amount of weight bearing permitted on fractured extremity
e. Use of isometric exercises (to diminish muscle atrophy and prevent development of disuse syndrome)
11. If client receiving anticoagulants, watch for signs of bleeding (easy bruising, bleeding gums, pale skin or mucous membranes, and decreased hemoglobin and hematocrit).

H. Pharmacologic and parenteral therapies: Client and family will state the purpose for and side effects of all medications.
1. During a closed reduction procedure, the following classifications of medications may be used: Local anesthetic, opioid analgesic,

muscle relaxant; sedative. Note: General anesthesia may be used during a closed reduction.
   a. Client-controlled analgesia: Morphine (Duramorph) and hydromorphone hydrochloride (Dilaudid)
   b. Epidural analgesia—monitor response to analgesia and client respiratory rate
2. Broad-spectrum antibiotics may be ordered to prevent or treat infections caused by pathogenic micro-organisms: Amoxicillin (Amoxil); erythromycin (Erythrocin).
3. Prevention of deep vein thrombosis is primary goal after open reduction and internal fixation of hip fracture; the following is used for clot prophylaxis:
   a. Low-molecular-weight heparin—enoxaparin (Lovenox)
   b. Warfarin (Coumadin)—prophylaxis and treatment of deep vein thrombosis
4. Stool softeners prevent constipation.
   a. Docusate sodium (Colace)
   b. Docusate calcium (Surfak)
5. Laxatives manage constipation due to impaired mobility, opioid analgesia.
   a. Magnesium hydroxide (Milk of Magnesia)
   b. Bisacodyl (Dulcolax)
6. Skeletal muscle relaxants—instruct client not to take with alcohol or other CNS depressants (effects may be additive):
   a. Methocarbamol (Robaxin)
   b. Carisoprodol (Soma)
7. IV fluids—monitor for signs of fluid volume overload (crackles in lung bases, dyspnea, tachypnea, tachycardia):
   a. Dextrose 5%/water (D5/W)—isotonic, hypotonic
   b. Lactated Ringer (LR)—isotonic
   c. Normal saline (NS; 0.9% NaCl)—isotonic

Rheumatoid Arthritis

I. Definition: Rheumatoid arthritis is a chronic, systemic, autoimmune disease characterized by inflammatory polyarthritis involving small and large peripheral joints and surrounding muscles, tendons, ligaments, and blood vessels. A potentially crippling disease, rheumatoid arthritis is marked by spontaneous remissions and unpredictable exacerbations often associated with increased physical or emotional stress. Although rheumatoid arthritis can occur at any age, the peak onset is between 35 and 50 years of age. Incidence is 3 times greater in women than in men.

II. Nursing process
A. Assessment
1. Assess for insidious onset of nonspecific symptoms.
   a. Fatigue
   b. Malaise
   c. Anorexia
   d. Persistent low-grade fever
   e. Weight loss
   f. Vague joint-related symptoms
2. As disease progresses, assess for more specific localized joint (articular) symptoms (commonly in fingers).
   a. Bilateral, symmetrical symptoms
   b. May extend to wrists, elbows, knees, ankles
   c. Warm, tender, edematous, painful joints with stiffness lasting longer than 30 min after arising
   d. Rheumatoid nodules
   e. Joint deformities, contractures
   f. Loss of sensation in fingers, numbness or tingling in feet, weakness
3. Assess for systemic effects.
   a. Cardiac manifestations—acute pericarditis, conduction defects, valvular insufficiency, and coronary arteritis
   b. Pulmonary manifestations—pleural effusion and interstitial fibrosis
   c. Neurologic manifestations—wrist drop, foot drop, carpal tunnel syndrome, and compression of spinal nerve roots
4. Assess for presence of deformities.
   a. Proximal interphalangeal joints hyperextend (Swan neck)
   b. Proximal interphalangeal joints flex (Boutonniere)
   c. Altered functional status
5. Observe for presence of difficulty with mobility and performance of activities of daily living.
6. Obtain diagnostic tests.
   a. CBC—decreased hemoglobin, hematocrit
   b. Rheumatoid factor—positive
   c. Erythrocyte sedimentation rate—elevated
   d. Synovial fluid analysis—turbid, yellow color; white blood cell count 2,000 to 75,000/mm^3; low viscosity
   e. X-rays
      (1) Hands, wrists: Marginal erosions of proximal interphalangeal, metacarpophalangeal, and carpal bones; generalized osteopenia
      (2) Cervical spine: Erosions producing vertebral subluxation

f. MRI—shows spinal cord compression resulting from C1-C2 subluxation and compression of surrounding vascular structures
g. Bone scan—shows "increased uptake" in involved joints
h. Synovial biopsy—may be done to rule out other causes of polyarthritis by noting the absence of other pathologic findings
i. Serum globulin levels—elevated

B. Analysis
1. Acute Pain related to inflammation
2. Chronic Pain related to joint inflammation, overuse of joint, and ineffective pain and/or comfort measures
3. Deficient Knowledge related to lack of information about disease process and treatment modalities
4. Fatigue related to discomfort, effects of prolonged mobility, and psychoemotional demands of chronic illness
5. Ineffective Role Performance related to chronic disease activity, long-term treatment, deformities, and stiffness
6. Ineffective Therapeutic Regimen Management related to complexity of chronic health problem, pain, and fatigue
7. Disturbed Body Image related to development of joint deformities

C. Planning
1. Promote increased comfort and decreased pain.
2. Facilitate attainment of highest degree of mobility within confines of the disease.
3. Use strategies to maintain skin integrity.
4. Encourage client to verbalize feelings about limitations.
5. Promote positive perception of well-being.
6. Schedule rest periods among periods of prolonged activity.
7. Aid in attainment of accurate body image.

D. Implementation
1. Administer prescribed medications.
2. Provide pain relief.
3. Promote self-care.
4. Promote client and family coping.
5. Promote adequate rest and sleep.
6. Encourage proper body alignment.
7. Discuss relaxation techniques.
8. Discuss maintaining optimal nutritional status.

E. Evaluation
1. Client reports increased comfort and decreased pain.
2. Client describes working toward attainment of highest degree of mobility within confines of disease.
3. Client is free from signs of skin breakdown.
4. Client verbalizes feeling about limitations.
5. Client verbalizes positive perception of well-being.
6. Client has periods of rest between periods of prolonged activity.
7. Client describes positive perception of body image.

CN

III. Client needs

A. Physiologic adaptation: Inflammatory process occurs in four stages.
1. Synovitis develops from congestion and edema of synovial membrane and joint capsule.
2. Pannus (thickened layers of granulation tissue) covers and invades cartilage, eventually destroying joint capsule and bone.
3. Fibrous ankylosis (fibrous invasion of pannus and scar formation) occludes joint space. Bone atrophy and misalignment cause visible deformities and disrupt the articulation of opposing bones, resulting in muscle atrophy, imbalance, and, possibly, partial dislocations (subluxations).
4. Fibrous tissue calcifies, resulting in bony ankylosis and total immobility.

B. Management of care: Care of the client with rheumatoid arthritis requires critical thinking skills and knowledge of assessment, and teaching and evaluation methods unique to the RN role. These skills cannot be delegated to an LPN or UAP.
1. Refer client to physical therapy and occupational therapy.
   a. Physical therapy program, including ROM exercises and individualized therapeutic exercises, forestalls loss of joint function.
   b. Occupational therapy program—helps maintain independence.
2. Be aware of potential problems in job, child care, maintenance of home, and social and family functioning that may result.
3. Refer to social worker or mental health counselor, as needed.
4. Refer client and family to the Arthritis Foundation, www.arthritis.org.
5. Consult dietitian—recommendations include reduction of overall fat intake, changing oils in the diet, and eating oil-rich, cold-water fish at least 2 times per week.
6. Consult with clinical psychologist to assist client in discussing changes caused by

illness, and separate physical appearance from feelings of personal worth, as well as behavior modification, biofeedback, and relaxation techniques.
7. Provide referral/consultation with sex therapist.
    a. Sexual problems/concerns can have a serious impact on body image.
    b. Include spouse/sexual partner in counseling to encourage communication.

C. Safety and infection control
1. To decrease likelihood of injury, encourage client's use of adjunctive aids including long-handled reacher, long-handled shoehorn, elastic shoelaces, Velcro fasteners, crutches, walker, and cane. Arrange for occupational therapist to teach correct use of braces, splints, and assistive mobility devices.
2. Help client obtain appropriate assistive devices (raised toilet seat, special eating utensils).
3. Use therapeutic guidelines with application of local heat or cold to affected joints.
    a. Apply heat or cold for 15 to 20 min 3 to 4 times per day.
    b. Avoid temperatures likely to cause skin or tissue damage by checking temperature of warm soaks or covering cold packs with a towel.
4. Arrange for physical therapist to teach correct use of adjunctive pain control measures.
    a. Transcutaneous electrical nerve stimulation unit
    b. Progressive skeletal muscle relaxation
5. Provide meticulous skin care.
6. Assess for sensory disturbances.

D. Health promotion and maintenance
1. Provide client and family teaching about disease, disease process, medication regimen, and need for continued follow-up care (see also pharmacologic and parenteral therapies).
2. Encourage use of splints to prevent contractures.
3. Encourage exercise consistent with degree of disease activity.
4. Encourage warm bath or shower in morning on arising to decrease morning stiffness and improve mobility.
5. Provide information on the support and services offered by the Arthritis Foundation.

E. Psychologic integrity
1. Identify significance of client's culture, religion, race, sex, and age on body image.
2. Assist client to discuss changes caused by illness.
3. Make referral to mental health professional, as needed.

F. Basic care and comfort
1. Monitor ability of client to follow self-care plan.
2. Establish a routine for self-care activities with rest periods to foster maximum independence with minimal fatigue.
3. Assist client in accepting dependency needs to ensure all needs are met; instruct family to encourage independence and intervene only when the client is unable to perform to promote independence.
4. Assess joint mobility, activity tolerance, and level of pain and discomfort; evaluate with client, family, and health care team, the effectiveness of past pain control measures used to assess what are the most useful measures.
5. Reduce or eliminate factors that precipitate or increase pain experience, such as fear, fatigue, and lack of knowledge, to minimize negative stimuli that may increase pain.
6. Teach use of nonpharmacologic techniques (relaxation, distraction, warm applications, and massage) before pain occurs or increases to promote muscle relaxation and decrease tension.
7. Provide prescribed analgesics, as appropriate, to help decrease pain, inflammation.
8. Supply adaptive devices such as a zipper-pull, easy-to-open cartons, lightweight cups.

G. Reduction of risk potential
1. Stress importance of laboratory follow-up while taking prescribed medications to monitor for potential adverse reactions:
    a. CBC and urinalysis while on gold and penicillamine (Cuprimine, Depen), a chelating agent
    b. Ophthalmologic examinations while taking hydroxychloroquine (Plaquenil)
    c. Liver function tests (aspartate aminotransferase, alanine aminotransferase) while taking etanercept (Enbrel)
2. Inform client of potential concurrent pathologic conditions such as pericarditis and ocular lesions, and need to promptly report these to physician.
3. If surgical intervention was required to correct connective tissue defect or remove loose bodies, follow postoperative orders of physician such as elevation of extremity; perform passive or active ROM, as appropriate; turn, cough, deep breathe at regular intervals; and participate in own self-care as soon as possible. Report numbness, paresthesias, and edema formation to surgeon.

H. Pharmacologic and parenteral therapies: Client will state the purpose for and associated side effects of all medications used to manage rheumatoid arthritis. Client teaching is as follows:
   1. Nonsteroidal anti-inflammatory drugs—used to relieve pain, inflammation (ibuprofen [Motrin]; naproxen [Naprosyn])
      a. Take with food to minimize GI upset.
      b. Report to physician increased ease of bruising and presence of tinnitus (ringing in ears).
   2. Disease-modifying antirheumatic drugs to reduce disease activity such as oral or injectable gold, hydroxychloroquine (Plaquenil), penicillamine (Cuprimine, Depen), leflunomide (Arava), and etanercept (Enbrel).
      a. Have liver enzymes (aspartate aminotransferase, alanine aminotransferase) checked every month for 12 months, then every 6 months thereafter.
      b. Withhold drug if infection develops; notify the physician.
      c. Report adverse effects to physician, such as hair loss, weight loss, GI distress, and rash or itching.
      d. Use reliable contraception.
   3. Corticosteroids—to reduce inflammatory process (prednisone [Deltasone], methylprednisolone [Medrol])
      a. Take drug exactly as directed; taper drug rather than stop abruptly (could cause serious withdrawal symptoms leading to adrenal insufficiency, shock, and death).
      b. Report adverse effects to physician, such as cushingoid effects (weight gain, moon face, buffalo hump, and hirsutism); may also mask signs and symptoms of infection and can elevate blood glucose level.
   4. IV fluids used:
      a. Normal saline (NS; 0.9% NaCl)—isotonic
      b. 5% dextrose/water (D5/W)—isotonic, hypotonic
      c. Lactated Ringer (LR)—isotonic

Osteoarthritis

I. Definition: Osteoarthritis, or degenerative joint disease, is the most common form of arthritis, and is characterized by progressive deterioration and loss of articular (joint) cartilage accompanied by proliferation of new bone and soft tissue in and around involved joints. Osteoarthritis may have a genetic basis in some clients; in others, the cause may be attributed to allergens or inflammation that can contribute to degeneration. Osteoarthritis is associated with aging, but not caused by it. Secondary causes include obesity, diabetes mellitus, congenital diseases of the bones, and trauma and injury. The disorder affects both sexes about equally, with onset usually after 40 years of age. If untreated, osteoarthritis leads to limited mobility, and in some cases, neurologic deficits are associated with spinal involvement.
   A. Osteoarthritis may be classified as primary or secondary.
      1. Primary idiopathic osteoarthritis refers to disorder when no underlying cause is apparent.
      2. Secondary osteoarthritis involves a predisposing factor such as trauma, congenital abnormality, or metabolic disorder.
   B. Osteoarthritis is characterized by site specificity, with certain synovial joints showing higher disease prevalence. These include:
      1. Weight-bearing joints (hips, knees).
      2. Cervical and lumbar spine.
      3. Distal interphalangeal, proximal interphalangeal (PIP), and metacarpophalangeal joints in the hands.
      4. Metatarsophalangeal joints in the feet (bunion deformity, or hallux valgus).
      5. Gender differences: Hips are more commonly affected in men, whereas hands are more commonly affected in women (especially after menopause).

II. Nursing process
   A. Assessment
      1. Perform a comprehensive physical assessment; assess for joint pain and stiffness—typically, these are most dominant symptoms and common reason for seeking medical evaluation.
         a. Onset of pain is insidious; client describes an "aching" asymmetric pain that increases with joint use, and is relieved by rest; as progresses, night pain or pain at rest is likely.
         b. Pain may increase with fall in barometric pressure that precedes inclement weather.
      2. Assess for additional signs and symptoms.
         a. Joint swelling or deformity
         b. Hard nodes on distal or proximal interphalangeal joints of fingers, known as *Heberden nodes* (when present on distal interphalangeal joints) and *Bouchard nodes* (when present on proximal interphalangeal joints)

c. Reduced ROM in joints
d. Leg-length discrepancy—possibly due to loss of joint space in advanced hip osteoarthritis
e. Muscle atrophy—in advanced disease secondary to joint splinting for pain relief
3. Obtain diagnostic tests.
a. X-rays of affected joints—show joint-space narrowing, osteophytes (bone spurs), and sclerosis
b. Bone scan—shows increased uptake in affected bones
c. Synovial fluid analysis—differentiates osteoarthritis from rheumatoid arthritis (by low cell count)
d. MRI—more sensitive than x-ray in marking progression of joint destruction

B. Analysis
1. Acute or Chronic Pain related to arthritic joint changes, and associated therapy
2. Impaired Physical Mobility related to musculoskeletal impairment and adjustment to new walking gait with an assistive device
3. Ineffective Sexuality Pattern related to pain, decreased joint function, or body image changes that interfere with sexual performance
4. Disturbed Sleep Pattern related to pain
5. Self-Care Deficit: Dressing/Grooming, related to joint deformity and pain with activity
6. Imbalanced Nutrition: More Than Body Requirements related to intake in excess of energy output
7. Chronic Low Self-Esteem related to changing physical appearance and social and work roles

C. Planning
1. Decrease pain and discomfort.
2. Promote physical mobility with aid of assistive devices, if needed.
3. Promote increased physical and psychologic comfort during sexual intimacy.
4. Provide optimal pain relief to promote likelihood of restful sleep.
5. Decrease self-care deficits.
6. Maintain nutritional balance.
7. Modify inaccurate perception of self.

D. Implementation
1. Administer prescribed medications.
2. Provide nonpharmacologic comfort measures.
3. Position to prevent flexion deformity.
4. Plan activities that promote optimal function and independence.
5. Prepare for surgical treatment, as indicated.
6. Provide balanced nutritional intake.

E. Evaluation
1. Client verbalizes decrease in pain.
2. Client demonstrates ability to perform some activities of daily living with minimal discomfort.
3. Client demonstrates appropriate use of assistive devices.
4. Client describes increased physical and psychologic comfort during sexual intimacy.
5. Client reports longer periods of uninterrupted rest and sleep.
6. Client requests assistance with self-care activities that joint deformity and pain do not permit.
7. Client attains and maintains balanced nutrition.
8. Client describes feelings of being socially engaged.

CN

III. Client needs

A. Physiologic adaptation: Osteoarthritis is managed with medications (see pharmacologic and parenteral therapies), along with the following:
1. Joint protection (total joint replacement may be considered if hips or knees are involved):
a. Rest affected joint during periods of acute inflammation; restrict weight bearing.
b. Apply splints or braces to maintain joint in functional position.
c. Limit joint immobilization for not more than 1 week; additional stiffness can result from prolonged rest.
2. Exercise and activity—ensure that regular exercise is performed; modify occupational and recreational activity to protect joint from stress.
a. Promote joint loading and mobilization to articular cartilage maintenance.
b. Prevent quadriceps muscle weakness, which can contribute to progressive articular damage.
3. Weight reduction, if needed, to improve arthritis symptoms and slow disease progression.

B. Management of care: Care of the client with osteoarthritis requires critical thinking skills and knowledge of assessment, and teaching and evaluation methods unique to the RN role. These skills cannot be delegated to an LPN or UAP.
1. Delegate responsibly those activities that can be delegated. All monitoring information is reported to the RN.

a. Monitor vital signs.
b. Assist with basic hygienic care.
c. Provide assistance with ambulation and other activity, as needed.
d. Provide application of heat or cold as prescribed.
e. Provide and set up food tray.
f. Assist with feeding, if needed.
g. Assist with use of assistive devices, as needed.

2. Provide client and family teaching regarding ways to protect joint and conserve energy (see safety and infection control) and adverse effects of medications (see reduction of risk potential).
3. Consult with physical therapist—may prescribe and implement modified weight-bearing exercises within client's tolerance level.
4. Consult with occupational therapist—may help with self-management strategies with use of assistive devices, as needed.
5. Consult with dietitian.
   a. If client is overweight, promote weight-reduction program (critical part of total treatment plan).
   b. Assist client and family to evaluate current diet to make appropriate changes.
6. Consult with orthopaedic surgeon, if needed.
7. Provide referrals to Arthritis Foundation, support groups.

C. Safety and infection control: Instruct client and family in ways to protect joint and conserve energy.
1. Use assistive devices, if indicated.
2. Avoid forceful repetitive movements.
3. Avoid positions of joint deviation and stress.
4. Use good posture and proper body mechanics.
5. Seek assistance with necessary tasks that may cause pain.
6. Modify environment to create less stressful ways to perform tasks.
7. Receive fluid intake of at least 2,500 ml of fluid per day.

D. Health promotion and maintenance
1. Instruct client to perform isometric exercises and graded exercises to improve muscle strength around involved joint.
2. Advise client to perform ROM exercises after periods of inactivity.
3. Suggest client perform important activities in the morning after stiffness has lessened, and before fatigue and pain become problems.
4. Advise client on lifestyle modifications such as wearing clothes that are less constrictive and without buttons, and using a tub or shower chair for bathing.
5. Assist client with acquisition of assistive devices (padded handles for utensils, grooming aids) to promote independence.
6. Encourage client to obtain adequate sleep and eat adequate meals to enhance general health.
7. Refer client for additional information and support to local chapter of Arthritis Foundation, www.arthritis.org.

E. Psychologic integrity
1. Identify significance of client's culture, religion, race, sex, and age on body image.
2. Assist to discuss changes caused by illness, and assist in separating physical appearance from feelings of personal worth.
3. Facilitate contact with other clients with similar changes in body appearance.
4. Provide referral or consultation with counselor, clinical psychologist, or sex therapist.

F. Basic care and comfort
1. Administer analgesics and anti-inflammatory drugs to relieve pain and inflammation.
2. Apply warm compresses to sore joints.
3. Massage surrounding muscles, but not overinflamed joints.
4. Promote adequate rest and reduction of stress.
5. Position client to promote comfort, but also prevent flexion deformity.

G. Reduction of risk potential
1. If prescribed nonsteroidal anti-inflammatory drugs, provide client and family teaching about the following measures:
   a. Use regularly for maximal effect.
   b. Have blood work to monitor renal function (creatinine, blood urea nitrogen), liver function (aspirate aminotransferase, alanine aminotransferase).
   c. Report the following to the physician:
      (1) Signs of bleeding (tarry stool, bruising, petechiae, nosebleeds)
      (2) Edema
      (3) Skin rashes, urticaria
      (4) Persistent headaches
      (5) Visual disturbances
2. If prescribed salicylates, provide client and family teaching regarding the following measures:
   a. Report to physician signs of bleeding, including tarry stools, bruising, petechiae, and nosebleeds.
   b. Take with food, milk, antacids as prescribed, or full glass of water.

c. Use enteric-coated aspirin (Ecotrin) to aid in prevention of gastric ulcer formation and GI bleeding.
d. Promptly report to physician presence of tinnitus and dizziness as these may be signs of aspirin toxicity.

3. If systemic corticosteroids prescribed, provide client and family teaching regarding the following measures:
   a. Do not abruptly stop medication; taper dose slowly (exacerbation of symptoms occurs with abrupt withdrawal).
   b. Report corticosteroid use to surgeon or dentist to avoid postoperative adrenal insufficiency.
   c. Instruct client that side effects of corticosteroid use are like those of Cushing syndrome:
      (1) Fluid retention
      (2) GI irritation
      (3) Osteoporosis
      (4) Insomnia
      (5) Hypertension
      (6) Steroid psychosis
      (7) Secondary diabetes mellitus
      (8) Acne
      (9) Menstrual irregularities in females
      (10) Hirsutism
      (11) Risk of antibiotic-resistant infection
      (12) Bruising
   d. Have the following monitored: Blood glucose level (can be elevated with chronic steroid use), CBC, and potassium level.
   e. Monitor BP and weight; limit sodium intake and report signs of infection.
4. If physician does intra-articular injections of corticosteroids, inform client:
   a. Joint may feel worse immediately after injection.
   b. Improvement lasts weeks to months following injection.
   c. Avoid overusing affected joint after injection.

H. Pharmacologic and parenteral therapies: Client will state the purpose for and associated side effects of all medications used to manage osteoarthritis. Client teaching is as follows:
1. Analgesics, with acetaminophen (Tylenol) first-line therapy; other analgesics such as nonsteroidal anti-inflammatory drugs and tramadol (Ultram) used to manage moderate to moderately severe pain. Monitor the following: CBC, hepatic function (aspartate aminotransferase, alanine aminotransferase), and renal function (creatinine, BUN).
2. Occasionally, opioid analgesics are needed: Oxycodone (OxyContin) with acetaminophen (Percocet) or with aspirin (Percodan), and hydrocodone (Hycodan) with acetaminophen (Vicodin) or with aspirin or acetaminophen (Lortab).
   a. Monitor for constipation; receive adequate fluids and fiber.
   b. Report signs of bleeding with aspirin-containing products.
   c. Have CBC and liver function tests (aspartate aminotransferase, alanine transferase).
   d. Report any CNS or respiratory changes; hold if respirations less than 12 per minute.
3. Topical analgesics: Capsaicin (Capsin) is especially beneficial for knee pain; may be used with other systemic medications.
   a. Avoid contact with eyes or broken/irritated skin.
   b. If applied with bare hand, wash immediately following application.
   c. Avoid tight bandages over areas of application of the cream.
   d. Monitor for increased incidence of cough with angiotensin-converting enzyme inhibitors.
4. IV fluids:
   a. Normal saline (NS; 0.9% NaCl)—isotonic
   b. Lactated Ringer (LR)—isotonic
   c. Dextrose 5%/water (D5/W)—isotonic, hypotonic
5. Complementary and alternative treatments:
   a. Herbal supplements such as ginger and tumeric have been shown to reduce pain and inflammation of osteoarthritis.
   b. Movement therapies provide low-impact form of exercise.
   c. Acupuncture has shown modest beneficial effects.

Amputation

I. Definition: Amputation is the total or partial surgical removal of an extremity. The extent of amputation is based on the level of maximal viable tissue available for wound healing.

A. Indications for amputation
1. Severe toxicity due to gangrene (typically caused by chronic arterial occlusion)
2. Malignant tumors
3. Severe osteomyelitis

4. Intractable limb pain from chronic infections or trophic ulcers
5. Chronic and severe functional impairment due to a damaged extremity from injury or congenital deformities
6. Chronic ischemia from extensive peripheral vascular disease

B. Therapeutic interventions
1. Below-the-knee amputation: Facilitates successful adaptation to prosthesis because of retained knee function; common in peripheral vascular disease.
2. Above-the-knee amputation: Upper extremity amputation; necessitated by trauma or extensive disease.
3. Upper-extremity amputation: Usually necessitated by severe trauma, malignant tumors, or congenital malformation.

C. Types of amputation
1. Open or guillotine: Performed on infected limb because it allows wound to drain freely; involves second surgery for residual limb revisions, and closure after infection has been eradicated.
2. Closed or flap: Performed when there is no evidence of infection and no need for draining.

II. Nursing process

A. Assessment
1. With advanced peripheral vascular disease, assess neurovascular status of involved extremity for:
   a. Pain
   b. Gangrene
   c. Chronic venous stasis ulcer
   d. Infected wound that fails to heal
   e. Dark red color when dependent
   f. Skin for subcutaneous tissue atrophy
2. Obtain a detailed health history to determine causative factors and health problems that can compromise recovery.
3. Obtain diagnostic tests.
   a. Doppler ultrasound—used to document lack of perfusion
   b. Transcutaneous oxygen pressure—offers most accurate assessment of blood supply; best prediction of residual limb healing potential
   c. Plethysmography—evaluates arterial flow through performance of segmental systolic BP measurements
   d. Angiography—aids in determination of level of amputation
   e. Fluorescein fluorometry—determines nutritive blood flow to area through monitoring by fluorometer after injection with fluorescein dye

B. Analysis
1. Disturbed Body Image related to loss of limb
2. Risk for Injury related to altered center of gravity, use of assistive devices, and prosthesis
3. Chronic Pain related to disruption of nerve endings
4. Risk for Disuse Syndrome related to severe pain and immobility secondary to amputation
5. Deficient Knowledge: Care of Residual Limb and Prosthesis, related to signs and symptoms of skin irritation and pressure necrosis
6. Impaired Physical Mobility related to altered center of gravity and use of assistive devices
7. Ineffective Coping related to disturbed body image and altered role performance
8. Risk for Deficient Fluid Volume related to insufficient intake and blood loss during surgery
9. Ineffective Tissue Perfusion: Peripheral, related to altered blood vessel integrity and function

C. Planning
1. Treat underlying health problem.
2. Maintain satisfactory pain control.
3. Facilitate maximum rehabilitation potential with use of prosthesis, if indicated.
4. Develop coping strategies to adjust to body image changes.
5. Enhance development of satisfying lifestyle adjustments.
6. Teach required care for residual limb and prosthesis.
7. Provide list of indications of pressure necrosis, irritation from shrinkage device/prosthesis.
8. Demonstrate components of prescribed exercise regimen.

D. Implementation
1. Administer prescribed medications.
2. Provide preoperative and postoperative interventions as indicated.
3. Assess for and intervene as necessary to prevent or control general postoperative complications; should hematoma form, assist surgeon with aspiration.

E. Evaluation
1. Client demonstrates adaptation to loss of limb and interest in resuming role-related responsibilities.
2. Client is free from signs and symptoms of injury.

3. Client's subjective perception of pain decreases as documented by pain intensity rating scale.
4. Client verbalizes understanding of prescribed exercise regimen and performs exercises independently.
5. Client is free from symptoms of contracture as evidenced by complete ROM of joints and maintenance of muscle mass.
6. Client verbalizes knowledge about care of residual limb, prosthesis, and independently demonstrates wrapping of residual limb.
7. Client verbalizes knowledge about indications of pressure necrosis and irritation from shrinkage device or prosthesis.
8. Client demonstrates physical mobility without loss of balance.
9. Client verbalizes coping strategies to adjust to altered body image and altered role performance.
10. Client has adequate fluid balance.
11. Client's peripheral tissues demonstrate adequate perfusion with warm temperature, and pink skin/mucous membrane color.

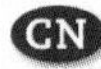

III. Client needs

A. Physiologic adaptation
1. Decrease edema by elevating residual limb for 12 to 24 hr; remove pillow after this to promote functional alignment and prevent contractures.
2. Prevent contractures with the following measures:
   a. Avoid positioning residual limb in externally rotated, abducted position.
   b. Adduct residual limb on regular schedule (to prevent abduction contractures).
   c. Initiate exercises as soon as possible (ideally, on the first or second postoperative day) including:
      (1) Active ROM exercises
      (2) Strengthening exercises
      (3) Hyperextension of residual limb
      (4) Position prone for several hours each day

B. Management of care: Care of the client undergoing amputation requires critical thinking skills and knowledge of assessment, and teaching and evaluation methods unique to the RN role. These skills cannot be delegated to an LPN or UAP.
1. Delegate responsibly those activities that can be delegated. All monitoring information is reported to the RN.
   a. Monitor vital signs.
   b. Monitor intake and output.
   c. Provide high-protein diet with vitamin and mineral supplements.
   d. Provide oral fluids.
   e. Inspect daily residual limb and all bony prominences for evidence of skin breakdown.
   f. Promote activity to help decrease phantom limb pain.
   g. Encourage self-care and independent mobility.
2. Provide client and family teaching regarding care for residual limb and prosthesis (see safety and infection control).
3. Consult with dietitian. Note: Clients with leg amputation expend more energy in ambulation than clients without an amputation.
   a. High biologic-value proteins—to promote healing
   b. Adequate carbohydrate intake—to provide sufficient energy
4. Consult with prosthetist for prosthesis fitting and adjustment; provide client care and teaching as indicated:
   a. Instruct client in crutch walking.
   b. Prepare client for fitting of stump for prosthesis.
   c. Instruct client in exercises to maintain ROM.
   d. Provide psychosocial support.
5. Promote follow-up visits with surgeon and prosthetist.
6. Provide referral to community health nurse to foster optimal physical and emotional adjustment.
7. Provide referral to Amputee Resource Foundation and Amputee Shoe and Glove Exchange.

C. Safety and infection control
1. If wound draining, send wound culture and sensitivity test, as ordered.
2. Recognize that increasing discomfort may indicate presence of hematoma, infection, or necrosis.
3. Promote re-establishment of balance (amputation alters distribution of body weight).
   a. Transfer to chair within 48 hr of surgery.
   b. Instruct and guard lower-limb amputee during balance exercises.
   c. Support plan developed by physical therapist.
4. Provide client and family teaching regarding care for residual limb and prosthesis:
   a. Never adjust or mechanically alter prosthesis without professional help.

b. Inspect and care for remaining limb.
c. Avoid applying creams and lotions (softens skin excessively) or alcohol (dries skin, leading to cracking) to residual limb.
d. Avoid putting adhesive bandages or tape on residual limb as these can irritate skin and cause lesions and infection when pulled off.
e. Inspect residual limb daily with mirror for redness,blistering, and abrasions.
f. Correctly wrap residual limb with elastic bandage to control edema and to form firm conical shape for prosthesis fitting.
g. Wash and dry limb thoroughly at least 2 times per day (removing all soap residue) to prevent skin irritation and infection; avoid soaking residual limb because this results in edema.
h. Wear residual limb sock to absorb perspiration and avoid direct contact between prosthetic socket or harness and skin; avoid wrinkles in residual limb sock to prevent potential pressure areas.
i. Wipe sock of prosthesis with damp cloth when prosthesis is removed for evening.
j. Have prosthesis checked periodically.
k. Protect remaining extremity from injury and secure prompt treatment of problems.

D. Health promotion and maintenance: Instruct client on residual limb conditioning:
1. Push residual limb against soft pillow.
2. Gradually push residual limb against harder surfaces.
3. Massage healed residual limb to soften scar, decrease tenderness, and improve vascularity.

E. Psychologic integrity
1. Support through psychologic acceptance of body image change; anticipate reactions such as anger, denial, withdrawal, and depression.
2. Obtain psychologic referral as indicated.
3. Use resources to help strengthen coping skills, such as social worker, clergy, and client family and friends.
4. Encourage participation in rehabilitation planning and self-care.
5. Observe for signs of depression, despondency (withdrawal, decreased appetite, excessive sleeping, loss of interest in others, activities).

F. Basic care and comfort
1. Provide proper positioning; prevent contractures.
2. Maintain skin integrity.
3. Believe client who reports phantom pain.
   a. Pain phenomenon is real to client.
   b. Medicate for pain, as ordered.
4. Involve client in activities of self-care to promote independence.

G. Reduction of risk potential
1. Monitor for signs of excessive blood loss—indicated by hypotension, widening pulse pressure, tachycardia, diaphoresis, restlessness, decreased alertness.
   a. Report excessive bleeding promptly to surgeon and regular physician.
   b. Keep tourniquet ready to apply to residual limb.
   c. Reinforce dressing as required, using aseptic technique.
   d. Maintain accurate record of bloody drainage on dressing (outline blood stains on dressings) and in drainage system.
   e. Observe every 10 min for 24 hr.
2. Maintain pressure dressing; reapply, if necessary using sterile dressing secured with elastic bandage.
3. Instruct client to avoid long periods in bed in one position to prevent dependent edema, flexion deformity, and skin pressure areas.
   a. Lower-extremity amputations—hip flexion contractures
   b. Upper-extremity amputations—postural abnormalities (encourage good posture)

H. Pharmacologic and parenteral therapies: Client will state the purpose for and associated side effects of all medications. Although opioids provide effective treatment of incisional pain, they may be ineffective for phantom limb sensation.
1. Beta-blockers (propranolol [Inderal])
2. Anticonvulsants (phenytoin [Dilantin])
3. Muscle relaxants (baclofen [Lioresal])
4. Tricyclic antidepressants (amitriptyline [Elavil])
5. Topical analgesic (capsaicin [Capsin])
6. IV fluids:
   a. Normal saline (NS; 0.9% NaCl)—isotonic
   b. Lactated Ringer (LR)—isotonic
   c. Dextrose 5%/water (D5/W)—isotonic, hypotonic
7. Hypertonic IV fluids—for excessive blood loss with extracellular fluid volume deficit: May cause dangerous intravascular volume

overload and pulmonary edema; administer slowly and with extreme caution.
   a. Lactated Ringer with 5% dextrose (D5/LR)
   b. 5% dextrose and normal saline (D5/0.9 NS)
   c. 5% dextrose and 0.45% normal saline (D5/0.45 NS)
   d. 3% normal saline (3% NS)
   e. 10% dextrose and water (D10/W)

Herniated Intervertebral Disk

I. Definition: The intervertebral disk is a semi-fluid-filled fibrous capsule that facilitates movement of the spine and acts as a shock absorber. Herniated intervertebral disk (also known as *ruptured* or *slipped* disk) is a disorder involving pressure on the vertebral disk that causes the nucleus pulposus (elastic material from center of the disk) to break (herniate) through the fibrous rim of the disk and impinge on spinal nerve roots. Herniation usually occurs posteriorly in the lumbar region or lumbosacral region, and can occur in any portion of vertebral column; if untreated, herniation may cause permanent neurologic dysfunction.
   A. Herniated intervertebral disk can result from:
      1. Degenerative disorders
      2. Trauma
      3. Congenital predisposition or malformation
   B. Risk factors include:
      1. Repetitive bending/lifting involving twisting motion
      2. Continuous vibration
      3. Smoking
      4. Poor physical condition
      5. Obesity
      6. Prolonged sitting
      7. Severe scoliosis
      8. Above-average height

II. Nursing process
   A. Assessment
      1. Assess for cervical herniation—involves pain or stiffness in:
         a. Head
         b. Neck
         c. Top of shoulders
         d. Scapular region
         e. Upper extremities
      2. Assess for lumbar and lumbosacral herniation.
         a. Low back pain with radiation into buttocks and down leg
         b. Positive straight-leg raising test
            (1) Radiation of pain below knee when leg is elevated 45 degrees from supine position indicates lumbosacral nerve root involvement.
            (2) Pain at lesser elevation may indicate worsening condition.
         c. Varying degrees of sensory and motor dysfunction resulting in weakness and decreased asymmetric reflexes
         d. Postural deformity of lumbar spine may be evident.
         e. Pressure on sciatic nerve can produce severe, sometimes debilitating, pain.
         f. Mobility often altered; involves:
            (1) Decreased ability to stand upright
            (2) Asymmetric gait
            (3) Limited ability to flex forward
            (4) Restricted side movement
      3. Obtain diagnostic tests.
         a. CTS or MRI—identifies herniated disk
         b. Myelogram—determines level of disk herniation
         c. Electromyogram—localizes spinal nerve involvement
         d. X-ray of spine—shows narrowing of vertebral interspaces in affected areas, loss of curvature of spine, and spondylosis
         e. Diskography—identifies degenerated or extruded disks by means of contrast medium injected into disk space using fluoroscopy
         f. Laboratory tests: Serum alkaline and acid phosphatase, glucose, calcium, erythrocyte sedimentation rate, and WBC count—rule out metabolic bone disease, metastatic tumors, diabetic mononeuritis, and disk space infection
   B. Analysis
      1. Acute or Chronic Pain related to nerve compression and irritation, and muscle spasms
      2. Impaired Physical Mobility related to pain (muscle spasms), therapeutic restrictions (bed rest, traction/braces), muscular impairment, and depression
      3. Deficient Knowledge related to treatment options
      4. Risk for Injury related to impaired physical mobility
      5. Ineffective Coping related to effects of chronic pain
   C. Planning
      1. Reduce or eliminate pain and muscle spasms.
      2. Promote resumption of previous level of mobility.
      3. Develop strategies to manage chronic pain.
      4. Promote adaptation to lifestyle changes.

5. Provide information about treatment options.
6. Prevent injury.
7. Identify effective coping strategies.

D. Implementation
1. Provide pain relief and conservative management as indicated (see basic care and comfort).
2. Provide perioperative and postoperative care, and ongoing assessments (see management of care).
3. Provide client and family teaching.
4. Promote client and family coping.

E. Evaluation
1. Client verbalizes relief of pain (rates pain as less than 4 on pain scale of 1 to 10).
2. Client describes effective methods of managing chronic pain.
3. Client demonstrates previous level of mobility.
4. Client describes acquired knowledge related to treatment options.
5. Client is free from signs and symptoms of injury.
6. Client returns to previous levels of work and lifestyle.

CN

III. Client needs

A. Physiologic adaptation: If signs of spinal cord compression are present (significant motor/sensory loss, loss of sphincter control), prompt surgical intervention is used; otherwise, surgery is considered only after symptoms fail to respond to conservative therapy (e.g., analgesics, muscle relaxants, weight reduction). Client is monitored postoperatively for signs of cord compression (medical emergency) caused by bleeding/hematoma.
1. Diskectomy with laminectomy—incision is made allowing removal of part of vertebra (laminectomy) permitting removal of herniated portion of disk (diskectomy).
2. Microdiskectomy—microsurgical techniques used to remove herniated portion of disk and small parts of lamina. Client may be out of bed in first day and discharged in 1 to 3 days. Microdiskectomy results in less tissue damage, less pain, fewer muscle spasms, and increased postoperative spinal stability than diskectomy.
3. Percutaneous lumbar disk removal—ultrasonic nucleotome cannula inserted in intervertebral space via fluoroscopy to allow fragmentation of disk and its aspiration. Local anesthesia used; may be performed on outpatient basis.
4. Spinal fusion—indicated for clients with recurrent low back pain, spondylolisthesis, or subluxation of vertebrae. Either donor bone or bone chips are harvested from iliac crest or tibia and placed between vertebrae in area of unstable spine to fuse and stabilize area; internal fixation may be necessary.
5. Other surgical procedures:
   a. Foraminotomy—surgical enlargement of intravertebral foramen to reduce tension and create additional room for nerve root
   b. Hemilaminectomy—removes part of lamina of vertebra to reduce pressure on an adjacent nerve
   c. Anterior cervical vertebrectomy with interbody fusion—may be necessary for multilevel cervical disk disease
   d. Intradiscal electrothermal treatment—uses an electrical probe to heat/shrink injured disk tissue
   e. Implantable spinal cord stimulators—aid in control of chronic pain

B. Management of care: Care of the client with a herniated intervertebral disk requires critical thinking skills and knowledge of assessment, and teaching and evaluation methods unique to the RN role. These skills cannot be delegated to an LPN or UAP.
1. Delegate responsibly those activities that can be delegated. All monitoring information is reported to the RN.
   a. Monitor vital signs.
   b. Provide basic hygienic care.
   c. Monitor intake and output.
   d. Assist with logrolling when moving client from side to side.
   e. Assist with activity as allowed.
2. If client had surgical intervention, provide postoperative care and client teaching:
   a. Assess strength, sensation, and movement of extremities.
   b. Promote measures to maintain adequate airway.
   c. Prevent infection.
   d. Maintain proper body alignment when in bed (provide firm mattress) and when turning (use logrolling).
   e. Encourage client to wear well-fitted, safe walking shoes when ambulating.
   f. Teach proper body mechanics to prevent injury.
   g. Caution to avoid slippery surfaces and activities that can involve sudden back movements.
3. Provide postoperative care for diskectomy with laminectomy; notify surgeon or

physician of significant assessment findings.
   a. Paralytic ileus
   b. Urinary retention
   c. Cerebrospinal fluid leakage
   d. Meningitis
   e. Hematoma at operative site
   f. Nerve root injury causing wrist drop or foot drop
   g. Postural deformity
4. Provide postoperative care for microdiskectomy; notify surgeon or physician of indications of complications such as bleeding at site, weakness, numbness in extremities.
5. Provide postoperative care for percutaneous lumbar disk removal and notify surgeon or physician of complications such as bleeding or weakness and numbness of extremities. Assess client for:
   a. Back stiffness
   b. Soreness
   c. Spasm
   d. Transient syncope
6. For spinal fusion:
   a. Provide postoperative care and assess the client for severity of pain at bone donor site (tibia, iliac crest).
   b. If client had anterior cervical fusion, assess for:
      (1) Difficulty swallowing, management of secretions
      (2) Hoarseness
      (3) Complaints of excessive pressure in neck or severe, uncontrolled incisional pain—may signal excessive bleeding
7. Provide postoperative care for other surgical procedures. Assess client for:
   a. Pain
   b. Drainage
   c. Numbness, tingling in extremities
   d. Loss of strength in extremities
8. Notify surgeon of postoperative wound infection indicated by:
   a. Edema around surgical site
   b. Discharge at surgical site
   c. Persistent redness
   d. Fever, local warmth at surgical site
   e. Unusual tenderness, pain at/near surgical site
9. Consult dietitian regarding client diet and information about food choices (high in calcium, vitamin D, C, and protein having high biologic value) as well as fluid intake.
10. Consult physical therapist to aid in client mobility (see also reduction of risk potential):
   a. Exercises to strengthen muscles
   b. Strategies to prevent skeletal muscle spasms
   c. Use and care of braces, immobilizers, cervical collars, and other assistive devices

C. Safety and infection control
1. Monitor for signs of infection (see management of care for indications).
2. Encourage client to use postsurgical activity restrictions as directed by physician and physical therapist; these may affect the following:
   a. Driving, riding in a car
   b. Returning to work
   c. Sexual activity
   d. Lifting, carrying
   e. Tub bathing
   f. Going up and down steps
   g. Amount of time spent in or out of bed
3. Instruct client to avoid watching wall-mounted television units because of risk of extension, rotation, and flexion of neck.

D. Health promotion and maintenance
1. Emphasize importance of complying with bed rest, use of cervical collar or back brace, and other conservative measures to reduce inflammation and heal disk herniation.
2. Instruct client who has had cervical disk herniation to avoid extreme flexion, extension, or rotation of neck and to keep head in a neutral position during sleep.
3. Encourage client to do stretching and strengthening exercises of extremities and abdomen after acute symptoms have subsided; start an aerobic program, such as walking; wear supportive shoes with moderate heel height when walking.
4. Instruct client about proper body mechanics to prevent recurrence:
   a. Use leg and abdominal muscles rather than the back.
   b. Bend knees on lifting.
   c. Carry load close to midtrunk.
5. Encourage good nutrition, avoidance of obesity, smoking cessation, and proper rest to reduce risk of recurrence.
6. Encourage follow-up with physical therapy as indicated for reconditioning.

E. Psychologic integrity
1. Explain factors that may contribute to development of maladaptive coping.
2. Communicate information and a caring attitude.
3. Discuss how to develop coping skills that enhance self-esteem and social interaction.

4. Encourage relaxation techniques such as imagery and progressive muscle relaxation.
5. Facilitate return to previous levels of work and lifestyle, or successfully adapt to lifestyle changes.

F. Basic care and comfort
1. Provide pain relief and conservative management as indicated.
   a. Enforce decreased activity to reduce paravertebral muscle spasms and resulting pain.
   b. Keep head of bed elevated 20 degrees and knee of bed flexed to reduce stress on lower back muscles.
   c. Apply moist heat or ice to lower back to reduce pain and muscle spasm.
   d. Administer analgesics, nonsteroidal anti-inflammatory drugs, and/or muscle relaxants as ordered; document effect to promote comfort and evaluate effectiveness.
   e. Instruct in appropriate exercises to increase muscle strength around spinal cord (pelvic tilts, straight-leg raises).
2. Prevent complications of immobility.
3. Promote self-care by encouraging active participation in self-care.

G. Reduction of risk potential
1. Monitor and report any sudden reappearance of:
   a. Radicular pain—may indicate nerve root compression from slipping of bone graft or collapsing of disk space
   b. Burning back pain radiating to buttocks—may indicate arachnoiditis
2. If receiving opioid analgesics for pain management, monitor:
   a. Respiratory rate
   b. Level of consciousness
   c. Effectiveness of pain relief
3. Encourage good, balanced nutrition, avoidance of obesity, smoking cessation, and proper rest to reduce risk of recurrence.
4. Advise client to avoid factors that enhance muscle spasms such as fatigue, chilling, anxiety, and staying in one position too long.
5. Advise client to avoid prolonged periods of sitting, which stresses the back.
6. Encourage client to use firm mattress and bed board to support normal spinal curvature.
7. Instruct client in technique for sitting up on bedside from supine position: Logrolling to side, then rising to sitting position by pushing against mattress with hands while swinging legs over side of bed.
8. Instruct client to report promptly to physician indications of worsening neurologic function:
   a. Muscle weakness
   b. Paralysis
   c. Bowel/bladder dysfunction

H. Pharmacologic and parenteral therapies: Drug therapy includes muscle relaxants, opioid or nonopioid analgesics, anti-inflammatory agents, and stool softeners or laxatives (if needed). Client and family will state the purpose for and associated side effects of all medications.
1. Muscle relaxants: Carisoprodol (Soma) and methocarbamol (Robaxin)—used to reduce muscle spasms.
   a. Monitor liver enzymes (aspartate aminotransferase, alanine aminotransferase).
   b. Monitor renal function (blood urea nitrogen, creatinine).
2. Analgesics
   a. Aspirin, acetaminophen (Tylenol)—administer sufficient medication to achieve pain relief and adequate pain reduction.
   b. Narcotics—used for acute pain episodes.
      (1) Monitor respiratory rate.
      (2) Hold if respirations less than 12 per minute.
      (3) Avoid using alcoholic beverages.
3. Nonsteroidal anti-inflammatory drugs: Celecoxib (Celebrex) and nabumetone (Relafen). For client with GI upset—cyclooxygenase-2-specific nonsteroidal anti-inflammatory drugs.
   a. Monitor liver function (aspartate aminotransferase, alanine aminotransferase).
   b. Monitor renal function (creatinine, blood urea nitrogen).
4. Corticosteroids: Dexamethasone (Decadron) and prednisone (Deltasone)—may be given for short period of time to reduce cord edema, if present.
   a. Do not stop abruptly.
   b. Taper off slowly to prevent corticosteroid insufficiency.
5. Stool softeners: Docusate sodium (Colace) and laxatives magnesium hydroxide (Milk of Magnesia)—prevent/treat painful constipation/straining.
   a. Withhold drug if diarrhea develops.
   b. Administer each dose with sufficient liquid; increase fluids throughout day.
6. IV fluids
   a. Normal saline (NS; 0.9% NaCl)—isotonic

b. Dextrose 5%/water (D5/W)—isotonic, hypotonic
c. Lactated Ringer (LR)—isotonic

Spinal Cord Injury

I. Definition: Injury to the spinal cord results from damage caused by fractures, contusions, or compression of the vertebral column. The spinal cord may be severed, lacerated, stretched, or compressed, and interrupt neuronal function and transmission of nerve impulses. Blood supply to the spinal cord may be interrupted as well.
   A. The segment of the population with greatest risk for spinal cord injury is young adult men between 16 and 30 years of age. Older adults are also at risk from falls.
   B. Injury is classified according to the following:
      1. Completeness of injury and motor/sensory function (American Spinal Injury Association)
         a. ASIA A = Complete: absent sensory and motor function at S4 to S5
         b. ASIA B = Incomplete; intact sensory but absent motor function below level of injury and includes level S4 to S5
         c. ASIA C = Incomplete; intact motor function distal to level of injury and more than half of key muscles distal to level of injury have muscle grade less than 3
         d. ASIA D = Incomplete; intact motor function distal to level of injury and more than half of key muscles distal to level of injury have muscle grade greater than or equal to 3
         e. ASIA E = Normal; intact motor and sensory function
      2. Cause
         a. Traumatic: Caused by injury such as a traumatic blow that may cause fracture, crushing injury, or dislocation of the vertebrae; or knife or gunshot wounds that can sever the spinal cord
         b. Nontraumatic: Caused by diseases such as arthritis or cancer, degenerative disease
      3. Site—level of spinal cord involved; the most common sites of injury are the cervical areas C5, C6, and C7, and the junction of the thoracic and lumbar vertebrae, T12 and L1.
      4. Mechanism of injury
         a. Compression
         b. Hyperflexion
         c. Hyperextension
         d. Rotational
         e. Penetrating
      5. Degree of spinal cord function loss
         a. Is lowest level in which motor function, sensation remain intact.
         b. When spinal shock occurs after injury, can be total loss of spinal cord function below level of injury.
            (1) Is no reflex activity.
            (2) Return of reflexes—1 to 6 weeks or longer (6 months or more).
         c. If no returning motor function after reflexes return—spinal cord considered irreversibly damaged.
         d. Immediate death—C1 through C3 spinal cord injury.
            (1) Respiratory muscle paralysis.
            (2) Survival requires ventilator for rest of life.
   C. Complications
      1. Shock
      2. Respiratory or cardiac arrest
      3. Thromboembolism
      4. Infections
      5. Autonomic dysreflexia

II. Nursing process
   A. Assessment
      1. Perform a comprehensive physical assessment; assess for common immediate signs and symptoms.
         a. Pain
         b. Paresthesias, loss of sensation
         c. Altered motor function—paresis/paralysis
         d. Level of consciousness
      2. Obtain a detailed health history, including possible history of cause for spinal cord injury (e.g., motor vehicle or sport-related injury).
      3. Assess for neurologic damage—depends on level of injury; edema may temporarily increase deficits.
         a. Below C4:
            (1) Loss of motor, sensory function from neck down.
            (2) Loss of independent respiratory function.
            (3) Loss of bowel, bladder control.
         b. Below C6:
            (1) Loss of motor, sensory function below shoulders.
            (2) Loss of bowel and bladder control.
            (3) Impaired intercostal muscle function.
         c. Below C8:
            (1) Loss of motor control.
            (2) Loss of sensation to parts of arms, hands.
            (3) Loss of bowel and bladder control.

d. Below T6:
   (1) Loss of motor control.
   (2) Loss of sensation below midchest but with motor control; sensation preserved in arms, hands.
   (3) Loss of bowel, bladder control.
e. Below T12:
   (1) Loss of motor control, sensation below waist.
   (2) Loss of bowel, bladder control.
f. Below L2:
   (1) Loss of motor control, sensation in legs, pelvis.
   (2) Loss of bowel, bladder control.
g. Below L4:
   (1) Loss of motor control, sensation in parts of thighs and legs.
   (2) Loss of bowel and bladder control.

4. Obtain diagnostic tests.
   a. X-rays of spinal column, including open-mouth studies for adequate visualization of C1 and C2—determines fracture.
   b. Spinal MRI—detects soft tissue injury, bony injury, hemorrhage, and edema.
   c. Nerve conduction testing and electromyogram—determine function of neural pathways.
   d. CTS—locates area of cord damage and searches for other injuries that often accompany spinal trauma.

B. Analysis
1. Impaired Urinary Elimination related to neurologic impairment and limited fluid intake
2. Risk for Injury related to immobility
3. Impaired Gas Exchange related to diaphragmatic fatigue or paralysis and retained secretions
4. Decreased Cardiac Output related to venous pooling of blood, bradycardia, and immobility
5. Impaired Skin Integrity related to immobility and poor tissue perfusion
6. Constipation related to neurogenic bowel, inadequate fluid intake, diet low in roughage, and immobility
7. Impaired Physical Mobility related to spinal cord injury, vertebral column instability, or forced immobilization by traction
8. Risk for Autonomic Dysreflexia related to reflex stimulation of sympathetic nervous system after spinal shock resolves
9. Imbalanced Nutrition: Less Than Body Requirements related to increased metabolic demand, GI hypomotility, and inability to eat independently
10. Risk for Ineffective Coping related to loss of control over bodily functions and altered lifestyle secondary to paralysis
11. Disturbed Body Image related to paralysis
12. Interrupted Family Processes related to change in function of ill family member

C. Planning
1. Maintain optimal level of neurologic functioning.
2. Prevent potential complications of immobility.
3. Provide client and family teaching.
4. Facilitate return to home and the community at an optimal level of functioning.
5. Promote client ability for self-care.

D. Implementation
1. Provide emergency treatment.
2. Administer prescribed medications.
3. Assist with immobilization and reduction of dislocations and stabilization of the cervical vertebral column.
4. Provide perioperative interventions.
5. Prevent complications of immobility.
6. Prepare client and family for ambulation and home maintenance management.
7. Teach signs and symptoms of impending autonomic hyperreflexia (dysreflexia) episodes that occur with cord lesions above T6 (see reduction of risk potential).
8. Promote normal bowel and bladder elimination.

E. Evaluation
1. Client is free from signs of respiratory distress.
2. Client is free from complications of immobility such as venous thrombosis or pulmonary emboli.
3. Client has optimal skin integrity.
4. Client produces a bowel movement at least every other day.
5. Client demonstrates ability to perform self-catheterization to empty bladder or to void with adequate emptying.
6. Client is free from complications of immobility.
7. Client exhibits no signs of dysreflexia, or receives immediate and appropriate nursing or medical interventions if it occurs.
8. Client has weight loss of less than 10%, with normal serum values of protein and albumin.
9. Client verbalizes ability to cope with effects of spinal cord injury.
10. Client expresses positive self-concept.
11. Client's family maximizes individual and collective strengths to meet client's needs.

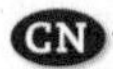

III. Client needs

A. Physiologic adaptation: Spinal cord swells in response to injury; edema plus hemorrhage can cause additional compression, ischemia, and compromised function. Neurologic deficits (from compression) may be reversible if resulting edema, ischemia do not lead to spinal cord degeneration, necrosis. Treatment for stages of injury is as follows:
  1. Immediate posttrauma phase (less than 1 hr)—immobilize client, including head, body, and hips.
  2. Acute phase (1 to 24 hr)
     a. Maintain pulmonary stability through intubation and mechanical ventilation or diaphragmatic pacing, if needed.
     b. Maintain cardiovascular stability, ensure perfusion of spinal cord by restoring BP and implementing localized cord cooling.
     c. Immobilize spinal cord with skeletal tongs.
     d. Promote surgical intervention to prevent further neurologic damage—may include decompression or stabilization with various hardware.
  3. Subacute phase (within 1 week)—Promote halo traction for cervical injuries (for up to 12 weeks).
  4. Chronic phase (beyond 1 week)—Emphasis on rehabilitation:
     a. Physical therapy
     b. Urologic evaluation
     c. Occupational therapy

B. Management of care: Care of the client with a spinal cord injury requires critical thinking skills and knowledge of assessment, and teaching and evaluation methods unique to the RN role. These skills cannot be delegated to an LPN or UAP.
  1. Delegate responsibly those activities that can be delegated. All monitoring information is reported to the RN.
     a. Monitor vital signs.
     b. Monitor intake and output.
     c. Encourage deep breathing and use of incentive spirometer.
     d. Observe for bleeding around fracture site.
     e. Measure circumference of calf, thigh; assist with application of thigh-high antiembolism stockings, as prescribed.
     f. Initiate measures to reduce pain.
     g. Assist with maintenance of adequate nutrition and a high-fiber diet.
     h. Maintain adequate fluid intake of 2,000 ml/day.
     i. Monitor skin integrity
     j. Encourage client to express feelings.
     h. Promote self-care.
  2. Promote skeletal traction with cervical injury (skeletal tongs such as Gardner-Wells tongs or Crutchfield tongs) or halo traction—applied by physician. Nurse responsibilities include:
     a. Ensure weights hang freely and do not interfere with traction; never remove weights.
     b. Clean tong insertion sites.
     c. Assess tong insertion sites for infection.
  3. Consult with social worker to locate and contact available community resources; work with support agencies to acquire, maintain needed assistive equipment.
  4. Provide information on alternative means for achieving sexual satisfaction; consult with certified sex therapist, if indicated.
  5. Promote rehabilitation among multidisciplinary team as appropriate.
  6. Provide a referral to the National Spinal Cord Injury Association.

C. Safety and infection control
  1. For client receiving skeletal traction, provide meticulous skin care at pin sites of skull tongs/halo device to prevent infection.
  2. Never attempt to reposition by grasping a halo or other stabilization device.
  3. For clients with high-level lesions, provide continuous monitoring and maintain patent airway; be prepared to intubate if respiratory fatigue/arrest occurs.
  4. Monitor results of ABG analysis, chest x-rays, and sputum cultures for respiratory infection.
     a. Provide fluids, humidified air/oxygen to loosen secretions.
     b. Implement chest physiotherapy to assist pulmonary drainage and prevent infection.
  5. Replace indwelling catheter with intermittent catheterization as soon as possible to minimize risk of infection.

D. Health promotion and maintenance: Provide client and family teaching about physiology of nerve transmission, and how spinal cord injury has affected normal function. Additional teaching includes the following:
  1. Reinforce to client that rehabilitation is lengthy and involves adherence to therapy to increase bodily function.

2. Explain that spasticity may develop 2 weeks to 3 months after injury and may interfere with routine care and activities of daily living; teach measures to manage spasticity:
   a. Maintain calm, stress-free environment.
   b. Allow plenty of time for activities.
   c. Perform ROM slowly and smoothly.
   d. Avoid temperature extremes.
3. Instruct client in ways to prevent pressure ulcers:
   a. Inspect skin frequently.
   b. Reposition regularly while in bed.
   c. Perform weight-shifting, lift-offs every 15 min while in wheelchair.
   d. Avoid friction and shearing forces.

E. Psychologic integrity
1. Evaluate ability of client and family to develop coping strategies; encourage new strategies, if needed.
2. Assess for prolonged use of inappropriate defense mechanisms, inability to accept current status, and refusal to use available support services.
3. Encourage client verbalization of concerns; offer support and assist with problem-solving.
4. Foster decision-making regarding care to increase feelings of control.
5. Encourage social interaction to foster sense of returning normalcy to life; spinal cord injury results in real loss, which requires adjustment.
6. Assess family dynamics related to roles and responsibilities to determine problematic areas, strengths.
7. Assist family members to understand client's feelings to strengthen client's feelings of worth.
8. Encourage open communication among family members regarding long-term planning to meet needs, including financial aspects.

F. Basic care and comfort
1. Administer prescribed medications (see pharmacologic and parenteral therapies).
2. Prevent complications of immobility:
   a. Perform passive ROM exercises on paralyzed limbs to maintain joint mobility.
      (1) Use high-top tennis shoes to prevent foot drop.
      (2) Apply trochanter rolls from iliac crest to midthigh of both legs to prevent external rotation of hip joints.
      (3) When turning every 2 hr, always maintain body alignment and use logrolling technique.
   b. Teach active ROM exercises to maintain/increase strength/mobility in arms.
   c. Prevent deep vein thrombosis, pressure ulcers, contractures, constipation, pneumonia.
3. Teach transfer skills, if appropriate.
4. Institute bowel-care program as early as possible to manage defecation.
   a. Advise to set schedule for defecation, preferably 15 to 20 min after meal.
   b. Provide warm fluids prior to bowel elimination attempt.
   c. Encourage client to obtain sufficient dietary roughage, adequate fluids.
   d. Encourage client to attempt defecation in sitting position.
5. Prevent stasis of urine to decrease likelihood of urinary tract infection.
   a. Schedule frequent times for voiding.
   b. Maintain adequate fluid intake, but avoid at bedtime.
   c. Perform intermittent bladder catheterization as appropriate.
6. Teach effective coughing and deep breathing.
7. Ensure adequate rest and discuss stress-management techniques.

G. Reduction of risk potential
1. Monitor for autonomic dysreflexia (medical emergency involving exaggerated autonomic response to stimuli below level of lesion in clients with lesions at or above T6); may result in seizures or death, without prompt treatment.
   a. Monitor for signs and symptoms such as:
      (1) Pounding headache
      (2) Profuse sweating
      (3) Nasal congestion
      (4) Piloerection (goose bumps)
      (5) Bradycardia
      (6) Severe hypertension
   b. Immediately place in sitting position to help lower blood pressure and diminish intracranial pressure. Remove possible causative stimuli such as:
      (1) Bowel or bladder distention caused by fecal impaction, urinary retention, or kinked indwelling catheter.
      (2) Abnormal skin stimulation such as lying on wrinkled sheets; hot or cold stimulation; or pain from constricted clothing.

(3) Distention or contraction of visceral organs such as gastric distention or emptying overdistended bladder too fast.
(4) Infection, especially of urinary tract.

c. Administer antihypertensive medication as ordered; monitor BP every 3 to 5 min until condition resolves.

2. Alert caregivers that autonomic dysreflexia is a complication that may occur for 5 to 6 years after a spinal cord injury. Teach indications, prevention, and emergency measures to implement (as previously noted).
3. Apply elastic support hose, sequential compression device, and administer anticoagulants as ordered to reduce risk of thrombophlebitis.
4. Encourage weight-bearing activity to prevent osteoporosis and risk of kidney stones.
5. Perform ROM exercises to prevent contractures and maintain rehabilitation potential.
6. Monitor BP with position changes when lesion above midthoracic area to prevent orthostatic hypotension.
7. Monitor neurologic changes; report to physician promptly:
   a. Change in skin sensation.
   b. Loss/gain of muscle strength.
8. With high-level lesions, continuously monitor respirations as client may develop respiratory fatigue/arrest.

H. Pharmacologic and parenteral therapies: Pharmacologic properties and drug metabolism are altered in spinal cord injury; therefore, drug interactions may occur. The differences in drug metabolism correlate with level and completeness of injury with greater change apparent in clients with cervical injury. Client and family will state the purpose for and side-effects of all medications.

1. High-dose corticosteroids—reduce disability if given within 8 hr of injury. Methylprednisolone (Medrol)—given intravenously as soon as possible to reduce spinal cord edema.
   a. Monitor kidney, liver function, thyroid function, CBC, electrolytes, weight, and total cholesterol.
   b. Monitor glucose—development of secondary diabetes.
   c. Monitor for signs and symptoms of Cushing syndrome (moon face, buffalo hump, abdominal distention, muscle weakness, ecchymoses).
2. GM-1 ganglioside sodium (Sygen) salt intravenously to enhance neuronal regeneration. Begin 72 hr after injury; continue for 18 to 32 days.
3. Histamine-2 receptor blockers: Cimetidine (Tagamet); ranitidine (Zantac)—prevent gastric irritation and hemorrhage.
   a. Monitor for bradycardia.
   b. Monitor for loss of bowel sounds.
   c. Monitor CBC and renal and liver function.
4. Anticoagulants given in small doses to reduce risk of thrombophlebitis, pulmonary emboli (low-dose heparin 5,000 units). Monitor petechiae formation and bleeding gums.
5. Muscle relaxants: Baclofen (Lioresal) and diazepam (Valium)—to manage spasticity.
   a. Monitor client ambulation.
   b. Monitor laboratory tests—renal, liver function tests, and glucose.
   c. Monitor for confusion, depression, and hallucinations.
6. Osmotic diuretics: Isosorbide (Ismotic); mannitol (Osmitrol); urea (Ureacin)—to reduce edema; monitor intake and output.
7. Hypertonic colloidal solution: Dextran (Hyskon)—prevents blood pressure from dropping; improves capillary blood flow. Monitor BP and hematocrit.

Bibliography

Altman, G. (2004). *Delmar's fundamental and advanced nursing skills* (2nd ed.). Albany, NY: Delmar.

American Spinal Injury Association. *International standards for neurological classification of spinal cord injury.* Retrieved June 6, 2008 from http://www.asia-spinalinjury.org

Ellis, J., & Hartley, C. (2005). *Managing and coordinating nursing care.* Philadelphia: Lippincott Williams & Wilkins.

Karch, A. (2008). *Lippincott's nursing drug guide.* Philadelphia: Lippincott Williams & Wilkins.

Purnell, L., & Paulanka, B. (Eds.). (2003). *Transcultural healthcare: A culturally competent approach.* Philadelphia: Davis.

Smeltzer, S. C., Bare, B. G., Cheever, K. H., & Hinkle, J. L. (2008). *Brunner and Suddarth's textbook of medical-surgical nursing* (11th ed.). Philadelphia: Lippincott Williams & Wilkins.

Taylor, C., Lillis, C., LeMone, P., & Lynn, P. (2006). *Fundamentals of nursing.* Philadelphia: Lippincott Williams & Wilkins.

Weber, J. R., & Kelley, J. (2007). *Nurses handbook of health assessment.* Philadelphia: Lippincott Williams & Wilkins.

Yarbro, C. H., Frogge, M., & Goodman, M. (2004). *Cancer symptom management* (3rd ed.). Sudbury, MA: Jones and Bartlett.

CHAPTER 31

Practice Test

Fractures

1. The nurse is caring for a client who is 30 years of age with a fracture of the right femur and left tibia. Both legs have casts. The nurse assesses the following: (i) respirations are 30 per minute and are rapid and shallow; (ii) presence of faint expiratory wheeze; and (iii) coughing produces thin pink sputum. The client is yelling at the nurse and wants to be released from the hospital; this is behavior unlike that previously reported. The last pain medication was administered 3 hr ago. The nurse should do which of the following?

☐ 1. Cut slits in the top of the casts.
☐ 2. Administer pain medication.
☐ 3. Contact the HCP.
☐ 4. Order a chest x-ray.

2. A client is being discharged following an open reduction and internal fixation of the left ankle, and is to wear a non-weight bearing cast for 2 weeks. The nurse should teach the client to do which of the following when using crutches?

☐ 1. Use a four-point gait.
☐ 2. Maintain two finger widths between the axillary fold and underarm piece grip.
☐ 3. Keep leg dependent when sitting.
☐ 4. Maintain balance by supporting body's weight on the axillae.

3. The nurse is caring for a client who is 35 years of age with a grade III compound fracture of the right femur; the client has been placed in skeletal traction. The intended outcome of the traction is to:

☐ 1. Prevent skin breakdown.
☐ 2. Prevent movement in the bed.
☐ 3. Preserve normal length of the leg.
☐ 4. Reduce and immobilize the fracture.

4. A client who is 75 years of age is admitted with a fracture of the femur. The nurse should first assess:

☐ 1. Ability to change positions.
☐ 2. Type of pain.
☐ 3. Mechanism of injury.
☐ 4. Extent of anxiety.

5. A client who has had his left arm crushed under a grain truck bed for 30 min without sustaining any bone fractures is being admitted to the hospital. The nurse should first:

☐ 1. Monitor for infection.
☐ 2. Promote physical mobility.
☐ 3. Prevent neurovascular compromise.
☐ 4. Prevent disuse syndrome.

6. AF The nurse is caring for a client with metastatic bone cancer. The goal of nursing care is to prevent pathologic fractures. Which of the following actions will assist with this goal? Select all that apply.

☐ 1. Monitor serum calcium levels.
☐ 2. Avoid bumping the client's bed.
☐ 3. Assist the client while ambulating.
☐ 4. Support joints when repositioning the client.
☐ 5. Review record of chemotherapy use.

7. Which of the following nursing strategies is most important for the nurse to implement following hip surgery?

☐ 1. Provide a trochanter roll to maintain alignment.
☐ 2. Provide regular monitoring of neurovascular function.
☐ 3. Provide passive ROM exercises to affected extremity.
☐ 4. Monitor client's elimination pattern.

8. A client had a total hip replacement for a left hip fracture 24 hr ago. The nurse should assist the client to maintain the left leg in which of the following positions?

☐ 1. Adduction and internal rotation.
☐ 2. Straight and elevated 20 degrees.
☐ 3. Adducted with the knee elevated.
☐ 4. Abduction and neutral rotation.

Rheumatoid Arthritis

9. A client with rheumatoid arthritis is taking high doses of nonsteroidal anti-inflammatory medications. The nurse should instruct the client to:

☐ 1. Take prescribed medication with food to lessen the likelihood of an upset stomach.
☐ 2. Not to stop taking the medication suddenly; the dose needs to be decreased gradually.
☐ 3. Use mouthwash to rinse the mouth after taking this medication.
☐ 4. Not to drive if dizziness occurs.

10. The nurse is planning an exercise program with a client who has rheumatoid arthritis. The goal is to maintain as much function as possible. Which of the following types of exercise will be most effective for this client?
- □ 1. Walking.
- □ 2. Recumbent bicycle.
- □ 3. Treadmill.
- □ 4. Aquatic exercises.

11. A client has an exacerbation of rheumatoid arthritis with joint tenderness, symmetrical joint edema, and subcutaneous nodules. Which of the following information is needed before the nurse can work with the client to plan care?
- □ 1. Therapies begun at the time of diagnosis.
- □ 2. Current resources being used.
- □ 3. Pulse, respirations, and BP.
- □ 4. Presence of fatigue, muscle weakness, and anorexia.

12. AF The nurse is reviewing laboratory reports for a client with rheumatoid arthritis. Which of the following laboratory tests will provide information about the extent of the client's immune response and degree of inflammation? Select all that apply.
- □ 1. Erythrocyte sedimentation rate.
- □ 2. C-reactive protein.
- □ 3. Antinuclear antibody titer.
- □ 4. Rheumatoid factor.
- □ 5. Amylase.
- □ 6. Lipase.

Osteoarthritis

13. AF A client with osteoarthritis is experiencing pain in the joints of the hands. To relieve the pain the nurse should do which of the following? Select all that apply.
- □ 1. Provide hand splints to reduce hand movement.
- □ 2. Administer acetaminophen as needed.
- □ 3. Encourage ROM exercises.
- □ 4. Provide a heat pack as prescribed.
- □ 5. Advise the client that weight loss will be helpful.

14. The nurse is instructing an overweight client with osteoarthritis about diet and nutrition. Which of the following statements best indicates that the client understands how to maintain adequate nutrition?
- □ 1. "I will eat six or seven small meals per day."
- □ 2. "I will eat a well-balanced, low-calorie diet."
- □ 3. "I will eat more chicken, fish, and lean red meat."
- □ 4. "I will eat a low-protein, low-carbohydrate diet."

Amputation

15. The nurse is developing discharge plans with a client with an above-the-knee amputation. In order to prepare the residual limb for prosthesis fitting, the nurse instructs the client to:
- □ 1. Use a figure-eight bandage wrapping technique.
- □ 2. Wrap the limb from the thigh to the stump.
- □ 3. Remove the bandage 3 times a day.
- □ 4. Keep the bandage tight to minimize phantom pain.

16. The nurse is evaluating a UAP who is providing care to a client who had a right below-the-knee amputation 1 day ago. The nurse should intervene on observing the client lying in which of the following positions?
- □ 1. Left side-lying position with pillows supporting both extremities in an extended position.
- □ 2. Positioned on back with left leg in full extension and right leg in extension and slightly elevated on a small pillow.
- □ 3. Positioned on back with both legs flexed and supported by pillows.
- □ 4. Positioned on back with both legs extended and two pillows under the head.

Herniated Intervertebral Disk

17. A client is discharged with the following prescription for severe back pain from a herniated intravertebral disk: Hydrocodone 5 mg acetaminophen 500 mg one-half to one tablet by mouth each 8 to 12 hr as needed. The nurse should instruct the client to:
- □ 1. Start with one-half tablet and take one every 12 hr.
- □ 2. Start with one-half tablet and take one every 8 hr.
- □ 3. Start with one tablet and then take one tablet every 8 hr.
- □ 4. Start with one tablet and then take one tablet every 12 hr.

18. AF The nurse is developing a care plan for a client with chronic low back pain caused by a herniated intervertebral disk. Which of the following are priorities in planning care for this client? Select all that apply.
- □ 1. Maintain bed rest.
- □ 2. Teach effective coping skills.
- □ 3. Promote mobility.
- □ 4. Assure adequate tissue perfusion.
- □ 5. Relieve pain.

Spinal Cord Injury

19. AF The nurse is providing care for a client with a spinal cord injury and urinary catheter

in place. The nurse finds the client in a recumbent position with a rapid increase in the BP; the client has a pounding headache and is damp from sweating. The nurse should do which of the following in priority order? Place in order from first to last.

_____ 1. Notify the HCP.
_____ 2. Loosen clothing.
_____ 3. Assist client to sitting position.
_____ 4. Check urinary catheter for kinks.

20. A client had a C6 spinal cord injury 4 hr ago. Which of the following nursing diagnoses is a priority?

- ☐ 1. Urinary retention.
- ☐ 2. Powerlessness.
- ☐ 3. Risk for impaired skin integrity.
- ☐ 4. Ineffective breathing pattern.

Answers and Rationales

1. 3 The nurse's first action is to notify the HCP because the client is likely experiencing a fat embolus. Fat emboli are associated with embolization of marrow or tissue fat or platelets and free fatty acids to the pulmonary capillaries, producing rapid onset of symptoms. Multiple fractures and fractures of the long bones or pelvis increase a client's risk for developing a fat embolus; in addition, young adults between 20 and 30 years of age are at a higher risk for fat emboli with fractures. When fat emboli do occur, hypoxia results; therefore, it is most important the nurse assess changes in level of consciousness and observe changes in behavior such as restlessness and irritability. The nurse does not cut the cast; there is no indication that the casts are obstructing circulation. ABGs are used to confirm the diagnosis, not chest x-ray. The client's behavior is a result of hypoxemia, not pain. (A)

2. 2 The nurse instructs the client to maintain two finger widths between the axillary fold and the underarm piece grip of the crutches to prevent pressure on the brachial plexus. The client is advised to use the three-point gait; in the four-point and two point-gait there is partial weight bearing of both feet. The client is also advised to keep the affected leg elevated when sitting to prevent swelling, and to use the arms, not the axillae, to maintain balance and support. (S)

3. 4 Skeletal traction is often used to regain normal length of the bone, but in this situation the main purpose of the traction is to reduce and immobilize the fracture. This type of traction allows the client to move in bed without dislocating the fracture. This client has an open fracture, but skeletal traction will not prevent further skin breakdown. (A)

4. 3 The nurse first assesses the mechanism of injury to help determine related injuries, tests needed, and potential treatment options. The next step is to assess the location, type, quality, and intensity of the pain. Neurovascular stasis of the injured site is assessed after pain; therefore, the nurse checks for functional ability or changing positions. Although the nurse can also determine the extent of anxiety while assessing the injury and can use communication strategies to minimize anxiety, it is not the first priority for assessing this client. (M)

5. 3 This client has sustained a compression injury; therefore, monitoring the neurovascular integrity of the injured extremity is essential. In this type of injury, compartment syndrome (increased tissue pressure causing hypoxemia) leads to permanent loss of function in 6 to 8 hr. If the skin is broken, the wound is treated and the client is monitored for infection. Because this client has had severe trauma, the nurse evaluates for hemorrhage and shock in the early stages of recovery. Preventing disuse syndrome and encouraging physical mobility are important interventions following the acute phase. (A)

6. 2, 3, 4 Metastatic bone disease is often a result of metastasis from a primary tumor such as breast, prostate, GI tract, lungs, kidney, ovary, and thyroid. Pathologic fractures at the site of metastasis are common because of weakening of the involved bone. Nursing care focuses on preventing pathologic fractures; these interventions include avoiding bumping the client's bed, assisting the client in ambulating, and supporting the joints when repositioning the client. The nurse guards the client against falls by encouraging the client to wear shoes and use proper lighting. Monitoring serum calcium levels and reviewing chemotherapy use do not contribute to the nursing goals for this client. (R)

7. 2 Surgical trauma and postoperative edema may compromise neurologic as well as vascular systems in the affected leg; this takes precedence over positioning, movement, and elimination. (R)

8. 4 The nurse assists the client in keeping the leg abducted and in neutral rotation to prevent stress on the prosthetic hip; pillows may be used to maintain this position, particularly when turning the client or assisting the client to stand and ambulate. The other positions do not maintain the prosthetic hip in proper alignment for healing. (S)

9. 1 Gastric upset is a side effect of nonsteroidal anti-inflammatory medications; taking medication with food minimizes this effect. Corticosteroids affect adrenal gland function and are discontinued by lowering the dose gradually, but this is not true of nonsteroidal anti-inflammatory medications. It is not necessary to rinse the mouth, as stomatitis is not a usual side effect. Dizziness is not an effect of this drug. (D)

10. 4 Individuals with rheumatoid arthritis need to maintain an active exercise program to strengthen and preserve muscle movement and ROM. Aquatic exercises are ideal because the water promotes buoyancy and the client can more easily obtain full ROM and muscle use. Walking, bicycling, and using a treadmill may be too painful, and do not strengthen the upper body muscles or provide sufficient ROM. (H)

11. 4 Rheumatoid arthritis may have no obvious symptoms when there is an exacerbation. The client may have unexplained weight loss, loss of appetite, fatigue, a persistent low-grade fever, general malaise, and muscle weakness. The nurse obtains a full understanding of the client's energy level, ROM, and appetite before developing a care plan with the client. It is not necessary to know the initial therapies at the time of diagnosis, as the nurse is planning care for the client's current state of health. Knowing the client's resources is helpful, but that information is not needed at this time to plan care. To know if the client has an elevated temperature is more important to plan care than to know the other vital signs. (A)

12. 1, 2, 3, 4 The erythrocyte sedimentation rate (ESR) indicates alteration of blood proteins by inflammatory and necrotic processes, and is an indicator of widespread inflammatory reaction by infection or autoimmune disorders. C-reactive protein (CRP) is a glycoprotein produced by the liver in response to acute inflammation. The CRP assay is a nonspecific test that determines the presence of inflammation. Antinuclear antibodies (ANA) are autoantibodies; their presence indicates immune complex diseases, among other conditions. Rheumatoid factor is a macroglobulin-type antibody that clients with rheumatoid arthritis harbor. Amylase and lipase are two enzymes secreted by the pancreas to aid in carbohydrate and fat digestion, respectively, and are not related to the inflammation of the RA. (A)

13. 2, 3, 4 ROM is important to maintain joint mobility; clients who are in pain often do not move the joints, which can lead to stiffness and functional impairment. Heat packs are prescribed to increase circulation to the affected area and to decrease pain; the client should also take pain medication as needed. Hand splints can lead to joint stiffness and functional impairment. Weight loss helps with pain in the large, weight-bearing joints, but it does not help pain in the hands. (H)

14. 2 The client may need to lose extra pounds to reach her "ideal weight," but she needs to maintain a well-balanced diet while doing so. Extra weight places extra stress and strain on affected weight-bearing joints. (H)

15. 1 Prior to discharge, the nurse instructs the client to wrap the residual limb with an elastic bandage using a figure-eight wrap. This will shape the limb and prepare it for prosthesis fitting. The client is instructed to wrap the bandage in a distal-to-proximal direction, and to wear the bandage at all times except for bathing. If the bandage is causing pain, the client can rewrap the bandage with a looser wrap; bandaging techniques do not affect phantom limb pain. (H)

16. 3 The affected extremity should be in full extension and may be elevated to prevent contractures or limit the ROM of the extremity. The client may be positioned on any side as well as the front or back as long as the legs are extended and the client is turned frequently. The nurse assists the UAP to reposition the client and provides additional direction about correct positioning. (M)

17. 1 The nurse instructs the client to start the prescription by taking the least amount of the medication. The client is advised to monitor pain level and adjust the dosage according to the amount of pain relief. (D)

18. 3, 5 Reliving pain and promoting physical mobility are the two priorities in caring for a client with low back pain. Unless there is a healing process required, bed rest is discouraged as it may significantly decrease the rate of recovery and increase pain and disability.

The client is encouraged to ambulate, perform back exercises, and participate in aerobic and strength-training exercises to maintain function. Promoting effective coping for chronic pain is important, but not a priority. Tissue perfusion is not a concern unless the disk is compromising circulation. (C)

19. 1, 3, 2, 4 The client is having autonomic dysreflexia. The nurse first notifies the HCP and assists the client to a sitting position; then, the nurse loosens the clothing and anything that might be constricting the client. Autonomic dysreflexia is often caused by obstruction in a catheter, pressure on the back from lying on an object, or from an impaction; therefore, the nurse's next action is to check the catheter for an obstruction and, if necessary, for other potential sources of pressure. (M)

20. 4 During the acute phase of a spinal cord injury, the nurse monitors the client's breathing pattern as the client is at risk for respiratory arrest from paralysis of the respiratory muscles. The client may have a neurogenic bladder and is at risk for urinary retention, but that is not a priority for the acute phase. The client will be at risk for impaired skin integrity because of immobilization; the nurse establishes plans to prevent skin breakdown, but this is not the immediate concern for this client. As the client moves into the subacute and chronic phases of the injury, the nurse can plan to assist the client to manage the sense of powerlessness. (A)

chapter 32

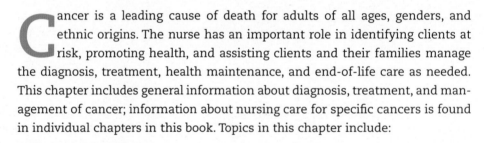

The Client With Cancer

Cancer is a leading cause of death for adults of all ages, genders, and ethnic origins. The nurse has an important role in identifying clients at risk, promoting health, and assisting clients and their families manage the diagnosis, treatment, health maintenance, and end-of-life care as needed. This chapter includes general information about diagnosis, treatment, and management of cancer; information about nursing care for specific cancers is found in individual chapters in this book. Topics in this chapter include:

- Diagnosis of Cancer
- Management of Cancer
- Oncologic Complications
- End-of-Life Care

Diagnosis of Cancer

I. Definition: Cancer is a class of diseases characterized by abnormal and uncontrolled cell division. These cells have the ability to invade other tissues through metastases, either directly or by the movement of cells to remote sites.
   A. Classification of cancer
      1. Carcinoma—malignant tumor beginning in epithelial cells of the organ; most common form of cancer. Types named for type of cell involved.
      2. Sarcoma—cancer beginning in connective tissue, such as cartilage, fat, muscle, or bone.
      3. Lymphoma—cancer of the lymphatic system.
      4. Leukemia—malignancies within the blood; types are named for dominant cell involved.
   B. Diagnostic testing
      1. Biopsy—gold standard for diagnosing
      2. X-ray
      3. Blood and/or urine tests
   C. Tumor staging and grading
      1. Staging—determines size of tumor and how far it has spread from the original site (metastasis); TNM system frequently used:
         a. Tumor (T)—extent of primary tumor
            (1) TX—primary tumor cannot be assessed
            (2) T0—no evidence of primary tumor
            (3) Tis—carcinoma in situ
            (4) T1, T2, T3, T4—increasing size and extent of primary tumor
         b. Nodes (N)—presence or absence of local lymph node involvement
            (1) NX—regional lymph nodes cannot be assessed
            (2) N0—no regional lymph node metastasis
            (3) N1, N2, N3—increasing extent of lymph node involvement
         c. Metastasis (M)—presence or absence of distant metastasis
            (1) MX—distant metastasis cannot be assessed
            (2) M0—no distant metastasis present
            (3) M1—distant metastasis present
      2. Grading—classification of tumor cells; determines how closely the tumor resembles the tissue it originated in; helps to predict behavior and prognosis of tumors.
         a. Grade I—well-differentiated tumor; closely resembles the tissue of origin
         b. Grade II—less differentiated
         c. Grade III—increasingly poorly differentiated
         d. Grade IV—poorly differentiated; does not resemble tissue of origin; tends to be less responsive to treatment
   D. Risk assessment and prevention
      1. Primary prevention: Reduce risk of cancer in healthy individuals.
         a. Promote dietary changes—decrease fat intake, increase fiber, increase fresh vegetables.
         b. Avoid known carcinogens (e.g., tobacco, ionizing radiation, asbestos, ultraviolet rays).
         c. Promote lifestyle changes (stop smoking, reduce alcohol intake, increase exercise).
         d. Initiate prevention programs for topics, including hazards of smoking, and dietary education.
      2. Secondary prevention
         a. Detect and screen for early diagnosis of cancer.
         b. Refer client to genetic counseling (cancers such as breast cancer and colon cancer have familial component).
         c. Initiate public awareness and health-teaching seminars for topics such as breast self exams and testicular self exams.
         d. Promote screening exams, including mammograms, colonoscopies, Pap smears, prostate-specific antigen blood tests, rectal exams, and skin assessments.
   E. Signs and symptoms of cancer
      1. Weight loss
      2. Cachexia
      3. Pallor (related to anemia)
      4. Fever (related to infection)
      5. Pain
      6. Other signals
         a. Lump or thickening in breast
         b. Changes in a mole
         c. Difficulty swallowing
         d. Unusual bleeding or discharge
         e. Persistent hoarseness
         f. Change in bowel or bladder patterns

Management of Cancer

I. Definition: The overall management of cancer involves removing cancer cells to the extent possible. The client, family, and health care team collaborate to determine realistic outcomes and appropriate types of treatment.

Chemotherapy

I. Definition: Chemotherapy is the use of drugs to destroy tumor cells.
  A. Uses
    1. Primary use in clients with leukemia
    2. Extends life expectancy in clients with lymphoma
    3. Can be used along with surgery to prevent some types of cancer from reoccurring
  B. Classification of agents used
    1. Alkylating agents
    2. Antimetabolites
    3. Plant alkaloids
    4. Antibiotics
    5. Hormones
  C. Administration: can be given PO, IM, or IV (see also section on pharmacologic therapies)
  D. Common side effects
    1. Mucositis
    2. Nausea
    3. Vomiting
    4. Diarrhea
    5. Anemia
    6. Myelosuppression
      a. Neutropenia
      b. Anemia (see Chapters 13 and 22)
      c. Thrombocytopenia (see Chapters 13 and 22)
    7. Hair loss
    8. Organ toxicities related to chemotherapeutic agent used (renal, cardiopulmonary, or neurologic)

II. Nursing process
  A. Assessment
    1. Conduct baseline health assessment.
    2. Assess client's readiness for chemotherapy.
    3. Assess client's physical response.
    4. Assess client's psychologic response.
  B. Analysis
    1. Deficient Knowledge related to treatment and side effects
    2. Risk for Infection related to altered immune system
    3. Risk for Injury related to thrombocytopenia
    4. Risk for Injury related to decrease in RBC
    5. Fluid Volume Deficit related to nausea, vomiting, and anorexia
    6. Disturbed Body Image related to side effects of chemotherapy
    7. Imbalanced Nutrition: Less Than Body Requirements related to nausea, vomiting, and anorexia
    8. Impaired Oral Mucous Membrane related to chemotherapy
    9. Impaired Tissue Integrity: Alopecia and/or Malignant Skin Lesions related to chemotherapy or cancer
    10. Chronic Pain related to cancer and side effects of cancer therapy
    11. Fatigue related to treatment, side effects, and/or anemia
  C. Planning
    1. Eradicate cancer.
    2. Eliminate or help subdue side effects.
  D. Implementation
    1. Provide client and family teaching (see management of care).
    2. Frequently assess client for signs and symptoms of infection.
    3. Avoid any invasive procedures during therapy, as possible.
    4. Restrict client activities if platelet count is less than 10,000.
    5. Avoid medications that increase chance of bleeding, such as aspirin.
    6. Instruct client to inform health care team of any increased bruising or increased bleeding times.
    7. Provide client with transfusion, if ordered.
    8. Administer antiemetics prior to receiving treatment to minimize nausea and vomiting.
    9. Monitor nutritional status. Suggest small, frequent meals with increased caloric content in order to ensure adequate nutrition. Ensure client receives dietary consult to assist with client meeting nutritional needs. Administer nutritional supplement meals if indicated.
    10. Assess client's weight frequently.
    11. Frequently assess client for pain; administer analgesics for pain from mucositis as necessary.
    12. Promote skin integrity.
      a. Frequently assess client's skin for signs of breakdown.
      b. Turn and reposition client if unable to do so on own every 2 to 3 hr to prevent skin breakdown.
      c. Provide client with appropriate dressings for skin breakdown and frequently assess change dressings.
      d. Monitor albumin level and nutritional intake to help prevent skin breakdown.
    13. Administer oxygen therapy, if indicated.
  E. Evaluation
    1. Client understands and verbalizes reasons for treatment and associated side effects.
    2. Client identifies ways to minimize or prevent side effects and when to notify health care team for assistance with symptom control.

3. Client remains free of infection.
4. Client remains free of injury.
5. Client remains free of fluid volume deficits.
6. Client does not suffer from any body image disturbances.
7. Client minimizes weight loss.
8. Client is free from mucositis.
9. Client's skin remains intact.
10. Client is free from pain or pain is well managed.
11. Client demonstrates ability to minimize fatigue.

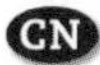

III. Client needs

A. Physiologic adaptation

1. Closely monitor the client for effectiveness of any treatment given.
2. Monitor laboratory values for effectiveness of treatment.
3. Monitor client for side effects of treatment.
4. Watch for signs and symptoms of reaction to blood transfusion, if indicated.

B. Management of care: Care of the client with cancer requires critical thinking skills and knowledge of assessment, and teaching and evaluation methods unique to the RN role. These skills cannot be delegated to an LPN or UAP.

1. Assess client for any signs of organ toxicity throughout treatment.
2. Frequently assess vital signs, ECGs, neurologic status.
3. Assess client's pain frequently throughout cancer treatment.
4. Provide client and family teaching about the following:
   a. Medications, length of treatment, and goals of therapy.
   b. Dietary restrictions or medication interactions associated with treatment.
   c. Potential side effects of therapy (nausea, vomiting, loss of appetite, stomatitis, alopecia, bleeding.
   d. Signs and symptoms of infection (temp greater than 101°F, or chills) and to notify HCP.
   e. Signs and symptoms of anemia, and to report any syncopal episodes, chest pain, palpitations, and/or dizziness to HCP.
5. Consult social services for client and family to assist with needs throughout therapy.
6. Consider physical therapy consult for client deconditioned from treatment and/or side effects.
7. Consult a dietician to assist client develop an adequate diet that helps to manage side effects.

C. Safety and infection control

1. Encourage client and family/friends to perform frequent hand hygiene to help prevent infection.
2. Prevent any trauma to client's skin to help prevent infection, including the use of catheters, enemas, suppositories, NG tubes, and rectal thermometers, unless necessary.
3. Advise myelosuppressed client and family on protective measures.
   a. Perform frequent hand hygiene.
   b. Use electric razor only.
   c. Protect skin from sun exposure.
   d. Provide frequent mouth care (using gentle toothbrush).
   e. Avoid exposure to individuals with colds or other contagious illnesses.
   f. Avoid animal excretion: Do not clean litter box or birdcage.
4. Avoid administering any live vaccines; prevent contact between client and individual who has received a live vaccine within 30 days.
5. Instruct neutropenic client and family to report any signs of infection, including temperature greater than 100.4°F, chills, dysuria, or dyspnea.
6. Implement bleeding precautions for client with thrombocytopenia.

D. Health promotion and maintenance: Provide client and family teaching.

1. Prevent dehydration by drinking 2 to 3 L of fluids per day; report signs and symptoms of dehydration (thirst, headache).
2. Prevent stomatitis with oral hygiene. Encourage client to frequently perform mouth care using soft-bristled brush; avoid use of mouthwashes containing alcohol or hydrogen peroxide. Use ice chips to keep client's oral mucosa moist. Keep lips well lubricated.
3. Promote ways to minimize hair loss, such as avoiding perms or coloring, and vigorous brushing or hair dryer use. Introduce to client the potential use of wigs, scarves, or hats when hair loss occurs. Reassure client that hair will return, although texture and color may be different.
4. Manage persistent symptoms of anemia such as fatigue and decreased activity tolerance; take frequent rest breaks and conserve energy if hypoxic.
5. For client with thrombocytopenia—have soft diet to avoid irritating digestive mucosal lining.
6. For client with nausea and vomiting—eat small, frequent meals and premedicate with antiemetics if necessary.

7. For client with diarrhea—eat bland foods that are low-roughage, low-fat, and are high in pectin; avoid alcohol and drinks with caffeine.
8. Prevent mucositis by eating a high-protein diet with adequate fluid intake (greater than 1,500 ml/day, unless contraindicated).
9. Minimize foods with excessive odors that can affect taste.
10. Void as frequently as possible.
11. Notify HCP if unable to keep food or fluids down.

E. Psychologic integrity
1. Acknowledge client's feeling of hopelessness and frustration with treatment and side effects.
2. Provide client experiencing alopecia support and introduce client to local cancer resources for additional support.
3. Introduce client to local places to find wigs, scarves, and the like.

F. Basic care and comfort
1. Eliminate fresh fruits and vegetables, raw meat, eggs, and fish from diet to help prevent chemotherapy-induced neutropenia.
2. Frequently turn and reposition client as necessary to help prevent against any pressure ulcers.
3. Reinforce need for meticulous hygiene in neutropenic clients.
4. Assess client with anemia for activity tolerance.
5. Weigh client weekly or as indicated to assess for nutritional deficits.
6. Perform strict monitoring of intake and output to help prevent hemorrhagic cystitis.

G. Reduction of risk potential
1. Monitor ANC serum calculation to assess for neutropenia.
2. Culture urine and any other suspected areas for infection to determine source in neutropenic client.
3. Obtain chest x-ray in neutropenic clients to help find source of infection.
4. Monitor blood cultures daily in neutropenic clients.
5. Monitor hemoglobin, hematocrit, RBC values frequently for clients with anemia.
6. Monitor platelets, hematocrit, and coagulation panel in clients with thrombocytopenia.
7. Assess electrolytes, vitamin levels, and albumin level for signs of adequate nutrition.
8. Assess BUN and creatinine levels throughout treatment to early identify kidney complications (particularly, hemorrhagic cystitis).

H. Pharmacologic and parenteral therapies: Client will state the purpose for and side effects of all medications used during treatment of cancer.
1. Antibiotics as ordered for the neutropenic client.
2. Oxygen therapy if anemic client becomes hypoxic.
3. Epoetin alfa as ordered to help improve hemoglobin level.
4. Stool softeners to prevent constipation and straining in clients with thrombocytopenia, as ordered.
5. Antiemetics as indicated.
6. Prophylactic antiemetics considered prior to chemotherapy for clients with acute nausea and vomiting.
7. Fluids and electrolytes replaced in clients with diarrhea.
8. Antidiarrheal medication as indicated.
9. Analgesics as indicated for pain.

Radiation Therapy

I. Definition: Radiation therapy is the use of high-energy rays to destroy cancer cells or interfere with ability to grow or multiply.

A. Uses
1. Curative—primarily used to treat Hodgkin lymphoma and uterine cancer.
2. Palliative—used to prevent pain and stop bone fractures occurring as a result of metastases.
3. Adjunctive—used along with chemotherapy and/or surgery.

B. Types
1. External—external machine that emits radiation.
2. Internal—source of radiation is radioisotopes, which emit radiation; isotopes placed where the main source of cancer is within the body.
3. Combination of both treatments used together.

C. Radiation protection principles
1. Distance—stay as far away as possible from radiation source; the further away from the source, the less exposure to radiation.
2. Time—spend as little time as possible near radiation source; the less time near the source, the less exposure to radiation.
3. Shielding—use available materials to shield self from radiation, such as lead shields.

D. Side effects of radiation therapy depend on location of tumor and site receiving therapy.
1. Anorexia, nausea, vomiting
2. Fatigue, malaise, headaches
3. Diarrhea

4. Skin reactions (burns and ulcerations); alopecia
5. Anemia
6. Urinary frequency, urgency, dysuria, and hematuria; cystitis, urethritis
7. Thick, tenacious sputum, loss of taste, dry mouth and tooth decay; mucositis
8. Pneumonitis; cough

II. Nursing process

A. Assessment
1. Conduct baseline health assessment.
2. Assess client's readiness for radiation therapy.
3. Assess client's physical response.
4. Assess client's psychologic response.

B. Analysis
1. Deficient Knowledge about administration and side effects
2. Impaired Skin Integrity related to potential breakdown or skin reactions
3. Risk for Injury related to displacement or loss of implant in internal radiation

C. Planning
1. Eradicate cancer or provide palliative relief.
2. Eliminate or help subdue side effects.

D. Implementation
1. Provide client and family teaching (see also management of care in client needs section).
   a. Optimize nutritional intake.
      (1) High calories, high protein, low fat
      (2) Adequate hydration
      (3) B_{12} supplements
      (4) Frequent, small meals
   b. Maintain NPO status 2 to 3 hr before radiation therapy and 2 hr after.
   c. Avoid vigorous washing of skin to help prevent breakdown.
   d. Ensure skin (including skin folds) is clean and dry at all times.
   e. Avoid any skin care products that contain heavy metal or perfume.
   f. Avoid sunlight as much as possible to not dry out skin further.
   g. If skin breakdown occurs (blistering or loss of outer layer of skin), cover with nonadherent dressing and use paper tape only.
2. Limit client activity during internal radiation.
3. Keep head of bed in semi-Fowler position or below during internal radiation.
4. During internal radiation, check implant frequently to avoid loss or displacement.

E. Evaluation
1. Client and family understand and verbalize how treatment works and which side effects to report to HCP.
2. Client's skin remains intact.
3. Client does not experience injury caused by implant.
4. Client and family can manage side effects.

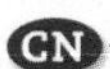

III. Client needs (see client needs for chemotherapy)

Bone Marrow and Stem Cell Transplant

I. Definition: Blood and marrow stem cell transplant is a procedure through which the client's bone marrow is destroyed via chemotherapy or radiation and then replaced with new bone marrow. The procedure is used for leukemia, aplastic anemia, and lymphoma; the process takes about 45 days from admission to discharge, with the majority of the time spent recovering after transplant.

A. Donor sources
1. Allogenic—genetically matched donor (can be relative or unrelated).
2. Autologous—client's own bone marrow.

B. Stages of the transplant process: Pretransplant, conditioning, transplant, posttransplant.

C. Potential side effects: Transplant reaction, infection, graft-versus-host disease.

Pretransplant Stage

I. Definition: Occurs prior to transplant once donor tissue has been located and matched

II. Nursing process

A. Assessment: Perform thorough evaluations to assess the current state of the disease:
1. Perform nutritional assessment.
2. Perform comprehensive physical examination.
3. Assess social support system.
4. Obtain diagnostic tests.
   a. Bone marrow biopsy
   b. Pulmonary function tests
   c. ECG
   d. Lab workup including CBC, RBC type
   e. Blood work to assess past exposures (e.g., HIV, syphilis, hepatitis, herpes)

B. Analysis
1. Deficient Knowledge related to procedure
2. Fear related to unknown outcomes

C. Planning
1. Provide client and family teaching.
2. Prevent infection.

D. Implementation
1. Provide client and family teaching (see also management of care in client needs section).
   a. Advise a low-bacteria diet.
   b. Assist and instruct client in implementing self-care procedures such as hand

hygiene, frequent mouth care, skin care, perineal care, strict intake and output, and nutrition.
2. Ensure an informed consent has been obtained for procedure.
3. Administer antibiotics to help decrease bacteria present in body.

E. Evaluation
1. Client has no adverse reactions; complications are managed.
2. Transplant is successful.

Conditioning

I. Definition: Use of radiation or chemotherapy to eradicate cancer cells from the client

II. Nursing process

A. Assessment
1. Assess for side effects of medication and/or procedure: Mucositis, hemorrhagic cystitis, diarrhea, liver toxicity, pancytopenia, nausea and vomiting, hepatic veno-occlusive disease (VOD).
2. Obtain diagnostic tests: CBC, platelet count, electrolytes, blood and urine cultures when indicated, ECG, and other tests as indicated.

B. Analysis
1. Deficient Knowledge related to procedure
2. Ineffective Tissue Perfusion: Cardiovascular, related to effects of medication
3. Imbalanced Nutrition: Less Than Body Requirements related to nausea and vomiting
4. Risk for Infection related to neutropenia

C. Planning
1. Eradicate all of client's own bone marrow.
2. Manage side effects.
3. Ensure fluid and nutritional balance; use central catheter for fluid administration as well as administering blood products and obtaining blood samples.

D. Implementation
1. Provide client and family teaching (see also management of care in client needs section).
   a. Advise a low-bacteria diet.
   b. Promote adequate hydration—4,000+ ml daily, unless contraindicated.
2. Administer IV fluids to supplement fluid intake, and before and after each chemotherapy treatment.
3. Weigh client daily.
4. Perform bladder irrigation as indicated.
5. Assess vital signs as ordered.
6. Closely monitor caloric intake.
7. Provide client with small, frequent meals.
8. Provide high-caloric, high-protein supplemental drinks as indicated.
9. Administer antiemetic as indicated.
10. Encourage client not to have frequent visitors because of exposure increasing risk of infection, but to maintain close contact with family and friends during procedure.
11. Closely monitor client for signs and symptoms of anxiety.
12. Keep client in strict isolation during therapy.
13. Ensure client wears a mask when leaving isolation room.
14. Ensure flowers and plants are not kept in client's room.
15. Ensure client is not using tap water unless bathing
16. Frequently assess skin integrity.

E. Evaluation
1. Client verbalizes understanding of procedures regarding bone marrow transplant.
2. Client does not experience any renal impairment (particularly hemorrhagic cystitis).
3. Client maintains weight.
4. Client is free from anxiety and demonstrates ability to use tools to relieve anxiety.
5. Client is free from signs of infection.

Transplant Stage

I. Definition: Infusion of bone marrow or peripheral stem cells

II. Nursing process

A. Assessment: Assess client for allergic reaction to bone marrow transfusion including fever, chills, hematuria, and chest pain.

B. Analysis: Risk for Excess Fluid Volume related to bone marrow infusion

C. Planning
1. Provide client and family teaching.
2. Replace client's bone marrow supply with new marrow.

D. Implementation
1. Administer marrow infusion according to procedure protocol (generally slowly, but within 4 hr).
2. Assess vital signs every 5 min throughout infusion and after infusion, every 15 min for 2 hr.
3. Frequently assess client for signs or symptoms of allergic reaction; if allergic reaction occurs:
   a. Administer medications as ordered.
   b. Never stop infusion; slow down rate and notify physician immediately.

E. Evaluation: Client does not experience fluid volume overload throughout infusion.

Posttransplant Stage

I. Definition: Follow up and management of complications

II. Nursing process

A. Assessment: During posttransplant stage, many complications can occur. Assess client for the following complications:
1. Signs of bleeding: Petechiae, bruising, occult blood
2. Signs of an infection
3. Graft-versus-host disease (GVHD)

B. Analysis
1. Risk for Injury related to thrombocytopenia
2. Deficient Knowledge related to posttransplant care
3. Risk for Infection related to immunosuppression
4. Fear related to unknown outcomes of transplant

C. Planning
1. Prevent infection.
2. Prevent renal failure.
3. Manage nausea, vomiting, mucositis.
4. Monitor client for graft-versus-host disease.

D. Implementation
1. Frequently assess platelet level, hemoglobin, hematocrit, and electrolytes.
2. Assess vital signs and neurologic status every shift.
3. Provide client with frequent mouth care and assess oral cavity for signs of bleeding.
4. Assess stool and urine for occult blood.
5. Avoid use of aspirin and NSAIDs.
6. Replete client with platelets as indicated.
7. Implement bleeding precautions: Use electric razor, use soft-bristled toothbrush, and avoid rectal temps or any medications rectally.
8. Provide client teaching about procedures and potential complications (see also management of care in client needs section).

E. Evaluation
1. Client has no signs of bleeding.
2. Client is free from infection.
3. Client's urinary output and kidney function are within normal limits.

III. Client needs (see client needs for chemotherapy)

Oncologic Complications

I. Definition: Oncologic complications can result because of the disease process and as untoward effects of cancer therapies. The nurse assesses the client for these complications and directs nursing care toward preventing them.

Superior Vena Cava Syndrome

I. Definition: Superior vena cava syndrome involves an obstruction of the superior vena cava caused by a tumor pressing against the superior vena cava. The condition is most commonly seen in lung cancer; symptoms can be gradual or arise suddenly.

II. Nursing process

A. Assessment
1. Assess for signs and symptoms including impaired venous drainage, cough, dyspnea, dysphagia, difficulty buttoning shirt because of tumor.
2. Obtain diagnostic tests.
   a. Chest x-ray
   b. Thoracic CT scan
   c. MRI

B. Analysis
1. Ineffective Tissue Perfusion: Cardiopulmonary, related to impaired venous drainage
2. Risk for Excess Fluid Volume related to impaired venous drainage

C. Planning
1. Alleviate symptoms with supportive therapy.
2. Treat underlying condition.

D. Implementation
1. Assess client's cardiovascular, respiratory, and neurologic systems frequently.
2. Assess client's level of consciousness per shift (at least every 8 hr) or as indicated.
3. Monitor vital signs every shift or as indicated.
4. Ensure client is on cardiac telemetry and monitor as indicated.
5. Administer corticosteroids as indicated.
6. Place client in semi-Fowler position to ease shortness of breath as necessary.
7. Encourage client to minimize activity to decrease oxygen demands.
8. Assess client for signs and symptoms of activity intolerance.
9. Administer oxygen therapy as indicated.
10. Assess client for signs and symptoms of edema.
11. Administer diuretics as indicated.
12. Closely monitor client's fluid intake and output.
13. Restrict fluids as necessary to prevent increased edema.

E. Evaluation
1. Client demonstrates adequate tissue perfusion.
2. Client has minimized edema.

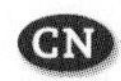

III. Client needs

A. Physiologic adaptation
1. Place client on cardiac monitor in order to monitor any cardiac disturbances or changes.

2. Frequently assess client for increased shortness of breath, trouble swallowing, visual changes, altered mental status, or increased edema.

B. Management of care: Care of the client with superior vena cava syndrome requires critical thinking skills and knowledge of assessment, and teaching and evaluation methods unique to the RN role. These skills cannot be delegated to an LPN or UAP.
   1. Provide client with frequent assessments including vital signs, neurologic assessments, and ECGs as indicated.
   2. Inform physician of any changes noted during each assessment.
   3. Monitor client for complications associated with chemotherapy and/or radiation therapy, if indicated.

C. Safety and infection control: Follow guidelines for chemotherapy/radiation therapy as indicated.

D. Health promotion and maintenance: Provide client teaching, including frequent updates with regard to treatment plan.

E. Psychologic integrity: Promote consults such as social services, as indicated.

F. Basic care and comfort
   1. Place client in semi-Fowler position in order to facilitate ease of breathing.
   2. Encourage client to decrease activity and take frequent rest breaks in order to minimize shortness of breath.
   3. Closely monitor client's fluid intake and output (ensure edema does not worsen).

G. Reduction of risk potential: Identify client as "at risk" and closely monitor for complication; client is at an increased risk to develop complication with lung cancer, lymphomas, and when metastases are present.

H. Pharmacologic and parenteral therapies: Client will state purpose for and side effects of medications used to treat superior vena cava syndrome.
   1. Radiation therapy to alleviate symptoms by decreasing tumor size.
   2. Chemotherapy to shrink tumor, if indicated.
   3. Corticosteroids, diuretics as indicated.
   4. Oxygen therapy as indicated.

Spinal Cord Compression

I. Definition: Compression of spinal cord and nerve roots as a result of tumor compression and may result in permanent neurologic problems.

II. Nursing process

A. Assessment
   1. Assess for signs and symptoms.
      a. Pain exacerbated by activity
      b. Sensory problems such as numbness and tingling in extremities
      c. Loss of positional sense
      d. Loss of motor function
      e. Bladder and/or bowel dysfunction
   2. Obtain diagnostic tests.
      a. Percussion tenderness at level of compression
      b. Abnormal reflexes
      c. MRI, x-rays, bone scan, and/or CT scan

B. Analysis
   1. Acute Pain related to tumor growth and cord compression
   2. Impaired Physical Mobility related to neuromuscular impairment

C. Planning
   1. Relieve compression on spinal cord.
   2. Treat underlying condition.

D. Implementation
   1. Assist client with performing active and passive range of motion as indicated.
   2. Consult physical therapist as indicated.
   3. Assist client with turning and repositioning every 2 hr or as needed.
   4. Encourage client to minimize activities to prevent vertebral fractures.
   5. Administer pain medication as needed.
   6. Advise client with regard to undertreating pain.
   7. Ensure client is premedicated, if necessary, before repositioning or working with physical therapy.

E. Evaluation
   1. Client verbalizes relief in pain.
   2. Client does not physically decompensate.

CN

III. Client needs

A. Physiologic adaptation
   1. Provide client with nursing management indicated for radiation therapy.
   2. Provide client with nursing management indicated for chemotherapy, if relevant.

B. Management of care: Care of the client with spinal cord compression requires critical thinking skills and knowledge of assessment, and teaching and evaluation methods unique to the RN role. These skills cannot be delegated to an LPN or UAP.
   1. Provide client with frequent assessments, including vital signs, and neurologic assessments as indicated.
   2. Inform physician of any changes noted during each assessment.

3. Monitor client for complications associated with chemotherapy and/or radiation therapy, if indicated.

C. Safety and infection control
1. Assess skin frequently for signs of breakdown from immobility.
2. Assess WBC count, as indicated, for signs of infection.

D. Health promotion and maintenance: Provide client teaching including frequent updates with regard to treatment plan.

E. Psychologic integrity: Provide client with support and consults from social services and psychiatry as indicated.

F. Basic care and comfort
1. Provide client with frequent repositioning to relieve pain.
2. Encourage client to cough and deep breathe because of client's immobility.
3. Provide client with range of motion exercises, passive or active as appropriate, to maintain muscle tone.
4. Consult physical therapist as indicated.
5. Provide client with intermittent catheterizations, if necessary.

G. Reduction of risk potential: Encourage client to remain on bed rest, if indicated, to help prevent a vertebral fracture.

H. Pharmacologic and parenteral therapies: Client will state the purpose for and side effects of all medications used to treat spinal cord compression.
1. Radiation therapy to decrease size of tumor.
2. Chemotherapy along with radiation therapy, if indicated.
3. Corticosteroid therapy to decrease inflammation at compression site.
4. Surgery in the case of vertebral fracture leading to further nerve damage.
5. Analgesics as indicated.

Hypercalcemia

I. Definition: Hypercalcemia is an increased level of calcium in blood that can be life-threatening. This oncologic complication results from bone destruction by tumor or tumors that promote calcium release.

II. Nursing process

A. Assessment
1. Assess for signs and symptoms including fatigue, weakness, confusion, slow reflexes, nausea, vomiting, and dehydration.
2. Obtain diagnostic tests: Elevated calcium in blood.

B. Analysis
1. Activity Intolerance related to generalized weakness
2. Constipation related to slowed intestinal mobility

C. Planning
1. Return calcium levels to baseline.
2. Treat underlying cause.

D. Implementation
1. Encourage client to maintain as much physical activity as possible.
2. Provide client teaching about reasons to maintain level of activity (e.g., prevent bone demineralization).
3. If client unable to tolerate much physical activity, assist client with active or passive range of motion exercises.
4. Assess client's ability to tolerate activities by vital signs, skin color, and client's report of any nausea, dizziness, or shortness of breath.
5. Consult physical therapist to ensure client maintains activity level.
6. Encourage client to increase fiber intake.
7. Administer laxatives as ordered.

E. Evaluation
1. Client maintains activity level.
2. Client does not suffer from constipation, or constipation resolves.

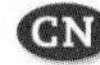

III. Client needs

A. Physiologic adaptation
1. Perform frequent assessments of serum calcium levels.
2. Administer IV fluids to dilute calcium levels and promote kidney excretion.

B. Management of care: Care of the client with hypercalcemia requires critical thinking skills and knowledge of assessment, and teaching and evaluation methods unique to the RN role. These skills cannot be delegated to an LPN or UAP.
1. Provide client with frequent assessments, including vital signs, and neurologic assessments as indicated.
2. Inform physician of any changes noted during each assessment.

C. Basic care and comfort
1. Encourage client to drink 2 to 3 L of fluids daily to help kidneys flush out increased levels of calcium, unless contraindicated.
2. Encourage client to remain active to prevent bone demineralization.

D. Health promotion and maintenance: Provide client teaching including frequent updates with regard to treatment plan.

E. Psychologic integrity: Provide client support and referral as needed.

F. Basic care and comfort: Assist client to maintain activities of daily living as needed.

G. Reduction of risk potential: Closely monitor client with cancer that involves an increased risk of causing hypercalcemia.

H. Pharmacologic and parenteral therapies: Client and family will state the purpose for and side effects of all medications used to treat hypercalcemia.
1. Radiation or chemotherapy to shrink tumor size.
2. Corticosteroids for some cancers to decrease bone demineralization.
3. Biphosphates administered via IV.
4. Inorganic phosphates (Neutra-Phos) to decrease calcium levels, preferably given PO or rectally.
5. Laxatives or stool softeners for constipation that can be caused by hypercalcemia.
6. Antiemetics as indicated.

Cardiac Tamponade (see also Chapter 20)

I. Definition: Cardiac tamponade is an accumulation of fluid in pericardial space, constricting the heart and decreasing the heart's ability to effectively pump blood throughout the body. The complication is usually a result of thoracic tumors or cancer treatments such as radiation therapy; onset can be gradual or rapid.

II. Nursing process

A. Assessment
1. Assess for signs and symptoms.
   a. Kussmaul sign (neck vein distention during inspiration)
   b. Pulsus paradoxus
   c. Distant heart sounds, rubs, and gallops
   d. Tachycardia
   e. Shortness of breath and tachypnea
   f. Chest pain, orthopnea, and diaphoresis
   g. Weakness, lethargy
2. Obtain diagnostic tests.
   a. ECG
   b. Chest x-rays
   c. CT scan

B. Analysis
1. Decreased Cardiac Output related to altered contractibility
2. Ineffective Tissue Perfusion: Cardiopulmonary, related to mechanical reduction of blood flow
3. Activity Intolerance related to imbalance between oxygen supply and demand

C. Planning
1. Eliminate or control cardiac effusions.
2. Treat underlying cause.

D. Implementation
1. Assess client for pulsus paradoxus, neck vein distention, tachycardia, and distant heart sounds.
2. Closely monitor client's fluid intake and output.
3. Assist physician with pericardiocentesis procedure as indicated.
4. Frequently assess client's vital signs and perform serial ECGs.
5. Frequently assess client's cardiac and respiratory status, including color of skin and capillary refill.
6. Assess client's level of consciousness.
7. Elevate head of bed to ease client's breathing.
8. Encourage client to minimize activity in order to reduce oxygen requirements.
9. Assist client in sitting up or transferring to a chair several times a day in order to decrease cardiac deconditioning.

E. Evaluation
1. Client demonstrates adequate cardiac output.
2. Client demonstrates adequate tissue perfusion.
3. Client does not experience any muscle deconditioning.

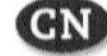

III. Client needs

A. Physiologic adaptation
1. Provide interventions during pericardiocentesis (aspiration of pericardial fluid by large-bore needle); only provides temporary relief in most cases caused by cancer; occasionally, a pericardial catheter is placed and sclerosing agents are injected to help prevent fluids from reaccumulating; openings in pericardium can be surgically made to drain fluid—done as a palliative measure.
2. Place client on cardiac monitor in order to monitor any cardiac changes.
3. Promote radiation therapy to shrink tumor size.
4. Assess client for pulsus paradoxus.
5. Perform ECG as indicated.

B. Management of care: Care of the client with pericardial cardiac tamponade requires critical thinking skills and knowledge of assessment, and teaching and evaluation methods unique to the RN role. These skills cannot be delegated to an LPN or UAP.
1. Provide client with frequent assessments, including vital signs, oxygen saturation levels, and neurologic assessments as indicated.
2. Inform physician of any changes noted during each assessment.

3. Frequently assess heart and lung sounds, neck vein distention, respiratory status, and cardiac perfusion.
4. Perform frequent assessments of level of consciousness.

C. Safety and infection control: When pericardial catheter is placed, ensure sterile dressing covers area.

D. Health promotion and maintenance: Provide client teaching, including frequent updates with regard to treatment plan.

E. Psychologic integrity: Reassure client and sit with client as much as needed to relieve anxiety.

F. Basic care and comfort
1. Monitor fluid intake and output.
2. Encourage client to minimize physical activity to minimize oxygen demands.
3. Elevate client's head of bed to promote ease of breathing.
4. Reorient client as needed.

G. Reduction of risk potential: Frequently assess lab results, including arterial blood gases and electrolytes as indicated.

H. Pharmacologic and parenteral therapies: Client will state the purpose for and side effects of all medications used to treat cardiac tamponade.
1. Chemotherapy to shrink tumor size and relieve pressure on heart.
2. Prednisone and diuretics to help with mild effusions.
3. Oxygen therapy as indicated.

Disseminated Intravascular Coagulation (see also Chapter 20)

I. Definition: Disseminated intravascular coagulation (DIC) is a clotting disorder resulting in increased clotting throughout the body. It is not a disease itself, but rather a sign of an underlying condition, and usually causes severe bleeding.

II. Nursing process

A. Assessment
1. Assess signs and symptoms
   a. Abnormal bleeding, usually sudden and severe, involving more than one system (bleeding most notable at sites of invasive procedures such as an IV, chest tube)
   b. Sudden bruising
   c. Clot formation (in clients with cancer, DIC develops more slowly, resulting in clot formation rather than bleeding)
2. Obtain diagnostic tests.
   a. Blood studies
   b. Elevated PT and PTT; decreased PT and PTT in cancer client with slowly forming DIC
   c. Decreased platelets
   d. High fibrinogen degradation products
   e. Low serum fibrinogen

B. Analysis
1. Ineffective Tissue Perfusion: Cardiopulmonary, related to interruption of flow to organs
2. Acute Pain related to tissue trauma
3. Anxiety related to emergent situation and threat of death

C. Planning
1. Identify underlying cause and control bleeding.
2. Monitor vital signs.
3. Replace clotting factors.
4. Provide anticoagulation therapy.

D. Implementation
1. Ensure IV access.
2. Administer fresh-frozen plasma as ordered.
3. Administer IV heparin, if indicated and as ordered.
4. Observe for signs of increased bleeding (especially at sites of invasive procedures) and apply pressure as necessary. Report any changes to physician.
5. Closely monitor vital signs (BP, temperature, pulse, respiratory rate) as ordered and report any changes in client's condition to physician.
6. Assess neurologic status as indicated and report any changes to physician.
7. Assess arterial blood gases.
8. Administer pain medications as indicated.
9. Maintain calm, nonstressful environment.
10. Reassure client as indicated.
11. Provide client and family with information regarding the condition and how it is being treated in easy-to-understand language.
12. Be attentive to client's nonverbal cues.
13. Provide client and family with clergy, social worker, as indicated.

E. Evaluation
1. Client's bleeding stops or is controlled.
2. Client has no new sources of bleeding.
3. Client verbalizes relief of pain.
4. Client and family demonstrate control over anxiety.

III. Client needs

A. Physiologic adaptation
1. Assess client for signs and symptoms of bleeding, particularly when risk factors are present.

2. Monitor client's lab values as indicated; note slow changes in coagulation for clients with cancer.

B. Management of care: Care of the client with DIC requires critical thinking skills and knowledge of assessment, and teaching and evaluation methods unique to the RN role. These skills cannot be delegated to an LPN or UAP.
   1. Provide client with frequent assessments, including vital signs, neurologic assessments, and ECGs as indicated.
   2. Inform physician of any changes noted during each assessment.

C. Safety and infection control
   1. Ensure aseptic technique throughout emergent event.
   2. Ensure sites of bleeding are cleaned properly, once controlled, and appropriate wound care is provided.

D. Health promotion and maintenance: Provide client teaching, including frequent updates with regard to treatment plan.

E. Psychologic integrity
   1. Identify client and family stressors associated with situation and help provide tools to alleviate them.
   2. Consult clergy and social services as indicated.

F. Basic care and comfort
   1. Provide pain relief as appropriate.
   2. Ensure client is comfortable; reposition in bed if necessary and provide clean, dry clothes.

G. Reduction of risk potential: Prevent bleeding, infection.

H. Pharmacologic and parenteral therapies: Client will state the purpose for and side effects of all medications used to manage DIC.
   1. Fresh-frozen plasma to replace clotting factors.
   2. IV heparin, if indicated, to prevent thrombosis.
   3. Other blood products, if needed.
   4. Analgesics for pain relief.
   5. Oxygen therapy, if indicated.

Syndrome of Inappropriate Antidiuretic Hormone

I. Definition: Certain types of cancers result in the uncontrolled release of antidiuretic hormone, leading to increased extracellular volume, hyponatremia, and water intoxication; increased fluid volume also results in the release of atrial natriuretic factor, which worsens the hyponatremia. SIADH is most frequently seen with small cell lung cancer, but several antineoplastics and morphine can also stimulate antidiuretic hormone secretion.

II. Nursing process

A. Assessment
   1. Assess for signs and symptoms including irritability; nausea and vomiting; weight gain; fatigue, lethargy, or confusion; seizure; abnormal reflexes; and coma.
   2. Obtain diagnostic tests.
      a. Decreased serum sodium level
      b. Increased urine osmolality
      c. Increased urine sodium level
      d. Decreased serum BUN and creatinine levels

B. Analysis
   1. Excess Fluid Volume related to compromised regulatory mechanism
   2. Disturbed Thought Processes related to hyponatremia
   3. Risk for Injury related to hyponatremia

C. Planning
   1. Regulate fluid volume.
   2. Maintain sodium levels within normal range.
   3. Treat underlying cause.

D. Implementation
   1. Assess lung sounds for crackles as indicated.
   2. Assess vital signs every 8 hr or as indicated.
   3. Monitor labs values including serum electrolytes, urine osmolality, and urine sodium.
   4. Closely monitor fluid intake and output.
   5. Perform daily weights.
   6. Implement fluid restrictions as ordered.
   7. Administer parenteral sodium replacement as indicated.
   8. Administer diuretics as indicated.
   9. Assess neurologic status and mental state frequently.
   10. Orient client as necessary to person, place, and time.
   11. Teach family and friends of client who are affected by personality changes, irritability, and other mental status changes, that changes are temporary.
   12. Minimize client's activity as indicated.
   13. Encourage client to ask for assistance when ambulating to prevent injury.
   14. Consult physical therapy to assist with client's activity intolerance.

E. Evaluation
   1. Client demonstrates balanced fluid levels.
   2. Client remains fully alert and oriented.
   3. Client remains free of injury.

CN

III. Client needs

A. Physiologic adaptation
   1. Place client on cardiac monitor in order to monitor any cardiac disturbances or changes.

2. Assess client for signs and symptoms of fluid overload.
3. Provide frequent assessment of serum electrolytes in order to identify more imbalances and the improvement or worsening of syndrome.
4. Frequently assess other lab values such as BUN, creatinine, and urinary sodium levels.

B. Management of care: Care of the client with SIADH requires critical thinking skills and knowledge of assessment, and teaching and evaluation methods unique to the RN role. These skills cannot be delegated to an LPN or UAP.
1. Provide client with frequent assessments, including vital signs, neurologic, cardiac, and respiratory assessments as indicated.
2. Inform physician of any changes noted during each assessment.
3. Maintain strict intake and output records, and daily weight will be recorded.

C. Safety and infection control: Ensure client is in safe environment in order to decrease risk for falls related to fatigue and lethargy.

D. Health promotion and maintenance: Provide client teaching, including frequent updates with regard to treatment plan.

E. Psychologic integrity: Promote consults such as social services as indicated.

F. Basic care and comfort
1. Restrict fluid intake to 500 to 1,000 mL/day to decrease fluid overload.
2. Encourage client to take frequent rest periods as appropriate.
3. Reorient client as necessary.

G. Reduction of risk potential: Closely monitor lab values in clients who have an increased risk of developing complications.

H. Pharmacologic and parenteral therapies: Client will state purpose for and side effects of all medications used to treat SIADH.
1. Demeclocycline if fluid restriction is not adequate for control; helps decrease fluid overload and therefore helps to regulate serum sodium level.
2. Diuretic therapy and/or IV sodium replacement for severe neurologic symptoms as indicated.

Tumor Lysis Syndrome

I. Definition: Tumor lysis syndrome is a complication associated with radiation therapy and chemotherapy in which degradation products of the cancer enter the bloodstream and result in electrolyte imbalances (hyperkalemia, hypocalcemia, hyperphosphatemia, and hyperuricemia). Tumor lysis syndrome can be fatal, and usually occurs with large tumors or rapidly growing cancers such as leukemia, lymphomas, and small cell lung cancer.

II. Nursing process

A. Assessment
1. Assess for signs and symptoms including weakness and lethargy; muscle cramps, tetany; nausea, vomiting, and diarrhea; numbness or tingling; and seizures, renal failure, dysrhythmias, and cardiac arrest.
2. Obtain diagnostic tests: Serum electrolyte imbalances.

B. Analysis
1. Activity Intolerance related to generalized weakness
2. Fatigue related to metabolic imbalances
3. Decreased Cardiac Output related to electrolyte abnormalities
4. Risk for Excess Fluid Volume related to excess fluid intake

C. Planning
1. Resolve electrolyte and uric acid abnormalities.
2. Prevent acute renal failure.
3. Treat underlying cause.

D. Implementation
1. Frequently assess serum labs for improving or worsening electrolyte abnormalities.
2. Assess urine pH to ensure urine is alkalinized as part of treatment therapy.
3. Administer medications such as diuretics, allopurinol, sodium polystyrene sulfonate (Kayexalate), dextrose, insulin, and phosphate-binding gels as indicated.
4. Instruct client to report any symptoms of electrolyte abnormalities, specifically hyperkalemia, hypocalcemia, hyperphosphatemia, and hyperuricemia.
5. Assess client's activity level and ability to tolerate activity.
6. Consult physical therapy to help client maintain activity level.
7. Encourage client to take frequent rest periods as needed.
8. Frequently assess client's vital signs, cardiac system, and neurologic status.
9. Frequently assess client for signs and symptoms of fluid overload resulting from aggressive hydration to flush out released metabolites from the tumor.
10. Monitor serum electrolytes and uric acid levels for signs of fluid volume overload.

E. Evaluation
1. Client maintains ability to tolerate activity.
2. Client's fatigue is resolved or managed.

3. Client's cardiac output is not altered.
4. Client maintains fluid volume balance.

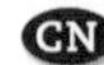

III. Client needs
- A. Physiologic adaptation
  1. Closely monitor electrolyte and uric acid laboratory levels.
  2. Assess client for signs and symptoms of fluid overload related to increased hydration.
  3. Ensure client is on cardiac monitoring.
- B. Management of care: Care of the client with tumor lysis syndrome requires critical thinking skills and knowledge of assessment, and teaching and evaluation methods unique to the RN role. These skills cannot be delegated to an LPN or UAP.
  1. Provide client with frequent assessments including vital signs, neurologic assessments, and ECGs as indicated.
  2. Inform physician of any changes noted during each assessment.
- C. Safety and infection control: Provide aggressive fluid hydration before and after chemotherapy to prevent renal failure.
- D. Health promotion and maintenance: Provide client teaching, including frequent updates with regard to treatment plan.
- E. Psychologic integrity: Promote consults such as social services as indicated.
- F. Basic care and comfort: Assist client with basic care as needed.
- G. Reduction of risk potential: Closely monitor client undergoing radiation therapy and chemotherapy for increased risk of tumor lysis syndrome.
- H. Pharmacologic and parenteral therapies: Client will state purpose for and side effects of all medications used to treat tumor lysis syndrome.
  1. IV fluids with sodium bicarbonate to increase urine pH and help prevent renal failure.
  2. Diuretics and allopurinol to help prevent renal failure.
  3. Sodium polystyrene sulfonate (Kayexalate) to treat hyperkalemia, if indicated.
  4. Dextrose and insulin administration to treat hyperkalemia, if indicated.
  5. Phosphate-binding gels to treat hyperphosphatemia, if indicated.
  6. Hemodialysis if client not responding to other therapies to regulate electrolytes and uric acid.

End-of-Life Care

I. Definition: End-of-life care occurs when treatment options are no longer successful. End-of-life care involves palliative care and community-based, hospice, and hospice-home care services. End-of-life care requires a multidisciplinary approach to care that includes the client, family, and friends.
- A. Palliative care: Palliative care aims to prevent or treat symptoms of disease or side effects connected to disease, and to provide psychologic, social, and spiritual care. The goal is not to cure the disease, but to relieve symptoms and improve quality of life.
- B. Hospice: The clients can receive palliative care by entering a facility that treats terminally ill clients or by setting up an interdisciplinary team to follow the client within the home setting.

II. Nursing process
- A. Assessment: Assess signs and symptoms of approaching death.
- B. Analysis
  1. Risk for Spiritual Distress related to impending death
  2. Anxiety related to impending death
  3. Risk for Complicated Grieving related to death
- C. Planning
  1. Assist client and family in accepting the course of their illness.
  2. Help client and family make appropriate plans.
- D. Implementation: Promote social visits for client; encourage client to interact with family and friends (see also psychologic integrity and basic care and comfort).
- E. Evaluation
  1. Client is able to discuss personal feelings with regard to dying.
  2. Client is free of anxiety.
  3. Client's family and friends are able to express their grief.

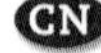

III. Client needs
- A. Physiologic adaptation
  1. Assess client for signs and symptoms of pain, both verbal and nonverbal cues.
  2. Assess client for signs of dyspnea.
  3. Auscultate client's lung sounds every shift or as indicated.
  4. Assess client's fluid balance.
  5. Assess client's skin color, temperature, and skin turgor.
  6. Assess client for constipation and/or intestinal obstruction.
  7. Assess client for any neurologic changes, as delirium can occur.
  8. Assess client for any signs of approaching death such as decreased food intake, urinary output decrease, increased somnolence, irregular breathing, decreased

circulation resulting in cyanotic extremities, and increased oral secretions.

B. Management of care: Care of the client receiving end-of-life care requires critical thinking skills and knowledge of assessment, and teaching and evaluation methods unique to the RN role. These skills cannot be delegated to an LPN or UAP.
    1. Encourage client and family to discuss advance directives and let their HCPs know of their wishes. Apply legal and ethical principles in the analysis of complex issues during end-of-life care.
    2. Provide client and family resources to help manage financial concerns.
    3. Promote consult with psychiatrist, if indicated, and chaplaincy consult if desired.
    4. Encourage client to begin funeral planning, and making final wishes known to friends and family.

C. Safety and infection control: Maintain asepsis and hand hygiene techniques to prevent infection.

D. Health promotion and maintenance: Assist client to have a comfortable death.

E. Psychologic integrity
    1. Assess client for signs of depression.
    2. Encourage client and family to discuss feelings and fears; allow time to grieve and mourn.
    3. Support client's family with their own acceptance and in assisting client to accept diagnosis.
    4. Identify the client's end-of-life priorities.
    5. Provide client and family with local support groups.

F. Basic care and comfort
    1. Ensure client is as comfortable as possible; frequently assess client and notify physician of any changes.
    2. Frequently assess client for pain; if client unresponsive, assess nonverbal cues and vital signs for indicators of pain.
    3. Assess client's ability to request pain medications. Other methods of pain relief may need to be used if client is unresponsive.
    4. Assess client's ability to breathe comfortably.
    5. Place client in semi-Fowler position to allow for lung expansion and ease of breathing.
    6. Assess client for ability to tolerate foods; encourage client to eat small, frequent meals; provide client with nutritional supplements as necessary.
    7. Provide client with frequent mouth care.
    8. Encourage adequate nutrition and hydration to prevent constipation.
    9. Assess client for ability to perform activities of daily living and assist as necessary.
    10. Assess client for activity intolerance.

G. Reduction of risk potential: Turn client frequently; prevent skin breakdown.

H. Pharmacologic and parenteral therapies: Client and family will state the purpose for and side effects of all medications used during end-of-life care.
    1. Analgesics as indicated.
    2. Appetite stimulants as indicated.
    3. Stool softeners as necessary.
    4. Oxygen therapy as needed.

Bibliography

Altman, G. (2004). *Delmar's fundamental and advanced nursing skills* (2nd ed.). Albany, NY: Delmar.

Ellis, J., & Hartley, C. (2005). *Managing and coordinating nursing care.* Philadelphia: Lippincott Williams & Wilkins.

Karch, A. (2008). *Lippincott's nursing drug guide.* Philadelphia: Lippincott Williams & Wilkins.

Purnell, L., & Paulanka, B. (Eds.). (2003). *Transcultural healthcare: A culturally competent approach.* Philadelphia: Davis.

Smeltzer, S. C., Bare, B. G., Cheever, K. H., & Hinkle, J. L. (2008). *Brunner and Suddarth's textbook of medical-surgical nursing* (11th ed.). Philadelphia: Lippincott Williams & Wilkins.

Taylor, C., Lillis, C., LeMone, P., & Lynn, P. (2006). *Fundamentals of nursing.* Philadelphia: Lippincott Williams & Wilkins.

Weber, J. R., & Kelley, J. (2007). *Nurses handbook of health assessment.* Philadelphia: Lippincott Williams & Wilkins.

Yarbro, C. H., Frogge, M., & Goodman, M. (2004). *Cancer symptom management* (3rd ed.). Sudbury, MA: Jones and Bartlett.

CHAPTER 32

Practice Test

Diagnosis of Cancer

1. AF The nurse is instructing a client about preventing skin cancer. Which of the following instructions are appropriate? Select all that apply.

- ☐ 1. Apply sunscreen 15 min before going in the sun.
- ☐ 2. Use 15 SPF or greater.
- ☐ 3. Avoid being in the sun between 10 a.m. and 4 p.m.
- ☐ 4. Use only licensed tanning parlors.
- ☐ 5. Take daily vitamin D.

2. A nurse is providing teaching for a woman who is trying to stop smoking because she is at high risk for breast cancer and is now pregnant. Which client statement indicates the teaching is effective?

- ☐ 1. "I should take the nicotine patch off while I smoke and replace it when done."
- ☐ 2. "Nicotine can go through breast milk, so I shouldn't smoke while nursing."
- ☐ 3. "I can chew as many pieces of nicotine gum a day as needed to decrease cravings."
- ☐ 4. "Smoking isn't harmful unless you smoke for more than 10 years."

3. A client has a carcinoembryonic antigen (CEA) blood level drawn. This test is used for which of the following reasons?

- ☐ 1. Differentiate between malignant and benign tissue cell growth.
- ☐ 2. Determine if metastasis of a primary tumor has occurred.
- ☐ 3. Evaluate the status of the client's immune system.
- ☐ 4. Identify the stage and grade of a malignancy.

4. A client had a fiberoptic bronchoscopy. The client can have liquids when he or she:

- ☐ 1. Has regular nondyspneic breathing.
- ☐ 2. Is oriented to time and place.
- ☐ 3. Can hold a glass.
- ☐ 4. Has a cough and gag reflex.

Management of Cancer

5. Which of the following teaching measures does the nurse include when teaching an elderly client receiving long-term oral prednisone therapy?

- ☐ 1. Anticipate occasional fevers.
- ☐ 2. Report neck or back pain.
- ☐ 3. Discontinue taking the drug if nausea occurs.
- ☐ 4. Take the drug only as long as necessary.

6. The RN is administering intravenous chemotherapy to a client with cancer. Which of the following is not an appropriate technique?

- ☐ 1. Taping all IV tubing connections.
- ☐ 2. Wearing gloves when handling the client's urine.
- ☐ 3. Disposing of chemotherapy waste as hazardous material.
- ☐ 4. Wearing a long-sleeved gown when administering chemotherapy.

7. The nurse is instructing a client about skin care while receiving radiation therapy to the chest. The nurse instructs the client to do which of the following?

- ☐ 1. Apply lotion if the skin becomes dry.
- ☐ 2. Shave the chest to prevent contamination from chest hair.
- ☐ 3. Wash the area with tepid water and mild soap.
- ☐ 4. Keep the area covered with a Teflon dressing between treatments.

8. A client is having a surgical biopsy to diagnose a tumor that may be cancerous. Which one of the following nursing interventions is appropriate in helping the client prepare for the surgery?

- ☐ 1. Reassure the client that the results of the biopsy could be negative.
- ☐ 2. Distract the client from worrying about the surgery.
- ☐ 3. Encourage the client to express fears about the surgery.
- ☐ 4. Tell the client not to worry about being apprehensive; all clients experience such feelings.

9. During the intravenous administration of a chemotherapeutic vesicant drug, the nurse observes that there is a lack of blood return from the intravenous catheter. Which of the following interventions does the nurse perform first?

- ☐ 1. Stop the administration of the drug.
- ☐ 2. Reposition the client's arm and continue with administration of the drug.

- □ 3. Irrigate the catheter with normal saline.
- □ 4. Continue to administer the drug and assess for edema at the IV site.

10. A client receiving chemotherapy for cancer has an elevated serum creatinine level. The nurse should next:
- □ 1. Cancel the next scheduled chemotherapy.
- □ 2. Administer the scheduled dose of chemotherapy.
- □ 3. Notify the HCP.
- □ 4. Obtain a urine specimen.

11. When preparing to administer a chemotherapeutic agent to a client, the nurse should take which of the following measures?
- □ 1. Recap all needles used to prepare agents.
- □ 2. Dispose of chemotherapy wastes in the client's bedside trash.
- □ 3. Use gloves and disposable long-sleeved gowns when handling agents.
- □ 4. Administer only prepackaged agents from the manufacturer.

12. A client who is receiving chemotherapy develops stomatitis. Which of the following actions is appropriate for the nurse to incorporate into the plan of care?
- □ 1. Rinse client's mouth with full-strength hydrogen peroxide every 4 hr.
- □ 2. Encourage client to use a soft-bristled toothbrush after each meal.
- □ 3. Provide hot tea with honey to soothe the client's painful oral mucosa.
- □ 4. Avoid using dental floss until the client's stomatitis is resolved.

13. A client with cancer is being considered for a bone marrow transplant. In considering a match for the recipient, which of the following is an ideal donor?
- □ 1. Parent.
- □ 2. Sibling.
- □ 3. Histocompatible (HLA-matched) donor.
- □ 4. Donor listed in the National Marrow Donor Program registry.

Oncologic Complications

14. A client with cancer who is receiving radiation therapy develops thrombocytopenia. The priority nursing goal is to prevent which of the following?
- □ 1. Pain related to spontaneous bleeding episodes.
- □ 2. Altered nutrition related to anemia.
- □ 3. Injury related to the decreased platelet count.
- □ 4. Skin breakdown related to decreased tissue perfusion.

15. A client who has been diagnosed with lung cancer complains of increasing shortness of breath and difficulty swallowing. The client has facial swelling and engorged jugular veins. The nurse assesses the client for which of the following?
- □ 1. Pulmonary emboli.
- □ 2. Cardiac tamponade.
- □ 3. Syndrome of inappropriate secretion of antidiuretic syndrome (SIADH).
- □ 4. Superior vena cava syndrome.

16. A client had a colon resection yesterday. The client's hemoglobin was 14.1 g/dl yesterday and today's hemoglobin level is 7.2 g/dl. The client's oxygen saturation is 87%. The nurse performs which of the following interventions first?
- □ 1. Assess the client.
- □ 2. Administer a 500 ml of normal saline intravenously.
- □ 3. Administer oxygen.
- □ 4. Administer two units PRBCs.

17. The nurse is caring for a client with metastatic bone disease. The client is complaining of excessive thirst and frequent urination. The nurse observes that the client's reflexes are hypoactive and the client appears confused. The nurse reviews the laboratory reports to determine the levels of which of the following?
- □ 1. Potassium.
- □ 2. Sodium.
- □ 3. Phosphate.
- □ 4. Calcium.

End-of-Life Care

18. The nurse is collaborating with the physician to develop a care plan to help control chronic pain in a client with cancer who is receiving hospice home care. Which one of the following plans is most appropriate for preventing and reducing the client's pain?
- □ 1. Administer analgesics on a regular basis with administration of additional analgesics for breakthrough pain.
- □ 2. Keep the client sedated with tranquilizers to prevent awareness of pain sensations.
- □ 3. Encourage the client to avoid intravenous pain medication until the condition has reached the terminal stage.
- □ 4. Administer analgesics when the client's vital signs indicate that the severity of the pain is increasing.

19. A nurse refers a client and his family to a hospice program. The primary goal of hospice care is to achieve which of the following outcomes?
- □ 1. Facilitate use of technology in the client's care.

☐ 2. Provide support for the client and his family.
☐ 3. Reduce the cost of care.
☐ 4. Teach the client to provide self-care.

20. A client who is near death is receiving hospice care to manage severe pain. The client is receiving a narcotic pain medication intravenously per a patient-controlled analgesia (PCA) pump. The client is lethargic and is sleeping much of the time. He has not complained of any pain for the last 12 hr. The nurse plans care based on the fact that the client:

☐ 1. Received too much medication through an overdose of medication administered through the PCA pump.
☐ 2. May be nearing death as specific dosages and time intervals for self-administration of the analgesic is programmed into the PCA machine to prevent overdose.
☐ 3. Has obtained sufficient pain relief because he has no pain for the last 12 hr.
☐ 4. Has an IV that has infiltrated and the analgesic has been injected into the subcutaneous tissues, thereby being absorbed faster than prescribed.

Answers and Rationales

1. 1, 2, 3 Skin cancer is the most common form of cancer. To prevent skin cancer, the nurse instructs the client to avoid overexposure to sun by applying sunscreen at least 15 min before going in the sun and using sun block with a sun protection factor of 15 or greater. The client is also instructed to avoid being in the sun at midday (10 a.m. to 4 p.m.). The client should not use sun lamps or tanning parlors because of the harmful rays. Use of vitamin D does not protect against skin cancer. (H)

2. 2 Nicotine enters breast milk freely and crosses the placenta. Pregnant and nursing mothers who continue to smoke cause risk of injury to their babies. Nicotine patches are worn throughout the day and taken off only at bedtime. Clients using nicotine patches are instructed to avoid cigarettes completely while on a transdermal nicotine-reduction program. Nicotine gum is limited to no more than 24 pieces per day in early therapy, then in decreasing amounts thereafter. Smoking is dangerous to health no matter how long a smoker has smoked. Health risks do increase in association with time and quantity. (D)

3. 1 Cancer cells cause an antigen reaction in blood serum, from proliferation of malignant tumor cells, which is measurable and is known as carcinoembryonic antigen (CEA). This test differentiates between malignant and benign cancer tissue cell growth. The test does not determine if metastasis of a tumor has occurred, identify the stage and grade of a malignancy, or evaluate the client's immune system. (M)

4. 4 Clients who have a fiberoptic bronchoscopy receive a topical anesthetic prior to the procedure, which decreases the cough and gag reflex. It is important to withhold liquids until the gag reflex returns in order to prevent aspiration. Regular nondyspneic breathing does not assure an adequate cough and gag reflex, nor does orientation to time and place or the ability to hold a glass of water. (R)

5. 2 Most clients receiving long-term glucocorticoid therapy have low bone mineral density; up to 25% sustain osteoporotic fractures. The nurse monitors the client for signs of compression fractures and instructs the client to notify the HCP with new-onset neck or back pain. Fevers are not normal and may indicate infection (clients taking glucocorticoids may have depressed immune functioning). The drug is never discontinued without a physician's order. (H)

6. 1 According to safety guidelines from the Occupational Safety and Health Administration and the Oncology Nursing Society, antineoplastic agents are administered using Luer-Lok fittings on all intravenous tubings to minimize the risk of exposure from needlestick injury. Additionally, nurses preparing and administering chemotherapy wear gloves and a disposable, long-sleeved gown. Antineoplastic agents are disposed of as hazardous material and gloves are always worn when handling the excretions of clients who have received chemotherapy. (S)

7. 3 Clients receiving radiation experience dryness or redness in the area of the radiation. The nurse instructs the client to wash the area with soap and water and keep the area dry. The client does not apply lotion, shave, or cover the area. (H)

8. 3 Allowing the client to express fears and concerns about the impending surgery allows him or her to explore feelings about surgery. Reassuring the client about positive results may provide false hope. Providing distraction does not allow the client to deal with the issue at hand, nor does telling the client not to worry. (P)

9. 1 An intravenous catheter with no blood return is most likely occluded and not patent. A chemotherapeutic vesicant drug extravasates into the surrounding skin tissue and causes tissue necrosis. The nurse stops administration of the drug immediately. Repositioning the arm does not improve patency. Irrigating the catheter may cause the medication to enter tissue. It is inappropriate to wait and see if the arm becomes edematous because of the vesicant action of the drug. (S)

10. 3 Nephrotoxicity of a chemotherapy agent is assessed by monitoring serum creatinine. Creatinine is the most sensitive indicator of proper kidney function. In this case the client is experiencing decreased kidney function, most likely due to the chemotherapy. The nurse consults the HCP for guidance. Administering the next dose of chemotherapy could potentially cause further kidney damage. It is inappropriate to cancel the chemotherapy without checking with the HCP or to tell the client that the cancer is spreading. A urine specimen will not provide other helpful information. (S)

11. 3 Chemotherapeutic agents are very toxic; therefore, precautions are taken such as the use of gloves and long-sleeved gowns when handling agents to prevent incidental contact with skin. Recapping needles is against universal precaution standards, and chemotherapy waste is disposed of in biohazard containers according to institution policy. Prepackaged agents can still be hazardous if not handled properly. (S)

12. 2 Stomatitis is an inflammation of the mucous membranes of the mouth resulting from chemotherapy. Using a soft-bristled toothbrush prevents further bleeding and irritation to the already irritated gums and mucous membranes. Hydrogen peroxide can further irritate the mouth. Fluids need to be lukewarm instead of hot; dental floss can be used if it is done gently. (C)

13. 3 Bone marrow transplants are performed with increasing frequency. If the client is not able to use his or her own marrow (autologous bone marrow transplantation), it is possible to use marrow from donors. The ideal donor is one who has identical HLA phenotypes to the recipient. Although this may be a parent or a sibling, exact matches do not always occur within families, or the family member may not be able to donate for various reasons. The National Marrow Donor Program maintains a registry of available donors with their marrow type, but being registered does not assure that the donor is a match.

14. 3 This client is at high risk for bleeding because of the decreased platelet count. The priority nursing goal is to prevent injury to this client by preventing bleeding occurrences. Spontaneous bleeding may cause pain but is not the priority. The client has a low platelet count, but not a low hemoglobin count such as exists in anemia. Skin integrity is a risk but not a priority. (S)

15. 4 Superior vena cava syndrome is a syndrome in which the superior vena cava is obstructed or compressed by tumor growth. Signs and symptoms result from a blockage of venous blood flow from the head, neck, and upper trunk and include difficulty breathing or swallowing, facial swelling, and jugular venous distention. The other selections do not refer to superior vena cava syndrome. (M)

16. 3 This client has decreased oxygen saturation and also decreased hemoglobin, which puts the client at great risk for cardiac ischemia. The nurse administers oxygen immediately. The other interventions are appropriate, but not the priority at this time. (M)

17. 4 Excessive thirst, frequent urination, hypoactive reflexes, and confusion are all signs of hypercalcemia, in which the client's serum calcium level is elevated. Hyperkalemia produces cardiac dysrhythmias and muscle weakness, hypernatremia produces altered cerebral function, and hyperphosphatemia produces signs of hypocalcemia such as muscle twitching, spasms, and cramps. (M)

18. 1 Maintaining a steady blood level of analgesics is beneficial for the client with chronic cancer pain. Administering analgesics on a regular basis helps to control pain more efficiently. It may also be necessary for the client to have additional doses of medication ordered to be administered for breakthrough pain. Keeping the client overly sedated may not help to control pain, and intravenous analgesics are more effective at controlling pain as they are more predictable in their distribution than many oral medications. Vital signs are not a reliable indicator of how much pain the client is experiencing. (M)

19. 2 The goal of hospice is to provide support for clients and families with end-stage terminal illness. Hospice care provides comfort and care during the final stages of a terminal illness. Although it may be easier to use technology in a hospice setting, that is not the primary goal. The exact cost of hospice care varies, and what is covered by private, state, or federal insurance programs also varies, but the cost is typically less than that of hospitalization; however, reducing the cost of care is not the goal of hospice programs. It is not an expectation that the client will learn to provide self-care in a hospice program, but the client is encouraged to assume as much responsibility for care as the client wishes or is able to assume. (C)

20. 2 The client is likely becoming more comatose and is not self-administering the pain medication. The client is not receiving too much medication because the PCA pump has controls to prevent overdose. The client is likely having pain, but is not able to recognize it. There is no indication that the IV has infiltrated. (D)

chapter

33 The Client Having Surgery

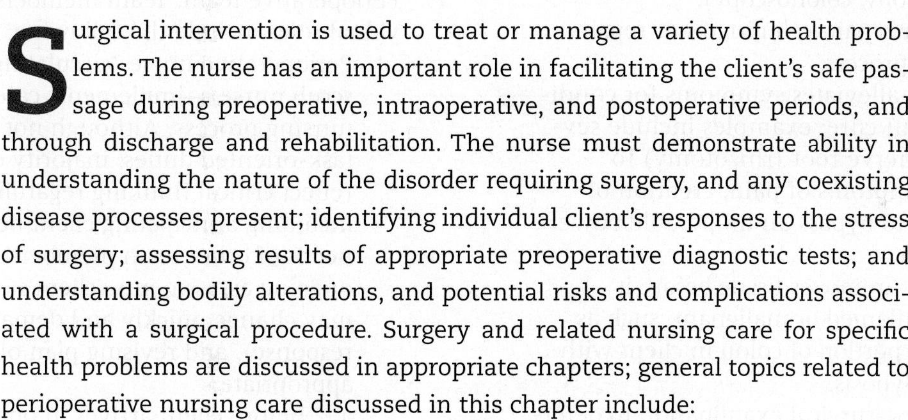

Surgical intervention is used to treat or manage a variety of health problems. The nurse has an important role in facilitating the client's safe passage during preoperative, intraoperative, and postoperative periods, and through discharge and rehabilitation. The nurse must demonstrate ability in understanding the nature of the disorder requiring surgery, and any coexisting disease processes present; identifying individual client's responses to the stress of surgery; assessing results of appropriate preoperative diagnostic tests; and understanding bodily alterations, and potential risks and complications associated with a surgical procedure. Surgery and related nursing care for specific health problems are discussed in appropriate chapters; general topics related to perioperative nursing care discussed in this chapter include:

- Surgery: Preoperative, Intraoperative, and Postoperative Periods
- Ethical and Legal Implications for the Client Having Surgery

Surgery: Preoperative, Intraoperative, and Postoperative Periods

I. Definition: Surgery is the branch of health care concerned with treating disorders, injuries, and deformities by operation and instrumentation. For further information, see Internet sites www.aorn.org and www.aspan.org.

A. Perioperative period—involves interaction among a client, surgeon, nurse, and health team members, and refers to entire surgical experience, including:
   1. Preoperative period—begins with decision to perform surgery.
   2. Intraoperative period—begins when client is received in operating room.
   3. Postoperative period—begins when client is admitted to post anesthesia care unit and extends through follow-up evaluation.

B. Purposes for surgery
   1. Diagnostic—determines presence or extent of pathology such as biopsy or "oscopies" (bronchoscopy, colonoscopy).
   2. Removal or repair—eliminates or repairs pathologic process.
   3. Palliative—alleviates symptoms for condition without cure; examples include severing of a nerve root (rhizotomy) to remove symptoms of pain, creation of colostomy to bypass an inoperable bowel obstruction.
   4. Preventive—removes tissue before it becomes inflamed or malignant, such as removal of portion of colon in client with familial polyposis.
   5. Explorative—surgical examination to determine nature or extent of disease (e.g., exploratory laparotomy).
   6. Cosmetic improvement such as repairing burn scar or changing breast shape.

C. Suffixes describing surgical procedures:
   1. -ectomy—excision or removal of (e.g., appendectomy)
   2. -lysis—destruction of (e.g., electrolysis)
   3. -orrhaphy—repair of (e.g., herniorrhaphy)
   4. -oscopy—looking into (e.g., endoscopy)
   5. -ostomy—creation of an opening into (e.g., colostomy)
   6. -otomy—cutting into or incision of (e.g., tracheotomy)
   7. -plasty—repair or reconstruction of (e.g., mammoplasty)

D. Categories of surgery
   1. Optional—performed at client's discretion (e.g., cosmetic)
   2. Elective—scheduled at client's convenience (e.g., removal of a cyst)
   3. Required—needed for conditions necessitating intervention within a few weeks (e.g., partial thyroidectomy)
   4. Urgent imperative—required for condition necessitating intervention within 24 to 48 hr (e.g., appendectomy)
   5. Emergency—performed immediately to sustain life or maintain function (e.g., craniotomy)

E. Surgical settings: Surgery may be a carefully planned event (elective) or may arise with unexpected urgency (emergency). Ambulatory surgery refers to same-day or outpatient surgery (usually take less than 2 hr and requires less than 3- to 4-hr stay in postanesthesia care unit). Both elective and emergency surgeries may be performed in a variety of settings (e.g., emergency department, endoscopy clinics, freestanding surgical clinics) based on:
   1. Complexity of surgery
   2. Potential complications
   3. General health status of client

F. Perioperative team: Team members and individual roles include the following:
   1. Perioperative nurse (circulating nurse, scrub nurse)—implements care based on nursing process. Although not limited to task-oriented duties, majority of behaviors reflect critical thinking regarding safe care, including anticipating client needs and needs of other team members, performing ongoing assessments (client's condition may change quickly and demand prompt response), and revising plan of care as appropriate.
      a. Before client arrives in operating room, nurse collaborates with members of surgical team to prepare client and operating room.
         (1) Serves as client and family advocate throughout intraoperative experience.
         (2) Determines additional needs or tasks to be completed before surgery to meet client's plan of care.
         (3) Provides preoperative education regarding upcoming experience and physical comfort measures.
         (4) Helps reduce client's anxiety via communication and touch.
         (5) Establishes time outs to ensure correct surgical site.
      b. While client in operating room, different functions may be assumed

that involve either sterile or unsterile activities:

(1) Circulating role—not scrubbed, gowned, gloved, and remains in unsterile field: Documents nursing care either electronically or by hand; this includes assessment and identification of clinical problems, nursing diagnoses, and interventions.

(2) Scrubbing role—follows designated scrub procedure, is gowned, gloved, in sterile attire, and remains in sterile field.

(a) Responsible for scrubbing for surgery.

(b) Sets up sterile tables and equipment.

(c) Assists surgeon and surgical technicians during surgical procedure.

2. Surgical technician or LPN can perform scrubbed function under RN supervision—assists surgeon by passing instruments and implementing other technical functions during surgical procedure.
3. Surgeon's physician (perioperative physician) may be client's primary physician or one selected by client's physician or the client. Surgeon's physician is responsible for the following:
   a. Collects preoperative medical history; performs physical assessment that includes the need for surgical intervention and choice of surgical procedure.
   b. Provides informed consent for surgical site.
   c. Manages preoperative workup.
   d. Oversees client safety in operating room.
   e. Manages postoperative care of client.
4. Surgeon's assistant—can be a physician who functions in an assistive role throughout a surgical procedure, or can be RN or nonphysician who functions in role under direct supervision of surgeon. Roles include the following *(NOTE: Hospital policy defines role of surgeon's assistant and physician responsibility when nonphysician fills role)*:
   a. Usually holds retractors to expose surgical area.
   b. Assists with hemostasis and suturing.
   c. May perform portions of operative procedure under direct supervision of surgeon.
5. RN's first assistant—works in collaboration with surgeon to produce optimal surgical outcome:
   a. Handles tissue.
   b. Usually holds retractors to expose surgical area.
   c. Assists with hemostasis and suturing.
6. Anesthesiologist or nurse anesthetist—administers anesthesia.
   a. Anesthesiologist: Medical doctor who has completed residency in field of anesthesia, is credentialed by the American Board of Anesthesiology, and is licensed as an anesthesiologist in state where practices.
   b. Nurse anesthetist: RN who has graduated from an accredited nurse anesthesia program, has successfully completed the national certification examination to become a certified registered nurse anesthetist, and is licensed as such in state where practices.
   c. Responsibilities of anesthesiologist or nurse anesthetist:

(1) Assesses client preoperatively to determine safest anesthesia for client's needs and anticipated operative procedure.

(2) Prescribes preoperative and adjunctive medications.

(3) Monitors cardiac and respiratory status.

(4) Monitors vital signs throughout surgical procedure.

(5) Administers anesthetic during surgical procedure and notifies surgeon if difficulties arise.

(6) Administers fluid and monitors electrolytes.

(7) Administers and monitors medications, blood and blood products throughout surgical procedure.

(8) Supervises recovery in postanesthesia care unit and documents recovery in first 24 hr.

7. Radiographic/cardiovascular technicians:
   a. Take x-ray images.
   b. Perform cardiovascular support services, as needed.
8. Postanesthesia care unit nurse:
   a. Supervises client's immediate recovery period.
   b. Collaborates between postanesthesia care unit nurse and anesthesiologist or nurse anesthetist; fosters a smooth transfer of care.
   c. Provides care for client until client recovers from effects of anesthesia, is

oriented, has stable vital signs, and shows no evidence of hemorrhage.
d. Facilitates discharge planning.

Preoperative Period

I. Definition: The preoperative period is the segment of the perioperative period that begins with the decision to perform surgery and ends with a client's transfer to the operating room table.
II. Nursing process
A. Assessment
1. Identify risk factors for surgery-related complications.
a. Client who is very young or very old is at risk for increased stress.
b. Compromised nutritional status has negative effect on recovery and wound healing.
(1) Obesity presents greater risk for postoperative pulmonary complications (hypoventilation, hypoxia); more likely to have coexisting cardiac, hepatic, biliary, endocrine, or metabolic problems.
(2) Pregnancy presents risk for unborn child.
(3) Chronic illness or condition may affect recovery (e.g., diabetes mellitus).
(4) Malnourished
2. Assess respiratory status to identify risk factors for postoperative complications.
a. Dyspnea, shortness of breath
b. Upper respiratory infection
c. Cough/wheezing
d. Copious mucus/sputum production
e. Chest discomfort/pain
f. History of smoking, including number of packs-per-day determination
g. Regular use of inhalants
h. Presence of clubbed fingers
3. Assess cardiovascular status.
a. Apical, radial pulse
b. BP
c. Electrocardiographic tracings
d. Presence, character of peripheral pulses
e. Skin color, temperature
f. Presence of sensation in fingers, toes
g. Presence of edema, staging of edema
h. Capillary refill in fingers, toes
4. Assess for and report evidence of fluid and electrolyte imbalance.
a. Extracellular fluid volume deficit (hypovolemia)
b. Extracellular fluid volume excess (edema, hypertension)
c. Prolonged vomiting, diarrhea, hemorrhage
d. Abnormal serum levels of sodium, potassium, magnesium, calcium, or pH level
5. Assess hepatic and renal function.
a. History of liver disease (cirrhosis, chronic alcohol abuse)
b. Complaints of dysuria, oliguria, anuria, incontinence, or urinary tract infection
c. Urinalysis results; serum creatinine, BUN levels
d. Serum liver enzyme levels:
(1) Aspartate aminotransferase
(2) Alanine aminotransferase
6. Examine record for endocrine and metabolic problems.
a. Could affect response to surgery.
b. Poorly managed diabetes mellitus may impair wound healing and recovery.
7. Assess immunologic and hematologic function.
a. History of allergies and manifestations of the allergies
b. Previous reactions to anesthetic agents, blood transfusion
c. Immunosuppression status
d. History of substance use/abuse
8. Assess neurologic function.
a. History of seizures, other neurologic disorders (Parkinson disease, myasthenia gravis)
b. Level of consciousness, orientation and mental status
c. Pupillary response to light, accommodation
9. Assess integumentary system.
a. Bleeding tendencies (ecchymosis, petechiae)
b. Contusions, abrasions, skin breakdown
c. Presence and quality of hair and nails
10. Evaluate medication history for drugs that increase operative risk by affecting coagulation time or interfere with anesthetics, such as:
a. Steroids—anti-inflammatory, immunosuppressive action
b. Diuretics—decrease intravascular fluid volume
c. Phenothiazines—strong sedation, hypotensive effects
d. Antidepressants—produce drowsiness, orthostatic hypotension
e. Antibiotics—may produce ototoxicity, nephrotoxicity
f. Anticoagulants—interfere with blood coagulation

g. Street drugs, alcohol—may potentiate or interfere with anesthesia

11. Assess for any type of prosthetic devices or metal implants.
    a. Artificial eye
    b. Hip or knee replacements
    c. Pacemaker, implantable cardioverter or defibrillator
    d. Lens implants
    e. Dentures or hearing aids
12. Assess client and family knowledge base to guide teaching.
13. Consider psychosocial factors that could affect response to surgery.
    a. Anxiety, fear
    b. Defense mechanisms including denial, regression, intellectualization, withdrawal, and anger
    c. Self-esteem, body-image concerns
14. Obtain preoperative laboratory tests.
    a. Urinalysis—assesses renal status, hydration, and presence of urinary tract infection or disease.
    b. Chest x-ray—assesses pulmonary disorders and cardiac enlargement.
    c. CBC: RBCs, hemoglobin, hematocrit, WBCs, WBC differential—assess for anemia, immune status, and infection.
    d. Electrolytes—assess metabolic status, renal function, and diuretic side effects.
    e. ABGs, oximetry—assess pulmonary function and metabolic function.
    f. Prothrombin or partial thromboplastin time—assesses bleeding tendencies.
    g. Blood glucose—assesses metabolic status and presence of diabetes mellitus.
    h. Creatinine—assesses renal function and skeletal muscle metabolism.
    i. BUN—assesses renal function and skeletal muscle metabolism.
    j. Electrocardiogram—assesses for cardiac disease and electrolyte abnormalities.
    k. Pulmonary function studies—assess pulmonary status and diffusing capacity.
    l. Liver function tests—assess liver function; aspartate aminotransferase and alanine aminotransferase levels.
    m. Type and crossmatch—assess blood availability for replacement. (Elective surgery clients may have own blood available.)
    n. Pregnancy test—assesses reproductive status.

B. Analysis
1. Fear related to upcoming surgical procedure
2. Anxiety related to prognosis and lack of knowledge
3. Disturbed Sleep Pattern related to anxiety
4. Risk for Injury related to altered level of consciousness
5. Deficient Knowledge: Surgical Procedure, Preoperative Routine, and Postoperative Care, related to lack of teaching

C. Planning
1. Reduce fear related to upcoming surgical procedure.
2. Decrease anxiety.
3. Maintain environment conducive for rest and sleep.
4. Prevent injury from drowsiness from preoperative medications.
5. Provide client and family teaching.

D. Implementation
1. Promote measures that help decrease anxiety for client and family.
2. Discuss surgical experience with client and family to minimize anxiety and increase knowledge.
3. Provide client and family teaching.
4. Perform preoperative skin preparation as appropriate.
5. Provide GI preparation as prescribed.
6. Assure client and responsible family member have provided informed consent for surgery.
7. Ensure safe transport of client to surgical suite.

E. Evaluation
1. Client exhibits and reports decreased anxiety concerning upcoming surgical experience.
2. Client's family reports decreased anxiety concerning upcoming surgical experience.
3. Client verbalizes understanding of surgical procedure, preoperative nursing care, and the expected postoperative course.
4. Client verbalizes understanding of postoperative pain relief, including how to use devices such as client-controlled analgesia pumps, if appropriate.
5. Client is free from signs and symptoms of injury.
6. Client obtains adequate rest and sleep.

CN

III. Client needs

A. Physiologic adaptation
1. Nutrition—review physician orders regarding NPO status (may vary per institutional protocol and age).
    a. Before surgery with general anesthesia: Solid foods and liquids withheld for 6 to 8 hr to prevent aspiration.
    b. Before surgery with local anesthesia: Solid foods and liquids withheld for 3 hr to avoid aspiration.

c. TPN administered to clients who are malnourished, have protein or metabolic deficiencies, or cannot ingest foods or fluids.

2. Elimination—with intestinal or abdominal surgery, enema or laxative prescribed evening before or morning of surgery; client voids immediately prior to surgery.

B. Management of care: Care of the preoperative client requires critical thinking skills and knowledge of assessment, and teaching and evaluation methods unique to the RN role. These skills cannot be delegated to an LPN or UAP.

1. Delegate responsibly those activities that can be delegated. All monitoring information is reported to the RN.
   a. Monitor vital signs.
   b. Maintain NPO status as prescribed.
   c. Assist with removal of all jewelry, nail polish, acrylic nails, hair pins, glasses, contact lenses, dentures, and, perhaps, hearing aids. *Note: Depending on policy, hearing aids and glasses may be left in place until removal becomes necessary in operating room. Send labeled containers to operating room for safe placement in case removal becomes necessary.*
   d. Administer enemas as prescribed.
   e. Assist with applying clean gown after removal of all clothes.
   f. Assist with basic hygienic care.
2. Consult with surgeon who is responsible for obtaining consent for surgery.
   a. Assure that client understands surgeon's explanation of surgery; witness client's signing of consent form.
   b. Document witnessing signing of consent form after client acknowledges understanding the procedure.
   c. Withhold sedation until client signs consent.
      (1) Minors may need parent/legal guardian to sign consent form.
      (2) Older clients may need legal guardian to sign consent form.
3. Consult with member of clergy.
   a. Respect and support spiritual beliefs of client and family.
   b. Assist in arranging for spiritual help.
4. Discuss and identify location of advance directives, living will, and durable power of attorney for health care.

C. Safety and infection control

1. Prepare client skin while client is on nursing unit.
   a. Use electric razor or clippers while shaving hair to prevent break in skin integrity.
   b. Apply antibiotic scrub to surgical area as ordered.
2. Instruct client to remain in bed after preanesthetic medication administered; if client must get up, assist as needed.
3. Ensure the following are completed and documented in client's record.
   a. History, physical examination
   b. Consultation requests
   c. Prescribed laboratory results
   d. Electrocardiogram and chest x-ray reports
   e. Blood screen, type, and crossmatch
4. Complete preoperative checklist before client is transferred to the operating room.
   a. Consents are signed.
   b. Nurse has instructed client about all phases involved in perioperative period.
   c. Prostheses removed, valuables stored in locker or with family.
   d. Time of premedication documented.
   e. Last time client ate or drank documented.
   f. Document that client voided before surgery.
   g. Monitor and document client's vital signs.
5. Ensure safe transport to surgical suite; assure stretcher has side rails and safety strap, and warm blankets provided.
6. Ensure client is wearing identification bracelet.

D. Health promotion and maintenance

1. Provide client and family teaching about the following measures:
   a. Deep-breathing and coughing exercises
   b. Relaxation techniques
   c. Postoperative exercises of extremities
   d. Turning and moving techniques
   e. Pain-management techniques
   f. Incentive spirometry use
   g. Splinting of incision:
      (1) Use when incision is abdominal or thoracic.
      (2) Place pillow over incision during deep breathing and coughing; press gently against incisional area to splint or support.
2. Inform client to expect some discomfort after surgery; teach importance of requesting medication for pain or using client-controlled anesthesia before pain becomes severe.

E. Psychologic integrity
  1. Answer any questions or concerns the client and family may have regarding surgery.
  2. Allow time for privacy for client to prepare for surgery psychologically.
  3. Be alert to level of anxiety; promote measures that help decrease anxiety for client, family:
    a. Assist client to identify and verbalize concerns that can affect surgical experience (e.g., fear of unknown, fear of death, loss of work or role).
    b. Discuss surgical experience including what happens from time being prepared for surgery to waking up in postanesthesia care unit.

F. Basic care and comfort: Perform standard preoperative procedures (see management of care for basic care procedures delegated to UAP or LPN)

G. Reduction of risk potential
  1. Carefully check written preoperative orders and clarify which medications are, or should not be, administered on day of surgery:
    a. In case of insulin—clarify the time and amount of last dose before surgery.
    b. Clarify whether routine cardiac, antihypertensive, and asthma medications should be taken on day of surgery.
  2. Provide client and family teaching about preoperative medications, including desired effects (see pharmacologic and parenteral therapies).
  3. Instruct client not to get out of bed following administration of preoperative medications, and to call for assistance if needed. Place call light within reach and raise side rails.

H. Pharmacologic and parenteral therapies: Client and family will state the purpose for and side effects of all medications used preoperatively.
  1. Frequently used preoperative medications:
    a. Benzodiazepines
      (1) Midazolam (Versed)—reduces anxiety
      (2) Diazepam (Valium)—induces sedation
      (3) Lorazepam (Ativan)—induces amnesia
    b. Narcotics
      (1) Morphine (Duramorph)—relieves discomfort and pain
      (2) Meperidine and fentanyl (Sublimaze)—provide analgesia and sedation
    c. Histamine H_2–receptor antagonists
      (1) Cimetidine (Tagamet)—increases gastric pH
      (2) Famotidine (Pepcid)—decreases gastric volume
      (3) Ranitidine (Zantac)—blocks gastric acid secretion
    d. Antacids: Sodium bicarbonate—increases gastric pH; neutralizes gastric acid
    e. Antiemetics
      (1) Metoclopramide (Reglan)—increases gastric emptying
      (2) Droperidol (Inapsine)—decreases nausea and vomiting
      (3) Ondansetron (Zofran)—prevents nausea and vomiting
    f. Anticholinergics
      (1) Atropine (Atropair)—decreases oral and respiratory secretions
      (2) Scopolamine (Hyoscine)—controls secretions
  2. Other medications that may be administered preoperatively:
    a. Antibiotics—may be administered throughout perioperative period for:
      (1) Client with history of congenital or valvular heart disease to prevent endocarditis
      (2) Client undergoing surgery in which wound contamination is potential risk (GI surgery), or in which wound infection could have serious postoperative complications (cardiac, joint replacement surgery)
    b. Eyedrops—administer as ordered and on time to adequately prepare eye for surgery.
    c. Routine prescription drugs—check written preoperative orders (see reduction of risk potential).
  3. IV fluids that may be initiated preoperatively:
    a. Normal saline (NS, 0.9% NaC1)—isotonic
    b. Lactated Ringer (LR)—isotonic
    c. Dextrose 5%/water (D5/W)—isotonic, hypotonic (use cautiously if client has diabetes mellitus)

Intraoperative Period

I. Definition: The intraoperative period begins when a client is received in the operating room and ends with admission to the postanesthesia care unit. It is imperative that the nurse promote client safety standards including right site, right procedure, and right person throughout the intraoperative period according to Universal Protocol established by the Joint Commission.

A. Universal Protocol
   1. Intended to achieve goal of safety for client having surgery
   2. Based on consensus of experts from clinical specialties and professional disciplines
   3. Endorsed by more than 40 professional medical associations and organizations

B. Steps of Universal Protocol for eliminating wrong site, wrong procedure, and wrong person during surgery include the following:
   1. Preoperative verification process
      a. Purpose—ensures all relevant documents and studies are:
         (1) Available prior to start of procedure; missing information or discrepancies are addressed before starting procedure
         (2) Reviewed and
            (a) Consistent with each other
            (b) Consistent with client's expectations
            (c) Consistent with team's understanding of intended client, procedure, and site and (as applicable), any complaints
      b. Process—an ongoing process of information gathering and verification.
         (1) Begins with determination to perform procedure
         (2) Continues through all settings and interventions involved in preoperative preparation of client up to and including "time out" just before the start of a procedure
   2. Marking the operative site
      a. Purpose—identifies unambiguously the intended site of incision or insertion
      b. Process—intended surgical site is marked such that the mark will be visible after client has been prepared and draped for procedures; used for:
         (1) Right or left distinction
         (2) Multiple structures (such as fingers and toes)
         (3) Multiple levels (as in spinal procedures)
   3. "Time out" immediately before starting the procedure
      a. Purpose—conducts a final verification of the correct client, procedure, site, and implants, if applicable
      b. Process—involves active communication among all members of the perioperative team:
         (1) Consistently initiated by a designated member of the team
         (2) Conducted in a "fail-safe" mode; the procedure is not started until any questions or concerns are resolved

II. Nursing process

A. Assessment
   1. Classify client's physical status for anesthesia in accordance with the American Society of Anesthesiologists (http://www.asa.org).
      a. P1—normal healthy client
      b. P2—client with mild systemic disease (mild cardiac disease, mild diabetes mellitus)
      c. P3—client with severe systemic disease (poorly controlled diabetes mellitus, pulmonary complications)
      d. P4—client with severe systemic disease that is a constant threat to life (severe renal, cardiac disease)
      e. P5—moribund client who is not expected to survive without the surgery (ruptured aortic aneurysm)
      f. P6—client declared brain-dead; organs are being removed for donor purposes
   2. Audit client's record for appropriate documentation.
      a. Current signed consent form
      b. Completed history, physical examination record
      c. Recent diagnostic and laboratory reports
      d. Evaluation of overall physiologic, psychologic, emotional status
   3. Verify known allergies.
   4. Validate client identification and correct surgery scheduled.
   5. Assess for special musculoskeletal and neurologic considerations or precautions.
   6. Assess pulse oximetry.
   7. Assess risk for accidental hypothermia or malignant hyperthermia during anesthesia administration and surgery.

B. Analysis
   1. Risk for Imbalanced Fluid Volume related to preparation for surgery
   2. Risk for Imbalanced Body Temperature related to cool temperature in operating room
   3. Risk for Infection related to intentional disruption of skin integrity
   4. Ineffective Tissue Perfusion: Cardiac, Respiratory, and Peripheral, related to lessened extracellular fluid volume

5. Risk for Injury: Positioning, related to sedation
6. Risk for Injury related to altered level of consciousness

C. Planning
1. Maintain fluid and electrolyte balance.
2. Maintain normothermia.
3. Prevent infection.
4. Promote tissue perfusion.
5. Prevent injury.
6. Prevent deep vein thrombosis.

D. Implementation (see basic care and comfort)

E. Evaluation
1. Client maintains adequate fluid balance throughout surgery.
2. Client has satisfactory body temperature on completion of surgery.
3. Client shows no signs or symptoms of systemic or wound infection.
4. Client arrives safely in postanesthesia care unit and exhibits adequate cardiac, respiratory, and peripheral circulation.
5. Client is free from signs of injury from chemical, electrical, or physical hazards from surgery.
6. Client remains free from injury.

CN

III. Client needs

A. Physiologic adaptation
1. Anesthesia introduced to produce four stages of anesthesia:
   a. Stage 1—client becomes drowsy, loses consciousness
   b. Stage 2—stage of excitement; client's muscles are tense, breathing may be irregular
   c. Stage 3—involves depression of vital signs, reflexes
   d. Stage 4—involves complete respiratory depression
2. Controlled hypotension used to decrease amount of expected blood loss by lowering BP during administration of anesthesia.
3. Controlled hypothermia is deliberate lowering of body temperature to decrease metabolism, reducing both demand for oxygen and anesthetic requirements.

B. Management of care: Care of the intraoperative client requires critical thinking skills and knowledge of assessment, and teaching and evaluation methods unique to the RN role. These skills cannot be delegated to an LPN or UAP.
1. Assume role of client advocate.
2. Verify identification of client in accordance with Universal Protocol to prevent wrong site, wrong procedure, and wrong person surgery.
3. Ensure that client is wearing identification bracelet.
4. Confirm operative procedure and operative site.
5. Involve client (or legally designated representative) in process to extent possible.
6. Ensure that ethnic/spiritual beliefs are respected.

C. Safety and infection control
1. Ensure client's safety in operating room.
   a. Maintain room temperature and humidity to prevent hypothermia.
   b. Remove any potential contaminants.
   c. Prevent unnecessary room traffic.
   d. Keep room noise and talk at a minimum.
   e. Assess electrical equipment for proper operation.
   f. Ensure necessary equipment and supplies are available, and instruments, sutures, and dressings are ready for use.
   g. Count and document sutures, needles, instruments, and sponges.
   h. Ensure that staff call client by name and provide individualized attention.
   i. Assist in transferring client to operating room table.
   j. Cover client with warm blanket and attach the safety strap.
   k. Remain at client's side during anesthesia induction.
   l. Verify proper client positioning to protect nerves, circulation, respiration, and skin integrity; always pad pressure areas.
   m. Ensure that newly requested items are quickly supplied to the anesthesia or scrub team by the circulating nurse.
2. Decrease risk of infection.
   a. Promote good hand hygiene among all sterile members of surgical team (scrub assistant, surgeon, and assistant); cleanse hands and arms by scrubbing with brush and detergent before entering sterile field.
   b. Use evidence-based practice principles of basic aseptic technique in operating room:
      (1) All materials that enter sterile field must be sterile; if sterile item comes in contact with unsterile item, sterile item becomes contaminated. Contaminated items are removed immediately from sterile field.
      (2) Sterile team members wear only sterile gowns and gloves.

(3) A wide margin of safety is maintained between sterile and unsterile field.
(4) Tables are considered sterile only at tabletop level.
(5) Edges of sterile packages are considered contaminated once packages are opened.
(6) Bacteria travel on airborne particles and enter sterile field with excessive air movement and currents; prevent by minimizing air movement.
(7) Bacteria travel by capillary action; contamination occurs through moist fabrics; prevent by keeping fabrics dry and/or changing moist fabrics as necessary.
(8) Bacteria harbor on client's and team members' hair, skin, and in respiratory tract; confine bacteria with appropriate attire.
(9) Apply sterile dressings to all wounds.
(10) Ensure nonscrubbed personnel refrain from touching or contaminating anything that is sterile.

D. Health promotion and maintenance: The anesthesiologist or nurse anesthetist and perioperative nurse accompany client to postanesthesia care unit; a report of client's status and the procedure performed is communicated. RN responsibilities include:
1. Monitor blood, fluid, and other drainage output.
2. Coordinate health team activities.
3. Monitor client's temperature continuously.
4. Monitor pertinent electrolyte values.

E. Psychologic integrity
1. Promote ethical behaviors (respect, confidentiality) in operating room.
2. Maintain a quiet, relaxing atmosphere; client can hear.
3. Provide privacy for client.
4. Identify and respect ethnic, spiritual, and other concerns of client that can affect surgical experience. Examples may include the following:
a. Jehovah's Witness—may refuse blood transfusions.
b. Islamic—left hand considered unclean; nurse uses right hand to administer drugs and treatments.
c. Native American—may request that surgically removed body tissue be preserved so that may be ritually buried.
5. Listen attentively; provide information that may allay concerns.

F. Basic care and comfort
1. Monitor client's response to stressors related to surgical experience.
2. Maintain asepsis in surgical environment (see safety and infection control).
3. Advocate for safe care of client.
4. Adjust operating room furniture so client is comfortable.
5. Maintain controlled temperature of operating room to facilitate client comfort under surgical drapes.
6. Provide privacy for client by restricting influx of hospital personnel.
7. Position client for comfort and so that operative area is accessible.
8. Assess client's level of consciousness, skin integrity, mobility, emotional status, and functional limitations.
9. Use plan of care that incorporates, respects client's value system, lifestyle, ethnicity, and culture; care plan reflects client's level of function and ability during perioperative period.

G. Reduction of risk potential
1. Recognize possibility for unanticipated intraoperative events that occasionally occur.
a. Anaphylaxis—most severe form of allergic reaction with life-threatening pulmonary and circulatory complications.
b. Allergies to latex (observe latex allergy protocols according to agency policy).
c. Malignant hyperthermia—rare metabolic disease characterized by hyperthermia with rigidity of skeletal muscles that can lead to death.
2. Prevent injury to sensitive skin from tape, electrodes, warming and cooling blankets, and dressings.
3. Provide careful transferring, lifting, and positioning of client. Special care required for older adults, clients with osteoporosis or osteoarthritis, injuries or other health problems for which positioning improperly could cause further injury or pain.
4. Use Universal Protocol for preventing wrong site, wrong procedure, wrong person surgery (see definition for steps).

H. Pharmacologic and parenteral therapies: Client and family will state purpose for and side effects of all intraoperative medications.
1. Anesthesia
a. General (inhaled or IV)—refers to drug-induced depression of central nervous system that produces analgesia,

amnesia, and unconsciousness (affects whole body)
(1) Inhalation anesthetics: Isoflurane (Forane); nitrous oxide
(2) IV barbiturates: Methohexital sodium (Brevital)—high lipoid affinity provides prompt effect on cerebral tissue
(3) IV, IM nonbarbiturates: Midazolam hydrochloride (Versed)—induces cataleptic state and produces amnesia for procedure

b. Conscious sedation—uses IV or nasal routes of sedation to depress consciousness, but maintains airway and ventilations.
(1) Midazolam (Versed); have reversal agent, flumazenil (Romazicon), available
(2) Ketamine (Ketalar)
(3) Fentanyl (Sublimaze); have reversal agent, naloxone (Narcan), available

c. Local—used to produce pain control without rendering client unconscious. Types include topical, spinal, nerve block, and epidural.
(1) Benzocaine (Americane): Topical
(2) Lidocaine (Xylocaine): Topical, spinal, nerve block, epidural
(3) Tetracaine (Pontocaine): Topical, spinal, nerve block
(4) Procaine (Novocain): Spinal, nerve block
(5) Bupivacaine (Marcaine): Epidural, nerve block
(6) Chloroprocaine (Nesacaine): Nerve block
(7) Mepivacaine (Carbocaine): Nerve block

2. Sedatives/hypnotics—used for clients experiencing anxiety-related situations, insomnia; available in oral, parenteral, and rectal preparations.
a. Barbiturates—amobarbital (Amytal); pentobarbital (Nembutal); secobarbital (Seconal)
b. Nonbarbiturates—chloral hydrate (Noctec); temazepam (Restoril)

3. Opioids—fentanyl (Sublimaze), meperidine (Demerol), morphine (Duramorph): Induces, maintains anesthesia; reduces stimuli from sensory nerve endings; provides analgesia during anesthetic recovery. Nurse protects airway in anticipation of vomiting.

4. Benzodiazepines—midazolam (Versed), diazepam (Valium), lorazepam (Ativan): Induces, maintains anesthesia; provides conscious sedation or sedation during local and regional anesthesia. Nurse assures reversal agent is available.

5. Neuromuscular blocking agents—facilitate endotracheal intubation; promote skeletal muscle relaxation (paralysis) to enhance access to surgical sites. Effects of nondepolarizing agents are usually reversed toward the end of surgery by administration of anticholinesterase agents.
a. Depolarizing agent—succinylcholine (Anectine)
b. Nondepolarizing agents—vecuronium (Norcuron), atracurium (Tracrium), pancuronium (Pavulon)
c. Anticholinesterase agents—neostigmine (Prostigmin), pyridostigmine (Mestinon), edrophonium (Enlon)

6. Antiemetics—ondansetron (Zofran), metoclopramide (Reglan), promethazine (Phenergan): Prevent vomiting with aspiration during surgery; counteract emetic effects of inhalation agents, opioids. Droperidol (Inapsine) most often used during surgery (others used postoperatively); administered with caution in clients with heart disease.

7. IV fluids
a. Normal saline (NS; 0.9% NaCl)—isotonic; need for administration of blood/blood products
b. Dextrose 5%/water (D5/W)—isotonic, hypotonic
c. Lactated Ringer (LR)—isotonic; used for fluid loss due to bleeding. Does not contain magnesium or phosphate.
d. *Hypertonic solutions* may be needed to increase the extracellular fluid volume.
(1) 5% dextrose in normal saline (D5/NS)
(2) 10% dextrose in water (D10/W)
(3) 3% sodium chloride (3% NaCl)
e. *Colloids* may be used as volume expander when treating hypovolemic shock from surgery or trauma.
(1) Albumin—major plasma protein
(2) Dextran—glucose solution with colloidal activity similar to albumin that expands plasma volume by pulling fluid from interstitial to intravascular space
(3) Hetastarch (Hespan, Hextend)—is a synthetic colloid made from cornstarch; expands plasma volume; used in shock precipitated by hemorrhage, trauma, burns, sepsis;

plasma volume expansion starts decreasing at about 24 hr.

f. *Blood* increases colloidal oncotic pressure within the intravascular space; increases overall blood volume.

Postoperative Period

I. Definition: The postoperative period begins immediately after surgery and continues through client rehabilitation (see individual sections below for more information on each stage of postoperative care).

Immediate Postoperative Stage

I. Definition: The immediate postoperative stage begins directly after completion of the surgical procedure and continues for up to 4 hr. Details regarding client transfer from operating room to postanesthesia room are as follows:
   A. Postanesthesia care unit
      1. Client's immediate recovery supervised by postanesthesia care unit nurse.
      2. Care unit located adjacent to operating room to minimize transportation of client immediately after surgery and provide ready access to anesthesia and surgical personnel.
      3. May involve areas designated for recovery depending on whether client had undergone general anesthesia; or local, regional, or conscious sedation.
   B. Admission to postanesthesia care unit
      1. Admission is joint collaborative effort between anesthesiologist or nurse anesthetist, and postanesthesia care unit nurse.
         a. Fosters smooth transfer of care
         b. Uses standardized approach to "hand off" communications, including opportunity to ask and respond to questions
            (1) Involves complete list of client's medications communicated to next provider of service when client is transferred to another service practitioner within organization
            (2) Involves at least two client identifiers
      2. Components of postanesthesia admission report:
         a. General client information
            (1) Name
            (2) Age, date of birth
            (3) Gender
            (4) Anesthesiologist or nurse anesthetist
            (5) Surgeon
            (6) Surgical procedure
            (7) Family and/or significant other presence
         b. Client history
            (1) Indication for surgery
            (2) Medical history, medications, allergies
         c. Intraoperative management
            (1) Anesthetic medications
            (2) Other medications received preoperatively or intraoperatively
            (3) Blood loss
            (4) Fluid replacement totals including blood transfusion(s)
            (5) Urine output
         d. Intraoperative course
            (1) Unexpected anesthetic events/reactions
            (2) Unexpected surgical events
            (3) Vital signs, monitoring trends
            (4) Results of intraoperative laboratory tests
         e. Postanesthesia care unit plan
            (1) Potential, unexpected problems (with plan for intervention)
            (2) Suggested postanesthesia care unit course
            (3) Acceptable parameters for laboratory test results
            (4) Postanesthesia care unit discharge plan

II. Nursing process
   A. Assessment: Assess client immediately on admission to postanesthesia care unit to obtain baseline data. Position client before assessment to ensure adequate airway.
      1. Respiratory system
         a. Monitor vital signs.
         b. Monitor airway patency and adequate ventilation (prolonged mechanical ventilation during anesthesia may affect postoperative lung function).
         c. Monitor for secretions.
         d. Observe chest movement for symmetry and use of accessory muscles.
         e. Monitor pulse oximetry and oxygen administration.
         f. Note rate, depth, and quality of respirations (expect rate more than 10 and less than 30 breaths per minute).
         g. Assess breath sounds.
         h. Monitor for signs of atelectasis, pneumonia, or pulmonary embolism.
      2. Cardiovascular system
         a. Assess skin and check capillary refill.
         b. Assess peripheral pulses and presence of edema.

c. Monitor for bleeding.
d. Assess pulse rate and rhythm.
e. Monitor for signs of hypertension and hypotension.
f. Monitor for cardiac dysrhythmias.

3. Musculoskeletal system
   a. Assess for ability of client to move extremities.
   b. Assess overall positioning.
4. Neurologic system
   a. Assess level of consciousness.
   b. Monitor body temperature.
5. Temperature control—monitor for signs of hypothermia that may result from anesthesia, a cool operating room, or exposure of skin and internal organs during surgery.
6. Integumentary system
   a. Assess surgical site, drains, and wound dressings.
   b. Monitor for and document any drainage or bleeding from surgical site.
   c. Assess skin for redness, abrasions, or breakdown that may have resulted from surgical positioning.
7. Fluid and electrolyte balance
   a. Monitor IV administration as prescribed.
   b. Monitor intake and output.
   c. Monitor for signs of hypocalcemia, hyperglycemia, and metabolic/respiratory acidosis or alkalosis.
8. GI system
   a. Monitor for nausea and vomiting.
   b. Monitor for abdominal distention.
9. Renal system
   a. Assess bladder for distention.
   b. Monitor color and quality of urine.
   c. Monitor intake and output.
10. Pain management
    a. Monitor subjective complaints of pain.
    b. Assess type of anesthetic used and preoperative medication administered.
    c. Monitor for objective data related to pain (facial expressions, body gestures, increased pulse rate, increased BP, increased respirations).
    d. If narcotic administered, assess every 30 min for respiratory rate and pain relief.
    e. Assess effectiveness of pain medication and noninvasive pain-relief measures (positioning, back rub).

B. Analysis
1. Ineffective Airway Clearance related to prolonged sedation
2. Risk for Aspiration related to reduced level of consciousness
3. Ineffective Breathing Pattern related to incisional pain
4. Risk for Deficient Fluid Volume related to inadequate intake, wound drainage, and gastric decompression
5. Risk for Infection related to surgical wound
6. Risk for Injury related to anesthesia, sedation
7. Acute Pain related to surgical incision
8. Urinary Retention related to effects of anesthesia
9. Risk for Ineffective Tissue Perfusion: Cardiovascular, related to effects of anesthesia and surgery

C. Planning
1. Maintain airway clearance.
2. Prevent aspiration of secretions.
3. Provide pain relief.
4. Promote effective breathing pattern.
5. Correct fluid volume deficit.
6. Prevent infection.
7. Prevent injury.
8. Promote adequate urine output.

D. Implementation
1. Assess client's cardiac, respiratory, urinary, neurologic, and neurovascular status, and document on postanesthesia care unit record.
2. Promote measures that address potential complications.
3. Maintain airway patency and optimal respiratory function.
4. Provide pain relief.
5. Promote measures that prevent complications of immobility.
6. Offer emotional support and reassurance.

E. Evaluation
1. Client has adequate tissue perfusion with stable cardiovascular, respiratory, urinary, neurologic, and neurovascular status.
2. Client exhibits clear lungs on auscultation.
3. Client reports pain relief with nursing interventions.
4. Client is free from complications from immobility.
5. Client maintains fluid balance.
6. Client remains free of infection.
7. Client is free from signs of injury.

CN

III. Client needs

A. Physiologic adaptation
1. Anesthesia depresses respiratory function.
2. Anesthesia and immobilization during surgery may result in circulatory compromise.
3. Medications and anesthetic agents depress central nervous system.
4. Incision provides portal for infection and need for wound care.

5. Use of equipment (drains and tubes) creates portal for infection and risk for obstructed drainage.
6. NPO status and use of anesthesia alters fluid and electrolytes.

B. Management of care: Care of the client in the immediate postoperative stage requires critical thinking skills and knowledge of assessment, and teaching and evaluation methods unique to the role of the postanesthesia care unit nurse. These skills cannot be delegated to an LPN or UAP.
   1. Provide interventions for client respiratory needs—maintain patent airway and optimal respiratory function.
      a. Position client on side until awake, unless contraindicated.
      b. Administer oxygen as necessary.
      c. Encourage turning, coughing, and deep breathing as soon as client is able.
      d. Use suction to clear secretions as needed.
      e. Elevate head of bed at least 30 degrees, unless contraindicated.
      f. Monitor pulse oximetry.
   2. Provide interventions for client circulatory needs.
      a. Monitor heart rate, rhythm, BP at frequent intervals; document every 15 min.
      b. Monitor peripheral circulation by noting color, temperature, capillary refill, presence of peripheral pulses, and pulse oximetry.
   3. Provide interventions for client neurologic needs.
      a. Monitor level of consciousness.
      b. Monitor motor and sensory status of extremities.
      c. Monitor pupillary blink and gag reflexes.
      d. Reorient client to time, place, and situation as needed.
   4. Provide wound care; note location of wound and drainage for color, odor, amount, and consistency. (Can delegate to LPN.)
   5. Monitor output of drains and patency of tubing. (Can be delegated to UAP or LPN.)
   6. Provide interventions for client fluid and electrolyte needs.
      a. Maintain IV therapy.
      b. Monitor intake and output.
      c. Monitor blood values and report abnormal values.
   7. Assess pain for location, intensity, duration, precipitating factors, and effectiveness of pain management (e.g., medications, postoperative activities such as coughing and deep breathing).
   8. Request consult with surgeon, anesthesiologist and nurse anesthetist, and perioperative nurse in operating room, as needed.
   9. Consult with IV therapist to aid in maintenance of IV fluid therapy.
   10. Consult with respiratory therapist to promote adequate ventilation.

C. Safety and infection control
   1. Avoid positioning client in supine position until pharyngeal reflexes have returned.
   2. Maintain patency of nasogastric tube, if present.
   3. Ensure client understands how to use client-controlled analgesia pump, if present.
   4. Reinforce dressings (surgeon may perform first dressing change).
   5. Administer prescribed IV antibiotics as ordered.

D. Health promotion and maintenance
   1. Encourage deep-breathing and coughing exercises as soon as possible.
   2. Monitor for signs of hypertension and hypotension.
   3. Encourage resumption of activity as allowed.

E. Psychologic integrity
   1. Offer emotional support and reassurance; allow client to verbalize feelings of anxiety.
   2. Provide calm, quiet, and restful environment.
   3. Explain all activities to client upon arrival in postanesthesia care unit to decrease anxiety, confusion. Explain the following:
      a. Surgery is completed
      b. Moved to recovery room
      c. Who is caring for client, and what is being done

F. Basic care and comfort
   1. Administer medications to manage pain; evaluate outcomes of pain management and document.
   2. Manage nausea and vomiting as needed; administer antiemetics if required; provide ice chips or fluids.
   3. Reposition client for comfort.
   4. Offer mouth care, bathing, and back care as needed.

G. Reduction of risk potential
   1. Identify actual or potential problems that may occur as result of anesthetic administration, surgical intervention; intervene

appropriately. Monitor for common postoperative problems such as:
a. Airway compromise (obstruction)
b. Respiratory insufficiency (hypoxemia, hypercarbia)
c. Cardiac compromise (hypotension, hypertension, arrhythmias)
d. Neurologic compromise (emergence delirium, delayed awakening)
e. Hypothermia
f. Pain
g. Nausea and vomiting

2. After initial assessment is completed, postanesthesia care unit nurse continues to apply nursing process; assess at least every 15 min or more frequently, depending on client's status:
a. Airway
b. Vital signs (every 5 min for three times; then, every 15 min)
c. General appearance
d. Level of consciousness, reflexes
e. Movement of extremities
f. Pain level
g. Urine output
h. IV or central line patency
i. Drain or catheter patency
j. Operative site, dressings for signs of hemorrhage or abnormal drainage
k. Functioning of cardiac, oxygen monitors
l. Signs/symptoms of hypovolemic shock
3. Monitor respiratory rate and pulse oximetry because of use of opioid analgesics.
4. Be aware that extubated clients who are lethargic may not be able to maintain an airway.
5. Be aware that stridor, wheezing, or crowing may indicate partial obstruction, bronchospasm, or laryngospasm; crackles or rhonchi may indicate pulmonary edema.
6. Recall that bounding pulse may indicate hypertension or fluid overload.
7. Prevent complications of immobility.
a. Assess for signs and symptoms of skin breakdown, respiratory difficulties, deep vein thrombosis, and bladder or bowel problems.
b. Encourage client to turn, cough, and deep breathe frequently.
c. Encourage client to perform passive and active ROM exercises frequently.

H. Pharmacologic and parenteral therapies: Client and family will state purpose for and side effects of all medications used in immediate postoperative phase.
1. Antibiotics: Ampicillin (Amcill), cefazolin (Ancef), ceftazidime (Fortaz)—prevent/treat infection.
a. Before first dose of antibiotic, assess for allergies and determine whether culture has been obtained.
b. After multiple doses of antibiotic, assess for superinfection (thrush, yeast infection, and diarrhea).
c. Assess IV access site for phlebitis.
d. Monitor WBC count.
2. Antiemetics: Ondansetron (Zofran), trimethobenzamide (Tigan), dimenhydrinate (Dramamine)—relieve nausea and vomiting.
a. Advise that antiemetic may cause drowsiness.
b. Measure emesis.
c. Maintain intake and output.
d. Monitor for dehydration.
3. Opioid analgesics: Codeine (Paveral), hydrocodone (Hycodan), hydromorphone (Dilaudid)—relieve moderate to severe pain.
a. Assess pain; medicate according to pain scale (0-10) findings.
b. Rule out any complications.
c. Institute safety measures (bed in low position, side rails up, call light within reach).
d. Evaluate effectiveness of pain medication in 30 min.
e. Monitor respiratory rate.
4. Parenteral therapies—monitor BP; hypertonic fluids may cause fluid shifting into intravascular compartment.
a. Normal saline (NS; 0.9% NaCl)—isotonic
b. Dextrose 5%/water (D5/W)—isotonic, hypotonic
c. Lactated Ringer (LR)—isotonic
d. Dextrose 5% in normal saline (D5/NS)—hypertonic
e. 3% sodium chloride (3% NaCl)—hypertonic

Intermediate Postoperative Stage

I. Definition: The intermediate postoperative stage begins 4 hr after completion of the surgical procedure on client discharge from the postanesthesia care unit; this stage continues for up to 24 hr.
A. Prior to discharging client from postanesthesia care unit: Nurse provides verbal report summarizing operative and postanesthetic period to receiving nurse on clinical unit.

B. On entrance to clinical unit: Nurse who receives client on clinical unit assists in transferring client from cart onto bed. IV lines, wound drains, dressings, and traction devices are protected.

II. Nursing process

A. Assessment

1. Record time of client's arrival on unit.
2. Assess baseline vital signs.
3. Assess airway and breath sounds.
4. Assess neurologic status, including level of consciousness and movement of extremities.
5. Assess wound, dressing, drainage tubes; note type and amount of drainage.
6. Assess color and appearance of skin.
7. Assess urinary status; check for bladder distention and catheter patency, if present.
8. Assess current pain intensity; note last type and dose of pain control.
9. Check IV infusion; check integrity of insertion site and size of catheter.
10. Determine emotional condition and support needs.

B. Analysis

1. Acute Pain related to surgical incision and reflex muscle spasm
2. Nausea related to GI distention and medication or anesthesia effects
3. Risk for Infection related to surgical incision, inadequate nutrition and fluid intake, presence of environmental pathogens, invasive catheters, and immobility
4. Ineffective Airway Clearance related to inability to clear tenacious secretions
5. Impaired gas exchange related to risk for hemorrhage due to ineffective vascular closure or alterations in coagulation
6. Ineffective peripheral tissue perfusion and thromboembolism related to dehydration, immobility, vascular manipulation, or injury
7. Risk for Urinary Retention related to horizontal positioning, pain, fear, analgesic and anesthetic medications, or surgical procedure
8. Risk for imbalanced fluid volume and paralytic ileus related to bowel manipulation, immobility, pain mediation, and anesthetics

C. Planning

1. Relieve pain.
2. Alleviate nausea.
3. Prevent infection.
4. Maintain patent airway.
5. Detect signs of hemorrhage.
6. Prevent thrombus formation.
7. Promote elimination of urine.
8. Prevent development of paralytic ileus.

D. Implementation (see health promotion and maintenance)

E. Evaluation

1. Client has optimal respiratory function.
2. Client is free from postoperative complications.
3. Client verbalizes relief of pain.
4. Client maintains optimal fluid and electrolyte status.
5. Client maintains optimal nutritional status.
6. Client demonstrates optimal bowel and bladder elimination patterns.
7. Client displays optimal wound healing.

CN

III. Client needs

A. Physiologic adaptation

1. Respiratory status is monitored closely because of anesthetic agents, sedation, and depression of central nervous system (see management of care).
2. Level of consciousness and responsiveness is monitored because of anesthetic agents and use of postoperative pain medications.
3. Break in skin integrity at surgical wound site is monitored because of incision and drains, if used.
4. Urinary status (last voiding and amount) is monitored because of potential effects of anesthesia and medications on kidney function.

B. Management of care: Care of the client during intermediate postoperative stage requires critical thinking skills and knowledge of assessment, and teaching and evaluation methods unique to the RN role. These skills cannot be delegated to an LPN or UAP.

1. Delegate responsibly those activities that can be delegated. All monitoring information is reported to the RN.
   a. Monitor vital signs.
   b. Monitor intake and output.
   c. Assist with turning, coughing, and deep breathing as ordered.
   d. Provide oral hygiene and lip care.
   e. Provide back care, if permitted.
2. Closely monitor respiratory status, including:
   a. Airway patency
   b. Rate, depth, and pattern of respirations
   c. Character of breath sounds
   d. Signs of peripheral or mucous membrane cyanosis
   e. Arterial blood oxygen level according to pulse oximeter determination
3. Monitor level of consciousness and responsiveness.

4. Consult with respiratory therapist, IV therapist, surgeon, and attending physician as needed.
5. Contact social services/discharge planning/case manager to arrange for services such as home health care, meal delivery, transportation assistance, and special equipment (wheelchair, walker, oxygen equipment) as needed.

C. Safety and infection control
1. Assess need for side rails to be up on bed.
2. Evaluate client's level of consciousness, responsiveness.
3. Assess neurovascular status in extremities to prevent injury.
4. Ascertain that correct IV solution is infusing, and at correct rate.
5. Keep call light within client's reach.
6. Assist with ambulation as needed.
7. Determine working condition of all equipment.
8. Note signs of infection at surgical site (redness, odor, drainage, warmth).
9. Keep sequential compression devices on or encourage foot pumps until client is ambulating.
10. Monitor temperature for elevation, indicating systemic infection.
11. Use clean/sterile technique (per agency protocol) when removing, irrigating, and changing surgical dressing.
12. Reduce risk of nosocomial infection by maintaining medical/surgical asepsis.

D. Health promotion and maintenance
1. Promote lung expansion.
   a. Use incentive spirometer as indicated.
   b. Progress mobility from ROM exercises to ambulation as tolerated.
      (1) Gradually increase exercise from lying, to sitting, to standing, and then to ambulating.
      (2) Provide assistance and encouragement.
      (3) Maintain safety precautions.
2. Promote measures to address potential complications (hypoxemia, hypovolemia, hemorrhage, pulmonary embolism, allergic drug reactions, cardiac arrhythmias).
3. Promote optimal fluid intake, and monitor and assess output; assess for urinary retention.
4. Promote normal voiding patterns.
5. Promote return to normal GI function—minimize abdominal distention from decreased peristalsis through exercise, ambulation, decreased opioid dosage/usage, or rectal tube placement.
6. Provide adequate nutrition—resume oral feeding as soon as gastric, bowel function returns.
7. Promote wound healing.
   a. Assess dressing and wound for signs and symptoms of infection.
   b. Use clean, no-touch technique for dressing changes, unless ordered otherwise.

E. Psychologic integrity
1. Assist with identification of effective coping strategies.
2. Discuss postoperative depression if appropriate.
3. Teach about grieving process; refer to support group as needed.

F. Basic care and comfort (see health promotion and maintenance)

G. Reduction of risk potential
1. Prevent pneumonia, encourage turning, coughing, deep breathing at least every 2 hr; progress mobility from ROM exercises to ambulation.
2. Minimize risk of deep vein thrombosis.
   a. Assess for early signs (redness, edema, tenderness along vein).
   b. Apply elastic hose, a sequential compression device, or administer low-dose heparin, as prescribed.
   c. Teach measures to prevent vessel constriction.
3. Intervene as appropriate to prevent postoperative depression, disorientation, psychosis.
   a. Orient postoperatively.
   b. Provide prescribed medication, close supervision.
   c. Contact mental health professional as required.
4. Prevent urinary tract infection.
   a. Encourage adequate fluid intake.
   b. Monitor fluid intake and output.
   c. Assess for urinary retention.
   d. Provide catheter care.
5. Prevent paralytic ileus and abdominal distention.
   a. Assess for bowel sounds and flatus every 8 hr.
   b. Encourage ambulation.
   c. Provide passive ROM; encourage client to do active ROM exercise, as permitted.

H. Pharmacologic and parenteral therapies (see medications used for immediate postoperative stage)

Extended Postoperative Stage

I. Definition: The extended postoperative stage begins when client is admitted to postanesthesia care unit and extends through follow-up evaluation. Nursing care for the client in the extended postoperative stage involves monitoring for and providing interventions to prevent postoperative complications.

II. Nursing process
  A. Assessment: Continue to assess body systems for complications.
    1. Respiratory complications—assess respiratory rate and patterns, pulse oximetry, and breath sounds.
    2. Cardiovascular complications—assess BP and heart rate and rhythm, skin temperature, and color of skin and mucous membrane.
    3. Urinary complications
      a. Assess urine quantity and quality, including color, amount, consistency and odor.
      b. Check indwelling catheter for patency.
      c. Assess ability of client to void within 6 to 8 hr after surgery; if no voiding occurs:
        (1) Inspect abdominal contour.
        (2) Palpate bladder.
        (3) Percuss bladder for distention.
    4. GI complications
      a. Auscultate abdomen in all four quadrants to determine presence, frequency, and characteristics of bowel sounds.
      b. If vomiting occurs, evaluate emesis for color, consistency, and amount.
    5. Surgical wound
      a. Assess wound type, drains inserted, and expected drainage.
      b. Assess for drainage change from sanguineous (red) to serosanguineous (pink) to serous (clear yellow); drainage should decrease over hours or days.
        (1) Purulent drainage indicates wound infection.
        (2) Sudden discharge of brown, pink, or clear drainage tends to precede wound dehiscence (separation, disruption of previously joined wound edges).
    6. Pain
      a. Observe for behavioral clues of pain such as wrinkling of face or brow, clenched fist, moaning, diaphoresis, and increased pulse rate.
      b. Assess for pain on a visual analogue scale (1-10) for objective measure.
    7. Temperature—observe for alterations to determine early signs of inflammation and infection; detect patterns of hypothermia and/or fever.
    8. Psychologic function
      a. Assess signs and symptoms of anxiety and depression.
      b. Assess for confusion and delirium due to:
        (1) Fluid and electrolyte imbalance
        (2) Hypoxemia
        (3) Effects of drugs
        (4) Sleep deprivation
        (5) Sensory alteration, deprivation, overload
        (6) Delirium tremens—results from alcohol withdrawal; assess for restlessness, insomnia, nightmares, tachycardia, apprehension, disorientation, irritability, and auditory or visual hallucinations.
  B. Analysis: Following surgery, the client may experience a variety of nursing problems. The nurse must gather data frequently and make appropriate nursing diagnoses individualized for each client. Common nursing diagnoses are listed here.
    1. Ineffective Airway Clearance related to postoperative pain
    2. Ineffective Breathing Pattern related to postoperative pain
    3 Deficient Fluid Volume related to NPO status
    4. Ineffective Tissue Perfusion: Cardiovascular, related to decreased blood flow
    5. Activity Intolerance related to pain or immobility
    6. Ineffective tissue perfusion: cardiopulmonary related to bedrest
    7. Impaired Urinary Elimination related to difficulty voiding
    8. Nausea related to use of anesthetics and pain
    9. Imbalanced Nutrition: Less Than Body Requirements related to loss of appetite or NPO status
    10. Ineffective tissue perfusion: gastrointestinal related to paralytic ileus from anesthesia
    11. Risk for Infection related to incision or drains
    12. Acute Pain related to incision
    13. Anxiety related to outcome of surgical procedure
    14. Disturbed Body Image related to surgery
  C. Planning
    1. Maintain respiratory status.
    2. Maintain adequate cardiac output.
    3. Maintain adequate fluid volume.
    4. Prevent thromboembolism.
    5. Promote elimination of urine.
    6. Maintain nutrition; offer high-protein foods.
    7. Prevent paralytic ileus.
    8. Prevent infection.

9. Promote wound healing.
10. Relieve pain.
11. Prevent pneumonia and atelectasis.
12. Prepare client for discharge.

D. Implementation
1. Provide interventions to prevent respiratory complications.
   a. Encourage coughing, deep breathing, and turning at least every 2 hr; splint abdominal incision with pillow to provide support, aid in coughing and expectoration of secretions.
   b. Encourage use of incentive spirometer 10 times every hour while awake.
   c. Assist with progressive ambulation.
   d. Provide regular, adequate analgesic medication.
   e. Ensure that incision does not separate.
   f. Provide adequate hydration (at least 2,000 ml/day).
2. Provide interventions to prevent cardiac complications.
   a. Document cardiac output.
   b. Monitor hematocrit, electrolytes.
   c. Monitor IV fluid replacement.
   d. Monitor IV access site for discomfort.
   e. Provide adequate, regular mouth care.
   f. Encourage leg exercises 10 to 12 times every 1 to 2 hr while awake.
   g. Assist with progressive ambulation as tolerated.
   h. When elastic stockings or sequential compression devices are used, must be removed, reapplied at least twice daily for skin care, inspection.
   i. Monitor body prominences for signs of increased pressure, breakdown.
   j. Prevent syncope by making position changes slowly.
3. Provide interventions to prevent urinary complications.
   a. Monitor intake and output to determine fluid balance.
   b. Percuss bladder routinely for 48 hr postoperatively to assess for distention.
   c. Position client in as normal position as possible for voiding.
   d. Use appropriate pain measures and provide privacy to reduce anxiety and promote ease in voiding.
4. Provide interventions to prevent GI complications.
   a. Provide oral intake as soon as gag reflex returns and bowel sounds present.
   b. Insert nasogastric tube to decompress stomach to prevent nausea, vomiting, and abdominal distention.
   c. When oral intake is allowed, provide clear liquids and advance to regular diet as tolerated.
   d. Encourage ambulation to stimulate peristalsis and expel flatus.
   e. If hiccoughs are due to partial obstruction of nasogastric tube, irrigate to restore patency.
5. Provide interventions to prevent complications involving surgical wound.
   a. Record drainage on dressing including type, amount, color, consistency, and odor.
   b. Assess effect of position changes on drainage.
   c. Use clean, no-touch technique when changing dressing unless ordered otherwise.
   d. Promote frequent careful examination of incision site; infection indicated by redness, edema, pain, fever, increased WBC count.
      (1) Area around sutures and staples—slightly reddened, edematous (expected inflammatory response)
      (2) Around incision—normal color, temperature
6. Relieve pain.
   a. Provide analgesics as ordered.
   b. Provide effective pain management to promote optimal healing.
   c. Monitor undesirable side effects including:
      (1) Constipation
      (2) Nausea, vomiting
      (3) Respiratory, cough depression
      (4) Hypotension
   d. Monitor epidural analgesia.
   e. Monitor client-controlled analgesia.
7. Provide interventions to prevent complications related to body temperature.
   a. Measure temperature every 4 hr.
   b. Maintain meticulous asepsis with regard to wound, IV site.
   c. Encourage airway clearance.
   d. Obtain wound, urine, blood cultures as ordered.
   e. Administer antibiotics, as prescribed.
   f. Use body-cooling blanket when fever rises above 103°F, if ordered.
8. Prevent complications as a result of psychologic factors (see psychologic integrity).

E. Evaluation
1. Client demonstrates effective airway clearance: Clear breath sounds, effective breathing pattern, and effective cough.

2. Client's blood gas analysis indicates adequate gas exchange.
3. Client demonstrates adequate cardiac output; BP and heart rate within normal limits; skin warm to touch; mucous membranes pink.
4. Client demonstrates ability to ambulate with no signs of dyspnea, muscle weakness, or skin moistness.
5. Client is free from signs and symptoms of thromboembolism.
6. Client voids an adequate amount of urine (about 500 ml in 8 hr) following surgery; free from signs of bladder distention on palpation or ultrasound of bladder.
7. Client verbalizes absence of nausea.
8. Client ingests adequate amount of food and fluid.
9. Client's bowel sounds are present with passage of flatus.
10. Client is free from hiccoughs.
11. Client is free from signs and symptoms of infection; wound edges are intact with no abnormal drainage present; body temperature is normal within 4 days.
12. Client reports decrease in level of pain using appropriate pain scale.
13. Client adapts to alterations imposed by surgical intervention.
14. Client has positive perception of body image.
15. Client actively participates in making informed decisions.
16. Client and family understand postsurgical care instructions.
17. Client is advised about home care services, and services are arranged as needed.

CN

III. Client needs

A. Physiologic adaptation: Encourage client use of pharmacologic and nonpharmacologic measures to manage discomfort and pain. As time progresses with continued wound healing, encourage increased use of nonpharmacologic measures (distraction, imagery, relaxation techniques, back rub).
   1. Promote effective airway clearance; establish effective breathing pattern; promote effective oxygenation; prevent pneumonia and atelectasis.
   2. Prevent thromboembolism—encourage client to move in bed; ambulate as possible; use antithromboembolic hose as ordered; encourage fluids.
   3. Manage nausea—offer high-protein foods.
   4. Prevent paralytic ileus—urge client to ambulate and pass gas; encourage bowel movement; encourage fluids.
   5. Promote wound healing—change dressing as ordered; encourage adequate nutrition; assess for signs of infection.

B. Management of care: Care of the client in the extended postoperative stage requires critical thinking skills and knowledge of assessment, and teaching and evaluation methods unique to the RN role. These skills cannot be delegated to an LPN or UAP.
   1. Delegate responsibly those activities that can be delegated. All monitoring information is reported to the RN.
      a. Monitor vital signs.
      b. Monitor intake and output.
      c. Assist with turning, coughing, and deep breathing.
      d. Assist with progressive activity as allowed.
      e. Assist with nutritional intake.
      f. Provide basic hygienic care.
   2. Consult the following, as indicated:
      a. Surgeon, attending physician, physician specialists
      b. Dietitian
      c. Client care coordinator; discharge planner to arrange for home health care, arrange for assistive devices
      d. Social worker
      e. Physical therapist
      f. IV therapist
   3. Consult with client care coordinator, discharge planner, and community-based supply business to arrange for home health care and assistive devices as needed, including:
      a. Elevated toilet seat
      b. Oxygen equipment
      c. Braces, splints, continuous–passive-motion machines
      d. Transportation services

C. Safety and infection control: Provide client and family teaching; administer verbal and written instructions for care in the home setting.
   1. Inspect wound at least twice each day; use mirror if unable to view completely.
   2. Notify physician when wound is reddened, irritated, or has any drainage or odor. Inspect dressing for bleeding and drainage.
   3. Clean wound as prescribed by physician.
   4. Take oral temperature twice daily; notify physician if greater than 101°F (remind client that low-grade fever not uncommon).
   5. Avoid putting any increased strain on wound; no lifting allowed for abdominal wound, and no walking for leg incision.
   6. Obtain activity level adequate to convalescent period.

D. Health promotion and maintenance
1. Instruct client on dietary information appropriate during convalescent period to promote healing.
   a. Protein: 1.2 to 2 g/kg body weight per day—promotes tissue healing.
   b. Calories: Based on body weight, sufficient to supply energy; spare protein for tissue building.
   c. Vitamins, minerals
      (1) Zinc—increases strength of healing wound (4 to 6 mg/day)
      (2) Vitamin C—required for collagen formation (500 to 1,000 mg/day)
2. Instruct client to consume at least 2,000 ml of noncaffeinated fluids per day.
3. Provide client with follow-up visit information.
4. Reinforce client need to take all prescribed medications; report any unusual or adverse effects to physician.
5. Encourage client to actively participate in prescribed rehabilitation program to promote optimal health.

E. Psychologic integrity
1. Provide adequate emotional support.
   a. Take time to actively listen.
   b. Offer explanations, genuine reassurance.
   c. Encourage presence, assistance of significant other(s).
2. Observe and evaluate behavior; monitor for fear, pain, and anxiety, which can effect recovery.
3. Discuss client's expectation of activity, assistance needed following discharge.
4. Include in discharge planning; provide information, support to make informed decisions.
5. Be alert to signs of alcohol withdrawal syndrome; report any unusual, disturbed behavior promptly (see assessment for signs and symptoms).

F. Basic care and comfort
1. Continue to assess client's body systems and monitor for signs of infection.
2. Encourage active ROM exercises every 2 hr.
3. Continue to encourage ambulation to promote peristalsis and passage of flatus; increase ambulation daily to increase muscle strength.
4. Encourage client to perform as many activities of daily living as possible.
5. Instruct client to maintain adequate diet and fluid intake (see health promotion and maintenance).

G. Reduction of risk potential
1. Provide continual monitoring for postoperative complications, and provide client and family teaching regarding care in the home setting (see safety and infection).
2. Monitor for drug toxicity, especially in older adult clients—indicated by decreased renal perfusion and reduced ability to eliminate drugs.
   a. Carefully assess renal and liver function.
   b. Emphasize to client prevention of drug overdosage and toxicity.
   c. Encourage client to ingest at least 2,000 ml of noncaffeinated fluids per day—unless contraindicated (heart failure, hypertension, or renal insufficiency).
3. Monitor for postoperative delirium associated with anesthetics—differentiate delirium from dementia by observing for alterations in level of consciousness; consider potentially reversible cause (e.g., infection, side effect of analgesic medication).
4. Manage pain; if untreated, pain can have negative effect on recovery. Provide client and family teaching regarding the following:
   a. Use analgesics as prescribed by physician.
   b. Avoid consumption of alcohol with analgesics as both depress central nervous system.
   c. Avoid operating machinery or driving until permitted, and know response to medication.

H. Pharmacologic and parenteral therapies: Client will state the purpose for and side effects of all medications used postoperatively, including antibiotics and anesthetics.

Ethical and Legal Implications for the Client Having Surgery

I. Definition: The client having surgery is protected by various laws and ethical responsibilities that also affect all HCPs. The nurse serves in the role of an advocate to speak on behalf of the client and protect the client's right to make decisions. Chapter 40 presents a broader scope of ethical and legal implications in regard to managing client care.

Ethical Implications for the Client Having Surgery

I. Definition: *Ethics* is the branch of philosophy concerned with the distinction between right and wrong based on a body of knowledge, and not solely on opinions. Ethics take into account a person's morals and value system. *Note: A nurse's religious or personal preference may allow refusal to assist in surgeries where a "dilatation, evacuation" is performed.* (See Chapter 40 for basic concepts of ethics.)

Legal Implications and Documents for the Client Having Surgery

I. Definition: Law and legislation protect both the client and nurse in terms of scope of acceptable practice and individual client rights.

II. Legal risk areas
- A. Assault—occurs when a person puts another person in fear of harmful or offensive contact. Involves victim fearing or believing that threat will result in harm.
- B. Battery—intentional touching of another's body without consent.
- C. Invasion of privacy—refers to violating confidentiality, intruding on private matters, or sharing client information with unauthorized persons.
- D. False imprisonment—occurs when restraining devices are used without appropriate clinical need.
- E. Malpractice—performance of care below the standard of care by a professional, resulting in injury to the client.
- F. Negligence—commitment of an act that a reasonable person would not have done, or omission of a duty a reasonable person would have performed.

III. Client rights
- A. Written document reflecting clients' rights to participate in health care, with emphasis on client autonomy.
- B. Some client rights include:
  1. Right to considerate, respectful care
  2. Right to know names, roles of persons involved in care
  3. Right to consent/refuse treatment
  4. Right to privacy
  5. Right to expect that hospital will provide necessary health services

IV. Organ donation and transplantation
- A. Client has right to decide to become organ donor or refuse organ transplant as treatment option (religious beliefs may play a role in decision).
- B. Criteria
  1. Uniform Anatomical Gift Act—lists who can provide informed consent for donation of deceased client's organs.
  2. United Network for Organ Sharing—sets criteria for organ donations.
- C. Religious beliefs
  1. Catholic Church—views organ transplantation as acceptable.
  2. Orthodox Church—discourages organ transplantation.
  3. Islam (Muslim)—discourages organ transplantation and removal of body parts.
  4. Jehovah's Witness—organ transplant may be accepted, but organ must be cleansed with nonblood solution before transplantation.
  5. Orthodox Judaism—all body parts removed during autopsy must be buried with body because it is believed that the entire body must be returned to earth. Organ transplantation may be allowed with rabbi's approval.
  6. Gypsies and Shintos—forbid followers to donate or receive organ(s).

V. Health Insurance Portability and Accountability Act (1996)
- A. Describes how personal health information may be used. Personal health information includes:
  1. Individually identifiable information that is related to client's past, present, or future health
  2. Treatment
  3. Payment for health care services
- B. Describes how client can obtain access to the information.

VI. Informed consent
- A. Consents and releases are legal documents that indicate client's permission (or that of client's legal representative) to perform surgery, perform a treatment, or give information to third party. Consent is obtained for all surgical/invasive procedures.
  1. In most states, when nurse is involved in informed consent process, the nurse is witnessing only the signature of client on informed consent form and is not responsible for explaining the procedure or assuring the client understands.
  2. Client is informed by the surgeon in understandable terms of:
     a. Risks and benefits of surgery or procedure
     b. Consequences for not receiving surgery or procedure
     c. Alternative options
     d. Name of physician performing surgery or procedure
  3. Client's questions about surgery or procedure must be answered before signing consent.

4. Consent must be signed freely by client without threat or pressure, and must be witnessed by another adult.
5. Legally, client must be mentally, emotionally competent to give consent. Client who has been medicated with sedating medications or any other medications that may affect cognitive abilities cannot be asked to sign consent.
6. Consent is required for use of restraints, photographing the client, the disposal of body parts during surgery, donating organs after death, or performing an autopsy.
7. Client may withdraw consent at any time before the procedure (withdrawal may be written or verbal).

B. Exceptions
1. Minors—client under legal age (as defined by state statute) may not give legal consent; consent obtained from parent or legal guardian.
2. Emancipated minor has established independence from parents through marriage, pregnancy, service in armed forces, or by court order; is considered legally capable of signing an informed consent.
3. Life-threatening emergencies

VII. End-of-life issues

A. Patient Self-Determination Act (1990)—states clients must be provided with information about their rights to identify written directions about care they wish to receive in event they become incapacitated and are unable to make health care decisions.

B. Advance directives are written documents recognized by state law; these provide directions concerning provision of care when client is unable to make own treatment choices, and may include health care proxy who will make health care decisions in the event of client's incapacitation. Types of advanced directives include:
1. Living will—specifies client's wishes for health care treatment, including the use of surgical procedures and use of resuscitation, should the client be unable to so direct.
2. Do-not-resuscitate (DNR) orders—written order by physician, following client's and family's wishes to limit extraordinary measures (such as CPR, drugs, intubation) when client has indicated desire to be allowed to die if stops breathing or heart stops beating.
   a. Client or legal representative must provide informed consent for do-not-resuscitate status.
   b. Do-not-resuscitate order must be defined clearly so that other treatment not refused by client will be continued.
   c. Physicians, nurses, and other health care personnel cannot witness the client's informed consent for DNR.
   d. Nurse who attempts to resuscitate when do-not-resuscitate order exists would be acting without client's consent, and committing battery.
3. Durable medical power of attorney is a document signed by the client designating a person to make health care decisions on the client's behalf should the client be unable to make such decisions.

C. Nurse's role in end-of-life documentation—the nurse follows agency policy addressing witnessing legal documents, and ensures completion and documentation of the following:
1. Client is provided with information about right to identify written directions about care client wishes to receive.
2. If advance directive exists, it is part of medical record.
3. Physician is notified of presence of advance directive.
4. Directions of advance directive are followed by all members of health care team.

Bibliography

Altman, G. (2004). *Delmar's fundamental and advanced nursing skills* (2nd ed.). Albany, NY: Delmar.

Ellis, J., & Hartley, C. (2005). *Managing and coordinating nursing care.* Philadelphia: Lippincott Williams & Wilkins.

Karch, A. (2006). *Lippincott's nursing drug guide.* Philadelphia: Lippincott Williams & Wilkins.

Smeltzer, S. C., Bare, B. G., Cheever, K. H., & Hinkle, J. L. (2008). *Brunner and Suddarth's textbook of medical-surgical nursing* (11th ed.). Philadelphia: Lippincott Williams & Wilkins.

Taylor, C., Lillis, C., LeMone, P., & Lynn, P. (2006). *Fundamentals of nursing.* Philadelphia: Lippincott Williams & Wilkins.

CHAPTER 33

Practice Test

Surgery: Preoperative, Intraoperative, and Postoperative Periods

1. AF Which of the following measures are nurse responsibilities when a client is undergoing surgery? Select all that apply.
□ 1. Develop an individualized plan of care.
□ 2. Serve as the client's advocate.
□ 3. Call "time out" if a potential error is observed.
□ 4. Communicate the outcome of the surgery to the family.
□ 5. Collaborate with the health care team.

2. A client is to have elective surgery. The nurse should plan with the client to schedule the surgery:
□ 1. If the client wishes to have the procedure done.
□ 2. At the client's convenience.
□ 3. Within the next 2 weeks.
□ 4. Within the next 2 days.

3. A client is to have NPO for at least 2 hr before same-day surgery. A nurse learns the client had half a glass of orange juice 3 hr prior to admission. The nurse should:
□ 1. Report the incident to the nursing supervisor.
□ 2. Inform the surgery department.
□ 3. Notify the anesthesiologist.
□ 4. Reschedule the surgery.

4. A client is anxious prior to surgery. The nurse should:
□ 1. Administer an antianxiety agent.
□ 2. Describe the entire intraoperative experience.
□ 3. Reassure the client about the capability of the surgeon.
□ 4. Encourage verbalization of feelings.

5. A client is receiving atropine sulfate (Atropair) prior to surgery. Which of the following is the intended outcome of this drug?
□ 1. Constricts pupils.
□ 2. Stimulates the central nervous system.
□ 3. Decreases cardiac output.
□ 4. Suppresses oral secretions.

6. The intended outcome of a client receiving cimetidine (Tagamet) prior to surgery is to:
□ 1. Decrease the volume of gastric secretions.
□ 2. Decrease the pH of gastric secretions.
□ 3. Reduce the amount of anesthetic needed.
□ 4. Dispel the memory of unpleasant factors associated with surgery.

7. A client arrives in the operating room wearing two post earrings on each eyebrow. The nurse should do which of the following?
□ 1. Ask client to remove the earrings and place them in a labeled container.
□ 2. Call a nurse on the medical-surgical clinical unit and request that he or she come to remove the earrings and give them to the client's family.
□ 3. Remind anesthetist to remove the earrings when the client is anesthetized.
□ 4. Secure the earrings with paper tape.

8. The nurse notices that a cart brought by an operating room transporter to transport a client has a nonfunctioning clasp on the safety belt. The nurse should do which of the following?
□ 1. Call the Safety/Security Department to report the problem.
□ 2. Use a draw sheet to secure the client during transport.
□ 3. Contact the Clinical Engineering Department to repair the clasp.
□ 4. Request that the transporter bring a different cart with a functional clasp.

9. A scrub nurse puts on the hair covering after putting on sterile gloves. The charge nurse should base a response to this nurse on which of the following?
□ 1. If a sterile item comes in contact with an unsterile item, it is contaminated.
□ 2. Contaminated items should be removed immediately from the sterile field.
□ 3. A wide margin of safety must be maintained between the sterile and unsterile field.
□ 4. Bacteria harbor on the client's and the team members' hair, skin, and respiratory tracts and must be confined by appropriate attire.

10. A scrub nurse in the operating room should do which of the following?
□ 1. Scrub for a minimum of 3 min.
□ 2. Scrub without mechanical friction.

□ 3. Scrub from the hands to the elbows.
□ 4. Hold the hands higher than the elbows.

11. In the operating room the surgeon is checking the x-ray of a client who is to have lobe of the left lung removed. The nurse notes that the name on the x-ray is not the same name as that of the client. The nurse should:
□ 1. Call the x-ray technician to take another x-ray.
□ 2. Call the surgeon aside to ask to have the x-ray checked.
□ 3. Look for the correct x-ray.
□ 4. Call a time out.

12. A client is receiving a large volume of PRBCs during surgery. The nurse should observe the client for hypocalcemia because?
□ 1. Extra calcium is needed during stressful events.
□ 2. Anesthesia causes hypocalcemia.
□ 3. Hypoperfusion to the parathyroid glands affects calcium levels.
□ 4. The preservative in PRBCs binds with calcium.

13. A client who had a partial gastrectomy 24 hr ago has a nasogastric tube in place. The expected outcome of using a nasogastric tube following a partial gastrectomy is to:
□ 1. Assess the pH of gastric secretions.
□ 2. Remove stomach contents.
□ 3. Delay peristalsis until initial healing takes place.
□ 4. Assess characteristics of drainage at anastomosis.

14. AF Three days after a cholecystectomy, a client states, "I feel like my stomach is going to burst." The client is taking a regular diet. After determining that vital signs are stable, in which order does the nurse do the following to assist the client?
_____ 1. Position client on right side.
_____ 2. Offer 120 ml of hot liquids.
_____ 3. Auscultate for bowel sounds.
_____ 4. Encourage ambulation.

15. The nurse assesses that a client is restless in the immediate postoperative period. The nurse should first:
□ 1. Administer a sedative.
□ 2. Offer ice chips.
□ 3. Administer oxygen.
□ 4. Apply wrist restraints.

16. A nurse auscultates a client's breath sounds on the fourth postoperative day and hears loud, low-pitched, rumbling sounds on expiration. The nurse should first:
□ 1. Administer oxygen.
□ 2. Encourage the client to cough.
□ 3. Request an order for incentive spirometry.
□ 4. Reposition the client to high-Fowler position.

17. During the extended postoperative period following an abdominal hysterectomy, a client has a urine output of 20 ml/hour. The nurse should:
□ 1. Consider this to be normal.
□ 2. Evaluate the client's fluid intake.
□ 3. Prepare to return the client to the operating room.
□ 4. Consult the urologist.

18. On the first day after abdominal surgery, the nurse auscultates a client's abdomen for bowel sounds; there are none. The nurse should first:
□ 1. Encourage a client to use the client-controlled analgesia pump more often.
□ 2. Ask another nurse to validate the absence of bowel sounds.
□ 3. Encourage the client to take more ice chips.
□ 4. Document assessment findings in the client's medical record.

Ethical and Legal Implications for the Client Having Surgery

19. Prior to nonemergency surgery, the client needs to give consent for the procedure. Which of the following measures is the responsibility of the nurse?
□ 1. Obtain informed consent.
□ 2. Explain the surgical procedure.
□ 3. Verify the client understands the consent form.
□ 4. Inform the client about surgical risks.

20. AF The nurse is verifying that the client has given consent for surgery. For consent to be valid prior to nonemergency surgery, there must be adequate disclosure of which of the following? Select all that apply.
□ 1. Nursing care plan in the postanesthesia care unit.
□ 2. Purpose of proposed treatment.
□ 3. Risk and benefits of the surgical procedure.
□ 4. Outcome of the surgery.
□ 5. Side effects of anesthetics.

Answers and Rationales

1. 1, 2, 3, 5 The perioperative nurse is an RN who implements client care based on the nursing process. The RN functions as the client's advocate throughout the intraoperative experience, and collaborates with the health care team to implement the plan of care. The nurse also assures safe passage during surgery by noting potential for error and asking for the health team to review actions before proceeding. It is the responsibility of the surgeon to communicate with the client's family about the outcome of the surgery. (M)

2. 2 Elective surgery is scheduled at the client's convenience. Optional surgery is scheduled if the client decides to have the surgery. Required surgery is scheduled within a few weeks, while urgent surgery is scheduled within 24 to 48 hr. (S)

3. 3 Restriction of fluids and food is designed to minimize the potential risk of aspiration and to decrease the risk of postoperative nausea and vomiting. A client who has not followed this instruction may have surgery delayed or cancelled, so it is vital that the surgical client understands and adheres to these restrictions. The nurse notifies the anesthesiologist/anesthetist; surgery may be rescheduled, but a HCP makes that determination. It is not necessary to report this incident to the supervisor. (R)

4. 4 Surgery is a frightening event, even when the procedure is considered relatively minor. A nurse who is aware of a client's perceived or actual stressors can provide support and sufficient information during the preoperative period so that anxiety will not become overwhelming. Nonpharmacologic interventions are used before using antianxiety agents that will depress the central nervous system. Describing the entire intraoperative experience may increase a client's anxiety. Reassuring the client does not help the client work through the anxiety. (P)

5. 4 Atropine sulfate (Atropair) is within the class of anticholinergics and is administered preoperatively to decrease oral and respiratory secretions. By blocking vagal impulses to the heart, the pulse rate and cardiac output increase. Atropair produces mydriasis (dilation of pupils) and selective depression of the central nervous system. (D)

6. 1 Cimetidine (Tagamet) decreases gastric acid secretion and raises the pH of stomach secretions by blocking H_2 receptors on parietal cells of the stomach. The drug has no effect on amount of anesthetic agents required or recollection of surgical experience. (D)

7. 1 All jewelry is removed prior to arrival in the OR as jewelry may be lost, can carry pathogens, and could conduct electrical current. If a client prefers not to remove a wedding ring, the ring must be taped securely to the finger to prevent loss. Asking a nurse from the clinical unit to come into the OR is an unnecessary influx of hospital personnel that may invade a client's privacy and/or introduce pathogenic micro-organisms from the outside environment. Removing jewelry is not part of the anesthetist's role. Securing the earrings with tape is not appropriate; the tape is not sterile and may also interfere with monitoring a client by the anesthesiologist or nurse anesthetist. (S)

8. 4 The nurse ensures client safety during transport and therefore requests another cart for transport. The other options do not ensure client safety. Method of transportation and person transporting the client are documented by the nurse responsible for the transfer. The clasp needs to be repaired. Contacting the security department is not appropriate. (S)

9. 1 A hair covering is not sterile. The sterile gloves came in contact with an unsterile item; therefore, the gloves are contaminated and no longer sterile. Bacteria reside on hair. The other principles are not reflecting violation with the action identified. (S)

10. 4 Holding the scrubbed hands higher than elbows allows micro-organisms/water to not contaminate scrubbed hands. A scrub nurse must follow the designated scrub procedure; some facilities may require longer than 3 min to scrub for surgery. Mechanical friction aids in removal of micro-organisms that reside on skin. (S)

11. 4 When the nurse or any other member of the surgery team notices a discrepancy or a potential error, a time out is called so all members of the surgical team can stop what they are doing and work as a team to solve the problem. The other actions do not promote client safety in the operating room, and are not sufficient to address the concern. (S)

12. 4 Clients who undergo multiple transfusions are at risk for developing electrolyte problems; these may include hyperkalemia, increased ammonia levels (because of cellular release from stored blood products), and hypocalcemia (because of chelation of calcium with citrate, a blood preservative). Extra calcium is not necessarily needed during stressful events. Anesthesia does not cause hypocalcemia; it depresses the central nervous system. Parathyroid hormone from the parathyroid glands raises the plasma calcium level by promoting the transfer of calcium from the bone to plasma. Hypoperfusion to the parathyroid glands does not affect calcium levels. (S)

13. 2 A nasogastric tube is used to decompress the remaining portion of the stomach to decrease pressure on the suture line, and to allow for resolution of edema and inflammation resulting from surgical trauma. It is not necessary to determine the pH of gastric secretions or to know characteristics of drainage at the anastomosis. A nasogastric tube has no effect on peristalsis being delayed. (A)

14. 3, 2, 1, 4 The nurse first auscultates the abdomen for bowel sounds to determine if peristalsis has resumed and is present. The nurse then administers hot liquids to stimulate peristalsis and promote expulsion of the gas that is causing the client to be uncomfortable. Positioning the client on the right side permits gas to rise along the transverse colon and facilitates its release. Abdominal distention may be minimized by early and frequent ambulation, which stimulates intestinal motility. The nurse also assists the client to ambulate. (C)

15. 3 Restlessness in the immediate postoperative period may be a sign of cerebral hypoxia as a result of depression of the central nervous system from anesthetic agents and sedatives. Administering sedatives would depress the central nervous system further. A client may aspirate ice chips when he or she is restless. Wrist restraints may increase agitation and cannot be used without justification. (S)

16. 2 Encouraging a client to turn, cough, and deep breathe postoperatively facilitates gas exchange and aids in removal of secretions to prevent formation of mucous plugs. Rhonchi are adventitious or abnormal breath sounds that are present when an airway is partially obstructed owing to secretions or mucosal edema. Administering oxygen and requesting an order for incentive spirometry may be helpful, but not the first intervention to be done. Elevation of the head of the bed promotes ease of breathing, but a high-Fowler position does not allow for complete descent of the diaphragm. (A)

17. 2 Low urine output (800 to 1,500 ml) in the first 24 hr after surgery may be expected, but this is too low (480 ml). Evaluation of a client's fluid status considers both total intake and output. By the second or third postoperative day, a client will have increasing urinary output after fluid has been mobilized and immediate stress reaction subsides. Acute urinary retention can occur in the postoperative period, especially after lower abdominal or pelvic surgery. To consult a urologist or prepare to return a client to the operating room is not an appropriate intervention at this time. (A)

18. 4 Bowel sounds are not present until the third or fourth postoperative day; the nurse documents assessment findings. Using narcotic analgesics in the client-controlled analgesia pump further decreases peristalsis. Too many ice chips may promote abdominal distention, especially if the client is not ambulating in the intermediate postoperative period. (A)

19. 3 The surgeon is responsible for explaining the surgery procedure, explaining the risks of the procedure, and obtaining the informed consent. A nurse may be responsible for obtaining and witnessing a client's signature on the consent form. The nurse is the client's advocate, verifying that a client (or family member) understands the consent form and its implications, and that consent for surgery is truly voluntary. (R)

20. 2, 3 Three conditions must be met for consent to be valid. First, there must be adequate disclosure of the diagnosis; the nature and purpose of the proposed treatment; the risks and consequences of the proposed treatment; the probability of a successful outcome; the availability, benefits, and risks of alternative treatments; and the prognosis if treatment is not instituted. Second, a client must demonstrate clear understanding and comprehension of the information being provided. Third, the recipient of care must give consent voluntarily. It is not necessary to inform the client of the specific nursing care plan after surgery. The exact outcome of the surgery cannot be predicted, nor can the client's reaction to the administration of drugs or anesthesia. (R)

chapter

34

The Client With Health Problems of the Integumentary and Sensory Systems

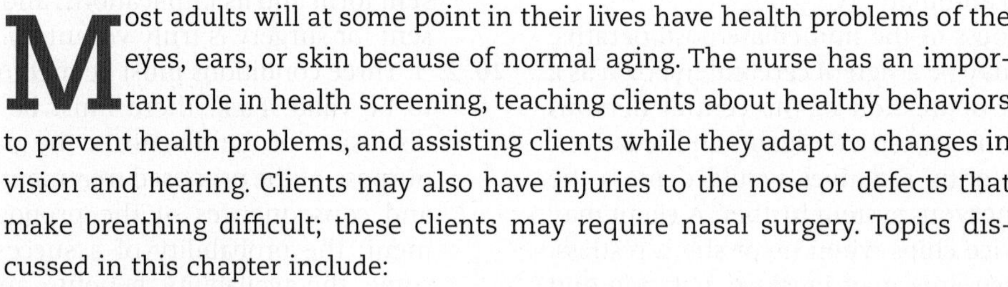

Most adults will at some point in their lives have health problems of the eyes, ears, or skin because of normal aging. The nurse has an important role in health screening, teaching clients about healthy behaviors to prevent health problems, and assisting clients while they adapt to changes in vision and hearing. Clients may also have injuries to the nose or defects that make breathing difficult; these clients may require nasal surgery. Topics discussed in this chapter include:

- Disorders of the Eye
- Disorders of the Ear
- Nasal Surgery
- Burns
- Pressure Ulcers

Disorders of the Eye

I. Definition: Health problems of the eye include cataracts, retinal detachment, glaucoma, and macular degeneration.
   A. A cataract is a clouding or opacity of the lens usually caused by degenerative changes. These changes cause an accumulation of water as well as alterations in the lens fiber structure; if untreated, a cataract leads to blindness.
   B. Retinal detachment is a separation of the sensory retina from the pigment epithelium in the eye; this may follow an injury to the eye, but is more often the result of degenerative changes in the vitreous chamber. If left untreated, detachment of the retina results in blindness.
   C. Glaucoma is a condition characterized by increased intraoptic pressure, optic nerve atrophy, and peripheral visual field loss. It is caused by an imbalance between the production and drainage of aqueous humor, and is a leading cause of blindness.
      1. Primary open-angle glaucoma (most common type) is caused by a decrease in the outflow of aqueous humor from obstructed drainage channels.
      2. Primary angle-closure glaucoma (acute glaucoma) is caused by a decrease in the outflow of aqueous humor when the angle is closed; this is usually the result of a bulging lens caused by aging.
      3. Secondary glaucoma is caused by blockage of the outflow channels by inflammatory processes or other ocular disorders.
   D. Macular degeneration is characterized by progressive deterioration of the maculae of the retina. The condition is often related to aging (age-related macular degeneration) and eventually results in blindness.
      1. Dry (atrophic) macular degeneration progresses slowly; this occurs when the macular cells have atrophied. Yellow-white spots (drusen) can be seen on ophthalmoscopic examination.
      2. Wet (exudative) macular degeneration occurs rapidly; degeneration is characterized by the development of abnormal blood vessels in the macula, which leak and scar.

II. Nursing process
   A. Assessment
      1. Obtain a detailed health history focusing on history of diabetes, hypertension, eye injuries, or infections; verify presence of family history of cataracts or glaucoma.
      2. Assess for signs and symptoms of changes in visual acuity.
         a. Cataract—abnormal color perception and glare (especially at night)
         b. Retinal detachment—light flashes, floaters, cobweb in field of vision, painless loss of vision "like a curtain coming down"
         c. Glaucoma—sudden, severe pain in eye with acute angle-closure glaucoma; tunnel vision, colored halos around lights, and blurred vision
         d. Macular degeneration—blurred vision, blind spots, distorted vision
      3. Measure visual acuity (legal blindness is 20/200).
         a. Distance with Snellen chart
         b. Near vision with Jaeger chart
      4. Assess pupillary response to light and accommodation.
      5. Test extraocular muscle function via corneal light reflex.
      6. Assess client's knowledge of pathophysiology and proposed treatment.
      7. Obtain diagnostic tests.
         a. Cataracts—tonometry to measure intraocular pressure; ophthalmoscopy to rule out retinal detachment; perimetry to determine visual field
         b. Retinal detachment—ophthalmoscopy to view retina; gonioscopy for magnification of lesion
         c. Glaucoma—tonometry to measure intraocular pressure; gonioscopy to view angle of the anterior chamber of the eye
         d. Macular degeneration—ophthalmoscopy for visualization; fluorescent angiogram
   B. Analysis
      1. Risk for Injury related to visual impairment
      2. Self-Care Deficit: Dressing or Grooming, related to visual impairment
      3. Disturbed Sensory Perception: Visual, related to diminished or absent vision
      4. Anxiety related to uncertainty of cause of disease and outcome of treatment
      5. Acute Pain related to physiologic process and surgical correction
      6. Deficient Knowledge related to disease process and treatment regimen
   C. Planning
      1. Prevent injury.
      2. Improve or maintain vision.
      3. Reduce anxiety.
      4. Relieve pain.
      5. Provide client and family teaching.
      6. Promote compliance with therapeutic regimen.

D. Implementation
  1. Perform visual assessments and document findings.
  2. Provide care to the client pre- and postoperatively in outpatient setting (see management of care).
  3. Teach client self-care strategies.
  4. Facilitate follow-up care.

E. Evaluation
  1. Client adequately explains health behaviors that protect vision.
  2. Client remains free of injury.
  3. Client demonstrates ability to perform activities of daily living.
  4. Client identifies adaptive coping strategies.
  5. Client shows improvement in visual acuity.
  6. Client reports minimal to no pain.
  7. Client expresses optimism regarding improved vision.
  8. Client verbalizes an understanding of the disease process and treatment plan.
  9. Client administers eyedrops as instructed.
  10. Client returns for scheduled follow-up appointments.

III. Client needs

A. Physiologic adaptation
  1. Treatment and procedures for disorders of the eye may include:
    a. Cataracts—intracapsular extraction, extracapsular extraction, intraocular lens implant surgery
    b. Detached retina—laser photocoagulation or scleral buckling procedure; photocoagulation—laser; and diathermy—high-frequency current
    c. Glaucoma
      (1) Open-angle glaucoma—trabeculoplasty, trabeculectomy, cyclocryotherapy
      (2) Angle-closure glaucoma—laser peripheral iridotomy; surgical iridectomy
    d. Macular degeneration—is a degenerative process; argon laser therapy may be used for age-related macular degeneration.
  2. General nursing care for the client undergoing treatment for an eye disorder is as follows:
    a. Maintain intraocular pressure low enough to prevent optic nerve damage.
    b. Preserve remaining vision with regular eye exams and early intervention.
    c. Prevent infection by using aseptic technique when administering eye medications and applying dressings.
    d. Optimize improvements in visual acuity postoperatively by stressing adherence to activity and positioning directives.

B. Management of care: Care of the client with an eye disorder requires critical thinking skills and knowledge of assessment, and teaching and evaluation methods unique to the RN role. These skills cannot be delegated to an LPN or UAP.
  1. Delegate responsibly those activities that can be delegated, including basic care needs and vital sign checks for the stable client. Instruct UAP in communication strategies appropriate to sight-impaired client. All monitoring information is reported to the RN.
  2. Provide interventions to treat the client with a cataract.
    a. Prepare client for cataract removal and intraocular lens implant surgery.
      (1) Instruct client to avoid food and fluids 6 to 8 hr preoperatively.
      (2) Administer prescribed mydriatic and cycloplegic eyedrops.
      (3) Administer topical corticosteroids.
      (4) Administer topical antibiotics.
      (5) Administer antianxiety agents.
    b. Teach postoperative lens implant care.
      (1) Use topical antibiotics and topical corticosteroid as prescribed.
      (2) Use mild analgesic as prescribed.
      (3) Use eye shield, especially at night.
      (4) Avoid activities that increase intraocular pressure, such as bending.
      (5) Report symptoms of complications to the physician, including intense pain in operative eye, purulent drainage, increased redness or decreased vision.
    c. Provide additional client and family teaching.
      (1) Provide information about vision aids such as strong reading glasses, use of bright light for near-vision activities.
      (2) Suggest client avoid driving at night.
      (3) Advise client that eyeglass prescription may need to be changed.
  3. Provide postsurgical interventions for retinal detachment.
    a. Administer topical antibiotic.
    b. Administer topical corticosteroid.
    c. Administer analgesics.
    d. Administer mydriatics.
    e. Position client to maintain intravitreal bubble.

f. Instruct client to avoid activities that increase intraocular pressure, such as bending.
4. Provide interventions for glaucoma.
   a. Open-angle glaucoma:
      (1) Administer medications used to manage glaucoma, including beta-adrenergic blockers, alpha-adrenergic agonists, cholinergic agents (miotics), and carbonic anhydrase inhibitors.
      (2) Provide preoperative instructions if surgery indicated (type of surgery, postoperative care will include elevating head of bed 30 degrees).
   b. Angle-closure glaucoma:
      (1) Darken the environment.
      (2) Apply cool compresses to forehead.
      (3) Provide quiet, private environment.
      (4) Administer medications including topical cholinergic agent and hyperosmotic agent.
   c. Provide preoperative instructions if surgery indicated (type of surgery, postoperative restrictions, if any).
5. Provide interventions for macular degeneration.
   a. Dry (atrophic)—identify low-vision assistive devices available to client; recommend that client drive in daylight only and at reduced speeds.
   b. (Wet) exudative—instruct client to avoid direct exposure to sunlight and other intense light sources for 5 days after photodynamic therapy.

C. Safety and infection control
1. Use sighted guide technique to assist client with ambulation.
2. Verbally describe environment when ambulating with client.
3. Initiate fall-prevention strategies, especially with older clients.
4. Apply contrasting color edging on stairs.
5. Identify methods to increase lighting, such as halogen lamps.
6. Orient client to immediate surroundings by identifying one object as focal point and orient other objects in relation to it.
7. Modify home environment by removing obstacles such as area rugs.

D. Health promotion and maintenance
1. Encourage client to follow guidelines for routine eye exams.
2. Teach client to use protective eyewear when indicated.
3. Suggest that the client wear sunglasses that block UV rays.
4. Remind client to consume the recommended amounts of antioxidant vitamins such as C and E.

E. Psychologic integrity
1. Evaluate community resources for partially sighted and blind clients.
2. Make eye contact with partially sighted clients.
3. Explain activities and noises in client's environment.
4. Allow client to express anger and grief.
5. Assist client in identifying fears and coping strategies.
6. Include family members in discussions, if acceptable to client.
7. Communicate with normal conversational tone and manner.
8. Address client directly rather than through a family member or caregiver.
9. Introduce self on entering room of partially sighted or blind client.
10. Verbalize "good-bye" on departure of room of partially sighted or blind client.
11. Refer client to transportation services to reduce potential for social isolation.

F. Basic care and comfort
1. Administer mild analgesics as indicated postoperatively.
2. Assist client with activities of daily living as needed.
3. Place items client will use regularly within easy reach.
4. Use positions of clock to describe items on tray or in room.
5. Offer use of optical devices such as magnifiers for vision enhancement.
6. Recommend approach magnification techniques, such as sitting closer to television.
7. Suggest contrast enhancement techniques.
8. Inform clients of large-print options.

G. Reduction of risk potential
1. Instruct older clients to apply pressure to the inner canthus when administering beta blocking eyedrops to prevent systemic absorption.
2. Be aware of contraindications for each category of eye medications.
3. Instruct client about risk for falls.

H. Pharmacologic and parenteral therapies: Client will state the purpose for and side effects of all medications used to treat disorders of the eye. See Table 34-1 for ophthalmic medications. Use the following eye medication administration techniques.
1. Prevent contact between the eye dropper or ointment tube and the eye.

Table 34-1 Ophthalmic Medications

Medication	Intended Outcome	Side Effects
Mydriatics Phenylephrine HCL (Neo-Synephrine, Mydfrin)	Dilates pupils.	Tachycardia and hypertension may result, especially in elderly. Limit systemic absorption with punctual occlusion.
Cycloplegic Agents Tropicamide (Mydriacyl, Tropicacyl); cyclopentolate HCL (Cyclogyl, Pentolair); homatropine hydrobromide (Isopto Homatropine); scopolamine (Isopto Hyoscine); atropine (Atropisol, Isopto Atropine)	Dilates pupils.	Used in refraction studies. Cyclopentolate has been associated with psychotic reactions in children.
Beta-Adrenergic Blockers Betaxolol (Betoptic); carteolol (Ocupress); levobunolol (Betagan); metipranolol (OptiPranolol); timolol maleate (Timoptic)	Decreases aqueous humor production.	Contraindicated in clients with asthma, COPD, and heart failure.
Alpha-Adrenergic Agonists Dipivefrin (Propine); epinephrine (Epifrin); apraclonidine (Iopidine); brimonidine (Alphagan); latanoprost (Xalatan)	Decreases aqueous humor production.	May cause redness and eye pain, tachycardia, and hypertension. Use punctual occlusion to limit systemic absorption.
Cholinergic Agents (miotics) Carbachol (Isopto Carbachol); pilocarpine (Isopto Carpine, Pilocar)	Facilitates aqueous humor outflow.	Decreases visual acuity, especially in bright light. Advise client to bring driver and sunglasses.
Carbonic Anhydrase Inhibitors Acetazolamide (Diamox); dichlorphenamide (Daranide); methazolamide (Neptazane); brinzolamide (Azopt); dorzolamide (Trusopt)	Decreases aqueous humor production.	May cause paresthesias, hearing impairment, tinnitus, and confusion. Cross-allergic response with sulfonamides possible. Do not give if client on high-dose aspirin therapy.
Hyperosmotic Agents Glycerin liquid (Ophthalgan, Osmoglyn Oral); isosorbide solution (Ismotic); mannitol solution (Osmitrol)	Reduces intraocular pressure by increasing extracellular osmolarity, thus moving fluid to extracellular and vascular spaces.	Do not give to clients with pulmonary edema or heart failure.

2. Avoid cross-contamination—never share medications between clients.
3. Wear gloves and use clean technique to administer medications.
4. Ask client to look up; approach the eye from the side to reduce blinking.
5. Place medication in conjunctival sac rather than directly on the cornea.
6. Apply pressure to the inner canthus to prevent systemic absorption.
7. Ask client to blink to distribute ointments.

Disorders of the Ear

I. Definition: Health problems of the ear increase with normal aging and include hearing loss and Ménière disease.

A. Hearing loss involves impairment of the transmission of sound waves, particularly conductive hearing loss and sensorineural hearing loss. Other types of hearing loss that are less common include presbycusis, (progressive hearing loss related to aging and involving high frequencies), impacted (caused by cerumen), ototoxic (cranial nerve damage caused by side effects of drugs), and otosclerosis (fixation of the stapes prevents sound transmission).

1. Conductive hearing loss—the conduction of sound from the outer to the inner ear is impeded by conditions such as impacted cerumen, middle ear disease, or otosclerosis.
2. Sensorineural hearing loss—the inner ear or auditory nerve is impaired by conditions

such as aging (presbycusis), noise trauma, or by systemic diseases.

B. Ménière disease is an inner ear disturbance that produces profound vertigo often accompanied by nausea and vomiting. Etiology is unknown but the condition results in accumulation of endolymph in the membranous labyrinth, causing it to rupture. Attacks of vertigo occur suddenly and vary from hours to days in length.

II. Nursing process

A. Assessment

1. Obtain history of middle ear infection, perforated tympanic membrane, and use of ototoxic medications or aspirin.
2. Question client regarding hearing loss, tinnitus, vertigo, ear pain, feeling of fullness or pressure, and use of hearing devices.
3. Observe client's behavior for signs of hearing loss such as tilting head toward speaker, asking for repetitions of comments or questions, and ignoring speaker if unable to see his or her face during communication.
4. Palpate external ear and mastoid area for tenderness and lesions.
5. Observe for nystagmus in lateral gaze.
6. Use otoscope to inspect tympanic membrane for clearness and light reflection.
7. Use tuning fork to determine type of hearing loss (Rinne and Weber tests).
   a. Weber test—in conductive loss there is sifting of sounds to ear with hearing loss; in sensorineural loss there is shifting of sounds to the better ear.
   b. Rinne test—in conductive loss the sound is perceived as longer by bone; in sensorineural loss the sound is perceived as longer by air conduction.
8. Obtain diagnostic tests such as audiometry to assess client's hearing ability.

B. Analysis

1. Risk for Injury related to hearing impairment
2. Risk for Falls related to vertigo
3. Disturbed Sensory Perception: Hearing, related to diminished or absent hearing
4. Anxiety related to uncertainty of cause of disease and outcome of treatment
5. Deficient Knowledge related to disease process and treatment regimen
6. Social Isolation related to inability to hear communication

C. Planning

1. Prevent injury.
2. Decrease vertigo.
3. Improve hearing.
4. Reduce anxiety.
5. Provide client and family teaching.

D. Implementation

1. Provide interventions for hearing loss.
   a. Encourage use of hearing protection devices.
   b. Instruct client how to use hearing aid.
   c. Recommend client learn speech reading.
   d. Use nonverbal communication such as hand gestures.
   e. Face client directly when speaking.
   f. Decrease noise and distraction in environment.
   g. Speak clearly in normal tone of voice into better ear.
   h. Use simple sentences.
   i. Avoid overenunciating or exaggerating facial expressions.
   j. Use written materials.
2. Provide interventions for Ménière disease.
   a. Promote bed rest in quiet, darkened room during acute attack.
   b. Administer antiemetics and sedatives as needed.
   c. Reassure client that condition is not life-threatening.
   d. Assist with ambulation when attack subsides.

E. Evaluation

1. Hearing loss
   a. Client verbalizes understanding of techniques to prevent injury.
   b. Client identifies techniques to enhance communication.
   c. Client demonstrates effective speech reading.
   d. Client expresses understanding of disease process and treatment plan.
   e. Client inserts and maintains hearing aid properly.
2. Ménière disease
   a. Client verbalizes understanding of nature of the disease.
   b. Client adheres to fall-prevention strategies.
   c. Client verbalizes decreased anxiety.
   d. Client identifies measures to reduce incidence and severity of vertigo.

CN

III. Client needs

A. Physiologic adaptation

1. Hearing loss—treatment involves preserving hearing with frequent audiometric exams to monitor loss and audiologic rehabilitation. Treatment may also involve use of hearing aid; stapedectomy or use of cochlear implants.
   a. Prevent further hearing loss with ear protection and avoidance of noisy environments.

  b. Improve hearing by removing impacted cerumen.
  c. Prevent hearing loss by using ototoxic medications sparingly.
2. Ménière disease—treatment involves management of symptoms.
  a. Manage symptoms of nausea and vomiting with antiemetics.
  b. Manage symptoms of vertigo with antihistamines.
  c. Manage accumulation of endolymph:
    (1) Low-salt diet
    (2) Diuretics
    (3) Endolymphatic shunt surgery

B. Management of care: Care of the client with an ear disorder requires critical thinking skills and knowledge of assessment, and teaching and evaluation methods unique to the RN role. These skills cannot be delegated to an LPN or UAP.
  1. Provide interventions for hearing loss.
    a. Evaluate community resources for hearing-impaired clients.
    b. Perform hearing assessments and document findings.
    c. Delegate responsibly those activities that can be delegated, including basic care needs and vital sign checks for the stable client.
    d. Instruct UAP in communication strategies appropriate to hearing-impaired client (see psychologic integrity).
    e. Evaluate client need for hearing aids, implantable devices, or speech reading.
    f. Refer client to rehabilitation services when indicated.
  2. Provide interventions for Ménière disease.
    a. Provide supportive therapy to minimize vertigo.
    b. Provide a safe environment.
    c. Encourage follow-up with physician.
    d. Instruct UAP to respond to call light immediately.

C. Safety and infection control
  1. Hearing loss
    a. Use aseptic technique when administering ear drops.
    b. Instruct client to refrain from inserting Q-tips to clean ears.
    c. Remind client to use ear protection in noisy environments.
  2. Ménière disease
    a. Keep side rails up and bed in low position during acute attack.
    b. Instruct client to call for assistance before ambulation.
    c. Remind client not to drive or operate heavy machinery after taking antinausea or antivertigo medication.

D. Health promotion and maintenance
  1. Hearing loss
    a. Control environmental noise.
    b. Encourage use of ear-protection devices in noisy environments.
    c. Promote hearing conservation programs in the workplace.
    d. Encourage MMR immunizations of vulnerable persons.
    e. Monitor clients who are receiving ototoxic medications for hearing loss.
    f. Advise clients to discuss aspirin use with their physician.
  2. Ménière disease
    a. Recommend use of medications such as meclizine (Antivert) or diazepam (Valium) to reduce vertigo.
    b. Advise client to avoid sudden head movements or position changes.
    c. Suggest avoidance of fluorescent or flickering lights and watching television.
    d. Remind client to avoid caffeine, nicotine, and alcohol.
    e. Advise client to participate in smoking-cessation program.
    f. Recommend low-salt diet and regular exercise.

E. Psychologic integrity
  1. Reassure client that symptoms of vertigo are not life-threatening.
  2. Use communication strategies appropriate to hearing-impaired client.
    a. Face client in good lighting when communicating with hearing-impaired individual.
    b. Use gestures and written materials to enhance communication.
    c. Speak with normal voice into client's better ear.
    d. Address client directly rather than through a family member or caregiver.
    e. Use touch appropriately to convey caring.
    f. Speak clearly without overenunciating.
  3. Re-establish social network for client with hearing impairment.
  4. Enable client with hearing impairment to communicate effectively with listening devices and other aids.

F. Basic care and comfort
  1. Hearing loss
    a. Control environmental noise.
    b. Practice effective communication strategies (see psychologic integrity).

2. Ménière disease
   a. Assign client to room in low-traffic area.
   b. Ensure that call bell is within reach and instruct client in its use.
   c. Close drapes and dim lights.
   d. Assist client to comfortable position.

G. Reduction of risk potential
1. Require use of ear-protection devices in noisy environments.
2. Establish hearing conservation programs in the workplace.
3. Restrict exposure to fluorescent or flickering lights and television for clients with Ménière disease.

H. Pharmacologic and parenteral therapies: Client will state the purpose for and side effects for all medications used to manage disorders of the ear. Medications for Ménière disease are intended to control symptoms of nausea and vomiting and vertigo; these include:
1. Antivertigo medications—meclizine (Antivert) and diazepam (Valium)
2. Diuretics (hydrochlorothiazide)
3. Antiemetics—promethazine (Phenergan) and prochlorperazine (Compazine)

Nasal Surgery

I. Definition: Nasal surgery is required to repair nasal fractures, correct a deviated septum, or correct nasal deformities. The most common types of nasal surgery are rhinoplasty (reconstruction is used to improve function from breathing obstruction or birth defects; and cosmetic improves appearance); septoplasty, which is used to straighten a deviated nasal septum; and nasal fracture reductions.

II. Nursing process

A. Assessment
1. Assess ability of client to breathe through each nostril.
2. Inspect for edema and hematoma formation.
3. Observe for bleeding from nostril.
4. Inspect for nasal deformities and septal deviation.
5. Observe for ecchymoses under eyes (raccoon eyes).
6. Watch for clear drainage from nostrils (could indicate skull fracture or punctured sinus).
7. Monitor respiratory status with pulse oximetry.

B. Analysis
1. Ineffective Breathing Pattern related to obstructed nostrils
2. Acute Pain related to facial injury or surgical intervention
3. Disturbed Body Image related to nasal deformity
4. Risk for Aspiration related to bleeding from nose
5. Risk for Infection related to cerebral spinal fluid (CSF) leak

C. Planning
1. Maintain clear airway.
2. Maintain oxygenation.
3. Manage pain.
4. Provide emotional support.

D. Implementation
1. Preoperative care
   a. Instruct client to avoid aspirin and nonsteroidal anti-inflammatory drugs (NSAIDs) for 2 weeks prior to surgery.
   b. Instruct client to consult with prescribing physician regarding risk versus benefit of stopping antiplatelet therapy.
2. Postoperative care
   a. Apply ice packs to reduce swelling.
   b. Elevate head of bed to reduce edema.
   c. Monitor client for bleeding.
   d. Use humidified air as needed.
   e. Offer mild narcotic to control pain.
   f. Reinforce dressing as ordered and assist in the removal of nasal packing 1 to 2 days postsurgery.
   g. Reassure client that nasal splints will be removed in 2 days.

E. Evaluation
1. Client does not experience aspiration.
2. Client maintains oxygen saturation above 92%.
3. Client states that pain is managed satisfactorily.
4. Client describes expected postoperative outcomes.
5. Client identifies signs and symptoms requiring physician's attention.

CN

III. Client needs

A. Physiologic adaptation: The client who has had nasal surgery recovers within several weeks. Immediately following surgery, the nurse monitors the client for complications such as bleeding, infection, or aspiration.

B. Management of care: Care of the client undergoing nasal surgery requires critical thinking skills and knowledge of assessment, and teaching and evaluation methods unique to the RN role. These skills cannot be delegated to an LPN or UAP.
1. Instruct client or family member in drip pad change procedure.

2. Delegate responsibly those activities that can be delegated, including basic care needs of stable client; instruct UAP to notify nurse of respiratory distress, choking, or bleeding.

C. Safety and infection control
1. Maintain elevation of head to prevent aspiration.
2. Monitor nasal drainage to prevent infection of CSF.
3. Instruct client not to blow his or her nose while packing or splints are in place.

D. Health promotion and maintenance: Instruct client how to recognize early and late complications.

E. Psychologic integrity
1. Discuss client's expectations of surgery.
2. Reassure client that swelling and ecchymosis will disappear.

F. Basic care and comfort
1. Manage pain.
2. Suction throat as needed to remove bloody drainage.
3. Provide humidified oxygen via face mask for clients who are mouth-breathing.

G. Reduction of risk potential
1. Instruct client to use protective sports equipment.
2. Institute fall-prevention strategies to avoid nasal injuries.

H. Pharmacologic and parenteral therapies: Client will state the purpose for and side effects of all medications used to manage pain following nasal surgery; this includes mild narcotics such as codeine phosphate, acetaminophen (Tylenol No. 3) or hydrocodone/APAP (Vicodin).

Burns

I. Definition: Burns involve injury to tissues as a result of heat, chemicals, electrical current, or radiation. The source of injury, location of the burn, burn depth, and extent of injury assist to determine the severity of the injury, and develop the nursing plan for care. Nursing care involves teaching clients at risk for burns (e.g., children and older adults, and those who work with toxic chemicals) about preventing burns and how to provide emergency treatment at the site. Nursing care also involves planning and coordinating care through all phases of burn management from prehospital care through rehabilitation.

A. Source of injury
1. Thermal burns—caused by contact with flames, scalding fluids, or hot objects.
2. Smoke and inhalation burns—caused by breathing in hot air or noxious chemicals.
3. Chemical burns—caused by corrosive substances such as acids and strong alkalines.
4. Electrical burns—caused by exposure to current, either lightening or wires and cables.

B. Location of burn
1. Face and neck involvement indicates possibility of smoke inhalation.
2. Hands, feet, joints, and eye involvement often lead to self-care deficits and delayed healing.
3. Ears and nose are more susceptible to infection because of poor blood supply.
4. Circumferential burns of chest are likely to restrict respiratory effort.
5. Circumferential burns of extremities cause damage to nerves and circulation; also can lead to compartment syndrome.

C. Burn depth
1. Partial thickness
2 Superficial (first degree)—erythema that blanches on pressure, such as sunburn; only involves epidermis.
3. Deep (second degree)—blisters filled with fluid; involves severe pain due to nerve injury and is accompanied by edema. Both epidermis and dermis are injured.
4. Full thickness (third and fourth degree)—leathery skin insensitive to pain as nerve fibers are destroyed; may involve muscles and bones.

D. Extent of burn injury (may be revised after edema subsides)—total body surface area based on Lund and Browder chart or rule of nines (see Figure 34-1).

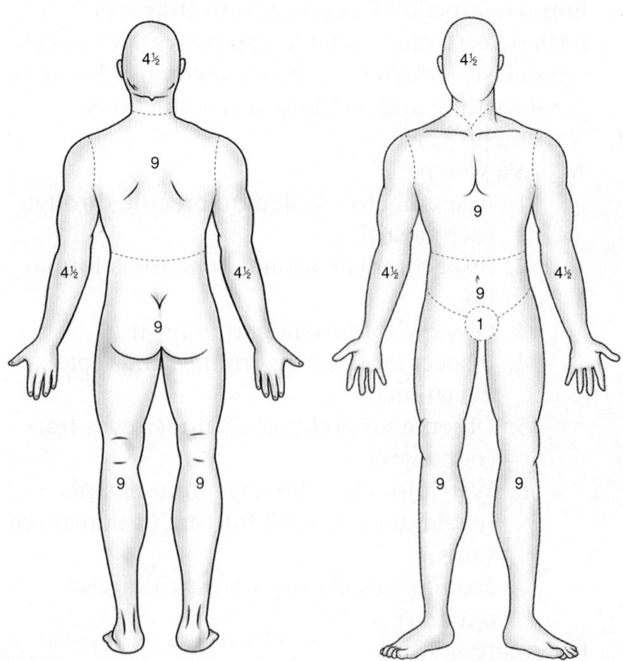

Figure 34-1. Total body surface area based on Lund and Browder chart or rule of nines.

II. Nursing process
   A. General assessment of client in a health care facility (see also Chapter 42).
      1. Determine if airway is patent. Assess victims of smoke inhalation for inhalation injury, including signs of carbon monoxide poisoning such as headache, confusion, nausea.
      2. Monitor oxygen saturation.
      3. Observe respiratory rate and effort.
      4. Monitor output.
      5. Weigh client daily.
      6. Measure BP.
      7. Monitor sodium and potassium levels.
      8. Measure temperature, pulse, and respiration.
      9. Observe circulation and sensation in affected extremities.
      10. Perform neurologic checks.
      11. Assess pain level with pain scale or by observing behavior.
      12. Assess location of burn (see definition).
      13. Determine depth of burn (see definition).
      14. Assess extent of burn injury based on Lund and Browder chart or rule of nines (see Figure 34-1).
      15. Observe appearance of wounds, including graft and donor sites.
      16. Monitor nutritional markers such as serum albumin and total protein.
      17. Assess client's level of anxiety.
   B. Analysis
      1. Risk for Deficient Fluid Volume related to plasma loss, fluid shift, evaporation
      2. Risk for Impaired Gas Exchange related to laryngeal edema due to smoke inhalation
      3. Risk for Imbalanced Body Temperature related to loss of skin and subcutaneous tissue
      4. Acute Pain related to burn injury and treatment measures
      5. Impaired Nutrition: Less Than Body Requirements related to increased caloric needs
      6. Risk for Infection related to impaired physical barrier and immune system
      7. Anxiety related to uncertain outcome
      8. Disturbed Body Image related to disfigurement
      9. Self-Care Deficit related to impaired mobility
   C. Planning
      1. Maintain adequate fluid volume.
      2. Maintain adequate gas exchange.
      3. Maintain body temperature.
      4. Relieve or manage pain.
      5. Maintain positive nitrogen balance.
      6. Prevent infection.
      7. Prevent contractures.
      8. Decrease anxiety.
      9. Promote positive body image.
      10. Teach self-care.
   D. Implementation (during acute phases of the burn injury)
      1. Insert large-bore IV catheter.
      2. Replace IV fluids based on Baxter formula.
      3. Insert indwelling urinary catheter.
      4. Administer tetanus prophylaxis.
      5. Administer analgesics IV as needed.
      6. Administer analgesic 30 min prior to debridement and other painful treatments.
      7. Clean and debride wound daily using aseptic technique.
      8. Initiate topical antibiotic therapy.
      9. Maintain patency of graft and donor sites.
      10. Use low-pressure beds and other devices to relieve pressure on compromised tissue.
      11. Position client to preserve range of motion.
      12. Encourage range of motion exercise.
      13. Apply measures such as elastic garments to reduce scarring.
      14. Apply emollient lotions to healing tissue to keep it supple and reduce itching.
      15. Administer enteral feedings until bowel sounds return.
      16. Offer progressive diet high in protein and carbohydrates as client is able to tolerate oral nutrition.
      17. Reassure client by explaining procedures and expected outcomes.
      18. Teach alternative methods of pain control such as guided imagery, relaxation.
      19. Administer antianxiety agents as indicated.
      20. Provide support to family members and friends.
      21. Assist clients with self-care activities as needed.
   E. Evaluation
      1. Client excretes minimum of 30 ml of urine per hour.
      2. Client sustains a systolic BP of at least 90.
      3. Client demonstrates sodium and potassium levels within normal range.
      4. Client maintains body temperature of 98°F.
      5. Client verbalizes relief in pain.
      6. Client maintains body weight within 10% of preinjury weight.
      7. Client's wounds remain free of exudates.
      8. Client demonstrates white cell count and temperature within normal limits.
      9. Client verbalizes realistic expectations.
      10. Client demonstrates ability to discuss changes in body image.
      11. Client demonstrates self-care within limits of changed abilities.

12. Client resumes relationship with family members and friends.

CN

III. Client needs

A. Physiologic adaptation: The goals of immediate treatment of burns are to stabilize the client's hemodynamic status, assure metabolic support, treat wounds, and prevent complications. Maintaining respiratory, cardiovascular, and renal stability are priorities during the emergent stage.

B. Management of care: Care of the client with burns occurs over several phases, each of which requires critical thinking skills and knowledge of assessment, analysis, planning, implementing, teaching, and evaluation methods unique to the RN role. These skills cannot be delegated to an LPN or UAP. Clients may be managed in a burn center and the nurse collaborates with an interdisciplinary team of health care professionals.

1. Prehospital phase
   a. Remove client from the source of the burn.
      (1) Extinguish flames.
      (2) Flush chemical burns with water.
      (3) Remove from source of electrical current.
   b. Cover small thermal burns with clean, cool, damp cloth.
   c. Care for large burns.
      (1) Maintain patent airway, breathing, and circulation.
      (2) Remove burned clothing.
      (3) Brush dry chemical from skin.
      (4) Prevent contamination of wound with clean, dry covering.
   d. Communicate circumstances of injury to medical personnel.
2. Acute/resuscitative—from burn onset and admission through resuscitation; begins with fluid loss and edema formation and ends with fluid mobilization and diuresis. Maintain respiratory, cardiovascular, and renal stability.
3. Intermediate/wound management and healing—may involve several weeks or months of care; begins with mobilization of fluid and diuresis and ends with wound healing or grafting. (See also implementation for acute burn injury.)
   a. Assist with wound cleansing, debridement, hydrotherapy, use of topical antimicrobials, wound care, and dressing changes as required by the type of burn and burn-management plan.
   b. Prepare client for surgery (excision and grafting) and manage postoperative care.
   c. Prevent infection—administer antibiotics as ordered.
   d. Prevent complications such as sepsis or pneumonia.
4. Rehabilitative—may involve several months of care; begins with wound healing or grafting, may involve multiple surgeries and reconstructive surgeries and continues until client is able to manage self-care.
   a. Delegate responsibly those activities that can be delegated. All monitoring information is reported to the RN.
   b. Refer client to physical therapy for recovery of joint function and ambulation.
   c. Refer client to counseling for emotional support.
   d. Refer client to occupational therapy for support with activities of daily living.
   e. Use dietician to provide nutritional support.
   f. Advise client and/or family to use self-help groups for support.
   g. Provide client and family teaching (see health promotion and maintenance).

C. Safety and infection control
1. Prevent infection by maintaining asepsis.
2. Maintain patency of grafts.

D. Health promotion and maintenance: Provide client and family teaching.
1. Teach client how to perform activities of daily living with new limitations.
2. Teach client how to identify signs to report to physician:
   a. Temperature greater than 100°F
   b. Duskiness or pallor of graft site
   c. Exudate from graft or donor site
   d. Increased pain
3. Instruct client and/or family member on wound care.
4. Remind client to use assistive devices to prevent contractures or scarring.
5. Provide anticipatory guidance related to changes in function or future treatment.
6. Advise client to apply emollient lotion to new skin regularly.

E. Psychologic integrity
1. Encourage expression of emotions, emphasize client's strengths and abilities, and foster positive self-esteem.
2. Encourage client to verbalize perceived change in body appearance; realistically discuss actual changes and losses.

3. Assist client in coping with lifestyle modifications.

F. Basic care and comfort
1. Provide pain control.
2. Maintain fluid balance.
3. Maintain positive nitrogen balance.
4. Preserve range of motion and functionality of joints.

G. Reduction of risk potential
1. Observe client risk for becoming burned.
   a. Occupational risk: Working with chemicals, heat, fire
   b. Age-related risk: Very young and very old, because of reaction time, judgment
   c. Environmental risk: Cooking over open fire; using space heaters; lack of adequate ventilation
2. Observe client risk for difficulty in recovery from burns.
   a. Age—very old or very young clients have impaired immune systems
   b. Pre-existing conditions: Cardiovascular, respiratory, or renal disease may complicate recovery; diabetes delays healing and may cause gangrene.
   c. Malnutrition or substance abuse may cause debilitation.
   d. Comorbidities such as head injury, fractures, put client at risk for recovery.
3. Develop burn-prevention programs for the home including:
   a. Conduct home safety assessments to identify risks.
   b. Set hot water heaters between 120°F and 130°F.
   c. Place smoke and carbon monoxide detectors in living areas and test yearly.
   d. Keep fire extinguishers in garage, kitchen, and basement; inspect and recharge yearly.
   e. Hold family fire drills on regular basis.
   f. Establish a meeting place in case of fire.
   g. Use space heaters and other appliances in accordance with manufacturer's recommendations.
   h. Keep number of local fire department displayed prominently near phone.
4. Develop burn-prevention programs for industrial settings.
5. Teach home care of minor burn injuries.

H. Pharmacologic and parenteral therapies: Client and family will state the purpose for and side effects of all medications used to treat burns.
1. IV fluid replacement during first 24 hr with crystalloids such as lactated Ringer solution, 5% dextrose and saline.
2. IV fluid replacement during second 24 hr with colloids such as dextran, albumin.
3. Wound cleansing with a surgical disinfectant.
4. Topical antibiotics such as silver sulfadiazine (Silvadene) over the wound to prevent infection.
5. Vitamins A, C, and E as well as zinc, folate, and iron to promote wound healing.
6. Analgesics such as morphine and fentanyl (Sublimaze) for pain relief.
7. Sedatives such as lorazepam (Ativan) and midazolam (Versed) to reduce anxiety.
8. Histamine blockers such as omeprazole (Prilosec) and lansoprazole (Prevacid) to prevent Curling ulcers.
9. Nystatin (Mycostatin) may be applied to oral mucosa to prevent overgrowth of *Candida albicans*.

Pressure Ulcers

I. Definition: Pressure ulcers (decubitus ulcers, bed sores) are ulcerations of the skin usually occurring over bony prominences; the ulcers can progress to subcutaneous tissue, muscle, and bone. Ulcers are caused from pressure or pressure in combination with friction or a shearing force that decreases blood flow to local areas. Staging (as defined by the National Pressure Ulcer Advisory Panel, 2007) is as follows:

A. Stage I: Intact skin; erythema; nonblanching macule; area may be painful, and may appear warmer or cooler compared to adjacent tissue.
B. Stage II: Breakdown of dermis, presenting as a shiny or dry shallow ulcer.
C. Stage III: Full-thickness tissue loss; breakdown into subcutaneous tissue.
D. Stage IV: Full-thickness tissue loss with exposed muscle, bone, or tendon. Slough or eschar may be present.
E. Unstageable: Full-thickness tissue loss with base of ulcer covered by slough and/or eschar in the wound; staging cannot be determined until the slough/eschar is removed.

II. Nursing process

A. Assessment
1. Assess client for risk factors.
   a. Poor nutrition
   b. Bowel or bladder incontinence
   c. Bed rest or immobility
   d. Pressure on area more than 2 hr
   e. Health problems such as edema, anemia, diabetes mellitus, or Alzheimer disease
   f. Age: Older adults; younger adults with neurologic impairment

g. Confusion
h. Client uses a wheelchair, or is confined to bed

2. Inspect skin frequently.
3. Document stage of pressure ulcer (see definition of stages).

B. Analysis
1. Impaired Skin Integrity related to pressure ulcer
2. Impaired Tissue Integrity related to pressure ulcer
3. Risk for Infection related to open wound
4. Acute Pain related to tissue damage

C. Planning
1. Prevent pressure ulcers.
2. Relieve pressure.
3. Protect open lesions.
4. Relive pain.
5. Prevent infection.

D. Implementation
1. Provide interventions for preventing pressure ulcers.
a. Turn client every 2 hr; prevent client from lying on hip bones; avoid pressure on legs, ankles, and heels; prevent contact between body parts.
b. Lubricate skin with lotion.
c. Relieve pressure with alternating-pressure mattresses or site-specific devices such as pads; avoid massaging area; do not use "donuts" or "rubber" rings as they cause pressure around the site.
d. Encourage client ambulation and sitting in different positions.
e. Maintain nutrition with adequate protein and fluid intake.
f. Keep sheets and clothing dry; change frequently.

2. Provide interventions for wound care.
a. Clean stage I ulcers with soap and water.
b. Clean stage II pressure ulcers with normal saline; do not use antiseptics or hydrogen peroxide.
c. Use wet-to-dry dressings as ordered for stage III and IV.
d. Cover wound with dressing as ordered (polyurethane film dressings, hydrocolloids, hydrogel dressings) for stage III and IV ulcers.
e. Prepare client for debridement (performed by health care provider)—usually for stage IV ulcers.
(1) Surgical debridement—involves removing necrotic tissue
(2) Nonsurgical debridement:
(a) Mechanical—involves use of high-pressure devices
(b) Enzymatic—involves use of topical enzymes
f. Prepare client for plastic surgery; skin grafts.

3. Provide interventions to prevent or manage infection.
a. Apply topical antibiotics as prescribed.
b. Use aseptic technique to prevent introduction of infection.

E. Evaluation
1. Client remains free of pressure ulcers.
2. Client's pressure ulcers heal and move from higher stages to lower stages.

CN

III. Client needs

A. Physiologic adaptation: Pressure ulcers heal by forming granulation tissue and then re-epithelialize. Pressure of 70 mmHg longer than 2 hr can cause tissue destruction. Shearing force, friction, and moisture contribute to skin breakdown.

B. Management of care: Care of the client with pressure ulcers requires critical thinking skills and knowledge of assessment, and teaching and evaluation methods unique to the RN role. These skills cannot be delegated to an LPN or UAP.
1. Delegate responsibly those activities that can be delegated, including basic care needs. All monitoring information is reported to the RN.
2. Evaluate care and assess client's skin and pressure ulcers frequently.
3. Use guidelines from the National Pressure Ulcer Advisory Panel to stage ulcers.
4. Use a multidisciplinary approach; consult with nurses and others with expertise in managing pressure ulcers.
5. Follow agency care standards for pressure ulcers.

C. Safety and infection control
1. Use safe measures for positioning, turning, and providing skin care to all clients.
2. Prevent skin breakdown.
3. Use aseptic technique when changing dressings.
4. Document and report changes in pressure ulcer; chart information about size, depth, color, odor, presence of necrotic tissue, and changes in exudate.

D. Health promotion and maintenance
1. Assess all clients for risk for pressure ulcers.
2. Promote optimal health and nutrition.
3. Prevent pressure ulcers as noted previously.

4. Promote smoking-cessation programs for client who smokes.

E. Psychologic integrity
   1. Pressure ulcers are debilitating; assist client adapt to changes in body image.
   2. Promote activity and social engagement.
   3. Provide support for client and family throughout long-term care.

F. Basic care and comfort
   1. Turn client frequently.
   2. Keep clothing and sheets clean and dry.
   3. Offer analgesia as needed.

G. Reduction of risk potential
   1. Identify clients at risk (see assessment).
   2. Initiate treatment as soon as pressure ulcer is identified.
   3. Prevent secondary infection.
   4. Prevent and identify complications such as sepsis, cellulitis, bone infection, and gas gangrene.

H. Pharmacologic and parenteral therapies: Medications for pressure ulcers are used to treat wound infections and/or dress the wound.
   1. Topical antibiotics
   2. Dressings
      a. Polyurethane film
      b. Hydrogel dressings

Bibliography

Altman, G. (2004). *Delmar's fundamental and advanced nursing skills* (2nd ed.). Albany, NY: Delmar.

Ellis, J., & Hartley, C. (2005). *Managing and coordinating nursing care.* Philadelphia: Lippincott Williams & Wilkins.

Karch, A. (2008). *Lippincott's nursing drug guide.* Philadelphia: Lippincott Williams & Wilkins.

National Pressure Ulcer Advisory Panel. Retrieved June 8, 2008 from http://www.npuap.org/

Purnell, L., & Paulanka, B. (Eds.). (2003). *Transcultural healthcare: A culturally competent approach.* Philadelphia: Davis.

Smeltzer, S. C., Bare, B. G., Cheever, K. H., & Hinkle, J. L. (2008). *Brunner and Suddarth's textbook of medical-surgical nursing* (11th ed.). Philadelphia: Lippincott Williams & Wilkins.

Taylor, C., Lillis, C., LeMone, P., & Lynn, P. (2006). *Fundamentals of nursing.* Philadelphia: Lippincott Williams & Wilkins.

Weber, J. R., & Kelley, J. (2007). *Nurses handbook of health assessment.* Philadelphia: Lippincott Williams & Wilkins.

CHAPTER 34

Practice Test

Disorders of the Eye

1. The nurse is teaching a client about health management for glaucoma. Which of the following statements indicates that teaching is effective?

□ 1. "I will limit the amount of water I drink during the day."
□ 2. "I will report any eye pain to my physician."
□ 3. "I will need to stay on the medication until the glaucoma is cured."
□ 4. "I will wear my sunglasses at all times."

2. The nurse is assessing a client with visual problems. Which of the following symptoms indicates need for immediate follow-up?

□ 1. Photosensitivity.
□ 2. Flashes of light.
□ 3. Redness of the sclera.
□ 4. Tearing.

3. AF The nurse is observing a student nurse administer eyedrops (see following figure).

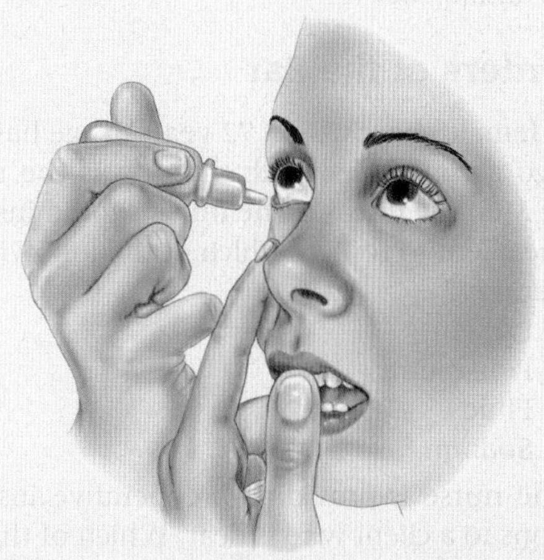

Which of the following instructions does the nurse provide to the student?

□ 1. Move the dropper to the inner canthus.
□ 2. Have the client raise her eyebrows.
□ 3. Administer drops in the center of the lower lid.
□ 4. Have the client squeeze both eyes after administering the drops.

4. A client with glaucoma is to receive 3 gtt of acetazolamide (Diamox) in the left eye. The nurse should do which of the following?
- □ 1. Ask the client to close the right eye while administering the drug in the left eye.
- □ 2. Have the client look up while administering the eyedrops.
- □ 3. Lift the eyebrows while the nurse positions the hand with the dropper on the client's forehead.
- □ 4. Wipe the eyes with a tissue following administration of the drops.

5. AF A client who had a cataract removed today will use eyeglasses after the surgery. The nurse should instruct the client about which of the following? Select all that apply.
- □ 1. The image will appear to be one-third larger.
- □ 2. Look through the center of the glasses.
- □ 3. The changes will be immediate.
- □ 4. Use handrails when climbing stairs.
- □ 5. Objects in the periphery will be smaller than they appear.

6. AF An adult client has bacterial conjunctivitis. The nurse should teach the client to do which of the following? Select all that apply.
- □ 1. Use warm saline soaks 4 times a day to remove crusting.
- □ 2. Apply topical antibiotic without touching the tip of the tube to the eye.
- □ 3. Perform hand hygiene after touching the eyes and surrounding areas.
- □ 4. Avoid touching the eyes.
- □ 5. Stay at home until the redness in the eye disappears.

Disorders of the Ear

7. A female client who is 72 years of age has vertigo accompanied with tinnitus as the result of Ménière disease. The nurse should instruct the client to restrict which of the following in her diet?
- □ 1. Protein.
- □ 2. Potassium.
- □ 3. Fluids.
- □ 4. Sodium.

8. The nurse is providing preoperative instructions to a client who is deaf. Which of the following strategies is most effective in assuring that the client understands the information?
- □ 1. Stand in front of the client and slowly explain the instructions.
- □ 2. Provide instructions to the spouse and have the spouse explain them to the client.
- □ 3. Give the client written material to read and follow up with time for questions.
- □ 4. Show the client a DVD with instructions.

9. A client who is prescribed by the health care provider (HCP) to take aspirin daily in order to prevent thrombus formation reports having ringing in the ears. The nurse advises the client to take which of the following measures?
- □ 1. Increase fluid intake.
- □ 2. Stop taking the aspirin.
- □ 3. Use acetaminophen instead.
- □ 4. Contact the HCP.

Nasal Surgery

10. The nurse is planning postoperative care for an adult client who has had nasal surgery for a deviated nasal septum. Which of the following measures does the nurse include in the plan?
- □ 1. Keep the bed flat for 24 hr after surgery.
- □ 2. Apply ice packs intermittently for 24 hr after surgery.
- □ 3. Change the nasal packing as needed.
- □ 4. Instruct the client to blow the nose to clear dried blood.

Burns

11. Which of the following indicates that fluid-replacement therapy is effective for a burn client in the emergent/resuscitative phase?
- □ 1. Decrease in wound exudate.
- □ 2. Increase in hemoglobin and hematocrit.
- □ 3. Sodium within normal range.
- □ 4. Urine output of 30 ml/hr.

12. A client with burns is progressing through the emergent/resuscitative phase of burn care into the acute stage. Which of the following is a priority for nursing care during the acute phase of burns?
- □ 1. Care for the burn wounds.
- □ 2. Promote client coping with altered body image.
- □ 3. Restore maximal functional ability.
- □ 4. Prevent hypothermia.

13. AF Which of the following assessment findings should the nurse anticipate in the first day or two following a major burn injury? Select all that apply.
- □ 1. Decrease in serum sodium.
- □ 2. Decreased urine output.
- □ 3. Elevated hematocrit.
- □ 4. Metabolic alkalosis.
- □ 5. Hypoglycemia.

14. A client sustained third-degree burns on his legs while he was burning leaves. In the emergency department, the nurse should anticipate an order for which of the following?
- □ 1. Administration of whole blood.
- □ 2. Compression stockings.

□ 3. Tetanus prophylaxis.
□ 4. Cortisone ointment application.

15. When a client has full-thickness burns, what measures are included in the care plan?
□ 1. Shave the burned areas of any hair growth at least weekly.
□ 2. Physically remove the eschar by scrubbing twice a week.
□ 3. Shower or bathe the client daily to remove loose, necrotic skin.
□ 4. Administer narcotic analgesics judiciously to avoid constipation.

16. The nurse is giving discharge instructions to a client who had third-degree burns on both legs. Which of the following teaching measures does the nurse provide?
□ 1. Wear elastic wraps on the legs for a least 1 year.
□ 2. Eat a low-calorie, low-protein diet.
□ 3. Avoid physical exercise for at least 3 months.
□ 4. Expose the burn areas to sunlight for faster healing.

17. An adult client is admitted with full-thickness burns on the front of both legs and lower abdomen. Using the rule of nines, estimate the extent of burns this client has sustained.
□ 1. 9%
□ 2. 18%
□ 3. 27%
□ 4. 36%

Pressure Ulcers

18. The nurse is assessing a client with a stage III decubitus ulcer on his coccyx. The nurse plans care based on the fact that the client will have which of the following?
□ 1. Erythema.
□ 2. Breakdown of the dermis.
□ 3. Full-thickness skin breakdown.
□ 4. Bone, muscle, and support tissue involvement.

19. The nurse is planning care for a hospitalized older adult client with a stage I pressure ulcer on his sacrum. In addition to turning the client every 2 hr, which of the following measures is involved in the care plan?
□ 1. Debride the area daily.
□ 2. Wash the area with soap and water as needed.
□ 3. Apply antibiotic cream twice a day.
□ 4. Rinse the area with normal saline every 4 hr.

20. Which of the following clients is at greatest risk for pressure ulcers?
□ 1. Client who is 70 years of age and ambulatory, but prefers lying in bed.
□ 2. Client who is 35 years of age with a T3 spinal cord injury.
□ 3. Client who is 72 years of age and undernourished, and has a left hip fracture.
□ 4. Client who is 80 years of age with Alzheimer disease.

Answers and Rationales

1. 2 Glaucoma is characterized by gradual loss of the visual field and usually does not cause pain; eye pain may indicate a medical emergency because of severely increased intraocular pressure. Glaucoma may be treated with diuretic therapy, but it is not necessary to restrict fluids. Treatment for glaucoma is ongoing and not "cured." Glaucoma may also be treated with miotics (i.e., cause pupil constriction), so sunglasses are not necessary. (H)

2. 2 Retinal detachment is characterized by visual disturbances such as blind spots and flashes of light; these symptoms indicate need for referral to an ophthalmologist. Photosensitivity, redness, and tearing can be a result of several health problems; the nurse refers the client to the HCP, but there is less urgency than with the indications of a retinal detachment. (A)

3. 3 The student has positioned the dropper and the client correctly to prevent injury to the client's eye. The nurse instructs the student to administer the drops in the center of the lower lid. Following administration of the eyedrops, the client is told to blink the eyes to distribute the medication. Squeezing or rubbing the eyes might cause the medication to drip out of the eye. (D)

4. 2 The nurse instructs the client to look up while eyedrops are instilled. Both of the client's eyes are kept open while the nurse administers the drug. If the client raises the eyebrows and the nurse positions the hand on the eyebrows, the movement of the forehead may cause the dropper to move and injure the eye. The client is told to gently blink the eyes after the eyedrops have been instilled; wiping the eyes could result in the tissue removing some of the medication. Excess fluid is removed with a cotton ball. (D)

5. 1, 2, 4 The use of glasses following cataract surgery does not totally restore binocular vision. Glasses cause images to appear larger and distort peripheral vision. The client is instructed to look through the center of the glasses and turn his or her head to view objects in the periphery; objects in the periphery are not smaller than they appear, but the client does need to turn to see them fully. The client is also instructed to use caution when walking or climbing stairs until he or she has adjusted to the change in vision. Changes in vision following cataract surgery are not immediate, and the nurse can instruct the client to be patient while adjusting to the changes. (A)

6. 1, 2, 3, 4 The client with conjunctivitis can use warm soaks to remove crusting; the nurse teaches the client to wrap soaks in a separate bag for disposal in order to avoid spread of the bacteria. Topical antibiotics are used to treat the infection; the client is instructed to avoid contaminating the tip of the medication dispenser. Bacterial conjunctivitis requires containing the spread of the infection; therefore, the nurse instructs the client to perform hand hygiene after touching the eyes and the surrounding area, but it is not necessary for the client to be isolated or stay at home. (R)

7. 4 Ménière disease is commonly seen in older women; the disorder is caused by pressure within the labyrinth of the inner ear as a result of excess endolympha resulting in swelling in the cochlea. Therefore, the nurse instructs the client about dietary restrictions of sodium to reduce fluid retention. Pharmacologic treatment includes antivertiginous drugs and diuretics. If the client is prescribed a diuretic, the fluid and electrolytes are monitored. The amount of protein does not have a direct influence in this disease process. (H)

8. 3 A client who is deaf benefits most from reading information and then having an opportunity to ask questions and follow up. Verbal communication, while appropriate, may not be sufficient. The spouse can be included in the teaching, but the nurse is responsible for ensuring that the client understands the instructions. DVDs may be helpful, but unless they have closed captioning, key points may be missed in the audio portion. (H)

9. 4 Because aspirin is ototoxic, the ringing in the ears is likely caused by long-term aspirin use. The nurse advises the client to contact the HCP; if the aspirin is to be discontinued, other drugs may be ordered. The client is not instructed to stop taking the drug without discussing the change with the HCP. Acetaminophen does not have the same antithrombotic properties as aspirin. Increasing fluid intake will not stop the ringing in the ears. (R)

10. 2 Following nasal surgery, the nurse uses intermittent ice packs to reduce edema. The head of the bed is elevated at all times to reduce swelling. The nurse does not change the nasal packing, but can change the drip pad under the nose. The client is instructed to not blow the nose; instead, the client can blot secretions with tissues. (C)

11. 4 In the emergent phase of burn therapy, massive amounts of fluid may be given to replace fluid that have or will shift to the interstitium. It is important that sufficient fluid is given to maintain urine output of at least 30 ml/hr. An increase in hemoglobin and hematocrit indicates hypovolemia; serum sodium is low in this phase because of loss in edema fluid and exudates and intracellular shift in exchange for potassium. (A)

12. 1 During the acute phase the nurse is primarily concerned with wound care and prevention of infection, although close monitoring of fluid and electrolytes is still necessary. During this stage clients may undergo wound debridement and/or skin grafts and may have complicated wound therapies. Although rehabilitation begins immediately in burn clients, body image and restoration of function (although critical) are of lesser priority in this stage. (A)

13. 1, 2, 3 Sodium will be low as it, along with fluid, shifts into the interstitium. Fluid shifts cause reduced renal perfusion and thus decreased urine output; sufficient fluids are given to maintain an output of at least 30 ml/hr. Likewise, as plasma is lost to the interstitium, hematocrit will rise. Because of decreased tissue perfusion, anaerobic metabolism will occur, causing metabolic acidosis. Stress causes release of adrenal corticoid hormones and catecholamines, which will result in a rise in blood sugar. (A)

14. 3 Contaminated wounds covering large areas of the body provide portals of entry for the tetanus bacillus, which is often present in soil. Unless the client is able to reliably report that tetanus vaccination is up to date, prophylactic dose is administered. Although the client receives large amounts of fluids in some combination of colloids and crystalloids, whole blood is not usually given unless the client is losing blood. Compression stocking are contraindicated with open wounds on the legs, and the legs are expected to swell. Cortisone ointment is not applied to the wounds; third-degree burns require debridement and very specialized wound care. (R)

15. 3 Full-thickness burns will not heal properly unless the dead tissues are removed daily. Showering or bathing the client daily assists with the process of dead tissue removal. In full-thickness burns, hair follicles are destroyed, so shaving is not necessary or appropriate. Cleaning the wounds only twice a week is too infrequent and could lead to infection. Although pain sensation may be minimal or absent in full-thickness burns, pain management includes analgesics as needed for the client to achieve adequate pain relief. (A)

16. 1 Elastic wraps or pressure stockings are worn over burned areas to prevent excessive skin growth and abnormal coloration following a burn injury. Postburn clients have high caloric and protein needs in order to continue healing, and are instructed to follow a high-calorie, high-protein diet. Burned areas are very susceptible to additional injury and are kept out direct sunlight for 1 year. (H)

17. 3 This client has been burned over approximately 27% of his body. The estimate is calculated with 9% for front of each leg and 9% for lower abdomen. (A)

18. 3 Stage III of pressure ulcer involves full-thickness skin breakdown. Erythema is observed in stage I and dermis breakdown in stage II. Bone, muscle, and supporting tissue are involved in stage IV. (A)

19. 2 Stage I pressure ulcers appear as non-blanching macules that are red in color; they are managed by washing the area with soap and water during daily care and as needed if the client is incontinent or perspiring. Stage II ulcers have breakdown of the dermis and are treated with normal saline. Stage III ulcers have full-thickness skin breakdown and may be treated with antibiotic cream as prescribed. In stage IV ulcers there is involvement of the bone, muscle, and supporting tissue; this may require debridement as performed by the HCP. (R)

20. 2 Clients at risk for pressure ulcers include those who are on bed rest or in a wheelchair; have bowel or bladder incontinence; are immobile, malnourished, or confused; and clients with health problems such as diabetes mellitus, edema, or anemia in which there is a risk for impaired skin integrity. Although older adults are at high risk, young adults who are immobile are also at high risk. The client who is 35 years of age with a T3 spinal injury will be immobile and unable to feel pressure on the areas below the injury; this client is at great risk for pressure ulcers. (R)

SECTION 3

Practice Test

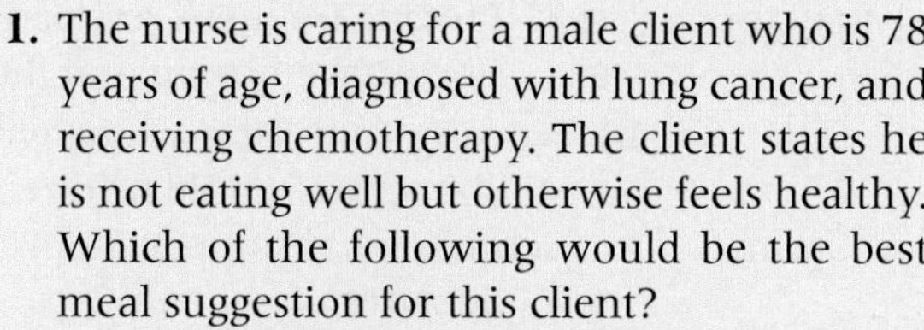

1. The nurse is caring for a male client who is 78 years of age, diagnosed with lung cancer, and receiving chemotherapy. The client states he is not eating well but otherwise feels healthy. Which of the following would be the best meal suggestion for this client?
   - ☐ 1. Cereal with milk and strawberries.
   - ☐ 2. Toast, Jello, and cookies.
   - ☐ 3. Broiled chicken, green beans, and cottage cheese.
   - ☐ 4. Steak, spinach, and french fries.
2. Following a lumbar puncture, which of the following findings should the nurse immediately report to the physician?
   - ☐ 1. Client's oral intake was 1,200 ml in the past 8 hr.
   - ☐ 2. Client required analgesia for headache.
   - ☐ 3. Moderate amount of serous fluid was noted on the lumbar dressing.
   - ☐ 4. Client is concerned about the test results.
3. **AF** A male client who is 68 years of age has been receiving monthly doses of chemotherapy for treatment of stage III colon cancer, and is now at the clinic for his fourth monthly dose. The nurse reports which of the following to the oncologist before administering the next dose of chemotherapy? Select all that apply.
   - ☐ 1. Hemoglobin 14.5 g/dl.
   - ☐ 2. Platelets 40,000/mm^3.
   - ☐ 3. BUN 12 mg/dl.
   - ☐ 4. WBC 2,300/mm^3.
   - ☐ 5. Temperature 101.2°F.
   - ☐ 6. Urine specific gravity 1.020.
4. The nurse is caring for a client 24 hr after an abdominal-perineal resection for a bowel tumor. The client's wife asks if she can bring him some home-made soup. Prior to determining if the client can have the soup, the nurse should first:
   - ☐ 1. Auscultate for bowel sounds.
   - ☐ 2. Ask the client if he feels hunger or gas pains.
   - ☐ 3. Consult with the dietician.
   - ☐ 4. Inquire about the ingredients in the soup.
5. **AF** The hospice nurse is caring for a woman with breast cancer and brain metastasis. The nurse is reviewing the laboratory results as noted below.

LABORATORY RESULTS

Test	Result
Potassium	4.0 mEq/L
Sodium	142 mEq/L
Chloride	100 mEq/L
Calcium	12.4 mg/dL

The nurse should:
   - ☐ 1. Document these results in the progress notes.
   - ☐ 2. Notify the HCP about the potassium level.
   - ☐ 3. Notify the HCP about the calcium level.
   - ☐ 4. Focus on comfort measures as a part of hospice care.
6. A woman receiving radiation therapy for lung cancer tells the nurse that she is having difficulty sleeping. Which of the following would be an appropriate action by the nurse?
   - ☐ 1. Suggest she stop watching TV before going to bed.

- □ 2. Assess the client's usual sleep patterns, amount of sleep, and bedtime rituals.
- □ 3. Tell the client this is expected with radiation therapy.
- □ 4. Suggest she stop drinking coffee until the therapy is completed.

7. A client returns to the recovery room following left supratentorial surgery for treatment of a brain tumor. The nurse should place the client in which of the following positions to facilitate venous drainage?

- □ 1. Lying flat without a pillow; head turned to the right.
- □ 2. Lying flat; head elevated on three pillows.
- □ 3. Head of the bed elevated to 30 degrees; head in neutral position.
- □ 4. Side-lying on the left side; head of bed elevated 10 degrees.

8. Which of the following clients is at highest risk for colorectal cancer?

- □ 1. Client who smokes.
- □ 2. Client who eats a vegetarian diet.
- □ 3. Client who has been treated for Crohn disease for 20 years.
- □ 4. Client who has a family history of lung cancer.

9. A female client who is 57 years of age, of Hispanic descent, and who does not speak English is being admitted for a lumpectomy. She is accompanied by her daughter who speaks English. In order to obtain admission information from the client the nurse should do which of the following?

- □ 1. Ask the daughter to serve as interpreter.
- □ 2. Ask one of the Hispanic nursing assistants to serve as interpreter.
- □ 3. Use limited Spanish known from high school and nonverbal communication.
- □ 4. Obtain a trained medical interpreter.

10. What instructions should the nurse give a client who is preparing for a cardiac catheterization?

- □ 1. "During the procedure you will have a general anesthetic and will be asleep."
- □ 2. "The test will use sound waves to detect if you have heart damage."
- □ 3. "You may be asked to cough or deep breathe during the procedure."
- □ 4. "You will be able to get up and walk immediately after the procedure."

11. When assessing a client who has cardiac tamponade, which finding is expected?

- □ 1. Elevated BP.
- □ 2. Warm, flushed skin.
- □ 3. Decreased pulse rate.
- □ 4. Distended neck veins.

12. When taking a history to determine the nature and strengths of a client's situational supports, which question would be most important for the nurse to ask?

- □ 1. How has your life changed because of your current situation?
- □ 2. Are you actively involved with others or groups in the community?
- □ 3. How have you handled crisis events in your life before?
- □ 4. How do you think this situation could have been avoided?

13. The nurse is assessing a client with a head injury. The intracranial pressure (ICP) is 18 mmHg. An appropriate nursing goal for this client is to:

- □ 1. Encourage the client to cough.
- □ 2. Position the client supine.
- □ 3. Provide frequent rest periods.
- □ 4. Encourage hourly oral fluids.

14. Nursing care for a client who has a basilar skull fracture should be directed toward preventing what complication?

- □ 1. Seizures.
- □ 2. Hyperglycemia.
- □ 3. Hypotension.
- □ 4. Infection.

15. Which of these nursing actions is most appropriate when caring for a client immediately following a transesophageal echocardiogram?

- □ 1. Place sand bags on the puncture site.
- □ 2. Check the gag reflex prior to offering fluids.
- □ 3. Assess the distal extremity for pulses.
- □ 4. Offer an oral analgesic for comfort.

16. When obtaining a health history from a client who has developed hepatic failure, which information should the nurse recognize as significant?

- □ 1. The client has a history of being a two-pack per day smoker for 20 years.
- □ 2. Because of headaches, the client takes acetaminophen frequently.
- □ 3. After returning from traveling outside the United States, the client had diarrhea.
- □ 4. The client routinely eats fresh-water salmon from the Pacific Northwest.

17. The nurse should include which of the following instructions in the teaching plan for a client who has a halo-traction vest?

- □ 1. Driving is possible as long as there is a passenger along.
- □ 2. Pins should be cleaned with hydrogen peroxide and rinsed with water.
- □ 3. The halo vest can be removed for no longer than 2 hr per day.

□ 4. The client, or family member, can tighten pins if they become loose.

18. The nurse is assessing a client who is in hypovolemic shock. Which of the following is expected?

□ 1. Hypertension.
□ 2. Tachycardia.
□ 3. Urinary diuresis.
□ 4. Bradypnea.

19. A client who has fractures of the pelvis and femur demonstrates shortness of breath, apprehension, and tachycardia. The nurse should recognize these symptoms as indicative of what complication?

□ 1. Compartment syndrome.
□ 2. Fat emboli.
□ 3. Wound sepsis.
□ 4. Hypovolemic shock.

20. Which statement, if made by a client who has received teaching about tetracycline, would indicate a need for further teaching?

□ 1. "I will continue taking the medicine until the entire bottle is complete."
□ 2. "I will take my medication with an antacid to reduce stomach upset."
□ 3. "I will plan to limit sun exposure while on this medication."
□ 4. "I will tell my doctor if I develop hives or other rashes."

21. Which statement made by a client who has been receiving combination antimicrobial therapy for 10 days indicates that the client is at risk for developing a superinfection?

□ 1. "My mouth is sore and I'm not interested in eating anything."
□ 2. "I have a headache that is throbbing and unrelenting."
□ 3. "There are reddened areas on my back and chest that look like a rash."
□ 4. "My urine looks darker and has some red spots in it."

22. A client with a cerebral concussion from a fall starts vomiting. What should the nurse do first?

□ 1. Report the finding to the physician.
□ 2. Assign a certified nursing assistant to sit with the client.
□ 3. Change the client to a liquid diet.
□ 4. Record the amount of the emesis in the chart.

23. A client suddenly develops an anaphylactic reaction to an antibiotic. Which finding is expected?

□ 1. Abdominal cramping, diarrhea, and nausea.
□ 2. Itching, hypertension, and polyuria.
□ 3. Bradycardia, muscle twitching, and diaphoresis.
□ 4. Wheezing, rash, and pallor.

24. A client receives an antihelminthic medication for a roundworm infection. The nurse evaluates the effectiveness of the drug when:

□ 1. The client's diarrhea is gone.
□ 2. Stool samples are negative for roundworms.
□ 3. Liver enzymes decrease.
□ 4. The client reports feeling better.

25. Which statement made by a client on IV aminoglycoside therapy indicates the client is experiencing an irreversible adverse effect of the drug?

□ 1. "I would like a laxative to help me pass stool."
□ 2. "I'm having a hard time hearing."
□ 3. "I'm not very interested in eating right now."
□ 4. "I feel tired and want to sleep all the time."

26. The nurse is developing a teaching plan for a client with a prosthetic heart valve replacement. The nurse should instruct the client to do which of the following?

□ 1. Sleep on the left side to avoid stress on the heart valve.
□ 2. Eat a low-fat, low-sodium diet that is rich in protein.
□ 3. Take the BP every day in the sitting position.
□ 4. Request prophylactic antibiotics prior to invasive surgery.

27. A nurse is providing discharge teaching to a client taking oral sulfonamides. Which statement by the client indicates the teaching was effective?

□ 1. "I should stop the drug as soon as it no longer burns when I urinate."
□ 2. "I will try to get out into the sunlight more often."
□ 3. "This medication should be taken after each time I urinate during day hours."
□ 4. "When I take this medication I will drink a full glass of water."

28. The nurse is teaching a client who is taking tetracycline. The nurse should instruct the client to avoid which of the following food groups?

□ 1. Meats.
□ 2. Dairy.
□ 3. Vegetables.
□ 4. Fruits.

29. AF A female client who is 25 years of age and nursing an infant who is 4 months of age is taking rifampin (Rifadin) to treat active tuberculosis. What should the nurse teach this client? Select all that apply.

- □ 1. "Your oral contraceptives may not work, so use an additional form of birth control."
- □ 2. "The drug may cause your urine and tears to have a blue color."
- □ 3. "Make sure that you wear sunglasses because of the side effect of photophobia."
- □ 4. "You will need to bottle-feed your baby while you are taking this drug."
- □ 5. "Report anorexia and jaundice to your HCP."

30. The nurse administers subcutaneous epinephrine to a client with wheezing and hives from a bee sting. What effect should the nurse expect?

- □ 1. Tachycardia.
- □ 2. Pupil constriction.
- □ 3. Hypotension.
- □ 4. Drowsiness.

31. AF The nurse is making follow-up telephone calls to a group of oncology clients. In which order should the nurse return the telephone calls?

_____ 1. Client receiving chemotherapy who has loss of appetite.

_____ 2. Client with a mastectomy 2 weeks ago who called for information on the American Cancer Society (ACS) Reach to Recovery program.

_____ 3. Client receiving spinal radiation for bone cancer metastases complaining of urinary incontinence.

_____ 4. Client with colon cancer who has questions about a high-fiber diet.

32. The nurse instructs the UAP to total the urinary intake and output on clients on the oncology unit at the end of the 8-hr shift. The nurse should instruct the UAP to do which of the following?

- □ 1. Ask clients if they are thirsty when totaling intake and output.
- □ 2. Inform the nurse if any client has less than 240 ml output.
- □ 3. Document intake and output on clients' medical records.
- □ 4. Write intake and output results on scrap paper for the nurse to give to the next shift.

33. Following a craniotomy for treatment of a malignant brain tumor in the occipital region, the client is transferred from ICU to a surgical unit. In reviewing the medication orders at the time of transfer, the nurse should question which one of these orders?

- □ 1. Ibuprofen (Motrin) 400 mg.
- □ 2. Naproxen (Naprosyn) 500 mg.
- □ 3. Morphine sulfate.
- □ 4. Acetaminophen (Tylenol).

34. The nurse is checking the laboratory results on a client with colon cancer who is 52 years of age and admitted for further chemotherapy. The client has lost 30 pounds since initiation of treatment. Which laboratory result should be reported to the HCP?

- □ 1. Blood glucose 95 mg/dl.
- □ 2. Total cholesterol 182 mg/dl.
- □ 3. Hemoglobin 12.3 mg/dl.
- □ 4. Albumin 2.8 g/dl.

35. AF The nurse is providing care for a client after a total laryngectomy for laryngeal cancer. Which of the following are important aspects of discharge teaching? Select all that apply.

- □ 1. Provide humidity at home to help keep secretions thin.
- □ 2. Follow a bland diet.
- □ 3. Use correct suction techniques.
- □ 4. Have communication rehabilitation with a speech pathologist.
- □ 5. Attend a smoking-cessation program.

36. AF A client who is 21 years of age has a bone marrow aspiration at a same-day surgery center. Which of the following statements made by the client demonstrates proper understanding of discharge teaching? Select all that apply.

- □ 1. "I will take Tylenol for pain."
- □ 2. "I do not need to inspect the puncture site."
- □ 3. "I will not be able to play basketball for the next 2 days."
- □ 4. "I will take aspirin if I have pain."
- □ 5. "I can apply an ice pack or a cold compress to the puncture site."

37. Which of the following clients is at greatest risk for skin cancer?

- □ 1. Physician who is 45 years of age.
- □ 2. High school student who is 15 years of age.
- □ 3. Butcher who is 30 years of age.
- □ 4. Mountain biker who is 60 years of age.

38. AF A client is discharged with the following prescription for chronic back pain:

Hydrocodone 5/acetaminophen 500 5 mg
1/2 to 1 PO each 8 to 12 hr as needed

The nurse should tell the client to do which of the following? Select all that apply.

- □ 1. Increase fluids to prevent constipation.
- □ 2. Maintain calories at 1,200 per day to avoid weight gain.
- □ 3. Use the least amount of the medication to prevent addiction.
- □ 4. Keep a pain diary to monitor the effectiveness of the medication.
- □ 5. Avoid driving until dosage is stabilized.

39. The most appropriate nursing action for a client with serum potassium of 2.8 mEq/L is to:
- □ 1. Monitor for flaccid paralysis.
- □ 2. Monitor for changes in level of consciousness.
- □ 3. Prepare for administration of cation exchange resin.
- □ 4. Notify the physician.

40. A client is scheduled for surgery and needs to sign the consent forms. The nurse should do which of the following?
- □ 1. Explain the operation in detail, including possible complications.
- □ 2. Witness the client's signature on the consent after the surgeon has explained the procedure.
- □ 3. Identify and mark the surgical site; record this information on the consent form.
- □ 4. Explain to the client why this particular surgery is necessary and provide other options if the client requests this information.

41. A client with bladder cancer has had a blood loss in the urine estimated at approximately 500 mL from the tumor. The hemoglobin is 8.0 g/dl, and a unit of packed cells is ordered. Which of the following represents an appropriate intervention by the nurse?
- □ 1. Attach the packed cells to the existing no. 19 gauge IV of 0.9% NaCl using a Y-tubing.
- □ 2. Start an additional no. 22 gauge IV site as the packed cells must be given in a separate line.
- □ 3. Attach the packed cells to the existing no. 22 gauge IV of 5% dextrose using a Y-tubing.
- □ 4. Start an additional IV access device that is a no. 22 gauge intracatheter.

42. A client returns from a bronchoscopy during which an oral topical anesthetic spray was used. What should the nurse do first?
- □ 1. Offer a warm, moist pack to soothe irritation.
- □ 2. Place the client in semi-Fowler position to reduce drug absorption.
- □ 3. Check for gag and swallowing reflex before offering fluids.
- □ 4. Monitor liver function tests for drug toxicity.

43. A client who is 65 years of age is admitted for hip replacement surgery. The nurse is implementing standing orders for administering pneumonia vaccine. The client states that he received a pneumococcal vaccine (Pneumovax) 3 years ago. The nurse should:
- □ 1. Document this information on the chart.
- □ 2. Administer the standing order.
- □ 3. Instruct the client to observe hand hygiene procedures.
- □ 4. Place the client in reverse isolation following surgery.

44. **AF** The nurse is performing nasotracheal suctioning for a client with pneumonia. In what order should the nurse perform the steps of the procedure? Place in order from first to last.

_____ 1. Apply suction.
_____ 2. Place the client in a sitting position.
_____ 3. Pass the catheter into the trachea.
_____ 4. Disconnect catheter from suction; apply oxygen with face mask.

45. The nurse is assessing a hospitalized older adult for the presence of pressure ulcers. The nurse notes that the client has an area 1 inch by 1 inch on his sacrum in which there is skin breakdown as far as the dermis. The nurse should note on the chart which of the following? The presence of:
- □ 1. Stage I pressure ulcer.
- □ 2. Stage II pressure ulcer.
- □ 3. Stage III pressure ulcer.
- □ 4. Stage IV pressure ulcer.

46. The nurse is instructing a client how to collect urine for a 24-hr urine study. The test begins at 8 a.m. and the client is instructed to save all urine for 24 hr. At 2 a.m., the client voids in the commode. After realizing that he was supposed to save his urine, he notifies the nurse caring for him. A total of 850 ml of urine has been collected. The nurse should:
- □ 1. Continue collecting the urine until 8 a.m.
- □ 2. Notify the nursing supervisor of the error.
- □ 3. Discard the entire amount collected thus far and begin again.
- □ 4. Continue collecting the urine, but collect an additional specimen after 8 a.m.

47. **AF** A client is admitted with a temperature of 103°F, dyspnea, and a productive cough. The nurse is planning care and reviews the physician admitting orders below:

PHYSICIAN ORDER

Bed rest
Oxygen at 2l/nasal cannula
Amoxicillin 500 mg intravenously q 8 h
Tylenol 2 tablets
Blood cultures stat

The nurse should first:
- □ 1. Administer antibiotics.
- □ 2. Administer acetaminophen (Tylenol) tablets.
- □ 3. Obtain the blood culture.
- □ 4. Conduct a nursing assessment.

48. A client is admitted to the recovery room following chest surgery. The client has an indwelling urinary catheter in place. After 1 hr, the nurse notes the urine output is 50 ml. The nurse should:
- □ 1. Notify the physician.
- □ 2. Check the patency of the catheter.
- □ 3. Continue to monitor urinary output.
- □ 4. Remove the catheter from the client.

49. A client has had a partial gastrectomy. On the first postoperative day the nurse is assessing the client's bowel sounds and determines that no bowel sounds are present. The nurse should:
- □ 1. Continue to monitor bowel sounds.
- □ 2. Notify the physician.
- □ 3. Offer hot fluids.
- □ 4. Administer an enema.

50. A client is scheduled for a hysterectomy in the morning. The evening before surgery, the client tells the nurse that she has changed her mind and doesn't want to have the surgery. An informed consent has been signed. The nurse should:
- □ 1. Notify the operating room supervisor so the operating room schedule can be changed.
- □ 2. Call the client's family to ask them to discuss this situation with her.
- □ 3. Tell the client that the signed consent indicates she must have the surgery.
- □ 4. Notify the physician about the client's change of mind.

51. A client with epilepsy is scheduled for surgery at 9 a.m. He takes phenytoin (Dilantin) every morning at 8 a.m. The nurse should:
- □ 1. Withhold all medication once the patient is NPO at midnight.
- □ 2. Administer the medication just prior to placing the patient on NPO status.
- □ 3. Administer the medication when the client returns from surgery.
- □ 4. Clarify with the physician how and if the drug should be administered.

52. Which of the following schedules represents the most appropriate schedule for medications to be administered "4 times a day"?
- □ 1. 0100 - 0800 - 1400 - 2000
- □ 2. 0300 - 0900 - 1500 - 2100
- □ 3. 0900 - 1300 - 1700 - 2100
- □ 4. 0800 - 1200 - 1800 - 2300

53. A client is to maintain NPO status for 8 hr prior to a diagnostic test. The client takes an antihypertensive and a cortical steroid daily. The nurse should do which of the following?
- □ 1. Instruct the client not to take the medications.
- □ 2. Tell the client to take the drugs with a sip of water.
- □ 3. Notify the physician and request clarification of how and when to take the medications.
- □ 4. Inform the client to take the medications after the test.

54. AF An older adult client has an IV of 1,000 ml infusing at 125 ml/hr over in 8 hr. The IV is at the 500 ml mark in 2 hr. The client has a headache, dyspnea, and tightness in chest. The nurse should do which of the following? Select all that apply.
- □ 1. Slow the IV to keep open rate.
- □ 2. Stop the IV.
- □ 3. Remove the IV.
- □ 4. Administer oxygen by mask.
- □ 5. Notify the physician.
- □ 6. Raise the head of the bed.

55. AF The nurse is initiating a venipuncture to administer IV fluids. Identify the vein that is most appropriate.

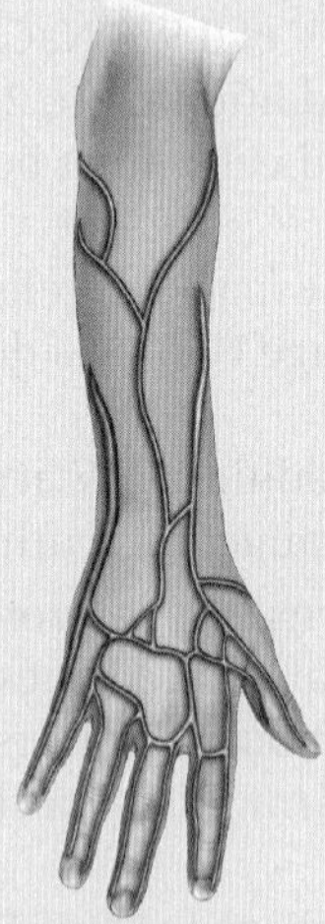

56. A client with a fractured hip is discharged:

Date: 28 August
Hydrocodone 5/acetaminophen 500 mg
One-half to one PO every 8 to 12 hr as needed
70
NO REFILLS

The nurse makes a home visit on August 30. The client is lethargic, with respirations of 10 per minute; BP 90/60. The bottle of pain

medication is on the kitchen counter. The nurse should do which of the following first?
- □ 1. Count the remaining pills in the bottle.
- □ 2. Call 911 for paramedics.
- □ 3. Ask the client to take deep breaths.
- □ 4. Contact the physician who prescribed the medication.

57. AF The nurse is assessing a client who had a craniotomy for a brain tumor. The client is receiving oxygen at 2 L/min, and the head of the bed is elevated 20 degrees. At 1000, the nurse finds that the client is opening eyes to pain, is making incomprehensible sounds, and has abnormal flexion with a Glasgow score of 7. The nurse checks the flow sheet below:

FLOW SHEET

Patient Care Flow Sheet

	Eye Opening	Verbal Response	Motor Response
0800	3	5	5
0900	2	4	4

The nurse should first:
- □ 1. Raise the head of the bed to 30 degrees.
- □ 2. Rub the client's sternum.
- □ 3. Notify the physician.
- □ 4. Increase oxygen flow to 4 L/min.

58. AF A client has been admitted with a history of abdominal pain in the right, upper quadrant for the past 2 weeks. The nurse should use which of the following data-collection instruments to understand the multifaceted nature of the client's pain experience? Select all that apply.
- □ 1. Visual Analogue Scale.
- □ 2. McGill-Melzack Pain Questionnaire.
- □ 3. Numerical Scale.
- □ 4. Initial Pain Assessment Scale.
- □ 5. FACES.

59. A client had a gastric bypass at 0800. It is now 1600. The nurse on the evening shift administered a dose of IV morphine at 1545. When should the evening nurse assess this client for postoperative pain on the evening shift?
- □ 1. Now (1600)
- □ 2. 1630
- □ 3. 1700
- □ 4. 1730

60. AF The nurse is providing care for a client with underwater-seal chest drainage, and recording the amount of drainage from the chest tube. The nurse should record the fluid in which of the chambers? Place an "X" on the correct chamber.

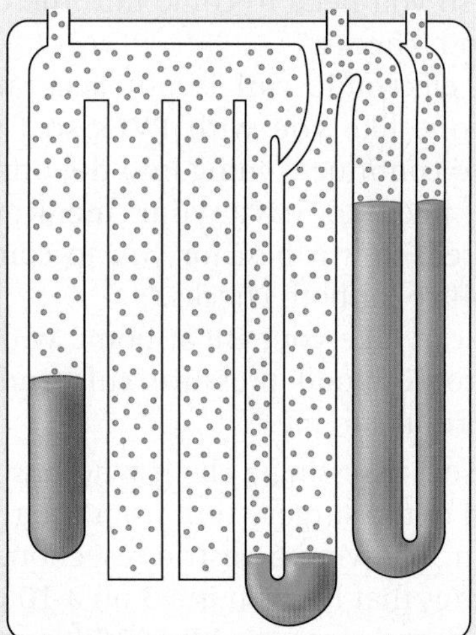

61. AF The nurse is monitoring a client after the removal of a lipoma from his shoulder. A low dose of the local anesthetic bupivacaine (Marcaine) with epinephrine was used to provide anesthesia. What information about Marcaine with epinephrine should the nurse keep in mind when monitoring the client's recovery? Select all that apply.
- □ 1. Blocks sensory nerves in preference to motor nerves.
- □ 2. Causes vasodilatation.
- □ 3. Has a long-lasting effect.
- □ 4. Is more toxic than lidocaine (Xylocaine).
- □ 5. Causes a local rash.

62. A client who is 70 years of age has his BP checked at BP Screening at the shopping center. The nurse reports a reading of 180/90. The client asks the nurse if he has hypertension. The nurse should tell this client:
- □ 1. "Yes, stage 2 hypertension exists when the systolic pressure is 180 mmHg or above and the diastolic pressure is 90 mmHg or above."
- □ 2. "Only a low-grade, stage 1 hypertension, which exists when the systolic pressure is 160 to 180 mmHg and the diastolic pressure is 80 to 90 mmHg."
- □ 3. "Not necessarily, hypertension does not exist until the systolic pressure is 200 mmHg and the diastolic pressure is 100 mmHg."
- □ 4. "One high reading does not constitute a diagnosis of hypertension, but you should have another checkup in 2 weeks."

63. A client with known premature ventricular contractions (PVCs) and hypertension asks the nurse if he can use his electronic BP cuff to take his BP instead of coming in to the clinic. Which is the nurse's best response?

☐ 1. "I like to check your pulse while you are here so you need to come into the office for both checks."
☐ 2. "The electronic cuff is not accurate in someone like you with PVCs so I need you to continue coming into the office."
☐ 3. "You need to have your medications checked, so it is best for you to come to the office for both checks."
☐ 4. "You can take your BP at home with the electronic blood pressure cuff and call your results to me."

64. The nurse is assessing a client who has been admitted to the surgery unit from the recovery room following a gastric resection. The client states that his pain is a 3 on a 10 point scale. The vital signs are BP 100/70; respirations 14; pulse 82. The client's pulse oximetry reading is 91%. The nurse administers oxygen by nasal cannula at a rate of 2 L/min as ordered. The expected outcome of administering the oxygen is:

☐ 1. Decreased pain.
☐ 2. Increased BP.
☐ 3. Improved arterial oxygen saturation.
☐ 4. Deeper respirations.

65. The nurse assessed an obese client's BP as 160/90 when he was in the office last week and asked the client to have his BP checked at home. The client calls the nurse reporting that his BP has been 190/94, 196/99, and 198/96 the past three readings. Which question is the most important one for the nurse to follow up on with the client?

☐ 1. "What size of the BP cuff are you using?"
☐ 2. "Are you experiencing any sensations of numbness or tingling?"
☐ 3. "What time of day did you take your BP?"
☐ 4. "Who took your BP?"

66. **AF** A client admitted to the hospital for GI bleeding has an artificial eye. How should the nurse maintain care of the eye prosthesis when the client is sedated for a gastroscopy? Select all that apply.

☐ 1. Ask the client how he cares for the prosthesis.
☐ 2. Remove the prosthesis as for any surgical procedure.
☐ 3. Assess the client's affected eye for infection and drainage.
☐ 4. Cover the eyes with protective eyewear.
☐ 5. Place tape over the prosthesis to secure it.

67. The nurse is assessing the exudate of a client's pressure sore as predominately thick and opaque tan to yellow in color. Which descriptor should the nurse document regarding the exudate in the chart?

☐ 1. Serosanguineous.
☐ 2. Serous.
☐ 3. Purulent.
☐ 4. Foul purulent.

68. **AF** The nurse is caring for a Hispanic female. Which approach demonstrates culturally sensitive nursing care? Select all that apply.

☐ 1. Touch the client when talking with her.
☐ 2. Talk with the client's assistive personnel about maintaining client modesty during morning care.
☐ 3. Assign female assistive personnel for the client's care.
☐ 4. Talk with the male of the family as the lead member of the family.
☐ 5. Ask the client about her preferences for care.

69. A nurse is checking a client's gastric tube before administering his medication through the tube. His last bolus feeding was 2 hr ago and the gastric residual at this time is 125 ml. The nurse should do which of the following first?

☐ 1. Clamp the gastric tube.
☐ 2. Lower the head of the bed to a medium Fowler position.
☐ 3. Flush the tube with 30 ml of water.
☐ 4. Administer the medication through the gastric tube.

70. **AF** The nurse is to administer a crushed pill into a feeding tube. The nurse should dissolve the finely crushed powder into at least how many milliliters of warm water?

_______________ ml

71. The nurse is applying 1 inch of a unit dose of nitroglycerin ointment on a marked paper on the client's skin. The nurse should do which of the following?

☐ 1. Keep the previous dose in place to avoid using the same site.
☐ 2. Apply the dose over an unshaved area to avoid infection from abrasions.
☐ 3. Massage the paper with the unit dose of medication after taped in place.
☐ 4. Date, initial, and note time on taped medication paper.

72. **AF** The nurse is instructing a client's wife about administering her husband's eyedrops after cataract surgery. Which instructions should be included? Select all that apply.

☐ 1. Clean dried crusts from outer to inner canthus.

□ 2. Hold eyedropper in dominant hand 1 inch above client's forehead.
□ 3. Have client close the eyes gently after the drop is applied.
□ 4. Ask client to hold pressure on inner canthus or inner corner of the eye after drop is applied.
□ 5. Have client use a tissue against the nasolacrimal duct.

73. The nurse is administering eardrops in both ears of an adult. Which interventions are appropriate?
□ 1. Warm refrigerated eardrops by holding the container under running warm water.
□ 2. Have client sit up straight so the nurse can access both ears.
□ 3. Pull the pinna down and back as the drops are placed in the ear canal.
□ 4. Have client place cotton in the ears after instilling the ear drops.

74. A client has a chest tube inserted for a pleural effusion. What color fluid should the nurse expect?
□ 1. Bright red.
□ 2. Serosanguinous.
□ 3. Pus.
□ 4. Straw-colored.

75. The nurse is administering a feeding through a gastric tube when the client suddenly complains of abdominal cramping. The nurse should first:
□ 1. Slow administration of the feeding.
□ 2. Stop administration of the feeding.
□ 3. Warm feeding solution.
□ 4. Contact the HCP.

76. AF The physician has prescribed nitrofurantoin (Macrodantin) 75 mg 4 times a day. The medication comes in an oral suspension of 25 mg/5 ml. How many milliliters should the nurse administer? ______________ ml

77. AF A client who is to receive "enemas until clear" states that she has "very poor control holding enemas." Which nursing interventions are appropriate for this client? Select all that apply.
□ 1. Position client on a bedpan in a dorsal recumbent position after administering the enema.
□ 2. Administer enema with the client sitting on the toilet.
□ 3. Repeat enemas until the client passes clear fluid free of fecal material.
□ 4. Notify the HCP if more than four consecutive enemas are needed.
□ 5. Keep the client NPO until the client is cleared of fecal material.

78. The nurse has placed a nasogastric tube for gastric decompression and is checking for correct placement. Which of the following is the best indicator of correct placement of the nasogastric tube?
□ 1. Aspirate pH of 4 or less.
□ 2. Saliva-appearing aspirate.
□ 3. The client can talk.
□ 4. The tube is visible in the back of the throat.

79. AF Which of the following assessment findings should alert the nurse that the client may be experiencing meningeal irritation? Select all that apply.
□ 1. Projectile vomiting.
□ 2. Positive Kernig sign.
□ 3. Positive Brudzinski sign.
□ 4. Nuchal rigidity.
□ 5. Photophobia.

80. When a client is admitted to the hospital with suspected bacterial meningitis, the nurse prevents spread of infection by instituting which of the following?
□ 1. Judicious hand hygiene.
□ 2. Neutropenia precautions.
□ 3. Reverse isolation.
□ 4. Droplet precautions.

81. A client is undergoing an edrophonium chloride (Tensilon) test. Which of the following responses indicates a positive Tensilon test reaction?
□ 1. Muscle twitching in the large muscles of the legs and arms.
□ 2. Decreased pain sensation.
□ 3. Temporary resolution of ptosis.
□ 4. Increase in the level of consciousness.

82. A client with myasthenia gravis is scheduled for surgery tomorrow. Because increased stress enhances the severity of symptoms of myasthenia, the nurse should monitor which of the following vital signs?
□ 1. Temperature.
□ 2. BP.
□ 3. Pulse.
□ 4. Respirations.

83. The nurse is assessing a female client who is receiving her second administration of chemotherapy for breast cancer. When obtaining the health history, the nurse should ask this client which of the following questions?
□ 1. Has your hair been falling out in clumps?
□ 2. Have you had nausea or any vomiting?
□ 3. Have you been sleeping at night?
□ 4. Do you have your usual energy level?

84. A client with acute renal failure has exhibited increasing mental confusion over the last two shifts. Which of the following laboratory tests would likely confirm the cause of the client's confusion?

- □ 1. BUN 22 mg/dl.
- □ 2. Calcium 10 mg/dl.
- □ 3. Creatinine kinase 50 mcg/ml.
- □ 4. Serum sodium 146 mEq/l.

85. A client's fluid intake has been restricted, and sodium polystyrene sulfonate (Kayexalate) enemas have been ordered. Because of the potential for electrolyte imbalances accompanying these measures, the nurse should assess the client for?

- □ 1. Muscle pain and cramping.
- □ 2. Dry mucous membranes.
- □ 3. Cardiac arrhythmias.
- □ 4. Orthostatic hypotension.

86. After abdominal surgery, a female client is voiding frequently, about 50 ml each time. Assessment reveals dullness in the suprapubic region on percussion. What action should be taken by the nurse?

- □ 1. Anchor a Foley catheter.
- □ 2. Encourage fluids.
- □ 3. Walk the client to the bathroom.
- □ 4. Notify the surgeon.

87. Which of the following nursing interventions would the nurse incorporate into a plan of care for a client who has acute glomerulonephritis?

- □ 1. Encourage rest during the acute phase.
- □ 2. Increase intake of dietary protein.
- □ 3. Decrease intake of carbohydrates.
- □ 4. Strain all urine.

88. A client had a fractured jaw repaired with the rigid plate fixation. Which of the following nursing interventions reduces the risk of aspiration in the first few hours postoperatively?

- □ 1. Administer the prescribed antiemetic.
- □ 2. Use wire cutters if vomiting occurs.
- □ 3. Irrigate the nasogastric tube every 2 hr.
- □ 4. Position the client supine with his head elevated at least 60 degrees.

89. Mycostatin suspension is ordered for a client with candidiasis esophagitis. How should the nurse instruct the client to self administer this medication?

- □ 1. Swallow and follow with water.
- □ 2. Swallow without any water.
- □ 3. Swish and then spit out.
- □ 4. Swish and then swallow.

90. A client has a nasoenteric tube to low intermittent suction requiring frequent irrigation to maintain patency. The nurse should irrigate as needed with which of the following solutions?

- □ 1. Half-strength normal saline.
- □ 2. Sterile water.
- □ 3. Tap water.
- □ 4. Normal saline.

91. The nurse is planning care for an acutely ill client with a continuous gastrostomy tube feeding. The nurse should plan to measure residual gastric contents:

- □ 1. Only when the client complains of discomfort.
- □ 2. Every 4 hr.
- □ 3. Twice a day.
- □ 4. Each time a new bag is hung.

92. A client has had a gastrostomy for 2 weeks and is receiving tube feedings. Nursing intervention for site care includes which of the following?

- □ 1. Apply antibacterial ointment twice daily.
- □ 2. Change dressing daily using sterile technique.
- □ 3. Cleanse site daily with soap and water.
- □ 4. Clean site every other day with iodine and alcohol.

93. A client is receiving TPN through the subclavian site, and the bag is empty. Another bag is not yet available from the pharmacy. The nurse should first:

- □ 1. Notify the physician.
- □ 2. Mix a new bag using supplies from the emergency cabinet.
- □ 3. Hang an IV of 10% dextrose in water until the new bag arrives.
- □ 4. Turn off the TPN and flush the catheter with normal saline.

94. A client hospitalized with a peptic ulcer suddenly vomits coffee ground emesis and complains of dizziness. His vital signs are BP 90/60; pulse 120; respirations 30. The stat hemoglobin and hematocrit report reveals a significant decrease, and the client's urinary output is decreased. The client is passing liquid black stools. What action should the nurse take first?

- □ 1. Elevate the client's head at least 60 degrees.
- □ 2. Give antacids per nasogastric tube and clamp.
- □ 3. Replace gastric output with IV fluids.
- □ 4. Send laboratory specimens for glucose and electrolytes.

95. A client hospitalized with diverticulitis complains of increasingly severe abdominal pain; assessment reveals the abdomen is rigid and tender. Vital signs are: temperature 101.6; pulse 120; BP 100/50. What action should the nurse take first?

- □ 1. Call the physician.
- □ 2. Administer prescribed PRN morphine.

- ☐ 3. Encourage fluids.
- ☐ 4. Administer prescribed PRN magnesium hydroxide (Dulcolax) suppository.

96. The nurse is evaluating the functioning of a new colostomy for a client who had surgery today. The nurse should anticipate that the client will be able to evacuate stool:

- ☐ 1. Immediately.
- ☐ 2. Within 24 hr.
- ☐ 3. Within 48 hr.
- ☐ 4. After 72 hr.

97. When planning care for the client with non–insulin-dependent diabetes mellitus, which of the following goals should the nurse identify as a priority?

- ☐ 1. Maintain a low-carbohydrate, high-fat diet.
- ☐ 2. Maintain ideal body weight.
- ☐ 3. Prepare for eventual daily insulin administration.
- ☐ 4. Include the family in the plan of care.

98. AF The nurse is to administer 3 ounces of a drug to a client. How many milliliters should the nurse administer? ____________ ml

99. The client has been instructed to save urine for 24-hr urine collection starting at 9:00 a.m. Which of the following statements indicates that the client has correctly understood the instructions?

- ☐ 1. "To start the test I will urinate at 9:00 a.m. and discard that urine."
- ☐ 2. "I must save all my urine in a sterile container."
- ☐ 3. "If I forget to save one urine, I will note that on the container."
- ☐ 4. "At the end of the test, I will urinate at 9:00 a.m. and discard that urine."

100. A client is undergoing peritoneal dialysis for the first time. The nurse notices blood-tinged fluid during the first few fluid exchanges. The nurse should:

- ☐ 1. Continue to monitor bleeding as this is an expected occurrence.
- ☐ 2. Take client's vital signs and notify the physician immediately.
- ☐ 3. Discontinue exchanges and request a serum hemoglobin be drawn.
- ☐ 4. Place client in a supine position and readjust the peritoneal catheter.

101. A client who is on continuous ambulatory peritoneal dialysis (CAPD) asks the nurse about special dietary measures that he should be following. Which one of the following information should the nurse include in the teaching plan?

- ☐ 1. Increase intake of carbohydrates.
- ☐ 2. Eat a high-protein diet.
- ☐ 3. Decrease intake of foods high in potassium.
- ☐ 4. Limit fluids to 1,500 ml a day.

102. A client with Parkinson disease is taking benztropine mesylate (Cogentin). The nurse should teach the client to anticipate which of the following problems as a result of this drug?

- ☐ 1. Blurred vision.
- ☐ 2. Diarrhea.
- ☐ 3. Dyskinesias.
- ☐ 4. Sudden freezing.

103. A client who has myasthenia gravis has forgotten to take the 12 noon dose of pyridostigmine (Mestinon) that is ordered every 4 hr. It is now 1 p.m. Which of the following instructions should the nurse give the client?

- ☐ 1. Skip the 12 noon dose but take two pills at 4 p.m.
- ☐ 2. Take the 12 noon dose immediately and another at 4 p.m.
- ☐ 3. Skip the 12 noon dose and resume the usual dose at 4 p.m.
- ☐ 4. Take two pills immediately and then skip the 4 p.m. dose.

104. A client had a cervical spine injury with complete motor and sensory loss below the level of injury. The nurse notices that the client's left calf feels very warm and it is slightly reddened. The nurse should:

- ☐ 1. Assess for the presence of Homans sign.
- ☐ 2. Assess tibial and peroneal nerve function.
- ☐ 3. Measure the circumference of both calves.
- ☐ 4. Palpate for pedal pulses bilaterally.

105. At 24 hr after surgery, a client who had surgery for a fractured hip has an elevated temperature of 101°F. Which of the following should the nurse do first?

- ☐ 1. Obtain an order for a urine culture and sensitivity.
- ☐ 2. Encourage deep breathing and coughing.
- ☐ 3. Obtain an order for culture and sensitivity of the incision site.
- ☐ 4. Increase the rate of the IV fluid.

106. When evaluating the care given by an LPN to a client who has just returned from an above-the-knee amputation, the RN knows that the LPN understands care when the LPN places the client's residual limb in which of the following positions?

- ☐ 1. Extension.
- ☐ 2. Abduction.
- ☐ 3. Flexion.
- ☐ 4. External rotation.

107. AF A client has a pressure sore on the sacrum and has orders for dressing changes. The wound culture revealed methicillin-resistant

Staphylococcus aureus (MRSA). Which action should the nurse take to prevent the spread of the organism to other clients? Select all that apply.

- □ 1. Wear a mask when having direct client contact.
- □ 2. Initiate contact precautions.
- □ 3. Instruct visitors to wear gowns over their clothing.
- □ 4. Wear a gown and sterile gloves with dressing changes.
- □ 5. Restrict visitors.

108. When caring for a client who is in the compensatory stage of hypovolemic shock, what is the nurse's first priority?

- □ 1. Position the client in the Sims position.
- □ 2. Assess pupillary response to light.
- □ 3. Monitor urine output.
- □ 4. Obtain liver enzymes.

109. A client takes 1/150 grain tablet of nitroglycerin sublingually at the onset of angina pain. Shortly afterward, he reports a throbbing headache and tingling under his tongue. The nurse should:

- □ 1. Report these findings to the physician.
- □ 2. Take client's BP every 10 to 15 min.
- □ 3. Suggest that client take only half a tablet next time.
- □ 4. Tell client that these are transient effects.

110. A client with COPD is experiencing shortness of breath and difficulty expectorating sputum. The nurse should advise the client to:

- □ 1. Take deep breaths and exhale forcefully 10 times every hour while awake.
- □ 2. Take several diaphragmatic breaths with pursed-lip exhalations before initiating a cough.
- □ 3. Take a deep breath and hold the volume as long as possible before coughing.
- □ 4. Take short shallow breaths before one rapid forceful exhalation.

111. AF The nurse is assessing the client's heart rate and rhythm on the cardiac monitor. The nurse notes the rhythm below.

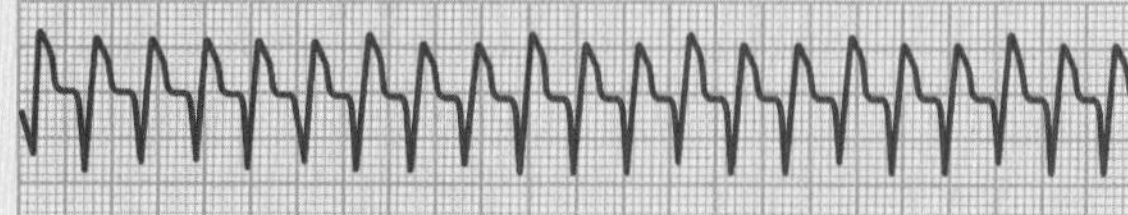

The nurse should do which of the following next?

- □ 1. Administer IV amiodarone (Cordarone).
- □ 2. Deliver a precordial blow and start CPR.
- □ 3. Call the rapid response team and prepare for defibrillation.
- □ 4. Administer sublingual nitroglycerine.

112. A client received 0.1 mL of PPD intradermally. After 72 hr, the nurse reads the area of redness and induration at the injection site as 13 mm. This nurse should interpret this to be:

- □ 1. A negative Mantoux test reaction.
- □ 2. Proof of active pulmonary tuberculosis.
- □ 3. A positive Mantoux test reaction.
- □ 4. A questionable test result and the test should be repeated.

113. A client with heart failure is started on digoxin (Lanoxin). Which of the following indicates that the drug is effective?

- □ 1. Increased heart rate.
- □ 2. Increased urine output.
- □ 3. Decrease in premature ventricular contractions.
- □ 4. Decreased BP.

114. Which statement by the client with Raynaud phenomenon will indicate to the nurse that teaching about health promotion has been effective?

- □ 1. "I will avoid chemical allergens such as red food dye."
- □ 2. "I will avoid shellfish like shrimp and crab."
- □ 3. "I will wear gloves to take things out of the freezer."
- □ 4. "I will make sure to drink plenty of water every day."

115. A client is on a continuous heparin infusion at 1,000 units/hr. The physician then writes an order that the client be started on warfarin (Coumadin) therapy. The nurse should do which of the following?

- □ 1. Question the order.
- □ 2. Administer both drugs as ordered.
- □ 3. Stop the heparin infusion and wait 4 hr before initiating Coumadin.
- □ 4. Give the first dose of Coumadin, wait 4 hr and then discontinue the heparin.

116. Following vein-stripping surgery, a client states that she is worried about varicosities returning in the future because of her excess weight. Which of the following is the most appropriate response by the nurse?

- □ 1. "The doctor is optimistic about the long-term results of your surgery."
- □ 2. "Weight reduction would help lessen the risk of future varicosities."
- □ 3. "It is not advisable to diet soon after surgery."
- □ 4. "Unfortunately, there is not much you can do to prevent varicosities."

117. A nurse is observing a UAP provide care for a client with *Clostridium difficile* infection.

Which of the following indicate the nurse should intervene? The UAP:

- □ 1. Leaves the client's door open when leaving the room.
- □ 2. Leaves a disposable stethoscope at the bedside.
- □ 3. Includes liquid stool on the intake and output record.
- □ 4. Wears a mask when in the client's room.

118. A client is returning to the unit after undergoing a subtotal thyroidectomy. When preparing to care for this client, the nurse should ensure that which of the following medications is available?

- □ 1. Terbutaline (Brethine).
- □ 2. Calcitonin-salmon (Calcimar).
- □ 3. Potassium iodide.
- □ 4. Calcium gluconate.

119. A client is admitted to the hospital for a total hip replacement. The client has been on prednisone therapy daily for the past 2 years for treatment of rheumatoid arthritis. Prior to surgery, which of the following should the nurse ensure?

- □ 1. The client receives the regular daily dose of prednisone.
- □ 2. The dosage of prednisone has been reduced.
- □ 3. The client discontinued prednisone therapy for at least 3 days prior to surgery.
- □ 4. Extra doses of cortisone have been ordered.

120. A male client who is 82 years of age has returned from the recovery room following his radical prostatectomy. To determine the client's need for PRN pain medication following surgery, the nurse should monitor the client for:

- □ 1. Cognitive impairment.
- □ 2. History of depression.
- □ 3. History of memory loss.
- □ 4. Previous history of trauma.

121. A client who takes levodopa/carbidopa (Sinemet) experiences worsening of symptoms about 1 hr after lunch. The nurse should assess which of the following?

- □ 1. Amount of fat in the diet.
- □ 2. Vitamin C supplementation.
- □ 3. Intake of dietary protein.
- □ 4. Carbohydrate intake.

122. Two weeks after a cervical cone biopsy, the nurse discovers the client did not keep the follow-up appointment for removal of the vaginal pack. The nurse should:

- □ 1. Instruct the client to remove the packing.
- □ 2. Apply gloves and remove the packing.
- □ 3. Instruct the client to go to the emergency department for removal of the packing.
- □ 4. Schedule an appointment for removal of the packing.

123. AF The nurse is assessing a client with a head injury. The client is experiencing bradycardia, severe hypertension, and a widening pulse pressure. The nurse should next assess the client for which of the following? Select all that apply.

- □ 1. Unequal pupil dilation.
- □ 2. Decreased urine output.
- □ 3. Seizure activity.
- □ 4. Tongue rolling.
- □ 5. Posturing.
- □ 6. Nuchal rigidity.

124. A nurse is assigned to four, day-of-surgery, postoperative clients. Which of the following clients should the nurse monitor most frequently? The client with a:

- □ 1. Repair of a rectocele.
- □ 2. Removal of a ruptured uterus.
- □ 3. Removal of a cancerous uterine tumor.
- □ 4. Embolization of a fibroid tumor.

125. A client with a subtotal gastrectomy is scheduled for discharge. To lessen the possibility of dumping syndrome, the nurse should instruct the client to:

- □ 1. Eat foods high in simple carbohydrates.
- □ 2. Walk for 30 min after each meal.
- □ 3. Avoid drinking fluids with each meal.
- □ 4. Lie down prior to the next meal.

126. An obese client is being given a high-dose steroid regimen as treatment for COPD. The client is extremely thirsty with 1,500 ml urine output during the 8-hr shift. The nurse should:

- □ 1. Evaluate the client's understanding of the high-dose steroid regimen.
- □ 2. Monitor the client for signs of hypervolemia.
- □ 3. Encourage the client to increase fluid intake to prevent fluid volume deficit.
- □ 4. Do a fingerstick blood glucose test and calculate the client's intake and output for 24 hr.

127. AF A client is to receive 1,000 ml of 5% dextrose in a 0.225% sodium chloride (NaCl) IV solution in an 8-hr period. The IV set delivers 15 drops per milliliter. The nurse should regulate the flow rate so it delivers how many drops of fluid per minute? ____________

128. When providing diet education for the client with diabetes mellitus, the nurse should:

- □ 1. Emphasize that the client eat only prescribed foods.

□ 2. Stress the importance of avoiding carbohydrates.
□ 3. Encourage the client to avoid eating in restaurants.
□ 4. Provide an opportunity for the client to practice food selection.

129. A client has dribbling, urgency, and an inability to get to the restroom before urination starts. Because of fear of having an "accident" in public, the client isolates herself in her room. The nurse should:
□ 1. Instruct client to intentionally urinate on a time schedule of every 2 hr.
□ 2. Encourage client to drink caffeinated beverages regularly.
□ 3. Move client's bed closer to her closet for fresh clothes.
□ 4. Instruct client to keep slippers on her feet.

130. The nurse is administering ondansetron (Zofran) to a client receiving chemotherapy. The nurse evaluates the drug is having the desired effect when the client says:
□ 1. "I don't have as much nausea as I did before."
□ 2. "The pain is better. My headache is almost gone."
□ 3. "I'm so much more alert now. I'm not so groggy."
□ 4. "The tingling in my feet is better."

131. Which of the following measures does the nurse include in the plan of care for a client with end-stage heart failure?
□ 1. Consult family independently to determine if life support should be withheld because the client's condition is deteriorating.
□ 2. Promote client and family encouragement by the health care team to withhold measures of life support because it appears that the client now has a poor quality of life.
□ 3. Provide client and family teaching on treatment options to determine preferences while the client is able to participate in decisions with end-of-life care.
□ 4. Offer the option of hospitalization or hospice care once the health care team has decided to discontinue treatment.

132. Which of the following clients is most at risk for coronary artery disease (CAD)?
□ 1. Female client who is 40 years of age, being treated for a new diagnosis of hypertension, has started an exercise program that includes walking 30 min per day, and has cholesterol level of 165 mg/dl.
□ 2. Male client who is 50 years of age, drinks two cups of coffee every morning, drinks alcohol in moderation during social events, and has triglyceride level of 110.
□ 3. Female client who is 60 years of age, has a continued history of smoking, reached menopause at 50 years of age, and high-density lipoprotein (HDL) of 35 mg/dl.
□ 4. Male client who is 70 years of age with no family history, low-density lipoprotein (LDL) of 100 mg/dl, and BP of 132/80.

133. AF A client with multiple sclerosis is experiencing constipation. The nurse should advise the client to do which of the following? Select all that apply.
□ 1. Add fiber in the diet.
□ 2. Increase fluid intake.
□ 3. Take daily enemas.
□ 4. Use laxatives.
□ 5. Use stool softeners.

134. A client is at high risk for hemorrhage following abdominal surgery. The nurse should do which of the following?
□ 1. Monitor for signs of thromboembolism.
□ 2. Apply antiembolism hose.
□ 3. Perform dressing change every 2 hr.
□ 4. Monitor for restlessness and a sense of impending doom.

135. A client who is taking multiple medications for CAD tells the nurse that she has a supportive family, but lives alone. She sometimes confuses her medications or forgets to take them. Discharge planning by the nurse should include:
□ 1. A caregiver living in the house.
□ 2. Placement in a skilled nursing care facility.
□ 3. Referral for a home health care nurse.
□ 4. Transfer to a special unit for dementia.

136. A client who had a cardiac catheterization 6 hr ago is having nausea and urine output is diminished. The client is receiving IV fluids that are to be discontinued when infused. There is 100 ml remaining in the infusion bag. The nurse should contact the physician, give the background information and current assessment, and then recommend:
□ 1. Continuing IV fluids.
□ 2. Inserting a Foley catheter.
□ 3. Encouraging a PO diet.
□ 4. Giving IV furosemide (Lasix).

137. AF The nurse is teaching a client at high risk for bladder cancer about strategies for preventing bladder cancer. The nurse should include which of the following in the teaching plan? Select all that apply.
□ 1. Prevent bladder calculi (stones).
□ 2. Prevent lower urinary tract infections (UTIs).

□ 3. Increase fluid intake to at least 3,000 ml/day.
□ 4. Quit smoking.
□ 5. Limit sexual activity.

138. The nurse is teaching a client with hypertension about the importance of compliance with taking ramipril (Altace) based on the knowledge that:
□ 1. Diastolic heart failure may be caused by decreased preload.
□ 2. ACE inhibitors decrease the contractile force of the heart.
□ 3. Systolic heart failure can develop from a prolonged increase in afterload.
□ 4. Cardioselective beta-blockers increase long-term survival.

139. The nurse is instructing an older adult female client with urinary incontinence how to improve bladder control. Which of the following indicates that the client has improved continence?
□ 1. Client performs Kegel exercises 3 times a day.
□ 2. Client uses an in-and-out catheter to prevent urinary retention.
□ 3. Client is continent for 18 hr.
□ 4. Client follows a schedule of voiding every 2 hr.

140. The nurse is assessing a client with a history of systolic heart failure who is receiving digoxin (Lanoxin), benazepril (Lotensin), metoprolol (Toprol-XL), and furosemide (Lasix). Assessment reveals bibasilar crackles, HR 68 bpm, atrial fibrillation, and potassium level of 3.1 mEq/L. The client is tired and reports having nausea, blurred vision, and seeing halos. The nurse should do which of the following first?
□ 1. Obtain a digoxin level.
□ 2. Request an order for a calcium channel blocker.
□ 3. Administer an extra dose of Lasix.
□ 4. Withhold the beta blocker.

141. A client is receiving TPN and lipids via a central line. There is an oozing of opaque fluid from around the central line site. The nurse should do which of the following first?
□ 1. Secure the Y-port where the lipids are infusing.
□ 2. Turn the client on left side and place the head lower than the feet.
□ 3. Confirm that the client is receiving broad-spectrum antibiotics.
□ 4. Using sterile technique, change the central line dressing.

142. The nurse is instructing a client with COPD about health promotion. The teaching plan should include which of the following key points?
□ 1. Obtain an annual influenza vaccine.
□ 2. Avoid the use of oxygen unless necessary.
□ 3. Limit exercise to activities in the house.
□ 4. Use only a corticosteroid medication.

143. When suctioning a tracheostomy tube, the nurse should:
□ 1. Apply suction when entering the tracheostomy.
□ 2. Continue advancing the catheter as far as it will go without resistance.
□ 3. Insert and remove catheter as quickly as possible.
□ 4. Suction while removing the catheter for maximum of 10 s.

144. A client with late-stage lung cancer is returning home with long-term oxygen therapy at 3 L via nasal cannula. The nurse should instruct the client to:
□ 1. Keep the oxygen away from heat sources.
□ 2. Remove the cannula while eating.
□ 3. Remain in the home when oxygen is on.
□ 4. Take the oxygen off when sleeping.

145. A client with stage II Parkinson disease is being discharged from the hospital. The nurse is reviewing home safety measures. Which of the following will be most effective in preventing falls for this client?
□ 1. Use aids for reaching.
□ 2. Sit in wheelchair.
□ 3. Use a soft recliner.
□ 4. Remove throw rugs.

146. A client is switching from using regular insulin to lispro insulin. The nurse should teach the client that:
□ 1. Lispro can be taken nasally.
□ 2. Regular insulin is taken with meals, lispro is not.
□ 3. Lispro works much faster than regular insulin.
□ 4. Hypoglycemia will not occur when taking lispro.

147. AF A client with anemia due to bleeding from ulcerative colitis is to receive 2 units of PRBCs. In what order should the nurse perform the following steps? Place in order from first to last.
_____ 1. Remain at client's bedside for 15 min.
_____ 2. Start an IV infusion.
_____ 3. Obtain informed consent for transfusion therapy.
_____ 4. Order laboratory studies for hemoglobin and hematocrit.

148. The nurse is assessing a client who is 75 years of age who has heart failure and is taking amiodarone (Cordarone) 400 mg/day maintenance dose. Which of the following indicates the client may have amiodarone toxicity?

- □ 1. Rales.
- □ 2. Leg cramps.
- □ 3. Slurred speech.
- □ 4. Vomiting.

149. The nurse is providing care for a client with acute coronary syndrome and observes a sudden change in the rhythm on the cardiac telemetry monitor. The nurse should do which of the following first?

- □ 1. Call the rapid response team.
- □ 2. Run a paper strip and document it in the chart.
- □ 3. Begin treatment with medications from the standing orders.
- □ 4. Assess the client's physical condition.

150. Which of the following clients is at greatest risk for dehydration?

- □ 1. Client with asthma who is 37 years of age.
- □ 2. Client with poorly managed diabetes who is 78 years of age.
- □ 3. Client with irritable bowel syndrome who is 56 years of age.
- □ 4. Client with lupus erythematosus who is 28 years of age and a runner.

Answers and Rationales

1. 3 The first substance used for energy is carbohydrates. Proteins are needed to maintain muscle mass, repair tissue, and maintain osmotic pressure in the vascular system. Fats, in a small amount, are needed for energy production. Answers 1, 2, and 4 have a large amount of carbohydrates, a small protein source, or a large amount of fat (french fries). Chicken, green beans, and cottage cheese are the best selection to provide a nutritionally well-balanced diet of carbohydrate, protein, and a small amount of fat. (H)

2. 3 For a lumbar puncture, a needle is inserted into the subarachnoid space to obtain a specimen of spinal fluid for diagnostic testing. Fluid on the lumbar dressing indicates cerebral spinal fluid (CSF) leakage, and must be reported immediately to the physician. The client is encouraged to drink fluids after a lumbar puncture to facilitate production of CSF. A mild headache is normal because of removal of CSF samples; this can be relieved by oral analgesics. The concerns of the client are discussed, but CSF leakage must be addressed immediately as a priority. (R)

3. 2, 4, 5 Chemotherapy causes bone marrow suppression and risk for infection. The platelets and WBC count are very low. High temperature is assessed further to rule out infection. BUN, hemoglobin, and specific gravity values are normal. (R)

4. 1 The nurse performs a thorough assessment of the abdomen and auscultates for bowel sounds in all four quadrants. Clients who have GI surgery may have a decreased peristalsis for several days after surgery. The client must be kept NPO until bowel sounds are present. The nurse checks the abdomen for distention, and inquires with the client and checks the medical record regarding passage of flatus or stool. If the client does not have bowel sounds, the nurse explains to the wife that it is too soon after surgery for her husband to eat. The ingredients in the soup are less important than being sure the client has bowel sounds and no longer needs to be NPO. (R)

5. 3 The normal calcium is 9.0 to 10.5 mg/dl. Hypercalcemia is often seen with malignant disease and metastases. The other laboratory values are normal. Hypercalcemia can be treated with fluids, furosemide (Lasix), or administration of calcitonin. Failure to treat hypercalcemia can cause muscle weakness, changes in LOC, nausea, vomiting and abdominal pain, and dehydration. The client will continue to receive palliative treatment, comfort measures, and risk reduction while in hospice care. (R)

6. 2 The nurse first assesses the client's usual sleep patterns, hours of sleep required before treatment, and usual bedtime routine. Assessment is required before any of the other options can be suggested. (H)

7. 3 The nurse elevates the head of the bed at 30 degrees to promote venous drainage and decrease intracranial pressure. The head is placed in midline position or neutral position. Clients with supratentorial surgery are positioned on the nonoperative side to prevent displacement of the cranial contents by gravity. (R)

8. 3 Clients over 50 years of age and who have a history of inflammatory bowel disease are at risk for colon cancer. Although the exact cause is not always known, other risk factors for colon cancer are presence of colon cancer in a first-generation relative and diet high in animal fats, including a large amount of red meat and fatty foods with low fiber. (R)

9. 4 A trained medical interpreter is required to ensure safety, accuracy of history data, and confidentiality of the client. The medical interpreter knows the client's rights and is familiar with the client's culture. Using the family member as interpreter violates the patient's confidentiality. Using the nursing assistant does not ensure accuracy of interpretation and translation back into English. (M)

10. 3 During a cardiac catheterization clients may be asked to cough or deep breathe to assist movement of the catheter in the arterial system. Fluoroscopic pictures, not sound wave images, are generated during the exam to document coronary disease. Local anesthetics are used during the procedure and clients are awake, although they may be drowsy from sedatives. After the procedure the client will remain supine while the puncture site is monitored for bleeding. (C)

11. 4 In cardiac tamponade, the client's blood volume is trapped in the pericardial sack, causing compression on the heart. The compressed heart is not able to expand to accept blood returning from the venous system. This causes blood to back up into major venous vessels such as those in the neck. The severely compromised heart is unable to adequately pump blood to the body, which causes a drop in BP, a compensatory increase in heart rate, and cool, pale skin. (A)

12. 2 Situational supports include people or groups that the client is actively involved with, or that are available to the client. Asking about how the client's life has changed, how crisis events have been handled in the past, or how the current situation could have been avoided will give the nurse additional information, but these questions do not help to directly identify situational supports. (P)

13. 3 Normal ICP is less than 15 mmHg; the client has increased ICP. The nurse clusters care and limits client interruptions in order to promote rest and avoid activities that will increase the ICP. Clients with increased ICP are positioned with the head of the bed elevated to facilitate reduction of cerebral edema. Because coughing can cause transient decreases in PaO_2, the client is not encouraged to cough. Encouraging oral fluids hourly provides additional stimulation and is not indicated. (A)

14. 4 In a basilar skull fracture, there is potential for an opening to be created between the normally sterile CSF surrounding the brain and the cavities of the unsterile nose and mouth. Preventing an infection involving the CSF and brain is of vital importance. There is no reason to suspect seizures, hyperglycemia, or hypotension in a client who does not have injury to the brain tissue itself. These are not associated with a basilar skull fracture. (A)

15. 2 The gag reflex may not be present immediately postprocedure. In order to prevent aspiration, it is essential to check for the return of the gag reflex prior to offering fluids. For this same reason, any oral medications are not offered until the gag reflex is verified. Because the procedure is done through a tube into the esophagus, there is no need to assess distal extremities or place sand bags. (A)

16. 2 Acetaminophen can cause liver damage and hepatic failure, especially in doses greater than 4 g/day. Smoking primarily causes cancer and respiratory disease. Diarrhea from international travel is most likely caused by parasites or other organisms. Fresh-water salmon is not known as a cause for hepatic failure. (S)

17. 2 Pin care is performed by cleaning around the pin sites with hydrogen peroxide-soaked cotton swabs and then repeating with water. Because of limitations in peripheral vision, clients in halo vests are not allowed to drive. The halo vest is never to be removed by the client as this could result in severe injury. The client is instructed to report any loose pins or signs of infection at pin sites to the HCP. (R)

18. 2 In hypovolemic shock, tachycardia occurs as a compensatory effort to deliver blood supply to tissues. Other symptoms of hypovolemic shock include hypotension, decreased urinary output, and tachypnea. (A)

19. 2 Long and large bone fractures can lead to the development of fat emboli within 24 to 48 hr after injury. Early symptoms include respiratory distress, chest pain, tachypnea, and apprehension. Symptoms of compartment syndrome are neurovascular in nature. Wound sepsis involves changes in color, fever, and other manifestations of infection. Clients with hypovolemic shock have tachycardia and hypotension. (A)

20. 2 Tetracyclines should not be taken at the same time as antacids because antacids can interfere with drug absorption. Taking the prescription until complete, limiting sun exposure because of photosensitivity, and reporting allergic symptoms such as rashes or hives are all appropriate actions. (R)

21. 1 Superinfections occur because of overgrowth of normal flora in the mouth or vaginal tract. The mouth can become sore, there may be loss of appetite, and furry black or white overgrowths can appear on the tongue. Headaches, skin rashes, and hematuria are not clinical manifestations of a superinfection. (S)

22. 1 The client with cerebral concussion demonstrates primarily lethargy and memory deficits. Other findings such as vomiting, unequal pupils, or seizures suggest additional pathology and are reported to the physician immediately. Assigning a CNA, changing the diet, and recording the emesis do not address the change in condition and potential need for emergency interventions. (M)

23. 4 Symptoms of anaphylaxis include wheezing, rash, and pallor. The client becomes hypotensive and tachycardic from peripheral vasodilation. Abdominal cramping, diarrhea, and nausea are common adverse effects from antibiotics but are not representative of anaphylaxis. (D)

24. 2 Antihelminthics are used to treat infestations caused by various types of worms such as flatworms, tapeworms, flukes, and roundworms. Stool examinations are monitored before therapy is started and for 1 to 3 weeks after treatment. Diarrhea, change in liver enzymes, and improvement in client well being do not directly suggest medication effectiveness. (D)

25. 2 Ototoxicity and renal toxicity are both potentially irreversible adverse effects from aminoglycoside therapy; these require frequent assessment and early management. Constipation, loss of appetite, and fatigue are not considered irreversible adverse effects. (D)

26. 4 The client with a prosthetic heart valve is at risk for endocarditis. The nurse instructs this client to request prophylactic antibiotics prior to any invasive surgery or procedure. The client is not required to sleep on the left side, follow a special diet, or monitor the BP unless otherwise indicated by health status. (D)

27. 4 Sulfonamides should be taken with sufficient fluid to maintain a urine output of at least 1,200 to 1,500 ml daily in order to prevent crystalluria and stone formation. The nurse instructs the client to continue taking antibiotics until the prescription is completed to prevent the development of resistant organisms. Sulfonamides can cause photophobia so clients should avoid unnecessary sun exposure. The pills should be taken on a scheduled basis, not in conjunction with voiding. (D)

28. 2 The absorption of tetracyclines may be reduced when taken with antidiarrheal agents, dairy products, or oral preparations. Meats, vegetables, and fruits are not known to cause reductions in tetracycline absorption. (D)

29. 1, 4, 5 Rifampin decreases the effectiveness of estrogens and hormonal contraceptive agents. The drug causes red/orange staining of the tears, urine, and other body fluids. Some contact lenses can be damaged from this staining. Photophobia is not an adverse effect of rifampin. Because rifampin crosses through the breast milk, mothers should not breast-feed while taking this medication. Hepatoxicity can occur with rifampin; the nurse instructs the client to report signs of hepatitis such as jaundice, anorexia, or abdominal pain. (D)

30. 1 Epinephrine stimulates the sympathetic nervous system, causing tachycardia, hypertension, and pupil dilation. The central nervous system can also be affected causing nervousness, restless, insomnia, and possible tremor. (D)

31. 3, 1, 4, 2 The nurse can use Maslow's hierarchy of needs to set priorities for responding to these clients. The client with bone cancer metastases to the spine may have spinal cord compression, damage, and severing of the spinal cord; the nurse contacts this client first to evaluate for urinary incontinence, paralysis, difficulty ambulating, and any weakness or loss of motor function. The nurse then contacts the client who has a loss of appetite to determine what the client is eating and if the client is losing weight, and to suggest strategies to improve the appetite. Next, the nurse calls the client with colon cancer to answer questions about diet. The client with a mastectomy does not appear to have physiologic needs, and the nurse can return this call last. (M)

32. 2 The RN has responsibility to describe to the UAP when to report to the RN a result that indicates a potential client problem with dehydration. The RN must assess and interpret results, as well as give concrete feedback to assistants on what is an expected situation or a specific result to report back to the RN. Urinary output should be at least 30 ml/hr, or 240 ml over the 8-hr shift. In most agencies, the UAP does not chart progress notes and would not need to record the results on scrap paper. Unless otherwise indicated, the UAP can offer fluids to clients who are thirsty. (M)

33. 4 Morphine is contraindicated because of depression of respiration. It may increase ICP if the client is not ventilating properly and there is an accumulation of CO_2, which is a potent vasodilator. Acetaminophen (Tylenol), ibuprofen (Motrin), and naproxen (Naprosyn) are not likely to mask symptoms of increased ICP or impact depression of respiration. (D)

34. 4 The nurse must recognize this albumin level indicates catabolism and potential for malnutrition. Normal albumin is 3.5 to 5.0 g/dl, and less than 3.5 indicates malnutrition. The other lab results are normal. (R)

35. 1, 3, 4, 5 Home care will include high-humidity environment, speech rehabilitation, smoking cessation, laryngectomy tube care, and suctioning. The client is not restricted to a bland diet. (M)

36. 1, 3, 5 Acetaminophen (Tylenol) is a safer analgesia than aspirin in order to avoid bleeding. Contact sports or trauma to the site are avoided. Cool compresses, not heat, limit swelling and bruising. The puncture is inspected every 2 hr for bleeding or bruising during the first 24 hr. (R)

37. 4 Basal cell carcinoma occurs most frequently in sun-exposed areas of the body. The incidence of skin cancer is highest in older people who live in the mountains or spend outdoor leisure time at higher altitudes because of the greater intensity of the rays of the sun. (H)

38. 1, 4, 5 Opiates such as hydrocodone can cause constipation; the nurse instructs the client to increase fluids and fiber in the diet. The client is also advised to record the medication dose used and the pain relief obtained. The client may experience dizziness and drowsiness while determining the most effective dosage, and is instructed to not drive while dizzy or drowsy. The prescription allows the client to make decisions about how much and how often to take the medication, and the client is encouraged to base those decisions on the amount of pain relief obtained. Although addiction is a concern, the client is using the drug to manage chronic pain. Hydrocodone does not cause the client to gain weight. (D)

39. 4 A potassium level of 2.8 mEq/L is extremely low (3.5 to 5.0 mEq/L is normal). This increases the client's risk for cardiac dysrhythmias. The nurse immediately notifies the HCP so replacement potassium can be administered. The client will not exhibit a change in level of consciousness or flaccid paralysis from the decreased potassium level. Cation exchange resins are used to decrease elevated potassium levels. (M)

40. 2 The nurse's responsibility for consent for surgery is to witness the client's signature. The surgeon explains the surgery, why the surgery is needed, the intended outcomes, as well as the risks and possible complications. Prior to receiving preoperative medication, the client identifies and marks the surgical site. (S)

41. 1 The packed cells are administered using a central catheter or no. 19 gauge needle. Blood is not compatible with dextrose as it may cause coagulation of the blood. Blood products are given with normal saline (NaCl). A Y-tubing is used and the saline can be used to keep the vein open when the blood is completed. A blood filter must be used for all blood products to filter out sediment from stored blood products. (D)

42. 3 Topical anesthetic sprays alter the gag and swallowing reflex; until the drug effect has dissipated, the client is at risk for aspiration. The gag and swallow reflex must be present before water, pills, or food are offered. A warm, moist pack will not help the irritation inside the throat area. Positioning does not alter topical drug absorption, and a single dose of a topical anesthetic will not likely cause any drug toxicity. (D)

43. 1 Pneumovax vaccine is effective for 10 years; therefore, the client does not need the medication at this time. The client has the right to refuse the vaccine; the nurse does not administer the drug as per standing order. The client should always observe hand hygiene practices, but it is not necessary to do so more than necessary. Reverse isolation is not necessary because the client is not at risk for pneumonia or other communicable diseases. (D)

44. 2, 3, 1, 4 Nasotracheal suctioning is used to remove secretions from the client who cannot cough up secretions. After explaining the procedure to the client, the nurse first assists the client to an upright position.

Next, the nurse passes the catheter into the trachea and assures catheter placement in the trachea by listening for air at the end of the catheter. The nurse then applies suction. After suctioning, the nurse disconnects the catheter from the suction source and administers oxygen by face mask. The nurse can repeat the procedure if needed and then withdraw the catheter while applying suction. (S)

45. 2 The nurse notes presence of stage II pressure ulcer as indicated by breakdown of the dermis, and stage III pressure ulcers as full-thickness skin breakdown. The nurse immediately initiates plans to relieve the pressure, assure good nutrition, and protect the area from abrasion. Stage I pressure ulcers appear as nonblanching macules that are red in color. Stage IV pressure ulcers involve the bone, muscle, and supporting tissue. (R)

46. 3 For an accurate 24-hr urine specimen, all urine must be collected during the 24-hr period; if the client does not save all urine, the test must be restarted. Extending the study for the client to give an additional urine specimen will not result in an accurate test. It is not necessary to notify the physician and supervisor. (M)

47. 3 The nurse first obtains the blood culture prior to administering antibiotics as the antibiotics will confuse the results of the blood culture, which is being obtained to identify the causative organism. The nurse can then administer the drugs and conduct the nursing assessment. (A)

48. 3 The urinary output of 50 ml in 1 hr is within normal limits; the nurse continues to monitor and record urinary output. It is not necessary to notify the physician. The catheter is patent as long as it continues to drain. The catheter is not removed until the client has recovered from anesthesia and is able to void. (A)

49. 1 The nurse continues to monitor bowel sounds as peristalsis will not return for 2 to 3 days after surgery. It is not necessary to notify the physician. Offering hot fluids and using enemas do increase peristalsis and the presence of bowel sounds, but are not appropriate at this point in the postoperative course. (A)

50. 4 The nurse notifies the physician about the client's change of mind. It is premature to inform the operating room personnel about a potential change in schedule. According to HIPPA laws, the nurse cannot discuss the client's situation with the family. The client has the right to refuse the surgery, and the nurse listens to the client's concerns and serves as an advocate by providing information for the client to make an informed decision. (P)

51. 4 The nurse clarifies with the physician if the client should still receive the medication. Drugs such as phenytoin (Dilantin) are administered on a regular schedule. The nurse does not withhold or administer the drug during the perioperative period unless instructed to do so by the physician. (D)

52. 3 QID means 4 times a day. The most practical schedule is to start the medication in the morning and continue throughout the day. Starting the medication at 0100 or 0300 will disrupt the client's sleep. Having a schedule that starts at 0800 is appropriate, but the client will need to stay up later in the evening to take the last dose. It is also important to space the doses as evenly as possible. (D)

53. 3 Drugs such as antihypertensives and steroids should not be discontinued abruptly. The nurse contacts the physician to clarify how and when the client should take the medications. (D)

54. 1, 5, 6 The client is experiencing circulatory overload from the rapid infusion of fluids. The client is at particular risk because of age. The nurse slows the IV infusion to a "keep open" rate and raises the head of the bed to facilitate breathing. The nurse also notifies the physician who can then determine next steps. (M)

55. The nurse starts the IV using a dorsal metacarpal vein. Using one of the metacarpal veins will allow the client to have range of motion in the hand; if there is a problem with these veins, the nurse then attempts to use the basilic or cephalic vein. (D)

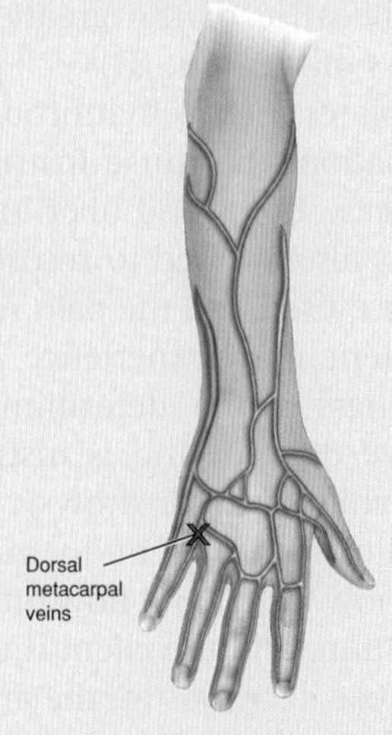

56. 2 The nurse first seeks medical assistance. The client may have taken an overdose of medication, but taking time to count the remaining pills, stimulating deep breathing, or contacting the physician will delay obtaining emergency support. (D)

57. 3 The client is experiencing a loss of consciousness. The Glasgow scale score has dropped from 13 at 0800 and is now 7. The change is significant and the nurse should therefore immediately notify the HCP before initiating other interventions such as raising the head of the bed or increasing oxygen. Sternal rub is used to assess response to painful stimuli and is not necessary as the client is responding to pain. (M)

58. 2, 4 The nurse uses the McGill-Melzack Pain Questionnaire and the Initial Pain Assessment Scale to obtain information on the multifaceted nature of pain for the initial history and physical data. The Visual Analogue Scale and Numerical Scale measure the client's physical intensity and psychologic distress of pain. The FACES scale is a visual analogue scale appropriate for children. (A)

59. 1 The AHCPR Clinical Guidelines for acute pain management recommend that the client's pain be assessed within 15 min after a pain medication is administered. The guidelines also recommend that clients with postoperative pain be assessed every 2 hr for the first 48 hr and every 4 hr thereafter. (C)

60. The nurse records drainage in the column that drains fluid from the client. (A)

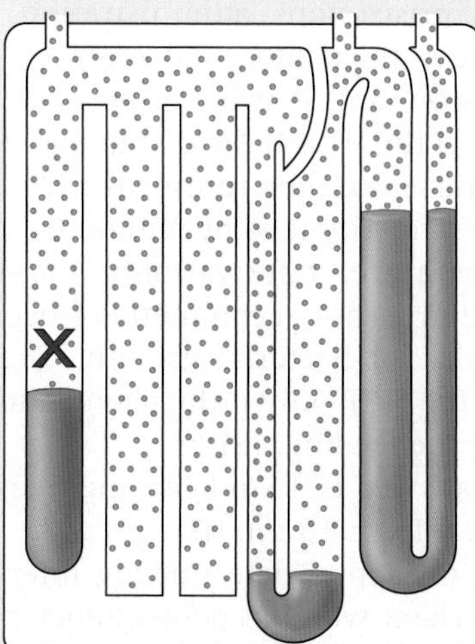

61. 1, 3, 4 A low dose of bupivacaine (Marcaine) blocks sensory nerves in preference to motor nerves, so this client may not experience motor weakness. Although Marcaine causes vasodilation, Marcaine with epinephrine causes vasoconstriction, which makes it stay at the local site and last longer. Marcaine lasts 4 to 8 hr; this is a longer duration than lidocaine (Xylocaine), which lasts around 2 hr. The client has received Marcaine with epinephrine, which means that the local effect is expected to last longer than 8 hr. Marcaine is 4 times more potent than lidocaine (Xylocaine) and about 4 to 6 times more toxic. Marcaine with epinephrine usually does not cause a rash. (D)

62. 4 The Joint National Committee on Prevention, Detection, Evaluation, and Treatment of High BP has identified the diagnosis of adult hypertension is based on the average of two or more readings that results in a high reading taken at each of two or more visits after the initial screening. Stage 2 hypertension is a systolic pressure of equal to or above 160 and a diastolic pressure equal to or above 100. Stage 1 hypertension is a systolic pressure of equal to or above 140 to 159 and a diastolic pressure equal to or above 90 to 99. (H)

63. 2 The best response is that electronic BP machines have a limitation and are vulnerable to error with clients who have dysrhythmias. The nurse may want to check the client's pulse or medications during the office visit, but doing these do not relate to the issue of using an electronic BP cuff. The client should not use an electronic BP cuff because of his dysrhythmia. (S)

64. 3 The client's arterial oxygen saturation is low, with 94% to 100% as normal range. The goal of administering oxygen is to improve oxygen saturation. The oxygen will not decrease the client's pain or increase the BP. The nurse assists the client take deep breaths to improve oxygenation, but adding the oxygen will not improve the depth of the respirations. (A)

65. 1 An appropriately sized BP cuff must be placed around the arm. A BP cuff that is too small will reflect an erroneously high recording compared to the baseline reading with a correctly sized cuff. Although the nurse may want to ask about aberrant sensations, the time of recordings, or who assessed the BP, the stem of this question presents information about a client's baseline BP and the three subsequent readings that are higher. (M)

66. 1, 3, 4 The nurse asks the client how he routinely cares for the eye prosthesis to determine compliance and knowledge of self-care. Unless the client's eye care provider specifies, the client's prosthesis is not removed unless the client complains of discomfort. Excess handling causes irritation and increased secretions. The client's eye is assessed for infection, drainage, tenderness, and odor. The client's eyes are covered with protective eyewear to prevent anything from falling into the eyes while the client is sedated for the procedure. It is not necessary to tape the prosthesis. (S)

67. 3 Exudate that is thick and opaque tan to yellow in color is purulent. Serosanguineous exudate is thin, watery, pale red to pink. Serous exudate is thin, watery, and clear. Foul purulent exudate is thick, opaque yellow to green, with an offensive odor. (S)

68. 1, 2, 3, 5 Hispanic clients, in general, are highly tactile, very modest, and usually want an HCP of the same sex. The oldest female of the family is considered the lead decision-maker of the family. Although the nurse should assess each client's preferences, it is important to be aware of the importance of the traditions in each culture; it is appropriate for the nurse to ask about the client's preferences. (H)

69. 1 The nurse clamps the gastric tube, keeps the head of the bed raised, withholds medication, and calls the physician. If the gastric aspirate is 100 ml or more, delayed gastric emptying has occurred. The client is at risk for gastric distention, esophageal reflux, and vomiting, which could lead to aspiration. The tube should not be flushed with another 30 ml of fluid. (M)

70. The answer is 30 ml. The nurse administers the crushed pill powder in at least 30 ml of warmed water to avoid occluding the tube. (D)

71. 4 The unit dose of marked paper on the client's skin is dated, initialed, and the time noted. The previous dose site is removed and cleaned before the new paper is applied to avoid overdosing the client. To increase absorption of medication through the skin, the area is clipped with a battery-powered or electric razor. The area is not shaved with a razor as this can cause nicks and increase potential for infection. The taped unit dose paper is not massaged because massaging can increase the blood supply to the area, causing increased absorption. This medication is designed to be absorbed over a period; increased absorption can lead to overdose. (D)

72. 3, 4, 5 After eyedrops are inserted, the client is instructed to close the eye gently to distribute the medication. The client is also advised to use a tissue to hold pressure against the nasolacrimal duct, located at the inner canthus, to prevent systemic absorption of the eyedrops. If dried eye crusts are present, a moist cotton ball or wash cloth is used to soak the crust and then clean the crust from the inner to the outer canthus. The eyedropper container is held in the dominant hand placed on the client's forehead so that the drops fall ½ to ¾ inches above the conjunctival sac. (D)

73. 1 The nurse warms eardrops that are stored in the refrigerator by holding the container under running warm water. The client is positioned in a side-lying position with the affected ear up, or in a sitting position with the ear up. After drops are instilled, the client stays in the side-lying position until the drops are absorbed; the nurse can then administer the drops in the other ear. The nurse pulls the pinna up and back as the drops are placed in the ear canal of an adult. It is not necessary to put cotton in the ears as some of the medication could be absorbed by the cotton. (D)

74. 4 Fluid from the chest tube inserted for a pleural effusion should be straw-colored. The fluid from the chest tube inserted from a recent chest surgery should be bright red at first and then gradually become serosanguinous and then serous. The fluid from the chest tube inserted into a pleural cavity with emphysema would have pus-colored drainage. (A)

75. 2 The nurse stops administration of the feeding; the abdominal cramping likely will stop, and it will not be necessary to contact the HCP. If the cramping does stop, the nurse can then resume the feeding at a slow rate. The feeding should be at room temperature, but warming the feeding solution is not recommended because of the risk of bacterial growth. The nurse calls the HCP only if the client cannot tolerate the feeding. (S)

76. The answer is 15 ml. 25 mg/5 ml = 75 mg/x ml:x = 15 ml. (D)

77. 1, 3, 4 An appropriate nursing intervention for a client who has poor sphincter control is to position the client on a bedpan in dorsal recumbent position after administering the enema. Do not administer the enema with the client sitting on the toilet as the curved rectal tubing can abrade the rectal wall. When an enema is ordered to be given until clear, the enema is to be repeated until the client returns clear fluid free of fecal material. After three consecutive enemas are administered, the client may experience a fluid and electrolyte imbalance; the nurse notifies the HCP if the client will need a fourth enema to be clear of fecal material. It is not necessary for the client to be NPO at this time, unless ordered by the HCP. (S)

78. 1 The only acceptable indicator of the correct placement of a nasogastric tube is a return aspirate pH of 4 or less using a gastric pH test. The client can talk when the nasogastric tube goes down the esophagus, but cannot talk when it is down the trachea. The nasogastric tube is soft and pliable, which allows it to easily coil in the back of the throat, so the nurse checks that the tube has not collected in the oral pharynx. The aspirate content of gastric juice is usually green and cloudy, not saliva-colored. (S)

79. 2, 3, 4, 5 Kernig and Brudzinski signs are indications of meningeal irritation. Kernig sign is evident when the client is lying with the thigh flexed on the abdomen and the leg cannot be fully extended because of pain. Brudzinski sign is evident when the client's neck is flexed, and flexion of the hips and knees occurs. Nuchal rigidity and photophobia are also signs of meningeal irritation. Projectile vomiting can indicate increased ICP. (A)

80. 4 In order to prevent the spread of the bacteria, droplet precautions are instituted until 24 hr after antibiotics are started. Hand hygiene is important, but the bacteria are spread by droplet. The client will not need neutropenia or reverse isolation as those are used to protect the immunosuppressed client from infection. (S)

81. 3 Edrophonium chloride (Tensilon) is a short-acting anticholinergic medication that temporarily alleviates the signs and symptoms of myasthenia gravis. Signs and symptoms temporarily reversed can include ptosis and respiratory and swallowing difficulties. Edrophonium chloride will have no effect on pain or level of consciousness. (A)

82. 4 Under stress, fatigue in muscles increases, including the muscles involved in respiration. Although it is important to monitor all vital signs, respirations are the most important in this case. (R)

83. 2 Chemotherapy agents typically cause nausea and vomiting when not controlled by antiemetic drugs. Antineoplastic drugs attack rapidly growing normal cells, such as in the GI tract. These drugs also stimulate the vomiting center in the brain. Hair loss, loss of energy, and sleep are important aspects of the health history, but not as critical as the potential for dehydration and electrolyte imbalance caused by nausea and vomiting. (D)

84. 1 Normal BUN value is 10 to 20 mg/dl; a rise in circulating BUN causes mental confusion. The calcium and sodium levels are normal and the creatinine (not the creatinine kinase) level would lend diagnostic information for renal failure. (A)

85. 3 Sodium polystyrene sulfonate (Kayexalate) enemas are used to lower serum potassium levels; cardiac arrhythmias are associated with hypokalemia. Muscle pain and cramping can be caused by hyperkalemia. Dry mucous membranes and orthostatic hypotension can be caused by dehydration. (D)

86. 3 The client's symptoms indicate urinary retention. The client is walked to the bathroom if able, as sitting on the toilet aids in urination. Dullness indicates a full bladder, and encouraging fluids will not help the client empty the bladder, but will cause increased distention. If the client still cannot void, the surgeon should be notified for a catheterization order. (R)

87. 1 Acute glomerulonephritis is an inflammatory disorder of the kidney usually preceded by a group A beta-hemolytic streptococcal infection of the throat; the most common signs are hematuria and proteinuria. The client is encouraged to rest during the acute phase (although prolonged bed rest has been shown to have little effect on outcomes). Dietary proteins will be restricted if the BUN is elevated, and carbohydrates are encouraged to prevent protein catabolism and provide energy. Straining urine is appropriate if the client has a kidney stone. (R)

88. 1 Administering prescribed antiemetics postoperatively is important in preventing vomiting, and thus aspiration. Wire cutters are kept at the bedside and are used if vomiting occurs. Vomiting increases the risk for aspiration—prevention is best. Irrigating the nasogastric tube is not indicated unless it is not draining; irrigation could cause nausea. The client should usually be positioned with the head elevated; however, if nausea and vomiting occur, position the patient on the side. (S)

89. 4 For fungal infections of the esophagus, nystatin (Mycostatin) is swished and then swallowed without water. Oral candidiasis can be treated with the swish-and-spit method. (D)

90. 4 Although tap water may be used, irrigating with normal saline can help prevent electrolyte loss that can be caused by use or absorption of large amounts of hypotonic solutions (such as tap water, sterile water, or half-strength saline). Normal saline is the best choice, especially if irrigating frequently or with large volumes. (A)

91. 2 Residual gastric contents are measured every 4 to 8 hr with continuous feedings, and the aspirated contents readministered to the client. If the residual is greater than 100 ml (200 ml with a nasogastric tube), the nurse suspects feeding intolerance. If this occurs twice, the physician is notified. (A)

92. 3 It is important to cleanse the site daily with soap and water to avoid skin breakdown from gastric juices that may leak around the tube; once the site is healed a dressing is usually not necessary. The dressing around a healed tube site is not sterile, and ointments are avoided. Iodine and alcohol may actually cause damage to healing skin. (A)

93. 3 An IV of 10% dextrose in water is hung to maintain patency of the line and prevent rebound hypoglycemia (TPN has high concentrations of glucose); the solution is not discontinued abruptly and, as the solution is commonly very complicated, is always mixed in the pharmacy. (D)

94. 3 The client is exhibiting signs of hypovolemia due to blood loss through the GI tract; fluids must be replaced quickly to prevent hypovolemic shock. When a client with a nasogastric tube begins to vomit, the tube is not clamped, and antacids are ineffective in treating active GI bleeding. The client who is vomiting is positioned either in high Fowler or side-lying position, depending on tolerance. Laboratory work may need to be done, but glucose and electrolytes are not a priority at this time. (R)

95. 1 The client is exhibiting signs that may be indicative of perforation or abscess secondary to diverticulitis; emergency surgical intervention may be indicated. Pain medication is indicated, but morphine is contraindicated as it can increase intraluminal pressure. The client is kept NPO. A suppository is not indicated and will be ineffective. (A)

96. 4 Stool is expected after 72 hr with a new colostomy. Peristalsis does not return until about 72 hr after abdominal surgery, and it is not realistic to expect the client to evacuate stool until then. (A)

97. 2 The greatest risk factor for non–insulin-dependent diabetes mellitus is obesity; therefore, maintaining ideal body weight is a priority when providing client care and teaching. A high-fat diet is contraindicated as it increases body weight and cardiovascular risk. A non–insulin-dependent diabetic can often control diabetes without insulin, especially if she loses weight. Including the family is important but is not the priority. (A)

98. The answer is 90 ml. One ounce has 30 ml. 30/ml/1 ounce = xml/3 ounces. X = 90 ml. (D)

99. 1 A 24-hr urine collection is started and finished with an empty bladder; the client is instructed to discard the first a.m. urine and collect all others for 24 hr (including the last one). The container for the urine is not sterile. Forgetting to save urine will necessitate beginning the test anew. (A)

100. 1 A few blood streaks (although not frank bleeding) in the fluid is normal for the first few exchanges after catheter insertion and should resolve. Continuing to monitor is the only action that is warranted at this time. (A)

101. 2 High protein loss occurs with CAPD; the client is instructed to eat a high-protein, well-balanced meal. The client starting on CAPD often gains weight and is advised to limit carbohydrate intake to help avoid excessive weight gain. Fluid, potassium, and sodium restrictions are usually not necessary. (H)

102. 1 Benztropine is an anticholinergic agent, and although these drugs are primarily selective for CNS cholinergic receptors, they can also block receptors in the periphery. This action leads to side effects of blurred vision and photophobia, dry mouth, urinary retention, and constipation. Side effects do not include diarrhea, dyskinesias, or freezing. (D)

103. 2 Pyridostigmine is a reversible cholinesterase inhibitor, which intensifies the effects of acetylcholine released from motor neurons, thereby increasing muscle strength. This drug has a duration of 2 to 4 hr so dosage intervals must be precise in order to prevent rapidly developing muscle weakness that can interfere with swallowing and breathing. Doses must never be skipped, but if they are, the client is instructed to take medication when he or she remembers. (D)

104. 3 Because of the warmth and redness of the extremity, the nurse determines if the client is experiencing deep vein thrombosis (DVT). It is important to monitor for unilateral edema by measuring calf circumference. Assessing for Homans sign or peripheral nerve functioning necessitates motor/sensory function, which is absent in this client. Pedal pulses are assessed, but will usually be present even with DVT. (R)

105. 2 The most likely cause of fever in the immediate postoperative period is atelectasis and stasis of secretions due to shallow breathing from pain, anesthesia, or opioid medications. The client must perform deep-breathing and coughing exercises to keep the lungs expanded and the airways clear. If fever persists, the physician is notified and may order cultures, increased IV fluids, or antibiotics. (R)

106. 1 Following amputation, the limb is placed in extension to prevent hip contracture; the foot of the bed may be elevated to prevent edema. Abduction, flexion, and external rotation must be avoided. (R)

107. 2, 3, 4 It is most important to initiate contact precautions as MRSA colonizes the skin, which then acts a reservoir of organisms that can be transmitted to others. MRSA is not transmitted through the air. The nurse should wear a gown and use sterile gloves if changing dressings; some agencies may require the use of a mask for dressing changes to protect the wound from potential droplet infection. It is not necessary to restrict visitors as long as they wear gowns. (S)

108. 3 In this stage of shock, the priority is assessing and maintaining tissue perfusion as blood will be shunted away from the skin, kidneys, and GI tract. Urine output will help determine the adequacy of volume replacement and the potential for volume overload. The client is maintained supine with the foot of the bed elevated to assist in cerebral perfusion. Assessing papillary changes is not the first priority in hypovolemic shock, but there may be neurologic changes associated with shock. Liver enzymes may eventually be drawn to assess organ damage, but the priority is resuscitation. (A)

109. 4 Sublingual nitroglycerin frequently causes these symptoms from vasodilatation; symptoms are transient, but some clients may need acetaminophen to relieve headache. No other action is necessary unless symptoms are severe or persist. It is never correct for the nurse to adjust the client's medication dose. (D)

110. 2 Taking several diaphragmatic breaths with pursed-lip exhalations before initiating a cough helps mobilize secretions into the major airways. Additionally, pursed-lip breathing prolongs exhalation, allowing more time for gas exchange to occur, and prevents collapse of alveoli at the end of exhalation. Other listed techniques are not effective. (A)

111. 3 The client is having ventricular tachycardia, a potentially lethal dysrhythmia. Because the nurse witnessed the event, the nurse should start CPR with a precordial blow. Amiodarone is not a first-line treatment; if the client is alert, the nurse can administer lidocaine (Xylocaine). Nitroglycerine is not an appropriate drug at this time as the client's heart is not having effective contractions. (R)

112. 3 Induration is an area that is hardened. Greater than 10 mm of induration and erythema is considered a positive Mantoux (greater than 5 mm in those at risk is considered significant), which indicates infection with *Mycobacterium tuberculosis.* Infection does not mean active disease. Vulnerable clients may soon develop active disease, or in healthy individuals the organism can lay dormant for years. Diagnosis of active TB is through sputum culture. (A)

113. 2 Digoxin exerts a positive inotropic effect on the heart; that is, it increases force of ventricular contraction, thereby increasing stroke volume and cardiac output. An increase in cardiac output will increase kidney perfusion and urine output. Digoxin enhances vagal effects in the heart, thereby slowing heart rate. BP may increase with increased cardiac output or may decrease as urine output increases, and is not the primary indicator of drug effectiveness. (D)

114. 3 Exposure of skin surfaces to cold in a susceptible client usually triggers the vasospastic episodes in the fingers or toes characteristic of Raynaud phenomenon; other triggers that may precipitate vasospasm are emotional stress and tobacco. This problem is not caused nor exacerbated by allergens (food dye, shellfish) or dehydration. (H)

115. 2 Heparin suppresses clotting by helping antithrombin inactivate thrombin and factor Xa, thus suppressing the formation of fibrin. Effects begin immediately after IV infusion and duration of action is brief. Warfarin (Coumadin) suppresses clotting by blocking biosynthesis of vitamin K-dependent clotting factors; because it has no effect on clotting factors already in circulation, initial response may not be evident for 8 to 12 hr after PO dose and the effect does not peak for several days. In order to ensure that the anticoagulation effect of Coumadin has occurred before discontinuing heparin, it will be started by overlapping with heparin until the INR is in an acceptable range (2 to 3). (D)

116. 2 Excess weight is a predominant predisposing factor in the development of varicosities. The client is referred to a dietician or nutritionist for advice with healthy weight loss, which can begin immediately. It is the role of the physician to inform the client about the success of the surgery. (H)

117. 4 *Clostridium difficile* is a serious infection usually secondary to antibiotic therapy and with high nosocomial potential. When normal intestinal flora is disrupted, this spore-forming bacterium can proliferate in the bowel, where it releases toxins into the bowel lumen causing diarrhea; in severe cases the client can develop pseudomembranous colitis. *Clostridium difficile* is transmitted on health care workers' hands, often after contact with contaminated equipment. Intensive cleaning and disinfection of equipment, along with Contact Precautions is necessary. Closing the door to a client's room is for prevention of airborne transmission and is not necessary with *C. difficile* infection, nor is wearing a mask. Disposable equipment will help prevent spread by contaminated equipment. Liquid stool should be recorded as output on the intake and output record. (S)

118. 4 The parathyroids may be accidentally removed during surgery, drastically affecting the client's serum calcium levels; tetany is a major complication requiring emergency administration of calcium gluconate. Terbutaline is a beta-agonist that causes relaxation of smooth muscle such as of the uterus or bronchioles. Calcitonin-salmon is a synthetic form of the thyroid hormone calcitonin and acts to maintain (lower) serum calcium by decreasing bone resorption and increasing calcium excretion. (S)

119. 4 The client needs extra cortisone in stressful situations such as surgery; the adrenals are unable to respond when the client has been receiving exogenous steroids over a period of time. Prednisone cannot be discontinued abruptly after long-term use as this could lead to an addisonian-like crisis (severe hypofunction of the adrenals). (R)

120. 4 Key components of assessing an older adult's pain include medical history, history of trauma, pain history, medications, previous pain experiences, and physical examination. Assessing history of other significant events can provide important information on client's pain experience, medications used, and tolerance to pain. Even though the older adult client may be cognitively impaired, the nurse takes the client's self-reported pain as serious because undertreating pain may be considered as a form of elder abuse. Medical history and physical examination are important components implementing effective pain management. History of depression and history of memory loss may be signs and symptoms of substance abuse or some other physiologic condition. (A)

121. 3 The absorption of levodopa/carbidopa (Sinemet) is impaired with protein and vitamin B_6. Fats, vitamin C, and carbohydrates are not known to interact with Sinemet. (D)

122. 3 Packing that occludes the cervix places the client at risk for a life-threatening infection. The packing should have been removed 24 hr after the procedure, and it needs to be removed as soon as possible. The nurse requires a written order from the HCP to remove the packing. The packing is commonly removed by the HCP. (S)

123. 1, 3, 5 Clients who have experienced a head injury often develop increased ICP. Cushing triad is a response to the increased ICP and is characterized by bradycardia, severe hypertension, and a widening pulse pressure. The nurse continues to monitor the client for other signs of increased ICP such as unequal pupil dilation, seizure activity, and posturing. Decreased urine output, tongue rolling, and nuchal rigidity are not signs of elevated ICP. (M)

124. 2 The nurse provides most frequent monitoring of the client with the least predictable or most unstable clinical pathway. Intraoperatively, the amount of trauma aligned with a rectocele, excision of a cancerous tumor, and embolization was controlled by the surgeon. Hence, the clinical pathway is likely to be more predictable than a ruptured uterus or the removal of tumors. (M)

125. 3 Dumping syndrome is a direct result of surgical removal of a large portion of the stomach and the pyloric sphincter. It is the rapid dumping of food into the jejunum without proper mixing and digestion. To minimize the occurrence of dumping syndrome, lying down after eating, eating a diet high in both fat and protein but low in carbohydrates, and no fluids with meals is suggested. (R)

126. 4 The client is at high risk for type 2 diabetes mellitus. Excessive thirst and excessive urination are signs of hyperglycemia, a manifestation of diabetes mellitus. Steroids may also increase carbohydrate metabolism, leading to hyperglycemia in the client with inadequate insulin. The nurse assesses the client's blood glucose. Because hyperglycemia places the client at risk for fluid volume deficit, the nurse calculates the client's fluid balance. Evaluating client understanding is important, but not a priority. Hypervolemia will not occur with excessive urination. Increasing the fluid intake may help prevent fluid volume deficit; however, unless the glucose level is decreased, the elevated glucose will cause continued osmotic diuresis. (A)

127. The answer is 31 gtt/min. (D)
Formula: Total volume × drip factor divided by total time in minutes:

$$\frac{1000 \times 15}{8 \times 60} = \frac{15{,}000}{480} = 31.2 = 31 \text{ drops/minute}$$

128. 4 It is most important the client is given the opportunity to demonstrate understanding of diet therapy by practicing food selection. The client must learn to choose foods that he or she likes and usually eats, but within the parameters of the prescribed diet. Carbohydrates will not be eliminated, but will be restricted. (H)

129. 1 A client with urinary incontinence is advised to maintain a regular, flexible schedule of urination (usually every 2 to 3 hr) while awake. Management of urinary incontinence includes instructing the client on consumption of an adequate volume of fluids and reduction/elimination of bladder irritants (particularly caffeine and alcohol) from the diet. Having quick access to clean, dry clothing does not improve urinary incontinence. Slippers on the feet are not part of normal attire, and may actually promote slipping on the floor, with subsequent falls and potential fractures. (A)

130. 1 Ondansetron (Zofran) is given to decrease the incidence and severity of nausea and vomiting associated with chemotherapy. Headaches and sedation are expected side effects. Neuropathies are not associated with Zofran therapy. (D)

131. 3 The health care team provides client and family teaching on the expected course and treatment options for heart failure, living will, and advance directive to determine preferences while the client is able to participate in treatment decisions. The client must be included in the decision-making process, not just the family. It is the role of the nurse and health care team to provide information about treatment options and issues to consider, but it is not appropriate to make recommendations; these are decisions the client and family must make. Suggesting hospice care is not appropriate until the client and family have made decisions about treatment options, but when appropriate, the nurse can provide information and facilitate a referral. (P)

132. 3 The risk for CAD increases significantly in women at menopause. Both active and passive smoking increase risk. Control of BP less than 140/90, cholesterol less than 200 mg/dl, LDL less than 130 mg/dl, HDL more than 40 mg/dl, and triglycerides less than 150 mg/dl reduces risk. Coffee may stimulate angina symptoms in a client with CAD, but this, as well as moderate alcohol intake, is not a risk factor. (H)

133. 1, 2, 5 Increasing fiber and fluids are effective interventions for constipation. Stool softeners and a bowel plan are also beneficial. Laxatives, suppositories, or enemas are used in moderation and only if needed. (H)

134. 4 Restlessness and a sense of impending doom are indicators of inadequate cerebral perfusion, and could indicate hemorrhage. Thromboembolism is not an indicator of hemorrhage. Applying antiembolism hose does not prevent hemorrhage. It is not necessary to change the dressing every 2 hr; if the dressing has drainage or bloody drainage, the nurse outlines the drainage on the dressing and/or reinforces the dressing. If the drainage increases in a short period of time, the nurse contacts the surgeon. (M)

135. 3 Interventions to facilitate and assure self-care behaviors at home can be provided by a home health care nurse; the nurse can assist the client to organize her medications, assess other home health care needs, and help the client and family maintain client independence. The problem of accuracy in providing medications does not indicate dementia or a need for constant care. (M)

136. 1 The nurse contacts the physician and, using S-BAR (situation, background, assessment, and recommendation), recommends continuing the IV fluids and requests an order for additional fluids. Adequate hydration is essential to assist in excretion of the radiopaque dye that can be toxic to the kidneys. Because the client is experiencing nausea and a decreased urine output, IV fluids are continued rather than forcing PO fluids. A Foley catheter could provide a better assessment of output, but is not indicated for a cardiac catheterization. Furosemide (Lasix) IV would further dehydrate the client and compromise renal function. (R)

137. 1, 2, 3, 4 The client with chronic recurrent stones (calculi, often bladder) and chronic lower urinary infections has an increased risk of squamous cell cancer of the bladder. The client who has indwelling catheters for long periods of time can develop these chronic conditions. Tobacco use is a risk factor for bladder cancer. Increasing daily fluid intake may aid in the development of stones (calculi) and prevent UTIs. Sexual activity does not need to be limited, but voiding after sexual intercourse aids in the prevention of UTIs, especially in female clients. (H)

138. 3 Hypertension is a major cause of heart failure and increases afterload, the resistance the ventricle has to pump against to eject blood. The "prils" are ACE inhibitors and decrease afterload, but do not affect myocardial contraction. Diastolic dysfunction results from a condition that causes the ventricle to become rigid and resistant to filling. (D)

139. 3 The ultimate goal is to promote urinary continence for 24 hr each day. The client is progressing toward the goal by achieving continence for 18 hr. Monitoring and managing urinary retention with in-and-out catheterization is important, but is not an outcome. Kegel exercises and following a voiding schedule are appropriate interventions to achieving the goal, but are not indicators that the goal has been attained. (H)

140. 1 The client has signs of digoxin toxicity, which can occur from a high digoxin and low potassium levels. Calcium channel blockers are contraindicated in the treatment of systolic heart failure. Potassium supplementation is required before any additional furosemide (Lasix) is given. There is no indication that the beta-blocker dose should be reduced; the adjustment period can cause fatigue, and the heart rate is normal. (D)

141. 2 A potential break in the central line places a client at risk for air embolism. The client is turned on the left side and the head is placed lower than the feet; the nurse also notifies the physician. Leakage is occurring at the IV insertion site, not the Y-port. There is no indication of catheter-related infection or septicemia; hence, broad-spectrum antibiotics are not needed. Sterile technique is used when changing a central line dressing; however, to change the central line dressing is not the most important action. The dressing could be removed later to assess the situation. Dressings covering the catheter site are changed according to institutional protocol; the site must be carefully observed for signs of inflammation and infection. The client receiving TPN is more susceptible to opportunistic infections. (D)

142. 1 Influenza vaccinations have been shown to decrease morbidity in clients with COPD. Exercise training improves symptoms of dyspnea and fatigue. Long-term oxygen therapy in hypoxic clients can prolong life. Bronchodilator medications are central to the symptomatic management of COPD. The addition of regular treatment with inhaled glucocorticosteroids to bronchodilator treatment is appropriate for symptomatic COPD patients with an FEV1 less than 50% predicted (stage III, severe COPD, and stage IV, very severe COPD) and repeated exacerbations. (H)

143. 4 Suction is applied when exiting the tube for 5 to 10 s. The suction catheter is advanced no more than 6 inches. Tissue damage and bleeding or advancing past the carina can occur with forceful advancement of the catheter until resistance is met. (R)

144. 1 The nurse instructs the client on home oxygen to keep the oxygen away from flame, sources of heat, and oil-based products. The client may experience shortness of breath with eating, so the nasal cannula should be left on during meals. The client can safely manage oxygen outside the home and should avoid social isolation. Oxygen may be required around the clock. (S)

145. 4 In clients with Parkinson disease, the gait is slowed and balance is altered because of the changes in posture. In addition, the client's gait shortens and the client shuffles; as a result, it is important that the environment is clear of hazards that can cause the client to stumble and fall. Bradykinesia and rigidity result in slow, jerky, and rigid movements so using a long-handled reacher may not be practical as this requires grasping and squeezing of the hands. The client is encouraged to wear shoes that can be slipped on, and have Velcro hook-and-loop. Activity is encouraged as long as possible to decrease the effects of muscle rigidity. Sitting in an upright chair with arms can help the client transfer from sitting to standing position. A soft recliner may offer additional challenges to a client with Parkinson disease. (S)

146. 3 The onset for subcutaneous lispro insulin is 15 min, while subcutaneous regular is 30 to 60 min. Lispro peaks in 30 to 90 min, while regular peaks in 2 to 4 hr. Lispro is only available by the subcutaneous route and should be taken 15 min before a meal. Both insulins cause significant decreases in blood sugar and can cause hypoglycemic reactions. (D)

147. 3, 2, 1, 4 Following hospital policy and procedure, the nurse first obtains informed consent and then obtains IV access using appropriate tubing with normal saline as the priming solution prior to retrieving blood from the blood bank. Next (after identifying the client at the bedside by confirming client name and identification number, blood bank identification band [if used], unit number, blood type, and expiration date), the nurse hangs the PRBCs, remains at the client's bedside during the first 15 min of transfusion therapy, and monitors vital signs per agency protocol. The last step is to obtain follow-up blood work to determine the client's response to transfusion therapy. (M)

148. 1 Rales, crackles, decreased breath sounds, cough, and shortness of breath are signs of pulmonary toxicity related to the use of the drug. The nurse should also assess the client for signs of dysfunction of the thyroid gland, resulting in lethargy and weight gain. Hypokalemia and hypomagnesemia may decrease the effectiveness of the drug. Leg cramps, slurred speech, or vomiting are not typical side effects of a maintenance dose of amiodarone (Cordarone). (D)

149. 4 The nurse always checks the client first to verify that the telemetry monitor is functioning accurately and, if so, to determine if the client is having symptoms to accompany the change in rhythm. Calling the rapid response team, administering medications, and documenting events may all be appropriate, but should not occur until the client is assessed and the necessary data are gathered. (A)

150. 2 Age and poorly managed diabetes are two major risks factors associated with dehydration. Asthma is treated with cortisone, which is likely to result in fluid retention. Irritable bowel syndrome is likely to result in dehydration, but the age of the client reduces the risks. Lupus erythematosus has nondefinitive clinical signs, which may or may not result in dehydration. (A)

SECTION 4

Nursing Care of Clients With Psychiatric Disorders and Mental Health Problems

chapter 35

Introduction to Nursing Care of Clients With Psychiatric Disorders and Mental Health Problems

Clients of all ages are at risk for psychiatric disorders and mental health problems. The role of the nurse for the client with situational mental illness such as the loss of a job or death of a spouse is to promote coping and mental health through use of effective communication strategies. Care for the client with chronic mental illness such as bipolar disorder involves a variety of interventions. Nursing care is based on ability to understand patterns of growth and development, and to assess a client's mental health status, promote mental health, and use nursing interventions to assist the client and family during illness and periods of crisis. Topics in this chapter include:

- Background Information
- Health Assessment
- Health Promotion
- Principles of Nursing Care Management

Background Information

I. Definition: Mental illness, as defined by the American Psychiatric Association, is "a clinically significant behavioral or psychologic syndrome or pattern that occurs in an individual and that is associated with present distress (e.g., a painful symptom) or disability (e.g., impairment in one or more important areas of functioning) or with a significantly increased risk of suffering death, pain, disability, or an important loss of freedom" (APA, 2000, p. xxxi).

A. While interpretation of behaviors is culturally defined, behavior that is considered other than normal within a cultural setting does not necessarily indicate a mental disorder (APA, 2000). Behavior is a dynamic, ever-changing state of being for an individual.
   1. Criteria that may indicate mental disorder include:
      a. Inability to meet basic needs.
      b. Inability to successfully communicate with others, resulting in unsatisfying relationships.
      c. Emotional instability.
      d. Ineffective coping with life events.
      e. Inability to adapt to change and cope with adversity.
      f. Lack of personal growth.
      g. Dissatisfaction with one's accomplishments.
   2. Additional elements that may affect mental health of a client include the following:
      a. Stress—a nonspecific internal response produced by a change in surroundings that is interpreted as threatening by the person.
         (1) Physiologic stressors include drugs, alcohol, heat, cold, trauma, infections, nutritional imbalance, and pain.
         (2) Psychosocial stressors include natural disasters, accident survival, death of friend/family, life crisis (e.g., unemployment), relationship conflicts (e.g., divorce), fear concerning world events, and failure.
      b. Anxiety—subjective psychologic distress sensation that occurs when person feels threatened and before a new experience. A feeling of uneasiness, tension, or apprehension that ranges from mild to panic levels (see Chapter 38).
      c. Experience of loss, grief, or dying (e.g., the client with cancer)
         (1) Loss includes both physiologic and emotional loss.
         (2) Grief is subjective and involves physiologic experiences associated with loss.
         (3) Mourning involves a psychologic process that occurs with an associated loss of something or someone with meaning to the person.
         (4) Dysfunctional grief can be manifested in various ways, such as absence of any grief response; prolonged grief with preoccupation of the deceased. Substance abuse, self-neglect, illness, and suicide are more common in those experiencing dysfunctional grief.

B. Misunderstanding of mental illness throughout the history of health care has resulted in fear of and ignorance toward individuals suffering from psychiatric and mental health problems; often, they were sent to prison or otherwise removed from society.
   1. 1800s—symptoms of mental health problems became understood as caused by an illness process, and provoked scientific research and care institutions (asylums). Linda Richards, a nurse, began teaching psychiatric concepts to nursing students (1880).
   2. 1950 to 1980—psychotropic medications were developed, and client rights for the mentally ill began to evolve. The Deinstitutionalization Movement began, and the Mental Health Centers Act of 1963 shifted treatment focus from in-patient to community-based care settings. Nursing theorist Hildegard Peplau (1952) developed *Interpersonal Relations in Nursing,* theory of nursing that focuses on the interpersonal processes that promote growth toward productive living.
   3. 1980 to present—community care focuses on mental health promotion. The 1990s are designated as the "decade of the brain," with research into all types of brain illnesses. Nursing focuses on the development of a therapeutic relationship, defined as a helpful and trusting relationship with a client. In many cultures there is still a stigma connected with mental illness.

C. Theories about growth and development provide a way to examine human behavior. According to theorists, mental illness occurs when there is disruption in the progression through the identified stages. See Table 35-1 for a summary of major theories related to growth and development.

Table 35-1 Growth and Development Theories Significant to Mental Health Nursing

Growth and Development Theory	Description of Theory	Developmental Stages	Application to Nursing
Freud's Psychoanalytic Theory	• Conscious: Experiences person is aware of. • Preconscious: Experiences that can be recalled and remembered. • Unconscious: Experiences not available to awareness.	• *Oral stage* (birth to 18 months): Infant deals with anxiety by gratification of oral needs. • *Anal stage* (18 months to 3 years): Toddler learns muscle and social control. • *Phallic stage* (3–6 years): Child establishes sexual identity. • *Latency stage* (6–12 years): Child establishes same-sex relationships. • *Genital stage* (12–18 years): Adolescent establishes relationships with opposite sex.	• All behavior has meaning, but it may be unconscious. • Nurse assesses client's anxiety level and use of defense mechanisms.
Erikson's Psychosocial Theory	• Ego development results from social interaction. • Developmental tasks must be completed in sequence.	• *Trust vs. mistrust* (infant): Views world as safe, relationships are nurturing. • *Autonomy vs. shame and doubt* (toddler): Achieves a sense of control. • *Initiative vs. guilt* (preschool): Learns to manage conflict; develops conscience. • *Industry vs. inferiority* (school age): Develops confidence in abilities. • *Identity vs. role confusion* (adolescence): Forms sense of self and belonging. • *Intimacy vs. isolation* (young adult): Forms adult relationships and attachments. • *Generativity vs. stagnation* (middle adult): Demonstrates creativity and productivity. • *Ego integrity vs. despair* (older adult): Accepts responsibility for self and life.	• Nurse assesses development and compares to expected norms. • Nurse encourages client to perform positive behaviors associated with appropriate life stage.
Sullivan's Interpersonal Theory	• Persons are shaped by parental approval and disapproval. • Anxiety occurs from conflict in relationships.	• *Infancy*: (birth to language): Need for bodily contact, sense of well-being if needs are met. • *Childhood* (language to 5 years): Parents give praise and acceptance; moderate anxiety leads to insecurity. • *Juvenile* (5–8 years): Thinks of self and others based on analysis of experiences; learns to negotiate needs; severe anxiety results in need for control. • *Preadolescence* (8–12 years): Develops same-sex friendships; moves away from family for satisfaction in relationships. • *Adolescence* (puberty to adult): Recognizes need for relationships with opposite sex; if healthy self-esteem has developed, person can then develop values, career decisions, social concerns.	• Learning to cope with anxiety is an important skill. • Nurse focuses interventions on dealing with current interpersonal issues.
Piaget's Cognitive Theory	• Persons develop thinking processes from infancy through adulthood.	• *Sensorimotor* (birth to 2 years): Develops sense of self separate from environment; object permanence. • *Preoperational* (2–6 years): Develops ability to express self with language; understands symbols. • *Concrete operations* (6–12 years): Starts to apply logic to thinking, applies rules. • *Formal operations* (12–15+ years): Learns to think and reason abstractly, develops logical thinking.	• Understanding how the client thinks allows the nurse to communicate in an age-appropriate manner. • Interventions and teaching are adapted to client's cognitive level.

(continued)

Table 35-1 Growth and Development Theories Significant to Mental Health Nursing (Continued)

Growth and Development Theory	Description of Theory	Developmental Stages	Application to Nursing
Maslow's Hierarchy of Needs Theory	• Focuses on the present behaviors and issues, as well as spiritual values. • Traumatic events can cause a person to regress to a lower level of motivation.	• Human needs are organized in a hierarchy: • Physiologic needs • Safety and security • Love and belonging • Self-esteem and esteem for others • Self-actualization	• Nursing care is prioritized to meet client needs from the lowest level (physiologic needs) through the higher levels. • Clients must have needs of lower levels met before they can focus on higher levels.

D. Theories to explain causes of mental illness may involve biologic, psychologic, or social-environmental factors.
   1. Biologic
      a. Biochemical influences (most popular)
      b. Hormonal influences
      c. Pregnancy environment
      d. Inherited (genetic) factors
   2. Psychologic
      a. Values/belief systems
      b. Perception of self
      c. Internal and external stressors
   3. Social-environmental (see previous point A)

Health Assessment

I. Definition: The client with a psychiatric or mental health problem requires cognitive and emotional assessments, a comprehensive physical examination, and a detailed risk assessment. The nurse must be skilled in interview techniques and age-related physical assessment techniques.
   A. Psychiatric history is obtained to identify patterns of functioning, risk factors of mental illness, coping mechanisms, and to ascertain cultural appropriateness of behaviors.
      1. General history information—assesses occupation, religious affiliation, marital status, and previous mental health data.
      2. Reason for seeking care—assesses recent difficulties, and changes in behavior or functioning.
      3. Presenting symptoms—assesses for feelings of depression and anxiety, suicidal ideation, changes in physical status such as weight change, and presence of sleep disturbance and headaches.
      4. Family history—assesses history of mental illness, family dynamics, and use of alcohol or drugs.
      5. Personal characteristics—assesses interests, hobbies, coping mechanisms, sexual patterns, and social relationships.
   B. Mental status examination is obtained to identify baseline and current, ongoing mental status to provide a format for the initiation of the nurse-client relationship. See Table 35-2 for general areas of assessment.
   C. Risk assessment for client safety involves assessing for self-harm (e.g., suicide ideation) and harm to others; this is a critical assessment for the client seen in any setting.
      1. Gains insight into the client's mental and emotional state, and into the possibility for harm to self or others.
      2. Is obtained by asking direct and specific questions.
      3. May affect medication choices in treatment (overdose potential and toxicity of medications).
   D. Mental illness diagnosis is based on the *Diagnostic and Statistical Manual of Mental Illness* (DSM-IV). This source provides criteria for each recognized mental disorder. Diagnosis is assigned to a system of five axises:
      1. Axis I: Clinical disorders.
      2. Axis II: Personality disorders and mental retardation.
      3. Axis III: Medical conditions.
      4. Axis IV: Psychosocial/environmental problems.
      5. Axis V: Global assessment of functioning (GAF) score ranging from 1 to 100 indicating level of impairment—the higher the number, the higher the functioning.

Table 35-2 Mental Status Assessment

Assessment Area	Assessment Data	Example Questions	Example Documentation
General Appearance	Gait, grooming and dress, behavior	Based on nurse's observations	"Overweight male who is unshaven with strong body odor, mismatched shoes, and unclean clothes. Gait is slow and exhibits poor eye contact."
Orientation	To person, place, time, situation	"Can you tell me what your name is? Where you are? What day and year it is? What season? Why you are here?"	"Client is oriented to person, place. Unable to identify date or reason for admission."
Mood and Affect	Subjective feelings, observed facial expressions	"Can you describe how you are feeling?" Affect is observed by nurse	"Client states feels 'numb and dead inside'. Affect is flat."
Speech	Type of pattern, pitch, volume	Observed by nurse	"Speech pattern is fast, pressured, and loud with flight of ideas."
Thought Processes	Ability and time needed to respond, connection of thoughts, abnormal thought patterns, thoughts of harm or fear, delusions, hallucinations, flight of ideas	"Are you hearing voices now? What are your thoughts now?"	"Client verbal responses are slow. Verbalizes a male voice telling him to 'hide the evidence' and 'don't tell the FBI.' Denies suicidal ideation or plan."
Cognition and Concentration	Recent and remote memory, basic knowledge, ability to assimilate new information	"Please remember the following three words: pencil, dog, balloon. I will ask you to repeat these words shortly." "What was the last holiday?" "Subtract 7 from 100 and keep subtracting 7 from your answer."	"Client is able to remember three items after 15 minutes. Identified last holiday as '4th of July' (current date is Feb 3). Unable to complete serial seven subtractions."
Abstract Reasoning and Comprehension	Ability to use abstract reasoning	"Can you explain the following: A penny saved is a penny earned?"	"Described the penny-saved proverb as 'somebody needs a better job if they only make a penny.'"
Insight and Judgment	Ability to understand accountability, illness and treatment	"What is your understanding of the reason your wife brought you to the hospital? What would you do if you saw a small child crying in the street?"	"I don't know why my wife brought me here; she is always saying that I am acting strange, but I am fine." "Client response to crying child was 'nobody should ever cry—the others will find you.' Became agitated when giving response."

Health Promotion

I. Definition: Mental health is affected by many factors, including illness or interpersonal factors. The goal of mental health promotion is to prevent illness and relapse. Therapeutic communication is the primary tool used by the nurse to deliver care to the client experiencing mental health problems.

A. Levels of mental health promotion

1. Primary prevention—prevent mental disorders and reduce disorders within a population: Activities include teaching alternatives to violence, and stress management; being active in preventive activities (e.g. gun control); and promoting self-esteem, parent-infant bonding, and respite care for caregivers.

2. Secondary prevention—identify mental health problems early to reduce duration of mental illness: Activities include promoting mental health screenings; providing referrals to mental health providers; and providing crisis intervention to individuals and communities after disasters (e.g., after flooding, tornadoes, or a bombing incident).
3. Tertiary prevention—focus on rehabilitation to minimize effects of mental illness: Activities include promoting support groups and social skill and vocational training for client and family.

B. Characteristics of therapeutic communication
1. Nurse's role
a. Assist client gain insight into feelings and behaviors.
b. Provide care that is goal-directed, open, concrete, and nonjudgmental.
c. Understand own values in order to be therapeutic.
2. Phases
a. Initial (introductory) phase—nurse builds trust, assesses client's feelings and actions, identifies primary problem, assesses anxiety level, and defines goals to achieve in conjunction with the client.
b. Working phase—nurse establishes and pursues specific objectives to achieve goals, focuses on and develops problem-solving and coping, explores feelings and emotions, and strives for client independence.

Table 35-3 Techniques for Therapeutic Communication

Therapeutic Communication Technique	Description	Example
Reflecting	Involves paraphrasing what the client has said to help identify the emotions involved.	Nurse: "What I hear you say is that you feel trapped in your current living situation. . . ."
Clarifying	Involves making sure the meaning of what the client has said is clearly understood.	Nurse: "You feel like your family is embarrassed by you?"
Broad Opening	Involves asking questions requiring more than a "yes" or "no" response.	Nurse: "Tell me what happened."
Summarizing	Involves summarization of discussion, or progress toward a goal to reinforce teaching.	Nurse: "The three things you have decided to do differently the next time your brother steals from you are . . ."
Using Silence	Can be supportive to demonstrate presence and acceptance of the client.	The nurse sits quietly by the client as she cries after talking about the death of her daughter.
Acknowledgment	Recognizes client's statement without imposing personal values.	Nurse: "You feel having an abortion is the best option for you?"
Confrontation	Restates mixed messages sent by client to promote discussion; this is an advanced skill that should be used cautiously.	Nurse: "You said you are angry that your son is ignoring you, but you refuse to take his phone calls."
Giving Information	Involves giving facts needed by the client.	Nurse: "Your group therapy has been moved to the day room this afternoon."
Exploring	Used to delve deeper into a topic without being intrusive.	Nurse: "Would you describe that statement more fully?"
Effective Use of Self-Disclosure	Used to help client open up—not to meet nurse's personal needs.	Nurse: "I remember feeling very tired and wondering if I would ever be able to sleep again when my children were very young. Do you have any friends or family that can help support you with your little ones?"
Establishing Boundaries	Protects client from actions that would impair recovery.	Nurse: "We are here to focus on your anger issues. This is not a time for talk about sexual issues."

c. Termination phase (goal is to terminate relationship)—nurse evaluates progress toward goals, discusses client's feelings about termination, and begins termination expectation in initial phase to foster independence in client.

3. Types of communication
   a. Verbal—involves spoken words.
   b. Nonverbal—communicates message using actions or behaviors; uses the five senses and includes tone of voice, pauses, body movement, gestures, dress, space, and touch.
4. Techniques
   a. Use active listening—involves being attentive and aware of cultural factors and nonverbal cues. See Table 35-3 for additional techniques to promote therapeutic communication.
   b. Avoid nontherapeutic communication—does not enhance the nurse-client relationship, creates a barrier to expressing feelings, and may hinder client progress. See Table 35-4 for nontherapeutic techniques.
   c. Recognizing client use of defense mechanisms—used to protect the person's ego from anxiety, guilt, and inadequacy; may be used unconsciously. See Table 35-5 for commonly used defense mechanisms.

II. General nursing interventions

A. Promote mental health—general principles include the following:

1. Form a therapeutic relationship with the client—set expectations and boundaries; develop trust; and provide consistency, respect, and a nonjudgmental attitude.
2. Provide goal-directed feedback to help the client move toward identified treatment goals and problem resolution.
3. Emphasize and reinforce progress toward positive results in client's thinking and behavior.
4. Promote safety for the client, other clients, and staff.
5. Identify physical needs—assess need for assistance with nutrition, activities of daily living, and elimination. Provide care for any current health issues (e.g., diabetes, infection, and hypertension).
6. Evaluate prescribed medications for appropriate drug, dose, timing, and route for the individual. Administer medications as prescribed. Assess for expected and adverse effects.
7. Provide client and family teaching regarding illness, treatment, and home care.
8. Promote coping skills (e.g., relaxation, nutrition, sleep, deep breathing, thought-stopping) to decrease stress and anxiety.
9. Evaluate client progress toward meeting identified goals—assess for improved functions in daily life as a result of nursing interventions. Progress evaluation may continue in a community-based care setting to assure ongoing absence of suicidal ideations or actions.

Table 35-4 Nontherapeutic Communication Techniques

Nontherapeutic Communication Technique	Description	Example
Closed-Ended Questions	Asking questions that can be answered with "yes" or "no" response.	Nurse: "Do you feel angry?"
False Reassurance	Suggesting there is no problem.	Nurse: "Don't worry. Lots of people have had this surgery with no problems."
Giving Advice	Making specific suggestions instead of offering information.	Nurse: "If I were you, I would . . ."
Changing Subject	Introducing a new topic to avoid a difficult or uncomfortable topic.	After client shares feeling of anger toward parent, the nurse says, "Are you ready for lunch?"
Challenging	Forcing a client to prove what he or she said.	Nurse: "How can you be the king of a country?"
Asking "Why"	Requesting rational explanation for irrational thoughts or behaviors.	Nurse: "Why did you think you could fly?"

Table 35-5 Commonly Used Defense Mechanisms

Defense Mechanism	Definition	Example
Repression	Unpleasant or unwanted experiences or emotions are kept from conscious awareness.	A victim of an assault does not remember anything about the incident.
Projection	Attributing person's own, unacceptable feelings to someone else.	A woman with a crush on her boss tells a coworker that the boss asked her for a date.
Displacement	Transferring feelings associated with one person or event to another person who is seen as less threatening.	After being reprimanded at work, a husband comes home and yells at his wife.
Denial	Unconscious refusal to believe a reality that is not what one wants or is too painful to face.	A client who has received a cancer diagnosis tells his family that all of the tests came back negative.
Rationalization	Trying to explain one's unacceptable behavior by presenting reasons that are meant to sound logical.	A client tells the nurse that if her husband were a better provider she would not use drugs.
Identification	Attempt to imitate someone else.	A teenager dresses like his favorite actor.
Introjection	Incorporation of values of an admired person into your own actions.	A young mother disciplines her child in the same manner as her grandmother.
Regression	Returning to an earlier level of functioning under stress.	A hospitalized child who is 7 years of age and does not wet the bed begins wetting the bed.
Undoing	Behavior to atone for previous actions.	A young woman volunteers at an orphanage after giving up a child for adoption.
Intellectualization	Using logical reasoning to separate from emotional involvement in situation.	After having a stillborn baby, a young mother describes the statistics related to infant mortality.
Reaction Formation	Behaviors that are the opposite of what is actually felt.	A person who dislikes elderly people volunteers at a nursing home.
Compensation	Striving for excellence in one area to compensate for a perceived weakness in another.	A worker with low self-esteem volunteers for double-shifts so the supervisor will like him or her.
Transference	Feelings and thought a client has toward nurse or other staff.	The client cries every time a certain nurse is on duty as the nurse reminds the client of his daughter, who died 3 years ago.
Countertransference	Feelings and thoughts a nurse or other staff has toward the client.	The client reminds the nurse of his father, who was an alcoholic who emotionally abused the nurse's mother.

B. Provide interventions specific to biologic, psychologic, and social-environmental factors contributing to mental health problem.
   1. Biologic interventions
      a. Encourage and assist with self-care activities.
      b. Promote sleep, activity, and exercise balance.
      c. Meet nutrition, hydration, and elimination needs.
      d. Provide pain management.
      e. Administer medications.
   2. Psychologic interventions
      a. Develop therapeutic relationship (see later discussion).
      b. Provide basic counseling.
      c. Develop conflict resolution skills.
      d. Follow through with behavior-modification therapy.
      e. Reinforce cognitive therapy strategies.

f. Provide health teaching to client and family.
g. Provide spiritual care as needed or requested.
h. Enhance relaxation skills.

3. Social interventions
a. Provide milieu therapy to foster growth.
b. Maintain safety.
c. Enhance group skills (e.g., encourage recreational activities).
d. Improve family interactions.
e. Promote communication skills.
f. Promote anger-management skills.

Principles of Nursing Care Management

I. Definition: Principles of managing care for the client with a psychiatric disorder or mental health problem include initiating appropriate treatment modalities, administering medications, and collaborating and communicating with the health care team.

II. Treatment modalities

A. Milieu therapy
1. Definition: Refers to the planned use of resources within the environment to promote client functioning, coping, and healing; and to allow the client to live outside the clinical setting.
2. Goal: Improves interpersonal skills, social functioning and activities of daily living.
3. Characteristics
a. Assists client manage with current reality.
b. Uses limit setting.
c. Involves client in decisions about care.
d. Supports client privacy.
e. Uses clear expectations for client.
f. Allows client to work toward treatment goal.
g. Allows client to receive feedback from treatment team.
4. Example: The client who exhibits an angry outburst in the dining room is escorted to her room to allow time to regain control. This action promotes an opportunity for the client to use coping skills and receive feedback from the treatment team, maintains limits set for behaviors, and protects fellow clients and staff.

B. Behavior modification
1. Definition: Behaviors involve responses to stimuli; because responses can be measured, behaviors can be changed. Therapy focuses on self-control, social skills training, and problem-solving.
2. Goal: Strengthens a desired behavior or response.
3. Characteristics
a. Positive reinforcement strengthens desired behavior.
b. Negative reinforcement (e.g., ignoring undesirable actions) decreases unwanted behavior.
c. Involves role modeling and teaching new behaviors.
d. Uses token economy system—client receives a reward for tokens earned from demonstrating positive behaviors.
e. Uses aversion (desensitization) therapy—involves teaching relaxation and coping mechanisms, and then exposing the client to low-anxiety situations in order to progress through higher anxiety-producing situations until the client can manage the anxiety.
4. Example: A group home has an established "token economy" system, where desired behaviors for each client are documented on a chart. At the end of the week, the client receives a token for each desired behavior, which can be traded in for snacks, free time, or some other reward.

C. Cognitive behavioral therapy
1. Definition: Aims to change patterns of thinking by helping the client recognize and replace negative thoughts with alternate patterns of thinking. Altered thinking leads to altered mood, which can then alter behaviors.
2. Goal: Changes negative distortions in thinking to provide relief of symptoms.
3. Characteristics
a. Thought-stopping uses a verbal or physical cue to stop a negative thought and replace it with a more positive one.
b. Cognitive restructuring has client turn a negative message into a positive one.
c. Positive self-talk changes the client's thinking about themselves from negative to positive.
d. Decatastrophizing focuses on learning to assess situations realistically rather than assuming the very worst will happen.
4. Example: When the client recognizes the thought of "I'm so stupid," he snaps a rubber band on his wrist while saying, "Stop!" The client then replaces the thought with, "I can solve this problem."

D. Crisis intervention
1. Definition: Seeks resolution of immediate crisis client can't handle alone.

2. Goal: Alleviates anxiety, reinforces positive coping and problem-solving, and identifies supports available to the client in order to return client to precrisis level of functioning.
3. Characteristics
   a. Maturational crisis: Involves developmental stages in life process such as leaving home or beginning a career.
   b. Situational crisis: Involves unanticipated events that threaten person's integrity, such as loss of spouse or employment.
   c. Adventitious crisis: Involves crisis outside the person's control, such as hurricane, riots, or a violent crime.
4. Example: A client is unable to make any decisions after the sudden death of her husband in an accident. The client's daughter helps her mother with important decisions during this period of crisis.

E. Group therapy
1. Definition: Brings together clients with common purposes (see characteristics).
2. Goal: Develops better relationships and coping through client learning new information and coping techniques, developing feelings of acceptance and hope, and gaining insight into consequences of behaviors.
3. Characteristics
   a. Psychotherapy groups focus on learning and altering behaviors.
   b. Family therapy focuses on communication and interactions among family members as they deal with family issues.
   c. Education groups provide information to group members on a specific topic (e.g., stress management or medications).
   d. Support groups help clients learn to cope.
   e. Self-help groups provide support; sessions may be led by a member of the group.
4. Example: A client's family members attend a monthly session to learn how to support the client's attempts to manage his addiction to pain medication.

F. Activity therapy
1. Definition: Uses various types of activities to enhance life skills of the client.
2. Goal: Assists client to develop coping skills, gain employment, and use positive, healthy means of expression.
3. Characteristics
   a. Occupational therapy enhances employment skills.
   b. Recreational therapy develops hobbies and interests.
   c. Music, art, pet, writing therapy increases coping, insight, and relaxation.
   d. Relaxation therapies decrease stress and anxiety, and increase coping.
4. Examples: The client attends groups that help him learn how to balance his checkbook, and improve his skills related to shopping, cooking, and relaxation.

G. Electroconvulsive therapy (ECT)
1. Definition: Uses pulses of small doses of electrical energy to one or both sides of the brain to cause a brief, controlled seizure to decrease depressive symptoms. This controlled seizure most likely modifies the neurotransmitters of the brain that affect mood.
2. Goal: Relieves mental illness symptoms.
3. Characteristics
   a. Indicated for severely depressed client nonresponsive to other treatments, pregnant client requiring treatment, and actively suicidal client when unable to wait for medication effects.
   b. Performed under anesthesia with continuous monitoring.
   c. Care is same for any procedure using anesthesia (NPO morning of treatment; void before procedure; remove dentures; apply hospital gown; and obtain signed consent).
   d. Nursing responsibilities involve providing emotional and educational support, preparing client for procedure, and monitoring and evaluating client response to procedure.
   e. Most common side effect is a temporary loss of short-term memory.
   f. Usually given in a series of two to three treatments per week for a period of 2 to 6 weeks.
4. Example: A client who is unable to tolerate side effects of antidepressants is becoming increasingly depressed with suicidal ideations. The treatment team determines the client will benefit from a course of ECT to relieve the depression.

H. Phototherapy
1. Definition: Used for the mood disorder, seasonal affective disorder.
2. Goal: Relieves symptoms of depression; most often used for seasonal depression (e.g., typically occurs in winter months).
3. Characteristics
   a. Therapy consists of using artificial light daily to affect serotonin and melatonin levels, which in turn affects mood.

b. A special, filtered light is used.
c. Side effects are rare.

4. Example: After noticing a pattern of depression occurring in December of each year, the client started receiving phototherapy each November to offset the effects of the shortened winter days.

III. Pharmacotherapy

1. Definition: Impacts the mental health of a client through use of medications.
2. Goal: Relieves symptoms of dysfunctional thoughts, moods, or actions.
3. Characteristics
   a. Close monitoring of clients is needed to assess side effects.
   b. Serum laboratory tests may be needed to monitor medication levels.
4. Example: A client's hallucinations are well controlled by the prescribed medication.

IV. General nursing interventions

A. Withdrawn client
1. Avoid punishment.
2. Limit isolation.
3. Plan time to be with client whether or not client chooses to speak.
4. Ask nonthreatening questions and wait for response.

B. Dependant client
1. Assess abilities of client to make decisions and perform activities of daily living.
2. Limit amount of assistance; provide only help that is needed.
3. Avoid making decisions for client—encourage problem-solving.
4. Show attitude of confidence in client's abilities.
5. Provide positive feedback when client does appropriate activities.
6. Promote involvement in activities.

C. Angry client
1. Encourage verbalization of feelings.
2. Identify and practice appropriate expressions of emotion.
3. Explore causes of emotions.
4. Consistently and nonjudgmentally reinforce unit rules if client acts out.
5. Protect safety of client and others.

D. Aggressive client
1. Assess for escalating behaviors or anger.
2. Do not avoid client.
3. Encourage verbalization of feelings as events occur.
4. Reduce stimuli or remove client from stimuli.
5. Follow agency policy related to unacceptable behavior.
6. Protect safety of client and others.
7. Speak slowly and softly.
8. Keep a comfortable distance from client—be prepared to move quickly.
9. Stay with client, but avoid touching or physical contact.

E. Suspicious or paranoid client
1. Give clear and straightforward explanations.
2. Keep appointments and commitments.
3. Use jokes with extreme caution as the client may not interpret correctly.
4. Assist client to correctly interpret environmental stimuli.
5. Project a kind, but neutral affect to client.
6. Warn about any changes, any side effects from medications, and any reasons for treatment delays.
7. Provide for client and others' safety needs.

F. Client experiencing grief and loss
1. Understand stages client and family experience during the death and dying process; Kübler-Ross stages of death and dying include the following:
   a. Denial—usually temporary, involves a denial of diagnosis or situation.
   b. Anger—client becomes angry at family and others.
   c. Bargaining—most bargains made with God specific to client religious beliefs; often involves requesting more time.
   d. Depression—client realizes cannot deny situation any longer; physical symptoms begin to appear.
   e. Acceptance—if allowed time and help to work through stages, client will reach a stage of readiness or peace about dying.
2. Support loss and grief throughout the lifespan.
   a. Infant-toddler (1 to 3 years of age)
      (1) Client has no real concept of death; reacts to separation and changes in rituals.
      (2) Nursing interventions: Encourage parental involvement; help parents deal with their feelings.
   b. Preschooler (3 to 5 years of age)
      (1) Client perceives death as sleep; finality of death not understood; illness and death seen as a punishment for actions.
      (2) Nursing interventions: Use play therapy to express thoughts regarding death; explain that death is not "sleep"; allow choice of attending funeral.
   c. School age (5 to 12 years of age)
      (1) Client may have fantasies of the unknown regarding what happens

to body after death; anxiety released by nightmares and superstitions.

(2) Nursing interventions: Answer questions regarding funerals, status of dead person; accept regression or angry behaviors; encourage verbalization of feelings.

d. Adolescent (12 to 18 years of age)

(1) Client has more mature understanding of death; may experience and show strong emotions; may ask questions regarding death.

(2) Nursing interventions: Encourage verbalization of fears and feelings (e.g., "Can you tell me how you are feeling?"); solicit support.

3. Investigate the meaning of the loss for the client. "How will your life be different now?"
4. Anticipate and support the client through the stages of grief. "Let me explain what the lab values mean."
5. Identify coping mechanisms useful for the client. "How have you handled stress in the past?"
6. Encourage review of client's strengths and capabilities despite changes. "What do you see as your strengths?"

V. Legal principles involved in planning care for the client with a mental health problem

A. Voluntary admission
1. Client voluntarily enters a treatment program without a court order.
2. Should client request discharge, the treatment team may agree to discharge the client, or initiate an involuntary admission process.

B. Involuntary admission
1. Client is admitted to a treatment program against his or her will.
2. Critical criteria to determine involuntary admission is based on client risk as danger to self or others; client gravely disabled; criteria varies in each state.
3. Client retains civil rights; involuntary admission does not automatically mean a person is incompetent.

C. Incompetence—determined by a court of law that a client is so impaired he or she is unable to make treatment and legal decisions. A client must have a representative for the legal proceedings to determine competence.

D. Restraints—physical or chemical (medication) methods of restricting a client's physical activity. Many health facilities follow a "no restraint" policy for care because of safety concerns for the client. Special care protocols and documentation must be followed when any type of restraint is used. The least restrictive means are used. Types of restraints are as follows:
1. Physical restraint: Devices such as vests, mittens, belts, or ties used to control physical movements to decrease risk for client self-harm and harm to others.
2. Chemical restraint: Medications used to sedate or calm disruptive or aggressive behaviors.
3. Seclusion: Involves isolating a client in a room from which he or she cannot leave. Relates to safety concerns for the client or others and acts to decrease stimuli and avoid property damage. Specific protocols must be followed.

E. Additional legal principles related to planning care include client rights, confidentiality, and informed consent (see Chapter 40).

VI. Legal principles related to liability for care for the client with a mental health problem (see also Chapter 40)

A. Malpractice—performance of care below the standard of care by a professional, resulting in injury to the plaintiff.

B. Negligence—commitment of an act that a reasonable person would not have done, or omission of a duty a reasonable person would have performed.

C. Invasion of privacy—violation of another person's right to be left alone and free from unwarranted contact.

D. Defamation of character—any untrue communication to another in written format (libel) or spoken (slander) that brings injury or damage of the reputation of another person.

E. False imprisonment—unjustifiable detention of a client.

F. Respondeat superior—acts of employees are attributable to employer, who will also be held responsible for injury to a plaintiff.

G. Battery—touching another without consent.

H. Assault—any action that causes a person to fear being touched without consent and in a way that is offensive.

VII. Ethical concepts related to nursing care involve philosophic viewpoints that deal with values of rightness and wrongness of actions. Ethical concepts of nursing care are presented in Chapter 40.

Bibliography

American Psychiatric Association. (2000). *Diagnostic and statistical manual of mental disorders* (4th ed., text revision). Washington, DC: American Psychiatric Association.

American Psychiatric Nurses Association www.apna.org

American Psychological Association. *Mental health patient's bill of rights.* Retrieved June 6, 2008 from http://www.apa.org/pubinfo/rights

Boyd, M. A. (2005). *Psychiatric nursing: Contemporary practice* (3rd ed.). Philadelphia: Lippincott Williams & Wilkins.

Canadian Federation of Mental Health Nurses. Canadian Standards of psychiatric nursing practice. Retrieved from www.cfmhn.org

Mohr, W. K. (2006). *Psychiatric-mental health nursing* (6th ed.). Philadelphia: Lippincott Williams & Wilkins.

Taylor, C., Lillis, C., & LeMone, P. (2005). *Fundamentals of nursing: The art and science of nursing care.* Philadelphia: Lippincott Williams & Wilkins.

U.S. Department of Health and Human Services, Centers for Medicare and Medicaid Services. *Regulations regarding use of seclusion and restraints.* Retrieved June 6, 2008 from http://www.cms.gov

Vidabeck, S. L. (2004). *Psychiatric-mental health nursing* (2nd ed.). Philadelphia: Lippincott Williams & Wilkins.

Zerwekh, J., & Claborn, J. C. (2006). *Illustrated study guide for the NCLEX-RN exam* (6th ed.). St. Louis: Mosby Elsevier.

CHAPTER 35

Practice Test

Background Information

1. The nurse is assessing the mental health status of a group of individuals. Which of the following individuals should the nurse determine to be mentally healthy?
- □ 1. Client who is 30 years of age and experiencing difficulty adapting to changes.
- □ 2. Client who is 40 years of age and demonstrates knowledge of self.
- □ 3. Client who is 25 years of age who has never had an interpersonal relationship.
- □ 4. Client who is 16 years of age who seeks isolation and seclusion.

2. The nurse is teaching a small group about mental illness. The nurse should teach the group to identify which of the following as being an important indicator of mental illness?
- □ 1. Ability to acknowledge problems in functioning.
- □ 2. Understanding that physical symptoms occur with mental symptoms.
- □ 3. Symptoms cause impairment in functioning.
- □ 4. Accepting the fact that medications are needed for the illness.

3. A client is admitted to the inpatient psychiatric unit. He states that his "anxiety is unmanageable." Which of the following activities is appropriate for this client?
- □ 1. Participating in a game such as Monopoly with other clients.
- □ 2. Daily walks with the nurse.
- □ 3. Bingo with a small group.
- □ 4. Softball game with two teams.

4. A client is exhibiting suspicious behavior and expresses a fear of sharing and asking for help. Using an Eriksonian model, the nurse would describe this client as being in which stage of development?
- □ 1. Initiative versus guilt.
- □ 2. Trust versus mistrust.
- □ 3. Generativity versus stagnation.
- □ 4. Identity versus role confusion.

Health Assessment

5. The nurse is conducting an initial assessment of a client with a mental health problem. Which statement made by the client is the client's chief complaint?
- □ 1. "I can always trust my wife."
- □ 2. "You never know who will turn against you."
- □ 3. "I've been hearing the voices of my dead parents and can't work."
- □ 4. "I wish I knew what I've done to deserve so much persecution."

6. AF The nurse is conducting an admission interview with a client and is assessing for risk factors related to the client's safety. The nurse should include which of the following in this targeted assessment? Select all that apply.
- □ 1. Suicide or self-harm ideation.
- □ 2. Incentives that motivate the client.
- □ 3. Recent use of substances of abuse.
- □ 4. Allergic reactions or adverse drug reactions.
- □ 5. Dietary preferences.

7. A client being admitted to the inpatient mental health unit for depression makes several comments about her husband, who died 4 years ago. She states she is getting tired of being alone and is anxious for him to come back and help her take care of all of the details at the house. What does this behavior suggest to the nurse?

- □ 1. The client is having a healthy grief reaction.
- □ 2. The client is experiencing dysfunctional grief.
- □ 3. The client is having delayed grief.
- □ 4. The client needs an immediate referral to a social worker.

8. The nurse is assessing an elderly client diagnosed with diabetes and chronic obstructive pulmonary disease (COPD) whose spouse died 3 weeks ago. Which of the following should the nurse address first?

- □ 1. Respirations of 16 to 20 per minute.
- □ 2. Expressed thoughts of being "better off dead."
- □ 3. Guilt about what was done at the time of the spouse's death.
- □ 4. A weight loss of 5 pounds in the last 2 weeks.

Health Promotion

9. The nurse has identified the client goal of: "Client will remain safe during hospitalization with the assistance of staff." Which nursing intervention is best related to this goal?

- □ 1. Offer high-calorie fluids as between-meal nourishment.
- □ 2. Assist client to identify three personal strengths.
- □ 3. Observe client for attendance at group sessions.
- □ 4. Implement suicide precautions.

10. A client who is receiving an antianxiety medication is reluctant to participate in group therapy. The client states, "I'm taking medicine to handle my stress. I don't need to talk about my problems." The nurse should base the response to the client on which of the following?

- □ 1. Group therapy is an immediate treatment for anxiety.
- □ 2. Medications relieve symptoms, but do not change the source of anxiety.
- □ 3. The client will need to attend group therapy only until the medication becomes effective.
- □ 4. The medications will not work unless the client participates in group therapy.

11. Which of the following actions is characteristic during the working phase of the therapeutic relationship between nurse and client?

- □ 1. The nurse evaluates the relationship.
- □ 2. The client expresses thoughts and feelings.
- □ 3. The nurse and client establish goals.
- □ 4. The nurse and client establish trust.

12. A client who is 67 years of age was widowed 8 months ago. Her family was amazed at her strength and calmness immediately after the funeral. Today, her son has brought her to the emergency department after she called him on the phone to say she was going to take an overdose of sleeping pills because she just realized she was all alone. Which defense mechanism has the client been using until now?

- □ 1. Denial.
- □ 2. Projection.
- □ 3. Introjection.
- □ 4. Reaction formation.

13. The parents of a dying child who is 2 years of age complain loudly about the care the child is receiving, and make constant requests of the nursing staff. What interventions by the nurse would be most appropriate?

- □ 1. Refer parents to the hospital clergy staff.
- □ 2. Ask parents if they would like to express their concerns to the physician.
- □ 3. Tell parents that if they cannot be quieter they will have to leave.
- □ 4. Allow parents to share their emotions about their child's impending death.

14. A client says to the nurse, "I don't know what to do. I can't decide if I should tell my son to move out unless he stops drinking. What do you think I should do?" What would be the best response by the nurse?

- □ 1. "I think you should ask your son to leave. You will feel better if you do."
- □ 2. "You are too tired to make a decision right now. Just wait awhile and things will probably work out anyway."
- □ 3. "I had a daughter that dropped out of college. I called her and told her she couldn't live at home anymore. You might try calling your son."
- □ 4. "I can help you look at the positives and negatives of the decision, but it is important that you make this decision."

Principles of Nursing Care Management

15. A female client who is 22 years of age and has diagnosis of borderline personality disorder is manipulative and very disruptive on the hospital unit. She is not dangerous to herself or others, but is clearly not making any therapeutic progress. She consistently refuses any medications. The nurse realizes that legally this client has which option?

- □ 1. Refuse treatment.
- □ 2. Receive forced treatment if the nursing team concurs.

□ 3. Be medicated if her family signs permission for treatment.
□ 4. Be guided to accept treatment recommendations by threatening loss of privileges.

16. A client has been involuntarily committed to a hospital because he has been assessed as being dangerous to self or others. The client has lost which of the following rights?
□ 1. The right to refuse medications and treatments.
□ 2. The right to send and receive uncensored mail.
□ 3. Freedom from seclusion and restraints.
□ 4. The right to leave the hospital against medical advice (AMA).

17. The risk-management nurse is doing a review of incident reports and recognizes that the theory of "respondeat superior" does not apply to which incident?
□ 1. A nurse who slapped a client while running an inpatient medication group.
□ 2. A nurse who had contact with and injured a client in the nurse's home.
□ 3. A nurse who made a medication error that resulted in the death of a client.
□ 4. A nurse who accidentally tripped and fell on an elderly client, resulting in a broken hip of the client.

18. A nurse hears a client state, "I've had it with this marriage. It would be so much easier to just hire someone to kill my husband!" What action should the nurse take?
□ 1. Since the client is still admitted to the hospital, the nurse must hold the statement in confidence.
□ 2. The nurse must start the process to warn the client's husband.
□ 3. An assessment of the client's response to treatment must be performed.
□ 4. The comment must be held in confidence because the client did not report the statement directly to the nurse.

19. A client states that she met a friend named Tony at the mall over the weekend while on a pass off of the mental health unit. Which response by the nurse would best encourage the client describe her relationship with Tony?
□ 1. "Isn't Tony the guy your friend is divorcing?"
□ 2. "Tell me more about what you did at the mall."
□ 3. "Tell me about you and Tony."
□ 4. "Weren't you supposed to go bowling on your pass?"

20. A client is taking olanzapine (Zyprexa). The client, who states he is being poisoned, refuses to take his scheduled medication. The nurse states, "If you don't take your medication, you will be put into seclusion." The nurse's statement is an example of which legal concept?
□ 1. Assault.
□ 2. Battery.
□ 3. Malpractice.
□ 4. Invasion of privacy.

Answers and Rationales

1. 2 Mental health is the ability to understand self, meet basic needs, assume responsibility for behavior, accurately interpret reality, and maintain relationships. Difficulty adapting, poor interpersonal relationships, and excessive seclusion do not indicate mental health. (H)

2. 3 Mental illness symptoms are determined by impairment of functioning, inability to adapt, excessive anxiety, fear, or suspiciousness, and withdrawal from society. This response must be beyond expected reaction to events and not a cultural response. Mental health occurs when the client can acknowledge the symptoms, understand that physical symptoms accompany mental health symptoms, and that medication may be needed to manage mental illness. (P)

3. 2 Taking walks with the nurse allows the client to develop trust in the nurse. Walking also allows an outlet for anxious energy. Monopoly, softball, and bingo are group activities that do not allow for the development of trust; the competitiveness of any game may also increase anxiety. (P)

4. 2 In the trust versus mistrust stage, the client is developing the ability to view the world as safe and develop trust in relationships. Being suspicious and not interrelating with others does not demonstrate that this stage has been mastered. Initiative versus guilt addresses managing conflict. Generativity versus stagnation addresses being creative and productive. Identity versus role confusion addresses developing a sense of belonging. (H)

5. 3 The reason a client seeks care is the chief complaint; in this case, the correct answer involves the client who hears voices. There are no data to indicate that not trusting a spouse or others and feeling persecuted have impaired the client's ability to function to cause the client to seek care. (H)

6. 1, 3, 4 When assessing client safety, the nurse assesses suicide thoughts or plan, recent use of illicit drugs (as they may cause impaired judgment or thought processes), and previously experienced allergic reactions and adverse reactions to medications. Note that safety involves many aspects of care. Incentives and diet preferences (allergies would be previously noted) are not directly related to safety, although they may be part of an overall assessment. (S)

7. 2 After 4 years, the client should rarely refer to her deceased spouse in the present tense. Continuing to do so, along with the hope he will come back home and the depression, are indications of dysfunctional grief. A healthy grief reaction may reflect sadness, but acknowledge the reality of the spouse being gone. Delayed grief would be more intense and the client would exhibit the typical stages of loss. A social work referral may be helpful, but does not address the client's lack of acceptance of the loss of her spouse. (P)

8. 2 A client who verbalizes thoughts about being "better off dead" is at high risk for suicide and should be referred for evaluation and intervention. This client has at least the depression risk factors of being elderly, recent loss, and underlying chronic illness. Respirations of 16 to 20 and occasional shortness of breath is to be expected with COPD. Guilt about events of a recent loss is not unusual as the person processes the event. Weight loss may be linked to the underlying illness or the depressive symptoms, but a 5-pound loss is not likely an immediate threat to health. (H)

9. 4 Suicide precautions are directly related to keeping a client safe while hospitalized. Between-meal snacks addresses nutritional needs and helps protect fluid and electrolyte status, but is not an immediate safety concern. Identifying personal strengths and attendance at group sessions assists the client with self-esteem and learning, but are not directly associated with immediate safety. (S)

10. 2 Taking antianxiety medications assists with the symptoms of stress and anxiety, but they do not change the underlying causes of the stress. Group therapy helps develop better relationships and coping skills, but there are many other possible causes of stress. Antianxiety medications tend to take effect quickly. The medications will decrease anxiety without group therapy, but long-term management of stress would include learning to recognize the sources and how to better manage them without medications in the future. (P)

11. 2 The working phase is used to establish and pursue specific objectives to achieve goals, develop and focus on problem-solving and coping, and explore feelings and emotions. Establishing goals and trust occurs in the initial or introductory phase. Evaluation occurs in the termination phase. (H)

12. 1 Persons in a state of denial do not acknowledge painful or unwanted events; once this mechanism no longer could be maintained by the client, she decompensated quickly. Projection is attributing one's own feelings to another. Introjection is incorporating values of an admired person into your own actions. Reaction formation is behavior that is the opposite of what is actually felt. (P)

13. 4 Facing the death of a child places great stress on parents, who may project their helplessness and anger onto caregivers. The nurse can help parents express their feelings and recognize their inability to prevent the death, thus becoming a partner in the process. Referring the parents to clergy may be helpful for spiritual distress, but does not directly address their feelings about the death. Telling the physician about the concerns separates the nurse from the parents, and does not allow the formation of a trusting bond. Threatening the parents with eviction if they are not quiet sets up a confrontational situation that is not therapeutic. (P)

14. 4 Therapeutically, the nurse assists the client make goals and decrease the anxiety of situations while encouraging appropriate responsibility by the client. Giving advice, encouraging the client to avoid difficult decisions, and inappropriate self-disclosure are not methods that promote growth in the client. (P)

15. 1 A client who is not gravely disabled, has not been deemed a danger to self or others, or who has not been declared incompetent retains the right to refuse treatment. Legal protocols need to be followed to initiate treatment against an adult client's wishes, even if the family wishes treatment to occur. Punitive threats of retaliation or loss of privileges are ethically unacceptable in administering treatment. (M)

16. 4 An involuntarily admitted client loses the right to leave the hospital until the condition is stable enough that the client no longer poses a danger to self or others. While hospitalized, the client retains all civil rights such as receiving mail, making phone calls, refusing treatment, and also receiving the least restrictive treatment. Should the involuntarily admitted client refuse treatment once admitted, he will be evaluated for the need to receive treatment against wishes in order to decrease the risk for self-harm or harm to others. (M)

17. 2 Respondeat superior refers to acts of employees that are attributable to the employer, who will also be held responsible for injury to a plaintiff. The nurse who saw a client in her own home was not acting as an agent of a larger system, the employer. Events that happened in the workplace would fall under this principle. (M)

18. 2 Based on the Tarasoff rule, confidentiality must be broken if there are credible threats made against another person's safety. Confidentiality does not override the safety of other persons. (M)

19. 3 Asking a broad question about the client and the other person is most likely to elicit comments about the relationship. Focusing questions on the other person gains information about the person, but not about the relationship. Asking what was done at the mall or what was done on the pass does not address the relationship. (P)

20. 1 The nurse's statement exemplifies assault, which is the threat of being touched in an offensive way without consent. Battery is touching another person without consent. Malpractice is care below the standard of care that results in injury. Invasion of privacy is a violation of a person's right to be left alone. (M)

chapter 36

The Client With Mood and Anxiety Disorders and the Client at Risk for Suicide

Mood disorders are characterized by disturbances in thinking or feelings that cause psychologic distress and behavioral impairment. These disturbances may occur along a continuum ranging from severe depression to elation, or mania. Approximately 18 million American adults have some type of mood disorder in a given year, and some may be at risk for suicide. Anxiety disorders are characterized by cognitive and psychologic symptoms such as fearfulness and dread, as well as physiologic symptoms such as increased cardiac and respiratory rates. Somatoform disorders, an anxiety-related disorder, involves experiencing physical symptoms for which there are no identified causes. Family and friends of those who have a mood disorder or suffer from anxiety or somatoform disorders are significantly impacted. The nurse has an important role in assisting the client and family to obtain early diagnosis, promoting mental health, and implementing plans for health maintenance. Topics discussed in this chapter include:

- Depression
- Bipolar Disorder
- Anxiety and Somatoform Disorders
- The Client at Risk for Suicide

Depression

I. Definition: Depression is a disorder defined by client experience of loss of interest in normal activities, and a depressed mood lasting for at least 2 weeks (see assessment signs and symptoms of depression). Depression often occurs in conjunction with other mental health diagnoses and is prevalent in clients with chronic illness or prolonged hospitalization.

A. Types
1. Dysthymic disorder is a milder depressive illness in which symptoms are chronic (at least 2 years' duration), but less severe than major depression.
2. Postpartum depression is a depressive episode occurring after childbirth (see also Chapter 7).
3. Seasonal affective disorder (SAD) involves recurrent depression at a particular time of year, especially when light is decreased (winter months).

B. Etiology: The exact causes of depression is not known; some contributing factors may include:
1. Genetic predisposition.
2. Neurochemical imbalances in the brain (dopamine, serotonin, and norepinephrine).
3. Effect of light on mood (e.g., SAD).
4. Medications and medical conditions.
5. Psychosocial influences (traumatic life event, dysfunctional family influences).

II. Nursing process

A. Assessment: Perform assessments in short segments if client exhibits underlying difficulty in concentration or energy.
1. Obtain a detailed health history and perform a comprehensive physical examination; assess the following:
   a. Presence of medical condition that may cause client condition (e.g., heart disease, stroke, diabetes, cancer, acquired immunodeficiency syndrome, hypothyroidism).
   b. Previous episode of depression.
   c. Gender—nearly twice as prevalent in females.
   d. Age—average age of onset is in the mid-20s.
   e. Marital status—single or widowed at higher risk.
   f. Current or past use of alcohol, illicit drugs, prescription drugs, over-the-counter drugs, and herbal drugs.
   g. Family history of mental illness.
   h. Psychologic factors—low self-esteem, guilt.
   i. Type of stressors or losses client currently perceives, including environmental or situational factors (e.g., stressful life event, lack of support).
   j. Suicidal ideation—critical assessment for all clients related to safety.
2. Assess for signs and symptoms.
   a. Affective—anxiety, anhedonia (loss of interest in pleasurable activities), sad or irritable mood
   b. Motivational—loss of interest in daily activities, feelings of hopelessness, suicidal thoughts or acts
   c. Cognitive—difficulty concentrating, sense of guilt, negative self-image
   d. Somatic (physical)—physical complaints of pain or discomfort
   e. Neurovegetative—decreased appetite, sleep disturbances, constipation, decreased interest in sex (decreased libido) slowed motor activity (psychomotor slowdown)
3. Obtain diagnostic tests.
   a. Mental status exam—standardized assessment tools (e.g., Beck Depression Inventory, Geriatric Depression Scale, Hamilton Rating Scale for Depression)
   b. Laboratory tests—often include checking electrolytes, CBC, and thyroid levels for imbalances
   c. Nutritional assessment including caffeine intake and vitamin deficiencies

B. Analysis
1. Risk for Self-Directed Violence related to depressed mood, feelings of hopelessness, suicide ideation or plan
2. Ineffective Coping related to lack of energy and inability to concentrate
3. Imbalanced Nutrition: Less/More Than Body Requirements related to decreased or increased intake
4. Disturbed Sleep Pattern related to stress and chemical imbalance (serotonin)
5. Anxiety related to situational or environmental stressors
6. Spiritual Distress related to terminal illness
7. Self-Care Deficit: Grooming, Feeding, and/or Hygiene, related to psychomotor retardation
8. Dysfunctional Grieving related to death of spouse
9. Social Isolation related to fear of animals
10. Chronic Low Self-Esteem related to lack of success in employment

C. Planning
1. Promote safety.
2. Promote verbalization of suicidal ideations, if present.
3. Promote self-care activities.

4. Promote coping strategies.
5. Promote adherence to medication regimen.
6. Promote adequate sleep pattern.
7. Initiate social interactions with staff, family, and friends.
8. Identify purpose and use of prescribed medications.

D. Implementation
1. Provide interventions to maintain safety: Monitor for self-harm risk and implement safety measures as needed (see safety and infection control).
2. Teach client about disorder and any treatments; instill hope through teaching.
3. Encourage social interactions; collaborate with other disciplines to develop plan for music, art, exercise therapy, and journal activities to express feelings.
4. Administer prescribed antidepressant medications; work with client to manage side effects of treatments or medications.
5. Promote adequate nutrition.
   a. Determine daily nutritional requirements—may need dietary consult.
   b. Record intake and output.
   c. Monitor weight.
   d. Offer small, frequent meals.
   e. Assist client to eat as needed.
   f. Monitor nutrition-related laboratory values (e.g., glucose, electrolytes, albumin levels).

E. Evaluation
1. Client remains safe from harm.
2. Client performs self-care activities.
3. Client attends prescribed therapy sessions.
4. Client demonstrates improved socialization and initiation of interactions.
5. Client exhibits desired effects from medications and is free from side effects of medications.
6. Client verbalizes decreased anxiety and increased ability to cope with current situation.
7. Client expresses plans for the future.
8. Client and support system use knowledge of disorder and medications to manage depression after discharge.

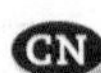

III. Client needs

A. Physiologic adaptation
1. Chemical imbalances cause neurovegetative signs in a person with depression—nurse assists in normalizing behavior and instilling hope.
2. Situational events may result in feelings of powerlessness, and alterations in sleep, and eating—nurse helps to identify situations within client's control and assists to maintain adequate nutrition and sleep.
3. Current medications increase the availability of neurotransmitters, which result in increased mood and energy—nurse provides teaching on proper medication administration, effects and side effects of medications.
4. Side effects of antidepressants affect many body systems—nurse provides close monitoring of cardiovascular status and promotes safety.
5. Client status may change rapidly—nurse frequently assesses client's mental status and risk.
6. Medical illnesses sometimes presents as depression—nurse monitors diagnostic tests and laboratory work for physical state, effects of medication, and therapeutic blood levels.

B. Management of care: Care of the client with depression requires critical thinking skills and knowledge of assessment, and teaching and evaluation methods unique to the RN role. These skills cannot be delegated to an LPN or UAP.
1. Delegate responsibly those activities that can be delegated, including promoting safety; providing therapeutic milieu and basic hygienic care; and monitoring of intake, output, and vital signs for the stable client. All monitoring information is reported to the RN.
2. Perform comprehensive physical assessments, medication therapy, and case management; provide milieu of unit client advocacy, and supervision of care by other members of the care team.
3. Lead selected group therapy sessions.
4. Assess for safety issues.
5. Provide information on client's status to members of the multidisciplinary team.
6. Collaborate with interdisciplinary team to provide optimal treatment plan for client. Includes physician, psychiatrist, nursing staff, recreational therapist, psychologist, social worker, dietician, and other specialties as indicated.
7. Make referrals to community resources.
8. Perform procedures related to admitting, transferring, or discharging a client.
9. Provide client and family teaching regarding rights and responsibilities. Document teaching performed and level of client and family understanding.
10. Receive and transcribe health care provider (HCP) orders.

11. Maintain client confidentiality.
12. Verify informed consent if prescribed ECT (electroconvulsive therapy).

C. Safety and infection control: Provide interventions to maintain safety. *Note: Client history of violence (suicide attempt) increases risk of current violence.*
   1. Monitor for self-harm risk—monitor for overt signs of self-harm indicators, including hopelessness, refusal to eat, refusal to take medications, giving away belongings, and inability to verbalize any future plans. Provide close monitoring during high-risk time for self-harm; these include:
      a. When client is going in or coming out of a depressive episode.
      b. Approximately 2 weeks after starting antidepressant medications, when client energy increases.
   2. Implement safety measures as needed.
      a. Promote "no-suicide" safety contract.
      b. Provide one-on-one monitoring.
      c. Take suicide precautions—remove harmful objects including cords from window blinds and phone; prevent extended time alone; place safety screens on windows.
      d. Observe client every 15 min.
      e. Restrict client to hospital unit (laboratory work and meals only on unit).
      f. Follow agency policy related to use of restraints or seclusion.

D. Health promotion and maintenance
   1. Teach awareness and avoidance of high-risk behaviors; promote lifestyle changes to include exercise, diet, moderation of alcohol.
   2. Recognize normal aging changes versus illness alterations.
   3. Reinforce need for medication use for prescribed length of time.
   4. Teach signs and symptoms of depression recurrence for early intervention.
   5. Reinforce community follow-up and referrals.
   6. Identify specific support persons and options (e.g., suicide hotline, crisis hotline).
   7. Identify barriers to learning.

E. Psychologic integrity
   1. Observe possible effects of cultural background of client experiencing depression; respect cultural differences of client within a safety framework.
      a. Client from Western culture may exhibit mood and cognitive symptoms (e.g., depressed mood and difficulty with concentration on tasks).
      b. Client from Asian culture may describe more somatic symptoms (e.g., fatigue and general body aches).
      c. Client from Middle East may describe having a problem of the "heart."
      d. Client who believes that depression is a sign of moral weakness or the work of evil spirits may feel more powerless to overcome the illness.
   2. Identify abnormal behaviors for client developmental age; recognize use of defense mechanisms—reinforce behavioral interventions as identified on client care plan; evaluate effectiveness.
   3. Evaluate client and significant others' response to treatment plan; use active listening and therapeutic communication techniques to increase client and family understanding of behaviors.
   4. Reinforce positive coping mechanisms of client, family; assist client to develop and use strategies to decrease anxiety. Provide a therapeutic environment and relaxation techniques as indicated (see basic care and comfort).
   5. Assist client in efforts to decrease chemical dependency.

F. Basic care and comfort
   1. Evaluate impact of illness on nutritional status and assist client as needed to meet nutrition needs (see implementation). Monitor client's hydration status; assess for constipation related to decreased activity and implement interventions as needed.
   2. Plan nursing measures to promote sleep.
      a. Identify sleep disturbance (difficulty falling asleep, difficulty staying asleep, sleeping too much as an escape).
      b. Identify and implement previous sleep rituals (e.g. bathe at night, quiet music).
      c. Limit caffeine intake in evening.
      d. Reinforce relaxation techniques (e.g., deep breathing, imagery, progressive muscle relaxation).
      e. Reduce environmental stimuli—television, radios, and lights.
      f. Administer medications as prescribed if other methods fail.
   3. Provide interventions for client with lack of energy and inability to concentrate.
      a. Assist client to meet activities of daily living (hygiene, eating), perform problem-solving, and maintain safety.
      b. Encourage client to focus on strengths rather than weaknesses; provide situations requiring simple decisions to increase confidence.

Table 36-1 Medications Used to Treat Mood Disorders

Classification	Generic/ Trade Name	Expected Outcomes	Reduction of Risk Potential	Management of Care
Tricyclic Antidepressants (TCA)	Amitriptyline (Elavil); doxepin (Sinequan); imipramine (Tofranil)	Elevates mood; increases activity level; stimulates appetite	• Evaluate suicide risk (related to cardiac toxicity potential). • Do not administer with an MAOI—need 14-day gap between these drug groups. • Promote safety—can cause sedation. • Dilute Sinequan concentrate with orange juice. • Avoid administration in clients with cardiovascular disease. • Narrow therapeutic index—can be lethal in overdose. • Monitor for drowsiness, dry mouth, blurred vision, weight gain, constipation, and orthostatic hypotension. • Monitor for adverse reactions: cardiac dysrhythmias, hypotension.	• Administer at bedtime if sedation occurs. • Teach client to avoid alcohol. • Teach client to rise slowly to prevent postural hypotension. • Advise use of sugarless candy, gum for dry mouth. • Advise fluids, fiber, and exercise to prevent constipation.
Selective Serotonin Reuptake Inhibitors (SSRI)	Fluoxetine (Prozac); sertraline (Zoloft); paroxetine (Paxil); citalopram (Celexa); escitalopram (Lexapro)	Elevates mood; increases concentration and energy	• Monitor for nausea, headache, insomnia, weight loss, skin rash, nervousness.	• Teach client therapeutic effective has delayed onset of up to several weeks. • Administer in the morning.
Monoamine Oxidase Inhibitors (MAOI)	Phenelzine sulfate (Nardil); tranylcypromine (Parnate)	Elevates mood; increases energy	• Avoid use with TCAs or SSRIs (risk for serotonin syndrome). • Avoid foods containing tyramine (aged cheese, red wine, beer, yeast, soy sauce, chocolate, processed foods and meats). • Avoid over-the-counter cold preparations and decongestants.	• Do not take with over-the-counter drugs without approval. • Teach signs of hypertensive crisis (elevation of BP, increased temperature, tremors, tachycardia).
Atypical Antidepressants	Bupropion (Wellbutrin); venlafaxine (Effexor); trazodone (Desyrel); duloxetine (Cymbalta)	Elevates mood; improves sleep and nutrition; improves concentration; has fewer side effects than TCAs and MAOIs; lowers seizure threshold related to (bupropion); both duloxetine and venlafaxine affect the neurotransmitters serotonin and norepinephrine	• Monitor for sedation, orthostatic hypotension, nausea, vomiting, priapism (trazodone), and dry mouth.	• Teach client therapeutic effect occurs in 2-4 weeks after initiation.

Classification	Generic/ Trade Name	Expected Outcomes	Reduction of Risk Potential	Management of Care
Mood Stabilizer (antimanic)	Lithium carbonate (Lithane, Lithobid)	Decreases activity level; improves sleep pattern	• Monitor lithium blood levels per protocol; typically level should be 0.5 to 1.5 mEq/L. Levels above 2 mEq/L considered toxic. • Monitor for increased thirst, increased urination, dry mouth, lethargy, muscle weakness, fine hand tremors. • Monitor for toxicity signs: vomiting, diarrhea, drowsiness, or lethargy, uncoordination, coarse hand tremors, muscle twitching. • Monitor for acute toxicity: seizures, coma, peripheral vascular collapse, death. • Prevent crushing, chewing, or breaking extended-release tablets.	• Encourage normal salt intake in diet, encourage fluid intake of 2-3 L/day. • Stress importance of ongoing serum drug levels to monitor for toxicity. • Teach symptoms of lithium toxicity.
Mood Stabilizer (originally anticonvulsant medications—used for those who do not respond or tolerate lithium carbonate)	Carbamazepine (Tegretol); valproic acid (Depakene) Divalproex sodium (Depakote) lamotrigine (Lamictal); oxcarbazepine (Trileptal)	Decreases activity level; improves sleep pattern	Carbamazepine: • Monitor for spots before eyes, drowsiness, dizziness, dry mouth, blood dyscrasias. • Monitor CBC frequently during initiation and regularly throughout treatment. Valproic acid: • Monitor for nausea, drowsiness, hepatotoxicity. • Monitor liver function studies. Lamotrigine: • Monitor for serious skin rash, do not stop abruptly. • Monitor for dizziness, suicidal ideation, hemorrhage. Oxcarbazepine: • Monitor for serious skin rash, cardiac failure, dizziness, sleepiness.	• Avoid tasks that require alertness until response known. • Stress importance of ongoing serum drug levels to monitor for toxicity.

c. Involve persons supportive to client.
d. Reinforce cognitive therapies that promote positive thinking.
e. Encourage expression of feelings and thoughts.

G. Reduction of risk potential
1. Decrease probability of relapse—provide client and family teaching about illness, medication follow-up care, and all treatments such as electroconvulsive therapy (ECT, see Chapter 35).
2. Monitor closely for suicide ideation, and signs and symptoms indicating relapse. Provide crisis intervention in suicidal clients.
3. Assess client for drug and alcohol dependencies or withdrawal.
4. Review risk factors for illness with client.
5. Instruct client of need for any laboratory work to monitor therapeutic level of medications. Interpret laboratory values and notify HCP as indicated.
6. Evaluate response to medications; assess client for side effects of medications. Check for potential interactions of medications with foods, fluids, other medications. (e.g., tyramine foods and MAOIs).

H. Pharmacologic and parenteral therapies: Client and family will state the purpose for and associated side effects of all medications used to treat depression (see Table 36-1). Document medication administration and client response to medication.

Bipolar Disorder

I. Definition: Previously known as manic-depressive disorder, bipolar disorder involves extreme mood swings from episodes of deep depression to mania (intense euphoria). A client in the depressive phase exhibits the same mood, behaviors, and needs characteristic of depression (see section on depression). The manic phase of bipolar disorder is discussed here, along with additional phases.

A. Episodes
   1. Mania—characterized by persistent and abnormally elevated, expansive, or irritable mood (see assessment for signs and symptoms).
   2. Hypomania—less severe than mania, and does not impair the person's functioning as severely as mania. Does include inflated self-esteem, attention-seeking behavior, decreased sleep, and risky behaviors.
   3. Bipolar I disorder—characterized by one or more manic episodes with one or more depressive episodes.
   4. Bipolar II disorder—less severe than bipolar I disorder; involves one or more hypomanic and depressive episodes.
   5. Cyclothymic disorder—resembles bipolar disorder with less severe symptoms; symptoms present at least 2 years in adults and 1 year in children and adolescents.

B. Etiology: The exact causes of bipolar disorder is not known; some contributing factors may include:
   1. Neurochemical imbalances in the brain (dopamine, serotonin, and norepinephrine).
   2. Genetic component.
   3. Acute episodes may be precipitated by psychosocial events such as trauma, loss, and stress.

II. Nursing process

A. Assessment: Observe challenges presented by the manic client related to distractibility and increased speech and motor behaviors; use secondary sources and continued observation as assessment tools.
   1. Obtain a detailed health history and perform a comprehensive physical examination; assess the following:
      a. Presence of neurotransmitter imbalances that cause client condition (e.g., hypo- or hyperthyroidism; hormone imbalances, glucose imbalances).
      b. Current or past use of alcohol, illicit drugs, prescription drugs, over-the-counter drugs, or herbal drugs.
      c. Family history of mental illness.
      d. Environmental factors.
      e. Psychosocial factors including ineffective coping, and denial of disorder.
   2. Assess for self-harm risk (critical assessment related to client's poor judgment, impulsive behaviors, and risk-taking).
   3. Assess for signs and symptoms of bipolar disorder—manic phase. Manic episode begins suddenly, rapidly escalates, and ends more abruptly than depressive episode. Symptoms include at least three of the following:
      a. Affective—involves sensations of euphoria, grandiose thoughts, agitated mood, and false sense of well-being; client alternates between tears and loud laughter (mood lability).
      b. Motivational—client exhibits high level of energy.
      c. Cognitive—involves poor judgment, rapid thoughts (flight of ideas) and speech (pressured), exaggerated self-esteem, and distractibility (client starts but does not complete projects).
      d. Behavioral—involves lack of sleep, decreased nutritional intake, high-risk activities (e.g., spending money, promiscuous sexual activity), greatly increased motor activity, flamboyant dressing, and anger if limits are set on behaviors.
      e. Somatic (physical)—client has difficulty meeting activities of daily living; may not sleep or eat for several days, and ignores personal hygiene.
   4. Obtain diagnostic tests.
      a. Laboratory tests—often include checking electrolytes, CBC, lithium, and thyroid levels for imbalances
      b. Nutritional assessment including caffeine intake and vitamin deficiencies

B. Analysis
   1. Risk for Self-Directed Violence related to deep sadness
   2. Risk for Other-Directed Violence related to poor anger management
   3. Imbalanced Nutrition: Less Than Body Requirements related to decreased food intake
   4. Ineffective Therapeutic Regimen Management related to failure to take medications as prescribed
   5. Self-Care Deficit: Grooming, Hygiene, and Feeding, related to low energy levels
   6. Disturbed Sleep Pattern related to hyperactivity
   7. Ineffective Role Performance related to situational or environmental stressors

C. Planning
   1. Prevent client harm to self or others.
   2. Promote balance of sleep and activity.

3. Promote self-care activities.
4. Promote adequate nutrition
5. Monitor intake and output.
6. Promote compliance with medication regimen.
7. Provide client and family teaching.

D. Implementation

1. Provide interventions to maintain safety: Monitor for self-harm risk, and implement safety measures as needed (see safety and infection control).
2. Provide client and family teaching about disorder and treatment needs.
3. Provide interventions to meet physiologic needs.
    a. Assist client to meet activities of daily living (hygiene, eating) and to maintain safety.
    b. Decrease environmental stimulation; establish a bedtime routine; offer sleep medications to promote sleep behaviors.
    c. Provide high-calorie, high-protein "finger foods" and snacks that client can eat while moving around.
    d. Monitor food and fluid intake, and hours of sleep.
4. Administer prescribed medications; work with client to manage side effects of treatments or medications.
5. Promote therapeutic communication (see psychologic integrity).

E. Evaluation

1. Client refrains from causing harm to self and others.
2. Client performs adequate self-care for grooming, sleep, and nutrition.
3. Client complies with treatment plan of medications and therapy.
4. Client realistically manages role performance needs.
5. Client shows desired effect from medications and is free from side effects of medications.
6. Client and support system use knowledge of disorder and medications to manage disorder after discharge.

CN

III. Client needs

A. Physiologic adaptation

1. Chemical imbalances in the brain lead to altered neurotransmissions, resulting in rapid thoughts, altered behaviors, and feelings of being invincible—nurse assists the client with safety needs.
2. Prescribed medications may impact health status—nurse monitors fluid balance and sodium intake for the client on lithium; and for adverse medication effects (e.g., blood dyscrasias, liver function, and toxic levels).
3. Prescribed medications may cause fluctuations of serum therapeutic levels—nurse monitors results of diagnostic tests for relationship to physical condition, and medication effects.
4. Client status can change rapidly—nurse documents procedures and treatments performed, and client response to treatment.

B. Management of care: Care of the client with bipolar disorder requires critical thinking skills and knowledge of assessment, and teaching and evaluation methods unique to the RN role. These skills cannot be delegated to an LPN or UAP.

1. Delegate responsibly those activities that can be delegated, including promoting safety; providing therapeutic milieu and basic hygienic care; and monitoring of intake, output, and vital signs for the stable client. All monitoring information is reported to the RN.
2. Perform comprehensive physical assessments; provide medication therapy, case management, milieu of unit, and client advocacy.
3. Direct noncompetitive physical activities such as walks, swimming, and painting.
4. Provide information on the client's status to members of the multidisciplinary team.
5. Resolve conflicts arising from client behaviors.
6. Collaborate with interdisciplinary team to provide optimal treatment plan for client, including physician, psychiatrist, nursing staff, recreational therapist, psychologist, social worker, dietician, and other specialties as indicated.
7. Make referrals to community resources.
8. Perform procedures related to admitting, transferring, or discharging a client.
9. Provide client and family teaching about rights and responsibilities; protect client rights and rights of other clients.
10. Document teaching performed and level of client and family understanding.
11. Maintain client confidentiality.

C. Safety and infection control: Plan interventions to prevent injury from self-harm, harm to others; implement safety measures as needed.

1. Promote "no-suicide" safety contract.
2. Provide one-on-one monitoring.
3. Institute suicide precautions—remove harmful objects including cords from window

blinds and phone; prevent extended time alone; place safety screens on windows.
4. Observe client every 15 min.
5. Restrict client to hospital unit (laboratory work and meals only on unit).
6. Follow agency policy related to use of restraints or seclusion.
7. Establish external controls and enforce nonjudgmentally; clearly identify acceptable and unacceptable behaviors.
8. Recognize safety needs related to impulsive behaviors, poor judgment; monitor behaviors frequently to avoid retaliation from others who are threatened or angered by client manic behaviors.

D. Health promotion and maintenance
1. Review risk factors related to illness and safety with client.
2. Assess client and family adaptation to illness process, and provide client and family teaching regarding ways to manage bipolar disorder; medication management and signs of toxicity; and high-risk behaviors.
3. Reinforce need for medication use even when feeling "well."
4. Teach signs and symptoms of relapse and need for early intervention.
5. Provide interventions to promote appropriate behaviors.
   a. Redirect need for movement to acceptable behaviors (e.g., walking, not running).
   b. Monitor client management of belongings and money to limit impulsive giving away of belongings or money.
   c. Reinforce personal boundaries by preventing client from being in public areas dressed inappropriately or intervening if client makes inappropriate personal advances toward other clients or staff.
   d. Provide distraction as needed to prevent inappropriate behaviors.
6. Reinforce community follow-up and referrals for client and family.
7. Identify barriers to learning.

E. Psychologic integrity
1. Respect cultural differences of client within a safety framework.
2. Recognize some clients resist stabilization of mania related to sense of accomplishment while in manic state.
3. Assess family dynamics for impact of illness and response to treatment plan; use active listening and therapeutic communication techniques to increase client and family understanding of behaviors.
   a. Use simple, clear sentences related to the client's short attention span.
   b. Ask client to repeat short messages to be sure they have processed them.
   c. Give printed information to reinforce unit expectations, schedules, and rules for behavior.
   d. Request client to repeat verbal messages more slowly if speech too rapid to understand.
   e. Set limits regarding taking turns to speak or meet with staff.
4. Reinforce positive coping mechanisms.

F. Basic care and comfort (see basic care and comfort for depression)

G. Reduction of risk potential
1. Interpret laboratory values and notify HCP as indicated; instruct client and family on need for laboratory work to monitor therapeutic level of medications, and effect on liver or blood system.
2. Monitor closely for suicide ideation, signs and symptoms indicating relapse.
3. Recognize use of caffeine and illicit drugs may increase mania.
4. Review applicable data prior to medication administration (e.g., allergies, serum lab results, client diagnosis, appropriateness of medication order for client).
5. Check for potential interactions of medications with foods, fluids, and other medications.

H. Pharmacologic and parenteral therapies: Client and family will state the purpose for and associated side effects of all medications used to treat bipolar disorder (see Table 36-1). Document medication administration and client response to medication.

Anxiety and Somatoform Disorders

I. Definition: Anxiety disorders encompass a group of conditions that have as a key feature excessive anxiety with the accompanying behavioral, physiologic, and emotional responses. The client with anxiety disorders experiences significant distress that often impairs daily routine, occupation, and/or social functioning. Four levels of anxiety were described by nursing theorist Hildegard Peplau. Table 36-2 shows levels and manifestations.

A. Types of anxiety disorders
1. Generalized anxiety disorder—involves at least 6 months of excessive and persistent anxiety and worry.

Table 36-2 Nursing Management of Anxiety

Level of Anxiety	Manifestations	Nursing Interventions
Mild	Increased alertness; able to learn new tasks	• Help client describe feelings. • Help client identify coping mechanisms to decrease anxiety.
Moderate	Focuses on immediate task; some difficulty maintaining attention; needs assistance to learn new tasks	• Help client understand cause of anxiety and to redirect activity to relieve tension (e.g., walking, music).
Severe	Feelings of dread; unable to focus attention, learn, or problem-solve; has physiologic symptoms of tachycardia, diaphoresis, chest pain	• Help client identify and alter anxiety-producing situations. • Do not take away coping mechanisms client is using without replacing with an alternate coping mechanism.
Panic	Complete inability to focus; unable to use coping mechanisms; can involve delusions and hallucinations	• Stay with client when levels of anxiety are severe or client is experiencing panic. • Give simple instructions, remove unnecessary stimulations. • Use quiet voice, relaxation techniques. • Medicate with prescribed antianxiety medication if needed.

2. Phobias—involve irrational fear of objects, animals, or situations; examples include:
   a. Agoraphobia—involves anxiety about or avoidance of places or situations from which help may not be available or from which escape may be difficult.
   b. Arachnophobia—fear of spiders.
   c. Social phobia—characterized by anxiety that occurs with certain kinds of social or performance situation; social phobias also lead to avoiding the situation or object that is feared.
3. Panic disorder—involves recurrent panic attacks that result in constant worry; panic attack—involves sudden onset of fearfulness, apprehension or terror accompanied with feelings of "impending doom."
4. Acute stress disorder—involves anxiety, dissociative, somatic, and other symptoms after experiencing a very traumatic stressor (lasts from 2 days to 4 weeks).
5. Posttraumatic stress disorder (PTSD)—occurs when a client experiences a reoccurrence of an extremely traumatic event, such as serving in a war, rape, bombing; client avoids stimuli associated with this event, has numb responses and persistent increased arousal. PTSD begins within 3 months to several years after the event and may last for a few months or for several years.
6. Obsessive-compulsive disorder—occurs when a client's thoughts, impulses, and images consume the client and the client is obligated to act out the behaviors. These behaviors interfere with the client's functioning, and the client becomes very anxious if unable to complete the ritual; with decreasing anxiety, the client reduces the amount of time spent on the rituals. Examples include the individual who washes hands after touching anything to the point of impaired social, personal, or occupational functioning.

B. Anxiety-related disorders: Dissociative disorders—a subconscious feature in which the client has a loss of memory, consciousness, identity, or environmental perception. Examples of dissociative disorders are:
   1. Dissociative fugue—client has episodes of leaving home or workplace without any explanation, traveling to another area and being unable to remember personal identity; client may assume a new identity.
   2. Dissociative amnesia—client has difficulty remembering essential personal information; amnesia is usually result of a stressful or traumatic event or nature.
   3. Dissociative identity disorder—client manifests two or more identities or personalities; client has no memory of another identity while in another identity. (This condition was formerly called *multiple personality disorder*.)
   4. Depersonalization disorder—client has a recurrent feeling of being removed from

personal body or mental processes; client cannot be psychotic or out of touch with reality. This condition occurs more often in clients with a history of childhood sexual or physical abuse.

C. Somatoform disorder—involves client's complaints that physical problems are present when diagnostic testing does not reveal physiologic cause. Psychologic conflicts and factors initiate symptoms and increase symptoms while client is not aware that symptoms exist.
   1. Conversion disorder—development of a symptom that appears to be caused by a disease and causes impairment in client's ability to carry out activities of daily living and/or to work.
   2. Hypochondriasis—involves fears of having a serious illness that are not supported by medical tests.

II. Nursing process

A. Assessment
   1. Assess the client with anxiety and anxiety-related disorders for:
      a. Restlessness.
      b. Irritability.
      c. Decreased attention span.
      d. Inability to control impulses.
      e. Feelings of apprehension, helplessness, or discomfort.
      f. Pacing and/or hyperactivity.
      g. Wringing of the hands.
      h. Difficulties with perceptual fields.
      i. Decreasing ability for verbal communication.
   2. Specifically assess the client with panic anxiety disorders for:
      a. Disorganized thought processes.
      b. Delusions.
      c. An inability to discriminate harmful situations or stimuli.
   3. Specifically assess the client with PTSD for the previous points and:
      a. Low self-esteem (many feel damaged by their experiences or unworthy).
      b. Nightmares or flashbacks of the event.
      c. Appearing terrified, crying, and screaming (during a flashback).
      d. Attempting to run away and/or hide (during a flashback).
      e. Experiencing intrusive thoughts of the traumatic event.
   4. Assess the client with dissociative disorders for:
      a. Confusion about own identity; assumption of new identity (dissociative fugue).
      b. Inability to recall painful/stressful/traumatic events (dissociative amnesia).
      c. Presence of two or more distinct identities; inability to recall details about personal life and life history (dissociative identity disorder).
      d. Feeling of being detached from thoughts or body (depersonalization disorder).
   5. Assess the client with somatoform disorders for irrational fears of disease; disease/illness behavior not supported by medical tests; frequent and multiple complaints of vague symptoms and illnesses.

B. Analysis: (Nursing diagnoses are based on specific data for specific anxiety, anxiety-related, and somatoform disorders).
   1. Anxiety related to mental health problem
   2. Ineffective Coping related to mental health problem
   3. Post-Trauma Syndrome related to mental health problem
   4. Chronic Low Self-Esteem related to mental health problem
   5. Powerlessness related to mental health problem
   6. Disturbed Sleep Pattern related to mental health problem
   7. Rape-Trauma Syndrome related to mental health problem
   8. Social Isolation related to mental health problem
   9. Ineffective Role Performance related to mental health problem
   10. Fear related to mental health problem

C. Planning
   1. Prevent client from harm to self and others.
   2. Decrease anxiety level.
   3. Promote healthy methods of dealing with stress.
   4. Introduce social support system in client's home community.
   5. Maintain adequate nutritional intake.
   6. Promote effective coping mechanisms.
   7. Promote adequate hours for sleep (at least 6 hr each night).

D. Implementation: Provide interventions to manage symptoms of anxiety, anxiety-related, and somatoform disorders (see also Table 36-2).
   1. Move client to a quiet area with decreased or minimal stimuli.
   2. Avoid requiring client to make choices.
   3. Use therapeutic communication; use clear, simple, and short statements.
   4. Administer prescribed PRN medications if delusions and/or disorganized thoughts are present.

5. Allow extra time for the OCD client to complete rituals until the client has reduced the amount of time and energy spent on rituals.

E. Evaluation
1. Client is able to manage stress and emotions and function in daily life.
2. Client verbalizes comfort and satisfaction with quality of life.
3. Client understands and adheres to medication regimen.
4. Client's episodes of anxiety are decreased in intensity and frequency.
5. Client's rituals are decreased in intensity and frequency.
6. Client does not injure self or others.
7. Client participates in support system in home community.
8. Client has adequate nutritional intake and receives at least 6 hr of sleep each night.

III. Client needs

A. Physiologic adaptation
1. Assess client's vital signs for generalized anxiety disorder/panic disorder in which vital signs may be elevated.
2. Monitor client's physiologic status during panic episodes.

B. Management of care: Care of the client with anxiety and somatoform disorders requires critical thinking skills and knowledge of assessment, and teaching and evaluation methods unique to the RN role. These skills cannot be delegated to an LPN or UAP.
1. Participate in interdisciplinary team conferences—nursing contributes data from 24-hr assessment and care.
2. Introduce client to community agencies such as halfway houses, for long-term care.
3. Provide and receive report on assigned hospitalized clients among health care team.
4. Act as a client advocate.
5. Maintain confidentiality.
6. Provide client and family teaching about signs and symptoms of anxiety disorders.

C. Safety and infection control
1. Discuss the home environment with the client/family member(s) of the OCD client to facilitate completion of rituals.
2. Provide care for self-inflicted wounds.

D. Health promotion and maintenance
1. Perform physical assessment on admission to psychiatric facilities and as per agency policy.
2. Provide long-term monitoring with medication histories to maintain compliance with anxiolytics or antidepressant medications.
3. Assist with planning for care in the home setting, including home health nurses and community health agencies.
4. Assist client with activities appropriate for preference and developmental age.

E. Psychologic integrity
1. Assess family dynamics; listen to client and family concerns about the specific anxiety disorders.
2. Assess cultural factors of the client with anxiety-related disorders.

F. Basic care and comfort
1. Allow enough time for the client with OCD to complete rituals.
2. Promote bowel elimination for client taking anxiety medications or antidepressants.
3. Provide nutrition for client whose anxiety disorder has an altered nutritional pattern.

G. Reduction of risk potential: Provide client and family teaching about medications and side effects.

H. Pharmacologic and parenteral therapies: Client and family will state the purpose for and associated side effects of medications. See Table 36-3 for medications used to treat anxiety and somatoform disorders. Document medication administration and client response to medication.

The Client at Risk for Suicide

I. Definition: Suicide is the intentional act of killing oneself.

A. Suicidal ideation refers to thoughts about suicidal acts, which are common to the client with a mood disorder.

B. Suicide plan is a specific strategy developed with the intent to kill oneself.

C. Suicide attempt is a suicidal plan that was acted on, but was not successfully completed.

II. Nursing process

A. Assessment
1. Obtain a detailed health history and perform a comprehensive physical exam; assess the following:
   a. Presence of chronic medical illness that may cause suicidal ideation (e.g., terminal stages of cancer; diseases in which death is the outcome, such as amyotrophic lateral sclerosis).
   b. Presence of mental illness (e.g., depression, bipolar disorder, schizophrenia, substance abuse, posttraumatic stress disorder, or borderline personality disorder).

Table 36-3 Common Medications for Clients with Anxiety and Somatoform Disorders

Classification	Generic/Trade Name Examples	Expected Outcomes	Reduction of Risk Potential	Management of Care
Anxiolytics—Benzodiazepines	Diazepam (Valium); alprazolam (Xanax); clorazepate (Tranxene); chlordiazepoxide (Librium); clonazepam (Klonopin); lorazepam (Ativan); oxazepam (Serax)	Relieves anxiety.	Instruct client to avoid CNS depressants such as alcohol or antihistamines; avoid caffeinated foods or beverages; do not stop taking drug abruptly; and use caution when driving.	Monitor postural hypotension. Encourage fluids.
Anxiolytics—Nonbenzodiazepines	Buspirone (BuSpar); meprobamate (Miltown, Equanil)	BuSpar has slow onset to relieve anxiety. Meprobamate has very rapid onset to relieve anxiety.	Instruct client to rise slowly from a sitting position; use caution when driving.	Advise client to take medications with food; report continuous agitation, restlessness or increased euphoria to HCP. Monitor postural hypotension.
Tricyclic Antidepressant	Clomipramine (Anafranil) for OCD; imipramine (Tofranil)	Reduces symptoms of OCD and anxiety, panic disorder, and agoraphobia.	Instruct client to use caution when driving.	Monitor postural hypotension.
SSRI Antidepressants	Fluoxetine (Prozac); fluvoxamine (Luvox) for OCD; paroxetine (Paxil); sertraline (Zoloft)	Reduces symptoms of panic disorder, OCD, generalized anxiety disorders, and social phobia.	Instruct client to use caution when driving. Monitor for dizziness, sedation, headache, insomnia, dry mouth and throat, vomiting, diarrhea, and sweating.	Encourage use of sugar-free hard candies or beverages. Encourage fluids. Administer if client is drowsy during daytime.
Antihistamines	Hydroxyzine (Vistaril, Atarax)	Relieves anxiety.	Instruct client to use caution when driving; avoid using these drugs with CNS depressants.	Avoid use in clients with history of hypertension.
Alpha-Adrenergic Agonist—Beta-Blocker	Propanolol (Inderal)	Reduces anxiety, panic disorder treatment, and generalized anxiety disorder.	Instruct client to use caution when driving. Monitor additive hypotension with other antihypertensives.	Monitor for orthostatic hypotension. Contraindicated in client with heart failure. Instruct client of side effects such as impotence, fatigue, and weakness.

c. Family history of mental illness and suicide attempts.
d. Any previous suicide attempts.
e. Current or past use of alcohol, illicit drugs, prescription drugs, over-the-counter drugs, or herbal drugs.
f. Gender
(1) Females more likely to attempt suicide.
(2) Males more likely to complete suicide because of tendency to use more lethal methods.
g. Type of stressors or losses client currently perceives, including environmental or situational factors (e.g., stressful life event, lack of support).

2. Assess self-harm risk (critical assessment related to suicide ideation and/or plan)—directly ask client, "Do you have any thoughts about hurting yourself or others?"
3. Assess lethality of suicide ideation.
a. Does client have a plan; if so, is plan specific?

b. Does client have the means to carry out the plan?
c. Is the plan likely to cause death if carried out?
d. Has client been giving away possessions or making a will?
e. Is there a specific time or date that is part of the plan?

4. Obtain diagnostic tests—laboratory tests:
   a. Drug screens—evaluates drug level in overdose
   b. Renal and liver function tests—evaluates damage from medications
   c. CBC—assesses amount of blood loss from traumatic attempts
   d. ABGs/pulse oximetry—assesses effect on oxygenation levels related to overdose

B. Analysis
   1. Risk for Self-Directed Violence related to mood disorder
   2. Risk for Suicide related to mood disorder
   3. Risk for Other-Directed Violence related to mood disorder
   4. Ineffective Coping related to mood disorder
   5. Anxiety related to mood disorder
   6. Spiritual Distress related to mood disorder

C. Planning
   1. Prevent client harm to self or others.
   2. Promote therapeutic nurse-client relationship.

D. Implementation
   1. Provide interventions to maintain safety (see safety and infection control). Monitor closely for suicide ideation, and signs and symptoms indicating increased suicide risk such as:
      a. Sudden change in client mood or affect (especially calm).
      b. Giving away belongings.
      c. Contacting or writing long letters to family and friends.
      d. Seeking opportunities to be alone without staff.
      e. Refusal to sign "no-suicide" contract.
      f. Verbal statements about being "gone".
   2. Provide interventions for suicide ideation or an attempt.
      a. Take control of crisis situation.
      b. Inform client that safety is top priority over other needs.
   3. Provide interventions to meet emotional needs.
      a. Recognize client feelings while protecting from harm.
      b. Avoid blaming client for feelings of hopelessness or pain.
      c. Assess resources available to client for ongoing emotional support.
      d. Promote positive self-characteristics.
      e. Identify possible solutions to perceived critical issues in person's life.

E. Evaluation
   1. Client and others remain safe from harm.
   2. Client identifies and verbalizes future plans.
   3. Client is compliant with treatment plan of medications and therapy.
   4. Client identifies immediate and future support systems.

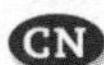

III. Client needs

A. Physiologic adaptation
   1. Client experiences hopelessness and is unable to see solutions to problems—nurse assesses client adaptation to life events leading to suicide ideation or plan.
   2. Client often needs support to ensure safety—nurse counsels family and client regarding ways to manage risk factors for suicide, medication regimen, treatments, and procedures.
   3. Client may attempt self-harm behaviors—nurse monitors applicable body system for injury after suicide attempt.
   4. Client's emotional status may change rapidly—nurse documents procedures and treatments performed, and response to treatment.

B. Management of care: Care of the client demonstrating suicidal ideation requires critical thinking skills and knowledge of assessment, and teaching and evaluation methods unique to the RN role. These skills cannot be delegated to an LPN or UAP.
   1. Delegate responsibly those activities that can be delegated, including promoting safety issues.
   2. Perform comprehensive assessments of client suicide ideation, plan, and lethality of plan.
   3. Direct crisis intervention, medication therapy, case management, and client advocacy.
   4. Provide ongoing assessment for safety issues.
   5. Provide information on the client's status to members of the multidisciplinary team; give and receive report on assigned clients.
   6. Maintain client confidentiality.
   7. Collaborate with interdisciplinary team to provide optimal treatment plan for client. Includes physician, psychiatrist, nursing staff, recreational therapist, psychologist, social worker, dietician, and other specialties as indicated.
   8. Make referrals to community resources.

9. Perform procedures related to admitting, transferring, or discharging a client.
10. Provide client and family teaching about rights and responsibilities; document teaching performed and level of client and family understanding.

C. Safety and infection control: Plan interventions to prevent injury from self-harm, harm to others; implement safety measures as needed.
1. Promote "no-suicide" safety contract.
2. Provide one-on-one monitoring.
3. Take suicide precautions—remove harmful objects, including cords from window blinds and phone; prevent extended time alone; place safety screens on windows.
4. Observe client every 15 min.
5. Restrict client to hospital unit (laboratory work and meals only on unit).
6. Follow agency policy related to use of restraints or seclusion.
7. Formulate a list of support persons so someone is always available to client (e.g., family and friends, church groups, mental health clinics or hotlines).

D. Health promotion and maintenance
1. Review risk factors related to illness and safety with client.
2. Intervene to protect client from high-risk behaviors during crisis phase.
3. Assess family structure for anger, shame, and grief associated with suicide attempts and completions; reinforce community follow-up and referrals for client and family.
4. Identify barriers to learning

E. Psychologic integrity
1. Respect cultural differences of client within a safety framework.
2. Reinforce behavioral interventions as identified on client care plan; evaluate effectiveness.
3. Evaluate client response to treatment plan.
4. Reinforce positive coping mechanisms.
5. Assess client for drug and alcohol dependencies or withdrawal.
6. Assess family dynamics.
7. Provide a therapeutic environment for client (see basic care and comfort for depression).
8. Use active listening and therapeutic communication techniques to increase client and family understanding of behaviors.

F. Basic care and comfort
1. Assist or provide client with basic hygiene and grooming as needed; evaluate ability of client to perform activities of daily living.
2. Incorporate complementary therapies into plan of care (e.g., music therapy, occupational therapy).

G. Reduction of risk potential
1. Review applicable data prior to medication administration (e.g., allergies, serum lab results, client diagnosis, appropriateness of medication order for client).
2. Check for potential interactions of medications with foods, fluids, other medications.
3. Safely administer prescribed medications using five rights.
   a. Monitor to be sure client has swallowed tablets or request change to liquid form of medication if available.
   b. Monitor packages and belongings for any home medications and keep in safe place.
   c. Monitor that client is not getting medications from other clients.

H. Pharmacologic and parenteral therapies: Client and family will state the purpose for and associated side effects of all medications used to treat mood disorders (see Table 36-1). Document medication administration and client response to medication.

Bibliography

American Psychiatric Association. (2000). *Diagnostic and statistical manual of mental disorders* (4th ed., text revision). Washington, DC: American Psychiatric Association.

Boyd, M. A. (2005). *Psychiatric nursing: Contemporary practice* (3rd ed.). Philadelphia: Lippincott Williams & Wilkins.

Centre for Suicide Prevention. http://www.siec.ca

Mohr, W. K. (2006). *Psychiatric-mental health nursing* (6th ed.). Philadelphia: Lippincott Williams & Wilkins.

Taylor, C., Lillis, C., & LeMone, P. (2006). *Fundamentals of nursing: The art and science of nursing care.* (6th ed.). Philadelphia: Lippincott Williams & Wilkins.

Videbeck, S. L. (2004). *Psychiatric-mental health nursing* (2nd ed.). Philadelphia: Lippincott Williams & Wilkins.

Zerwekh, J., & Claborn, J. C. (2006). *Illustrated study guide for the NCLEX-RN exam* (6th ed.). St. Louis: Mosby Elsevier.

CHAPTER 36

Practice Test

Depression

1. The nurse working in a community clinic is asked to help screen all clients for depression. Which of the following questions by the nurse is best to initiate this screening?
   - □ 1. "You look sad. Is something wrong?"
   - □ 2. "Are you depressed about this illness?"
   - □ 3. "How are you feeling today?"
   - □ 4. "Tell me how things have been going lately."
2. During admission, the client describes feeling depressed, "for as long as I can remember." The nurse understands this symptom is indicative of what type of depression?
   - □ 1. Major depression.
   - □ 2. Postpartum depression.
   - □ 3. Dysthymic disorder.
   - □ 4. Seasonal affective depression.
3. The nurse is updating the chart of a client who is 53 years of age and at the gynecology clinic. Assessment reveals a weight loss of 15 pounds (6.8 kg) since her appointment the year before. The client states, "I haven't felt like eating lately. I feel so tired all the time and I just don't have the energy to do any of my hobbies anymore." Based on the assessment of this client, what is the best action by the nurse?
   - □ 1. Suggest that the client be started on an antidepressant.
   - □ 2. Refer the client for evaluation of depression.
   - □ 3. Suggest a dietary consult for ways to improve her appetite.
   - □ 4. Inform the client that the nurse can only discuss her gynecologic care.
4. AF The nurse is assessing a client who is being admitted to an inpatient unit with a diagnosis of depression. Which of the following are expected findings? Select all that apply.
   - □ 1. Pacing during the admission process.
   - □ 2. Alteration in weight.
   - □ 3. Loss of interest in activities previously enjoyed.
   - □ 4. Extreme fear of a specific object.
   - □ 5. Nightmares of a traumatic event.
   - □ 6. Inability to sit still and focus on tasks.
5. The nurse is performing a depression screening at the site of a senior citizen meal program. What is an appropriate response from the nurse when a meal worker asks why depression in older adults is often undiagnosed and untreated?
   - □ 1. Older adult depression is often seen as part of normal aging.
   - □ 2. Older adults usually die before the onset of depression.
   - □ 3. Older adults are less likely to express their sadness.
   - □ 4. Older adults do not enter the health care system as often as younger adults.
6. The nurse is admitting a client diagnosed with seasonal affective disorder (SAD). Based on the underlying cause of this illness, which treatment does the nurse anticipate will be initiated for this client?
   - □ 1. Electroconvulsive therapy.
   - □ 2. Phototherapy.
   - □ 3. Relaxation therapy.
   - □ 4. Group therapy.

Bipolar Disorder

7. An HCP has prescribed valproic acid (Depakene) for a client with bipolar disorder who has achieved limited success with lithium carbonate (Lithane). The nurse should instruct the client about which of the following?
   - □ 1. Follow-up blood tests are necessary while on this medication.
   - □ 2. The extended-release tablet can be crushed if necessary for ease of swallowing.
   - □ 3. Tachycardia and upset stomach are common side effects.
   - □ 4. Consumption of a moderate amount of alcohol is safe if the medication is taken in the morning.
8. The nurse is caring for a client who completed an electroconvulsive therapy (ECT) procedure this morning. For what common side effect does the nurse assess?
   - □ 1. Temporary memory loss.
   - □ 2. Bruising and pain.
   - □ 3. Unstable BP.
   - □ 4. Elevated temperature.

9. AF The nurse performs which of the following interventions to prepare a client for ECT? Select all that apply.
- □ 1. Maintain NPO status.
- □ 2. Verify consent is signed.
- □ 3. Orient client to place and time.
- □ 4. Remove dentures.
- □ 5. Request client to void.
- □ 6. Assess client vital signs every 30 min.

10. The nurse is providing care for a client admitted to an inpatient unit who is experiencing a manic episode. What is a priority nursing intervention for this client?
- □ 1. Order all medications in a liquid form.
- □ 2. Base family visits on attendance at therapy groups.
- □ 3. Closely monitor the client's eating and sleeping habits.
- □ 4. Encourage the client to keep a journal about feelings and emotions.

11. The nurse is planning care for a client who has been experiencing a manic episode for 6 days and is unable to sit still long enough to eat meals. Which of the following will best meet the client's nutritional needs at this time?
- □ 1. Offer a green salad topped with chicken pieces.
- □ 2. Offer a peanut butter sandwich.
- □ 3. Offer a bowl of vegetable soup.
- □ 4. Offer to have the family bring in favorite foods.

Anxiety and Somatoform Disorders

12. A client is admitted to the psychiatric inpatient unit for constant hand-washing rituals. The client states that she washes her hands at least 30 times each day. The nurse notices in the admission assessment that the client's hands are red, cracked, and dry. What is the priority goal for this client?
- □ 1. Reduce the number of hand washings during a day.
- □ 2. Eliminate hand washing for 3 days.
- □ 3. Suggest floor scrubbing instead of hand washing.
- □ 4. Use another form of anxiety reduction.

13. Hildegard Peplau saw nursing as an interpersonal process with the nurse-client relationship at its core. Which nursing intervention based on this theory would be most beneficial for the nurse to use when interacting with clients?
- □ 1. Recognize self-esteem of the client.
- □ 2. Recognize safety needs of the client.
- □ 3. Look at reinforcements as consequences.
- □ 4. Focus on communication with the client.

14. A client is admitted to the inpatient unit for obsessive-compulsive disorder (OCD). This client performs a hand-washing ritual many times a day. Which intervention should the nurse include in the client's care plan?
- □ 1. Allow free-time for 10 hr of the day.
- □ 2. Place the client in time-out each time the client washes the hands.
- □ 3. Hold a structured schedule throughout the day and early evening hours.
- □ 4. Have intense therapy for the client including 5 hr of group therapy per day.

15. The nurse is assessing a client with anxiety; which of the following observations is the most important?
- □ 1. The nurse's own anxiety.
- □ 2. The client's tongue movements.
- □ 3. Pill-rolling motion by the client.
- □ 4. The client's family history.

16. A client is seen in the clinic for anxiety related to a diagnosis of social phobia. What behavior would the nurse expect this client to exhibit?
- □ 1. Unwillingness to attend the wedding of a close family member.
- □ 2. Confidence in situations with unfamiliar people.
- □ 3. Outgoing nature when meeting new people.
- □ 4. Excitement toward attending a "welcome to the neighborhood" party.

The Client at Risk for Suicide

17. A client says to the nurse, "You are my favorite nurse. I want you to remember me when I am gone." "What is the most appropriate response by the nurse?"
- □ 1. "All of the nurses here are good to all of the clients."
- □ 2. "Thank you. You are one of my favorite clients, too."
- □ 3. "I don't care if you like me or not, you still need to take your medication."
- □ 4. "Are you having thoughts of suicide or hurting yourself?"

18. The charge nurse is reviewing staff assignments for the upcoming shift. Which client requires a staff for one-to-one observation (nurse stays by the client at all times)?
- □ 1. A clinically depressed client who has previously attempted suicide but denies current suicide ideation.
- □ 2. The client who admits to being suicidal but has no plan on how to accomplish the act.
- □ 3. The client who admitted to being suicidal after a phone call, but later states, "I was just angry."

□ 4. The client who admits to being suicidal and has a plan on how to do it.

19. A client approaches the nurse and states he just wants to be dead. The nurse initiates a no-suicide contract with the client. What should the nurse request of the client when initiating a no-suicide contract?

□ 1. A formal agreement to discuss any suicide thoughts immediately with a staff member.
□ 2. An agreement to discuss alternative coping strategies.
□ 3. An agreement to postpone suicidal actions until treatment is tried.
□ 4. An agreement to discuss suicidal plans with the physician.

20. AF A wife brings her husband to the emergency department with a bleeding gunshot wound to the leg. The wife tells the nurse that her husband was trying to commit suicide. The nurse should do which of the following in order of priority?

_____ 1. Assess current suicide risk.
_____ 2. Ensure constant observation.
_____ 3. Remove potentially harmful objects from the area.
_____ 4. Assess the gunshot wound.

Answers and Rationales

1. 4 A broad-opening statement is best to open the topic of how a client is doing; this allows the client to direct the conversation without being guided by the nurse. Statements that interpret the client's feelings may not allow the person to tell what his or her feelings actually are; limiting a question to feelings from only today may not allow the client to explain how things are going on most days. (P)

2. 3 Dysthymic disorder is a chronic feeling of depression present for at least 2 years. Postpartum depression occurs in the period after childbirth. Major depression is a more severe depression that is present for a shorter period before being diagnosed. Seasonal affective disorder occurs cyclically, usually when light is decreased. (P)

3. 2 The nurse refers the client for evaluation of depression. Suggesting to the client that she needs medication is not within the nurse's scope of practice. Offering ways to improve the client's diet does not deal with the client's depressive symptoms (feeling tired with a loss of interest in activities). Ignoring the comments because they are not related to a gynecology concern ignores the psychosocial part of the client's assessment; also, many women only have contact with health care through a gynecology exam, so an opportunity to improve the quality of life for the client would be lost. (H)

4. 2, 3 A depressed mood, loss of interest in activities, sleep disturbance, feelings of guilt, decreased energy, decreased concentration, appetite changes, and thoughts of suicide are symptoms of depression. Pacing and inability to sit still can be related to medication effects or mania; extreme fear of an object is indicative of a phobia; nightmare is a traumatic event and is indicative of posttraumatic stress disorder. (P)

5. 1 Depression can have an onset at any age, but is seen as normal in older adult clients related to the multiple losses associated with aging. Older adults express sadness just as at any other age, but may need to be asked. Older adults are in the health care system more often than younger ages as chronic illness develops. (H)

6. 2 SAD is depression linked to the shortened days of fall and winter. Phototherapy increases the exposure to light and increases mood of the client. Electroconvulsive therapy is used for clients who cannot use or are nonresponsive to antidepressants in major depression. Relaxation therapy is used in anxiety disorders. Group therapy is used to increase coping and understanding in many disorders. (P)

7. 1 Valproic acid can cause hepatotoxicity, so regular liver function tests are needed while taking this medication; other than hepatotoxicity, side effects include nausea and drowsiness. The nurse instructs the client to not crush or split tablets as this can change absorption, and to avoid alcohol in order to maintain therapeutic blood levels. (D)

8. 1 Temporary memory loss is a common side effect of ECT treatments. Bruising, unstable BP, and elevated temperature are not expected side effects of this treatment. (A)

9. 1, 2, 4, 5 NPO status, a signed consent, removal of dentures, and preprocedure voiding are all preparations prior to a procedure involving anesthesia, such as ECT. Orientation and frequent assessment of vital signs occur after the procedure. (R)

10. 3 Manic clients often do not take time to eat or sleep as they are too distracted and disorganized. The nurse carefully monitors the need for intervention in these areas to prevent exhaustion and malnutrition. Liquid formulations of medications are indicated only if the client cannot or will not swallow tablets. Manic clients may not be good candidates for group therapy as they often tend to be disruptive in group; also, visits from the family should not be connected to the client's behavior. The client is not likely to be able to concentrate and complete journal entries at this time. (P)

11. 2 Giving the client finger foods that have protein, carbohydrates, and calories supplies energy and allows the client to eat while on the move. A salad or soup is very difficult for the client to eat while moving and may not supply the nutrients needed. Favorite foods from home may or may not be appropriate to eat while walking. (C)

12. 1 The desired outcome is to decrease the number of hand washings. To eliminate the hand-washing rituals for 3 days would increase anxiety. At this time, the client is using hand washing to reduce anxiety, and limiting the hand washing or switching to another type of anxiety reduction may increase anxiety. (P)

13. 4 Peplau's theory focuses on the interpersonal interactions a nurse has with a client, with therapeutic communication aiding the client in growth. Self-esteem is associated with most developmental theories; recognizing safety needs is associated with Maslow's hierarchy of needs; and reinforcements as consequences is part of behavioral therapy. (P)

14. 3 A structured schedule for the client with rituals reduces anxiety by methods other than hand washing. A schedule with 10 hr of free-time in a day allows the client to continue the hand-washing ritual. Negative reinforcement increases guilt and anxiety. An intense therapy program is not indicated for the OCD client's rituals. (P)

15. 1 The nurse should be cognizant of her or his own personal anxiety. Anxiety from the nurse is conveyed to the client. Symptoms such as the tongue movements and pill-rolling motions by the client may be related to neuroleptic administration and are not related to the anxiety of the client. The client's family history may be significant, but the nurse is assessing the client at this moment and in the current setting. (P)

16. 1 The client with a social phobia has a marked, persistent fear of social situations. The client is afraid of unfamiliar people and concerned with being under possible analysis by those who are familiar; therefore, this client would not likely attend the wedding of a close family member. Persons with social phobia are not confident and cannot present themselves in an outgoing manner in situations with unfamiliar people. This client would not be likely to attend a "welcome to the neighborhood" party as the guests would not be familiar. (P)

17. 4 In order to address client safety, the nurse makes a direct assessment of the state of mind of any client who makes a direct or indirect comment indicating possible self-harm. Commenting that all nurses are good deflects the client's more direct comment. Commenting that a client is liked more than others sets up a possible manipulation scenario and crosses therapeutic boundaries. Discounting the client's comment does not give the nurse an opportunity to explore the thoughts of the client and decreases the focus from the client to the tasks the nurse needs to perform. (P)

18. 4 The client who admits to being suicidal and has a plan is at the highest risk for suicide. A client who denies feeling suicidal or has no plan is less of a risk and requires monitoring but not 1:1 observation. (M)

19. 1 The contract gives the staff time to explore alternatives at a critical time for the client as the client is having suicide thoughts. Discussing alternative coping at a crisis time is not the best way to ensure client safety. Postponing suicide thoughts or plans does not provide immediate safety. The physician may not be available for immediate intervention with the client. (S)

20. 4, 3, 2, 1 The nurse first assesses and treats the bleeding gunshot wound. Next, the nurse removes any objects the client could use to harm himself, and ensures that the client will have constant observation. The nurse then assesses the client's immediate risk for suicide, and bases subsequent decisions on the level of risk. Once the client is safe and the wound is treated, the nurse contacts the crisis intervention team. (R)

chapter

37

The Client With Schizophrenia and Related Psychotic Disorders, Cognitive Disorders, Psychosexual Disorders, and Mental Health Disorders in Children and Adolescents

The client with mental illness such as schizophrenia and psychoses may have distorted thought processes, hallucinations, and a variety of psychomotor disturbances that disrupt the ability to effectively communicate with others. The nurse has an important role in assisting the client with a mental illness to obtain health care services and assuring ongoing health care for these chronic health care problems. Topi this chapter include:

- Schizophrenia and Related Psyc
- Cognitive Disorders
- Psychosexual Disorders
- Mental Health Disorders in Adolescents

Schizophrenia and Related Psychotic Disorders

I. Definition: Schizophrenia is a serious and persistent mental condition in which the client suffers from distorted thought processes, emotions, and perceptions, as well as impaired reality testing and behaviors. The condition is a syndrome of disease processes rather than a single condition, and presents differently in each individual client. Related psychotic disorders (see following for types and definitions) involve psychotic conditions that are other than schizophrenia, and are differentiated in terms of level of impairment and presenting symptoms.
   A. Symptoms of schizophrenia are categorized as positive or negative (see assessment).
      1. Positive (hard) symptoms—clearly obvious signs of psychotic behavior such as hallucinations and delusions (see later discussion).
      2. Negative (soft) symptoms—less obvious, but more pervasive signs such as lack of interest, monotone voice, and inability to feel pleasure (see later discussion).
   B. According to the *Diagnostic and Statistical Manual of Mental Disorders* (DSM-IV-TR), there are five types of schizophrenia (American Psychiatric Association, 2000).
      1. Paranoid schizophrenia—serious and persistent mental schizophrenia condition involving positive symptoms; client is suspicious, paranoid, distrusting, and can exhibit aggressive and hostile behaviors.
      2. Disorganized-type schizophrenia—involves primarily negative symptoms; client has very inappropriate affect or flat affect, loose associations, incoherence, and disorganized behavior.
      3. Catatonic-type schizophrenia—involves primarily negative symptoms; client shows marked psychomotor disturbance (either motionless or continuous motor activity); immobility may be manifested by waxy flexibility/catalepsy or stupor.
      4. Undifferentiated schizophrenia—client speech and behavior indicate the psychoses of schizophrenia, but fail to meet the criteria of catatonic, paranoid, or disorganized types.
      5. Residual schizophrenia—client does not have positive symptoms, but continues to manifest negative symptoms.
   C. Psychotic disorders
      1. Schizophreniform disorder—involves symptoms of schizophrenia within short duration; symptoms last at least 1 month, but less than 6 months.
      2. Schizoaffective disorder—involves a period of illness with mood episode (depressive, mixed, or manic), along with symptoms of schizophrenia; often misdiagnosed as schizophrenia.
      3. Delusional disorder—involves nonbizarre (believable) delusions of at least a month's duration. Functioning is not impaired outside the delusion; can be persecutory somatic, grandiose, erotomaniac, or jealous delusions.
      4. Brief psychotic disorder—involves at least one of the following symptoms: delusions, hallucinations, disorganized or catatonic behavior and/or disorganized speech for duration of less than 1 month.
      5. Shared psychotic disorder—involves sharing of a delusion with another delusional person; this disorder is not caused by a substance use, another thought disorder, or other general medical condition.
      6. Substance-induced psychotic disorder—psychosis induced by substances such as alcohol, drugs, or other medical conditions.

II. Nursing process
   A. Assessment
      1. Assess for positive (hard) symptoms.
         a. Ambivalence—seemingly contradictory viewpoints or feelings about the same person, event, or situation.
         b. Associative looseness—fragmented or weakly related ideas.
         c. Delusions—fixed false beliefs (no basis of reality); client may be aggressive toward others or self.
         d. Echopraxia—imitation of the movements or gestures of another person.
         e. Flight of ideas—continued flow of conversation; client jumps from one topic to another.
         f. Hallucinations—false sensory perceptions that do not exist in reality; client fails to make eye contact and mumbles constantly.
         g. Ideas of reference—feelings that external events have special meaning.
         h. Perseveration—persistent clinging to a single idea or topic; verbal repetition of sentences, words, or phrases (echolalia); client resists attempts to change the subject.
      2. Assess for negative (soft) symptoms.
         a. Alogia—lack of speech.
         b. Anhedonia—feelings related to lack of pleasure from life, relationships, or activities.
         c. Apathy—lack of feeling toward people, events, or activities.

d. Avolition—lack of will, drive, or ambition to accomplish tasks; client lacks energy to perform daily tasks.
e. Blunted affect—restricted emotional ranges of moods, tones, and feelings.
f. Catalepsy (also called *waxy flexibility*)—client's limbs remain in the position in which they are placed for an indefinite period of time; occurs in catatonic clients.
g. Catatonia—psychologically induced immobility occasionally marked by periods of agitation or excitement; client acts as if in a trance.
h. Flat affect—absence of expressions indicating emotions or mood (especially facial); client may have feelings of isolation.

3. For client with related psychotic disorder, assess the following:
   a. Presence of delusions, hallucinations, disorganized speech, and/or catatonic behavior.
   b. Substance use; related thought disorder (chronic organic delusional disorder, chronic organic hallucinogenic disorder, or other organic disorders), or general medical condition.
   c. Duration of symptoms—question client and family.
4. Obtain diagnostic tests: Abnormal Involuntary Movement Scale (AIMS)—assesses movement disorders related to antipsychotic medications.

B. Analysis
1. Risk for Other-Directed Violence related to mental health problem
2. Risk for Suicide related to mental health problem
3. Disturbed Sensory Perception related to mental health problem
4. Disturbed Thought Processes related to mental health problem
5. Impaired Verbal Communication related to mental health problem
6. Self-Care Deficits related to mental health problem
7. Social Isolation related to mental health problem
8. Ineffective Health Maintenance related to mental health problem
9. Deficient Diversional Activity related to mental health problem
10. Ineffective Therapeutic Regimen Management related to mental health problem

C. Planning
1. Prevent client from injuring self and others.
2. Assist client to make reality statements.
3. Foster a trusting relationship with the client.
4. Promote positive behaviors within group setting.
5. Encourage verbalization of thoughts and feelings in a safe and socially acceptable manner.
6. Promote adherence to prescribed therapeutic interventions.
7. Promote adequate routines for sleeping and food and fluid intake.
8. Promote independence related to self-care activities.

D. Implementation
1. Administer medications as ordered.
2. Promote social skills training.
3. Administer AIMS assessments (see assessment).

E. Evaluation
1. Client does not injure self or others.
2. Client exhibits grasp on reality as evidenced by citation of reality statements.
3. Client demonstrates a trusting relationship with the nurse.
4. Client reacts appropriately with others in the environment.
5. Client expresses thoughts and feelings in a safe and socially acceptable manner.
6. Client's symptoms are stabilized as a result of adherence to medication regimen, group therapy sessions, and participation in social skills training.
7. Client is free from untoward side effects of medications.
8. Client maintains adequate routines for sleeping and food and fluid intake.
9. Client adequately performs self-care activities.

CN

III. Client needs

A. Physiologic adaptation
1. Substance abuse and schizophrenia frequently occur as comorbid conditions—nurse assesses for presence of substance abuse.
2. Client at risk for depression and suicide—nurse assesses risk factors for suicide (see assessment).
3. Paranoid schizophrenia may involve refusal to eat (client may feel food is poisoned)—nurse monitors food intake.
4. Schizophrenia often accompanied by other medical conditions such as cardiovascular conditions, hypertension, diabetes, and dental issues—nurse assesses and provides care for concomitant physical health problems.

B. Management of care: Care of the client with schizophrenia or related psychotic disorder requires critical thinking skills and knowledge of assessment, and teaching and evaluation methods unique to the RN role. These skills cannot be delegated to an LPN or UAP.
   1. Participate in interdisciplinary team conferences—nursing provides data from 24-hr assessment and care.
   2. Introduce client to community agencies such as halfway houses, for long-term care.
   3. Assess client for depression and risk of suicide, including presence of chronic illness with frequent relapses, frequent hospitalizations, negative attitude toward treatment, and self-harm attempts (see also Chapter 36).
   4. Lead or colead individual and group therapy sessions.
   5. Provide and receive reports from the mental health care team.
   6. Act as a client advocate.

C. Safety and infection control
   1. Provide physical assessment for wounds, diabetic ulcers, and dental issues as indicated.
   2. Provide client and family teaching about safety in the home setting; for example, removing objects that could be used for self-harm or triggers for an anxiety attack.

D. Health promotion and maintenance
   1. Provide long-term monitoring to maintain compliance with medications.
   2. Assist client obtain home health nurses; encourage client participation in community health agencies.
   3. Assist client with leisure activities appropriate to developmental level.

E. Psychologic integrity
   1. Respect cultural differences of client within a safety framework.
   2. For paranoid client, be aware of client's personal space; avoid touching the client until he or she develops trust in the nurse.

F. Basic care and comfort: Assist with activities of daily living for client who is not able to complete personal care.

G. Reduction of risk potential
   1. Monitor for signs of suicide potential.
   2. Monitor for aggression aimed at others.

H. Pharmacologic and parenteral therapies: Client and family will state the purpose for and associated side effects of all medications. See Table 37-1 for common medications used for clients with thought disorders, including typical and atypical antipsychotics. Clients with schizoaffective disorders commonly receive antidepressant medications or mood stabilizers, as needed.

Cognitive Disorders

I. Definition: Cognitive disorders are characterized by a deficit or disruption in the ability of the client to learn and/or think.
   A. Delirium—cognitive dysfunction and disruption in consciousness with rapid onset. Delirium may also be called acute brain syndrome, ICU psychosis, acute confusion, and/or acute toxic psychosis.
   B. Dementia—characterized by continued deficits in cognition and memory. Types of dementia include:
      1. Alzheimer disease dementia (involves stages of condition).
      2. Vascular dementia.
      3. HIV dementia.
      4. Parkinson disease dementia.
      5. Substance-induced persistent dementia.
      6. Dementia due to Huntington disease.
      7. Dementia due to head trauma.
      8. Dementia due to medical condition (e.g., infections).

II. Nursing process
   A. Assessment
      1. Differentiate between dementia and other conditions that could cause cognitive deficiencies such as:
         a. Withdrawal from drugs.
         b. Endocrine disorders.
         c. Metal toxicities.
         d. Infections (e.g., HIV/AIDS, viral hepatitis, encephalitis).
         e. Metabolic disturbances (fluid and electrolyte disruptions, hepatic encephalopathy, hypoxia, hypotension, COPD, uremia).
         f. Neoplastic conditions.
         g. Trauma.
         h. Nutritional (malnutrition, deficiency of vitamin B_{12}, folate, thiamine).
         i. Pain.
         j. Seizures.
         k. Sensory deficits or overload.
      2. Assess for differentiating symptoms from Alzheimer disease, Pick disease, Huntington chorea, Wernicke-Korsakoff syndrome, and/or vascular dementia.
      3. Assess for delirium—sudden change in consciousness with fluctuation between lethargy and agitation; confusion, disorientation to time, person, place; lack of mental focus and concentration; changes in level of

Table 37-1 Common Medications for Clients With Thought Disorders

Classification	Generic/Trade Name	Expected Outcomes	Reduction of Risk Potential	Management of Care
Typical Antipsychotic Aliphatic Phenothiazines	Chlorpromazine (Thorazine); trifluoperazine (Stelazine)	Provides immediate relief of agitation from schizophrenia symptoms.	Increase dose until optimum dose achieved. Monitor for side effects including drowsiness; insomnia; EPS; dry mouth; salivation and drooling; nausea and vomiting; anorexia; constipation; hypotension; anemia; urinary retention; photophobia and photosensitivity; blurred vision; and urticaria.	Ensure client uses sunscreen when outdoors. Monitor bowel elimination. Monitor AIMS. Provide client teaching about side effects to prevent noncompliance with medication regime.
Piperazine Phenothiazines	Trifluoperazine (Stelazine); fluphenazine (Prolixin); thiothixene (Navane)	Trifluoperazine (Stelazine) relieves agitation from schizophrenia symptoms at most effective dose. Fluphenazine (Prolixin); may take 6 weeks to 6 months to achieve full therapeutic effects. Prolixin Decanoate (Prolixin D) provides symptom relief for clients for 3 to 4 weeks when administered IM; and is especially helpful for clients who are medication-noncompliant. Thiothixene (Navane) provides immediate relief with IM administration.	For client taking Trifluoperazine (Trilafon), monitor for drowsiness, pseudoparkinsonism, dystonia, and akathisia. For client taking Prolixin, prevent sudden death due to asphyxia or cardiac arrest. For client taking Navane, monitor for discolored urine (from pink to reddish brown), photophobia, and nasal congestion.	Monitor for side effects. Navane is sedating with a half-life of 34 hr. After administration, clients will not respond to questions for a considerable length of time.
Piperidine Phenothiazines Butyrophenone Dibenzoxazepine	Thioridazine (Mellaril); mesoridazine (Serentil); haloperidol (Haldol) loxapine (Loxitane); molindone (Moban)	Thioridazine (Mellaril) relieves agitation from schizophrenia symptoms at most effective dose. Haldol is sedating with a half-life of 21–34 hr with oral administration; also administered via Haldol Decanoate (Haldol D) alternate method to provide half-life of 3 weeks.	Monitor for side effects: drowsiness; insomnia; EPS; dry mouth; salivation and drooling; nausea and vomiting; anorexia; constipation; hypotension; urinary retention; photophobia and photosensitivity; blurred vision; urticaria. Mellaril can cause urine to be discolored from pink to reddish brown. Haldol can cause cough reflex suppression.	Monitor for side effects. Mellaril is sedating with a half-life of 10–20 hr. After administration, clients will not respond to questions for a considerable length of time. Monitor the client receiving Haldol for aspiration (related to cough reflex suppression). Monitor for sedation, orthostatic hypotension. Monitor client for dizziness, extrapyramidal effects such as weakness, agitation, torticollis, myoclonic twitches, shuffling gait.

(continued)

Table 37-1 Common Medications for Clients With Thought Disorders (Continued)

Classification	Generic/Trade Name	Expected Outcomes	Reduction of Risk Potential	Management of Care
Atypical Antipsychotic	Clozapine (Clozaril)	Relieves symptoms at optimum oral dose.	Monitor for side effects: weight gain, sedation, salivation, seizures, agranulocytosis, and sexual dysfunction.	Indicated in clients with TD. Check baseline and weekly WBC counts throughout treatment and for 4 weeks after discontinuation. Be alert if client develops fever and sore throat as this can be a symptom of agranulocytosis (medication stopped immediately).
Atypical Antipsychotic	Risperidone (Risperdal)	Provides some immediate relief; more when dose meets peak.	Monitor for side effects: agitation, anxiety, insomnia, nausea and vomiting, and neuroleptic syndrome (severe EPS and high fever).	Monitor side effects such as dizziness, orthostatic hypotension, dry mouth, drowsiness.
Atypical Antipsychotic	Olanzapine (Zyprexa)	Relieves symptoms when therapeutic dose is achieved.	Monitor for side effects: dizziness, somnolence, neuroleptic malignant syndrome (NMS), postural hypotension, fever, constipation, and weight gain.	Do not exceed 20 mg/day. Be alert to side effects, especially drowsiness/sleepiness. Evaluate for diabetes II in client experiencing side effect of weight gain.
Atypical Antipsychotic	Quetiapine (Seroquel)	May be sedating (especially initially).	Monitor for side effects: drowsiness, NMS, and orthostatic hypotension.	Observe for side effects.
Atypical Antipsychotic	Ziprasidone (Geodon)	Provides high sedation rate.	Monitor for side effects: drowsiness, somnolence, headache, dysrhythmias, nausea, dyspepsia, constipation, and fever.	Prevent noncompliance with medication regimen by explaining side effects to client (especially large weight gain).
Atypical Antipsychotic	Aripiprazole (Abilify)	Provides moderate sedation.	Monitor for side effects: headache, NMS, insomnia, anxiety. nausea and vomiting, lightheadedness, tremor, cough, orthostatic hypotension, constipation or diarrhea, rhinitis, and seizures.	Observe for side effects.

consciousness; drowsiness. In older adults, delirium can be mistaken for dementia.

4. Obtain diagnostic tests: Screening tests to rule out dementia.
   a. WBC—infection.
   b. CBC with differential; Hgb—anemia.
   c. ESR— infection or vasculitis.
   d. Urinalysis and toxicology test.
      (1) Sugar and acetone—diabetes.
      (2) Barbiturates and other toxic substances.
      (3) Leukocytes—infection.

(4) Albumin—renal failure.
(5) Heavy metals—heavy metal intoxication.

e. BUN and creatinine—renal failure.
f. Chest and/or skull x-rays—check tumors and/or trauma.

B. Analysis
1. Self-Care Deficit: Dressing and Grooming, related to motor and cognitive impairments
2. Risk for Injury related to cognitive impairment and wandering
3. Chronic Confusion related to cognitive impairment
4. Disturbed Sensory Perception related to cognitive impairment
5. Disturbed Thought Processes related to cognitive impairment
6. Impaired Verbal Communication related to cognitive impairment
7. Social Isolation related to cognitive impairment
8. Ineffective Health Maintenance related to cognitive impairment
9. Deficient Diversional Activity related to cognitive impairment
10. Ineffective Therapeutic Regimen Management related to cognitive impairment
11. Decisional Conflict related to cognitive impairment
12. Risk for Caregiver Role Strain related to demands of care for family member
13. Interrupted Family Processes related to ongoing change in family dynamics and need for care for the client
14. Imbalanced Nutrition: Less than Body Requirements, related to increased activity or inability to remember to eat

C. Planning
1. Promote client achievement of physical requirements.
2. Prevent injury.
3. Eliminate or reduce episodes of agitation.
4. Promote psychosocial support for client and family.
5. Promote adequate food and fluid intake.

D. Implementation
1. Assist with activities of daily living as client condition warrants; establish routines for meals, grooming, and leisure.
2. Assist client and family to express feelings and fears about the diagnosis, as well as role and health status changes.
3. Promote safety in home setting—remove household clutter and create predictability; instruct family to lock doors to outdoors/garages.
4. Describe options for care such as daycare and full-time nursing home care.

E. Evaluation
1. Client and family verbalize feelings about the diagnosis.
2. Client is free from injury as a result of measures to create safe environment.
3. Client demonstrates ability to function in the environment.
4. Client and family make plans for future care.
5. Client's family demonstrates effective coping related to changes in roles and client's health.

III. Client needs

A. Physiologic adaptation: Delirium has an underlying cause such as head trauma, endocrine imbalances, exposure to toxins—managing delirium involves treating or eliminating the cause. Untreated delirium can result in irreversible neurologic damage.
1. Client at risk for depression (especially with initial diagnosis) and may attempt suicide—nurse assesses risk factors for suicide (see management of care).
2. Client may have difficulty identifying food, or may forget to eat—nurse monitors food intake and provides adequate nutrition.

B. Management of care: Care of the client with a cognitive disorder requires critical thinking skills and knowledge of assessment, and teaching and evaluation methods unique to the RN role. These skills cannot be delegated to an LPN or UAP.
1. Participate in interdisciplinary team conferences—nursing contributes data from 24-hr assessment and care.
2. Introduce client and family to community agencies such as home health nursing and case-manager.
3. Assess client for depression and risk of suicide, including presence of chronic illness with frequent relapses, frequent hospitalizations, negative attitude toward treatment, and self-harm attempts (see also Chapter 36).

C. Safety and infection control
1. Provide physical assessment for wounds and diabetic ulcers as indicated.
2. Because older adult clients may not show usual symptoms of infections (e.g., fever in respiratory, urinary tract) monitor for changes in behavior.
3. Maintain a safe environment—remove objects that could cause danger; remove rugs that could cause the client to trip and fall; restrict client's driving as needed.

Table 37-2 Common Medications for Clients With Cognitive Disorders

Classification	Generic/Trade Name	Expected Outcomes	Reduction of Risk Potential	Management of Care
Cholinesterase Inhibitor	Tacrine (Cognex)	Slows progress of dementia; does not effect overall course of disease.	Monitor enzymes for toxic effects to liver.	Monitor for flulike symptoms.
Cholinesterase Inhibitor	Donepezil (Aricept)	Slows progress of dementia; does not affect overall course of disease.	Monitor for nausea, loose stools, and insomnia.	Monitor for guaiac stools.
Cholinesterase Inhibitor	Rivastigmine (Exelon)	Slows progress of dementia; does not affect overall course of disease.	Monitor for abdominal pain, nausea, and vomiting.	Monitor for loss of appetite.
Cholinesterase Inhibitor	Galantamine (Razadyne)	Slows progress of dementia; does not affect overall course of disease.	Monitor for loss of appetite, nausea, and vomiting.	Monitor for dizziness and syncope.

D. Health promotion and maintenance
   1. Promote long-term observation to maintain compliance with medication regimen.
   2. Assist client maintain orientation to time, place, and person; use clocks, calendars, familiar objects.

E. Psychologic integrity: Respect cultural differences of client within a safety framework.

F. Basic care and comfort
   1. Assist with activities of daily living for client who is not able to complete personal care; use clothes with Velcro and elastic that are easy for client to put on; keep client oriented to activities to perform; provide short, simple, and repeated directions.
   2. Provide calendars and clocks.
   3. Keep room well lit.
   4. Keep head of bed elevated.

G. Reduction of risk potential
   1. Monitor for signs of suicide potential.
   2. Monitor for aggression aimed at others.
   3. Monitor side effects of medications.

H. Pharmacologic and parenteral therapies: Client and family will state the purpose for and associated side effects of all medications used to treat cognitive disorders, including atypical antipsychotics, typical antipsychotics, and antidepressants, as indicated by individual client needs (see Table 37-2).

Psychosexual Disorders

I. Definition: Psychosexual disorders are mental health problems in which a client has difficulty relating to the opposite sex or responding in appropriate ways to interactions with others in social settings.

A. Sexual dysfunction—defined as an alteration in the sexual response cycle or by pain with intercourse. Disorders may involve the following:
   1. Desire—hypoactive sexual desire and sexual aversion disorder.
   2. Arousal—male erectile disorder and female hypoactive sexual disorder.
   3. Orgasm—male and female orgasmic disorders and premature ejaculation.
   4. Pain—dyspareunia (male or female) or vaginismus not attributed to a general medical condition.
   5. Other—medical condition or induced by use of medicinal and illegal substances.

B. Paraphilias
   1. Fetishism—fantasies, behaviors, or urges resulting in sexual arousal.
   2. Frotteurism—intense recurrent sexual arousal, fantasies, urges, or behaviors involving rubbing against or touching a nonconsenting person.
   3. Exhibitionism—intense recurrent sexual arousal from exposing genitals, usually to an unsuspecting stranger.
   4. Pedophilia—sexual arousal from sexual activity with children 13 years or younger.
   5. Masochism—sexual arousal from being made to suffer (e.g., act of being bound, abused, or beaten).
   6. Sadism—sexual arousal from inflicting suffering on others.
   7. Transvestic fetishism—heterosexual male achieving sexual arousal from cross-dressing.

8. Voyeurism—sexual arousal from watching someone who is disrobing, naked, or engaging in sexual activity.

C. Gender identity disorder—involves a strong and persistent identification with the opposite sex; the client has marked distress or impaired occupational, social, or other functioning because of the gender identity disorder.

II. Nursing process

A. Assessment: General assessments for psychosexual disorders include:

1. Anxiety.
2. Complaints of decreased sexual desire.
3. Complaints of absent or delayed orgasm.
4. Depression.
5. Body image disturbance.
6. Frustration.
7. Inability to maintain erections.
8. Coping skills.
9. Complaints of pain with intercourse.
10. Complaints of a premature ejaculation.
11. Isolation (social).
12. History of surgical procedures such as perineal prostatectomy, ileostomy, colostomy, radical cystectomy, abdominal perineal colon resection.

B. Analysis

1. Sexual Dysfunction related to psychosexual disorder
2. Chronic Low Self-Esteem related to psychosexual disorder
3. Impaired Social Interaction related to psychosexual disorder
4. Situational Low Self-Esteem related to psychosexual disorder

C. Planning

1. Promote client feelings of self-worth.
2. Promote methods to increase satisfaction with sexuality.

D. Implementation

1. Establish a therapeutic relationship—involves sharing intimate and sometimes embarrassing information that may be withheld unless a relationship of trust is achieved.
2. Observe personal attitudes regarding sex or psychosexual alterations.
3. Provide information for the client regarding sexuality and expressions.
4. Promote verbalization of fear, concerns, and health issues.
5. Provide client teaching about medical and/or surgical treatments (e.g., vacuum devices, penile implants).
6. Provide instruction about medications—sildenafil citrate (Viagra), alprostadil (Caverject), estrogen (Premarin), testosterone, for example.

E. Evaluation

1. Client adheres to treatment for sexual dysfunction.
2. Client achieves satisfying sexual intimacy.
3. Client verbalizes concerns and feelings about sexuality and listens and responds to needs of partner.
4. Client expresses sexuality in a healthy and socially acceptable manner.

CN

III. Client needs

A. Physiologic adaptation

1. For the male older adult client, the refractory period after ejaculation lengthens, resulting in a less firm erection, longer time to achieve an erection, and occasionally inability to achieve an erection.
2. For the female older adult client, there is a loss of lubrication and dyspareunia.
3. Medication use (such an antihypertensives, antidepressants, anti-Parkinson agents) and certain conditions (such as diabetes) may cause impotence and decreased libido.
4. The client who has sexual reassignment surgery requires hormone treatment as well as reconstructive surgery.

B. Management of care: Care of the client with a psychosexual disorder requires critical thinking skills and knowledge of assessment, and teaching and evaluation methods unique to the RN role. These skills cannot be delegated to an LPN or UAP.

1. Provide encouragement to discuss feelings about sexual dysfunction.
2. Assess and address self-esteem issues.
3. Refer client for counseling as needed; encourage marital or couples therapy for couples with difficulty with sexual expression.
4. Provide pre- and postoperative care for client receiving reconstructive sexual surgeries or having surgery that will involve sexual health.

C. Safety and infection control: Provide client teaching regarding susceptibility to sexually transmitted diseases and pelvic inflammatory disease for the client with multiple sexual partners.

D. Health promotion and maintenance: Inform client about side effects of medications that will impact sexual health as impotence; promote adherence to medication regimen.

E. Psychologic integrity

1. Promote active listening for statements of self-worth; allow the client to explore ideas about how sexual performance relates to self-esteem.
2. Differentiate feelings (e.g., loneliness, sadness) from negative self-esteem ("I am not lovable.").

3. Encourage client to focus on strengths and to increase time and energy spent on activities in these areas.
4. Encourage client with psychosexual concerns to describe all personal attributes, not only sexual performance.
5. Respect cultural differences of client; observe personal biases and concerns.

F. Basic care and comfort
1. Anticipate sexual concerns during life events, such as after a myocardial infarction (MI).
2. Assess for conditions client may hesitate to ask about such as dyspareunia, vaginismus, and priapism.

G. Reduction of risk potential (see safety and infection control).

H. Pharmacologic and parenteral therapies: Client will state purposes for and associated side effects of all medications used to treat psychosexual disorders, including male and female hormones and anti-impotence agents such as sildenafil citrate (Viagra) or vardenafil (Levitra).

Mental Health Disorders in Children and Adolescents

I. Definition: The child with a mental health disorder is more difficult to identify, as children often lack the ability to complete detailed abstract thinking as well as the verbal skills necessary to explain their thoughts. As a result of constant change and development, children experience difficulty discriminating between unusual and unwanted symptoms from normal sensations and feelings. Also, normal child behaviors vary from age to age and in terms of developmental level (see Chapter 9). Types of child and adolescent psychiatric disorders are as follows:

A. Mental retardation—involves less than average intellectual functioning accompanied by limits in the areas of communication and social functioning, education, self-care, safety, and health.
1. Causes may include factors such as a fragile X chromosome syndrome; Tay-Sachs disease; trisomy 21; maternal alcohol intake; fetal malnutrition, hypoxia, trauma, lead poisoning, or infections; and environmental influences such as deprivation of stimulation or nurturance.
2. The degree of difficulty a child experiences with cognitive disability is based on IQ and labeled as:
a. Mild—IQ ranges from 50 to 70.
b. Moderate—IQ ranges from 35 to 50.
c. Severe—IQ ranges from 20 to 35.
d. Profound—IQ is less than 20.

B. Learning disorders—suspected when a child's ability in mathematics, reading, or writing is below that for the education, age, and intelligence of the child, who is often poor in social skills and has low self-esteem. The child with a learning disability requires early assessment and intervention to prevent the disorder from continuing into adulthood.

C. Pervasive developmental disorders—characterized by all-encompassing and, most often, severely impaired social skills. Another name for this group of disorders is *autism spectrum disorders*. Two common pervasive developmental disorders include:
1. Autism—condition is identified in children no older than 3 years of age, and improves with treatment when child starts to speak and communicate with others. Unusual behaviors may increase in adolescence and are thought to be related to hormonal changes and increased social demands. Children with autism are "mainstreamed" into the classrooms at this time. Adults with autism may be given the diagnosis of schizoid personality disorder, mental retardation, or obsessive-compulsive disorder, and usually lack the social skills to allow independent functioning. Characteristics of the child with autism are as follows:
a. Displays little to no eye contact with others.
b. Fails to make attempts to communicate or relate to parents or peers.
c. Frequently appears to lack enjoyment; displays no emotional affects or moods.
d. Speech is often not understood by others.
e. Frequently engages in repetitive motor behaviors such as head-banging, body-twisting, or hand-flapping.
2. Asperger disorder—the child with this disorder displays impairments of social interaction and stereotyped behaviors as seen in the child with autism, but there is neither the language nor the cognitive delays of the autism client. Asperger disorder is generally lifelong.

D. Attention-deficit hyperactivity disorder (ADHD)—characterized by overactivity, impulsiveness, and inattentiveness. ADHD is a common disorder; occurs more frequently in boys (75%) and accounts for the majority of mental health referrals for school-aged children (3% to 5%) (Videbeck, 2004, p. 485). Diagnosis given once other psychiatric problems are ruled out, including bipolar disorder and inadequate parenting and home stressors when a child exhibits problems in the classroom. Specific characteristics of the disorder by age are as follows:

1. Infant—often fussy and has poor sleeping patterns.
2. Toddler—constantly active and may destroy objects such as toys.
3. School-aged child—has difficulty sitting in class and may make noise in class; this child is also distracted by sounds in the classroom and frequently fails to complete assignments or follow directions for homework.
4. Adolescent—occurs in two thirds of adolescents with ADHD in childhood; client exhibits manifestation of symptoms such as adopting high risk-taking behaviors, getting speeding tickets, and class cutting; and having difficulty maintaining interpersonal relationships. Thirty percent to 50% of these clients have ADHD in adulthood; client continues to experience higher rates of impulsivity, high-risk behaviors, and personality disorders (Videbeck, 2004, p. 485).

E. Conduct disorder—characterized by antisocial behavior in children and adolescents. This disorder involves aggression toward animals and people, deceitfulness, serious rule violations, and property destruction; very little empathy toward others and low self-esteem; temper outbursts and a poor frustration tolerance; and destructive behaviors at an early age, including sexual engagement, drinking, smoking, and illegal substance use.

F. Oppositional defiant disorder (ODD)—involves a long-term pattern of defiant, hostile, and uncooperative behavior. Client experiences fears, guilt, and anxiety about education, sex, and health; irregular or deficient learning patterns and numerous hypochondriac complaints; poor relationships with peers and is unable to delay personal gratification; and inability to socialize and assume autonomy.

G. Tourette disease—involves motor and one or more vocal tics; the complexity of tics change as time progresses. The child has impairment in social, academic, and occupational areas; has feelings of shame; and is self-conscious about the tics. This condition is sometimes relieved in early adulthood or sometimes is a lifelong problem for the client.

H. Encopresis—involves passage of feces in inappropriate places by a child over 4 years of age (chronologically or developmentally); disorder may be involuntary or intentional.

1. Involuntary encopresis usually accompanied with constipation.
2. Intentional encopresis usually accompanied with ODD or conduct disorder.

I. Enuresis—involves repeated voiding of urine by child at least 5 years of age (chronologically or developmentally); if intentional, enuresis is usually connected with a disruptive behavior disorder.

II. Nursing process

A. Assessment: Assess the child or adolescent with a mental health disorder by interviewing the parents, daycare providers, and/or teachers for presence of:

1. Infant—fussiness.
2. Toddler—hyperactivity.
3. School-aged child:
   a. Overactive, thrill-seeking, or dangerous behavior.
   b. Inability to pay attention to what is said.
   c. Achievement of developmental milestones (frequently lags behind others).
   d. Labile moods (tantrums and/or verbal outbursts).
   e. Becoming resistant or angry when adult attempts to redirect the child.
   f. Attention span short.
   g. Lack of judgment (e.g., may run in street).
   h. Disturbed relationships with peers.
4. Adolescent:
   a. Destruction of property.
   b. Deceitfulness or theft.
   c. Serious disobedience of rules (running away, staying out all night, truancy).
   d. Extreme appearance for age (tattoos, body piercing, clothing, hair).
   e. Slouching during interview.
   f. Use of profanity, name-calling, disparaging remarks about authority figures.
   g. Moodiness.
   h. Intact thought processes.
   i. Intellectual capacity (impaired only in mental retardation), but grades may be low.
   j. Low self-esteem.
   k. Unplanned pregnancies and/or STDs.

B. Analysis

1. Risk for Injury related to mental health disorder
2. Impaired Social Interaction related to mental health disorder
3. Compromised Family Coping related to mental health disorder
4. Ineffective Role Performance related to mental health disorder
5. Risk for Other-Directed Violence related to mental health disorder

6. Ineffective Coping related to mental health disorder
7. Chronic Low Self-Esteem related to mental health disorder
8. Noncompliance related to mental health disorder

C. Planning
1. Prevent injury to self and others.
2. Promote social skills appropriate for the child's developmental age.
3. Administer medications as indicated.
4. Promote adherence to treatment regimen.
5. Promote age-appropriate behaviors when interacting with peers and/or adults.
6. Promote self-esteem.
7. Promote effective problem-solving and coping skills.

D. Implementation
1. Ensure safety (see safety and infection control).
2. After gaining client's full attention, provide short, clear instructions.
3. Provide specific positive feedback when the client meets specific directions.
4. Provide a structured daily routine.
5. Set limits on unacceptable behavior; use "time outs" to regain self-control; show acceptance of client even when behavior is not acceptable.
6. Have client with conduct disorder keep a diary to identify and express feelings; role model and teach social skills to this client.
7. Teach parents effective age-appropriate expectations such as curfews, household assignments, and limit-setting with appropriate consequences.

E. Evaluation
1. Client makes progress toward appropriate behaviors.
2. Client's hyperactivity and impulsivity is reduced with medications.
3. Client exhibits improved sociability, attention span, academic achievement, and peer relationships.
4. Client is free from injury to self and others.
5. Client does not infringe on boundaries of others.
6. Client completes assigned tasks and demonstrates ability to follow directions.
7. Client adheres to prescribed treatment.
8. Client uses age-appropriate acceptable behaviors when interacting with peers and/or adults.
9. Client makes positive, age-appropriate statements about himself or herself.
10. Client demonstrates effective problem-solving and coping skills.

III. Client needs

A. Physiologic adaptation: The child with a mental health disorder may also have other health problems that require concurrent treatment. The goal is to treat the child's developmental needs as well as to promote physiologic and mental health. Treatment is considered effective when the child or adolescent has behavior that is legal and positive.

B. Management of care: Care of the child or adolescent with a mental health disorder requires critical thinking skills and knowledge of assessment, and teaching and evaluation methods unique to the RN role. These skills cannot be delegated to an LPN or UAP.
1. Participate in interdisciplinary team conferences—nurse provides data from 24-hr assessment and care.
2. Introduce client to community agencies such as halfway houses for long-term care.
3. Provide and receive report on the assigned hospitalized client from and among health care team members.
4. Act as a client advocate.
5. Set limits on unacceptable behavior—instruct all staff members to provide consistent limit enforcement.

C. Safety and infection control
1. Provide client and family teaching about specific mental health disorders and safety issues in the home, such as need to protect child from injury from malfunctioning equipment or electrical hazards.
2. Instruct parents on developmental milestones regarding safety.

D. Health promotion and maintenance
1. Perform physical assessment on admission to psychiatric facilities and as per agency policy.
2. Provide long-term monitoring of growth to maintain compliance with stimulant medications for the ADHD client.
3. Assist client to obtain home care, including home health nurses and community health agencies.
4. Assist client with activities appropriate for preference and developmental age.

E. Psychologic integrity
1. Provide active listening for the client and family regarding difficulties with adjusting to the mental health disorder.
2. Assess cultural factors affecting client care.
3. Provide a therapeutic milieu—make environment as quiet as possible, with minimal distractions.

Table 37-3 Medications for Children and Adolescents With ADHD

Classification	Generic/Trade Name Examples	Expected Outcomes	Reduction of Risk Potential	Management of Care
Stimulant	Methylphenidate (Ritalin)	Decreases impulsiveness and hyperactivity and improves attention span.	Monitor client for decreased appetite or delays in growth.	Administer after meals.
Sustained Release Stimulants	Methylphenidate (Ritalin SR, Concerta, Metadate CD)	Decreases impulsiveness and hyperactivity and improves attention span.	Monitor for insomnia.	Administer last dose in the early afternoon.
Stimulant Sustained Release Stimulants	Dextroamphetamine (Dexedrine) Dexedrine SR	Decreases impulsiveness and hyperactivity and improves attention span.	Monitor for decreased appetite.	Inform client and family this medication may take 2 days to take effect.
Amphetamine Sustained Release Amphetamine	Amphetamine (Adderall) Adderall XR, pemoline (Cylert)	Decreases impulsiveness and hyperactivity and improves attention span.	Monitor for liver function test elevation and decreased appetite.	Inform client and family this medication may take 2 weeks to achieve full effect.

4. Participate in group sessions with the client and family.
5. Use therapeutic communication techniques to assist the client and family to gain an understanding of the disorder.

F. Basic care and comfort
1. Evaluate the child on stimulant medication for ADHD weight and growth patterns.
2. Assist with activities of daily living.
3. Incorporate alternative and complementary therapies into plan of care (e.g., play therapy, art therapy).
4. Provide interventions for the client with ADHD regarding alteration in nutritional intake.
5. Provide therapies for comfort and treatment of injuries obtained in impulsive episodes to the client/parents/caregivers as needed.

G. Reduction of risk potential
1. Administer SNAP-IV Teacher and Parent Rating Scale to parents and/or teachers as an initial tool for ADHD, ODD, depression, and conduct disorder.
2. Identify client at risk for abuse.
3. Identify the need to institute suicide precautions; implement and maintain suicide precautions as needed.
4. Perform a risk assessment for injuries related to impulsiveness.

H. Pharmacologic and parenteral therapies: Antidepressants (imipramine [Tofranil]) are used with children with enuresis. See Table 37-3 for medications used with children and adolescents with ADHD. Client and family will state the purpose for and associated side effects of all medications used to manage specific mental health disorder.

Bibliography

American Psychiatric Association. (2000). *Diagnostic and statistical manual of mental disorders* (4th ed., text rev.). Washington, DC: Author.

Mohr, W. K. (2006). *Psychiatric-mental health nursing* (6th ed.). Philadelphia: Lippincott Williams & Wilkins.

Videbeck, S. L. (2004). *Psychiatric-mental health nursing* (2nd ed.). Philadelphia: Lippincott Williams & Wilkins.

CHAPTER 37

Practice Test

Schizophrenia and Related Psychotic Disorders

1. While the nurse is performing an admission assessment, the client stops talking in the middle of a sentence, tips his head to the side, and listens carefully. Which of the following is the client most likely experiencing?

□ 1. Somatic delusions.
□ 2. Pseudoparkinsonism.
□ 3. Delusions of reference.
□ 4. Auditory hallucinations.

2. AF The nurse is developing a care plan with a client who is receiving ziprasidone (Geodon) and has stopped taking the drug. The nurse should discuss which of the following side effects that may occur and be a reason the client is noncompliant with taking this medication? Select all that apply.

□ 1. Somnolence.
□ 2. Weight gain.
□ 3. Urticaria.
□ 4. Constipation.
□ 5. Headache.

3. When a client is receiving antipsychotic medications, the nurse monitors the results of which of the following tests?

□ 1. CAGE.
□ 2. AIMS.
□ 3. DSM-IV-TR.
□ 4. GDS.

4. The nurse is reviewing laboratory values of a client receiving clozapine (Clozaril). Which of the following laboratory values does the nurse immediately report to the primary care provider?

□ 1. WBC of 3,500.
□ 2. Hemoglobin of 11.2 g/dl.
□ 3. Sodium level of 136 mEq/L.
□ 4. Hyaline casts in the urinalysis.

5. The nurse should assess a client who believes that everyone is against him for which of the following?

□ 1. Hallucination.
□ 2. Illusion.
□ 3. Flight of ideas.
□ 4. Delusion.

Cognitive Disorders

6. During a home visit, a client who is 75 years of age tells the community health nurse, "Lately I'm getting forgetful about things. For one thing, I cannot remember names. Do you think I am getting Alzheimer disease?" Which of the following responses by the nurse is the most therapeutic?

□ 1. "It is normal for people your age to forget things such as names."
□ 2. "I do the same thing. Sometimes I cannot remember someone's name either."
□ 3. "Tell me more about your forgetfulness. It isn't unusual for forgetfulness to occur."
□ 4. "Most people your age have this problem. It's not Alzheimer."

7. A client is admitted with a diagnosis of dementia (Alzheimer type). Which nursing intervention is the priority when caring for this client?

□ 1. Ensure client meets other clients on the unit to prevent isolation.
□ 2. Ensure client completes own activities of daily living to prevent dependence.
□ 3. Ensure environment is safe to prevent injury.
□ 4. Ensure client receives food to prevent malnourishment.

8. A client admitted with a diagnosis of dementia tells the nurse, "We will have fireworks tonight. We always have fireworks on July 4th." Which response by the nurse is the most therapeutic for this client?

□ 1. "Today is November 9. We will have dinner soon and then your daughter is coming to visit."
□ 2. "Do not be silly. It is not the 4th of July."
□ 3. "What else are you planning for the 4th?"
□ 4. "I will bring your medication now."

9. A client is admitted with a diagnosis of dementia (Alzheimer type) and becomes agitated, violent, and has bizarre thoughts. The nurse is reviewing the client's medication record. Which of the following medications is ordered for the client with the expected outcome of reducing agitation?

□ 1. Tacrine (Cognex).
□ 2. Ergoloid (Hydergine).

□ 3. Diazepam (Valium).
□ 4. Risperidone (Risperdal).

10. The nurse is planning care for a client admitted for vascular dementia. Which of the following is most appropriate in assisting the client with activities of daily living?
□ 1. Perform activities for the client during hospitalization.
□ 2. Document all activities the nurse expects the client to complete during the shift.
□ 3. Inform client that if morning care is not completed by 8:30 a.m., the UAP will complete it.
□ 4. Encourage client to complete as many activities as possible and provide ample time to complete them.

Psychosexual Disorders

11. The nurse is counseling a male client receiving hormonal therapy prior to a breast augmentation for a sex-change surgery. The client expresses a concern about going home and telling his friends and family about his treatment and that he would like to be thought of as a woman. Which nursing diagnosis is the priority for this client?
□ 1. Social Isolation related to distance between client and family.
□ 2. Ineffective Role Performance related to inability to define role.
□ 3. Dysfunctional Family Processes related to fear.
□ 4. Disturbed Body Image related to gender identity disorder.

12. A couple informs the nurse that they have been having some "problems in the bedroom." The most appropriate response by the nurse is:
□ 1. "I can refer you to a therapist."
□ 2. "I need to obtain your admission history first."
□ 3. "What are your concerns?"
□ 4. "Let me refer you to a marriage counselor."

13. A client who is admitted to the adult unit of a mental health care facility with depression tells the nurse that he has pedophilia. The nurse should:
□ 1. Be aware of personal opinions and views.
□ 2. Recognize that because the client is depressed, the client will not be able to discuss the pedophilia.
□ 3. Ensure that the client is never alone with other clients on the unit.
□ 4. Refer the client to group therapy.

14. A client and her partner come to the clinic stating they have been unable to have sexual intercourse. The female client states she has pain and her "vagina is too tight." The client was raped at age 15 years of age. Which nursing diagnosis is appropriate for this client?
□ 1. Dysfunctional Grieving related to loss of self-esteem because of lack of sexual intimacy.
□ 2. Risk for Trauma related to fear of vaginal penetration.
□ 3. Vaginismus related to vaginal constriction.
□ 4. Sexual Dysfunction related to sexual trauma.

15. A client with erectile disorder is taking sildenafil (Viagra). The nurse should instruct the client to do which of the following?
□ 1. Take the medication 8 hr before having intercourse.
□ 2. Use nitroglycerine if chest pains occur during intercourse.
□ 3. Take up to three tablets within 24 hr.
□ 4. Expect an erection that lasts up to 4 hr.

Mental Health Disorders in Children and Adolescents

16. A child who is of preschool age is diagnosed as having severe autism. The most effective therapy involves which of the following?
□ 1. Antipsychotic medications.
□ 2. Group psychotherapy.
□ 3. 1:1 Play therapy.
□ 4. Social skills group.

17. A child who has received an order for pemoline (Cylert) for ADHD should be monitored for which of the following?
□ 1. Elevated WBC count.
□ 2. Decreased thyroid levels.
□ 3. Elevated liver function tests.
□ 4. Decreased hemoglobin levels.

18. AF A child is admitted to the child psychiatric unit for ADHD assessment. The nurse would expect to see which of the following symptoms? Select all that apply.
□ 1. Excessive climbing and running.
□ 2. Excessive fidgeting.
□ 3. Pouting behaviors.
□ 4. Cannot wait to take turns.
□ 5. Easily distracted.

19. AF The nurse is assessing a child with Asperger disease. Which of the following are expected findings for this child? Select all that apply.
□ 1. Delayed language development.
□ 2. Lack of social interaction.
□ 3. Cognitive delays for age.
□ 4. Lack of enjoyment.
□ 5. Repetitive motor behaviors.

20. A child with aggressive and impulsive behaviors is admitted to the child psychiatric unit with a diagnosis of a conduct disorder. Which of the following interventions is appropriate?

□ 1. Allow autonomy.
□ 2. Elicit feelings descriptions.
□ 3. Set limits.
□ 4. Teach assertiveness.

Answers and Rationales

1. 4 When the client is listening to the voices, it is most likely an auditory hallucination. Somatic delusions are false beliefs about the functioning of the client's own body. Pseudoparkinsonism is another name for the extrapyramidal symptoms of the medications. Delusions of reference involve events within the environment. (P)

2. 1, 2, 4, 5 Ziprasidone (Geodon) can cause somnolence, drowsiness, weight gain (can be excessive), constipation, and headache; these side effects may preclude noncompliance with this medication. Urticaria is not a common side effect of ziprasidone (Geodon). (D)

3. 2 The AIMS (Abnormal Involuntary Movement Scale) is used to test for extrapyramidal symptoms that occur as a side effect of typical antipsychotic medications such as chlorpromazine (Thorazine), trifluoperazine (Stelazine), haloperidol (Haldol), and fluphenazine decanoate (Prolixin). Extrapyramidal side effects may occur with some atypical antipsychotic medications, but not as frequently as with typical antipsychotic medications. The CAGE test is used to evaluate drug and alcohol use. DSM-IV-TR is the *Diagnostic and Statistical Manual*, 4th edition, and the GDS is the Geriatric Depression Scale. (D)

4. 1 A side effect of clozapine is leukopenia. A WBC count is drawn every week and if it starts to drop, the primary care provider is notified. Slightly low hemoglobin levels (11.2 g/dl) or a normal sodium of 136 mEq/L are not significant. Hyaline casts occur because of protein in the urine, and a small amount is normally found in the urine, especially after exercise. (D)

5. 4 A delusion is a false belief. A hallucination is a false perception of the senses. Flight of ideas involves jumping from one idea to the next. An illusion is a false interpretation of a sensory stimulus (such as seeing a fountain in the desert when the object is actually a cactus). (P)

6. 3 The therapeutic communication technique of asking the client to describe the forgetfulness seeks clarification and provides the client an opportunity to tell more about the problem. A client who is 75 years of age may take a prolonged time to remember as a result of normal cognitive changes of aging, but telling the client it is normal to forget is diminishing the importance of the comment. Referring to the nurse's self is also diminishing the importance of the client's concern. It is not the nurse's role to indicate that the client does or does not have Alzheimer disease; the nurse uses communication techniques that obtain sufficient information to determine if a referral is needed. (P)

7. 3 Client safety is a priority for a dementia client. With the characteristic forgetfulness, the client may not remember the other clients on the unit. Depending on the client's status, the client may not be able to complete activities of daily living. Providing for safety takes priority over promoting food intake. (S)

8. 1 By informing the client of the date and providing time frames, the nurse helps the client become oriented to time and place. Calling the client "silly" and telling the client that it is not the 4th of July is nontherapeutic and demeaning to the client. Asking the client what else he or she is planning to do is going along with the delusion and also not therapeutic. The response of bringing medication is not a therapeutic conversation and does not give the client an opportunity to say anything else. (P)

9. 4 Risperidone (Risperdal) is ordered for severe agitation and has a rapid response. Ergoloid (Hydergine) and tacrine (Cognex) stabilize and may improve the cognitive functioning of clients with dementia. Diazepam (Valium) is an antianxiety agent that would not have the desired effect on the severe agitation, violence, and bizarre thoughts. (D)

10. 4 By fostering independence and providing as much time as possible, the nurse is helping the client to continue to complete as many tasks as possible. Performing activities for the client is counterproductive. A list may cause the client to become frustrated if the list is not completed or if it becomes lost. Informing the client that the UAP will complete activities may be perceived as a threat. (P)

11. 4 As the client is first seeking counseling for his disorder and expresses a concern about informing his family about the decision, he is risking having the family reject him. Social isolation is an appropriate nursing diagnosis if the family should reject him. Ineffective role performance would be an appropriate diagnosis if the client had expressed a concern after having started the surgeries. (M)

12. 3 Asking the couple about their concerns is an open-ended question. Telling the clients that admission history is needed first gives the client the impression that the issue is not important; the couple may not want to bring the subject up in the future. Referring the client to a therapist or marriage counselor is appropriate only after determining the nature of the problem. (P)

13. 1 The nurse must be aware of personal opinions and views when caring for clients with psychosexual disorders. The care plan for the client will be developed to manage both the depression and the pedophilia. It is not necessary to restrict the client's interactions with others on this adult mental health unit. The physician will determine the type of therapy that will be most appropriate for this client. (P)

14. 4 Sexual dysfunction is the nursing diagnosis that is the most appropriate. Dysfunctional grieving because of lack of intimacy is not correct as the couple may have emotional intimacy. The trauma occurred when the female client was 15 years of age. Vaginismus is a medical diagnosis. (P)

15. 4 An expected outcome of taking sildenafil (Viagra) is an erection that can last up to 4 hr. The nurse instructs the client to take the medication 1 hr before having intercourse as an erection will occur within 1 hr, and to take only take one tablet in 24 hr. The nurse advises the client to avoid taking the drug if he takes nitrate therapy, such as nitroglycerine. (D)

16. 3 The preschool-aged child with severe autism will benefit from one-on-one play therapy. The therapist can develop a rapport with this child with nonverbal play. Antipsychotic medications are not indicated for the autism client. The child has difficulty with interpersonal relationships; therefore, group psychotherapy and social skills groups would not be effective. (P)

17. 3 Clients who take pemoline (Cylert) are monitored for elevated liver function tests. Other laboratory tests are not altered with this medication. (D)

18. 1, 2, 4, 5 A child with ADHD will manifest excessive climbing and running, excessive fidgeting, inability to take turns, and distractibility. This child does not exhibit pouting or moody behaviors. (P)

19. 2, 4, 5 The child with Asperger disease manifests many of the same symptoms as the child with autism, with exception of the delays in language and cognitive development. The child with Asperger disease displays a lack of social interaction, lack of enjoyment, and may exhibit repetitive motor behaviors. (P)

20. 3 The nurse promotes consistent limit-setting for the client with the aggressive and impulsive behaviors of a conduct disorder. It is not appropriate for the nurse to allow autonomy or elicit a description of feelings; assertiveness classes are also inappropriate. (P)

chapter

38

The Client With Personality Disorders, Substance Abuse and Addiction, and Eating Disorders

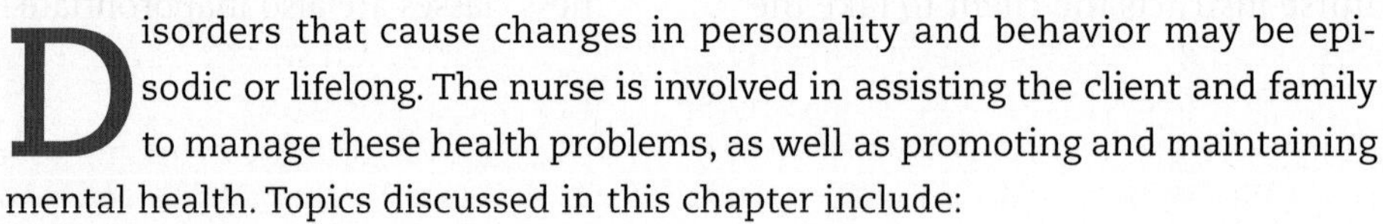

Disorders that cause changes in personality and behavior may be episodic or lifelong. The nurse is involved in assisting the client and family to manage these health problems, as well as promoting and maintaining mental health. Topics discussed in this chapter include:

- Personality Disorders
- Substance Abuse and Addiction
- Eating Disorders

Personality Disorders

I. Definition: Personality disorders involve lifelong patterns of behavior wherein personalty traits become rigid and fixed; the client experiences behavioral and personal distress that affect multiple areas of the client's life.

A. Personality disorders are listed under Axis II in the American Psychiatric Association's *Diagnostic and Statistical Manual of Mental Disorders,* 4th edition, Text Revision (DSM-IV-TR). According to the DSM-IV-TR, a diagnosis of personality disorders can be made when there are symptoms in two or more of the following areas:

1. Affect—intensity, range, and appropriate emotions.
2. Cognition—perceiving and meaning assignment to self, others, and events.
3. Interpersonal behavior.
4. Control of impulses (American Psychiatric Association, 2000).

B. Types of personality disorders are grouped into clusters (see assessment).

II. Nursing process

A. Assessment: Assess personality disorder type and cluster.

1. Cluster A: Client behavior is eccentric or odd.
   a. For paranoid personality disorders:
      (1) Preoccupied with distrust and suspicion of others; doubts the trustworthiness of friends or associates.
      (2) Secretive.
      (3) Interprets motives of others as evil.
      (4) Holds grudges.
   b. For schizoid personality disorders:
      (1) Detached from social relationships.
      (2) Restricted rage of emotions, especially in social settings.
   c. For schizotypal personality disorders:
      (1) Pervasive pattern of interpersonal and social deficits manifested by discomfort with reduced capacity for close relationships, as well as eccentric behavior.
      (2) Ideas of reference, magical thinking, odd thought patterns, suspiciousness, and an inappropriate affect.
      (3) Few close friends or confidants.
      (4) Social anxiety that does not subside with increased familiarity.
2. Cluster B: Client behavior is emotional, dramatic, or erratic.
   a. For antisocial personality disorders:
      (1) Persistent pattern of disregard toward, and violation of, the rights of others.
      (2) Failure to abide by the laws of multiple levels of authority.
   b. For borderline personality disorders:
      (1) Pervasive pattern of unstable interpersonal relationships, and an unstable self-image and affect.
      (2) Marked impulsivity and avoids abandonment (whether real or imagined), and manifests impulsivity in at least two self-harming behaviors (substance abuse, spending, and/or sex).
      (3) Recurrent suicidal gestures, threats, or self-harm.
      (4) Chronic feelings of emptiness.
      (5) Client polarizes between groups of staff, and others—"splitting."
   c. For narcissistic personality disorders:
      (1) All-consuming pattern of grandiose fantasies or behaviors, and a strong need for admiration.
      (2) Feelings of self-importance.
      (3) Demonstrates arrogance, haughtiness, and lack of empathy.
   d. For histrionic personality disorders:
      (1) Pattern of excessive emotional and attention-seeking behaviors.
      (2) Uncomfortable when not at the center of attention.
      (3) Exhibits sexually inappropriate behaviors.
      (4) Uses physical appearance to draw attention of others.
      (5) Considers relationships to be more intimate than they really are.
      (6) Speech is excessive, self-dramatizing, and theatrical and often is an expression of exaggerated emotions.
3. Cluster C: Client behaviors are anxious or fearful.
   a. For avoidant personality disorders:
      (1) Feels inadequate; socially inhibited; hypersensitive to any negative evaluations.
      (2) Avoids activities that involve interpersonal contact.
      (3) Exhibits inappropriate anger and shows restraint with intimate relationships because of a fear of being ridiculed or shamed.
   b. For dependent personality disorders:
      (1) Demonstrates need to be taken care of, leading to clinging and submissive behavior.
      (2) Fears separation; client experiences discomfort when alone because of exaggerated fears.

(3) Has difficulty making everyday decisions without receiving advice from others; needs for others to assume responsibility, and has difficulty initiating projects on own.

c. For obsessive-compulsive personality disorders:

(1) Exhibits a preoccupation with perfectionism, orderliness, and rigidity; these preoccupations often exist at the expense of flexibility, competence, and candor.

(2) Has difficulty being effective in occupational and social roles.

B. Analysis

1. Fear related to personality disorder
2. Social Isolation related to personality disorder
3. Risk for Other-Directed Violence related to personality disorder
4. Risk for Self-Directed Violence related to personality disorder
5. Chronic Low Self-Esteem related to personality disorder
6. Ineffective Coping related to personality disorder
7. Defensive Coping related to personality disorder
8. Impaired Social Interaction related to personality disorder
9. Ineffective Therapeutic Regimen Management related to personality disorder
10. Impaired Adjustment related to personality disorder
11. Powerlessness related to personality disorder

C. Planning

1. Identify behaviors that preclude hospitalizations.
2. Promote client functioning within therapeutic milieu.
3. Prevent client from harm to self and others.
4. Promote methods to deal with frustration and stress.
5. Promote client functioning in social environment.
6. Promote client ability to have functional relationships.
7. Promote client problem-solving skills.

D. Implementation

1. Discuss with the client the actions that precipitated hospitalizations.
2. Provide positive feedback for honesty and acceptable behaviors (for antisocial personality disorder client).
3. Identify unacceptable behaviors (e.g., stealing, using profanity), and develop consequences for unacceptable behaviors involving withholding an activity the client enjoys; inform client of consequences.
4. Provide consistent and thorough completion of the care plan.
5. Encourage identification of frustration sources, how dealt with previously, and the consequences that resulted from the actions.
6. Discuss feelings of frustration with coworkers when dealing with clients with personality disorders.
7. Avoid taking personally any severe criticism or unjustified flattery from the borderline personality client.

E. Evaluation

1. Client maintains a job with acceptable performance.
2. Client meets parenting responsibilities.
3. Client restrains from self-harm.
4. Client avoids committing immoral and illegal acts.
5. Client has stable personal relationships.
6. Client experiences a decrease in crises.

CN

III. Client needs

A. Physiologic adaptation: Personality disorders are managed with medication and therapy. The nurse provides supportive therapy with life-threatening situations such as suicide attempts (see Chapter 36 for discussion of suicide).

B. Management of care: Care of the client with a personality disorder requires critical thinking skills and knowledge of assessment, and teaching and evaluation methods unique to the RN role. These skills cannot be delegated to an LPN or UAP.

1. Communicate client's behaviors among staff members to set limits and reduce "splitting" and manipulation of staff. Assess staff for the following:
   a. Frustration level while working with clients.
   b. Emotional response to clients.
2. Participate in interdisciplinary team conferences—nursing contributes data from 24-hr assessment and care.
3. Introduce client to community agencies such as halfway houses for long-term care.
4. Provide and receive report on the assigned hospitalized clients among health care team.
5. Act as a client advocate.
6. Provide client and family teaching about the personality disorder.

C. Safety and infection control

1. Provide wound care for client with self-injury.

2. Provide client and family teaching about home safety issues, especially wound care for borderline personality.

D. Health promotion and maintenance
1. Perform physical assessment on admission to psychiatric facilities and as per agency policy.
2. Provide long-term monitoring with community mental health agencies to maintain compliance with psychotropics and psychotherapy.
3. Provide client and family teaching about home management of the personality disorder; assist with planning for care in the home setting, including home health nurses and community health agencies.
4. Assist client with activities appropriate for preference and developmental age.
5. Institute and monitor a contract with personality disorder client regarding rigidity and self-harm.

E. Psychologic integrity
1. Assess family coping mechanisms and facilitate client and family coping with diagnoses and crisis management.
2. Encourage client to participate in group sessions in both hospital and community settings.
3. Use therapeutic techniques of communication to help client understand behavior.
4. Maintain consistency for treatment plan on the nursing unit.

F. Basic care and comfort: Assist with activities of daily living for client who is not able to complete personal care.

G. Reduction of risk potential
1. As appropriate, assess the borderline personality client for risk for drug/alcohol dependency.
2. Assess self-harm attempts for lethality; provide wound care for harm attempts.

H. Pharmacologic and parenteral therapies: Common medications for the client with a personality disorder are the same as those ordered for comorbid conditions such as antidepressants for depressed clients (see Table 36-1) or for clients with anxiety (see Table 36-3). Client and family will state the purpose for and associated side effects of all medications.

Substance Abuse and Addiction

I. Definition: Substances involved in abuse and addiction include alcohol and drugs (see later discussion for specific types). Abuse and addiction are differentiated in that abuse involves the repeated use of substances, which leads to functional problems. Addiction occurs when functional problems become a part of daily living as a result of continued substance use. Substance abuse and addiction are illnesses.

A. Alcohol: Alcohol is a central nervous system depressant that is absorbed rapidly in the bloodstream.

B. Amphetamines/stimulants (includes amphetamine, benzphetamine, Benzedrine, dextroamphetamine) increase alertness, relieve fatigue, and increase feelings of decisiveness; they are also used for feeling "down" from tranquilizers and alcohol.

C. Cocaine (may also be classified as a stimulant or narcotic) produces euphoria, relaxation, and a feeling of being carefree or in control; effects last between 5 and 20 min.

D. Inhalants (may also be called stimulants) include substances such as butyl nitrite, amyl nitrite, gasoline, and toluene vapors (such as correction fluid, marking pens, or glue).

E. Cannabis (marijuana, tetrahydrocannabinol, hashish) cause a sense of a euphoria followed by lowered inhibitions, relaxation, and an increased appetite.

F. Hallucinogens and phencyclidine such as LSD, mescaline, peyote, psilocybin, and designer drugs such as ecstasy. Phencyclidine is also classified as a hallucinogen and includes PCP and angel dust. These drugs distort perceptions of reality and produce symptoms including hallucinations (usually visual) and depersonalization.

G. Opioids such as opium, morphine, heroin, codeine, hydromorphone, meperidine, and methadone cause euphoria, respiratory depression, drowsiness, constricted pupils (pinpoint pupils).

H. Sedatives, hypnotics, and anxiolytics include barbiturates, methaqualone, tranquilizers, chloral hydrate, and glutethimide; these cause anxiety reduction and sensory alteration and/or intoxication.

II. Nursing process

A. Assessment
1. Obtain information from client and family to discern which drug and how much, if known, was taken by the client.
2. Assess client for symptoms of intoxication or overdose.
   a. Alcohol
      (1) Intoxication: Unsteady gait; lack of coordination; slurred speech; impaired concentration, attention, memory and judgment; possible lack of inhibitions or aggressive behaviors.

(2) Overdose: Vomiting, unconsciousness, and respiratory depression.

b. Amphetamines/stimulants

(1) Intoxication: Increased alertness and energy level, dilated pupils, excessive perspiration, decrease in appetite, loss of coordination, dizziness, anxiety, restlessness and/or delusions, and increased vital signs (sometimes causing an unusually high heart rate).

(2) Overdose: Tremors, restlessness, hyperreflexia, confusion, increased respirations, arrhythmias, circulatory collapse.

c. Cocaine

(1) Intoxication: State of euphoria and relaxation; may also manifest in severe mood swings and irritability; and increased BP and heart rate.

(2) Overdose: May result in death from just one use.

d. Inhalants

(1) Intoxication: Loss of muscle control, slurred speech, loss of consciousness or drowsiness, excessive secretions from the nose and watery eyes.

(2) Overdose: May cause brain and lung damage; may result in death from just one use.

e. Cannabis

(1) Intoxication: Inappropriate laughter; impaired motor coordination, impaired short-term memory and judgment, distorted sense of time and perception.

(2) Overdose: Anxiety, panic, decreased attention, decreased motor skills and reaction time.

f. Hallucinogens and phencyclidine

(1) Intoxication: Anxiety, depression, ideas of reference, paranoid ideation, and sometimes life-threatening behaviors such as jumping from a window. Intoxication may also cause an increase in pulse, BP, and temperature; hyperreflexia, dilated pupils; perspiration; palpitations with tachycardia; blurred vision; lack of coordination and tremors.

(2) Overdose: Often referred to as a "bad trip" causes intense "flashbacks" and frightening dreams; overdose can result in severe psychosis or death.

g. Opioids

(1) Intoxication: Euphoria, respiratory depression, drowsiness, and constricted pupils (pinpoint pupils).

(2) Overdose: Shallow, slow breaths; clammy skin; convulsions; coma and death.

h. Sedatives, hypnotics, and anxiolytics

(1) Intoxication: Impaired judgment, slurred speech, loss of motor coordination.

(2) Overdose: Respiratory depression, coma, and death.

3. Assess client for withdrawal of a particular drug.
   a. Alcohol: Noted by 4 to 12 hr after stopping drinking; symptoms include hand tremors, elevated pulse, and BP, sweating, insomnia, nausea, and vomiting.
   b. Amphetamines/stimulants: Involve dysphoria with unpleasant dreams and difficulty sleeping or lack of sleep.
   c. Cocaine: Symptoms are the same as for amphetamines.
   d. Inhalants: Symptoms are unspecific; however, sometimes client who uses inhalants describes a psychologic craving for the drug.
   e. Cannabis: Unspecific.
   f. Hallucinogens and phencyclidine: Nonspecific as drug is not addictive.
   g. Opioids: Include dilated pupils, anxiety, restlessness, yawning, sweating, tearing.
   h. Sedatives, hypnotics, and anxiolytics: Symptoms depend on the half-life of the drug and are the opposite of the desired effect of the drugs; this includes autonomic hyperactivity (elevated vital signs), tremors, anxiety, insomnia, nausea, and agitation. Hallucinations and seizures are rarely seen with benzodiazepine withdrawal.
4. Obtain diagnostic tests.
   a. Obtain blood samples for blood alcohol levels (BAL); above 0.08% is considered intoxicated in most states while a BAL of 0.05% is not considered under the influence of alcohol.
   b. Obtain urine specimen for drug levels in the client suspected of using drugs.

B. Analysis

1. Ineffective Coping related to substance abuse
2. Ineffective Denial related to substance abuse
3. Risk for Injury related to impaired judgment from substance abuse
4. Ineffective Health Maintenance related to substance abuse

5. Risk for Other-Directed Violence related to substance abuse
6. Imbalanced Nutrition: Less Than Body Requirements related to substance abuse
7. Chronic Low Self-Esteem related to substance abuse

C. Planning
1. Promote abstinence from drug and/or alcohol use.
2. Promote coping strategies.
3. Establish a successful aftercare plan.
4. Promote adequate nutrition.
5. Protect client from injury to self or others.

D. Implementation
1. Assess the client for dependency.
2. Identify drug-seeking behaviors.
3. Provide health teaching—including dispelling myths and misconceptions about alcohol and drug use.
4. Promote coping skills for the client and the family.
5. Address family issues about alcoholism and drug use as an illness of the family.
6. Provide support to the family members who are codependent to decrease codependent behaviors; provide role-playing to discern how client and/or family handle difficult situations.
7. Set realistic goals such as remaining sober today; avoid long term-goals such as, "I will remain sober for a year."
8. Assess client's physical problems such as inadequate nutrition and sleep disturbances.

E. Evaluation
1. Client abstains from the substance.
2. Client demonstrates stable role performance(s) as a spouse, parent, and employee.
3. Client expresses satisfaction with the quality of life.
4. Client has adequate nutrition.
5. Client accepts the consequences of behaviors.
6. Client use nondrug or nonalcohol alternatives to deal with difficult situations or stress.
7. Client expresses feelings directly and openly.

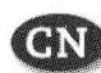

III. Client needs

A. Physiologic adaptation
1. Client who drinks or uses drugs may be malnourished—nurse assesses nutritional status.
2. Client with long-term use of alcohol can develop Wernicke encephalopathy, Korsakoff psychosis, cardiac myopathy, pancreatitis, esophagitis, hepatitis, peripheral neuropathy, cirrhosis, leucopenia, thrombocytopenia, and ascites of the abdomen—nurse uses precautions to manage/prevent complications of the client with the long-term effects of alcohol use.
3. Client with long-term use of inhalants experiences persistent dementia, anxiety, psychosis, or mood disorders—these are treated symptomatically.

B. Management of care: Care of the client experiencing substance abuse or addiction requires critical thinking skills and knowledge of assessment, and teaching and evaluation methods unique to the RN role. These skills cannot be delegated to an LPN or UAP.
1. Participate in interdisciplinary team conferences—nursing contributes data from 24-hr assessment and care.
2. Introduce client to community agencies such as halfway houses for aftercare.
3. Provide and receive report on the assigned hospitalized client among health care team.
4. Act as a client advocate.
5. Document procedures and treatments and the response to treatments.

C. Safety and infection control
1. Provide client and family teaching about home safety issues; especially symptoms of GI bleeding.
2. Assess the skin of the client with alcoholic neuropathy.
3. Use precautions to prevent injury when dealing with the client who is under the influence of drugs or alcohol.
4. Monitor for signs of infection in the alcoholic client with leukopenia.
5. Monitor for bleeding in the alcoholic client with thrombocytopenia.

D. Health promotion and maintenance
1. Perform physical assessment on admission to psychiatric facilities and as per agency policy.
2. Provide long-term monitoring of laboratory results regarding liver values, albumin levels, amylase level (for pancreatitis), and WBC count (for leucopenia) to maintain abstinence.
3. Provide assistance for client to obtain home care including home health nurses and introduction to community health agencies.

E. Psychologic integrity
1. Assess client's interpersonal relationships for strain; provide client and family information about support agencies such as AA, NA, and ACOA.
2. Assess spiritual factors affecting the care of the chemically dependent client.
3. Facilitate client coping with lifelong diagnosis of alcoholism; assist client with appropriate nonalcoholic or nondrug use activities as a substitute coping mechanism.

4. Encourage participation in group sessions teaching the alcoholic client effects of using drugs and/or alcohol, nutrition, and medications regimen.
5. Assess client for rationalizing use of substances.

F. Basic care and comfort
1. Assist with activities of daily living for the client with complication of alcoholism such as Wernicke encephalopathy or Korsakoff psychosis.
2. Provide nutritional supplements.

G. Reduction of risk potential
1. Monitor the alcohol-overdose client on the ventilator.
2. Perform gastric lavage for overdose victims.
3. Monitor for signs of delirium tremens (life-threatening complication).

H. Pharmacologic and parenteral therapies: Client and family will state the purpose for and associated side effects of all medications used to treat substance abuse and addiction. See Table 38-1 for common medications used for clients with substance abuse problems.

Table 38-1 Common Medications for Clients With Substance-Abuse Problems

Classification	Generic/Trade Name Examples	Expected Outcomes	Reduction of Risk Potential	Management of Care
Anxiolytic Sedative/ Hypnotic	Lorazepam (Ativan); chlordiazepoxide (Librium)	Eases alcohol-withdrawal symptoms.	Instruct client to avoid alcohol use; use with caution when driving or operating heavy machinery.	Monitor global assessments for effectiveness and vital signs. Monitor for dizziness or drowsiness.
Alcohol Deterrent	Disulfiram (Antabuse)	Maintains abstinence from alcohol.	Instruct client to avoid alcohol use—can cause serious illness or death.	Teach client to read labels to avoid products containing alcohol.
Heroin Deterrent	Methadone (Dolophine)	Maintains abstinence from heroin.	Monitor for nausea and vomiting.	The client has exchanged an addiction to heroin for an addiction to a legal drug, methadone; nurse teaches client that client will continue to need monitoring.
Opiate Deterrent	Levomethadyl (Orlaam)	Maintains abstinence from opiates.	Instruct client to avoid use on consecutive days.	Do not send this drug home with the client.
Opiate Blocking Agent	Naltrexone (ReVia, Trexan)	Reduces alcohol cravings; blocks effects of opiates.	Instruct client to take with milk or food.	Instruct client that he or she may not respond to the narcotics in cough medications; may cause restlessness or irritability, headache.
Antihypertensive; Adrenergic Agent	Clonidine (Catapres)	Eases opiate-withdrawal symptoms.	Prevent additive effect by instructing client to avoid use of alcohol and antihistamines, sedatives, hypnotics, and opioid pain medicines.	Take BP before each dose; hold if client has a low BP.
Vitamin Supplement	Thiamine (vitamin B_1)	Treats Wernicke-Korsakoff syndromes.	Not applicable	Instruct client about adequate nutrition.
Vitamin Supplement	Folic acid (folate); cyanocobalamin (vitamin B_{12})	Treats nutritional deficiencies.	Not applicable	Instruct client that urine may be dark yellow in color with folic acid; teach about proper nutrition.

Eating Disorders

I. Definition: An eating disorder is a severe disturbance in eating behavior. Types of eating disorders include the following:
   A. Anorexia nervosa—condition in which the client starves himself or herself and refuses to maintain an appropriate weight. Anorexia is characterized by emaciation, a disturbed body image, and an extreme fear of being obese; if untreated, the condition can be fatal.
   B. Bulimia nervosa—manifested by binge eating, followed by attempts to eliminate the body of the excess food (purging). The severity of the disorder is difficult to ascertain as the client performs these activities secretly. Damage is related to the frequency of the cycles and the physical complications of the condition.
   C. Binge eating disorder (BED)—condition is a less severe form of an eating disorder (affects 2% adults, 40% of them men) in which the client engages in recurrent episodes of binge eating and then has regular use of compensatory behaviors such as purging, excessive exercise, or laxative use. The client feels guilty, shameful, and disquieted about the purging and experiences marked psychologic distress.

II. Nursing process
   A. Assessment
      1. Assess client for eating attitudes, using assessment tools such as the Eating Attitudes Test.
      2. Assess the client with anorexia nervosa for:
         a. Amenorrhea (and infertility).
         b. Fatigue.
         c. Loss of sex drive.
         d. Body image disturbance.
         e. Decreased blood volume (low BP and orthostatic hypotension).
         f. Electrolyte imbalance (weakness or arrhythmias).
         g. GI complications (constipation).
         h. Need to achieve and please others.
         i. Rituals regarding food.
         j. Perfectionist attitude.
         k. Refusal to eat.
      3. Assess the client with bulimia nervosa and BED for:
         a. Episodes of binging and purging.
         b. Anxiety.
         c. Constant preoccupation with food.
         d. Avoiding conflict.
         e. Dental abnormalities—eroded teeth.
         f. Dissatisfied with personal body image.
         g. Feeling helpless.
         h. Extreme need for approval and acceptance.
         i. Frequent lying or making excuses to explain behavior.
         j. Guilt.
         k. Irregular menses.
         l. Perfectionist.
         m. Russell sign (bruised knuckles that occurs after inducing vomiting).
         n. Pharyngitis.
         o. Salivary and parotid gland swelling.
         p. Using amphetamines, and the like, to control hunger.
         q. Excessive exercise (sporadic sometimes).
   B. Analysis
      1. Altered body image related to eating disorder
      2. Anxiety related to eating disorder
      3. Imbalanced Nutrition: Less Than Body Requirements related to malnutrition from eating disorder
      4. Powerlessness related to eating disorder
      5. Chronic Low Self-Esteem related to eating disorder
      6. Deficient Fluid Volume related to eating disorder
      7. Constipation related to eating disorder
      8. Fatigue related to eating disorder
      9. Activity Intolerance related to eating disorder
      10. Risk for suicide related to depression
   C. Planning
      1. Establish satisfactory nutritional eating patterns.
      2. Eliminate use of purging behaviors.
      3. Promote effective coping behaviors (other than eating-focused).
      4. Promote client verbalization of feelings.
      5. Promote acceptance of body image.
   D. Implementation
      1. Establish nutritional eating patterns—should sit with client during eating times; closely monitor client for 1 to 2 hr after meals and snacks.
      2. Follow treatment plan guidelines regarding restrictions.
      3. Provide liquid protein supplements when unable to eat meal.
      4. Monitor client weight; use same amount of clothing.
      5. Observe for attempts to discard or hide food, or to make weight appear heavier (e.g., wearing additional clothing).
      6. Assist client to describe feelings.
      7. Help client to keep a self-monitoring journal as a nonfood coping strategy.
      8. Assist with relaxation techniques.

9. Assist client with recognizing benefits of a near-normal weight than the one they are striving for (emaciated).
10. Help client to identify personal strengths, talents, and interests.
11. Assist client and family to take control of the nutritional requirements independently.
12. Inform client and family about warning signs of the harmful effects of eating disorders, such as cardiac arrhythmias, muscle weakness, seizures.

E. Evaluation
1. Client maintains a body weight within 5% to 10% of ideal body weight.
2. Client refrains from purging behaviors and is free from medical complications from purging or starvation.
3. Client demonstrates improvement in eating disorder as evidenced by the Eating Attitudes Test.
4. Client is comfortable eating in a social setting.
5. Client verbalizes feelings of anger, anxiety, and guilt, and uses effective coping behaviors other than eating-focused.
6. Client verbalizes positive body image.

CN

III. Client needs

A. Physiologic adaptation: Because of the inadequate intake of food and fluids the client is at risk for starvation and will exhibit changes in blood chemistries and electrolytes. The goal is to restore the client to an adequate nutritional state.
1. Client has low temperature, pulse, and BP—nurse monitors vital signs.
2. Client may develop osteopenia or osteoporosis—nurse observes bone density exams.
3. Client may experience dehydration and edema in the lower extremities—nurse monitors hydration.

B. Management of care: Care of the client with an eating disorder requires critical thinking skills and knowledge of assessment, and teaching and evaluation methods unique to the RN role. These skills cannot be delegated to an LPN or UAP.
1. Participate in interdisciplinary team conferences—nurse provides data from 24-hr assessment and care.
2. Introduce client to community agencies such as halfway houses for long-term monitoring.
3. Provide and receive report on the assigned hospitalized client with health care team.
4. Act as a client advocate.

C. Safety and infection control: Provide client and family teaching about eating disorder and safety in the home setting, especially because of weakened bones and risk for fractures.

D. Health promotion and maintenance
1. Perform physical assessment on admission to psychiatric facilities and as per agency policy.
2. Provide long-term monitoring with lab tests to maintain compliance with nutrition.
3. Assist client obtain home care such as home health nurses, and participate in community health agencies.
4. Assist client with activities appropriate for preference and developmental age.
5. Document weight to monitor treatment procedures.

E. Psychologic integrity
1. Assess family dynamics (frequently there is a dominant mother and distant father); use therapeutic communication techniques and promote active listening.
2. Assess client for alcohol- or drug-related dependencies.
3. Provide a therapeutic milieu.
4. Participate in group sessions.
5. Respect cultural differences of client within a safety framework.

F. Basic care and comfort
1. Monitor client's weight (check agency policy—some facilities recommend client weighed with eyes facing away from the scale readout).
2. Assist the client who is too weak to complete personal care with activities of daily living.
3. Monitor for malnutrition.
4. Provide client nutrition through tube feedings, if warranted.
5. Provide skin care—especially over bony prominences in the cachexia victim.

G. Reduction of risk potential
1. Provide cardiac monitoring for client with low potassium level.
2. Identify suicidal tendencies and institute and maintain suicide precautions as needed.
3. Identify risk for pressure ulcers and provide skin care as needed.

H. Pharmacologic and parenteral therapies: Medications for the client with an eating disorder include those used for anxieties and depressive episodes (see Tables 36-1 and 36-3).

Bibliography

American Psychiatric Association. (2000). *Diagnostic and statistical manual of mental disorders* (4th ed., text rev.). Washington, DC: Author.

Mohr, W. K. (2006). *Psychiatric-mental health nursing* (6th ed.). Philadelphia: Lippincott Williams & Wilkins.

Videbeck, S. L. (2004). *Psychiatric-mental health nursing* (2nd ed.). Philadelphia: Lippincott Williams & Wilkins.

CHAPTER 38

Practice Test

Personality Disorders

1. AF A client with a diagnosis of borderline personality disorder is admitted with self-inflicted scratches on her forearms. The nurse is assessing the client's suicidal plan. It is important to assess which of the following? Select all that apply.
- □ 1. Presence of a suicidal plan.
- □ 2. Access to the means for enforcing the suicidal plan.
- □ 3. Expressions that her life "isn't worth anything."
- □ 4. Female gender.
- □ 5. Self-harm behaviors of razor blade cuts.

2. AF The nurse is developing a care plan for a client with a diagnosis of a borderline personality disorder. Which of the following would be most effective to help the client cope and control emotions? Select all that apply.
- □ 1. Assist client identify with emotions.
- □ 2. Decrease impulsivity.
- □ 3. Have client keep a journal of emotions and coping techniques.
- □ 4. Encourage client to delay gratification.
- □ 5. Use confrontation techniques.

3. A client diagnosed with borderline personality disorder is admitted to an inpatient unit. Which statement by the client describes a violation of the boundaries between the nurse and the client?
- □ 1. "You are better than the doctor and all the other nurses."
- □ 2. "Can you help me with my schedule for today?"
- □ 3. "What is this medication and why do I need it?"
- □ 4. "I just can't stop myself from hurting myself."

4. A client with a diagnosis of a borderline personality disorder tells the nurse, "You are the only one who understands me. Neither the doctor nor any of the other nurses really understand my situation." The *best* response by the nurse would be:
- □ 1. "Why would you say something like that? Everyone here understands you."
- □ 2. "I am interested in helping you just as much as the other staff members on this unit."
- □ 3. "You should really look at what you mean by 'understand.' You are really asking a lot from the staff."
- □ 4. "Everyone feels like that sometimes. Don't worry about it; it will get better."

5. AF The nurse is developing a care plan for a client with a borderline personality disorder who is being admitted to an acute care facility. Which of the following should be included in the plan? Select all that apply.
- □ 1. Develop a no self-harm contract.
- □ 2. Instruct client in "thought-stopping."
- □ 3. Express doubt about client's delusions.
- □ 4. Assist client to develop social skills.
- □ 5. Assist client to delay gratification.
- □ 6. Explain to client rules on the acute care unit.

6. A client is attending a group therapy meeting. He continues to dominate the conversation saying he had the "worst problems" of anyone on the unit. A female client is crying about her husband's death 6 months ago, but the client redirects the group to discuss his issues. This domineering client is demonstrating behaviors consistent with which disorder?
- □ 1. Antisocial personality disorder.
- □ 2. Histrionic personality disorder.
- □ 3. Narcissistic personality disorder.
- □ 4. Borderline personality disorder.

7. A nurse is documenting behaviors of a client with borderline personality in the progress notes. Which of the following progress notes indicates improvement?
- □ 1. Informs staff members on the evening shift that they are wonderful and the day shift staff is "terrible."
- □ 2. Cries in her room for 30 min when the roommate is not interested in attending a recreational activity with this client.
- □ 3. Yells at a group member when the other client points out that she is monopolizing the group.
- □ 4. Informs the nurse that she is anxious and having thoughts of hurting herself.

Substance Abuse and Addiction

8. AF Which of the following symptoms are expected indications that a client has alcohol withdrawal delirium? Select all that apply.
 - □ 1. Tachycardia.
 - □ 2. Tachypnea.
 - □ 3. Dry, flushed skin.
 - □ 4. Thirst.
 - □ 5. Hypertension.
 - □ 6. Abdominal cramping.

9. The nurse is planning care for a client with substance abuse. Which of the following approaches will be most effective?
 - □ 1. Group therapy with other substance abuse clients.
 - □ 2. Psychodynamic individual therapy.
 - □ 3. Group therapy with clients diagnosed with personality disorders.
 - □ 4. No self-harm contractual therapy.

10. A client who is about to be fired from his job because of his drinking signs himself into an alcohol-detoxification program. The nurse should assess which of the following first?
 - □ 1. Frequency and type of drinks used in the past week.
 - □ 2. Time and amount of drinks taken in the past 24 hr.
 - □ 3. Amount and type of substances taken in the past 30 days.
 - □ 4. Signs and symptoms of previous alcohol withdrawal events.

11. AF A client admitted for alcohol detoxification is taking disulfiram (Antabuse). The nurse should instruct the client to avoid ingestion of which of the following? Select all that apply.
 - □ 1. Aged cheeses.
 - □ 2. Beer.
 - □ 3. Communal wine at church.
 - □ 4. Chocolates.
 - □ 5. Cough syrup.

12. A client is admitted to the emergency department with suspected opiate abuse. The nurse should assess this client for which of the following symptoms?
 - □ 1. Pinpoint pupils.
 - □ 2. Calmness.
 - □ 3. Watery eyes.
 - □ 4. Mood swings.

13. AF A client is admitted to the emergency department having just used cocaine. The nurse should assess this client for which of the following? Select all that apply.
 - □ 1. Mood swings.
 - □ 2. Feeling of euphoria.
 - □ 3. Constricted pupils.
 - □ 4. Increased BP.
 - □ 5. Tachycardia.

14. The nurse is assessing a client with alcohol abuse. Which of the following indicates the client is having alcohol withdrawal?
 - □ 1. Elevated BP.
 - □ 2. Hyperactivity.
 - □ 3. Hypervigilance.
 - □ 4. Hypothermia.

Eating Disorders

15. AF A teenage client is admitted to the acute admission unit with both bulimia nervosa and anorexia nervosa. Which of the following are appropriate initial interventions for this client? Select all that apply.
 - □ 1. Assign a staff member to accompany the client when using the bathroom.
 - □ 2. Have the client keep a self-monitoring journal as a coping strategy.
 - □ 3. Weigh the client in same amount of clothing and facing away from scale readout at daily scheduled intervals (e.g., 0645 on Tuesdays and Fridays).
 - □ 4. Inform the client that parenteral nutrition will be necessary if the client does not gain weight.
 - □ 5. Assign a staff member to sit with client during meals and for 1½ hr after meals.
 - □ 6. Provide liquid protein supplements when client is unable to eat meals.

16. A client with an eating disorder is admitted to the acute admission unit of the psychiatric hospital. The nurse is scheduling the weights for Monday and Thursday mornings. In order to obtain an accurate weight, the nurse should do which of the following?
 - □ 1. Weigh the client at the same time between breakfast and lunch.
 - □ 2. Allow the client to go to the bathroom unattended before the procedure.
 - □ 3. Have the client wear the same type of underwear with each weight.
 - □ 4. Observe for attempts to put weights into clothing or body.

17. A young adult female who was admitted to the psychiatric hospital 2 months ago with an eating disorder is being discharged. Which of the following indicates the client understands discharge instructions?
 - □ 1. Client returns to the same living situation as she had prior to hospitalization.
 - □ 2. Client attends a social club at her local church.
 - □ 3. Client returns to the lab for routine lab tests.
 - □ 4. Client enrolls in a health club.

18. AF The nurse is reviewing the following laboratory work for a client who is admitted to the acute psychiatric admission unit for an eating disorder.

LABORATORY RESULTS

Test	Result
Albumin level	2.8 g/dl
Sodium level	145 mEq/L
Hemoglobin level	10.8 g/dl
Potassium level	2.7 mEq/L
Hematocrit level	37%

Which of the following findings does the nurse report to the HCP? Select all that apply.

☐ 1. Albumin level.
☐ 2. Sodium level.
☐ 3. Hemoglobin level.
☐ 4. Potassium level.
☐ 5. Hematocrit level.

19. A female client who is hospitalized for an eating disorder weighs 15 pounds less than ideal body weight. Which goal is a priority for this client?

☐ 1. Client attends all eating disorder support groups.
☐ 2. Client eats bigger meals at breakfast.
☐ 3. Client gains 1 pound per week.
☐ 4. Client reports an improved self-image.

20. A nurse is teaching a client who is diagnosed with bulimia how to use self-monitoring. The nurse should:

☐ 1. Have client keep a journal of feelings and experiences related to food and dietary intake.
☐ 2. Refer client to a dietician to develop weekly meal plans.
☐ 3. Teach techniques that help the client ignore feelings related to food.
☐ 4. Teach client how to calculate calorie content of various foods and liquids.

Answers and Rationales

1. 1, 2, 3, 5 The presence of a suicidal plan, having access to enacting the suicidal plan, and the self-harm behaviors are all important assessments for the borderline personality-disorder client. The expression that life "isn't worth anything" is also a concern when completing a suicidal assessment. Male clients are more likely to complete a suicide than female clients. (P)

2. 1, 2, 3, 4 To help the client with a borderline personality cope with and control emotions, the nurse assists the client to identify which emotions he or she is experiencing, plans to decrease the number of impulsive acts the client completes, and promotes client use of a journal in which emotions and coping techniques can be recorded. The nurse also encourages the client to delay immediate gratification of impulses. The nurse may use confrontation, but this is a component of the development of a therapeutic relationship, and does not help the client cope and control emotions. (P)

3. 1 When the client is flattering the nurse, it is a boundary violation. The other questions do not violate nurse-client boundaries. (P)

4. 2 The best response by the nurse implies caring and is clear that the boundaries are being violated in the flattering statement. Asking the client "why" he or she would say something like that can make the client defensive. Telling the client to look at what he or she is saying and telling the client that everyone feels like that sometimes are nontherapeutic responses. (P)

5. 1, 2, 4, 5, 6 The nurse develops a no self-harm contract for the client with borderline personality disorder; and instructs the client how to perform "thought stopping," a technique whereby the client alters the process of negative or self-critical thought patterns such as "I cannot do anything okay." The nurse also teaches social skills, such as appropriate boundary lines; assists the client to delay gratification of the id needs; and promotes limit-setting directives such as unit rules. The client with a diagnosis of borderline personality disorder would not experience delusions so the nurse does not need to express doubt with delusions. (P)

6. 3 The client who lacks empathy for others and has an inflated view of himself has a narcissistic personality disorder. The client diagnosed with antisocial personality exhibits irresponsibility, failure to honor obligations, and lack of guilt and empathy. The client with histrionic personality disorder manifests a great fluctuation in emotions, attention-seeking behaviors, and dramatic speech. The client with borderline personality disorder exhibits self-harm behaviors, impulsive behaviors, and has intense relationships (feel people are "all good" or "all bad"). (P)

7. 4 The client with borderline personality who informs the staff member that she is having anxious feelings and is having thoughts of self-harm is improving and has met a portion of her self-harm contract. The client who informs the evening shift that they are wonderful and the day shift staff is terrible is exhibiting splitting behaviors. The client who is crying for 30 min when her roommate does not want to go to recreation with her is being dramatic and having feelings of abandonment. When a client yells at a group member for pointing out that she is monopolizing the group, the client is exhibiting lack of remorse or guilt. (P)

8. 1, 2, 5 When a client is developing impending alcohol-withdrawal delirium, the initial symptoms are a fast pulse and respiratory rate, and an elevated BP. Red, flushed, dry skin and complaints of thirst occur with diabetic ketoacidosis. Abdominal cramping and severe diarrhea are symptoms of opiate withdrawal. (P)

9. 1 The most widely accepted therapy for the substance-abuse client is group therapy with other substance abusers. Psychodynamic individual therapy is indicated for anxiety disorders and for some personality disorder clients. A no self-harm contractual therapy is indicated for the borderline personality client. Group therapy for clients diagnosed with personality disorders would not be indicated for substance-abuse clients. (P)

10. 2 For the client admitted into alcohol detoxification unit, the amount, type, and time the substances were taken in the past 24 hr is the most important data to obtain in order to plan for care during withdrawal. The nurse can later obtain additional information about the client's history of drinking, such as type and frequency, use of other substances, and history of withdrawal events. (S)

11. 2, 3, 5 The client who is taking disulfiram (Antabuse) is advised to avoid all forms of alcohol including beer, communal wine at church, and cough syrup; these can trigger a serious physical reaction. Aged cheeses and chocolate are to be avoided by the client taking monoamine oxidase inhibitors. (D)

12. 1 The client with opiate abuse will have constricted (pinpoint) pupils. The client who has ingested sedatives will experience calmness. The client who has used inhalants will exhibit "watery eyes," and the client with cocaine ingestion will experience mood swings. (D)

13. 1, 2, 4, 5 The client who has used cocaine experiences mood swings, a feeling of euphoria, and an elevation in heart rate and BP. The client with cocaine use will have dilated pupils. (D)

14. 1 Tremulousness, sweating, and an elevated BP are all signs of alcohol withdrawal. Hyperactivity, hypervigilance, and hypothermia are not typically related to alcohol withdrawal, but may be associated with withdrawal of other substances. (A)

15. 1, 2, 3, 5, 6 Interventions for the client with both bulimia nervosa and anorexia nervosa involve assigning a staff member to accompany the client to the bathroom; promoting a self-monitoring journal as a nonfood coping strategy; providing daily weight measurement in the same clothing at the same times of the week, while facing the client away from the scale readout; assigning a staff member to sit with the client during meals and stay with the client for 1½ hr after meals; and providing liquid protein supplements when the client is unable to eat meals. Telling the client that parenteral nutrition will be necessary may be perceived as a threat and is not an appropriate initial intervention. (M)

16. 4 Prior to weighing the client, the nurse observes for attempts to add weight such as putting items in clothing or on the body. The client is weighed at the same time each week before breakfast, and wearing minimal clothing (usually just underwear) to prevent hiding of weighted items in clothing to increase weight. The nurse does not allow the client to go to the bathroom unattended prior to weighing, or the client may attempt to drink a large amount of water to increase water weight. (P)

17. 3 The client with an eating disorder is instructed to receive regular lab tests to monitor nutritional compliance. Frequently, the living situation from before hospitalization was dysfunctional, and returning to the situation can result in recurrent health problems. Social club is not a priority for the client, and enrolling in a health club could result in the client exercising excessively. (P)

18. 1, 3, 4 The normal albumin level is 3.5 to 5 g/dl; the normal hemoglobin level is 12 to 16 g/dl; and the normal potassium is 3.5 to 5 mEq/L. These levels are all low. The client is likely not eating a sufficient amount of protein; therefore, the albumin and hemoglobin are low. The potassium level would be low if the client was purging. The sodium level is normally 136 to 145 mEq/L, so this is in the normal range; however, it can be high in a client with an eating disorder. The normal hematocrit level is 37% to 47% in an adult. (A)

19. 3 The actual desired weight gain of 1 pound per week is the most measurable goal for the client. Attending all eating disorder support groups is a goal, but is not as important as actual weight gain. The client can eat a larger meal at breakfast and then not eat sufficient food and overexercise for the remainder of the day. The client's improved self-image is important, but actual weight gain is again a priority. (P)

20. 1 Bulimia can be related to internal and external stressors. Keeping a journal of feelings and experiences assists the client to identify patterns that trigger bulimic episodes. Developing meal plans and calculating calories does not address the underlying emotional link to eating and purging. Ignoring feelings related to food does not allow the client to develop insight into the underlying reasons why the behavior is occurring. (H)

chapter 39

Abuse and Mental Health Crises

The client who experiences events such as abuse and mental health crises may have a severe emotional response in which normal coping mechanisms are not sufficient to maintain mental health. Such events are difficult to identify, particularly in the pediatric client who does not have verbal skills to explain concerns. The nurse has an important role in identifying the client at risk, reporting evidence to appropriate authorities, and assisting the client to secure a safe environment. The nurse also is involved in assisting the client and family, and local community to develop healthy behaviors and promote and maintain health. Topics discussed in this chapter include:

- Abuse: Physical, Sexual, and Psychologic
- Crisis

Abuse: Physical, Sexual, and Psychologic

I. Definition: Abuse is defined as the "wrongful use and maltreatment of another person" (Videbeck, 2004, p. 210). Victims of abuse are found across the lifespan; this may be a spouse or significant other, a child, or an older adult.

A. Abuse of a spouse or significant other involves mistreatment of one person within an intimate relationship; abuse can be psychologic, physical, sexual, or a combination of these types. Fifteen to 25% of women experience violence while pregnant.

1. Psychologic or emotional abuse involves belittling, screaming, name-calling, destroying property, and making threats.
2. Physical abuse involves many activities from pushing and shoving to sever battering and choking that can result in breaking limbs and ribs, internal bleeding, brain damage, and even homicide.
3. Sexual abuse involves physical contact such as rape, molestation, or any sexual conduct with a person who does not consent or lacks the mental capacity to consent. Rape is defined as the "perpetration of an act of sexual intercourse with a female against her will and without her consent, whether her will is overcome by force, fear of force, drugs, or intoxicants" (Videbeck, 2004, p. 220). Frequently, the woman who is raped may also be physically beaten.

B. Child abuse is described as maltreatment or injury to a child; abuse can be physical, sexual, psychologic, involve neglect, or be a combination of these types of abuse. Domestic violence victims are children 27% of the time.

1. Physical abuse often results from unreasonably severe physical punishment to children, but can occur with intentional assaults onto children such as burning, biting, cutting, twisting limbs, and/or scalding the child with hot water. Children who have experienced physical abuse often have old injuries (scars, untreated fractures, and bruises in various stages of healing). Physical abuse is suspected if the history of an injury given by the caregivers or the parents does not fully explain the child's condition.
2. Sexual abuse involves sexual acts performed by an adult on a child under 18 years of age. This abuse includes rape, sodomy, or incest by the perpetrator or by an object. It may involve oral-genital contact between the child and the perpetrator or exposing the adult's genitals to the child. An additional form of this abuse involves exploitation of the minor—such as pornography.
3. Psychologic or emotional abuse involves verbal assaults on the child, family disagreements (constant), and withholding of affection. This type of abuse also often accompanies other types of abuse, such as physical or sexual abuse.
4. Neglect is the most prevalent type of child abuse, involving parent or guardian withholding of physical, educational, or emotional necessities for a child's well-being; this includes refusal to seek health care for the child, abandonment, inadequate supervision, reckless disregard for the safety of the child, spousal abuse in the child's presence, and school truancy permission.

C. Abuse of an older adult usually occurs by caretakers or family members; the abuser may be a guardian of finances, resulting in financial exploitation, and refusal to provide adequate medical treatment. Abuse of an older adult may also include physical and sexual abuse, psychologic abuse, and neglect. The majority of elder abuse clients are 75 years of age or older, and 60% to 65% are women. Abuse is suspected if malnourishment or dehydration occurs that is not linked to a specific illness.

II. Nursing process

A. Assessment

1. Assess victim of physical abuse for:
   a. Safety in the home.
   b. Injury with no reported history of trauma (child).
   c. Delay in attaining medical treatment for a serious injury.
   d. Inconsistencies given in the history during admission (e.g., reported cause versus condition—parent says child fell off couch and child has injuries of *shaken baby syndrome*).
   e. Unusual injuries for the age of the child (i.e., black eyes two times before the child is 6 months old).
   f. Fractures (and other old injuries) not treated (child).
   g. Multiple ecchymotic areas caregiver or parent cannot adequately explain (child, older adult client).
2. Assess victim of sexual abuse for:
   a. Increased incidence of UTIs; red, bruised, or swollen genitalia; bruising or tears of the rectum or vagina.
   b. Reluctance to get medical attention for injuries or denying injuries.

c. Details of event for rape survivors (inquire gently and with care).
d. Comprehensive physical examination by HCP for rape survivor before client has showered, brushed teeth, douched, changed clothes, or had anything to drink.
e. Safety in the home.

3. Assess victim of psychologic abuse and neglect for:
   a. Disorientation indicating medication misuse (older adult client).
   b. Hesitance to talk openly.
   c. Unusual activity in the client's bank account or missing of valuable belongings—not simply misplaced (older adult client).
   d. Unusual concern by caregiver over expense of medical care.
   e. Caregiver of older adult client not allowing client to have visitors or see anyone without the caregiver's presence.

B. Analysis
1. Rape-Trauma Syndrome related to sexual abuse/rape
2. Disturbed Sleep Pattern related to abuse
3. Ineffective Coping related to abuse
4. Post-Trauma Syndrome related to abuse
5. Chronic Low Self-Esteem related to abuse
6. Powerlessness related to abuse
7. Sexual Dysfunction related to abuse
8. Spiritual Distress related to abuse
9. Social Isolation related to abuse

C. Planning
1. Prevent injury.
2. Promote stress management.
3. Establish a social support system in the area the client lives.
4. Decrease anxiety, depression, and withdrawn behaviors.
5. Decrease stress-related symptoms.

D. Implementation
1. Assess client's vital signs in the emergency department.
2. Stay with the rape or violence victim in the emergency department.
3. Administer medications as necessary (e.g., antihypertensive therapies, pain medications, antibiotics, anxiolytics).
4. Provide caring, listening, and nurturing to the abuse-rape survivor client.
5. Assess client's potential for self-harm or suicide (see Chapter 36).
6. Assist client to a safe place such as safe houses and shelters or with trusted friends and family.
7. Assist client to identify feelings; be accepting of client's feelings.
8. Use grounding techniques for the client who is experiencing flashbacks or is dissociating after a traumatic event.

E. Evaluation
1. Client demonstrates ability to function in daily life.
2. Client demonstrates ability to protect himself or herself.
3. Client is free from injury from self and others.
4. Client demonstrates healthy and effective methods of stress management.
5. Client expresses emotions in a nondestructive manner.
6. Client participates in a social support system.
7. Client demonstrates decreased anxious, depressed, or withdrawn behaviors.
8. Client demonstrates a decrease in stress-related symptoms.

CN

III. Client needs

A. Physiologic adaptation: The client who is a victim of abuse has physiologic responses as well as psychologic responses to the event, and coexisting factors may compound the event. The nurse must facilitate adaptation to and set priorities for both types of responses.
1. Victims of physical abuse who are pregnant frequently experience miscarriage and stillbirth.
2. Date rape has been shown to increase with consumption of alcohol.
3. Abuse of older adults occurs more often when the elderly client has multiple chronic mental and physical health problems and when the client is dependent on family members for care.

B. Management of care: Care of the client who is a victim of abuse requires critical thinking skills and knowledge of assessment, and teaching and evaluation methods unique to the RN role. These skills cannot be delegated to an LPN or UAP.
1. Participate in interdisciplinary team conferences—nurse provides data from 24-hr assessment and care.
2. Introduce client to community agencies such as women's shelters for safety.
3. Provide and receive report on the assigned hospitalized clients with abuse, neglect, and rape.
4. Act as a client advocate.
5. Supervise the care provided to the rape-abuse client by LPN or UAP such as assistance with self-care and assessment of vital signs.

6. Maintain privacy and confidentiality.
7. Comply with state and federal reporting regulations for reporting abuse and neglect.

C. Safety and infection control
1. With incidences of rape or assault, stay with the client in the emergency department; at times the assailant will harm the client worse if it is discovered the client has reported the crime.
2. Obtain the assistance of hospital security, if necessary, to provide safety for the victim.
3. Protect the client from injury; assess home situation and provide the client and family teaching on safety issues.
4. During initial stages after the assault, the survivor may need specific directions and guidance from the nurse with procedures the client would normally be able to complete.
5. Provide the client and family with information and referrals to resources about diagnosis and treatment for STDs and pregnancy.

D. Health promotion and maintenance
1. Perform physical assessment and complete rape kit on admission to emergency department.
2. Identify barriers to learning by the rape/abuse survivor.
3. Assist client with obtaining care from shelter or community resources.

E. Psychologic integrity
1. Assess coping skills of the victim and family, and assist with coping.
2. Provide support and respect for the client's cultural practices and beliefs during the crises.
3. Use therapeutic communication to provide support for the client and/or family in the emergency department or in the hospital facility.
4. Recognize rape and abuse are highly underreported crimes—frequently related to the victim's feelings of guilt and shame; fear of further injury; and the belief that as a victim, there is no support from the legal system. The nurse supports the client's decision to report or not report the crime.
5. Assess for characteristics of violent families, including social isolation, abuse of control and power, and frequent association with alcohol and other drugs.
6. Assess family with violent characteristics for a pattern of violence perpetuated from one generation to future generations (occurs through role modeling).
7. Recognize violence occurs in all racial, ethnic, age, and sexual orientation, national origin, religious, and socioeconomic backgrounds; one population particularly at risk is immigrant women.

F. Basic care and comfort
1. Assist rape victim with a shower and oral care *after* initial examination is completed.
2. Provide client and family teaching about pain management.
3. Assess older adult client who is victim of abuse for bruises or fractures, lack of hearing aids or glasses, and fluid deficiency.
4. Provide therapies for comfort and treatment of injuries obtained during the abuse to the client as needed.

G. Reduction of risk potential
1. Provide client teaching regarding rape—date rape is also called *acquaintance rape* and may occur on the first date or after the couple has known each other for a period of time.
2. Identify suicidal tendencies and institute and maintain suicide precautions.
3. Identify client's risk for self-neglect following the trauma.
4. Maintain care for the abuse survivor; provide ventilator and cardiac monitoring support as needed because of the extent of the abuse and injury.

H. Pharmacologic and parenteral therapies: Medications for the victim of abuse and violence include those used for resulting anxieties and depressive episodes (see Tables 36-1 and 36-3).

Crisis

I. Definition: A "crisis" is an event (turning point) in a client's life that produces a devastating emotional response from which the client cannot effectively rely on usual coping mechanisms.

A. Stages of a crisis as defined by Caplan in 1964 include the following (Videbeck, 2004):
1. Stage 1—client is exposed to a stressor, develops anxiety, and attempts to use usual coping techniques.
2. Stage 2—usual coping techniques are ineffective, producing increased anxiety.
3. Stage 3—client makes additional efforts to deal with the stressor, including new methods of coping.
4. Stage 4—significant distress and disequilibrium develop when new coping methods fail.

B. Types of crises
1. Maturational crisis (also called *developmental crisis*) involves predictable events in the course of normal life, such as getting

married, the birth of a baby, and leaving home for the first time.

2. Adventitious crisis is precipitated by an unexpected event. Examples include terrorist attacks, riots, violent crimes such as murder or rape, and natural disasters such as tornadoes, floods, and hurricanes.
3. Situational crises are unexpected events that disrupt the client's psychologic integrity such as a death in the family, an emotional or a physical illness within the family, or the loss of a job.

C. Categories of crisis intervention
1. Authoritative intervention assesses the client's status and promotes problem-solving, such as offering information, raising the client's self-awareness, and directing the client's behavior by offering suggestions or directions.
2. Facilitative interventions have as a goal to provide compassionate understanding and encourage the client to recognize and discuss feelings; this involves listening to the client and affirming the client's self-worth.

II. Nursing process

A. Assessment—at the time of crisis, the nurse assesses the client for:
1. Perception of the crisis
2. Coping skills
3. Feelings the client is experiencing
4. Potential for self-harm

B. Analysis
1. Anxiety related to crisis
2. Ineffective Coping related to crisis
3. Situational Low Self-Esteem related to crisis
4. Disturbed Thought Processes related to crisis
5. Social Isolation related to crisis
6. Impaired Social Interaction related to crisis

C. Planning
1. Promote a trusting relationship.
2. Identify the exact problem.
3. Reduce negative perceptions of the crisis.
4. Promote use of healthy coping mechanisms.
5. Promote client's self-esteem.
6. Relieve anxiety.

D. Implementation
1. Provide listening, caring, and nurturing to the client in crisis.
2. Assess client's isolation and withdrawal; communicate with client's family and significant others.
3. Discuss coping techniques; discuss feelings that interfere with coping, and assist the client to develop healthy coping skills.
4. Assist client to focus on the problem and to develop goals to its resolution.
5. Provide lists of community resources and services.

E. Evaluation
1. Client develops trusting relationship with nurse.
2. Client demonstrates healthy coping mechanisms.
3. Client has positive self-esteem.
4. Client verbalizes relief of anxiety.
5. Client receives support from family and friends.

III. Client needs

A. Physiologic adaptation: Crisis can cause physiologic changes or aggravate existing health problems. The health care team must manage physiologic changes, monitor vital signs, and administer medications to treat concurrent health problems. At completion of the crisis (usually considered 4 to 6 weeks), the client has regained a usual level of functioning.

B. Management of care: Care of the client experiencing crisis requires critical thinking skills and knowledge of assessment, and teaching and evaluation methods unique to the RN role. These skills cannot be delegated to an LPN or UAP.
1. Participate in interdisciplinary team conferences—nurse provides data from 24-hr assessment and care.
2. Introduce client to community agencies such as halfway houses for long-term care.
3. Provide and receive report on the assigned hospitalized client.
4. Act as a client advocate.
5. Supervise care provided by LPN or UAP such as vital sign monitoring or provision of basic care and safety measures.
6. Maintain privacy and confidentiality.
7. Comply with state and federal reporting regulations for abuse and neglect.

C. Safety and infection control
1. With incidences as rape or assault, *the nurse stays with the client* in the emergency department—at times the assailant will inflict more severe harm if it is discovered that the client has reported the crime; obtain assistance of hospital security if necessary to provide safety for the victim.
2. Provide client and family teaching about safety issues in the home setting, especially handicap accessibility for the accident victim needing additional rehabilitation.
3. Prepare for and implement emergency response plans if crisis warrants.
4. If injury occurred in home setting, protect client from additional injury.

5. During initial stages after a crisis, provide specific directions for self-care or next steps of procedures that need to be completed.

D. Health promotion and maintenance
1. Perform physical assessment on admission to facilities per agency policy.
2. Identify barriers to learning by the client in crisis.
3. Assist client obtain home care such as home health nurses, and participate in community health agencies.
4. Provide healthy client and family community interactions.

E. Psychologic integrity
1. Prior to client discharge, dissolve the nurse-client partnership, and discuss how the client will deal with future crisis.
2. Identify suicidal tendencies and institute and maintain suicide precautions.
3. Identify client's risk for neglect to self and others during time of the crisis.
4. Assess family dynamics; promote coping mechanisms, communication, structure, and bonding; provide client and family with information about crisis processes and management; use therapeutic communication.
5. Encourage client to participate in crisis-management group sessions.
6. Provide client with a therapeutic milieu.
7. Provide support and respect for the client's cultural practices and beliefs during the crises.

F. Basic care and comfort
1. Assist client who is not able to complete personal care with activities of daily living.
2. Provide therapies for comfort and treatment of injuries obtained in the crisis to the client as needed.
3. Incorporate complementary and alternative therapies into care plan.
4. Educate client and family about pain management; administer medications as necessary (e.g., antihypertensive therapies, pain medications).

G. Reduction of risk potential
1. Provide ventilator and cardiac monitoring support as required by coexisting health problems.
2. Monitor for signs of dehydration or malnutrition for severe crisis victims.

H. Pharmacologic and parenteral therapies: Medications for the client experiencing crisis include those used for anxiety, thought disorders, and/or depression based on symptoms occurring after the crisis (see Tables 36-1 and 36-3).

Bibliography

American Psychiatric Association. (2000). *Diagnostic and statistical manual of mental disorders* (4th ed., text rev.). Washington, DC: Author.

Mohr, W. K. (2006). *Psychiatric-mental health nursing* (6th ed.). Philadelphia: Lippincott Williams & Wilkins.

Videbeck, S. L. (2004). *Psychiatric-mental health nursing* (2nd ed.). Philadelphia: Lippincott Williams & Wilkins.

CHAPTER 39
Practice Test

Abuse: Physical, Sexual, and Psychologic

1. AF The nurse is assessing an infant who is 6 months of age and has a black eye; the infant is brought by his mother to the quick-care clinic. The mother reports that the daycare provider told her the child "fell down the steps with his walker." The nurse should do which of the following in order of priority?

_____ 1. Report the incident to the social services department.
_____ 2. Document findings accurately.
_____ 3. Ask the mother for details about the incident and the daycare center.
_____ 4. Place an ice bag on the infant's eye.

2. A client comes to the clinic with complaints of abdominal pain; her significant other accompanies her and proceeds to answer all questions. The client avoids eye contact with everyone, sits away from the clinic staff, and has a bland affect. The nurse assesses that this client may be:

☐ 1. In too much pain to respond.
☐ 2. Suffering from depression.
☐ 3. A victim of intimate partner abuse.
☐ 4. Extremely tired.

3. A client comes into the emergency department after having been raped in the parking ramp of her apartment building. The client is very upset and crying. The nurse should first respond to the client by saying:

- □ 1. "Is that what you were wearing?"
- □ 2. "Have you showered and douched?"
- □ 3. "I will stay with you."
- □ 4. "Why did you wait an hour to come to the hospital?"

4. **AF** A female client is experiencing severe premenstrual syndrome (PMS) resulting in expressions of anger. The spouse expresses concerns about the safety of the children. In what order should the nurse perform the following?

_____ 1. Assess the female.
_____ 2. Notify child services.
_____ 3. Examine the children.
_____ 4. Notify the immediate supervisor.

5. **AF** The nurse is assessing a client who is 2 years of age and in the emergency department for burns on both feet, both lower legs, and the buttocks. The only area not burned from the waist down is the inside of the back of the knee. The parents inform the nurse that the child stepped into the bathtub and then sat down in the water when the water was too hot. The nurse should do which of the following in order of priority?

_____ 1. Provide fluid resuscitation and pain medications.
_____ 2. Assess burn depth in the different areas.
_____ 3. Document parent-child interactions.
_____ 4. Report incident to the authorities.

6. **AF** The nurse is assessing a client who is 4 years of age and admitted for a subdural hematoma that was determined to be caused by abuse. Nursing diagnoses for this child would include which of the following? Select all that apply.

- □ 1. Fear related to physical abuse.
- □ 2. Disturbed Thought Processes related to psychologic abuse.
- □ 3. Anxiety related to physical abuse.
- □ 4. Self-Care Deficit: Feeding, related to cerebral trauma.
- □ 5. Sleep Deprivation related to head injury.

7. The nurse is instructing a client about the cycle of violence. At what point in the cycle should the client be most concerned for her safety?

- □ 1. Honeymoon phase.
- □ 2. Tension-building phase.
- □ 3. Contrition phase.
- □ 4. Violent behavior phase.

8. The nurse is assessing a group of children in a daycare center. Which of the following children warrant further assessment?

- □ 1. Child who is 12 months of age who has bruises on one side of the head.
- □ 2. Child who is 3 years of age with a spiral fracture of the ulna whose mother does not know how the injury occurred.
- □ 3. Child who is 4 years of age who wears the same clothes to the center every day.
- □ 4. Child who is 2 years of age who has frequent episodes of untreated conjunctivitis.

9. Which of the following statements is true about women remaining in battering relationships with their husbands?

- □ 1. If the woman would meet her husband's needs faster, the violence would end.
- □ 2. The woman provokes the battering incidents by her behavior.
- □ 3. The woman deserves the battering as she is dependent and subservient to her husband.
- □ 4. If the woman did try to leave, she and/or her children would be at increased risk of violence.

10. A client who is being abused by her husband complains of insomnia, nervousness, and loss of appetite. The client states that she has been drinking lately and has been having difficulty with her job and her children. Once the nurse provides a diagnosis of Ineffective Coping related to the multiple stressors, which of these short-term outcomes is appropriate?

- □ 1. Client uses community support systems.
- □ 2. Client demonstrates a decrease in anxious behaviors.
- □ 3. Client verbalizes realistic future plans.
- □ 4. Client verbalizes an understanding of aggressive behavior.

Crisis

11. A single mother is diagnosed with multiple sclerosis. She is concerned that she will not be able to work and support her family and begins to drink heavily every evening. The nurse assesses that this client is experiencing a/an:

- □ 1. Alteration in perception.
- □ 2. Situational crisis.
- □ 3. Internal crisis.
- □ 4. Distortion in reflection.

12. The nurse is establishing a relationship with a client who has just lost her spouse suddenly in a work accident. The priority goal for this client is to:

- □ 1. Develop trust in the nurse.
- □ 2. Assess support from the family and friends.

□ 3. Listen to the nurse's directions.
□ 4. Identify appropriate community resources.

13. AF The nurse is counseling a parent whose son was just killed in an accident. The nurse should do which of the following at this time? Select all that apply.
□ 1. Listen to the client.
□ 2. Discuss feelings with the client.
□ 3. Obtain an order for medication for depression.
□ 4. Assess support systems.
□ 5. Discuss coping techniques the client is using.

14. The nurse is assessing a client who has just experienced a crisis. The nurse should first assess the client for which of the following behaviors?
□ 1. Capability of effective problem solving.
□ 2. Increased level of anxiety.
□ 3. Shortened attention span.
□ 4. Seeks help from others.

15. A client who had a cardiac arrest is admitted via ambulance to the emergency department. A family member comes to the emergency department, starts to cry, and asks the nurse what is happening with the client. The nurse explains what has happened, what resuscitative efforts have been done, and what the client responses to the attempts have been. What crisis intervention procedure did the nurse perform?
□ 1. Offers information.
□ 2. Encourages a discussion of feelings.
□ 3. Offers suggestions.
□ 4. Promotes problem-solving.

16. A client is brought to the emergency department after being raped. Which type of crisis is this client experiencing?
□ 1. Situational crisis.
□ 2. Developmental crisis.
□ 3. Maturational crisis.
□ 4. Adventitious crisis.

17. AF The nurse is assessing a client who is upset because her husband died suddenly. The nurse should assess the client for which of the following? Select all that apply.
□ 1. Perception of the crisis.
□ 2. Coping skills.
□ 3. Vital signs.
□ 4. Support systems.
□ 5. Feelings.
□ 6. Anxiety.

18. AF The nurse is working with a family in crisis. The nurse should do which of the following in priority order? Place in order from first to last.
_____ 1. Make a plan for managing the crisis.
_____ 2. Develop strategies to reduce symptoms.
_____ 3. Assess the family's resources.
_____ 4. Identify the family member in crisis.

19. AF The nurse is managing the care for a client in a disaster shelter who broke a femur and has lost her family home in a hurricane. The nurse should take which of the following measures? Select all that apply.
□ 1. Supervise the care provided to the client during the crisis.
□ 2. Obtain an order for antipsychotic medications for the client.
□ 3. Act as a client advocate for the client in crisis.
□ 4. Discuss with the interdisciplinary team available community resources for the client.
□ 5. Obtain accurate identification including name, age, address, contact information, and names of relatives.

20. A client experiences a crisis. After being unable to make decisions, the nurse assigns the nursing diagnosis of Disturbed Thought Processes related to crisis. Which of the following informs the nurse that the client has resolved the crisis?
□ 1. The client uses a coping strategy that is agreed on by the client and the nurse.
□ 2. The client realizes his personal capabilities.
□ 3. The client has a realistic interpretation of the crisis event.
□ 4. The client reports a decrease in feelings of anxiety.

Answers and Rationales

1. 4, 3, 2, 1 The nurse first assesses and manages the physical effects of the eye injury by placing an ice pack on the eye to reduce swelling. Next, the nurse obtains as much information about the situation and the day-care center as possible. The nurse documents all physical assessment findings and information provided by the mother. Because an infant who is 6 months of age should not be in a walker unattended, and black eyes do not occur from falls with walkers, this is a potential child abuse incident;

therefore, the nurse reports the incident as such using the agency's reporting structure (usually social services department reports the incidents to the authorities). (M)

2. 3 Frequently the abuse victim is depressed, withdrawn, and avoids eye contact. When the partner is answering all questions, he could be preventing her response in fear of what she might say. The client is most likely coming to the clinic for physical complaints such as the abdominal pain, and is very likely afraid of the abuser and depressed; but there are no assessment data to support these concerns as priority assessments. (S)

3. 3 The priority of the nurse is to provide for the client's safety. The rapist could have told the client that if she reported the rape, he would come back again and kill her. Asking the client if the clothing she is wearing is what she wore during the rape is part of the assessment, but could also be construed by the client as being a suggestive outfit. The question about the shower and douche does make a difference in the rape kit, but is not the priority that the client's safety is. Asking why the client waited an hour before coming to the hospital could put the client on the defensive. (P)

4. 1, 3, 4, 2 Nursing actions are based on assessment. The nurse first assesses the female client because she is the primary source of data and because of the nondefinitive clinical profile of PMS. The nurse then examines the children for obvious signs of abuse, and notes the nature of interactions between the children and the mother. After investigating appropriate avenues, the nurse notifies the immediate supervisor because of the potential risks to the children as well as the sensitivity of the issue. Lastly, if warranted, the nurse notifies child services officials after consulting with the supervisor. (S)

5. 2, 1, 3, 4 When a child steps into hot water, he or she does not sit down in it. This child was held in the scalding water and when he was held in the water, he abducted his knees (hence the areas not burned behind the knees). The nurse first assesses the extent of the burn and then assures fluid resuscitation and pain relief as needed. The nurse also documents what the parents report as well as the parent-child interaction. The burns appear to be from child abuse and must be reported to the authorities, which the nurse can do when the child is stable. (S)

6. 1, 3 The nursing diagnoses for the child who is a survivor of child abuse includes diagnoses of fear and anxiety. The client with delusions or hallucinations tends to have disturbed thought processes, and there are no data to indicate that the child is having hallucinations or delusions. The nurse assesses the child's level of consciousness related to the head injury, but there are no indications that the child will have difficulty eating or sleeping. (A)

7. 4 The violent behavior phase includes battering or violence; the nurse instructs the client to take measures to protect herself. In the honeymoon phase (and in the period of remorse or contrition), the abuser expresses regret, apologizes, and promises the victim it will never happen again. The tension-building phase is accompanied by arguments, silence, and complaints from the abuser about the victim. (P)

8. 2 Signs of child abuse include injury with a history that is inconsistent with the nature of the injury, or unusual injuries for the age of the child. A spiral fracture of a child is always investigated as potential child abuse as this injury is often due to twisting of an extremity. It is not unusual for a child who is learning to walk to have bruises. Wearing the same clothes is not an indication of abuse or neglect. The child with conjunctivitis requires health care, but having frequent episodes is not an indication of abuse or neglect. (P)

9. 4 The woman who is in a battering relationship is at risk for increased violence when she leaves the batterer. The woman does not deserve to be beaten. Her behavior does not provoke the beating, and the batterer will find an excuse for the battering. (P)

10. 2 A short-term outcome for the client with a nursing diagnosis of Ineffective Coping is to demonstrate a decrease in anxious behaviors. The goal of using community support systems and verbalizing realistic future plans are long-term goals. The goal of verbalizing an understanding of aggressive behavior would be appropriate if the woman were the aggressive person (e.g., the abuser). (P)

11. 2 The client is experiencing a situational crisis. An internal crisis is a stressor that is not as obvious to the outside observer. The client is not experiencing an alteration in perception or a distortion in her reflections on this situation. (P)

12. 1 The priority goal in the beginning of intervention is for the client to develop trust in the nurse. Support of family and friends is assessed as the relationship develops. The nurse's directions are not a priority goal for the client, and identifying community resources is an intervention, if needed, which occurs later in the relationship. (P)

13. 1, 2, 4, 5 When providing care for a client who experienced a recent death in the family, the nurse provides listening and discusses feelings with the client. The nurse also assesses the client's support systems and discusses the coping skills the client is using. There is no indication at this time that the client is depressed or needs an order for an antidepressant medication. (P)

14. 2 During the first phase of a crisis, the client exhibits elevated levels of anxiety. If the client is able to use problem-solving capabilities, there is no crisis. A shortened attention span is a characteristic of the fourth phase of the crisis. Reaching out to others for help is indicative of the third phase of a crisis. (P)

15. 1 When the nurse at the emergency department desk provides information about the client's status, she provides the family member with information. The information may have promoted problem-solving, but the data do not support that the family member did any problem-solving. The nurse did not offer suggestions to the family member or encourage a discussion of feelings. (P)

16. 4 An adventitious crisis is precipitated by an unexpected event. A rape is an example of this type of crisis. Situational crises are unexpected events that disrupt the client's integrity (e.g., death in the family). Maturational crises occur as predictable events in the course of normal life. (P)

17. 1, 2, 3, 4, 5 During a crisis, the nurse assesses the client's perception of the crisis, coping skills used in past crises, client's vital signs, support available to the client from family and friends, and feelings the client states she is feeling. Anxiety is a diagnosis. (P)

18. 4, 2, 3, 1 The nurse must first identify which member is exhibiting crisis symptoms. Next, the nurse identifies strategies to reduce the most severe symptoms. The nurse then assesses the family's resources. The family member in crisis may have such overwhelming feelings that he or she is unable to identify or describe the feelings. (M)

19. 1, 3, 4, 5 The nurse who is managing the care of the client in a disaster shelter provides for the management of care by supervising the care for the client in crisis. In a disaster, the nurse also must be sure that the client is identified and contact information about the client is documented. The nurse also acts as a client advocate for the client in crisis and discusses available community resources for the client with the interdisciplinary team assigned to this client. There are no data to indicate that antipsychotic medications are needed for this client at this time. (M)

20. 4 The client who is reporting a decrease in anxiety is experiencing an ability to think clearly and make logical decisions. Using an agreed-on coping strategy (problem-solving) is not a goal relevant to disturbed thought processes—it is a goal of ineffective coping. The ability to describe a realistic interpretation of the crisis is not as helpful a criterion for evaluation of the disturbed thought processes as is the reduced anxiety. (P)

SECTION 4

Practice Test

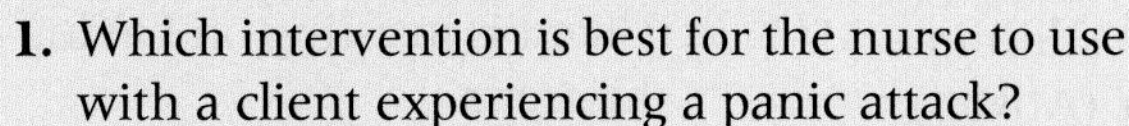

1. Which intervention is best for the nurse to use with a client experiencing a panic attack?

- ☐ 1. Encourage the client to verbalize feelings.
- ☐ 2. Teach the client relaxation techniques.
- ☐ 3. Remain with the client.
- ☐ 4. Initiate music therapy.

2. The nurse is preparing a care plan based on cognitive theory principles for a client diagnosed with depression. The nurse understands that the focus of this theory is based on which of the following principles?

- ☐ 1. The way in which the client thinks about himself and the world.
- ☐ 2. All behavior has meaning.
- ☐ 3. Loss may predispose client to lower functioning.
- ☐ 4. Problems with behavior can be resolved through interpersonal relationships.

3. The nurse is assessing a client who is taking tranylcypromine sulfate (Parnate). The nurse should report which of the following findings to the HCP?

- ☐ 1. A fever of 100°F.
- ☐ 2. BP of 170/100 mmHg.
- ☐ 3. Diarrhea.
- ☐ 4. Insomnia.

4. AF The nurse has received report about a group of clients admitted to the emergency department. In which order does the nurse assess the following clients? Place in order from first to last.

_____ 1. Client who is 20 years of age, a primipara in premature labor, and 1 cm dilated.

_____ 2. Client who is 7 months of age with RSV who is receiving a nebulizer treatment; temperature is 99°F and respirations are 20.

_____ 3. Client who is 40 years of age who takes olanzapine (Zyprexa), with a temperature of 101°F, pulse of 100, and BP of 160/100.

_____ 4. Client who is 30 years of age with shoulder pain following a skiing accident; client has stable vital signs and is waiting for an orthopaedic surgeon to assess the injury.

5. A client is admitted to an inpatient unit with severe depression. The client has noticeable poor personal hygiene from symptoms of decreased energy and interest in daily activities. The nurse suggests the client shower and change clothes. The client states, "I can't." What action should the nurse take next?

- ☐ 1. Wait until the client demonstrates trust in the nurse before bringing up the topic again.
- ☐ 2. Matter-of-factly assist the client to shower and dress in clean clothes.
- ☐ 3. Tell the client that it is a requirement to shower once medications take effect.
- ☐ 4. Explain that family members will not want to visit if the client is not clean.

6. A client with symptoms of mania is to be admitted to a nursing unit. What is the most appropriate room assignment for this client?

- ☐ 1. A single room near the unit fire escape door.
- ☐ 2. A single room near the nurse's station.
- ☐ 3. A double room shared with a client with mania.
- ☐ 4. A double room shared with a client with schizophrenia.

7. The nurse is providing care to a client who tells of a plan for suicide by crashing a car into a tree. The nurse should ask which of the following questions first?

- ☐ 1. "What effect would that have on your family?"
- ☐ 2. "Do you have access to a car?"
- ☐ 3. "Have you tried to hurt yourself in the past?"
- ☐ 4. "Isn't your medicine helping you?"

8. A client is having a manic episode in the dayroom of the nursing unit. The nurse should do which of the following?

- ☐ 1. Escort the client to a quiet area.
- ☐ 2. Engage the client in a game of volleyball with other clients.
- ☐ 3. Allow the client to do an activity of his choice until he is more stable.
- ☐ 4. Have the client play a card game of solitaire.

9. A client with bipolar I disorder takes lithium carbonate (Lithium) and lorazepam (Ativan). Which type of therapy would be most appropriate for this client?

- ☐ 1. Phototherapy.
- ☐ 2. Electroconvulsive therapy (ECT).
- ☐ 3. Psychoanalysis.
- ☐ 4. Group therapy.

10. A client is to have ECT. The nurse instructs the client about what effect after the procedure?

- ☐ 1. There may be some memory deficit of events just prior to the procedure.
- ☐ 2. Memory will be enhanced after the procedure.
- ☐ 3. There is commonly a long period of lethargy after the procedure.
- ☐ 4. Long-term memory will be lost.

11. What is the most appropriate nursing goal for a client hospitalized in an acute manic episode?

- ☐ 1. Client participates in unlimited recreation therapy to expend as much energy as possible.
- ☐ 2. Client participates in daily music therapy.
- ☐ 3. Client adequately expresses feelings throughout the day.
- ☐ 4. Client interacts appropriately with other clients on the unit.

12. AF The nurse is assessing a client who is admitted to the hospital and is experiencing a depressive episode. Which of the following are expected for this client? Select all that apply.

- ☐ 1. Sleeping much more than usual.
- ☐ 2. Loss of appetite.
- ☐ 3. Increased physical activity.
- ☐ 4. Decreased ability to concentrate.
- ☐ 5. Actively hallucinating.
- ☐ 6. Fear of being enclosed.

13. The nurse determines that the client understands the teaching regarding tranylcypromine sulfate (Parnate) when the client makes which of the following statements?

- ☐ 1. "I will need to follow a low-fat diet while taking this medication."
- ☐ 2. "I will need to increase my fluid and fiber intake while taking this medication."
- ☐ 3. "I should not eat any dairy products while on this medication."
- ☐ 4. "I should not eat salami and aged cheese while on this medication."

14. A mother brings her toddler into the clinic and states, "He doesn't act like my other children at this age." The nurse observes the child. Which of the following indicate the nurse should initiate a referral to a HCP?

- ☐ 1. Client is playing alone and quietly with toys.
- ☐ 2. Client is insisting on having all the toys for himself.
- ☐ 3. Client demonstrates early language development.
- ☐ 4. Client demonstrates lack of response when hugged by family members.

15. A client on an inpatient unit walks to the nurse's station at 0200 and requests another sleeping tablet after complaining of inability to sleep related to the bright light in the hall and noise from the kitchen area. The nurse should:

- ☐ 1. Administer a sedative medication as needed.
- ☐ 2. Move the client to another room.
- ☐ 3. Escort the client back to his room and partially close the door.
- ☐ 4. Allow the client to sit in the dayroom and read for an hour.

16. Three weeks ago, a client who was depressed and suicidal started taking a tricyclic antidepressant. What is the major concern of the nurse while assessing this client at a follow-up clinic appointment?

- ☐ 1. Promote regular lab work to monitor medication levels.
- ☐ 2. Review with the client diet restriction of foods containing tyramine.
- ☐ 3. Closely assess suicide risk for the client related to overdose toxicity of the medication.
- ☐ 4. Closely assess the client regarding the need for a medication to offset side effects of the medication.

17. The nurse is reviewing lab results for a client who is taking lithium carbonate (Lithium). The nurse should notify the HCP about which of the following lithium levels?

- ☐ 1. 0.5 mEq/L.
- ☐ 2. 0.7 mEq/L.

□ 3. 1.0 mEq/L.
□ 4. 2.0 mEq/L.

18. The nurse is caring for a client who is taking haloperidol (Haldol). The client complains of restlessness and inability to sit still during group therapy. The nurse should contact the HCP for an order for which of the following?
□ 1. An additional dose of haloperidol (Haldol).
□ 2. Benztropine (Cogentin).
□ 3. Propranolol (Inderal).
□ 4. Trazodone (Desyrel).

19. During the admission interview, a client firmly states that he believes the news reporter is talking about events that happened to him. This is an example of which type of thought process?
□ 1. Flight of ideas.
□ 2. Pressured speech.
□ 3. Ideas of reference.
□ 4. Paranoia.

20. AF The nurse is assessing a client with schizophrenia. Which of the following are expected positive symptoms of schizophrenia? Select all that apply.
□ 1. Delusions.
□ 2. Ambivalence.
□ 3. Hallucinations.
□ 4. Lack of volition.
□ 5. Flight of ideas.
□ 6. Anhedonia.
□ 7. Flat affect.

21. The nurse is completing discharge teaching for a client who has been prescribed clozapine (Clozaril). The nurse should:
□ 1. Teach the client about related diet restrictions.
□ 2. Have the client record a daily weight after discharge.
□ 3. Remind the client to use sunscreen when outside.
□ 4. Emphasize the importance of having regular lab work completed.

22. A client who has been taking fluphenazine (Prolixin) for 3 days suddenly cries out, his neck turns abruptly to one side, and his eyes roll up. The nurse should administer which of the following medications?
□ 1. Fluphenazine (Prolixin).
□ 2. Haloperidol (Haldol).
□ 3. Diphenhydramine (Benadryl).
□ 4. Chlorpromazine (Thorazine).

23. A client has been prescribed lorazepam (Ativan) for his anxiety. Prior to administering the first dose, the nurse should determine which of the following?
□ 1. Client's financial resources.
□ 2. Client's family support and monitoring.
□ 3. Client's use of alcohol.
□ 4. Client's typical food intake.

24. The nurse is teaching a client about the use of naltrexone (ReVia). Which statement by the client indicates the teaching is effective?
□ 1. "Using this drug will make me sleepy."
□ 2. "This medication is a good choice as it will only counteract street drugs."
□ 3. "This medication will block the effects of any opioid medication I take."
□ 4. "It is safe to use this medication with any over-the-counter medications."

25. AF The nurse is evaluating the weight gain of a client with anorexia. The client is to gain 10% of her weight within 6 months. At admission the client weighed 90 pounds. At 6 months, how much should this client weigh?

______________ pounds.

26. A client who came to the family practice clinic with a complaint of sore throat reports to the nurse that she takes a drink of alcohol every morning to "settle my nerves and keep my hands from trembling." The nurse recognizes that the client is at risk for which condition related to her alcohol use?
□ 1. A neurologic disorder.
□ 2. An anxiety disorder.
□ 3. Physical dependence.
□ 4. A personality disorder.

27. A nurse is providing care for a client with la belle indifférence related to her conversion disorder. What behavior would the nurse observe?
□ 1. Extreme concern related to the physical symptom with insistence for frequent lab tests.
□ 2. Manipulation of the staff in connection with her symptoms.
□ 3. Indifference or ignoring of the physical symptom.
□ 4. Delusions related to the cause of the behavior.

28. A client comes to the emergency department with sudden blindness. During the interview, the nurse recognizes that the client has achieved what primary gain from the blindness?
□ 1. A coworker has been assigned to do the major presentation the client was to do today.
□ 2. The client's spouse is giving the client attention by bringing the client to the hospital.
□ 3. The client's office sent a bouquet of flowers to the hospital.
□ 4. The client receives needed attention from health care personnel.

29. The nurse is assessing a client who is demonstrating severe anxiety. What technique should the nurse use?
- ☐ 1. Postpone assessment until the client is calmer.
- ☐ 2. Review the chart to identify current anxiety.
- ☐ 3. Ask broad, open-ended questions to validate the client's feelings.
- ☐ 4. Ask specific, direct questions.

30. The nurse is assessing a child who has been on a stimulant for several years for treatment of ADHD. The nurse should specifically assess which of the following?
- ☐ 1. Weight gain.
- ☐ 2. Insomnia.
- ☐ 3. Growth suppression.
- ☐ 4. Memory loss.

31. The nurse notes that a client diagnosed with anorexia nervosa has lost 0.5 pounds in the past week despite eating all meals and snacks. What is the most appropriate action for the nurse to take?
- ☐ 1. Notify the HCP with a request for an increase in medications.
- ☐ 2. Consult the dietitian and increase the caloric intake by 500 calories a day.
- ☐ 3. Schedule the client for cooking group to increase access to snack foods.
- ☐ 4. Monitor client activity for 2 hr after all meals and snacks.

32. AF The nurse should teach a client who is taking phenelzine sulfate (Nardil) to avoid which of the following foods? Select all that apply.
- ☐ 1. Beer.
- ☐ 2. Ice cream.
- ☐ 3. Pepperoni pizza.
- ☐ 4. Oranges.
- ☐ 5. Cheddar cheese.
- ☐ 6. Beef.

33. AF The nurse is assessing a child recently diagnosed as having ADHD. Which of the following behaviors indicate that the treatment plan is not yet effective? Select all that apply.
- ☐ 1. Moody.
- ☐ 2. Sullen.
- ☐ 3. Easy distractibility.
- ☐ 4. Does not wait to take turns.
- ☐ 5. Long periods of isolation.
- ☐ 6. Excessive fidgeting while sitting.
- ☐ 7. Interrupts others frequently.

34. A client who has been on antidepressant medication for 3 weeks tells the nurse, "My feelings of depression have decreased. I feel much better now." The nurse understands what about this client's risk for suicide?
- ☐ 1. Client at risk for suicide only in a community setting.
- ☐ 2. Client is no longer at risk for suicide.
- ☐ 3. Client is at greater risk for suicide than when she was more depressed.
- ☐ 4. Client is not at risk for suicide because there was no direct mention of suicide.

35. A client is taking a psychotropic drug. The nurse assesses which of the following is related to the client's ability to adhere to the medication regimen?
- ☐ 1. Client's support in the home setting related to taking medications.
- ☐ 2. Client's history of successfully taking these medications.
- ☐ 3. The number of other medications the client is currently taking.
- ☐ 4. The education and information about the medications that the client has received.

36. The nurse is evaluating the care plan for a client with obsessive-compulsive disorder. What is the best data for the nurse to gather related to the client's response to nursing interventions?
- ☐ 1. Suggestions of the nursing care team about which interventions are working.
- ☐ 2. The observation and documentation of client behaviors.
- ☐ 3. The client's family reports of how the client is changing in a positive fashion.
- ☐ 4. Group meetings between the client and the care team.

37. AF The nurse is admitting a client to the inpatient mental health unit. What characteristics does the nurse document under the general appearance section of the mini mental status exam? Select all that apply.
- ☐ 1. Memory.
- ☐ 2. Gait.
- ☐ 3. Grooming.
- ☐ 4. Ability to understand treatment.
- ☐ 5. Subjective feelings.
- ☐ 6. Eye contact.
- ☐ 7. Behavior.

38. AF A client who is 14 years of age and unresponsive is being admitted to the emergency department. The emergency personnel report that other teenagers with the client stated the client had been "huffing" toluene. The nurse should assess this client for which of the following? Select all that apply.
- ☐ 1. Spray paint around mouth.
- ☐ 2. Watery eyes.
- ☐ 3. Loss of motor coordination.
- ☐ 4. Constricted pupils.
- ☐ 5. Increased heart rate.

39. A client who recently emigrated from China is admitted to an inpatient unit. Neither the client nor the client's spouse speaks the English language. What action should the nurse take when admitting this client?
- ☐ 1. Ask the teenage son of the client to act as interpreter.
- ☐ 2. Use a picture board and hand motions to determine the client's needs.
- ☐ 3. Contact the hospital services department and request an interpreter be present.
- ☐ 4. Contact the client's clergy for assistance in translating for the client.

40. The client requests no visitors or phone calls except from a designated family member. The nurse should:
- ☐ 1. Understand that the client is concerned because the client does not have adequate insurance coverage for mental health care.
- ☐ 2. Accept the client's concern that those outside the hospital will think less of the client as a result of having a mental illness.
- ☐ 3. Support the client's request because too many visitors will disrupt the treatment program.
- ☐ 4. Allow family members to speak with the client, but restrict friends and coworkers.

41. A client with antisocial personality disorder is admitted to the inpatient psychiatric unit. The courts informed the client that if he voluntarily admitted himself for treatment, he could avoid serving a jail sentence. Following hospitalization, the client will most likely:
- ☐ 1. Continue treatment with a psychotherapist.
- ☐ 2. Seek admission to another facility for long-term care.
- ☐ 3. Return to the same behaviors as before the hospitalization.
- ☐ 4. Become a productive citizen in the community.

42. A client with anxiety disorder is taking buspirone (BuSpar). The nurse should provide which of the following instructions to the client and family?
- ☐ 1. Medication can cause headache.
- ☐ 2. Take medication before driving.
- ☐ 3. Rise slowly from a sitting position.
- ☐ 4. Take on an empty stomach.

43. AF A client is to receive olanzapine/fluoxetine (Symbyax) 6 mg/50 mg capsules. The client has 3 mg/25mg capsules on hand. How many capsules should the client take to achieve the desired dose?

_______________ capsules.

44. A client is admitted with a diagnosis of schizophrenia—catatonic type, and is in the excited phase. The client paces continuously and shouts when people speak to him. A short-term goal for this client is:
- ☐ 1. Client sleeps through the night.
- ☐ 2. Client attends all unit social activities.
- ☐ 3. Client maintains admission weight.
- ☐ 4. Client performs self-grooming activities daily.

45. AF A client is admitted to an inpatient unit under the influence of methamphetamine ingestion. The nurse would assess for which signs related to withdrawal of this substance? Select all that apply.
- ☐ 1. Fatigue.
- ☐ 2. Increased appetite.
- ☐ 3. Suicidal ideation.
- ☐ 4. Sweating.
- ☐ 5. Aching legs.

46. A client is being admitted to an inpatient unit with a diagnosis of bipolar I disorder. While being admitted, the client stands up, starts pacing, and yells, "Stop doing this! Don't you know who I am?" What is the best action for the nurse?
- ☐ 1. Continue to ask assessment questions of the client.
- ☐ 2. Teach relaxation techniques.
- ☐ 3. Provide a safe environment for the client and staff.
- ☐ 4. Administer prescribed medications to sedate the client.

47. AF A client with a tendency to become violent is admitted to the acute admission unit of a psychiatric hospital. Which of the following incidents could precipitate an angry outburst in this client? Select all that apply.
- ☐ 1. A client with Alzheimer disease is yelling about wanting to go home.
- ☐ 2. A staff member asks the client if he would like a snack during the activity.
- ☐ 3. The nurse notices that he is pacing and asks him if he is upset.
- ☐ 4. Another person takes the client's clothes from the clothes dryer and takes them to his own room.
- ☐ 5. The client is informed it is time for physical therapy, to which the client had been attending readily.

48. A client is attending anger-management classes. Which of the following indicate that the training has not been effective?
- ☐ 1. The client states that he is aware of the feelings, behaviors, and the thoughts that occur prior to being angry.

□ 2. The client has gained an awareness of the consequences of his behavioral and emotional anger responses.
□ 3. The client now sees situations where he is aroused angrily as a problem calling for a solution.
□ 4. The client has achieved the ability to delay the aggressive responses until the late stages of anger arousal.

49. The nurse is teaching the client prescribed a monoamine oxidase inhibitor (MAOI) about foods containing tyramine that will need to be avoided. Which statement indicates the client needs further teaching?
□ 1. "I'm glad I can continue to eat my favorite food, pepperoni pizza."
□ 2. "I can eat all of my favorite vegetables while on this medication."
□ 3. "I should not drink any beer while on this medication."
□ 4. "I can eat cottage cheese salad while on this medication."

50. AF The nurse is developing the nursing care plan for a college student who is admitted to the acute admission unit for an eating disorder. Which of the following nursing diagnoses are appropriate for this client? Select all that apply.
□ 1. Anxiety related to the eating disorder.
□ 2. Situational Low Self-Esteem related to the eating disorder.
□ 3. Disturbed Body Image related to the eating disorder.
□ 4. Imbalanced Nutrition: Less Than Body Requirements, related to the eating disorder.
□ 5. Activity Intolerance related to the eating disorder.
□ 6. Constipation related the eating disorder.

51. A client initially admitted to the neurology unit for paralysis is transferred to the inpatient acute psychiatric unit; the client is unable to walk because of the paralysis. The client had no injuries or infections preceding the paralysis. When questioned about the paralysis, the client showed a lack of concern. How would the nurse document this lack of concern?
□ 1. Hypochondriasis.
□ 2. La belle indifférence.
□ 3. Body dysmorphic disorder.
□ 4. Generalized anxiety disorder.

52. A client is admitted to the adolescent admission unit at a psychiatric facility for an eating disorder. The nurse is developing the care plan for the client. Which of these nursing interventions is an appropriate example of behavior modification for the client with an eating disorder?
□ 1. Provide high-protein, high-calorie meals and snacks.
□ 2. Encourage client to attend exercise groups in the recreation area.
□ 3. Provide medication for any complaints the client has.
□ 4. Allow the client to use the telephone to call her friends once she has gained 3 pounds.

53. A client is admitted to the psychiatric unit for PTSD. The client had served as a soldier in a war 30 years ago and is recently reliving a traumatic event that occurred during the war. Which of the following mental health problems is the client demonstrating in order to avoid remembering this event?
□ 1. Agoraphobia.
□ 2. Dissociation.
□ 3. Compulsions.
□ 4. Repression.

54. A client who is 30 years of age has insomnia; her son died 3 months ago of leukemia, and her mother died in a car accident 1½ years ago. The client makes the statement to the nurse, "I cannot stand it." The nurse should first ask the client:
□ 1. "Are you taking any antianxiety medications?"
□ 2. "Do you have any thoughts of killing yourself?"
□ 3. "How are you coping with the loss?"
□ 4. "What is your husband doing for you?"

55. The client with schizophrenia is taking clozapine (Clozaril). Teaching is understood as effective when the client states:
□ 1. "I'll contact my doctor if I get a sore throat."
□ 2. "I'll get my blood drawn once every 3 months."
□ 3. "I could develop diarrhea while on this medication."
□ 4. "I will have no problems taking my antihistamines."

56. Which of the following is an emphasis of milieu therapy?
□ 1. Expectations are mediated by staff authority.
□ 2. Clients have a formal relationship with staff.
□ 3. Staff pressure normalizes adaptation by the clients.
□ 4. Group and social interactions are fostered.

57. The nurse is developing a nursing care plan for a client diagnosed with borderline personality disorder. Which of the following is an appropriate short-term goal for this client?

- □ 1. Client functions within therapeutic milieu.
- □ 2. Client develops nondrug alternatives to stress management.
- □ 3. Client experiences a decreased anxiety level.
- □ 4. Client identifies methods to meet personal needs that are not infringing on others' rights.

58. A child is seen in the outpatient clinic with anxiety. The child becomes anxious when he touches a door handle or an item in a store that has been touched by another individual. What is the most appropriate nursing intervention for this child?

- □ 1. Explain the symptoms and treatment of this disorder to the parents.
- □ 2. Instruct the child to avoid all door handles and store items.
- □ 3. Teach cognitive behavioral approaches to anxiety.
- □ 4. Ask the child why he thinks he cannot touch these items when others do without incident.

59. A young mother who comes to the outpatient clinic is pacing, complaining of being restless, and having difficulty concentrating on the admission data form; she states that she has been unable to sleep lately and subsequently is tired all of the time. She worries about her children when they play with other children that they will be hurt. This client is experiencing:

- □ 1. Generalized anxiety disorder.
- □ 2. Posttraumatic stress disorder.
- □ 3. Panic disorder.
- □ 4. Body dysmorphic disorder.

60. A client is brought to the emergency department with a severe headache. The client has had numerous brain scans, CT scans, and MRIs, and no abnormalities or defects were found. Also, the client has had tests for abdominal pain, back pain, and generalized aching, which did not reveal any abnormalities. Which nursing diagnosis for this client would the nurse assign to this client?

- □ 1. Knowledge Deficit related to understanding the diagnostic studies.
- □ 2. Noncompliance related to following directions for preparation for the diagnostic studies.
- □ 3. Acute Pain related to headache.
- □ 4. Health-Seeking Behaviors related to need for attention.

61. AF A nurse is evaluating the outcomes of care for a client with anorexia nervosa. The client had been maintaining her weight for over a year at 110 pounds. She appears tired and weak during this visit to the health center. Her weight has dropped to 102 pounds. The nurse reviews the laboratory results below.

LABORATORY RESULTS

Test	Result
Hemoglobin	12.8 g/dl
Sodium	148 mEq/L
Potassium	2.5 mEq/L
Blood urea nitrogen	15 mg/dl

Which of the following interventions does the nurse perform first?

- □ 1. Notify the HCP about the potassium level.
- □ 2. Suggest the client increase iron in her diet.
- □ 3. Refer the client to a dietitian for diet planning with increased calories and protein.
- □ 4. Discuss with the client the consequences of using laxatives and diuretics.

62. A client with paranoid schizophrenia is admitted for observation. The client refuses to eat the food on the unit. The nurse should:

- □ 1. Prepare to insert a nasogastric feeding tube.
- □ 2. Call the physician for an order for total parenteral nutrition.
- □ 3. Have the client prepare food on the unit with the nurse.
- □ 4. Inform the client that the food is not poisoned here.

63. AF A client with paranoid schizophrenia is admitted to the inpatient unit after a failed suicide attempt. The nurse should do which of the following? List in order from first to last.

_____ 1. Question the patient about the method and plan for self-harm.
_____ 2. Complete the physician's admission orders.
_____ 3. Assign one staff member to be with the client at all times.
_____ 4. Assess the injuries the client has from the suicide attempt.

64. A client with a childhood trauma is experiencing dissociation. Which of the following questions is appropriate for the nurse to use to assess this client?

- □ 1. "Can you read the words in this book?"
- □ 2. "How are you feeling?"
- □ 3. "Do you feel your feet on the floor?"
- □ 4. "How many people are in this room?"

65. A client with schizophrenia is admitted to the inpatient psychiatric unit. The client states that he is experiencing hallucinations. Which of the following hallucinations is a priority for the nurse to report to the health care team?

- □ 1. Smelling another client's blood.
- □ 2. Sensations of bugs crawling on the skin.
- □ 3. Visualizing a frightening creature.
- □ 4. Hearing voices demanding the client to burn the left leg.

66. A client with anorexia nervosa is receiving the following medications. Which prescription would the nurse question for this client?

- □ 1. Fluoxetine (Prozac).
- □ 2. Acetaminophen (Tylenol).
- □ 3. Naproxen (Naprosyn).
- □ 4. Daily multivitamin.

67. AF A client who is withdrawing from alcohol is to have 1,000 ml of normal saline infused in 8 hr. Using an infusion set that has a drip factor of 15 gtt/min, how many drops per minute should the nurse infuse the normal saline?

______________ gtt/min.

68. AF The nurse is developing a care plan for a client with an anxiety disorder. The client describes a 10-pound weight loss in the last month. Outcomes that are appropriate for this client include which of the following? Select all that apply.

- □ 1. Client reports a decreased anxiety level.
- □ 2. Client develops a social system within home community.
- □ 3. Client demonstrates healthy methods of stress management.
- □ 4. Client expresses emotions in a nondestructive manner.
- □ 5. Client meets personal needs without infringing on others.
- □ 6. Client re-establishes an adequate nutritional intake.

69. A paranoid client is having a delusion. The nurse should:

- □ 1. Assist the client to relieve anxiety.
- □ 2. Ask the client why he or she feels this way.
- □ 3. Present reality when asked about the delusion.
- □ 4. Allow expressions of anger in appropriate ways.

70. A client is admitted to the inpatient psychiatric unit for cutting his wrists; his lacerations required several stitches, and he stated he did not remember cutting himself. The client is diagnosed with dissociative identity disorder. Which of the following is the priority short-term outcome for this client?

- □ 1. Client discusses what happened as a child when he became anxious.
- □ 2. Client develops an exercise program to deal with anxiety.
- □ 3. Client assumes decision-making role for personal health care needs.
- □ 4. Client notifies staff if he has the need for self-harm.

71. The nurse is developing a nutrition plan for a client with generalized anxiety disorder. The nurse should instruct the client to avoid which of the following?

- □ 1. Coffee, colas, energy drinks.
- □ 2. Salad greens, broccoli, zucchini.
- □ 3. Milk, cheese, yogurt.
- □ 4. Beans, lentils, Kashi.

72. A client with a histrionic personality disorder is admitted to a halfway house. What is an appropriate short-term goal for this client?

- □ 1. Client refrains from threatening others.
- □ 2. Client uses discussion as an alternative option to deal with anger.
- □ 3. Client recognizes patterns of isolating behavior.
- □ 4. Client responds to direction by staff without boundary violations.

73. A client with borderline personality disorder is admitted to the inpatient psychiatric unit for self-mutilation behaviors. Which of the following outcomes is the priority for this client?

- □ 1. Client describes a sense of control over intrusive thoughts.
- □ 2. Client constructs an exercise program.
- □ 3. Client refrains from self-mutilation.
- □ 4. Client demonstrates effective coping skills.

74. A client who is experiencing an anxiety disorder asks the nurse at the mental health clinic, "What will I do if I lose my job? I feel that I could lose it." What is the most therapeutic response by the nurse?

- □ 1. "I am sure things will be fine."
- □ 2. "What has happened that is worrying you?"
- □ 3. "You seem to be worrying about nothing."
- □ 4. "Maybe you should look for another job with greater security."

75. The physician prescribed lorazepam (Ativan) for a client in the outpatient clinic with an anxiety disorder. Which of the following statements by the client indicates that the nurse should give additional instruction?

- □ 1. "I can drive my truck route tonight."
- □ 2. "I need to avoid coffee for a while."
- □ 3. "If I want to stop this drug, I will contact my doctor."
- □ 4. "I will need to stay away from alcohol while I am on this medication."

Answers and Rationales

1. 3 Remaining with the client during a panic attack provides support, reassurance, and protection from harm. Relaxation techniques are ineffective at the panic level of anxiety; it is unlikely the client will be able to focus enough on feelings or music therapy for these interventions to be effective during a panic attack. (P)

2. 1 Cognitive theory examines the thinking processes of a client and his interpretation and perceptions related to those thoughts. Psychoanalysis focuses on the meaning that behaviors have. Maslow's hierarchy identifies that lower physiologic and emotional needs must be met to progress towards self-actualization. Interpersonal theory focuses on conflict in relationships. (P)

3. 2 A client taking an MAOI antidepressant is advised to report to the physician an increase in BP. Hypertensive crisis is the most serious adverse reaction of this class of medications. Fever and diarrhea are generally not side effects of this class of medications, but the nurse instructs the client to inform the HCP if they persist. Insomnia is a side effect but is not a priority at this time. (D)

4. 3, 2, 1, 4 The nurse first assesses the client receiving olanzapine (Zyprexa) with the fever and elevated BP; this client most likely has neuroleptic malignant syndrome, a potentially fatal syndrome, and requires close monitoring. The nurse then evaluates the client who is 7 months of age and receiving a nebulizer treatment; treatment indicates the child will most likely be discharged from the emergency department once this is completed. Next, the nurse assesses the woman who is 20 years of age and in premature labor for the progression of labor, and determines if the cervix is further dilated. Last, the nurse assesses the client with the ski injury for changes in vital signs and pain level. (M)

5. 2 Slowed thinking and difficulty concentrating make organizing simple tasks difficult for the severely depressed client. The nurse initiates tasks of daily living such as hygiene and eating as the client may be unable to complete even simple tasks due to intense feelings of despair, low self-worth, and fatigue. Waiting until trust has been established or for medications to take effect may result in a long gap of unmet personal needs. Coercing or threatening a client to complete desired activities is not appropriate. (C)

6. 2 A manic client often does not sleep and can be intrusive and agitated with others; therefore, the nurse assigns this client to a private room. A room near the nurse's station promotes closer observation of the client and monitoring of safety issues. Rooming with another client is likely to result in conflict because of high activity and impulsiveness. The nurse does not place the client in a room near an exit because of impulse behavior and concern for safety. (M)

7. 2 After assessing that the client is suicidal and has a plan, the nurse next assesses if the client has the means to commit suicide. Emotional effects of suicide on others are not a client priority at this point. Previous attempts increase the risk of suicide, but access to a viable way of committing the act now is more urgent. Asking the client about medicine does not focus on the immediate suicide threat. (R)

8. 1 Having the client in a quiet area will decrease external stimuli the client is dealing with; this allows for more of a sense of control and provides safety for the client and other clients on the unit. Competitive activities tend to increase the manic activity level. Certain limits may need to be given to the client to prevent self-harm and harm to others or their property. It is unlikely the client would be able to sit still long enough to play a quiet activity such as a card game or puzzle. (P)

9. 4 Group therapy can assist the client to improve interactions and emotional responses. Phototherapy is appropriate for seasonal affective depression. ECT is appropriate for major depression. Psychoanalysis is not appropriate for clients in a manic episode as they lack the ability to focus on personal insight. (P)

10. 1 There may be short-term memory loss after ECT, which resolves for most clients. Memory is not enhanced. There is no lingering lethargy after recovery from the anesthesia, and long-term memory is not affected. (R)

11. 4 The client in a manic episode needs to have boundaries and unit rules enforced, along with decreased stimuli. The nurse helps the client to maintain boundaries when interacting with others. Unlimited recreation will not aid the client in decreasing the expenditure of energy. It is unlikely the client will be able to participate in music therapy or express feelings in the acute phase. (M)

12. 1, 2, 4 The hospitalized client who is experiencing a depressive episode experiences sleep disturbance; loss of interest in activities of daily living, including appetite changes; guilt; decreased energy, concentration, and motor movement; and suicidal thoughts. Increased activity is seen in a manic episode. Hallucinations are associated with thought disorders such as schizophrenia. Extreme fear of specific objects or things is associated with phobias. (H)

13. 4 Foods with tyramine interact with MAOIs such as tranylcypromine and can cause hypertensive crisis. The nurse instructs the client to avoid foods that are processed, aged cheeses, wine and beer, and chocolate because of the level of tyramine in these foods. A low-fat diet is not necessary for this drug class. Increased food and fluids are appropriate for the anticholinergic effects of tricyclic antidepressants. Not all dairy products have tyramine. (D)

14. 4 Autistic children frequently show little emotion or response to contact with others. A normal toddler may play alone and quietly or want all of the toys to himself. Early language development is not related to autism. (H)

15. 3 Partially closing the door to decrease external stimuli is a noninvasive, quick intervention to aid with sleep disturbance. Other nonpharmacologic methods may also be tried before administering a medication. Moving the client to another room may be disruptive to other clients. Allowing the client to read decreases the amount of time available to sleep. (C)

16. 3 As a client improves on antidepressant medication, the risk for suicide increases as the client now has the energy to carry out a suicide plan. Tricyclics are cardiotoxic and can be lethal when an overdose is taken. Regular lab work is indicated for the mood stabilizer class of drugs. Diet restrictions are related to MAOIs. Antipsychotics more commonly require medications to manage side effects. (D)

17. 4 Maintenance serum level for lithium in most labs is 0.5 to 1.5 mEq/L. A level greater than 2.0 mEq/L is considered in the toxic range; the nurse provides close monitoring for this client and notifies the HCP. (R)

18. 2 The client is having Parkinson-like effects from taking haloperidol; the nurse notifies the HCP about the **S**ituation, provides **B**ackground information, reports the **A**ssessments, and makes a **R**ecommendation for additional medication (SBAR). Benztropine (Cogentin) will offset the Parkinson-like effect of the traditional antipsychotics such as haloperidol (Haldol). Giving additional haloperidol will only worsen the symptoms for the client. Propranolol is a beta blocker used for tremor and BP control; trazodone may have sedative side effects, but will not address the dopamine response this client is having. (D)

19. 3 Clients exhibiting ideas of reference personalize events and feel everything refers directly to them. Flight of ideas is exhibited by disconnected verbalization of thoughts and it is difficult to see a connection between each statement. Pressured speech refers to fast, disjointed, nonstop talking. Paranoia is exhibited when a client feels that he is being followed by others (usually an authority figure) or that others are out to harm him. (P)

20. 1, 3, 5 Positive symptoms of schizophrenia include delusions, hallucinations, ambivalence, flight of ideas, ideas of reference, and disordered thinking. Negative symptoms of schizophrenia include flat affect, ambivalence, anhedonia, apathy, and lack of volition or drive to take action. (P)

21. 4 An adverse effect of clozapine is agranulocytosis; it is important that the nurse emphasize the need to have regular lab work in order to monitor for this potential effect. Dietary restrictions are related to MAOI drugs. Measuring daily weight is not necessary. Sunscreen is important to use with antipsychotics. (D)

22. 3 The client is exhibiting signs of extrapyramidal symptoms (EPS), which is treated with diphenhydramine. Fluphenazine, haloperidol, and chlorpromazine can all cause the adverse effect of EPS, and additional medication from this class would worsen the symptoms. (D)

23. 3 As a benzodiazepine, lorazepam and alcohol are a very high-risk combination. The nurse determines the client's use of alcohol and instructs the client to avoid alcohol and alcohol products (e.g., cough syrup). Financial resources and family support are important for all clients, but do not specifically link to this drug class. Concerns about food are more linked with clients prescribed the MAOI drug class because of the risk of hypertensive crisis when ingested with tyramine. (D)

24. 3 Naltrexone blocks the effects of all opioids, which includes analgesics that may be needed in an emergency situation—a medic alert bracelet may be recommended. Drowsiness is not an expected side effect. Over-the-counter cough, cold, or antidiarrheal medications that contain opioids will have a decreased response when used with this medication. (D)

25. 99 pounds. 10% of 90 = 9. 90 + 9 = 99. (A)

26. 3 Needing an alcoholic drink first thing in the morning is a sign of withdrawal after a period of nonuse (sleep). A neurologic, anxiety, or personality disorder would be present throughout the day and would have additional symptoms if present. (H)

27. 3 La belle indifférence is manifested by a client's lack of concern over physical symptoms. Extreme concern over physical symptoms is related to hypochondriasis. Manipulation of staff is more associated with personality disorders. Delusions are associated with thought or mood disorders. (H)

28. 1 Primary gains are the direct external benefits from illness that a person receives, such as escape from an anxiety- or stress-producing situation. Secondary gains are internal benefits the person receives from being ill, such as attention from family or coworkers, and comfort measures such as a massage or special foods. (H)

29. 4 The anxious client has difficulty focusing and concentrating, so short, direct questions are better to gather information. Assessment data need to be gathered in order to plan interventions, and waiting to gather information may put the client at risk for harm. A current assessment is needed for current data, not data from a chart review. Open-ended questions are difficult for the anxious client to focus on, and are not used until the anxiety is better managed. (H)

30. 3 Growth suppression is a concern for children on stimulants, especially since the medication is prescribed throughout the growing years. Weight loss may occur related to stomach discomfort, causing the child to eat less. Insomnia can occur, but is managed by adjusting the time of the doses, and so does not have a lasting effect on the child. Memory loss is not seen with use of this class of medications. (D)

31. 4 The nurse monitors the activity of the client with anorexia nervosa who is losing weight while in treatment to assure that exercising or purging is not occurring until nutrients are absorbed. Some antidepressants used in anorexia (SSRIs) can cause a decrease in appetite; it is inappropriate to increase medications without knowing what medications the client is currently prescribed. Increasing caloric intake will not increase weight if the client does not retain the calories, or if she increases activity to compensate. Participation in a cooking group does not assure the intake of nutrients. (P)

32. 1, 3, 5 Beer, pepperoni, and cheddar cheese all contain tyramine related to yeast or aged meats and cheeses. The nurse instructs all clients taking MAOIs to avoid tyramine in order to reduce the risk of hypertensive crisis. The other foods are not restricted related to the use of this drug class. (D)

33. 3, 4, 6, 7 Common signs of ADHD include being easily distracted and forgetful, not waiting to take a turn, high activity levels and fidgeting, and interrupting others while talking. Because the child is still demonstrating these behaviors, the treatment plan is not yet effective. Being moody, sullen, or isolating self are indicative of depression in this age group. (A)

34. 3 With the depression lifted, the client may now have the energy to carry out suicide. This risk is present in all settings, not just in the community. Specific assessments are performed on depressed clients related to suicide ideation and plans, whether the client mentions suicide or not. (P)

35. 4 Understanding the rationale and anticipated results of medications increases the client's insight into the importance of adhering to the medication regimen. While support and previous success may help the client to be compliant, information about use and effects of the drug is more important to the client's likelihood of taking the drugs. The number of medications is not significant to compliance, but the nurse does determine if any other medications will have adverse interactions with the psychotropic drug. (D)

36. 2 Evaluation based on direct observation of objective patient data and the patient's subjective report is most accurate. Suggestions from staff and family members do not include input from the client. Group meetings with the client may be seen as threatening by the client, and accurate data may not be shared. (M)

37. 2, 3, 7 The nurse documents gait, grooming, and behavior as a part of the general appearance assessment. The nurse also assesses the client's level of orientation. Memory, hallucinations, and delusions are all part of the cognitive assessment of a client. Ability to understand treatment and accountability are part of insight assessment. Subjective feelings are included in the affect/mood assessment. Eye contact, speech, and psychomotor movement are part of the behavior assessment. (P)

38. 1, 2, 3, 5 The client who inhales toluene (from spray paint, correction fluid, glues, or paint thinner) may exhibit spray paint in the facial area and watery eyes; and have a loss of motor coordination, dilated pupils, and an increase in heart rate, respiratory rate, and BP. (A)

39. 3 The nurse requests an approved interpreter to assist in gathering medical information and explaining procedures. Clergy and family may gain information they need not know about the person, and may filter the interpretation through their own bias. A picture board and hand motions do not convey the needed information for a health history and development of a treatment plan. (M)

40. 2 The mental health client frequently carries social stigmas regarding how others will think and act towards him or her. A lack of insurance and loss of work may cause concern, but are not related to confidentiality. Visitors can be approved and given times that do not interfere with treatment. (P)

41. 3 The client with antisocial behaviors does not experience remorse for his or her behaviors; once admitted, this client usually returns to prehospitalization behaviors. The client does not continue therapy once out of the hospital environment. If this hospitalization was an alternative to a jail sentence, the client would not be assigned to another psychiatric facility. The client's lack of shame and guilt combined with a tendency to lie do not contribute to the option of becoming a productive citizen. (P)

42. 3 When the client takes nonbenzodiazepines such as buspirone (BuSpar), the client may develop postural hypotension; therefore, the nurse instructs the client to rise slowly from a sitting position. The nurse advises the client to be cautious when driving heavy machinery, and to take this medication with food. When SSRIs are taken, the client may experience a headache. (D)

43. 2 capsules. Two 3 mg/25 mg capsules is equivalent to 6 mg/50 mg. (D)

44. 3 It is important that the client with hyperactivity maintain admission weight and receive adequate nutrition. The client during the excited phase of catatonic type schizophrenia is susceptible to losing calories and fluid from constant movement. Providing finger foods (or foods the client can carry) may provide needed calories and fluids. Ultimately, the nurse can establish goals with the client to obtain adequate sleep, participate in social activities, and take care of self-grooming; the greatest risk during the excited phase is obtaining adequate nutrition. (P)

45. 1, 2, 3 Fatigue, increased appetite, suicidal ideation for several days, and depressive symptoms are associated with stimulant withdrawal. Sweating is more common with alcohol and cannabis withdrawal. Aching legs and back is associated with opioid withdrawal. (D)

46. 3 Safety for clients and staff is the priority concern for a client in a manic episode. Relaxation training is of little help at this stage of the illness; continuing to ask questions does not address the emergent safety concerns; medications may be a part of the treatment plan, but safety overrides the administration of medications. (S)

47. 1, 4 A client with a tendency to become angry and aggressive could become angry for several reasons, including anger at another client who is continually yelling on the unit, or if another client takes some of this client's personal belongings to his own room. Giving the client a snack would not precipitate a violent outburst. The nurse's assessing that the client was upset and clarifying the assessment with him would not precipitate an outburst. The client would not necessarily precipitate an aggressive episode. (P)

48. 4 The client who delays the aggressive responses until the later stages of the anger arousal is continuing to use the aggressive responses. The client who is aware of the feelings, behaviors, and the thoughts that occur prior to being angry is an indication that the anger management is effective. Another goal of anger management is for the client to gain an awareness of his behavioral and emotional anger responses. The anger-management classes have been effective when the client sees situations where he is aroused angrily as a problem calling for a solution. (P)

49. 1 Tyramine is contained in aged and processed foods, such as aged cheeses, meats, and yeast-containing foods and beverages, such as pepperoni pizza. Vegetables and cottage cheese (a fresh cheese) are safe to eat. Beer and beverages containing yeast should be avoided. (D)

50. 1, 3, 4, 5, 6 The nursing diagnoses for the client with an eating disorder include Disturbed Body Image, Anxiety, Imbalanced Nutrition: Less Than Body Requirements, Activity Intolerance, and Constipation. The client with a crisis has situational low self-esteem. The client with an eating disorder has a chronic low self-esteem. (P)

51. 2 When a client experiences a conversion disorder, such as paralysis, and demonstrates a lack of concern for the traumatic experience (such as being unable to walk), it is called la belle indifférence. Hypochondriasis occurs when the client is preoccupied with fears of having a medical condition. In body dysmorphic disorder the client is concerned with an imagined defect in appearance. In generalized anxiety disorder, the client is excessively worried or anxious for at least 6 months. (P)

52. 4 An example of behavior modification for the client with an eating disorder is to provide positive reinforcement for goals achieved such as telephone use for weight gain. Eating high-calorie, high-protein foods is not seen as positive by the client with an eating disorder. The client with an eating disorder will complete excessive exercise to keep weight off. Frequently, clients will elicit medication-seeking behaviors. (P)

53. 4 Repression is the inability to remember a traumatic event. It is a common defense mechanism used by clients with PTSD. Agoraphobia is the fear of having a panic attack when there is no easy way to escape. Dissociation occurs when the client demonstrates more that one personality or identity. Compulsions are repetitive behaviors that are performed in response to an obsessive thought. (P)

54. 2 The priority assessment of the client who has had multiple losses is assessment for suicidal thoughts. Assessing for use of antianxiety medications and present coping skills is important, but takes place after the suicidal assessment. Asking the client what her husband is doing for her is an assessment of coping, but could risk changing the subject and not being able to make the priority assessment of suicidal thoughts. (P)

55. 1 The nurse instructs the client taking clozapine (Clozaril) to contact the physician if he or she develops a sore throat as this may indicate a sign of infection. CBCs are drawn weekly for the first 6 weeks of treatment and then biweekly during the therapy. Clients taking clozapine frequently develop constipation. Taking antihistamines with clozapine may increase the anticholinergic properties of the antihistamines. (D)

56. 4 In milieu therapy, there is an emphasis on group and social interaction. Rules and expectations on the unit are mediated by peer pressure. Milieu therapy includes informal relationships with staff. In milieu therapy, there is an emphasis on interdisciplinary participation and goal-oriented, clear communications. (P)

57. 1 An appropriate short-term goal for the client with a borderline personality disorder is to be able to function within the therapeutic milieu. The client should also have a no self-harm contract and, as therapy progresses, demonstrate increasing problem-solving skills. The goal for a client with antisocial behavior is to identify methods to meet personal needs without infringing on the rights of others. Goals for a client who is chemically dependent include developing nondrug alternatives to managing stress. The goal for a client with an anxiety disorder is to experience a decrease in the level of anxiety. (P)

58. 3 Cognitive behavioral therapy is effective for treating anxiety disorders. The group identifies the target symptoms and examines the circumstances associated with the symptoms. The therapist and the client devise strategies to change the behaviors or the thoughts about the fears. Explaining the symptoms and treatment to the parents are not actively helping the child. No one can function in society by not touching door handles; thus, giving instructions to avoid all door handles and/or store items is unrealistic. Asking why can make the client defensive. (P)

59. 1 The client who experiences excessive worry is experiencing generalized anxiety disorder. The data presented do not give the impression that the client has had a traumatic event in the past that triggered the condition. With panic disorder, the client has a sudden onset of physical symptoms that are distressing to the client. With body dysmorphic disorder, the client is preoccupied with an imagined appearance defect. (P)

60. 4 The client with the multiple visits to the health care system is exhibiting health-seeking behaviors. The data do not support a knowledge deficit by the client or noncompliance with physician's orders. With the multiple visits to the emergency department, acute pain is not indicated with this client. (P)

61. 2 The client with a potassium level of 2.5 is at risk for cardiac consequences, including fatal arrhythmias, and may need to be hospitalized for an infusion of IV potassium. The elevated sodium level is most likely due to dehydration, and the hemoglobin level could also be due to dehydration. After the client receives parenteral fluids, other electrolytes and hemoglobin will be balanced.

Referring the client to a dietitian or discussing the consequences of using laxatives and diuretics is a later nursing intervention, but not a priority at this time. (A)

62. 3 Allowing clients to prepare food with the nurse or other staff on the unit allows the client to make choices and see the food. Preparing to insert an NG tube may seem like a threat to the client, resulting in further paranoia and distrust. TPN is not appropriate for the client, and the statement that the food is not poisoned communicates that the nurse does not believe the client's delusions. (P)

63. 4, 1, 3, 2 The nurse first assesses the injuries from the suicide attempt to prevent possible disruption of vital functions. The nurse then assesses the client's plans for self-harm. The third intervention is a 1:1 assignment if the client remains suicidal (as the nurse has been with the client since he arrived on the unit). While completing the physician's admission orders (immediate orders and documentation) is very important, this task is performed when all of the client's care is stabilized. (M)

64. 3 The nurse should ask the client who is experiencing dissociation questions regarding what is experienced through the senses. Questions such as, "What are you feeling?"; "Do you feel your feet on the floor?"; and "What are you touching?" are questions about feeling. The questions, "How are you feeling?"; Can you read?"; or asking the client to count people do not pertain to the client's senses and will not help the nurse assess the extent of the dissociation. (P)

65. 4 The nurse shares with the health care team the presence of a command hallucination, which is a voice demanding the client to take an action to perform self-harm. The tactile hallucination of feeling bugs crawling on the skin, and hallucination of seeing frightening creatures are very annoying to the client, but are not the priority. Smelling another person's blood is also very uncomfortable for the client, but is not as dangerous as a command hallucination. (S)

66. 1 Fluoxetine (Prozac) can cause weight loss and decreased appetite. Acetaminophen, naproxen, and multivitamins are not contraindicated in this client. (D)

67. 1,000 ml/8 hr = 125 ml/hr.
125 ml/60 min ×15 gtt/1 ml = 31 gtt/min. (D)

68. 1, 2, 3, 4, 6 The goals for the client with an anxiety disorder are to report a decreased level of anxiety, develop a social system within his or her home community, and demonstrate healthy methods of stress management. The client with an anxiety disorder is also expected to express emotions in a nondestructive manner and to re-establish an adequate nutritional intake. A goal for the antisocial personality disorder client is to meet his or her personal needs without infringing on the rights of others. (P)

69. 3 When a client asks the nurse about the delusion, the nurse presents reality and reinforces the client that he or she does not hear the voice or other delusion. The paranoid client is delusional related to anxiety, but is not able to manage the anxiety at this moment. Allowing expressions of anger may be harmful to the client or others. The nurse avoids "why" questions as these may cause the client to become defensive. (P)

70. 4 The priority outcome for the client with dissociative identity disorder who does not remember cutting himself is to inform the staff when he feels an urge to cause self-harm. Discussing anxiety-provoking activities from his childhood, developing an exercise program for anxiety reduction, and assuming the decision-making role for personal health care needs are not priorities at this time. (P)

71. 1 The client with generalized anxiety disorder is instructed to avoid foods containing caffeine and nicotine such as coffee, colas, and caffeinated energy drinks. Fruits, beans and grains, vegetables, and milk products will not affect the client with anxiety. (H)

72. 4 The client with histrionic personality disorder often displays poor boundaries with the staff; an appropriate short-term goal for this client is for him or her to respond to redirection by the staff. A client with antisocial personality disorder will threaten other clients, and responds to a goal of how to deal with anger. A client with antisocial personality disorder may need a goal to use interactions with staff to discuss alternative options to deal with anger. Clients with schizoid personality disorder will isolate themselves and may need to work on a goal to recognize isolating behaviors. (P)

73. 3 A priority goal for the client with borderline personality disorder is to refrain from self-mutilation. A goal for the client with anxiety disorder is to construct an exercise program and demonstrate effective coping skills. The client with obsessive-compulsive disorder has intrusive thoughts. (P)

74. 2 The nurses asks a question regarding what happened that is worrying the client in order to elicit the most comments from the client. The nurse's comments are caring and questions are open-ended. The nurse does not promote certainty that things will turn out fine for the client; this response is not therapeutic and does not elicit any further dialogue from the client. Telling the client that she is worrying about nothing gives the client the impression that her concerns are not important to the nurse. Telling the client to look for another job is giving advice and is not therapeutic. (P)

75. 1 When a client receives a benzodiazepine such as Ativan, he or she must be careful with driving heavy machinery. The client is instructed to avoid caffeinated foods and beverages, avoid stopping these drugs abruptly, and to avoid alcohol and other CNS depressants while on these drugs. (D)

SECTION 5

Management of Care

chapter 40

Managing Client Care Delivery

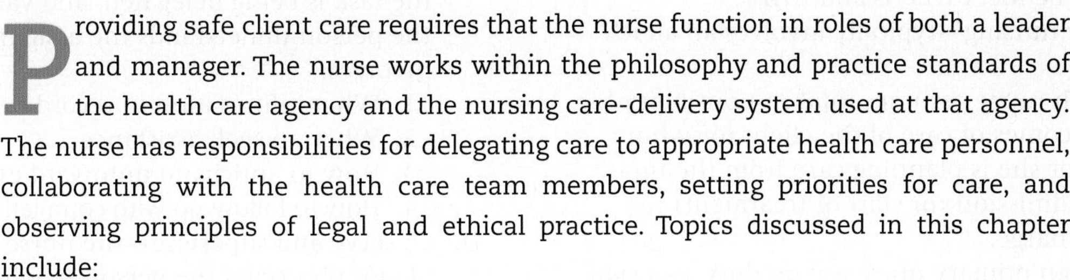

Providing safe client care requires that the nurse function in roles of both a leader and manager. The nurse works within the philosophy and practice standards of the health care agency and the nursing care-delivery system used at that agency. The nurse has responsibilities for delegating care to appropriate health care personnel, collaborating with the health care team members, setting priorities for care, and observing principles of legal and ethical practice. Topics discussed in this chapter include:

- Nursing Care Delivery Systems
- Delegation
- Setting Priorities for Care
- Ethical and Legal Implications for Managing Client Care

Nursing Care Delivery Systems

I. Definition: Nursing care is organized and delivered in a variety of ways. The type of delivery system used depends on the mission, philosophy, and preference of the health care institution, needs of client, intended outcomes of care, and qualifications and availability of staff.

II. Types of care delivery systems: The most common modes of delivering client care are team nursing, primary nursing, and functional nursing. Other types include total client care and case management. Care delivery systems may also be a combination of any of these, or designed uniquely to serve a particular group of clients or setting.

   A. Team nursing—led by RN; team members may include other RNs, LPNs, or UAP.
      1. Each team member works within his or her scope of practice and is accountable to the team and client for the outcomes of care. Working as a team requires coordination and collaboration as well as trust and respect.
      2. Team coordinates care with other health professionals such as respiratory therapists, physical therapists, occupational therapists, and home health personnel.
      3. Used when level of care required by client can be met by LPNs and UAPs.
   B. Primary nursing—typically involves an all RN staff.
      1. Each nurse assumes total responsibility for outcomes of care of the client for whom he or she is planning care from the time of admission (or start of treatment) to discharge.
      2. When primary nurse not on duty, associate nurses adhere to care plan developed by the primary nurse.
      3. Often used in intensive care units where care planning decisions are frequent and require the skill level of an RN.
   C. Functional nursing—an RN plans care to be delivered by staff.
      1. Care delegated according to education and skill level (see also guidelines for delegation).
         a. UAP bathes client.
         b. LPN administers medication.
         c. IV nurse starts and maintains all IV infusions.
      2. Personnel assigned to complete tasks rather than provide care for specific client.
      3. Used when a client requires care from health care personnel with specialized skills; for example, stoma specialist or diabetic educator. Often used in combination with team nursing or primary care.

Delegation

I. Definition: In order to achieve organizational goals, RN assigns selected nursing tasks and responsibilities to others as appropriate to education, training, and competency level.

II. Delegation process

   A. Assess—involves identifying the most qualified person(s) based on client needs, and official job description expectations within the agency and within the state nurse practice act (see principles of delegation). Capabilities of the person to whom the assignment is to be delegated is determined by:
      1. Observing personnel.
      2. Using checklists to identify strengths and limitations.
      3. Using competency assessment systems that document competency for all personnel.
   B. Plan—effective planning ahead takes into account:
      1. Client needs and expected outcomes.
      2. Available resources.
      3. Time frame for implementation.
   C. Communicate—the nurse provides clear directions and information to the person to whom the task is being delegated, and validates that the person understands the assignment. This involves:
      1. What information to record or report.
      2. When to seek assistance.
      3. How to anticipate untoward events.
      4. How to follow up with completion of the task.
   D. Observe and supervise—the nurse is responsible for observing the person to whom the task has been delegated, and supervising and guiding the implementation of the task as needed. Once assured that the person to whom the task has been delegated is capable, the nurse also empowers the team member and promotes autonomy within the scope of practice.
   E. Evaluate—the nurse must evaluate the completion of the delegated task and the outcome or result of client care. Evaluation requires that the nurse:
      1. Provide both positive and corrective feedback to the person to whom the task has been delegated.
      2. Follow up on care that is not in accordance with policy or standards of care.

III. Principles of delegation

   A. RN is responsible for the assessment, planning, implementation, and evaluation of nursing care. The nurse may delegate any of the components of the nursing process, but not the process itself.

B. RN must observe the six rights of delegation: (1) The right task, (2) at the right time, (3) under the right circumstances, (4) with the right directions and information, (5) under the right supervision, and (6) with the right follow-up and evaluation.

C. RN must delegate tasks to others only if they have the knowledge and skill to carry out the task.

D. RN must promote two-way communication—the person to whom the task is being delegated must have an opportunity to seek clarification, confirm understanding of the task, and report client outcomes to the RN.

E. RN must make decisions about delegation based on:
   1. Client needs.
   2. Competence of the person to whom the task is being delegated.
   3. Nature of the supervision required to complete the task.
   4. Policies and procedures of the health care institution, state nurse practice acts, and state boards of nursing—these govern what can be delegated and to whom.

F. RN must acknowledge individual as well as institutional accountability for delegation.
   1. Institution accountable for providing sufficient staffing and staff mix; as well as hiring, training, and developing competent staff.
   2. Nurse accountable for client care and outcomes when nursing tasks are delegated; if the nurse determines that client safety is in jeopardy by delegating a task, the nurse should not delegate the task.

IV. Guidelines for delegation

A. The nurse must be familiar with agency policy, but in general, the following can be delegated:
   1. LPN—dressing changes, urinary catheterization, administration of medications, and suctioning.
   2. UAP—skin care, bath and hygiene, transfers to bed or wheelchair, use of assistive devices, transportation, range of motion exercises, ambulation, and offering food (feeding as needed) and oral fluids.

B. The following can be delegated to another RN:
   1. Assessment, planning, implementation, and evaluation of care.
   2. Complex skills such as starting IVs and interpreting ECGs.
   3. Client teaching and staff education; serving as a client advocate.
   4. Communication with health care providers and other health team members and families when information requires nursing judgment.
   5. Other nursing activities within the scope of practice or requiring specialized training.

Setting Priorities for Care

I. Definition: Determines tasks to be accomplished and places in order of importance in order to provide safe and effective health care.

A. Involves determining the order in which clients are provided care, and which nursing actions for a client should be performed immediately.

B. Developed, when possible, in collaboration with the client and family.

II. Principles for setting priorities

A. In emergency situations, use principles of triage (see Chapter 42): airway, breathing, circulation, and disabilities.

B. In less emergent situations, use Maslow's hierarchy of needs to set priorities: physiologic needs; safety, love/belonging, self-esteem, and self-actualization.

C. Consider resources of time and equipment when setting priorities.

D. Set priorities based on nursing activities that have time requirements such as administering medications on a schedule or changing IV infusions.

E. Address actual and short-term needs prior to managing potential and long-term needs.

Ethical and Legal Implications for Managing Client Care

I. Definition: Clients are protected by various laws and ethical responsibilities that also affect all health care providers (HCPs). The nurse serves in the role of an advocate to speak on behalf of the client and protects the client's right to make decisions.

Basic Concepts of Ethics

I. Definition: *Ethics* is the branch of philosophy concerned with the distinction between right and wrong based on a body of knowledge, and not solely on opinions. Ethics take into account a person's morals and value system. *Note: A nurse's religious or personal preference may allow refusal to assist in surgeries where a "dilatation, evacuation" is performed.*

A. *Ethical principles* are codes that direct or govern nursing actions:
   1. *Autonomy*—respect for client's right to self-determination.

2. *Nonmaleficence*—obligation to do or cause no harm to another.
3. *Beneficence*—duty to do good to others and to maintain a balance between benefits and harms.
4. *Justice*—the equitable distribution of potential benefits and tasks; determining the order in which clients are provided care.
5. *Veracity*—the obligation to tell the truth.
6. *Fidelity*—the duty to do what one has promised.

B. *Ethical codes*—provide broad principles for determining and evaluating client care; ethical codes are not legally binding, but in most states the board of nursing has authority to reprimand nurses for unprofessional conduct that results from violation of ethical codes.
1. Code for Nurses—developed by International Council of Nurses
2. American Nurses Association Code of Ethics

C. *Ethical dilemma*—occurs when there is conflict between two or more ethical principles; no correct decision exists; may occur as result of differences in cultural or religious beliefs.

D. *Ethical reasoning*—process of thinking through what one ought to do in an orderly and systematic manner.

E. *Morality* is behavior in accordance with customs or traditions usually reflecting personal or religious beliefs.

F. *Values* are beliefs and attitudes that may influence behavior and the process of decision-making.

G. *Values clarification* is the process of analyzing one's own values to understand better what is truly important.

Basic Legal Implications and Documents

I. Definition: Law and legislation protect both the client and nurse in terms of scope of acceptable practice and individual client rights.

II. Regulation of nursing practice

A. The Nurse Practice Act is a series of statutes enacted by each state legislature to regulate practice of nursing in that state. The act also addresses licensure requirements for protection of the public.
1. Setting educational requirements for nurses
2. Distinguishing between nursing and medical practice
3. Defining the scope of nursing practice

B. Standards of care
1. Legal concept that describes professional behavior for nurses. Nurses' performance compared to competent nurse in same specialty practicing in a similar situation.
2. Sources of standards of care
   a. State Nursing Practice Acts
   b. American Nurses Association
   c. Healthcare Accrediting Agencies
   d. Nursing Specialty Organizations
   e. Case law
   f. Textbooks, journals
   g. Health care agency policies and procedures

C. Employee guidelines
1. Respondent superior—employer held liable for any negligent acts of employee if occurred during employment relationship.
2. Contracts—employee responsible for carrying out terms of contractual agreement. Nurse-employee relationship governed by established employee handbooks, and client care policies and procedures that create obligations, rights, and duties between parties.
3. Institutional policies—policies detail how nurses are to perform their duties (policies are not laws).

D. Floating
1. Nurses in floating situation do not assume responsibility beyond their level of experience or qualification.
2. Nurses required to inform supervisor of any lack of experience in caring for type of clients in area outside level of experience or qualification.

III. Legal risk areas

A. Assault—occurs when a person puts another person in fear of harmful or offensive contact. Involves victim fearing or believing that threat will result in harm.

B. Battery—intentional touching of another's body without consent.

C. Invasion of privacy refers to any of the following:
1. Violating confidentiality
2. Intruding on private matters
3. Sharing client information with unauthorized persons

D. False imprisonment—occurs when restraining devices are used without appropriate clinical need.
1. Use of restraints requires an order from the health care provider indicating type of restraint and time limits for use.
2. Clients or family members must give permission for restraint use.
3. The least restrictive restraint should be used.
4. Restraints must be removed regularly to prevent pressure and to provide care.

5. Use of restraints for managing behavioral emergencies is used when less restrictive measures have failed and the client or others is or will be in danger.
6. Chemical restraints are controversial and there is a fine line between using drugs as treatment and using drugs to control behavior.

E. Malpractice—performance of care below the standard of care by a professional, resulting in injury to the client.

F. Negligence—commitment of an act that a reasonable person would not have done, or omission of a duty a reasonable person would have performed.

G. Defamation of character—any untrue communication to another, written (libel) or spoken (slander), that brings injury or damage of the reputation of another person.

H. Respondeat superior—acts of employees are attributable to employer, who will also be held responsible for injury to a client.

IV. Client rights

A. Written document reflecting client's right to participate in health care with emphasis on client autonomy.

B. Some client rights include:
1. Right to considerate and respectful care
2. Right to know names, roles of persons involved in care
3. Right to consent or refuse treatment
4. Right to privacy
5. Right to expect that hospital will provide necessary health services

V. Organ donation and transplantation

A. Client has right to decide to become organ donor or refuse organ transplant as treatment option.

B. Criteria
1. Uniform Anatomical Gift Act—lists who can provide informed consent for donation of deceased client's organs.
2. United Network for Organ Sharing—sets criteria for organ donations.

C. Religious beliefs
1. Catholic Church—views organ transplantation as acceptable.
2. Orthodox Church—discourages organ transplantation.
3. Islam (Muslim)—discourages organ transplantation and removal of body parts.
4. Jehovah's Witness—organ transplant may be accepted, but organ must be cleansed with nonblood solution before transplantation.
5. Orthodox Judaism—all body parts removed during autopsy must be buried with body because it is believed that entire body must be returned to earth. Organ transplantation may be allowed with rabbi's approval.
6. Gypsies and Shintos—forbid followers to donate or receive organ(s).

VI. Informed consent

A. Consents and releases are legal documents that indicate client's permission (or that of client's legal representative) to perform surgery, perform a treatment, or give information to third party.
1. In most states, when nurse is involved in informed consent process, the nurse is only witnessing the signature of client on informed consent form and is not responsible for explaining the procedure or assuring the client understands.
2. Client is informed by the surgeon in understandable terms of:
   a. Risks and benefits of surgery or procedure.
   b. Consequences for not receiving surgery or procedure.
   c. Alternative options.
   d. Name of physician performing surgery or procedure.
3. Client's questions about surgery or procedure must be answered before signing consent.
4. Consent must be signed freely by client without threat or pressure, and must be witnessed by another adult.
5. Legally, client must be mentally, emotionally competent to give consent. Client who has been medicated with sedating medications or any other medications that may affect cognitive abilities cannot be asked to sign consent.
6. Client may withdraw consent at any time before the procedure (withdrawal may be written or verbal).

B. Type of consents
1. Surgical consent
   a. Obtained for all surgical/invasive procedures and diagnostic tests.
   b. Physician, surgeon, or anesthesiologist who performs operative or other procedure is responsible for explaining procedure, its risks and benefits, and possible alternative options.
2. Special consents—required for use of restraints, photographing the client, the disposal of body parts during surgery, donating organs after death, or performing an autopsy.

C. Exceptions
1. Minors—client under legal age (as defined by state statute) may not give legal consent; consent is obtained from parent or legal guardian.

2. Emancipated minor has established independence from parents through marriage, pregnancy, service in armed forces, or by court order; is considered legally capable of signing an informed consent.
3. Life-threatening emergencies.

VII. Health Insurance Portability and Accountability Act (1997)

A. Describes how personal health information may be used. Personal health information includes:
   1. Individually identifiable information that is related to client's past, present, or future health.
   2. Treatment.
   3. Payment for health care services.

B. Describes how client can obtain access to the information.

VIII. Incident reports

A. Incident reports record unusual or unexpected incidents as a means of identifying risk situations and improving client care. Incidents may include:
   1. Accidental omission of ordered therapies.
   2. Circumstances that led to injury/risk for client injury.
   3. Client falls.
   4. Medication administration errors.
   5. Needlestick injuries.
   6. Procedure-/equipment-related accidents.
   7. Visitor having symptoms of illness or sustaining an injury.

B. Incidents must be documented and the reports retained according to agency policy and procedure.
   1. Report form is not copied or placed in client's record.
   2. Report form is not referenced in client's record.

IX. Legal Implications of client and family teaching

A. Provide complete instruction in language that client/family can understand.

B. Document teaching, what was taught, evaluation of understanding, and who was present during teaching.

C. Inform client what would happen if information shared during teaching is not followed.

X. End-of-life issues

A. Patient Self-Determination Act (1990)—states clients must be provided with information about their rights to identify written directions about care they wish to receive in event they become incapacitated and are unable to make health care decisions.

B. Advance directives are written documents recognized by state law; these provide directions concerning provision of care when client is unable to make own treatment choices, may include health care proxy who will make health care decisions in the event of client's incapacitation. Types of advanced directives include:
   1. Living will—specifies client's wishes for health care treatment, including the use of surgical procedures and use of resuscitation, should the client be unable to so direct.
   2. Do-not-resuscitate (DNR) orders—written order by physician, following client's and family's wishes to limit extraordinary measures (such as CPR, drugs, intubation) when client has indicated desire to be allowed to die if stops breathing or heart stops beating.
      a. Client or legal representative must provide informed consent for do-not-resuscitate status.
      b. Do-not-resuscitate order must be defined clearly so that other treatment not refused by client will be continued.
      c. Physicians, nurses, and other health care personnel cannot witness the client's informed consent for DNR.
      d. Nurse who attempts to resuscitate when do-not-resuscitate order exists would be acting without client's consent and committing battery.
   3. Durable medical power of attorney is a document signed by the client designating a person to make health care decisions on the client's behalf should the client be unable to make such decisions.

C. Nurse's role in end-of-life documentation—the nurse follows agency policy addressing witnessing legal documents, and ensures completion and documentation of the following:
   1. Client is provided with information about right to identify written directions about care client wishes to receive.
   2. If advance directive exists, it is part of medical record.
   3. Physician is notified of presence of advance directive.
   4. Directions of advance directive are followed by all members of health care team.

Bibliography

Documentation in action. Ambler, PA: Springhouse.

Ellis, J., & Hartley, C. (2007). *Nursing in today's world*. Philadelphia: Lippincott Williams & Wilkins.

Grossman, V. (2003). *Quick reference to triage.* Philadelphia: Lippincott Williams & Wilkins.

Hood, L., & Pepper, S. (2005). *Leddy and Pepper's conceptual bases of professional nursing.* Philadelphia: Lippincott Williams & Wilkins.

Marquis, B., & Huston, C. (2005). *Leadership roles and management functions.* Philadelphia: Lippincott Williams & Wilkins.

National Council of State Boards of Nursing and American Nurses Association Joint Statement on Nursing Delegation. Retrieved June 6, 2008 from http://ana.org/pressrel/2006/PRjoint_NCSBN-ANA_j092606.pdf

Nurses legal handbook. Philadelphia, Lippincott Williams & Wilkins.

CHAPTER 40

Practice Test

Nursing Care Delivery Systems

1. A nurse is considering employment on a nursing care unit that uses a primary care nursing care delivery system. The nurse should understand that she or he will be working in a situation in which:

□ 1. There will be a team of RNs and LPNs delivering care.
□ 2. The RN will be assigned a specific task such as starting IV infusions to perform for all clients.
□ 3. There will be a UAP available to whom the nurse can delegate selected nursing activities.
□ 4. The staffing model will consist of RNs who will implement nursing care and evaluate outcomes for assigned clients.

2. A nurse is planning staffing for a nursing unit in which the primary need of the clients is for learning how to manage their health problem. Which of the following would be the ideal mix of staff for this unit?

□ 1. Three RNs.
□ 2. One RN and two LPNs.
□ 3. One LPN and two UAPs.
□ 4. One RN, one LPN, and one UAP.

Delegation

3. Which of the following activities would be appropriate to delegate to an unlicensed assistant for a client with coronary artery disease who is now free of chest pain?

□ 1. Assist client with identifying risk factors for CAD.
□ 2. Provide teaching on a low-fat diet to the client.
□ 3. Assess if the client's urine output is sufficient.
□ 4. Record the client's fluid intake during the shift.

4. Which client should the nurse assign to an unlicensed assistant?

□ 1. Client having a bronchoscopy performed at the bedside.
□ 2. Client who had a pneumonectomy without a chest tube yesterday.
□ 3. Client newly diagnosed with lung cancer receiving chemotherapy.
□ 4. Client who requires assistance with activity 4 days after a pulmonary wedge resection.

5. When taking a client's vital signs on the first postoperative day, the UAP reports to the nurse that the oral temperature is 100°F. The nurse should delegate which of the following to the UAP?

□ 1. Apply an ice cap to a client's forehead.
□ 2. Bathe the client with cool water.
□ 3. Place a hyperthermia blanket on the client's bed.
□ 4. Do nothing now, but continue to monitor a client's temperature.

6. AF A nurse is working with an unlicensed assistant. Which of the following clients should the nurse assign to the UAP? Select all that apply.

□ 1. Adult client newly diagnosed with diabetes who is learning to administer insulin.
□ 2. Older adult client who had hip replacement surgery and needs to walk in the hall with a walker.
□ 3. Adult client who had abdominal surgery yesterday and requires a dressing change.
□ 4. Young adult client who requires tube feedings.
□ 5. Adult client who had a hysterectomy 3 days ago and requires vital sign checks every 4 hr.

7. The UAP reports to the nurse that a newly diagnosed client with type 1 diabetes mellitus has a fingerstick blood sugar (FSBS) of 483 dl/ml. The nurse should first:

- □ 1. Assess the client.
- □ 2. Repeat the procedure.
- □ 3. Notify the HCP.
- □ 4. Ask the UAP to repeat the procedure.

8. Which of the following should the nurse delegate to the UAP when caring for a client with Guillain-Barré syndrome?

- □ 1. Assess weakness with range of motion exercises.
- □ 2. Reposition client every 2 hr.
- □ 3. Suction the endotracheal tube.
- □ 4. Show the client how to do deep-breathing exercises.

9. The nurse should instruct the UAP to allot more time for which of the following clients?

- □ 1. Client with calcium (Ca++) per IV infusion.
- □ 2. Client with albumin per IV infusion.
- □ 3. Client with sodium (Na) free per IV infusion.
- □ 4. Client with TPN via a central line.

Setting Priorities for Care

10. Which of the following clients should be seen by the nurse first? A client with:

- □ 1. Inguinal hernia repair having incisional pain.
- □ 2. Diabetes insipidus with hyponatremia.
- □ 3. A thyroidectomy with a heart rate of 112 beats/min.
- □ 4. Acromegaly with a history of heart failure.

11. The home health nurse should schedule the first appointment with which of the following clients?

- □ 1. Client recently diagnosed with psoriasis.
- □ 2. Client recently diagnosed with lung cancer.
- □ 3. Client recently diagnosed with tuberculosis.
- □ 4. Client discharged after a vaginal hysterectomy.

12. AF A nurse is caring for the following group of clients. After receiving shift report, the nurse should make rounds on the clients in which of the following order? Place in order of the highest to lowest priority.

_____ 1. Female client who is 34 years of age and just returning from the recovery room following an abdominal hysterectomy; IV running at 50 drops per minute with 100 ml remaining.

_____ 2. Client who is 50 years of age and diagnosed with diabetes mellitus 3 days ago who is learning to administer insulin.

_____ 3. Client who is 75 years of age with a fractured hip of 4 days who needs to be turned frequently.

_____ 4. Client who is 79 years of age 2 days postsurgery for removal of cancer of the colon who has had a tracheotomy for 4 years.

13. AF A client is brought to the emergency department with myasthenia crisis. The nurse should do which of the following in priority order? Place in order from first to last.

_____ 1. Check if the client missed a dose of medication.

_____ 2. Assess the client for signs of infection.

_____ 3. Check the gag reflex.

_____ 4. Prepare for intubation.

14. Four hospitalized clients have hypokalemia. Which client should the nurse see first?

- □ 1. Client with tachycardia and cirrhosis.
- □ 2. Client with inverted P wave and polyuria.
- □ 3. Client with decreased GI motility and increased thirst.
- □ 4. Client with type 2 diabetes mellitus and taking digoxin (Lanoxin).

15. A nurse who normally works with clients with heart disease is assigned to take care of a client who is receiving chemotherapy. Prior to taking care of the client, the nurse plans to review the standard of care for this client. Which of the following is the most appropriate source for standards of care in this situation?

- □ 1. Oncology Nursing Society.
- □ 2. American Nurses Association.
- □ 3. Hospital accreditation manual.
- □ 4. Agency policy and procedure manual.

16. A home health nurse is establishing priorities for home visits to a group of clients. Which one of the following clients can be seen later on in the week?

- □ 1. Client recently diagnosed with terminal cancer with metastasis to the brain.
- □ 2. Female client recently diagnosed with human immunodeficiency virus (HIV).
- □ 3. Client who is to demonstrate the ability to perform an insulin injection.
- □ 4. Client with acquired immune deficiency syndrome (AIDS) with CD4+ less than 200 cells/mm^2.

Ethical and Legal Implications for Managing Client Care

17. A client recently diagnosed with type 1 diabetes refuses to accept the diagnosis. The nurse should do which of the following?

- □ 1. Explain why the client has an ulcer on his leg.
- □ 2. Listen while the client continues to find reasons why the diagnosis is incorrect.
- □ 3. Give the client learning materials focusing on management of type 1 diabetes mellitus.
- □ 4. Review serum BUN and creatinine, and the BUN and creatinine ratio, to show the client the seriousness of the disease.

18. A client is scheduled for surgery. He is confused and shows signs of dementia. The nurse should ask which of the following persons to sign the consent for the client?

- □ 1. Minister.
- □ 2. Nursing supervisor.
- □ 3. Attorney.
- □ 4. Spouse.

19. A charge nurse asks a newly graduated RN who normally works on a medical-surgical nursing unit to take care of two clients in the coronary care unit. The nurse has not had experience with taking care of clients on monitors or using the medications that these clients are taking. The new nurse should do which of the following?

- □ 1. Accept the assignment and ask the nurses in the coronary care unit to administer the medications for these clients.
- □ 2. Explain to the charge nurse about his or her level of experience and express concerns about this assignment.
- □ 3. Tell the charge nurse that the assignment was to the medical-surgical unit and refuse to go to the coronary care unit.
- □ 4. Ask the charge nurse if the assignment can be reduced to taking care of one client.

20. A hospitalized client with end-stage heart failure has indicated that he does not want to be resuscitated. The physician has written the do-not-resuscitate (DNR) order on the chart. The client has a cardiac arrest, and the wife tells the nurse she wants the client to be resuscitated, and asks the nurse to "do something." The nurse should:

- □ 1. Begin CPR.
- □ 2. Call a "code."
- □ 3. Page the physician.
- □ 4. Assist the wife to manage her grief.

Answers and Rationales

1. 4 In primary nursing, the clients are cared for by RNs who assess, plan, implement, and evaluate nursing care for the clients to whom the nurse is assigned. Team nursing involves a team of RNs and others such as LPNs and UAP; the RN will delegate nursing care activities to others within the scope of their practice. Functional nursing involves assigning task(s) to one person who performs the task for all clients. (M)

2. 1 The ideal staffing for a nursing unit focused on client teaching and learning is to have three registered nurses. It is within the scope of practice for the RN to assess, plan, implement, coordinate, and evaluate client learning. It is not within the scope of practice for LPNs and UAP to provide client teaching. (M)

3. 4 UAPs are able to measure and record intake and output. The nurse is responsible for client teaching and evaluating the data collected about the client. (M)

4. 4 The nurse assigns the unlicensed assistant to the client who requires assistance with activity. The client undergoing a bronchoscopy requires interventions to be performed by the nurse, such as medications and monitoring. A client with a pneumonectomy on the first postoperative day requires close monitoring by the nurse. The client receiving chemotherapy will require assessment and intervention that can only be done by a nurse. (M)

5. 4 Temperature variation in the postoperative period provides valuable information about a client's status. Fever may occur at any time during the postoperative period. A mild elevation (up to 100.4°F) during the first 48 hr usually reflects the surgical stress response. After the first 48 hr, a moderate to marked elevation (higher than 99.9°F) is usually caused by infection. It is not appropriate to do any of the other options to lower a client's temperature at this time. (M)

6. 2, 5 The UAP can assist clients ambulate and take vital signs. It is within the RN scope of practice to teach the client to administer insulin, change dressings, and administer tube feedings. (M)

7. 2 When the nurse delegates tasks to others, the nurse must follow up and evaluate the accurate completion of the task. Since treatment decisions will be based on information about the fingerstick blood sugar, the nurse repeats the procedure to confirm the finding. The nurse also gathers additional information about the health status of the client prior to contacting the HCP. (M)

8. 2 Assessments, teaching, and suctioning are roles of the nurse. Basic care with frequent positioning is the most appropriate to delegate to the UAP. (M)

9. 1 Administration of calcium IV can be life-threatening and could result in postural hypotension and seizures. The BP is measured frequently, the client is kept on bed rest, and seizure precautions are placed. Administration of albumin, sodium-free solutions, and TPN do not place the client at the same risk. (M)

10. 3 Because the client with a thyroidectomy may be experiencing a thyroid storm or thyroid crisis, which can be immediately life-threatening, the nurse sees this client first. There is no evidence that the clients with incisional pain, hyponatremia, and heart failure are experiencing potential emergencies. (M)

11. 3 Tuberculosis places the community and family members at risk. The nurse needs to assure the client is taking medications appropriately. Psoriasis poses no specific risks. Recent diagnosis of lung cancer can cause significant emotional disturbance, but not necessarily physical risks. (M)

12. 1, 4, 3, 2 The nurse establishes priorities based on airway, breathing, circulation, and disability as well as immediacy of client needs. The client who is just returning from surgery needs to be assessed; the nurse will also need to check the IV. The client with cancer of the colon also needs to have vital signs, pain, and dressings checked; the tracheotomy is established, and in the report there was no mention of distress. The client with the fractured hip is at risk for pressure ulcers and should be seen next. The nurse should then make rounds on the client with diabetes and schedule the time to continue teaching injection technique at that time. (M)

13. 4, 3, 2, 1 Clients with myasthenia crisis have severe muscle weakness that may result in respiratory failure requiring mechanical ventilation. The nurse's first action is to focus on assuring an adequate airway by preparing for intubation. The nurse can then assess for a gag reflex for risk of aspiration. Once the airway and risk for aspiration are assured, the nurse can assess the client for infection and medication schedule. (M)

14. 4 The client with type 2 diabetes mellitus who is taking digoxin (Lanoxin) presents with two major risk factors for hypokalemia. Hypokalemia can increase sensitivity to digitalis, resulting in excessive cardiac force and decreased rate. Decreased potassium can result in decreased release of insulin, resulting in life-threatening serum glucose levels. Oral hypoglycemics increase the release of insulin. Decreased potassium affects the T waves. Presence of tachycardia and cirrhosis are not significant risks. Decreased GI motility and increased thirst are signs and symptoms of hypokalemia. (M)

15. 4 The policy and procedure manual at the health care agency will provide the most specific information about the standard of care for the client at that institution. Nursing professional organizations such as the Oncology Nursing Society develop broad standards that can be tailored for specific agencies and client situations. The American Nurses Association Standards of Care pertain to general nursing practice and professional behavior. Health care accreditation standards address standards from an institutional perspective and may not provide sufficient detail for managing nursing care in this situation. (M)

16. 2 Female clients with HIV are at risk for acquiring the papillomavirus, which predisposes them to cancer. This client needs to have regular Pap smears. Visiting this client could be delayed. Because of the safety risks and the need for pain management, the nurse sees the client with brain metastasis as soon as possible. A diabetic who may not inject insulin properly will be at great risk, and the nurse should plan to visit this client early as well. Because the client with CD4+ is at great risk for a fulminating infection, the nurse does not postpone the appointment. (M)

17. 2 Following the initial diagnostic period, clients often respond by denying the diagnosis. It is important for the nurse to use therapeutic communication skills to help the client manage grief experiences. This intervention will be the most effective because the potential for total management of the disease will be affected. Assessment of the renal status and the status of the lower limbs is relevant to the client needs, but since monitoring the glucose level is managed by the client, the nurse places the greatest emphasis on the client's phase of adjustment. If clients are assisted in managing emotional responses, they will be better able to learn about the disease and prevent complications. (M)

18. 4 The wife, or other responsible family member, may sign the consent form for a client with dementia. The minister, supervisor, and attorney cannot provide legal consent for surgery for this client. (M)

19. 2 The nurse should not accept an assignment to "float" to another nursing unit for which the nurse does not have experience or adequate preparation. The first step is to discuss the situation with the person making the assignment; if the situation is not resolved, the newly graduated nurse should ask to speak with the supervisor. (M)

20. 4 The nurse must respect the wishes of the client who has indicated that he does not wish to be resuscitated and not initiate CPR. Nurses who resuscitate clients who have directed otherwise may be considered to be battering the client. In this situation the physician has written the DNR order, and it is not necessary for the nurse to page the physician to reconsider the order. The nurse can assist the wife deal with her grief. (M)

chapter

41 Managing Client Safety

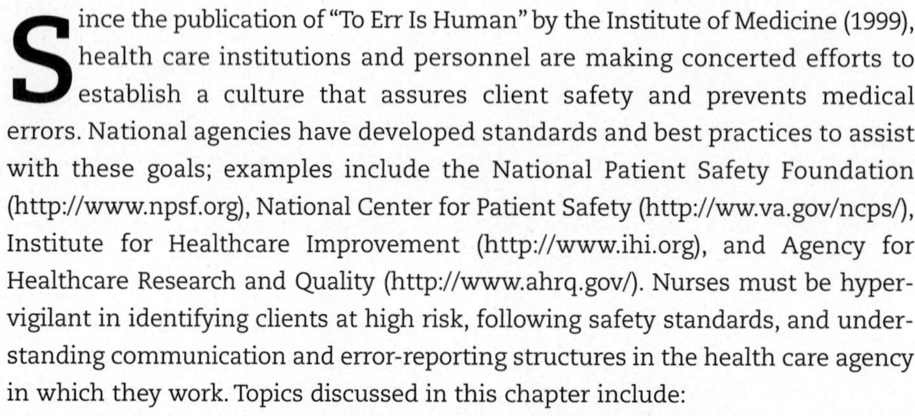

Since the publication of "To Err Is Human" by the Institute of Medicine (1999), health care institutions and personnel are making concerted efforts to establish a culture that assures client safety and prevents medical errors. National agencies have developed standards and best practices to assist with these goals; examples include the National Patient Safety Foundation (http://www.npsf.org), National Center for Patient Safety (http://ww.va.gov/ncps/), Institute for Healthcare Improvement (http://www.ihi.org), and Agency for Healthcare Research and Quality (http://www.ahrq.gov/). Nurses must be hypervigilant in identifying clients at high risk, following safety standards, and understanding communication and error-reporting structures in the health care agency in which they work. Topics discussed in this chapter include:

- Safe Administration of Medications
- Safe Administration of IV Fluids
- Rapid Response Teams
- Communication
- High-Risk Situations

Safe Administration of Medications

I. Definition: Medication errors (e.g., incorrect medication, duplicating orders, or administering incorrect medications) account for the most instances of death and disability to clients (Institute of Medicine, 2006). Safe administration of pharmacologic agents involves taking measures to avoid medication errors.

II. Methods to avoid medication errors

A. Observe Rights of Medication Administration: Involves right medication to right client at right time with right dose and right documentation.

1. Client also has the right to refuse the medication.
2. Nurse must use two sources of identification when administering medications to the client (usually the name identification band and medical record number). The following are not acceptable sources of identification:
   a. Client's room number—room can change frequently in care facilities.
   b. Calling client by name—hospitalized clients may be unconscious or receiving medications that may cause sedation.

B. Follow agency procedure for administering high-alert drugs: Includes drugs that, when administered in error, have an increased likelihood for causing harm or death, such as drugs that affect the heart rate, rhythm, and BP, anticoagulants, narcotics, and insulin. (See Box 41-1 for a list of high-alert drugs.)

1. Nurses must be vigilant when administering high-alert drugs.
2. Nurse must follow agency policy for administration (e.g., some agencies require that two nurses verify the dose prior to administration).

C. Follow agency procedures for reconciliation of medication orders: Refers to the process of avoiding medication error while the client is transitioned across care facilities, health care providers, or from facility to return home. Client's medication orders are reviewed at the time of each admission/transfer/discharge and compared with the orders being considered for the new setting of care.

1. Each agency establishes its own processes and procedures for medication reconciliation. Most often this process involves the pharmacist, health care provider (HCP), or nurse.
2. The nurse must assure that medication reconciliation procedures have occurred at each transition point in the client's care.

Box 41-1. High-Alert Drugs

Amiodarone
Anesthetics
Antiarrhythmics—lidocaine
Anticoagulants—heparin, warfarin (Coumadin)
Antineoplastic drugs
Dobutamine/dopamine
Electrolyte solutions with potassium and sodium
Insulin
Narcotics/opiates
Sedatives
Vasodilators—sodium nitroprusside (Nipride)

Safe Administration of IV Fluids

I. Definition: As with administering medications, the nurse has responsibility for safe administration of IV fluids to the right client, at the right time, with the right fluid/solution, at the right infusion rate. The nurse must follow all agency policies and procedures related to IV administration of blood and blood products as well as administration of high-alert medications.

II. Procedures for safe administration

A. Use standardized IV administration equipment across the entire clinical agency.

B. Reset "smart" infusion pumps (pumps with computer settings) when client is transferred or moves in bed.

C. Identify the client using TWO identifiers (e.g., asking client to state name, checking hospital identification number). Electronic scanning devices may also be used for bar codes and armbands. Do NOT identify client by room number or by calling the client's name.

D. Label IV bag with client's name, drug, date, time; label the pump chamber with the drug, concentration, and rate; label the distal tubing with drug, concentration, and rate.

E. Develop and follow policies, procedures, and guidelines for safe administration of IV infusions.

F. Collaborate with pharmacy; consult with pharmacists about drug and dose.

G. Do not hesitate to confirm or question any part of the medication administration process for correctness (includes drug, dose, potential for drug interactions, and client identification).

H. Double-check high-alert drugs (see Box 41-1); confirm with second licensed personnel as needed.

Rapid Response Teams

I. Definition: Rapid Response Team (RRT), also called *Medical Emergency Team* and *Urgent Response Team*, is a team of health care professionals who are designated to respond to a change in a client's status that may result in serious complications or death if additional changes occur. The goal of the RRT is to assure client safety and prevent error or untoward outcomes by bringing expertise to the clients' bedside in a timely manner.

II. Uses of RRTs
- A. Imminent or impending cardiopulmonary arrest.
- B. Changes in vital signs indicating potential shock, rapidly rising body temperature, increasing intracranial pressure, or respiratory distress; intuitive sense that the client is having or will have difficulty.

III. Members of RRTs
- A. Health care providers, residents, nurses, respiratory therapists; others as assigned.
- B. As opposed to "code teams," RRTs involve a less hierarchical approach (going through "channels") to initiating the team.

IV. Role of the nurse
- A. Identify clients who may require rapid response from a RRT.
- B. Serve on the RRT.

Communication

I. Definition: Communication involves transmitting accurate and organized information from one person (the sender) to another (the receiver). Clear communication is essential for assuring client safety and preventing error.

II. Types of communication
- A. Client status reports: Communication about the client's status may occur in face-to-face encounters, by telephone, or by written or electronic records, while protecting client privacy according to Health Insurance Portability and Accountability Act (HIPPA) standards.
- B. Shift reports
  1. Given at change of shift to ensure continuity of care by sharing important information about the client to the oncoming individual or team who will be caring for the client.
  2. Include current goals and priorities, changes in client's status, current or new treatments and medications, medications that have not been administered or, as important, when the next dose of a medication is to be administered, status of teaching plans, and progress toward discharge.
- C. Transfer reports
  1. Given each time the client changes location within the health care system (e.g., to/from surgery and recovery room; from critical care unit to step-down unit; from hospital to care facility or home).
  2. Include name, hospital identification number, current vital signs, medications, treatments given and to be given; status of drains, dressings, and intake and output; infusions and rate; laboratory results or laboratory results to be obtained; equipment in place/being used or to be obtained; advance directives/resuscitation status; and infection precautions.
  3. The nurse giving the transfer report must give the recipient of the communication an opportunity to ask questions.
- D. Reports to physician or health care provider
  1. Given to report change in client's condition, or request an order for medication, procedures, diet change.
  2. Nurse uses SBAR (Situation, Background, Assessment, Recommendation) to guide reporting. Include relevant data including vital signs, results of laboratory tests, action requested.
  3. If communication with physician or HCP results in an order over the telephone:
     - a. The physician or HCP must confirm the verbal order when the nurse repeats the order to the physician.
     - b. The nurse must have two nurses listen to the order and sign the chart according to agency policy when the order is transcribed by the nurse.
- E. Time outs
  1. Called when there is confusion on the part of *any* health team member that requires a discussion to clarify or modify plans. "Time outs" are called to:
     - a. Confirm identification of client.
     - b. Confirm correct site for a procedure.
     - c. Confirm all heath team members understand the sequence of actions that are about to occur.
  2. Called by the nurse or any health care team member. All team members must be present when information is reviewed.
- F. Discharge instructions
  1. Given to the client and family when the client is discharged from the care facility to another care facility or to home.
  2. Include information about the health problem and treatment regimen, medications,

diets, dressing changes, exercises, and activity level. The nurse verifies the client and family:
a. Understand when to take medications and what side effects to expect and/or report.
b. Are willing and able to administer drugs, treatments, or use special equipment.
c. Understand signs and symptoms to report to the health care provider, and who to contact for questions and problems.
d. Understand what to do in an emergency (e.g., bleeding, severe pain; changing levels of consciousness) and where and how to seek emergency assistance.
e. Are aware of availability of home care services and community resources.
f. Understand when and where to obtain follow-up care.

High-Risk Situations

I. Definition: Clients at high risk are those who have health care problems, age-related risks, or are receiving medications or treatments that increase risk for infection or injury. The nurse must identify clients at risk and observe nursing care standards to prevent or manage risk situations.

II. Types of high risks: Examples of risks include falls, pressure ulcers, infection, medication error, or surgical procedure error. (Falls, pressure ulcers, and infection are discussed here.)

A. Falls: Hospitalized clients are at high risk for falls; it is estimated that between 16% and 52% of clients may fall one or more times during hospitalization.

1. Risk factors
   a. Medications such as hypotensive drugs, psychotropic medications, sedatives, or narcotics
   b. Alcohol use
   c. Vision or hearing problems
   d. Gait or mobility problems
   e. Cognitive deficits
   f. Nocturia or incontinence
   g. Fear of falling
   h. History of previous falls
   i. Confusion or dizziness
2. Prevention
   a. Maintain safe environment in the client's room.
      (1) Put a sticker on the room door and place arm identification band to identify client as being at risk for falls.
      (2) Place bedside table and light switch in client's reach.
      (3) Assure client is able to get out of bed on his or her stronger side; keep bed in the low position; maintain safe use of side rails and per agency policy.
         (a) Full side rails are not used to prevent falls—use is considered a restraint and can contribute to injury and death if the client attempts to climb over the rail or becomes trapped between the rail and the bed.
         (b) Split side rails are used when the rail at the head of the bed is used for the client to pull up on, and the rail at the foot of the bed is in the down position.
      (4) Keep room well lit and remove clutter.
      (5) Assure bathroom is easily accessible and equipped with handrails and transfer devices as needed.
   b. Assist client with ambulation.
      (1) Use nonslip shoes or slippers except when walking on carpet.
      (2) Instruct client on using assistive devices and handrails as needed.
      (3) Orient the client to surroundings.
      (4) Have personnel walk with the client as needed.
   c. Collaborate with occupational therapists and physical therapists as needed to assess client's risk for fall and to develop individualized fall prevention plans.

B. Pressure ulcers: Refers to area of skin that breaks down because of pressure on the area usually as a result of client being on bed rest or spending increased time in a chair or wheelchair (see also Chapter 34). Pressure ulcers occur over bony prominences such as the sacrum, heels, back, hips, or elbows.

1. Risk factors
   a. Bed rest or increased time in wheelchair
   b. Increased age (older adult clients)
   c. Inability to move (e.g., spinal cord injuries, Guillain-Barré syndrome)
   d. Malnourished or underweight
   e. Dementia
   f. Incontinence
2. Prevention
   a. Relieve pressure using pillows, cushions, or air pressure mattresses.

b. Provide frequent turning.
c. Avoid friction.
d. Maintain hydration and nutrition.
e. Keep area at risk clean and dry.

C. Infections: Caused by a pathogen (virus, bacteria, fungus, protozoa, parasite).
1. Risk factors
a. Age: Very young and very old
b. Compromised immune system
c. Poor circulation
d. Invasive procedures such as surgery
e. Impaired skin integrity
f. Malnourished
g. Repeated exposure to pathogen
2. Prevention: Follow guidelines for Isolation Precautions—preventing transmission of infectious agents in healthcare settings (Centers for Infectious Disease Research and Policy and Centers for Disease Control).
a. Perform hand hygiene after touching blood, body fluids, secretions, excretions, and contaminated items, both immediately after removing gloves and between client contacts.
b. Establish personal protective environment to include gloves for touching blood, body fluids, secretions, excretions, contaminated items, mucous membranes, and nonintact skin; and gown during client procedures and activities involving contact of clothing or exposed skin with blood or body fluids, secretions, and excretions.
c. Use mask, eye protection (goggles), and face shield during procedures such as suctioning or endotracheal intubation that are associated with splashes or sprays of blood, body fluids, secretions. A fit-tested N95 or higher respirator is worn for clients with suspected or proven infections transmitted by respiratory aerosols, such as SARS.
d. Handle soiled equipment, textiles, and laundry to prevent transfer of microorganisms to others and to the environment (wear gloves if visibly contaminated and perform hand hygiene).
e. Follow procedures for routine care, cleaning, and disinfecting environmental surfaces, especially frequently touched surfaces in client care areas.
f. Do not recap used needles, or those bent, broken, or manipulated by hand. Use only a one-handed scoop technique when recapping is required. Use safety features when available; place used "sharps" in a puncture-resistant container.
g. For client resuscitation, a mouthpiece, resuscitation bag, and other ventilation devices are needed to prevent contact with the mouth and oral secretions.
h. Assign single rooms for clients at increased risk for transmission, who are likely to contaminate the environment, who do not maintain appropriate hygiene, and/or who are at increased risk of acquiring infection or having an adverse outcome following infection.
i. Institute respiratory hygiene and cough etiquette to include source containment of infectious respiratory secretions in symptomatic clients, starting with emergency triage and reception areas and clinician offices. Instruct the client who is sneezing or coughing to cover the mouth and nose, use tissues, and dispose of them in no-touch receptacles, practice hand hygiene after soiling the hands with respiratory secretions, and wear surgical masks or keep more than 3 feet away from others.

Bibliography

Agency for Health Care Research and Quality. *Glossary.* Retrieved June 6, 2008 from http://www.psnet.ahrq.gov/glossary.aspx#medicalemergencyteam

Center for Infectious Disease Research and Policy. www.cidrap.umn.edu
Centers for Disease Control. www.cdc.gov

Institute of Medicine. (1999). *To err is human.* Retrieved June 6, 2008 from http://www.iom.edu

Institute of Medicine. (2006). *Preventing medication errors: Quality chasm series.* Retrieved June 6, 2008 from http://www.iom.edu

CHAPTER 41

Practice Test

Safe Administration of Medications

1. AF The nurse is administering indomethacin (Indocin) to a neonate. To assure that the nurse has identified the neonate correctly, the nurse should do which of the following? Select all that apply.
   - □ 1. Ask parents to confirm that this is their baby.
   - □ 2. Ask another nurse to confirm that this is the neonate for whom the medication has been prescribed.
   - □ 3. Check neonate's identification band against the medical record number on the chart.
   - □ 4. Verify date of birth from the medical record with the date of birth on the client's identification band.
   - □ 5. Compare the number on the crib with the number on the client's identification band.

2. While preparing to administer medications to a client, the nurse compares the medication in the medication box with the physician's orders and discovers that the physician ordered prednisone 15 mg PO for a client with cirrhosis and the medication in the client's medication box is prednisolone 5 mg. The nurse should next do which of the following?
   - □ 1. Call pharmacy for prednisone 15 mg.
   - □ 2. Notify the charge nurse or supervisor.
   - □ 3. Call the physician for clarification.
   - □ 4. Contact the pharmacy about the discrepancy.

3. The nurse should seek clarification about which of the following medication orders?
   - □ 1. Give 5,000 units bolus dose of heparin IV push.
   - □ 2. Give 200,000 units heparin by IV drip, and infuse over 24 hr.
   - □ 3. Give 40,000 units of heparin by IV drip, and infuse over 24 hr.
   - □ 4. Give 500 units of heparin IV piggyback every 4 to 6 hr.

4. A client has accidentally received twice the normal dose of a medication that was administered on the previous shift. What should the nurse who discovers the error do first?
   - □ 1. Call the person who made the error and request that an incident report be completed.
   - □ 2. Observe the client and note any changes in condition.
   - □ 3. Call the physician to obtain an order for additional IV fluids to dilute the drug.
   - □ 4. Administer a drug antidote per standing order.

Safe Administration of IV Fluids

5. A neonate is to have an IV infusion of normal saline running at a keep-open rate. The nurse is setting the alarms on an IV infusion pump. The nurse should set the alarms:
   - □ 1. At 5% above and 5% below the keep-open rate.
   - □ 2. Within a 15% range of the keep-open rate.
   - □ 3. To sound when the infusion is infiltrating.
   - □ 4. At the exact drip rate as prescribed.

6. AF A teenager is receiving an IV infusion of D5W administered by an infusion pump. The nurse should verify the alarm settings on the infusion pump at which of the following times? Select all that apply.
   - □ 1. When the infusion is started.
   - □ 2. At the beginning of each shift.
   - □ 3. When the client returns from x-ray.
   - □ 4. When the client plays computer games.
   - □ 5. After a visit from friends.

7. AF A client who is receiving a blood transfusion suddenly experiences chills and a temperature of 101°F. The client also has a headache and appears flushed. The nurse should do which of the following? Place in order from first to last.
   - _____ 1. Obtain a blood culture from the client.
   - _____ 2. Send the blood bag and administration set to the blood bank.
   - _____ 3. Stop the blood infusion.
   - _____ 4. Infuse normal saline to keep the vein open.

8. AF A client is receiving TPN. The charge nurse observes a traveling staff nurse change the central line dressing with clean gloves and sterile dressings. The charge nurse should do which of the following? Select all that apply.
   - □ 1. Contact the IV therapy department.
   - □ 2. Place a mask on the client.

□ 3. Contact the nurse supervisor.
□ 4. Inform the traveling nurse that sterile technique must be used to change central line dressings.
□ 5. Report the incident to the infection control department.

Rapid Response Teams

9. The nurse on a postsurgical nursing unit is caring for a client who had a colectomy 2 days ago. The client has a recent history of coronary artery disease. The client's vital signs suddenly change, with the BP dropping to 84/86 and the heart rate increasing to 110. The client is short of breath and complains of pain in his chest. The nurse should do which of the following first?
□ 1. Reassess vital signs in 5 min.
□ 2. Call for a stat ECG.
□ 3. Notify the client's surgeon.
□ 4. Call the rapid response team.

10. AF A task force is planning to establish an RRT. Which of the following are appropriate members to include on this team? Select all that apply.
□ 1. RN who works in the ICU.
□ 2. Intensivist.
□ 3. On-call ICU resident.
□ 4. Respiratory therapist.
□ 5. RN from a temporary agency.
□ 6. LPN charge nurse.
□ 7. Critical care nurse practitioner.

Communication

11. AF A neonate is in the operating room having surgery to correct a ventricular-septal defect. There is confusion about the extent of the defect on the echocardiogram. The nurse calls a "time out." Surgery can continue only when which of the following occur? Select all that apply.
□ 1. The surgeon verifies the correct procedure.
□ 2. The surgeon verifies correct surgical site.
□ 3. The nurse re-establishes the sterile field.
□ 4. The surgical team identifies the client using two sources of identification.
□ 5. Another echocardiogram is obtained.

12. AF The physician is calling in a telephone order for ampicillin. The nurse should do which of the following? Select all that apply.
□ 1. Write down the order.
□ 2. Ask the physician to come to the hospital and write the order on the chart.
□ 3. Repeat the order to the physician.
□ 4. Ask the physician to confirm that the order is correct.
□ 5. Ask the nursing supervisor to cosign the telephone order as transcribed by the nurse.

13. The nurse is receiving results of a blood glucose level from the laboratory over the telephone. The nurse should:
□ 1. Write down the results, read back the results to the caller from the laboratory, and receive confirmation from the caller.
□ 2. Repeat the results to the caller from the laboratory, write the results on scrap paper, and then transfer the results to the chart.
□ 3. Indicate to the caller that the nurse cannot receive results from lab tests over the telephone, and ask the lab to bring the written results to the nurses' station.
□ 4. Request that the laboratory send the results by e-mail to transfer to the client's electronic record.

14. AF A client is being transferred from the recovery room to the medical surgical nursing unit. The nurse from the recovery room should report which of the following to the nurse in the medical surgical unit? Select all that apply.
□ 1. Type of surgery.
□ 2. Name of insurance provider.
□ 3. Current vital signs.
□ 4. Names of all surgeons participating in the surgery.
□ 5. Amount of blood loss.
□ 6. Fluids infusing including rate and type of fluid.
□ 7. Medications ordered.

15. A client who had a myocardial infarction 3 days ago is being transferred from the cardiac ICU to the cardiac step-down unit. Which of the following information is most important for the nurse in the ICU to transmit to the nurse in the cardiac step-down unit?
□ 1. When the client had the last bowel movement.
□ 2. The current heart rate and rhythm.
□ 3. The infusion rate for the "keep-open" IV infusion.
□ 4. The client's level of chest pain.

16. AF A client with a history of myocardial infarction 3 years ago was admitted at 7 a.m. for a cholecystectomy scheduled at 9 a.m. The client has been NPO since midnight. At 8:30 the client complains of chest pains. At 7 a.m. the client's vital signs were pulse, 80; respirations, 14; BP, 110/70. At 8:30 a.m. the nurse takes the vital signs again: pulse is 110; respirations, 20; BP, 90/60. The nurse calls the surgeon. The nurse should discuss which of the following? Select all that apply.

□ 1. That the client has remained NPO.
□ 2. The previous history of myocardial infarction.
□ 3. The change in vital signs.
□ 4. The type of surgery scheduled.
□ 5. Request for ECG.
□ 6. Request to administer nitroglycerine tablet.
□ 7. Presence of chest pains.

High-Risk Situations

17. A client is admitted to the emergency department with sneezing and coughing. The client is in the triage area, waiting to be seen by a physician. To prevent spread of infection to others in the area and to the health care staff, the nurse should do which of the following?
□ 1. Place the client in an isolation room.
□ 2. Ask the others in the area to move away from the client.
□ 3. Give the client a surgical mask to wear.
□ 4. Ask the client to wash his hands before being examined.

18. AF Which of the following clients are at risk for falling? Select all that apply.
□ 1. Client who is 45 years of age, in hospice with terminal cancer, and receiving morphine every 2 hr.
□ 2. Client who is 70 years of age, hospitalized for lung biopsy, and receiving no medications.
□ 3. Client who is 62 years of age, recovering from breast biopsy in outpatient surgery, and has a fear of falling.
□ 4. Client who is 80 years of age and in a locked facility for clients with cognitive impairment.
□ 5. Client who is 75 years of age and recovering at home from hip replacement surgery on the left hip.

19. A UAP is preparing for bed a client who has had knee surgery 2 days ago. As the nurse makes rounds, which of the following requires the nurse to intervene?
□ 1. The call light is pinned to the head of the bed in the client's reach.
□ 2. The night light is dimmed, giving low-level lighting to the room.
□ 3. There is a clear path to the bathroom.
□ 4. The side rails on the head and foot of the bed are in the up position.

20. AF A female client who is 70 years of age and on bed rest has become incontinent of urine. To prevent pressure ulcers, the nurse should do which of the following? Select all that apply.
□ 1. Apply perineal pads and change frequently.
□ 2. Institute a turning schedule.
□ 3. Inspect the groin for wetness.
□ 4. Wear incontinence briefs.
□ 5. Anchor a Foley catheter.

Answers and Rationales

1. 3, 4 The nurse uses at least two sources of identification prior to administering medication to any client, such as the medical record number and the client's date of birth. It is not safe practice to ask the parent or a nurse to verify the correct client. It is also not safe to use the room number or crib number as a source of identification as clients' locations in the hospital are frequently changed. (S)

2. 3 The nurse calls the physician for clarification. The nurse must be vigilant when comparing medication in the medication box to the physician orders; prednisolone, for example, is 3 to 5 times more potent than prednisone. The nurse cannot make a pharmacy substitution change without prescriptive authority. The prednisolone is not returned until a clarification order is obtained to determine the substitution drug and dosage is correct. It is not necessary to contact the charge nurse or supervisor, as the nurse must first clarify the order with the physician. The nurse reports the incident according to agency policy, and notifies all involved of the change in the medication order. (D)

3. 2 200,000 units of heparin is too large of a dose. Heparin may be given in a 5,000-unit bolus dose IV; then 20,000 to 40,000 units infused over 24 hr with a dose adjusted to maintain desired APTT, or 5,000 to 10,000 units IV piggyback every 4 to 6 hr. (D)

4. 2 In any situation that involves a medication error, the nurse first assesses the client immediately to determine any changes in condition and the need for urgent interventions. Calling the physician and/or administering an antidote is not done until the client is assessed and the necessary data are gathered. The nurse finding the error can complete an incident report after the client's safety is established and any emergency treatments are completed. (D)

5. 1 Although agency procedures and policies may vary, national patient safety guidelines recommend that alarms on infusion pumps are set at 5% above and 5% below the prescribed infusion rate. A wider range is not safe. The alarms must be set to indicate a change in the drip rate, not infiltration. Setting the alarms for the exact drip rate will cause the alarms to trigger when the client moves, and this exact range is not needed to alert the nurse to an unsafe rate. (S)

6. 1, 2, 3 The settings on infusion pumps are verified at the time the infusion is started, at the beginning of each shift, and when the client is moved or transported. The client can move in bed, for example, as occurs when the client is playing a computer game or visiting with friends; but if the alarm is triggered, the nurse verifies the settings. (S)

7. 3, 4, 1, 2 The client is experiencing a septic reaction to the blood transfusion. The nurse's first action is to stop the infusion and notify the HCP and blood bank. The nurse then uses an infusion of normal saline to keep the vein open. Next, the nurse obtains a sample of the client's blood for a blood culture, and last, the nurse sends the blood bag and the administration set to the blood bank for culture. (M)

8. 2, 4 Prior to changing a central line dressing, the nurse places a mask on the client to decrease the chance of airborne contamination (the nurse must also wear a mask). Sterile technique is used to change central line dressings because the client is very susceptible to opportunistic infection. Many clients receiving TPN also are receiving chemotherapy, corticosteroids, or antibiotics that can mask signs of infection. The hyperglycemia that is a metabolic complication of TPN is ideal for the promotion of growth of micro-organisms; septicemia can be an outcome. Not all institutions use the specialized IV team from the IV department to manage central line therapy. The nurse supervisor's role does not include direct supervision of a central line dressing change. The nurse supervisor may be consulted with a complex situation related to central line management. It is not necessary to notify the infection control department. (M)

9. 4 The nurse activates the RRT. Although the client has not had a cardiac arrest, the change in vital signs and the presence of chest pain are indications that other adverse events may follow. The purpose of the RRT is to respond to a situation in which rapid intervention may prevent untoward outcomes. An ECG will be helpful for assessing the nature of the change in vital signs and the chest pain, but it is not sufficient. Although the nurse can ask the unit clerk or other personnel to call the surgeon after notifying the RRT, the surgeon may not be able to respond in a timely manner. (M)

10. 1, 2, 3, 4, 7 The RRT is composed of health care professionals who have critical care skills required to assess the client and respond to the incident. The team also includes members who are onsite, available to respond, and do not have competing priorities. The team can include nurses with critical care experience—either RNs or advanced practice nurses; physicians, including residents; physician assistants; intensivists or hosptialists; and respiratory therapists. LPNs do not have the requisite skills. Unless the nurse from the temporary agency has the requisite skills and is very familiar with the specific policies and procedures of the agency and works full time at the hospital, that nurse is not the most appropriate member for this team. (S)

11. 1, 2, 4 When a time out is called prior to surgery, the surgical team must read back all orders, verify the correct site, reidentify the client, and double-check the echocardiogram. The sterile field has not been disrupted and does not need to be set up again. It is not necessary to obtain another echocardiogram as long as the confusion is clarified and the surgical team is satisfied all are ready to begin the surgery. (S)

12. 1, 3, 4 To assure client safety while obtaining telephone orders, the order must be received by the RN. The nurse writes the order, reads the order back to the physician, and receives verbal confirmation from the physician that the order is correct. It is not necessary for the physician to come to the hospital to write the order on the chart, or to have the nursing supervisor cosign the telephone order. (S)

13. 1 To assure client safety, the nurse first writes the results on the chart, then reads them back to the caller and waits for the caller to confirm that the nurse has understood the results. The nurse may receive results by telephone; and although electronic transfer to the client's electronic record is appropriate, the nurse can also accept the telephone results if the laboratory has called the results to the nurses station. (S)

14. 1, 3, 5, 6, 7 Transfer reports must include information about the client's surgery, all current treatments and medications, vital signs, including pain level, fluid status including blood loss, and current IV infusions. It is not necessary to identify the surgeons who were present during the surgery or report the name of the insurance provider. (M)

15. 2 While all of the information presented in this report can be conveyed during the transfer report, the nurse from the cardiac intensive care unit must be certain that the receiving nurse is aware of the client's current heart rate and rhythm. If the IV infusion is running at a keep-open rate, the receiving nurse will time the rate and note it on the chart. The nurse assesses the client's current level of chest pain, rather than receive information about the level of pain prior to transferring from the intensive care. The nurse can assess the status of the client's bowel movement on an ongoing basis. (M)

16. 2, 3, 5, 6 Using SBAR (situation, background, assessment, recommendation) the nurse informs the physician of the current situation (chest pains), the background (history of myocardial infarction), and assessment (chest pains, vital signs changes, likelihood of having a myocardial infarction). The nurse also discusses recommendations and suggestions for orders such as the ECG and nitroglycerine tablet. (S)

17. 3 In order to prevent infections in hospitals, the nurse institutes measures to contain respiratory secretions in symptomatic clients. The nurse gives the client a mask to wear, and tissues; the nurse instructs the client to dispose of used tissues in a no-touch receptacle. It is not necessary to place the client in isolation. It is not appropriate to ask others to move away from the client, but the nurse can ask the client to keep 3 feet away from others in the waiting room, if there is room. The nurse instructs the client to perform hand hygiene after blowing his nose or touching his nose or face, but doing so is not a prerequisite for being examined by the HCP. The nurse and HCP also use hand hygiene practices when caring for this client. (S)

18. 1, 3, 4, 5 Clients who are at risk for falling include the client taking narcotics, the client with a known fear of falling, the client with cognitive impairment, and the client with gait problems. Age and setting are not necessarily risks for fallings. (S)

19. 4 Side rails are considered restraints and are not used at both the head and foot of the bed. Using side rails at the head of the bed will aid the client in sitting up and are safe, but using side rails at both the head and the foot of the bed presents risks for a client who might become wedged between the rail and the bed or attempt to climb over them. The nurse discusses side rail use with the UAP and lowers the side rail at the foot of the bed. The nurse assures the bed is placed in low position. The accessible call light, dim lighting, and clear path to the bathroom are factors that contribute to fall prevention. (S)

20. 2, 3, 4 This client is at risk for pressure ulcers because of her age, because she is on bed rest, and because of her incontinence. The nurse assesses all pressure points and the groin area, assures the client changes positions every 2 hr, and has the client wear incontinence pads containing absorbent material (specially designed to absorb many times its weight in water) or disposable incontinence briefs. Feminine hygiene pads (perineal pads) are not designed to contain/absorb urine. Anchoring a Foley catheter increases the risk for infection. (R)

chapter

42 Managing Emergencies and Disasters

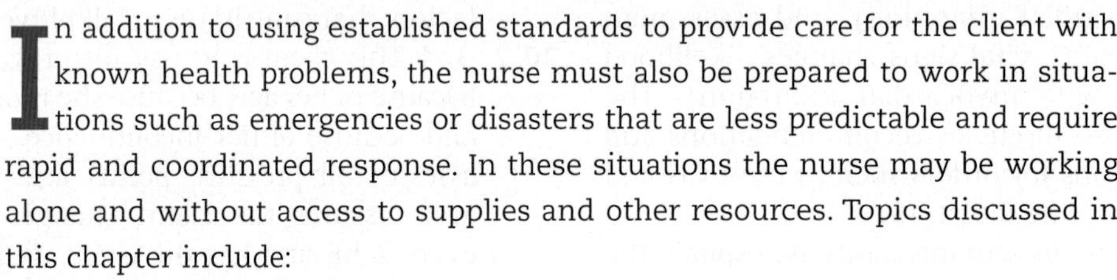

In addition to using established standards to provide care for the client with known health problems, the nurse must also be prepared to work in situations such as emergencies or disasters that are less predictable and require rapid and coordinated response. In these situations the nurse may be working alone and without access to supplies and other resources. Topics discussed in this chapter include:

- Managing Emergencies
- Managing Disasters

Managing Emergencies

I. Definition: An emergency is a situation that poses an immediate threat to human life or serious damage to property or the environment.
   A. Emergencies require coordinated and rapid response; delayed treatment could result in further injury or death.
   B. Emergency situations occur in both hospital and community settings and may include cardiopulmonary arrest, airway obstruction, injury to the head or spine, burns, dehydration, shock, poisoning, environmental (spill or release of hazardous material that affects water, air, or land, and threatens the health of citizens), animal bites, sexual assault, complications of pregnancy, violence, suicide, and biologic/chemical events (spill or release of chemicals or biologic agents that threaten the health of citizens).
   C. Emergencies may be managed at the site with first aid until medical treatment can be provided by rescue units or in the emergency department when the client is transported to a general or specialized (e.g., Burn Center) facility.

II. Nurse role
   A. Triage: Refers to sorting or placing of emergency (or disaster) victims in categories according to the urgency and level of care needed.
      1. Each emergency department establishes its own triage system involving categories or levels. (See Box 42-1 for example of triage levels.)
      2. Principles of triage include the following:
         a. Conduct assessment quickly and efficiently.
         b. Use A (airway), B (breathing), C (circulation), D (disability) as a guide for assessing clients; once categorized, place tag on the victim with identifying information including triage category, name and age (if known), medication and/or treatment administered at the scene.
         c. Communicate with client—follow established lines of command and

Box 42-1. Priorities of Care and Triage Categories

Standardized triage categories are usually developed within each emergency department. Most common triage systems consist of five levels of acuity.

Triage Level I—Resuscitation
Conditions requiring immediate nursing and physician assessment. Any delay in treatment is potentially life- or limb-threatening. Includes conditions such as:
- Airway compromise
- Cardiac arrest
- Severe shock
- Cervical spine injury
- Multisystem trauma
- Altered LOC (unconsciousness)
- Eclampsia

Triage Level II—Emergent
Conditions requiring nursing assessment and physician assessment within 15 min of arrival. Conditions include:
- Head injuries
- Severe trauma
- Lethargy or agitation
- Conscious overdose
- Severe allergic reaction
- Chemical exposure to the eyes
- Chest pain
- Back pain
- GI bleed with unstable vital signs
- Stroke with deficit
- Severe asthma
- Abdominal pain in clients older than 50 years of age
- Vomiting and diarrhea with dehydration
- Fever in infants younger than 3 months of age
- Acute psychotic episode
- Severe headache
- Any pain greater than 7 on a scale of 10
- Any sexual assault
- Any neonate age 7 days or younger

Triage Level III—Urgent
Conditions requiring nursing and physician assessment within 30 min of arrival. Conditions include:
- Alert head injury with vomiting
- Mild to moderate asthma
- Moderate trauma
- Abuse or neglect
- GI bleed with stable vital signs
- History of seizure, alert on arrival

Triage Level IV—Less Urgent
Conditions requiring nursing and physician assessment within 1 hr. Conditions include:
- Alert head injury without vomiting
- Minor trauma
- Vomiting and diarrhea in client older than 2 years of age without evidence of dehydration
- Earache
- Minor allergic reaction
- Corneal foreign body
- Chronic back pain

Triage Level V—Nonurgent
Conditions requiring nursing and physician assessment within 2 hr. Conditions include:
- Minor trauma, not acute
- Sore throat
- Minor symptoms
- Chronic abdominal pain

Adapted from Nettina, S. M. (2005). *Lippincott manual of nursing practice* (8th ed.). Philadelphia: Lippincott Williams & Wilkins.

communication; report facts and accurate information.

d. Manage anxiety in self, coworkers, and victims.

e. Consider the family.

f. Recognize the impact on nurse conducting triage—difficult when dealing with clients, neighbors, family known to the nurse; when large numbers of deaths; or when decisions need to be made continued treatment of victims whose death is imminent.

B. Assessment: Also review information about specific emergent situations in related chapters in this book.
  1. Initial—Airway, Breathing, Circulation, Disability (as stated previously).
  2. Secondary—brief but complete assessment including vital signs, pulse oximetry, neurologic assessment, history of the event or injury, emotional assessment, and family presence.

C. Intervention
  1. Assure open airway.
  2. Initiate CPR as needed.
  3. Stop bleeding as needed.
  4. Start IV infusion.
  5. Insert gastric tube as needed.
  6. Draw blood for laboratory studies (blood type and crossmatch; hemoglobin/hematocrit; electrolytes; blood alcohol, toxicology screens).
  7. Manage pain; provide comfort measures.
  8. Explain procedures to client and family.

Managing Disasters

I. Definition: A disaster is a man-made or natural event that results in massive destruction with disruption of infrastructure and services. The end result of a disaster is the potential for mass casualties with resulting demands on the health care system.

A. Occurrence may involve a facility (such as a health care facility) and be relatively contained, or may encompass a large geographic area (e.g., natural disaster such as a flood or hurricane). Cause may involve the following:
  1. Adverse weather conditions such as floods, blizzards, ice and snow storms, tornadoes, or hurricanes.
  2. Release of hazardous materials such as toxic gases, chemicals, or pathogens.
  3. Outcome of intentional acts of destruction such as bombs, release of pathogens, fires, or gunshots.

B. Levels
  1. Level I: Significant damage to an area—declared by the president; federal government involved in coordinating regional, state, and national resources.
  2. Level II: Moderate disaster—emergency designated by president/or governor; require state and federal assistance.
  3. Level III: Minor disaster with minimal and contained damage—state of emergency declared by president or state and local officials.

C. Phases
  1. Mitigation: Involves assessing risk and reducing or minimizing the effects of the disaster.
  2. Preparedness: Involves developing plans for evacuation; training personnel, stockpiling supplies and provisions.
  3. Response: Involves activating plans to save lives, reduce further damage, manage priorities (triage); and treat casualties.
  4. Recovery: Involves restoring infrastructure and establishing stability.

II. Nurse role

A. Prepare
  1. Self-preparation—nurse's first action is to take care of self and family; have a 3- to 5-day supply of food, water, power sources, and communications capabilities.
  2. Become educated—understand types of disasters and supplies and use of personal protective equipment (PPE).
  3. Protect clients—be familiar with the clinical facilities' evacuation plan.

B. Plan
  1. Know agency disaster plan.
  2. Plan for receiving a rapid influx of clients.
  3. Develop evacuation plans, particularly for fires (see Box 42-2).
  4. Know who is in charge—identify incident command structure to organize staff into

Box 42-2. Fire Response Procedures: R.A.C. E

Rescue—Attempt to rescue anyone in the immediate vicinity of the fire.

Alarm—Turn in the alarm by using the fire alarm pull station. Be prepared to give your name, title, extension number, location, and extent of the fire.

Confine—Close all doors and windows to confine the fire to the smallest area possible. Do not lock any door.

Extinguish—Evacuate per agency policy. Put out the fire if you have been trained in the use of a portable fire extinguisher and are comfortable in doing so. If not, close the door to the area and assist in the evacuation of the area.

leadership and functional roles; integrate agency plans with community-wide disaster plans.
5. Train personnel.
6. Conduct "mock disaster" drills, including fire drills.
7. Develop plans to care for the caregivers.

C. Manage: Disasters are managed by federal, state, local governments, and agencies such as the American Red Cross. The nurse works within plans established and implemented by these agencies.
1. Participate in agency disaster-management plans and those within the community.
2. As first responder, care for victims, participate in triage activities, and collaborate with rescue teams.
3. Preserve forensic evidence.

D. Triage (see definition and principles in management of emergencies): Triage definitions vary for war, community disasters, and planning in emergency departments (see Box 42-1).

Bibliography

Ellis, J., & Hartley, C. (2007). *Nursing in today's world.* Philadelphia: Lippincott Williams & Wilkins.

Grossman, V. (2003). *Quick reference to triage.* Philadelphia: Lippincott Williams & Wilkins.

Hood, L., & Leddy, S. (2005). *Leddy and Pepper's conceptual bases of professional nursing.* Philadelphia: Lippincott Williams & Wilkins.

Marquis, B., & Huston, C. (2005). *Leadership roles and management functions.* Philadelphia: Lippincott Williams & Wilkins.

Nettina, S. M. (2005). *Lippincott manual of nursing practice* (8th ed.). Philadelphia: Lippincott Williams & Wilkins.

Springhouse. (2005). *Rapid response to everyday emergencies: A nurse's guide.* Ambler, PA: Springhouse.

CHAPTER 42 Practice Test

Managing Emergencies

1. An employee at an industrial factory is splashed with acids. What should the nurse do first?
- □ 1. Apply ice packs to the areas burned.
- □ 2. Cover the affected area with dry, sterile dressings.
- □ 3. Apply an alkaline solution to buffer the acids.
- □ 4. Flush large amounts of water over the burned area.

2. A client is admitted to the emergency department following an overdose of barbiturates. What should the nurse do first?
- □ 1. Assess and assist ventilation.
- □ 2. Monitor the BP.
- □ 3. Prepare to administer blood products.
- □ 4. Place the client in the Trendelenburg position.

3. A male client who is 76 years of age comes to the emergency department with sudden onset of severe pain in his back, flank, and abdomen. He reports feeling weak and his BP is 68/31. Urine output is absent. Bilateral leg pulses are weak, although bruit and pulsation are noted at the umbilicus. The nurse should first:
- □ 1. Obtain a consent for emergency surgery.
- □ 2. Assess leg pulses with a Doppler test.
- □ 3. Palpate the abdomen for presence of a mass.
- □ 4. Start an IV infusion.

4. An alert client is admitted to the emergency department with a severe laceration of his arm with heavy bleeding. What action should the nurse take first?
- □ 1. Apply a tourniquet above the wound.
- □ 2. Assess pulse and nerve functioning of the arm.
- □ 3. Cover the wound with a dressing and apply firm pressure.
- □ 4. Start an IV infusion.

5. A small airplane has crashed in a neighborhood of 10 houses. One of the victims appears to have a cervical spine injury. First aid for this victim includes which of the following?
- □ 1. Establish an airway with head tilt.
- □ 2. Immobilize the spine.
- □ 3. Logroll the victim to a side-lying position.
- □ 4. Elevate the feet 6 inches.

6. AF Several clients come to the emergency department suspected contamination by the Ebola virus. The nurse should do which of the following? Select all that apply.
- □ 1. Call in extra staff to assist with the possibility of more clients with the same condition.

□ 2. Isolate all the suspected clients in the emergency department in one area.
□ 3. Obtain diluted household bleach from housekeeping services.
□ 4. Restrict visitors from the emergency department.
□ 5. Request that the emergency department be closed to other clients.

7. The nurse in the immediate care clinic is assessing a client who is 80 years of age and lives with his son's family. The client has scald burns on his hands and both forearms (10% first- and second-degree burns). The nurse should first:
□ 1. Cleanse the wounds with warm water.
□ 2. Apply antibiotic cream.
□ 3. Call for transport to a burn center.
□ 4. Cover the burns with sterile dressing.

8. **AF** The following clients have been admitted to the emergency department. In which order does the nurse assess these clients? Place clients in order from first to last.
_____ 1. Client who is 12 years of age with a fractured tibia.
_____ 2. Client who is 8 years of age with lacerations to legs and arms.
_____ 3. Client who is 16 years of age with a "sore throat."
_____ 4. Client who is 6 months of age with diarrhea and dehydration.

9. A client who is 16 years of age is seen in an emergency department following a rape. The management of a rape victim should primarily be directed toward:
□ 1. Relieving physical discomfort.
□ 2. Maintaining self-esteem.
□ 3. Assessing for sources of infection resulting from the rape.
□ 4. Teaching the victim how to prevent further attacks.

10. A client has a cerebral concussion from a fall. The nurse should assess the client for which of the following?
□ 1. Lethargy.
□ 2. Vomiting.
□ 3. Unequal pupils.
□ 4. Seizures.

Managing Disasters

11. There is a suspected outbreak of anthrax transmitted by skin exposure. A client is admitted to the emergency department with lesions on his hands. The physician has prescribed antibiotics and sent the client home. The nurse should do which of the following? Select all that apply.
□ 1. Instruct client to take the antibiotics for as long as prescribed.
□ 2. Inform client to avoid contact with others during the treatment.
□ 3. Remind client to wear a mask for 60 days.
□ 4. Tell client that skin lesions will clear up within 1 to 2 days.

12. There is a suspected SARS epidemic in a community of 10,000 people. As clients with SARS are admitted to the hospital, the nurse should use personal protective equipment (PPE) for which of the following?
□ 1. Respiratory.
□ 2. Enteric.
□ 3. Contact.
□ 4. Blood.

13. **AF** There has been a train derailment and 30 people are injured. In which order should the following clients be treated? Place in order from first to last.
_____ 1. Client who is 20 years of age, unresponsive, and has a C3 injury to his spinal cord.
_____ 2. Client who is 80 years of age with a compound fracture of the arm.
_____ 3. Client who is 10 years of age with a laceration on his leg.
_____ 4. Client who is 25 years of age with a sucking chest wound.

14. **AF** There has been a fire in an apartment building and it has spread to seven apartment units. Victims have suffered burns, minor injuries, and broken bones from jumping from windows. Which persons can be safely treated at the scene and transported to a health care facility after victims with more emergent problems have been transported first? Select all that apply.
□ 1. Female client who is 5 months pregnant with no apparent injuries.
□ 2. Middle-aged male client with no injuries, rapid respirations, and coughing.
□ 3. Client who is 10 years of age with an apparent simple fracture of the humerus.
□ 4. Client who is 20 years of age with first-degree burns on hands and forearms.
□ 5. Client who is 75 years of age with second-degree burns on both legs.

15. There has been a shooting in a shopping mall. Three victims with gunshot wounds are brought to the emergency department. The nurse should take which actions to preserve forensic evidence?
□ 1. Cut around blood stains to remove clothing.
□ 2. Place each item of clothing in a separate paper bag.

☐ 3. Place all wet clothing in a plastic bag.
☐ 4. Refrain from documenting client statements.

16. AF A client who was a victim of a gunshot wound and treated in the emergency department died. The nurse should delegate to the UAP to do which of the following during postmortem care? Select all that apply.

☐ 1. Remove all tubes and IV lines.
☐ 2. Cover the body with a sheet.
☐ 3. Notify the family.
☐ 4. Transport the body to the morgue.
☐ 5. Inform the coroner about the cause of death.

17. AF There has been an airline crash with mass casualties. The nurse is directing personnel to tag all victims. Which of the following information should be placed on the tag? Select all that apply.

☐ 1. Triage priority.
☐ 2. Identifying information as possible (name, age, address).
☐ 3. Medications and treatments administered.
☐ 4. Description of jewelry and valuables.
☐ 5. Next of kin.

18. There has been a car accident involving four vehicles on a remote interstate. The nearest emergency department is 15 min away. Which of the following victims should be transported by helicopter to the nearest hospital?

☐ 1. Client who is 10 years of age with simple fracture of the femur, who is crying and cannot find his parents.
☐ 2. Middle-aged female client with cold, clammy skin; heart rate of 120; and is unconscious.
☐ 3. Middle-aged male client with severe asthma, heart rate of 120, and is having difficulty breathing.
☐ 4. Client who is 70 years of age with severe headache, but conscious.

19. AF Several clients who work in the same building were brought to the emergency department complaining of similar clinical manifestations: fever, headache, a skin rash over their entire body, and abdominal pain with vomiting and diarrhea. On initial assessment, the nurse found all to have a low BP and all developed petechiae in the area where the BP cuff had inflated. Which of the following isolation precautions should that nurse initiate? Select all that apply.

☐ 1. Contact isolation with double-gloving and shoe covers.
☐ 2. Respiratory isolation with positive pressure rooms.
☐ 3. Strict hand hygiene.
☐ 4. Protective eye wear.
☐ 5. Enteric precautions.

20. AF The nurse notices a fire in a wastebasket in a client's room. The nurse should do which of the following in priority order? Place in order from first to last.

_____ 1. Confine the fire by closing the door to the client's room.
_____ 2. Extinguish the fire.
_____ 3. Remove the client from the room.
_____ 4. Pull the fire alarm at the alarm pull station.

Answers and Rationales

1. 4 Chemical-burned areas are immediately flushed with water to remove any remaining acids and prevent further destruction. Ice may cause vasoconstriction and further tissue damage. Dressings are not applied until after the acids are flushed from the areas. Alkaline solutions are also capable of causing burns and are avoided. Following emergency care, the client is instructed to seek additional care as needed. (M)

2. 1 Barbiturates can cause significant respiratory depression. The nurse's first action is to immediately assess the respiratory status and assist in ventilation as needed. Monitoring the vital signs is important, but respiratory care takes precedence over the BP. Without other injury, blood products are not necessary. Placing the client in the Trendelenburg position will put pressure from the abdominal contents onto the diaphragm and further impair breathing. (M)

3. 4 The symptoms noted are classic symptoms of leaking abdominal aneurysm and shock; the client needs immediate fluid volume replacement. Assessing the pulses with a Doppler will be of no additional diagnostic value. Palpating the abdomen with suspected abdominal aneurysm is strictly contraindicated and could lead to rupture. After emergency resuscitation, consent for surgery is needed. (M)

4. 3 The priority action is to stop blood loss by direct, firm pressure to the wound; a tourniquet can cause neurovascular damage to the extremity and is used as a last resort. Assessing pulse and nerve functioning and starting an IV are critically important, but not until bleeding is controlled. (M)

5. 2 The victim of a neck injury is immobilized and moved as little as possible. It is also important to assure an open airway; this is accomplished with a jaw thrust without tilting the head. The nurse does not logroll the victim to a side-lying position or elevate the feet; both actions could cause additional injury to the spinal cord. (M)

6. 2, 3, 4 The nurse isolates all suspected clients in the emergency department in one area and restricts visitors from the emergency department to minimize exposure to others. There is no indication at this time that extra staff is needed, so the nurse does not call in extra staff and minimizes exposure to other health care workers. The nurse obtains diluted (1:100) household bleach to decontaminate areas suspected of being in contact with the virus. It is not known how many more victims there are at this time, so it is not necessary to close the emergency department. (S)

7. 3 The nurse has the client transported to a burn center. The client's age and the extent of the burns require care by a burn team. Additionally, the nurse considers that the client may be a victim of geriatric abuse and investigates further as needed. The nurse refrains from cleansing the wound, applying cream, or covering the area. (M)

8. 4, 1, 2, 3 The infant who is 6 months of age with diarrhea is seen first because of risk for further dehydration; the nurse immediately starts an IV infusion. The client who is 12 years of age is seen next; this child is considered to require urgent care, but can wait several hours. The client who is 8 years of age can be seen next; he is considered to require nonurgent care and will respond to assessment and first aid. The last client to receive care is the client who is 16 years of age; this client is considered nonurgent and likely will not require the services of the emergency department. (M)

9. 2 Rape is a demeaning event in a person's life. Helping maintain self-esteem is a priority. The nurse will also be involved in promoting comfort, conducting the physical exam, and promoting safety; but during the emergency department visit, the nurse can be a client advocate and preserve the client's dignity and self-respect. (P)

10. 1 Symptoms such as lethargy and change in memory or attention span are common following a concussion and may last from several weeks to several months. Vomiting, unequal pupils, and seizures are not expected with a concussion and may suggest additional pathology. (A)

11. 1 Anthrax is treated with antibiotics, and the client must continue the prescription as prescribed, even if symptoms do not persist. The client with anthrax is not contagious and does not need to follow isolation procedures at home. Anthrax from skin exposure is not transmitted by respiratory contact and the client does not need to wear a mask. The client may have skin lesions at the point of contact with macula or papule formation; the eschar will fall off in 1 to 2 weeks. (S)

12. 1 SARS is transmitted by respiratory spread; the nurse wears a mask (N95), gloves, gown, and eye protection. SARS is not spread by body fluids (diarrhea, emesis, blood) or by contact. (S)

13. 4, 2, 3, 1 During a disaster, the nurse must make difficult decisions about which persons to treat first. The guidelines for triage offer general priorities for immediate, delayed, minimal, and expectant care. The client with a sucking chest wound needs immediate attention and will likely survive. The client who is 80 years of age with a compound fracture is classified as delayed; emergency response personnel can immobilize the fracture and cover the wound. The client who is 10 years of age has minimal injuries and can wait to be treated. The client with a spinal cord injury likely will not survive and should not be among the first to be transported to the health care facility. (M)

14. 1, 3, 4 The pregnant woman is not in imminent danger or likely to have a precipitous delivery. The client who is 10 years of age is not at risk of infection and can be treated in an outpatient facility. First-degree burns are considered less urgent. The male client with respiratory distress and coughing is transported first as he is likely experiencing smoke inhalation. The client who is 75 years of age with second-degree burns is also transported to a burn center or emergency department. (M)

15. 2 Preserving forensic evidence is essential for investigative purposes following injuries that may be suspected as having criminal intent. The nurse places each item of clothing in a separate paper bag and labels it; wet clothing is hung to dry. The nurse does not cut or otherwise unnecessarily handle clothing, particularly clothing with evidence such as blood or body fluids. The nurse documents carefully the clients' description of the incident and uses quotes around the clients' exact words where possible; documentation will become a part of the clients' records and can be subpoenaed for subsequent investigation. (M)

16. 2, 4 Deaths resulting from injuries such as gunshot wounds are considered reportable deaths; all evidence including tubes and IV lines must remain intact until the coroner has been contacted. The UAP can cover the body and transport the body to the morgue. The HCP is the one to notify the family and discuss details with the coroner. (M)

17. 1, 2, 3 Tracking victims of disasters is important for casualty planning and management. All victims must receive a securely attached tag indicating the triage priority, any available identifying information, and if any care has been given, along with time and date. It is not necessary to document presence of jewelry or next of kin. Tag information is recorded in a disaster log and used to track victims and inform families. (M)

18. 2 The middle-aged female client is likely in shock; she is classified as a triage level I, requiring immediate care. The child with moderate trauma is classified as triage level III, urgent, and can be treated within 30 min. The man with asthma and the man with the severe headache are classified as emergent, triage level II, and can be transported by ambulance and reach the hospital within 15 min. (M)

19. 1, 3, 4 The nurse institutes treatment for hemorrhagic fever viruses, which includes contact isolation with double-gloving and shoe covers, strict hand hygiene, and protective eye wear. The nurse starts respiratory isolation with negative pressure rooms, not positive pressure rooms. Enteric precautions are not appropriate in this situation. (M)

20. 3, 4, 1, 2 The nurse uses the RACE procedure to manage a fire: Rescue, Alarm, Confine, Extinguish. (S)

SECTION 5

Practice Test

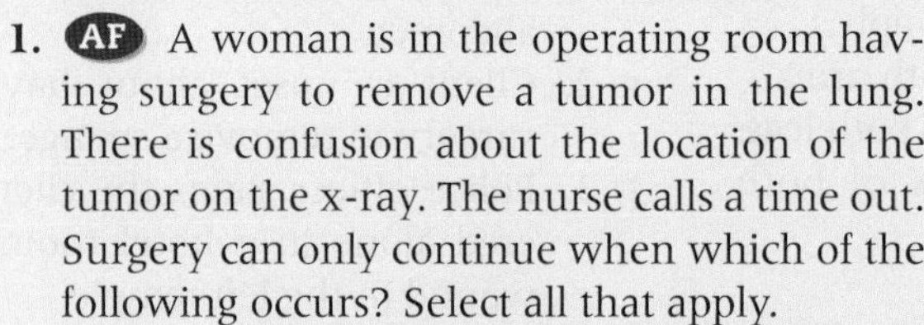

1. AF A woman is in the operating room having surgery to remove a tumor in the lung. There is confusion about the location of the tumor on the x-ray. The nurse calls a time out. Surgery can only continue when which of the following occurs? Select all that apply.
   - □ 1. The surgeon verifies the correct procedure.
   - □ 2. The surgeon verifies the x-ray.
   - □ 3. The nurse re-establishes the sterile field.
   - □ 4. The surgical team verifies the client using two sources of identification.
   - □ 5. The client confirms the marking of the site for the incision.

2. Which of the following clients can be assigned to UAP?
   - □ 1. Client with stable pulmonary artery pressures after a mitral valve replacement.
   - □ 2. Client on bed rest with bathroom privileges and negative troponin and CK-MB levels.
   - □ 3. Client admitted with chest pain to rule out a myocardial infarction.
   - □ 4. Client requiring discharge and wound care teaching after coronary artery bypass surgery.

3. AF The nurse received shift report at 0730 on the following clients. In which order of priority should the nurse make rounds on these clients? Place in order from first to last.
   - _____ 1. Postoperative client scheduled to receive an IVPB antibiotic at 0800.
   - _____ 2. Client with discharge orders for 1200.
   - _____ 3. Client with a BP of 78/32 and pulse of 104.
   - _____ 4. Postoperative client who is complaining of incisional pain.

4. After abdominal surgery, a female client is voiding frequently, about 50 ml each time. Assessment reveals dullness in the suprapubic region on percussion. What action should be taken by the nurse?
   - □ 1. Anchor a Foley catheter.
   - □ 2. Encourage fluids.
   - □ 3. Walk the client to the bathroom.
   - □ 4. Notify the surgeon.

5. Because of a temperature elevation of 104°F that is unresponsive to antipyretics, the nurse places a client in septic shock on a hypothermia blanket. What should the nurse instruct the UAP to perform?
   - □ 1. Turn the client every 2 hr.
   - □ 2. Document dietary intake.
   - □ 3. Report appearance of skin.
   - □ 4. Wrap the client's hands and feet.

6. A client was in an explosion at the factory where she works. Several of her coworkers and she were hurt in the explosion, with four people dying as a result of their injuries. Which statement by the client demonstrates that she is coping with the trauma of the crisis?
   - □ 1. "I have been going to a support group that helps. I can now eat better."
   - □ 2. "I keep having nightmares of the explosion. It is hard to take."
   - □ 3. "I will not ever go back to work again."
   - □ 4. "I often think about the fact that I survived and others did not."

7. AF There has been a fire in an apartment building. All residents have been evacuated,

but many are burned. Which of the following clients should be transported to a burn center for treatment? Select all that apply.

□ 1. Client who is 8 years of age with 10% third-degree burns.
□ 2. Client who is 20 years of age who inhaled smoke from the fire.
□ 3. Client who is 50 years of age and diabetic, with first- and second-degree burns on his left forearm (about 5% burned area).
□ 4. Client who is 30 years of age with 9% second-degree burns on the back of his left leg.
□ 5. Client who is 40 years of age with second-degree burns on his right arm (about 10%).

8. AF There has been an explosion at a chemical plant, producing flames and smoke. More than 20 persons have burn injuries. Which of the victims should be transported to a burn center immediately? Select all that apply.

□ 1. Victim with chemical spills on both arms.
□ 2. Victim with third-degree burns of both legs.
□ 3. Victim with first-degree burns of both hands.
□ 4. Victim in respiratory distress.
□ 5. Victim with first-degree burns around both knees, who is agitated.

9. The staffing office notified the charge nurse that one of the nurses scheduled to work has called in sick. The available staff now includes one RN and two UAP for a team of eight clients. Which of the following clients should be reassigned to the RN?

□ 1. Client diagnosed with Addison disease 2 days ago.
□ 2. Client with chronic renal failure who is to be discharged.
□ 3. Client admitted at 2000 yesterday with dehydration related to diarrhea.
□ 4. Client admitted today at 1100, with hypokalemia and first-degree heart block.

10. Which of the following incident reports is documented incorrectly?

□ 1. After a thorough search, nursing staff were unable to locate client's lower dentures.
□ 2. Client fell out bed while reaching for cane. The bed was at the lowest level.
□ 3. Because of short staffing, phenytoin (Dilantin) 100 mg IV was given instead of Dilantin 100 mg PO.
□ 4. T. Downs, RN. discovered client lying on floor next to bed. Client stated, "I got dizzy."

11. A client with a gastrostomy feeding tube has become confused and restless, and is attempting to remove the tube. The UAP has placed soft ties on the client's wrists. The RN should do which of the following first?

□ 1. Leave the restraints in place.
□ 2. Ask the UAP to remove the restraints.
□ 3. Obtain hand mitts instead of the soft ties.
□ 4. Request an order for restraints from the physician.

12. AF Because of religious beliefs, a seriously ill client refuses a blood transfusion. In what order should the nurse perform the following? Place in order from first to last.

_____ 1. Notify the physician.
_____ 2. Assess client's current status.
_____ 3. Inform client about other options for blood transfusions.
_____ 4. Explain the potential outcomes of the client's decision.

13. Which of the following is not an appropriate documentation of adverse events?

□ 1. Client states his wife stabbed him in the abdomen.
□ 2. Client is upset about having a second surgery to remove a sponge.
□ 3. Police officer states the client was discovered alone in a hotel room with a small wound in the left temple.
□ 4. Client was shot in the chest by a police officer while attempting to rob a department store.

14. A client tells the charge nurse that the IV narcotic analgesics on the first shift are significantly more effective than those given at night. The charge nurse suspects the night nurse may be injecting the clients with something other than the prescribed drugs. What should the charge nurse do next?

□ 1. Meet with the immediate supervisor about the suspicions.
□ 2. Communicate the clients' statements to the second shift nurse.
□ 3. Meet with the immediate supervisor about the client's statements.
□ 4. Assess the client comfort levels during shifts when the nurse is absent.

15. A nurse working on the first shift is frequently late, resulting in the charge nurse having to provide client care. Since the only source of information is the recorded shift report, the nurse must call the second-shift nurse at home. What is the most effective intervention for this situation?

□ 1. Assess the impact of the tardiness on client care.
□ 2. Tell the second-shift nurse to remain until the nurse arrives.
□ 3. Tell the nurse to avoid calling the second-shift nurse at home.
□ 4. Help the nurse determine the cause/s of the frequent tardiness.

16. An adult client has a severe nosebleed. The nurse should assist the client to assume which of the following positions?

- □ 1. Upright with neck hyperextended.
- □ 2. Trendelenburg position.
- □ 3. Supine with head to the side.
- □ 4. Upright with head tilted forward.

17. AF A client is admitted to the hospital for total knee replacement. The nurse is reconciling the medications the client takes at home with those ordered by the physician for use in the hospital. The nurse should do which of the following? Select all that apply.

- □ 1. Document all medications the client brought to the hospital.
- □ 2. Verify medications dispensed by the hospital are the same as those the client takes at home.
- □ 3. Ask client if he takes medications other than those he brought with him.
- □ 4. Report to the pharmacist discrepancies between what medications the client brought to the hospital and what is currently ordered.
- □ 5. Only administer medications prescribed by the physician for use during hospitalization.

18. The nurse has administered a preoperative medication to a client scheduled for surgery. The nurse charts the medication after the administration and then realizes that medication was charted on the wrong client record. The nurse should:

- □ 1. Erase the mistake and document the medication on the correct record.
- □ 2. Write the word "error" next to the mistake and initial it.
- □ 3. Draw a line through the mistake, write the word "error," and initial it.
- □ 4. Notify the nursing supervisor so a witness to the error can be documented.

19. A nursing unit secretary is answering the telephone. The charge nurse realizes that the secretary needs further instruction when the secretary states:

- □ 1. "If a physician calls, I can give information about the client."
- □ 2. "If a client's priest calls, I can give information from the client's record."
- □ 3. "If the primary nurse calls, I can give information about the client."
- □ 4. "Under no circumstances should I give information about a client to a family member or friend."

20. A client has had a suprapubic catheter in place for 2 days. Which of the following activities can the nurse delegate to the UAP?

- □ 1. Clean the area around the catheter.
- □ 2. Determine adequacy of the output.
- □ 3. Instruct the client how to care for the catheter.
- □ 4. Change the catheter.

21. A client relates a past history of swelling and wheezing after being stung by a bee. The nurse should instruct the client to carry an emergency kit containing which of the following medications?

- □ 1. Diphenhydramine (Benadryl).
- □ 2. Ephedrine.
- □ 3. Epinephrine.
- □ 4. Hydrocortisone.

22. A child had cleaning fluid splashed in his eye and is screaming and holding the eye. What should the nurse tell the mother to do first?

- □ 1. Apply a light bandage over the eye so the child cannot rub it.
- □ 2. Calm the child so that emergency treatment can be started.
- □ 3. Hold the child's head under the faucet and let water run over the eyeball.
- □ 4. Take the child and the cleaning fluid to the emergency department.

23. Following a disaster, the triage nurse should instruct the client-transporters to place which of the following clients in the only vacant treatment room?

- □ 1. Ambulatory client with a hairline fracture of the humerus.
- □ 2. Semicomatose client with a large bruise on the abdomen.
- □ 3. Client in a wheelchair with pressure dressings on both thighs.
- □ 4. Ambulatory client with first- and second-degree burns on the upper limbs.

24. During surgery, the nurse should call a "time out" on observing another nurse do which of the following?

- □ 1. Move instruments from a sterile towel to a sterile bowl.
- □ 2. Place a sterile drape in position from front to back.
- □ 3. Keep sterile, gloved hands below waist level.
- □ 4. Discard sterile supplies into a waste receptacle.

25. The nurse is admitting a client in respiratory distress to the emergency department. The client has several bruises on both arms. It is appropriate for the nurse to ask the client which of the following questions during the admission process?

- □ 1. If you become unable to make the decision, do you want to be resuscitated?

□ 2. Would you like us to tell someone that you are here?
□ 3. If you become unable to make decisions, do you want the agency to handle your legal affairs?
□ 4. Are you now or have you ever been physically abused by person or persons that live with you?

26. A client with severe chest trauma is admitted to the emergency department. What should the nurse do first?
□ 1. Obtain an explicit description of the cause.
□ 2. Determine the extent of the injuries to the chest.
□ 3. Identify the client's ability to communicate.
□ 4. Determine history of allergic reaction.

27. A client with a history of chronic renal failure had an abdominal hysterectomy and a bilateral oophorectomy. The client will take hormone-replacement therapy on discharge from the hospital. The nurse can delegate which of the following activities to the LPN?
□ 1. Make a referral to an exercise program.
□ 2. Explain the relationship between renal failure and decreased estrogen levels.
□ 3. Provide client teaching about side effects associated with estrogen and progesterone.
□ 4. Change the client's dressing.

28. A HCP instructs the nurse, who is having difficulty placing a catheter in the bladder of a client with benign prostate hypertrophy (BPH), to use a stylet. The nurse should:
□ 1. Refuse to comply.
□ 2. Perform the procedure.
□ 3. Offer to assist the HCP.
□ 4. Contact the immediate supervisor.

29. During shift change report, the nurse receives the following information about assigned clients. Which of the following clients should the nurse see first? The client with:
□ 1. Hydronephrosis, scheduled for surgery tomorrow morning.
□ 2. Possible pelvic inflammatory disease, admitted 1 hr ago.
□ 3. Transurethral resection of prostate (TURP) with bladder irrigation.
□ 4. Radical mastectomy who does not know if the excised tissue is cancerous.

30. Four clients need attention immediately. The nurse could delegate which of the following to the LPN?
□ 1. Suction the airway of a client with a tracheotomy with copious drainage.
□ 2. Reinforce an abdominal dressing that has moderate serous drainage.
□ 3. Take the BP of a client during a severe hypertensive crisis.
□ 4. Teach a client refusing a procedure about the expected outcome of the procedure.

Answers and Rationales

1. 1, 2, 4 When there is a time out called prior to surgery, the surgical team must read back all orders, verify the correct procedure, verify the site, double-check the x-ray, and reidentify the client. The sterile field has not been disrupted and does not need to be set up again. The client has received preoperative medication and cannot make decisions at this time. (S)

2. 2 The client with negative troponin and CK-MB levels rule out an MI and can be safely cared for by the UAP. The client with a pulmonary artery catheter requires close monitoring by a nurse. The client with chest pain requires close monitoring and interventions by a nurse. Client teaching is performed by the nurse. (S)

3. 3, 4, 1, 2 The client with marginal BP is assessed first; this client also has mild tachycardia and could be at risk for bleeding or shock. The client with pain is assessed second, and pain medication administered if necessary. The nurse next administers the scheduled antibiotic to the postoperative client, keeping in mind there is a window of time before and after the scheduled dose time that is approximately 1 hr. The client with the discharge scheduled for noon is seen next so that the nurse can complete the client's teaching and paperwork in time for discharge. (M)

4. 3 The client's symptoms indicate urinary retention; the client is walked to the bathroom if able, as sitting on the toilet aids in urination. Dullness indicates a full bladder, and encouraging fluids will not help the client empty the bladder, but rather will cause increased distention. If the client still cannot void, the surgeon is notified for a catheterization order. (R)

5. 4 The most appropriate intervention for a temperature elevation that is unresponsive to antipyretics is a hypothermia blanket. The hands and feet of a client lying on a hypothermia blanket are wrapped to prevent frostbite. A fever of 104°F that is nonresponsive to antipyretics is a potentially life-threatening risk. Repositioning, dietary intake, and monitoring for a rash will not contribute to lowering body temperature. (M)

6. 1 The client is using the support group as a coping mechanism. Continuing to have nightmares is not an improvement of her condition. To never go to work is not coping with the trauma. Survival guilt is not effective coping. (P)

7. 1, 2, 3 When the nurse is triaging burned clients, the following clients are transferred to a burn center: children under 10 years of age or adults over 50 years of age with 10% or greater second- and third-degree burns; clients between 11 and 49 years of age with 20% second- and third-degree burns; clients of any age with more than 5% third-degree burns; clients with smoke inhalation; and clients with chronic diseases such as diabetes, heart, or kidney disease. (M)

8. 4, 1, 2 Victims with chemical burns, second- and third-degree burns more than 20% of body surface, and those with inhalation injury are transported to a burn center. The victim with first-degree burns of the hands, and the agitated client with first-degree burns around the knees can be treated with first aid on the scene and referred to a health care facility. (M)

9. 4 The client with hypokalemia combined with neck pain requires assessment and intervention by an RN. The UAP can take care of the other clients with assistance from the RN as required. (M)

10. 3 "Short staffed" is subjective and difficult to define and it implies cause of incident. Recording of the incident report should include objective information that can be substantiated. The other examples of documentation are appropriate. (M)

11. 4 The client indicates need for restraints from dislodging the gastrostomy tube. Prior to using restraints, the nurse must obtain an order from the HCP. The use of restraints is reevaluated frequently. (S)

12. 2, 3, 4, 1 The nurse first assesses the client's physical status and obtains details about the reasons for refusing the blood transfusion. Next, the nurse informs the client about other options as appropriate, such as synthetic plasma expanders, and then informs the client about consequences of a decision to not accept a transfusion. Last, the nurse can notify the HCP, explain the client's decision, and give the nurse's recommendations. (M)

13. 4 Documentation includes information needed to promote management of care for the client and the source of any information communicated to the nurse. (H)

14. 3 To follow protocol, the nurse reports objective data rather than personal interpretation. Since it is possible that clients' rights may be violated, the nurse must be cautious in communicating information to the possible culprit. Assessment of comfort at night is outside the first-shift nurse's boundaries of responsibility. (M)

15. 4 Discussing the problem of tardiness with the nurse directly addresses the problem. If the transfer of duties is not complete, risks to the client are obvious. Having the second-shift nurse remain does not resolve the problem, is unfair, and it is not cost-effective. Because quality nursing care requires a complete database, the first-shift nurse has to make the calls. (M)

16. 4 The client with a nosebleed is assisted into an upright position with the head tilted forward. This prevents aspiration and assists the blood in clotting. Supine with the head to the side and upright with the neck hyperextended could contribute to aspiration, and Trendelenburg position could make it difficult for the client to breathe. (S)

17. 1, 2, 3, 5 Medication reconciliation involves documenting all medications prescribed for the client, verifying with the client or family that all medications the client takes at home are being administered while the client is in the hospital (unless changed or contraindicated). The nurse also asks the client if he is taking any other medications. Discrepancies in orders are reported to the HCP who is ordering the medications. The nurse administers only drugs that are ordered to be administered in the hospital. (S)

18. 3 Charts are legal documents requiring the nurse to provide accurate information. If a charting error occurs, the nurse draws a line through the error, writes the word "error," and includes initials. Erasing charting is not acceptable. It is not sufficient to write the word "error"; the nurse must also draw the line through the error. A supervisor does not need to witness a charting error. (S)

19. 2 According to client privacy laws, information can be shared only with health care personnel. No information can be provided to religious advisors, family, friends, or business associates. (S)

20. 1 The nurse can delegate the UAP to clean the area around the catheter. The nurse makes judgments about the urine output and teaches the client about catheter care. The catheter should not require changing this soon after surgery, and the nurse contacts the HCP if the catheter does need to be changed at this time. (M)

21. 3 The client with allergies to bees is instructed to carry epinephrine (Adrenalin) in order to prevent the development of anaphylactic shock. The nurse instructs the client to know how and when to administer the drug and to seek medical attention after injecting. None of the other listed medications are effective; although an antihistamine such as Benadryl may be somewhat useful, it will not work quickly enough. (S)

22. 3 The priority is to flush the offending solution from the child's eye; this is best accomplished by letting water from a faucet run over the eyeball. The mother should attempt to calm the child, but delaying the eye flush can lead to permanent eye damage. After copious flushing, the parent is instructed to seek medical attention immediately. (S)

23. 2 Before decisions can be made about the client needs, the status of these clients requires further investigation. A hairline fracture poses no immediate risks. The client in a wheelchair has received first aid, and pressure dressings have been applied. Burns will cause severe pain and predisposes the client to infection, but reduced level of consciousness and a bruised abdomen indicate more serious injury. (M)

24. 3 Keeping sterile gloved hands below the waist level is considered a break in surgical aseptic technique. Moving instruments from a sterile towel to a sterile bowel, placing a sterile drape in position from front to back, and discarding sterile supplies into a waste receptacle are all considered acceptable surgical technique. All personnel involved must stop what they are doing and re-establish the sterile field. (S)

25. 1 On admission to the emergency department, the nurse asks the client about advanced directives. The client has rights to privacy and may not want others to know about the admission to the emergency department; however, the nurse can ask the client an open-ended question to determine if someone is with him, or if he wants someone present. The nurse does not suggest methods for handling legal affairs; open-ended questions are appropriate, such as, "Should you become unable to decide, how do you want your legal affairs handled?" The nurse does assess the client further for the cause of the bruises, but there is not sufficient evidence at this point to ask directly about abuse. (M)

26. 2 Decisions about client's care are based on assessment of the primary problem. Knowledge of the cause will contribute to the clinical picture, but does not need to be done before determining current client status. Immediate care can be performed without input from the client. Knowledge of allergies will be needed prior to administering medications. (M)

27. 4 It is within the scope of practice for the LPN to change the client's dressing. Providing client teaching or explaining about the relationship of renal failure and estrogen levels, as well as making referrals, are with the scope of practice for the RN. (M)

28. 4 Using a stylet to insert a catheter is not within the scope of nursing practice; the nurse does not assume this responsibility. The nurse can offer to assist the HCP; this action will meet the goal of relieving the client's distended bladder and have the nurse work within the scope of nursing practice. Refusing to carry out the order will not solve the client's problem. The nurse first tries to resolve the problem with the HCP, and then if unresolved, contacts the supervisor. (M)

29. 1 The client the nurse knows the least about is seen first. Effective time management is more efficient if the planning evolves from an appropriate database. The other options present definitive diagnoses. (M)

30. 2 The nurse can delegate the LPN to reinforce the dressing; it is the simplest procedure and requires the least amount of decision-making, as well as the least risk. Airway maintenance with copious drainage requires complex decision-making about oxygenation. Monitoring serial BP during a hypertensive crisis requires immediate complex decision-making and action after collecting the data. Teaching a client about a procedure, explaining the outcome, and reducing anxiety and fear are not within the scope of practice for the LPN. (M)

PART THREE

Postreview Tests

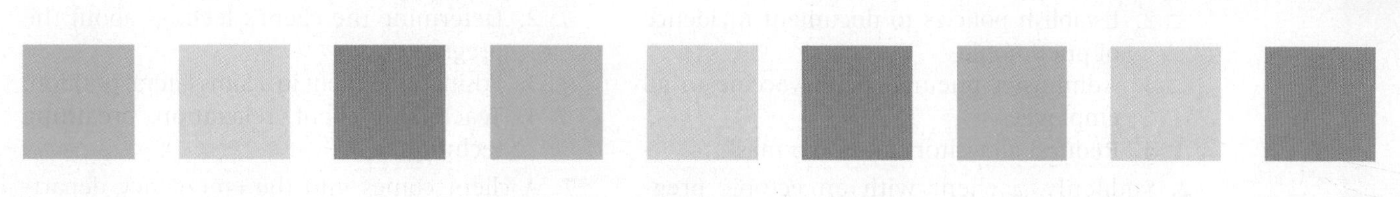

Comprehensive Practice Test 1

1. Which of the following will be most effective in reducing pneumonia in clients in long-term care facilities?
- □ 1. Require all clients to have pneumococcal vaccine prior to admission.
- □ 2. Establish policies to document incidence of pneumonia.
- □ 3. Administer pneumococcal vaccine to all employees.
- □ 4. Request all visitors to wear a mask.

2. Suddenly, a client with an ectopic pregnancy no longer meets criteria for administration of methotrexate therapy because the size of the ectopic pregnancy has increased. The client is hospitalized for a salpingostomy and experiencing abdominal pain and a drop in BP to 90/60. Heart rate is 110 and respirations are 22. What should the nurse do first?
- □ 1. Administer oxygen.
- □ 2. Place the client in Trendelenberg position.
- □ 3. Measure abdominal girth.
- □ 4. Determine the level of pain.

3. A mother tells the nurse that her infant who is 1 week of age has excessive amounts of saliva in the mouth and occasionally appears to turn dusky when taking a bottle. What should the nurse advise the mother?
- □ 1. Come to the health care facility today.
- □ 2. Enlarge the holes in the nipple.
- □ 3. Try smaller, but more frequent feedings.
- □ 4. Be sure she is "burping" the baby after every ounce of formula.

4. AF A hospital is instituting a medication safety program with an emphasis on medication reconciliation. Medication reconciliation should take place on which of the following occasions? Select all that apply.
- □ 1. When client is admitted.
- □ 2. When client moves from one room to another on same unit.
- □ 3. When client transfers from ICU to an ICU step-down unit.
- □ 4. At the change of shift.
- □ 5. At the time of discharge.

5. What diet is advisable for a preschooler with gastroenteritis once rehydration has been achieved?
- □ 1. BRAT diet (bananas, rice, applesauce, and toast or tea).
- □ 2. Full liquid diet.
- □ 3. Clear liquid diet.
- □ 4. Regular pediatric diet.

6. A pregnant woman arrives for her first prenatal visit. In preparing the client for a pelvic exam the nurse should:
- □ 1. Ask the client if she needs to empty her bladder.
- □ 2. Determine the client's feelings about the pregnancy.
- □ 3. Position the client in a Sims lateral position.
- □ 4. Teach the client relaxation breathing techniques.

7. A client comes into the emergency department having used cocaine. The nurse is assessing the client. How long should the nurse continue to assess the client for a cocaine "high"?
- □ 1. 5 to 20 min.
- □ 2. 21 to 40 min.
- □ 3. 41 to 60 min.
- □ 4. 61 to 75 min.

8. A client with human immunodeficiency virus (HIV)/acquired immunodeficiency syndrome (AIDS) who is receiving fluoxetine (Prozac) experiences an intolerable level of nervousness and anxiety. The nurse should:
- □ 1. Request prescription for anxiety.
- □ 2. Schedule an assessment of serum CD4+ levels.
- □ 3. Instruct the client to request another antidepressant.
- □ 4. Ask the client if a new stressor is causing the problems.

9. An infant who is 10 months of age has had a cleft lip repair. Immediately following surgery the nurse should do which of the following first?
- □ 1. Initiate chest physiotherapy.
- □ 2. Place the infant in the prone position.
- □ 3. Give the infant a pacifier.
- □ 4. Apply elbow restraints.

10. A child has wax in one ear canal. The parents should:
- □ 1. Observe the child for hearing impairment.
- □ 2. Teach the child to clean the ear with a Q-tip and tap water on weekly basis.
- □ 3. Do nothing; ear wax is helpful in that it removes dirt from the ear canal.
- □ 4. Apply ear drops daily for at least 3 days to soften the wax.

11. Following delivery, a client tells the nurse, "Since I delivered, I cannot get enough to drink." The nurse recognizes this is a physiologic response resulting from:
- □ 1. Excessive hormone fluctuations.
- □ 2. Fluid shifts associated with diuresis.

- □ 3. Increasing blood volume.
- □ 4. Slowed GI function.

12. AF The school nurse is teaching a substance-abuse seminar to school-aged children. The nurse should be sure the children know that which of the following drugs can cause death in school-aged children with first use? Select all that apply.
- □ 1. Inhalants.
- □ 2. Cannabis.
- □ 3. Cocaine.
- □ 4. Alcohol.
- □ 5. Hallucinogens.

13. The nurse observes a UAP helping a client with venous stasis put on antiembolism stockings. Which of the following indicates the UAP needs further instruction?
- □ 1. UAP asks the nurse to look at the client's legs prior to applying stockings.
- □ 2. UAP gets the client out of bed to ambulate after applying stockings.
- □ 3. Client's legs are elevated while sitting in the chair.
- □ 4. Client is sitting in a chair while the UAP applies stockings.

14. A pregnant woman has been in labor for 10 h. She is now 4 cm dilated, 100% effaced, plus 1 station. Contractions palpate mild to moderate in intensity and occur every 3 to 5 min. The nurse concludes that the client is in which phase of labor?
- □ 1. Active phase.
- □ 2. Antepartal phase.
- □ 3. Latent phase.
- □ 4. Transition phase.

15. In the postanesthesia care unit the nurse should do which of the following while a client recovers from general anesthesia used for abdominal surgery?
- □ 1. Place client in Trendelenburg position.
- □ 2. Keep client NPO.
- □ 3. Encourage deep breathing and coughing.
- □ 4. Withhold analgesics.

16. AF The nurse is teaching a client with acute renal failure about managing nutrition. Which of the following should the nurse include in the teaching plan? Select all that apply.
- □ 1. Drink at least 3,500 ml of fluids each day.
- □ 2. Have an adequate protein intake using high biologic-value proteins.
- □ 3. Eat foods that are high in potassium, such as beef broth or bananas.
- □ 4. Restrict phosphate intake.
- □ 5. Include foods high in sodium in the diet.

17. A nurse asks a coworker to change dressings on a client because the nurse believes that the client does not like the nurse and will refuse the needed care. Which of the following responses from the coworker is most appropriate to promote behavioral changes in the nurse?
- □ 1. "OK. He doesn't give me any problems. I will do you this favor."
- □ 2. "I'd like to, but I'm behind on my meds, and I will need to have a break today."
- □ 3. "I will ask another nurse to do this for you because I am busy right now. We should try to share his care with everyone."
- □ 4. "I'd like to help, but I think it is important for you to deal with him. He's done this to others because he has been allowed to."

18. The nurse is reviewing the health record of a child who is of school age. He has a hearing loss of 60 dB. The nurse should inform the child's teacher that this child has difficulty hearing which of the following?
- □ 1. Very loud noises.
- □ 2. Normal conversation.
- □ 3. Fire alarms.
- □ 4. Shrill sounds.

19. AF A primigravid client is admitted for an induction of labor. The nurse reviews the following progress notes:

PROGRESS NOTES

Date	Time	Progress Notes
3/11/09	2400	Client is receiving intravenous oxytocin (Pitocin), at 3 mU/hr. The latest vaginal exam revealed 2 cm dilation, 70% effacement, minus 2 station. An epidural was placed 3 hours ago. Client is experiencing no discomfort and is resting quietly. ~Nancy Hopper, RN

The nurse should do which of the following first?
- □ 1. Assess bladder fullness.
- □ 2. Discontinue oxytocin (Pitocin).
- □ 3. Discontinue epidural infusion.
- □ 4. Rupture the amniotic membrane.

20. After the third stage of labor is complete, the nurse should do which of the following?
- □ 1. Administer methylergonovine (Methergine).
- □ 2. Administer oxytocin (Pitocin).
- □ 3. Massage the uterus.
- □ 4. Perform McRoberts maneuver.

21. AF Which of the following instructions should the nurse provide a client who is

taking isoniazid (INH) 5 mg/kg PO daily? Select all that apply.

- □ 1. Take medication with meals.
- □ 2. Expect to be disease-free after 6 weeks.
- □ 3. Avoid ingestion of tyramine-containing foods.
- □ 4. Take pyridoxine (vitamin B_6) while taking the drug.
- □ 5. Use of alcoholic beverages may cause liver damage.

22. AF Two days following surgery for an abdominal hysterectomy, the client is having pain of 9 on a 10-point scale. The client has received the narcotic pain medication as ordered every 3 hr, but relief (3 on a 10-point scale) only lasts for 2 hr. The nurse has taught the client relaxation techniques, but these do not relieve the pain. The client is refusing to ambulate because of the abdominal pain and the fact that she still has an IV infusion. The nurse plans to contact the physician. Which of the following should the nurse discuss with the physician? Select all that apply.

- □ 1. Medication, dose, frequency of administration, last dose.
- □ 2. Client vital signs, including pain.
- □ 3. Effectiveness of relaxation techniques.
- □ 4. Client's refusal to ambulate.
- □ 5. Request for use of different medication(s) for pain.
- □ 6. Rate of infusion of the IV fluids.

23. A father has sprinkled cornmeal on the hospital floor under his daughter's bed. He tells the nurse not to touch it because it serves as a source of strength for his child. The nurse should:

- □ 1. Leave the cornmeal on the floor as he instructed.
- □ 2. Call housekeeping to clean the floor to prevent ants or bugs.
- □ 3. Explain that cornmeal has no such properties.
- □ 4. Ask the child whether she has noticed any effects.

24. Which of the following interventions would be most effective in preventing suicide of an adolescent who has already made two suicide attempts?

- □ 1. Refer client to peer counseling.
- □ 2. Help client learn better problem-solving.
- □ 3. Teach parents to keep medicine in a locked cabinet.
- □ 4. Help client locate a close friend at school.

25. A client in her third trimester of pregnancy is having nocturnal leg cramps. The nurse should instruct the client to:

- □ 1. Elevate lower extremities frequently during the day.
- □ 2. Perform full leg-extension exercises twice a day.
- □ 3. Increase milk consumption to one quart per day.
- □ 4. Relax in the hot tub in the evening.

26. To relive a child's feeling of thirst immediately after tonsillectomy, the nurse should offer:

- □ 1. Milk.
- □ 2. Juice.
- □ 3. Ice chips.
- □ 4. Ginger ale.

27. AF The nurse is to administer 35 mg of a drug that is dispensed in an ampoule with 25 mg/ml. The nurse should administer how many milliliters? ______________ml.

28. A child with allergic rhinitis is using a nasal antihistamine spray. When teaching the parents about the use of such sprays, the nurse should advise the parents to expect:

- □ 1. A permanent increase in nasal secretions.
- □ 2. A decrease in histamine release after an initial increase.
- □ 3. An increase in nasal secretions after an initial decrease.
- □ 4. Reflux of gastric contents into the esophagus.

29. AF A child has had a kidney transplant. The nurse is reviewing the results of the client's laboratory tests.

LABORATORY RESULTS

Test	Result
BUN	85 mg/dl
White cell count	14,000/mm3
Serum potassium	3.8 mEq/L
Red cell count	4,000/mm 3

Which of the following data suggests that the transplanted kidney is not functioning well?

- □ 1. BUN.
- □ 2. White cell count.
- □ 3. Serum potassium.
- □ 4. Red cell count.

30. A client who is in labor has been in a Fowler position for 2 hr. After palpating the contractions at moderate intensity, the nurse repositions the client to a left lateral side-lying position. An expected outcome for this nursing intervention is to:

- □ 1. Decrease fetal heart rate.
- □ 2. Increase contraction frequency.

☐ 3. Increase maternal BP.
☐ 4. Increase uterine blood flow.

31. AF A client is admitted with antisocial personality disorder. Which of the following are important interventions for the nursing staff? Select all that apply.
☐ 1. Assist client to develop new responses to behavior as they arise.
☐ 2. Ascertain that all staff members on the unit understand the plan of care.
☐ 3. Set limits for behavior with clear consequences.
☐ 4. Make expectations and consequences for behavior clear to the client.
☐ 5. Change staff assignments per client request.

32. The nurse is counseling a teenager who is sexually active. A male partner has genital herpes. To prevent spread of the infection to the female partner, the couple should:
☐ 1. Use a condom during intercourse.
☐ 2. Delay intercourse until 10 days after penicillin is begun.
☐ 3. Apply acyclovir (Zovirax) topically prior to intercourse.
☐ 4. Avoid intercourse until a Papanicolaou test is negative.

33. An otherwise healthy adolescent has not had a menstrual cycle for 3 months. The nurse should first:
☐ 1. Schedule a Pap smear.
☐ 2. Schedule a mammogram.
☐ 3. Review the dietary and exercise history.
☐ 4. Obtain a specimen for serum estrogen level.

34. A child has severe diarrhea and poor skin turgor. His body temperature has increased 3°F. The nurse should give which of the following fluids first?
☐ 1. Chicken broth.
☐ 2. Apple juice.
☐ 3. Jell-O.
☐ 4. Oral rehydration therapy.

35. AF A client who is 17 years of age writes a suicide note and then swallows aspirin. Which of the following factors are frequently associated with adolescent suicide attempts? Select all that apply.
☐ 1. Client is identified by others as a "loner."
☐ 2. Client states he has been feeling sad lately.
☐ 3. Client took only six aspirins, so he has some left.
☐ 4. Client's parents were recently divorced.
☐ 5. Client recently broke up with his girlfriend.

36. The laboring client tells the nurse that the pain with her contractions is located primarily in her lower back. To relieve pain, the nurse should first:
☐ 1. Administer analgesia.
☐ 2. Allow rest between contractions.
☐ 3. Apply counterpressure in the area.
☐ 4. Contact the health care provider (HCP) to administer epidural pain medication.

37. When providing teaching for parents of children with sickle cell disease, the nurse should stress the importance of which of the following?
☐ 1. Diet high in iron and vitamin C.
☐ 2. Restricting the use of antibiotics.
☐ 3. Avoiding environmental allergens.
☐ 4. Maintaining a high fluid intake.

38. A client who is 14 years of age is admitted to the hospital a second time for treatment for anorexia nervosa. Her response to questions are either yes, no, or no response. The primary nursing goal in caring for this adolescent is to:
☐ 1. Encourage client to eat a nutritious diet.
☐ 2. Develop rapport with client, leading to a trusting relationship.
☐ 3. Decrease client anxiety as soon as possible.
☐ 4. Relieve client anger so she can respond to questions.

39. A client who is 6 years of age is being evaluated for possible hyperactivity. His mother reports that he is just "all boy." Which of the following data would be most important to assess to help evaluate his behavior?
☐ 1. Whether he was breast- or bottle-fed as an infant.
☐ 2. Family medical history for circulatory illnesses.
☐ 3. A review of the boy's typical day.
☐ 4. Past medical history for communicable diseases.

40. A client with high cholesterol is taking fenofibrate (TriCor). The nurse should teach the client about which of the following?
☐ 1. Take the medication with food.
☐ 2. Report increased gallbladder attacks.
☐ 3. Have regular liver function laboratory tests.
☐ 4. Take cholestyramine (Questran) and fenofibrate (TriCor) concurrently.

41. A child who is 7 years of age is admitted to the hospital for a fractured femur. He has skeletal traction applied. Which of the following would be most effective in preventing muscle atrophy in his unaffected leg?
☐ 1. Passive range-of-motion exercises.
☐ 2. Quadriceps-setting exercises.
☐ 3. Kicking a balloon at the foot of the bed.
☐ 4. Massaging the leg every 4 hr.

42. A client is taking phenytoin (Dilantin) 100 mg PO 3 times a day for a seizure disorder. The nurse should instruct the client about which of the following?

- □ 1. The urine may turn pink.
- □ 2. There may be abnormal bruising.
- □ 3. Client can continue normal activities.
- □ 4. Client should withhold medication if GI disturbance occurs.

43. Immediately following surgery, a client who had a prostatectomy is experiencing pain unrelieved by oral analgesics. The client has a catheter with continuous bladder irrigation. The nurse should:

- □ 1. Increase tension on the catheter.
- □ 2. Examine the dressing for bleeding.
- □ 3. Decrease the rate of the continuous irrigation fluid.
- □ 4. Administer oxybutynin (Ditropan) 5 mg PO.

44. **AF** A client is brought to the emergency department with an intentional overdose of meperidine (Demerol). The nurse should assess the client for which of the following? Select all that apply.

- □ 1. Rapid respirations.
- □ 2. Hypertension.
- □ 3. Convulsions.
- □ 4. Slurred speech.
- □ 5. Clammy skin.

45. The morning after a lumbar puncture, a client reports a severe headache. The nurse should assess the client for which of the following?

- □ 1. Decreased tendon reflexes.
- □ 2. History of sinus headaches.
- □ 3. Headache ceases when client lies down.
- □ 4. Widened pulse pressure with hypotension.

46. **AF** At 0700, prior to planning care for a client with increasing ICP, the nurse reviews the progress notes below.

PROGRESS NOTES

Date	Time	Progress Notes
5/19/09	0600	Client was restless all night. Glasgow coma score decreased from 12 at 2400 to 6 at 0600. Vital signs = T = 99, P = 110, R = 22, BP = 150/85. Codeine 30 mg per mouth at 0200 relieved headache. IV of Normal Saline infusing at 125 gtts/minute. ~Donna Scott, RN

The nurse should do which of the following first?

- □ 1. Decrease IV infusion rate.
- □ 2. Lower head of the bed.
- □ 3. Administer oxygen as ordered.
- □ 4. Give codeine 30 mg PO as needed for headache.

47. Five months following a tubal ligation, a client who is also taking an oral contraceptive reports that her menstrual period is 5 weeks late and she has been spotting. The nurse should do which of the following first?

- □ 1. Tell client to stop taking the oral contraceptive.
- □ 2. Assess client's emotional response to her delayed period.
- □ 3. Determine client's sexual activity since the tubal ligation.
- □ 4. Assess amount of spotting and characteristics of the drainage.

48. **AF** The nurse is assessing the anterior fontanelle of an infant who is 2 months of age. Where should the nurse place the fingers to palpate the anterior fontanelle?

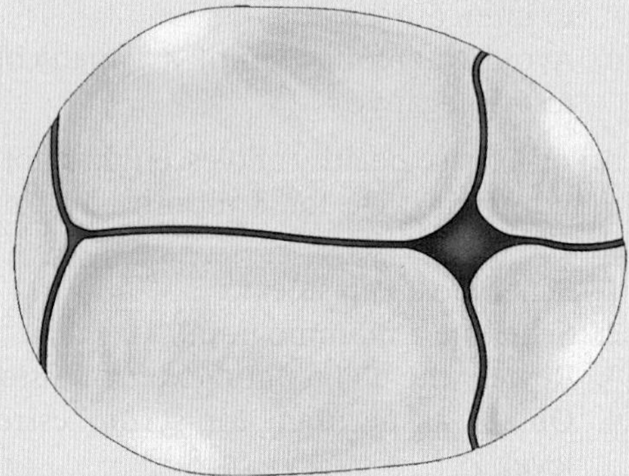

49. A client who is 35 years of age has multiple sclerosis. Which of the following are realistic goals for this client? The client will:

- □ 1. Adapt to the irreversible immobility.
- □ 2. Take hot showers and sunbathe if desired.
- □ 3. Experience recovery with each remission.
- □ 4. Attend regular therapy sessions to manage suicidal thoughts.

50. Prevention of social isolation is a goal on the care plan of a client with human immunodeficiency virus (HIV)/acquired immunodeficiency syndrome (AIDS). Which of the following interventions will have the best success in meeting this goal?

- □ 1. Refer client to a HIV/AIDS support group.
- □ 2. Enlist assistance of family and friends.
- □ 3. Help client learn to be self-sufficient.
- □ 4. Refer client for counseling.

51. A client is recently diagnosed with thromboangiitis obliterans (Buerger disease).

Changing which of the following behaviors will be most important for this client?
- □ 1. Client wears open-toed shoes.
- □ 2. Client uses acetaminophen (Tylenol) every 4 hr to manage pain.
- □ 3. Client goes to the beach without sunscreen.
- □ 4. Client is a tobacco smoker.

52. A client is hospitalized for exacerbation of COPD. The nurse is preparing the client for discharge. Which of the following is a realistic outcome for this client?
- □ 1. Client sleeps without pillows.
- □ 2. Client has decreased sputum production.
- □ 3. Client plans activities within respiratory limitations.
- □ 4. Client maintains ABGs within normal limits.

53. A client is scheduled to receive amphotericin B 0.3 mg/kg IV daily and digoxin (Lanoxin) 0.25 mg PO daily. The nurse should:
- □ 1. Monitor hepatic function.
- □ 2. Monitor for an allergic reaction.
- □ 3. Request a prescription for a potassium supplement.
- □ 4. Schedule the drugs to be given to the client so that pharmacokinetics do not overlap.

54. Following surgery for a fractured femur, an adult client returns home. Which of the following goals should be included in the care plan?
- □ 1. Client refrains from using analgesics.
- □ 2. Client demonstrates ability to use an immobilizing device.
- □ 3. Client understands that bone healing will take 3 to 6 months.
- □ 4. Client reports swelling and discoloration remaining after 48 hr.

55. A committee of RNs is developing a plan to reduce the incidence of sepsis at their health care facility. Which of the following topics is appropriate for a staff-development program for the UAP at this facility?
- □ 1. Subtle signs of infection in the older adult.
- □ 2. Relationship between fever and infection.
- □ 3. How hand hygiene can interrupt the infection chain.
- □ 4. Policies regarding infection control.

56. When performing perineal care for a multigravida who is at 42 weeks' gestation, the client's membranes rupture. The nurse notices meconium-stained fluid. What priority nursing action should be taken?
- □ 1. Begin an amnioinfusion.
- □ 2. Monitor fetal heart tones.
- □ 3. Notify the physician.
- □ 4. Place the fetal scalp electrode.

57. Which one of the following clients is at the greatest risk for melanoma?
- □ 1. Asian client who is 22 years of age with multiple nevi.
- □ 2. White client who is 45 years of age with family history of melanoma.
- □ 3. White client who is 33 years of age with a history of tanning bed use.
- □ 4. Native American client who is 67 years of age and living in the high desert.

58. A client with compartment syndrome is scheduled for a fasciotomy. Which of the following is the priority nursing goal following surgery?
- □ 1. Relieve pain.
- □ 2. Manage anxiety.
- □ 3. Promote tissue perfusion.
- □ 4. Improve nutrition.

59. A client is scheduled for an emergency appendectomy. Prior to transport to the operating room, agency policy requires a second staff signature on the informed consent form. After signing the form, the nurse should ask which of the following individuals to sign the form?
- □ 1. Family member in the room with the client.
- □ 2. Unit UAP who is a notary.
- □ 3. Religious advisor who is present.
- □ 4. LPN.

60. A client with type 2 diabetes mellitus is having difficulty with dietary management. Which of the following approaches will be most effective in helping the client follow the diet?
- □ 1. Determine client's food preferences.
- □ 2. Help client identify the problem with dietary management.
- □ 3. Ask client to develop a meal plan for a 2-week period.
- □ 4. Have client monitor daily fingerstick blood sugar levels.

61. The nurse is instructing a woman who is having hot flashes about the advantages and disadvantages of hormone-replacement therapy, but determines the client's religious beliefs prohibit the use of hormone-replacement therapy. The nurse can assist the client by doing which of the following?
- □ 1. Teach client about the characteristics of ginseng.
- □ 2. Explore the religious beliefs interfering with health maintenance.
- □ 3. Explain that estrogen is produced by the body and is not a foreign substance.

□ 4. Advise that pyridoxine (vitamin B_6) may be used for hot flashes.

62. An infant has undergone cleft palate repair. The nurse should instruct the parents to do which of the following when feeding their infant?
- □ 1. Hold infant semiupright while feeding.
- □ 2. Position infant on the abdomen after feeding.
- □ 3. Avoid burping infant during feeding.
- □ 4. Remove metal appliance taped to the cheeks during feeding.

63. The nurse is teaching a pregnant client who is 37 years of age about managing her severe bilateral leg varicose veins. The nurse concludes that the client understands the instruction when the client says she will avoid which of the following?
- □ 1. Vitamin C intake.
- □ 2. Exercising.
- □ 3. Standing for prolonged periods.
- □ 4. Wearing antiembolism hose.

64. A client is receiving an oral narcotic for chronic back pain. Which statement indicates that the client is following a realistic, positive pain-management plan?
- □ 1. "I will continue to have pain between my pain medication dosages."
- □ 2. "I should wait until I begin to feel pain before I take the next dose of pain medication."
- □ 3. "When I go home I should be able to perform my daily activities of care without being limited by pain."
- □ 4. "When I go home, if my pain stops me from doing my daily activities of care, I should decrease my activities."

65. A client with heart failure is receiving digoxin (Lanoxin) as ordered. The client's serum potassium is 3.2 mEq/L. The nurse interprets the serum potassium level as:
- □ 1. This is an expected finding.
- □ 2. The client is at increased risk for digitalis toxicity.
- □ 3. The client may have had a myocardial infarction.
- □ 4. The digoxin dose may need to be increased.

66. A client is admitted with third-degree heart block. The nurse can evaluate client teaching regarding the anticipated treatment as being effective when the client says which of the following?
- □ 1. "I understand I will be going for an angiogram so the doctor can look for blockages."
- □ 2. "I understand I will be given pills to keep my heart beat regular."
- □ 3. "I understand the doctor will put in a pacemaker to keep my heart rate normal."
- □ 4. "I understand that I will not need treatment unless my heart rate goes above 120."

67. A primigravida has been in labor for 12 hr. She is 8 cm dilated with profuse bloody show, 100% effaced, and has contractions every 2 to 3 min lasting 90 s. The client is irritable and complains, "I can't do this anymore!" The nurse concludes the client is:
- □ 1. About to have a precipitous delivery.
- □ 2. Having titanic contractions.
- □ 3. Hemorrhaging.
- □ 4. Making expected progress.

68. During a physical assessment of a client diagnosed with amyotrophic lateral sclerosis 6 months ago, the nurse should expect to find:
- □ 1. Absence of reflexes.
- □ 2. Impaired cognitive function.
- □ 3. Muscle atrophy.
- □ 4. Sensory loss.

69. The nurse is counseling a pregnant woman who smokes. Which of the following plans of care would be most effective?
- □ 1. Ask the physician to order transdermal nicotine.
- □ 2. Report the client to Child Protective Services.
- □ 3. Support the client to reduce cigarette consumption daily.
- □ 4. Tell the client she must stop smoking immediately.

70. The nurse is planning care for a client with heart failure. A nursing intervention to decrease preload is to:
- □ 1. Have client lift the arms above the head.
- □ 2. Elevate the head of the bed.
- □ 3. Position client flat in left lateral position.
- □ 4. Elevate the client's feet.

71. The nurse is assessing a client who is 54 years of age with a history of coronary artery disease and hypertension. The nurse palpates the point of maximal impulse (PMI) at the sixth intercostal space lateral to the midclavicular line. The nurse should interpret this finding as which of the following?
- □ 1. PMI is in the normal location.
- □ 2. Client may have left ventricular hypertrophy and dilation.
- □ 3. Client has age-related displacement of the heart.
- □ 4. Nurse should reassess PMI during sustained expiration.

72. A gravid client in her third trimester asks the nurse if she can travel "so we can have a little vacation before the baby is born." Which of the following responses is the most important for the nurse to determine now?
- □ 1. How do you plan to travel?
- □ 2. How long do you plan to be gone?
- □ 3. Will we need to reschedule your appointment?
- □ 4. Who is going with you?

73. AF The nurse is providing care for a client who had a myocardial infarction. The nurse observes on the client's cardiac monitor that ECG changes from a normal sinus rhythm to the following pattern.

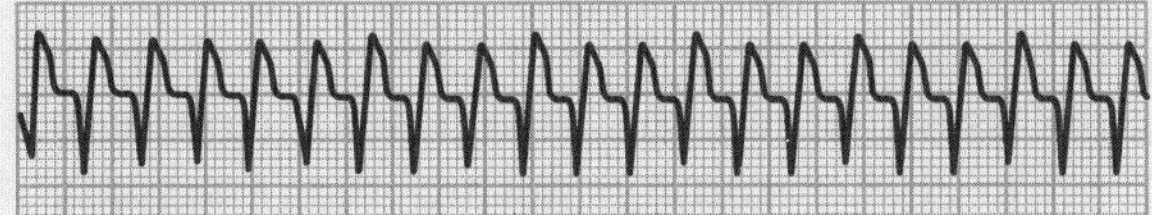

The client is alert. The nurse should do which of the following first?
- □ 1. Give a precordial thump.
- □ 2. Page the code team.
- □ 3. Administer lidocaine (Xylocaine) bolus as ordered.
- □ 4. Start CPR.

74. The nurse is assessing a client's ECG strip. The measurement of the QRS complex is 0.14 s. Which is the correct interpretation by the nurse?
- □ 1. Atrial conduction is normal.
- □ 2. Hypokalemia is present.
- □ 3. It meets the criteria for normal sinus rhythm.
- □ 4. Ventricular depolarization is prolonged.

75. The nurse is preparing a client who was hospitalized with heart failure for discharge to the home setting. The client currently is up ad lib, ambulating for short periods in the hallway. The nurse should instruct the client to do which of the following?
- □ 1. Limit walking to inside the house to avoid shortness of breath.
- □ 2. Start with the current level of walking and increase to 60 min/day within 3 weeks.
- □ 3. Increase walking to 45 min/day within 2 weeks.
- □ 4. Increase the pace and distance until able to walk 3 to 5 times per week for 45 min.

76. A client has acute pancreatitis. Which of the following is the nursing goal priority?
- □ 1. Maintain tissue integrity.
- □ 2. Relieve pain.
- □ 3. Reintroduce oral feedings.
- □ 4. Fluid replacement.

77. A client with a myocardial infarction is taking 0.81 mg of aspirin. The expected outcome of this medication is an:
- □ 1. Analgesic effect.
- □ 2. Antiplatelet effect.
- □ 3. Antipyretic effect.
- □ 4. Acidotic effect.

78. A client is admitted to the hospital with peripheral arterial occlusive disease with severe claudication. To relieve the claudication the nurse should:
- □ 1. Apply ice packs.
- □ 2. Administer heparin.
- □ 3. Encourage use of an oxygen mask.
- □ 4. Administer pentoxifylline (Trental).

79. A client is pacing rapidly on the unit. He is wringing his hands and sweating, complaining of palpitations and nausea, and is having difficulty focusing on what others say to him. The client states he feels he is having a heart attack and feels like he could die. The nurse should develop a care plan based on the fact that this client is experiencing which level of anxiety?
- □ 1. Mild.
- □ 2. Moderate.
- □ 3. Severe.
- □ 4. Panic.

80. The nurse is providing instructions for the use of the Blom-Singer voice prosthesis to a client who had a transesophageal puncture. The nurse teaches the client to perform which of the following when speaking with this prosthesis?
- □ 1. Place a vibrating device on the neck.
- □ 2. Block the stoma to redirect expired air into the esophagus.
- □ 3. Use air forced into the esophagus to create sound when releasing.
- □ 4. Speak on inspiration.

81. A client with a total laryngectomy has an oxygen saturation of 90%. Which of the following is the best delivery device for supplemental oxygen?
- □ 1. Nasal cannula.
- □ 2. Non-rebreather mask.
- □ 3. Tracheostomy collar.
- □ 4. Venturi mask.

82. A client who is 6 years of age has a severe nosebleed. The nurse should instruct the caregiver to do which of the following?
- □ 1. Pack the nose with gauze.
- □ 2. Have the child lie down.
- □ 3. Bring the child to the emergency department.
- □ 4. Pinch the nares for 15 min.

83. A client is becoming inappropriate by flirting with the nurse. The nurse should confront the behavior by taking which of the following measures?
- □ 1. Identify the behavior and define boundaries of appropriate behavior.
- □ 2. Tell the client the nurse cannot provide care if the behavior continues.
- □ 3. Ignore the behavior and leave the room.
- □ 4. Share the information in shift report and request a team conference.

84. A client is recovering from abdominal surgery. She persists in shouting for the nurse instead of using the call light, as she has been repeatedly asked to do. The other clients are disturbed by her shouting. Which of the following responses is most appropriate for the nurse to make?
- □ 1. "Please stop shouting for me instead of using your light."
- □ 2. "You must stop shouting because you are disturbing others."
- □ 3. "When you shout for me instead of using your light, I feel very frustrated because I want to take care of you as well as the other clients."
- □ 4. "I'm sorry that I can't get to your room as soon as I'd like. Please try to use the light instead of shouting for me."

85. The nurse is planning with a middle-aged client with newly diagnosed diabetes to follow a diet for management of the diabetes. Which of the following statements is least accurate regarding making the behavior change that will be required to follow this diet?
- □ 1. The client will change eating habits if the nurse provides accurate, understandable written information.
- □ 2. The nurse and client should define and solve the problem together.
- □ 3. The client's beliefs, values, and behavior will influence the ability to make effective changes in eating patterns.
- □ 4. The client will probably have difficulty changing present eating habits regardless of what information the nurse provides.

86. The nurse is attempting to help a client with cancer develop healthy coping skills. Which of the following behaviors on the part of the client indicates that she is acquiring the coping skills?
- □ 1. Client directs anger at herself instead of at her husband.
- □ 2. Client avoids contact with the nurse.
- □ 3. Client cries frequently when alone.
- □ 4. Client openly expresses feelings to her daughter.

87. A client who is admitted for a mastectomy states, "I don't want my husband to see me like this. I can't see how he can look at me with only one breast." A facilitating response from the nurse is:
- □ 1. "I know how you feel; all women feel that way at first."
- □ 2. "Don't let it bother you; you know he loves you."
- □ 3. "You're worried because you think you won't be attractive anymore."
- □ 4. "You'll have time to adjust; be patient."

88. A client is being admitted for an exploratory laparotomy for possible ovarian cancer. The goal of communication during the admission assessment for this client is for the nurse to:
- □ 1. Assert control during the assessment interview.
- □ 2. Determine what the client knows regarding health care procedures.
- □ 3. Establish a collaborative relationship with the client.
- □ 4. Convey hope for a positive outcome from the surgery.

89. AF A client is admitted to the emergency department with suspected amphetamine overdose. The nurse should assess this client for which of the following? Select all that apply.
- □ 1. Lack of coordination.
- □ 2. Agitation.
- □ 3. Seizures.
- □ 4. Elevated temperature.
- □ 5. Clammy skin.

90. The nurse is attempting to complete an admission assessment for a client. The client looks afraid, speaks in short quick sentences, and is pacing in the hall outside his room. Which intervention by the nurse will assist the client with anxiety?
- □ 1. Call the HCP for a sedative order.
- □ 2. Ask about medications the client is presently taking and check vital signs.
- □ 3. Make an introduction to the client and explain the need for information.
- □ 4. Assign a staff person to sit with the client until he is able to do the admission assessment.

91. A client is admitted following a suicide attempt. The client cut the inside of her arm from the antecubital fossa to the hand. She informed the staff that she has had multiple episodes of self-harm and has several visible scars on both arms. Based on the client's

history, diagnosis of which personality disorder does the nurse anticipate the client to receive?
- □ 1. Antisocial.
- □ 2. Dependent.
- □ 3. Passive-aggressive.
- □ 4. Borderline.

92. The hospital is following national patient safety guidelines to prevent pressure ulcers in clients. Which of the following will be most helpful?
- □ 1. Identify the risk level for each client on admission.
- □ 2. Use pressure mattresses on all beds.
- □ 3. Serve high-protein meals.
- □ 4. Establish a schedule to turn each client.

93. AF The nurse is assessing a client with long-term alcohol use. Which of the following are expected findings? Select all that apply.
- □ 1. Pancreatitis.
- □ 2. Hallucinations.
- □ 3. Depression.
- □ 4. Esophagitis.
- □ 5. Tremors.

94. On noting early decelerations on the fetal monitor tracing, the nurse concludes:
- □ 1. Client needs to have a cesarean section.
- □ 2. Fetal head is being compressed.
- □ 3. Physician must be notified.
- □ 4. Umbilical cord is being compressed.

95. AF The nurse is teaching a client with newly diagnosed diabetes mellitus. The client will be taking an oral antidiabetic agent. The nurse should include which of the following information about hypoglycemia in the teaching plan? Select all that apply.
- □ 1. Have three meals and a bedtime snack.
- □ 2. Hypoglycemia will not occur unless the client is taking insulin.
- □ 3. Symptoms of hypoglycemia can include irritability, hunger, shaking, and sweating.
- □ 4. Eat a carbohydrate snack before engaging in strenuous exercise.
- □ 5. Alcohol consumption can increase the incidence of hypoglycemia.

96. A client with septic shock received drotrecogin alfa (Xigris) 24 mcg/kg/hr. The nurse should teach the client to:
- □ 1. Eat a well-balanced diet.
- □ 2. Plan activities within energy levels.
- □ 3. Report if toothbrushing causes bleeding.
- □ 4. Report signs/symptoms of infection such as fever.

97. AF A client is admitted for posttraumatic stress disorder (PTSD). Which of the following are expected? Select all that apply.
- □ 1. Nightmares.
- □ 2. Low self-esteem.
- □ 3. Delusions.
- □ 4. Terrified appearance during a flashback.
- □ 5. Attempts to run away during flashbacks.
- □ 6. Intrusive thoughts of trauma.

98. The nurse is assessing a client who is 3 years of age who has been admitted to the emergency department with localized wheezing on auscultation. The nurse obtains a history from the child's mother. Which statement by the mother should the nurse follow up with further questioning?
- □ 1. She gives the child hard candy as an afternoon treat.
- □ 2. The child has two cousins who have many allergies.
- □ 3. The child was playing with a friend who had pneumonia 1 week ago.
- □ 4. The child was eating peanuts yesterday.

99. A client who is 14 weeks pregnant has her first prenatal visit. The following orders are written on her chart. Which order should the nurse clarify with the health care provider?
- □ 1. Schedule abdominal ultrasound.
- □ 2. Administer MMR vaccine.
- □ 3. Schedule amniocentesis.
- □ 4. Prenatal vitamins daily.

100. A hospital has established a goal of reducing methicillin-resistant *Staphylococcus aureus* (MRSA) infections. The most effective way to reduce the spread of MRSA in the hospital is by doing which of the following?
- □ 1. Restrict visitors to clients with known infections.
- □ 2. Isolate clients with known infections.
- □ 3. Use respiratory precautions.
- □ 4. Require all hospital personnel to use hand hygiene procedures.

Answers and Rationales

1. 1 The most effective way to reduce the spread of pneumonia at long-term care facilities is to require that all clients admitted have a vaccine for pneumonia. This measure prevents newly admitted clients from exposing other clients. Documenting the incidence of pneumonia provides information about the extent of the illness, but does not reduce spread. Employees will benefit from having the pneumonia vaccine, but the most effective measure is to assure that none of the clients is carrying the bacteria. It is not necessary for all visitors to wear a mask; however, the nurse can suggest that those visitors with upper respiratory infections observe hand hygiene precautions, use and properly dispose of tissues, and consider not visiting while ill. (M)

2. 1 The client is in shock and the primary goal is to reduce the threat of hypoxia; therefore, the nurse administers oxygen. Lowering the head of the bed increases blood flow to the head and may increase abdominal pressure. Measuring abdominal girth and assessing pain are relevant, but does not assist in meeting the client's immediate needs. (S)

3. 1 Any infant who has an excessive amount of frothy saliva in the mouth or difficulty with secretions and unexplained episodes of cyanosis is suspected of having an esophageal atresia/tracheoesophageal fistula and referred immediately for medical evaluation. Suggesting other alternatives is not appropriate in this circumstance.(A)

4. 1, 3, 5 The nurse checks the client's medications and medication orders on admission; all medications that the client is currently taking are reconciled with those prescribed to take in the hospital. Medications are reconciled again if the client transfers from one unit to the next as the medication orders may change; and then again at discharge to home or another health care facility. It is not necessary to perform medication reconciliation procedures when the client moves to a different room on the same nursing unit, or at the change of shift. (M)

5. 4 In older children, a regular diet can generally be offered after rehydration is achieved. Early reintroduction of nutrients is desirable. Continued feeding or early reintroduction of a normal diet has no adverse effects and actually lessens the severity and duration of the illness. A diet of easily digestible foods such as cereals, cooked vegetables, and meats is adequate for the older child. A BRAT diet is contraindicated because the diet has little nutritional value (low in energy and protein), is high in carbohydrates, and is low in electrolytes. (H)

6. 1 The nurse offers the client the opportunity to empty her bladder prior to the pelvic exam. An empty bladder will decrease pelvic pressure and discomfort experienced during the exam. Determining the client's feelings about the pregnancy and teaching the client about relaxation breathing techniques are not interventions that will facilitate the pelvic exam. The female client needs to be in the lithotomy position for the exam. (M)

7. 1 The "high" from the cocaine lasts from 5 to 20 min. The nurse needs to monitor the client during that time as the client could die. (D)

8. 3 Nervousness and anxiety are common side effects of antidepressants. If the client finds the experience intolerable, the nurse instructs the client to request another medication. Altered CD4+ levels place the client at risk for infection, but not necessarily related to fluoxetine (Prozac). Since the known information indicates the drug is the problem, the drug is eliminated first. If a new stressor is causing the problem, the drug is not effective. (D)

9. 4 The major efforts in the postoperative period are directed toward protecting the operative site. Elbow restraints are used to prevent the infant from rubbing or disturbing the suture line and are applied immediately after surgery. It is important to remove the elbow restraints one at a time periodically to exercise the arms and to provide relief from the restrictions and to observe the skin integrity. (S)

10. 3 No action is needed as ear wax rarely leads to hearing impairment. Excess removal can interfere with its function of removing dirt from the ear canal. It is not necessary to clean the ear with a Q-tip or apply ear drops. (H)

11. 2 The rapid diuresis and diaphoresis that occur during the second to fifth postpartal days result in a weight loss of approximately 5 pounds. Women often feel thirsty during this period and want additional fluid. Although hormone fluctuations occur after delivery, these fluctuations do not have an affect on the client's thirst. Blood volume decreases after delivery. GI function returns to normal activity once delivery is accomplished. (A)

12. 1, 3 For children of school age, the drugs that most often cause death on first use include inhalants and cocaine. Both of these drugs may cause heart problems and collapse. (D)

13. 4 Venous pooling and edema occur when the feet are placed in a dependent position with standing or sitting. Application of antiembolism stockings before getting out of bed prevents the veins from becoming engorged. Stockings are removed periodically to inspect the skin. The client's legs can be elevated in bed to promote venous return. (M)

14. 1 In the active phase of labor the cervical dilation ranges from 3 to 7 cm. During the latent phase of labor, cervical dilation ranges from 0 to 3 cm, and during the transition phase from 7 to 10 cm. Effacement and descent occur as the fetus descends into the maternal pelvis. Complete effacement (cervical thinning) is 100%. Zero station is engagement, plus 1,2,3,4 stations indicate where the presenting part is located in relation to the maternal ischial spines. (M)

15. 3 While the client is in the postanesthesia care unit, the nurse encourages deep breathing and coughing. The nurse also elevates the head of the bed to a semi-Fowler position to promote ventilation of lungs with descent of the diaphragm. Deep breathing and coughing facilitates gas exchange and promotes return to consciousness. Maintaining NPO status is not necessary once the client is conscious and the gag reflex has returned. The client can have pain medication as ordered. (A)

16. 2, 4 The challenge of nutritional management in renal failure is to provide adequate calories to prevent catabolism despite the restrictions required to prevent electrolyte and fluid disorders, and azotemia. If the client does not receive adequate nutrition, catabolism of body protein will occur. This process causes increased urea, phosphate, and potassium levels. To absorb calcium from the GI tract, activated vitamin D must be present. Only functioning kidneys can activate vitamin D, allowing absorption to occur. Phosphate is released from bone when hypocalcemia occurs. Elevated serum phosphate levels are also a result of its decreased excretion by the kidneys. When urinary output decreases, fluid retention occurs; encouraging a high fluid intake is not recommended. A nurse does not encourage foods/fluids high in potassium; the serum potassium levels are already increased because the normal ability of the kidneys to excrete the majority of the body's potassium is impaired. Excessive intake of sodium is avoided because this can lead to volume expansion, hypertension, and heart failure. Water excess can lead to cerebral edema. (H)

17. 4 The nurse can encourage behavioral change in a colleague by expressing support for the colleague's feelings and providing information about the client. The other responses allow the client's behavior to continue and do not help the nurse deal with the behavior. (P)

18. 2 Normal conversation is conducted at about 50 dB, and thus the child will not be able to hear normal conversation or whispering. The child has a hearing loss that will need to be treated. The nurse follows up with the audiologist to be sure the child is receiving care. The child will be able to hear fire alarms, loud noises, and shrill sounds, but will require follow-up care for his hearing loss. (H)

19. 1 A full bladder can impede fetal descent; the nurse encourages the client to void every 2 to 4 hr. If the client demonstrates inability to void and the bladder becomes distended, she may need to be catheterized. Oxytocin (Pitocin) is used to cause labor contractions, leading to delivery of the infant. The epidural infusion relaxes the client and may cause the uterine contractions to fade; the Pitocin keeps the contractions continuing. Rupturing amniotic fluid is not within the scope of the practice for the nurse. (M)

20. 2 Oxytocin (Pitocin) is given to stimulate uterine contractions after delivery of the placenta (third stage) to reduce uterine bleeding. Methergine is available (when Pitocin is ineffective) for uterine atony, subinvolution, leading to risk for hemorrhaging. Massage to the uterus would be appropriate if the uterus was not responding to the oxytocic medicines. The McRoberts maneuver is used to assist with labor dystocia. (D)

21. 3, 4, 5 Ingesting tyramine-containing foods with INH may result in a hypertensive crisis. INH is vitamin B_6-depleting. Ingestion of alcoholic beverages on a regular basis may compound the risk of hepatotoxicity. INH should be taken on an empty stomach. Clients are considered disease-free after negative sputum specimens, which may take 6 to 9 months. (D)

22. 1, 2, 3, 4, 5 The nurse provides the HCP with information about the Situation, Background, Assessment, and Recommendation (SBAR). The nurse informs the HCP that the client is refusing to get out of bed because of the pain and the lack of pain relief. The nurse reports vital signs so the HCP can determine that respirations, which could be depressed by narcotic pain medication, are adequate. The nurse also provides information about the history of pain relief from medications and relaxation. The nurse can recommend that the HCP collaborate with the client and nurse to try another approach to pain relief. The rate of infusion of the IV is irrelevant in this situation. (M)

23. 1 Respecting cultural traditions and beliefs is a major component of culturally competent care. The other actions do not demonstrate respect for the father's belief that cornmeal will give strength to his child. The nurse should respect client's requests to implement traditions and beliefs as long as they are not harmful to the client, other clients, or the health care team. (P)

24. 2 Suicide is a solution when there does not appear to be any other solution. Helping an adolescent learn better problem-solving can help prevent a second attempt. The other options do not deal with the underlying problem and are short-term solutions. (P)

25. 1 Elevating lower extremities improves circulation and helps relieve muscle cramps during pregnancy. Full leg-extension exercises such as stretching with toes pointed should be avoided. Reducing milk consumption to 1 pint per day and supplementing with calcium lactate can help reduce the phosphorus levels in the body. Pregnant women should avoid hot tubs as it can cause hyperthermia, which can interfere with fetal cell metabolism. (C)

26. 3 Immediately after surgery the nurse offers the child ice chips. Milk clings to the back of the pharynx so it is difficult to swallow. Juice can sting the surgical site. Ginger ale bubbles can be irritating. Ice chips are soothing. (C)

27. 1.4 ml. 35 mg/xml = 25mg/1ml x = 1.4 (D)

28. 3 Nasal antihistamine sprays reduce inflammation at first; after 3 days they actually cause inflammation, and are therefore used on a short-term basis. The sprays do not cause reflux of gastric contents into the esophagus. (D)

29. 1 An elevated BUN indicates the kidney is not excreting nitrogenous wastes from the body. This is an undesirable finding for a client with a recent renal transplant. An elevated white cell count is a sign of an infection. The serum potassium is normal. The red cell count is normal. (A)

30. 4 The left lateral side-lying position causes the heavy uterus to tip forward, away from the vena cavae, allowing free blood return from the lower extremities and adequate placental filling and circulation. Assuming this position decreases maternal BP. Positioning the client is a comfort measure; decreasing fetal heart rate and increasing contraction frequency are not goals of positioning. (C)

31. 2, 3, 4 The client with an antisocial personality disorder is frequently manipulative. The nurse develops the care plan to describe expectations of the client and consequences for behaviors; and makes certain the client and all unit staff understand the components of the care plan. Client assessment before developing the care plan is complete enough that no new behaviors would need to be described. Stable staff assignments are important when dealing with a client with this personality disorder. (P)

32. 1 Condoms provide protection against the spread of sexually transmitted diseases as well as acting as a contraceptive. Penicillin is used to treat syphilis. Applying acyclovir (Zovirax) prior to intercourse will not prevent the spread of the herpes. A Papanicolaou test is done to identify cervical cancer. (H)

33. 3 Adolescents often eat improperly and exercise vigorously to reach weight control goals. Because an adequate amount of body fat is necessary for ovulation, the nurse first determines dietary intake and exercise patterns. Since this age group is not at risk for cancer, the Pap smear would not be the next step. The most common sign/symptom of uterine cancer is vaginal bleeding. The density of breast tissue is similar to the density of cancerous tissue in the breast; therefore, mammograms are not an effective diagnostic tool for this age group. Since estrogen contributes to the development and maintenance of secondary sex characteristics, the client would need to present with deficits in this area to justify assessment of the hormone level. (H)

34. 4 Infants and children with acute diarrhea and dehydrations are first treated with oral rehydration therapy; this is more effective, safer, less painful, and less costly than IV rehydration. Fruit juices and gelatin have high carbohydrate content, very low electrolyte content, and high osmolarity. Chicken broth is not given because it contains excessive sodium and inadequate carbohydrates. (A)

35. 4, 5 Adolescents are at high risk for suicide. Suicide is often the result of a loss such as a girlfriend, a parent, or self-esteem. The divorce of the client's parents and the breakup with the girlfriend represent losses that will be permanent and puts the client at risk again. Adolescents may be "loners" or feel sad, but are generally not at risk for suicide. The nurse instructs the caregiver to create a safe environment by removing drugs that can be dangerous if swallowed, but the underlying problem of the loss and how the adolescent is dealing with it must be addressed immediately. (P)

36. 3 The nurse first tries nonpharmacologic approaches to pain management. Using the palm of the hand to apply counterpressure to the client's lower back often helps to relieve back pain during labor. If this does not help, the nurse can administer analgesics as prescribed. Resting between contractions is used during the second stage of labor if the fetus is experiencing signs of distress. The nurse can contact the HCP for an epidural if the client chooses this method of pain management. (C)

37. 4 A high fluid intake decreases blood viscosity and the likelihood that sickled cells will occlude capillaries, precipitating sickle cell crisis. A diet high in iron is not necessary although patients should take daily folic acid supplements to aid in erythropoiesis. Clients with sickle cell disease are at increase risk for infection and frequently need antibiotic therapy. Environmental allergens do not play a role in sickle cell disease. (H)

38. 2 Children with eating disorders may have low self-esteem, yet high expectations for themselves. Therapy to reverse their feelings about themselves begins with establishing a trusting relationship with HCPs. (P)

39. 3 The nurse evaluates the child's behavior by taking a careful history and documenting attention span and activities. Type of feeding and history of circulatory illness or communicable diseases do not contribute to hyperactivity. (A)

40. 1 Taking the medication with food increases gastric transit time, resulting in increased absorption. Because the drug may cause cholelithiasis, it is contraindicated in gallbladder disease. The client should have regular liver function tests. Bile acid sequestrants bind with the drug and decrease its effectiveness. (D)

41. 3 Children who do not feel sick are usually interested in active games to prevent boredom and preserve strength and prevent atrophy in unaffected muscles. Kicking a balloon is one way to engage the child in needed active exercises. Passive range of motion and massage do not require muscle movement needed to prevent atrophy. Quadriceps-setting exercises are muscle-specific, and this child should use all of the muscles in his unaffected leg. (H)

42. 2 A major side effect of phenytoin (Dilantin) is reduction in red blood cells and platelets; the client may bruise easily. Typically, there is no change in the color of urine. Drowsiness may occur initially, so the client is instructed to avoid activities requiring precision until this side effect subsides. Abrupt withdrawal may result in significant increase in seizure activity. (D)

43. 4 Pain unrelieved by analgesics immediately following a prostatectomy is usually associated with bladder spasms; to relieve spasms, the nurse first tries administering the oxybutynin (Ditropan). Placing tension on the catheter may be used to treat bladder spasm, but is generally adjusted by the surgeon. The nurse assesses dressing for bleeding, but pain is not related to bleeding. The nurse does not decrease the rate of the bladder irrigation as the irrigation fluid is used to prevent obstruction of the catheter. (D)

44. 3, 4, 5 The client with a meperidine (Demerol) overdose will have convulsions, slurred speech (if able to speak), and clammy skin. Respirations will be slow and shallow. BP will be low. (D)

45. 3 Spinal headaches following a lumbar puncture can occur if the client stands up, and tends to be reduced or alleviated when the client lies down. The client is instructed to remain in bed with the head slightly elevated for 24 hr after a lumbar puncture. A blood patch is the primary treatment for spinal headaches. Because it is common to have spinal headaches after a lumbar puncture, unless findings indicate otherwise, the headaches are not likely related to sinus problems. Decreased deep tendon reflexes are associated with spinal cord injuries or increased intracranial pressure. Widened pulse pressure and hypotension is associated with increased intracranial pressure. The nurse assesses the client for spinal headache before addressing more serious side effects. (A)

46. 3 The priority for the client with increasing ICP is to avoid hypoxia. The nurse assures the client maintains fluid and electrolyte imbalance. Codeine is commonly prescribed for headache related to increased ICP, but the nurse has not assessed the client's need for pain medication, and pain is not the priority at this time. Lowering the head of the bed could increase ICP; the nurse elevates the head of the bed 30 degrees and keeps the client's head and shoulders in alignment to maintain venous return. (A)

47. 3 The nurse first determines if the client has had sexual activity since the tubal ligation. If the client has been sexually active, the use of contraceptives is suspended to protect the fetus. If the client has had spotting, the nurse determines extent of the spotting to assess if the client has had an abortion. Addressing emotional concerns would depend on the intensity of the client's concerns. Physical protection of the fetus takes priority. (R)

48. The nurse palpates the fontanelle for size and shape. Normal fontanelles are flat and soft. Bulging fontanelles can indicate hydrocephalus, while depressed fontanelles can indicate dehydration. (A)

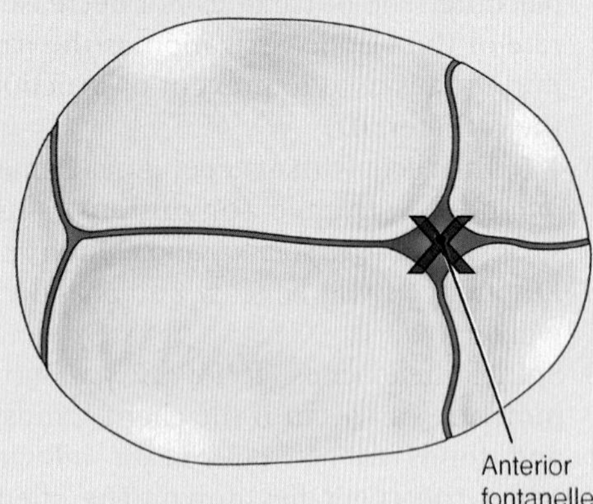

49. 4 Suicide is 7.5 times higher in clients with multiple sclerosis than the general population of the same age. Immobility is reversible. Hot showers and sun tanning would increase problems with fatigue. The extent of recovery during remissions gradually decreases. (H)

50. 1 The client is likely to benefit from a support group as a result of interacting with individuals with similar needs. Social isolation is less likely to occur if established relationships are maintained. Many clients with HIV/AIDS lack close relationships with family and friends. The client could learn to be self-sufficient, but a sense of belonging is an important need. (P)

51. 4 Smoking results in vasoconstriction; stopping smoking alone often relieves the pain associated with thromboangiitis obliterans. The client can use acetaminophen (Tylenol) for pain on a regular basis because pain can significantly reduce quality of life. Because of decreased circulation, healing of injury to the feet is slow and could result in infection; while the nurse instructs the client to wear protective shoes, promoting smoking cessation is the priority. The client is also advised to wear sunscreen. Most clients report extreme sensitivity to cold temperatures, and the client likely enjoys being in warm environments. (H)

52. 3 Before the client returns to the home setting, an understanding of how to manage activities within the limits imposed by the hypoxia is important. The client with COPD commonly sleeps with the head elevated to promote ease of breathing. Decreased sputum production may indicate recovery, but is also related to the extent of disease as well as the ability to expectorate. Blood gases will not return to normal limits, but the client can adapt to the physiologic limitations. (A)

53. 3 Amphotericin B causes hypokalemia. Hypokalemia can contribute to digoxin toxicity. The nurse requests a prescription for a potassium supplement. Neither drug is hepatotoxic. The nurse assesses all clients for allergic reactions, but typically neither of these drugs causes allergic reactions. Since both drugs are prescribed daily, the therapeutic dose levels are likely to be maintained for 24 hr. (D)

54. 3 In the healthy adult, complete bone healing occurs within 3 to 6 months. The client can use analgesics as prescribed for pain; pain will diminish in several weeks. Immobilizing devices used on fractures of the femur are not generally removed and replaced by the client. Resolution of swelling and discoloration will take longer than 48 hr. (A)

55. 3 In forming the staff-development program, the nurses consider the level of education and information appropriate to the role of the audience (UAP) and the type of information that will address the goals of the plan. The nurses provide information about hand hygiene and the importance of hand hygiene to reduce the incidence of sepsis. A staff education program about the subtle signs of infection in older adults is limited to only one sector of the population at the agency. Teaching about the relationship between fever and infection may not provide sufficiently concrete information. UAPs are not involved in setting infection control policies. (M)

56. 2 When the amniotic bag of waters ruptures (artificially or spontaneously), the priority nursing action is to monitor fetal heart tones. The greatest risk for the infant is for the cord to prolapse into the vaginal opening, which would cut off the blood supply to the fetus. The amnioinfusion is helpful to thin out meconium-stained fluids, and placing a fetal scalp electrode provides direct fetal monitoring; but these interventions require a physician's order. Once fetal heart tones are monitored, the nurse notifies the physician of changes in the client's status, including the fetal heart rate, dilation, and presence of meconium-stained fluids with ruptured membranes. (R)

57. 2 The client most at risk for melanoma is the white client (greatest risk is fair-skinned individuals) who is 45 years of age (risk highest between 20 and 45 years of age), with a first-degree family history. The nurse provides health information to the other clients, who are also at risk. (H)

58. 3 Compartment syndrome is caused by inadequate tissue perfusion. Because of the risks to the tissue, the priority goal for the nurse is to promote tissue perfusion after the fasciotomy. The nurse also develops plans to manage nutrition, anxiety, and pain; but maintaining oxygenation to the tissues is a priority. (A)

59. 4 Informed consent is a legal document and must be signed by a licensed staff member on the unit. Family members, UAPs, and religious advisors cannot sign the informed consent. (M)

60. 3 Asking the client to develop a meal plan promotes client learning and assures safety until the client understands how to plan meals. Once the client has developed the plan, the nurse helps to identify if there are problems with the plan and provides feedback. Food preferences are addressed as the meals are planned, but the more effective approach is to integrate the food preferences into a dietary plan. The client may not be able to identify the problem with dietary management, and doing so does not give the client the needed direction for long-term meal planning. Monitoring glucose levels does not directly address the client's need of learning to follow a diet. (M)

61. 4 The nurse must respect the client's religious beliefs. Pyridoxine is a proven alternative to hormone-replacement therapy, specifically for relief of hot flashes. Ginseng is commonly used for insomnia. Soybean rather than ginseng is the herb known to provide natural hormone replacement. It is not necessary for the client to further explain her beliefs, and the nurse should not attempt to convince the client to use estrogen by explaining that it is not a foreign substance. (H)

62. 1 Following surgery, the infant will have to alter an established pattern of breathing and adjust to breathing through the nose. The nurse instructs the parents to position the infant in a semiupright position while feeding to provide the infant with the most comfort. The nurse advises the parents not to place the infant on the abdomen as this will put pressure on the suture line. The parents are instructed to burp the infant frequently, and to not remove the metal appliance for feeding. (S)

63. 3 Standing for prolonged periods of time causes pooling of blood and distention of blood vessels. Women are also cautioned to not sit with legs crossed or wear knee-high hose or garters. Vitamin C may be helpful in reducing the size of varicosities because it is necessary for the formation of blood vessel collagen and endothelium. Exercising stimulates venous blood return and is effective in alleviating varicosities. Elastic support stockings such as TED hose are recommended for relief of varicosities. (H)

64. 3 The client should have realistic goals for pain management. The plans should be developed by the client and health care team so that the pain can be controlled and maintained at the clients' desired level of pain and functioning. A realistic goal for this client is that the client is free from pain, uses analgesia that relieves pain between doses of the medication, takes the medication before the onset of pain, and can perform daily activities of care without limitations. The nurse instructs the client to not wait for pain to develop before requesting pain medication. The client is advised to call the HCP if prescribed pain medication is not sufficient to control pain for performance of basic daily activities of self-care. (H)

65. 2 Low potassium levels potentiate the effect of digitalis preparations, as do low magnesium levels. The client with hypokalemia is more prone to digoxin toxicity. The potassium level is maintained within the normal range of 3.5 to 5 mEq/L and the digoxin level within the therapeutic range of 0.5 to 1.1 ng/ml (levels greater than 2 ng/ml are toxic). (D)

66. 3 In third-degree heart block, completely independent depolarization of the atria and ventricles occurs and results in loss of effective cardiac output. Temporary or permanent pacing will restore cardiac output by reproducing cyclic depolarization of atria and ventricles. Depending on the underlying condition, the client may undergo angiogram but angiogram is not necessary for insertion of a pacemaker, and the problem may or may not be coronary artery blockage. The drug of choice to try and reverse third-degree heart block is IV atropine sulfate; if atropine is unsuccessful, the client is symptomatic (low heart rate and signs of decreased cardiac output), and/or the client shows signs/symptoms of an acute MI, pacing will be done. (A)

67. 4 The client is making expected progress. The transition phase of stage one labor is from 7 to 10 cm dilation, with contractions 2 to 3 min apart, lasting 70 to 90 s. The client may become fatigued and irrational during this phase; her statements are typical. The client is not hemorrhaging; as the cervix effaces and dilates, cervical capillaries rupture, causing profuse bloody show to be seen. Precipitous delivery takes place in less than 3 hr. Titanic contractions are prolonged contractions lasting between 100 and 180 s. (A)

68. 3 Muscle atrophy occurs with the progressive motor neuron degeneration. There is no sensory deficit or cognitive impairment. Deep tendon reflexes become overactive. (A)

69. 3 While the ultimate goal for this client is total smoking cessation, supporting the client to reduce her cigarette consumption is a start to better health for both mother and infant. Asking the physician for a nicotine patch is helping with the physical effects of smoking, but not taking into consideration the psychologic effects of the habit. Although the fetus is at risk, the nurse is not required to report this to Child Protective Services. The nurse will not gain the client's trust and cooperation by directing the client to stop smoking. (H)

70. 2 Preload is increased by venous return to the heart. By placing the client in high Fowler position, preload is decreased. Positioning the client flat or elevating the feet or arms will increase venous return. (A)

71. 2 The client with a history of coronary artery disease and hypertension is at risk for heart failure, causing cardiac remodeling with hypertrophy and dilation of the left ventricle prior to the client experiencing symptoms. The PMI is normally located on the left anterior chest at the fifth intercostals space, midclavicular line. The location of the PMI in this client is not related to age. It is not necessary to assess the PMI when the client exhales as the PMI will not change. (A)

72. 1 If traveling by automobile during pregnancy in the third trimester, the nurse instructs the client to plan for frequent rest or stretch periods, preferably every hour, but at least every 2 hr. This break will relieve stiffness and muscle ache and improve lower extremity circulation, helping to prevent varicosities, hemorrhoids, and thrombophlebitis. Airlines do not permit women who are more than 7 months' pregnant to fly, or may require written permission from the woman's primary care provider. Although the nurse's responses regarding the length of time the client will be away and whether the next appointment needs to be rescheduled are helpful in keeping the client involved in her plan of care, these are not the most important responses. Asking the client who is going with her is not as important as the method of travel during the third trimester. (H)

73. 3 The client has ventricular tachycardia, a life-threatening dysrhythmia. Since the client is still alert and the nurse witnessed the change of rhythm, the nurse first administers lidocaine. After administering the lidocaine, the nurse notifies the HCP. If the rhythm does not revert to normal, the HCP will consider performing a cardioversion. It is premature to administer a precordial thump or start CPR when the client is still alert. (A)

74. 4 The QRS complex represents ventricular depolarization. The normal QRS complex is 0.4 to 1.0 s. Low potassium can cause depression of the ST segment, a flat or inverted T wave, and presence of U wave. Hyperkalemia can cause the QRS to widen. (A)

75. 4 Exercise is individually tailored based on tolerance and capability. Exercise is gradually increased over 1 to 3 months as the client is able. The client is advised to not limit exercise, but to stop if there is shortness of breath, and is reminded to observe safety measures, such as walking with someone and monitoring symptoms as exercise increases. Walking at a moderate pace 3 to 5 times per week for 30 to 45 min is an appropriate goal. (H)

76. 2 The client with acute pancreatitis experiences excruciating pain, which interferes with management of other health maintenance activities. Because steatorrhea is common with acute pancreatitis the rectal tissue may become irritated, but this is not as significant as the severe pain. Gradual reintroduction of oral intake is important, but will not occur if the client is experiencing severe pain. (H)

77. 2 Aspirin decreases platelet aggregation and blood clot formation. It reduces mortality significantly when started promptly after a suspected myocardial infarction, and is given as a daily dose. Aspirin is used for other conditions related to its analgesic and antipyretic properties. It does not increase or decrease acidity. (D)

78. 4 Exercise and pentoxifylline (Trental) are interventions to decrease claudication. Trental increases erythrocyte flexibility and reduces blood viscosity to improve blood supply to the muscle. The goal is to reestablish blood flow in areas of ischemia; applying ice packs will cause vasoconstriction. Heparin is an IV anticoagulant and not used as a treatment for claudication. There are no data to support the use of oxygen therapy for this client. If arterial disease becomes severe, bypass surgery may be needed. (D)

79. 4 The client who is having physiologic changes feels like he is going to have a heart attack and die, and cannot focus is experiencing panic level anxiety. Other lower levels do not include the physiologic changes. (P)

80. 2 A transesophageal puncture is a small opening between the trachea and the esophagus where a one-way valve is inserted through the stoma. By blocking the stoma, air expired from the lungs is forced into the esophagus through the valve and words are formed in the mouth to produce sound. A mechanical larynx is a vibrating device used to speak. Esophageal speech uses belching action transformed into speech as air is expelled. On inspiration, air goes from the stoma directly to the lungs and cannot produce speech. (H)

81. 3 After a total laryngectomy, the client breathes through a permanent stoma formed from the trachea and can no longer breathe through the nose and mouth. A tracheostomy collar is the only means to apply oxygen. (A)

82. 4 The highest priority for a nosebleed is to maintain adequate oxygenation and prevent aspiration. Pinching the nares for 10 to 15 min and using ice compress to the nose are sufficient methods to stop bleeding for most children. Placing the client in a flat position may compromise the airway and increase bleeding. Severe epistaxis or posterior bleeding may require packing by the HCP. The caregiver can try first aid measures such as applying pressure to the nares before bringing the child to the emergency department. (R)

83. 1 The nurse has the responsibility to confront the client's behavior. Confrontation involves asserting one's rights without violating the rights of others. Telling the client the nurse cannot continue to provide care or ignoring the client does not address the issue of behavior and does not provide opportunity for the client to change his behavior. While a team conference may be appropriate in the long term, the client's behavior must be addressed at the moment. (P)

84. 3 In option 3, the nurse identifies the behavior and the response it produces in the nurse. Confrontation points out aggressive behavior, and explanation of feelings promotes a working relationship with the client rather than a defensive reaction. To tell the client to stop shouting does not provide information about acceptable behavior. Apologies as indicated in option 4 do not communicate to the client the impact of behavior on others (the nurse). (P)

85. 1 It cannot be assumed that acquisition of knowledge alone will induce the client to change her eating habits. To have the nurse and client define and solve the problem together is a true statement. The client's beliefs, values, and behavior will influence her ability to make changes, and the client will have difficulty making those changes in her eating patterns. (P)

86. 4 Open expression of feelings is a healthy coping skill. Directing anger at self, avoiding contact with the nurse, and crying when alone are not as healthy coping behaviors and indicate the need for further work in managing feelings. (P)

87. 3 The best response involves the nurse acknowledging the client's feelings and the underlying cause. Responding that fears of unattractiveness cause worry, reflect on and clarify client feelings. Stating that the nurse knows how the client feels is false as the nurse does not know how another feels. To inform the client that she should not let the physical changes bother her because he loves her provides potentially false reassurance. The comment that the client has time to adjust does not address how the client feels at the time the statement is made. (P)

88. 3 The goal of communication with this client is to establish a therapeutic relationship in which the nurse is collaborating with the client to address needs identified by the client. The nurse does not assert control, nor convey hope. Although the nurse can explain health care procedures to the client if she asks for information, the goal of the initial client-nurse encounter is to establish a collaborative relationship. (P)

89. 2, 3, 4 The client with suspected amphetamine overdose would exhibit agitation, convulsions, and an increase in body temperature. The client could die with this overdose. Lack of coordination is a symptom of overdose of cannabis. Clammy skin is a symptom of overdose of sedatives or anxiolytics. (D)

90. 3 The nurse's goal is to establish the nurse-client relationship; therefore, the nurse has the client sit, and explains why the hospital needs the information from the admission assessment. Calling the physician for a sedative order or having a staff member assigned to the client before the nurse has made any attempt to establish a nurse-client relationship are not priority nursing interventions. Checking the vital signs and asking about medications the client is taking is not the first step in developing a therapeutic relationship. (P)

91. 4 Self-mutilation is characteristic of the client with borderline personality disorder. The antisocial personality disorder client is manipulative and has a history of criminal behaviors. The dependent personality disorder client needs to be taken care of and has clinging behavior. The passive-aggressive behavior client avoids responsibility until it becomes problematic and then provides an aggressive response to criticism. (P)

92. 1 On admission, each client is assessed for risk of pressure ulcers, and then receives an individualized plan developed by the nurse. The plan may include nutritional management, use of special mattresses, and turning schedule. Not all clients will require the use of each ulcer-prevention strategy. (M)

93. 1, 3, 4 The client with chronic alcoholism can develop pancreatitis and esophagitis, and is often depressed. Hallucinations and delusions are associated with delirium tremens and alcohol withdrawal. (A)

94. 2 Early decelerations are viewed as a normal labor pattern indicating periodic decreases in the fetal heart rate resulting from pressure on the fetal head during contractions. Variable decelerations indicate compression of the cord. There is no indication that the client needs to have a cesarean section, nor that the physician needs to be notified. (A)

95. 1, 3, 4, 5 Regular meals and snacks are encouraged to prevent hypoglycemia. Symptoms of hypoglycemia vary, but include irritability, hunger, shaking, sweating, confusion, and headache. Because strenuous exercise can cause hypoglycemia, the nurse teaches the client to eat a carbohydrate snack before exercising. Alcohol consumption can cause hypoglycemia. Hypoglycemia can occur with oral diabetic agents even when the client is not taking insulin. (R)

96. 3 Drotrecogin alfa (Xigris) is an anticoagulant-antithrombotic and can cause clinically significant bleeding 28 days after administration ceases; therefore, the nurse instructs the client to report if toothbrushing causes bleeding Eating a well-balanced diet is needed for health maintenance, but is not related to the drug. Avoiding fatigue is an important part of re-establishing health after septic shock, but is not directly related to Xigris therapy. Generally, infections resulting in septic shock are not likely to recur. (D)

97. 1, 2, 4, 5, 6 The client with PTSD will experience nightmares and flashbacks of the traumatic event. This client may have a low self-esteem, or appear terrified during a flashback, and may attempt to run away and/or hide during flashbacks. The client will also experience intrusive thoughts of the trauma. Delusions are experienced by the client with a thought disorder and the client with panic disorder. (P)

98. 4 Localized wheezing suggests only a small portion of a lung is involved, such as occurs following aspiration. The nurse should gather additional information about the incident and refer the client to a HCP. Eating hard candy would not cause the child to wheeze. Allergies are not contagious and do not generally present with wheezing. Exposure to a child who is recovering or has recovered from pneumonia will not cause disease, and pneumonia does not present with wheezing. (R)

99. 2 Live virus vaccines such as the MMR are contraindicated during pregnancy because they may transmit the viral infection to a fetus. The abdominal ultrasound and prenatal vitamins are considered normal orders for a pregnant client. Amniocentesis, if required, may be performed at 14 weeks' gestation when an adequate amount of amniotic fluid is available. (M)

100. 4 MRSA infections are increasing in the hospital and in the community. The organism is carried on the skin and is spread by physical contact; if the organism invades the lungs, it can be transmitted by droplet spread. Carriers of MRSA are difficult to identify, and currently not all hospitalized clients are tested for the presence of a MRSA infection. Hand hygiene is the most effective, practical, and widespread method to reduce the spread of MRSA for all persons who are in the hospital. Visitors do not need to be restricted, but they should be instructed to perform hand hygiene. Clients with identified MRSA infections are isolated and, if necessary, respiratory precautions can be used. (S)

Comprehensive Practice Test 2

1. The nurse notices blood on the blanket of an infant born 12 hr ago. The umbilical cord is bleeding. What nursing action should the nurse take first?
- □ 1. Notify the physician.
- □ 2. Place another clamp on the cord.
- □ 3. Remove the umbilical clamp.
- □ 4. Administer another vitamin K injection.

2. AF The nurse is assessing a client who is taking lithium carbonate (Lithium). Which signs and symptoms should the nurse assess related to lithium toxicity? Select all that apply.
- □ 1. Diarrhea.
- □ 2. Fever.
- □ 3. Seizures.
- □ 4. Hypotension.
- □ 5. Tachycardia.
- □ 6. Lethargy.

3. The nurse is assessing a client who has been in a motor vehicle accident and admitted to the emergency department. Which finding would require immediate follow-up by the nurse?
- □ 1. Tachycardia with occasional premature atrial contractions.
- □ 2. Elevated temperature of 100.2°F.
- □ 3. Blood-tinged, amber urine.
- □ 4. Absent lung sounds on the left.

4. A multigravid client has undergone an emergency cesarean section under general anesthesia. The nurse should monitor the client for which of the following complications during the postpartal recovery period?
- □ 1. Flatus.
- □ 2. Gastric reflux.
- □ 3. Sore throat.
- □ 4. Uterine atony.

5. The nurse is planning teaching about hand hygiene for a cognitively impaired child who is 5 years of age. Which of the following teaching methods would be most effective?
- □ 1. Explain why clean hands are good.
- □ 2. Demonstrate how to wash hands.
- □ 3. Play a game.
- □ 4. Show child a 5-min DVD.

6. Which one of the following adolescents is at risk for alcoholism? An adolescent who:
- □ 1. Changed schools and misses having close friends.
- □ 2. Avoids unfamiliar people.
- □ 3. Has a family history of alcoholism.
- □ 4. Exhibits rapid mood swings.

7. In the intermediate postoperative period following a hemorrhoidectomy, a nurse should assess the client for which complication?
- □ 1. Paralytic ileus.
- □ 2. Pneumonia.
- □ 3. Thromboembolism.
- □ 4. Difficulty voiding.

8. A new mother brings her daughter who is 2 weeks of age to the clinic for her scheduled 2-week well visit. The mother tells the nurse, "I don't think my breast milk is sufficient, she is always fussy after feedings and sucks on her fist." Which piece of information is most important for the nurse to determine at this time?
- □ 1. "Does she have a bowel movement at least twice a day?"
- □ 2. "Have you increased your calorie intake?"
- □ 3. "How long does she nurse at each breast?"
- □ 4. "How many diapers does she wet in 24 hr?"

9. An older adult client is admitted for an evaluation after becoming increasingly forgetful and at times becoming disorientated. Which of the following is a reversible cause of disorientation?
- □ 1. Vascular dementia.
- □ 2. Electrolyte imbalances.
- □ 3. HIV dementia.
- □ 4. Multiple sclerosis.

10. A toddler has a tympanic membrane that is bulging. On visualization, the nurse notes that the membrane is discolored orange and immobile, and there is presence of a few air bubbles behind the membrane. The toddler is afebrile and the mother reports the child has been sleeping well. The nurse should:
- □ 1. Tell the mother to administer acetaminophen (Tylenol) that is appropriate for weight.
- □ 2. Discuss how an otitis media with an effusion is typically monitored.
- □ 3. Have the mother administer ibuprofen that is appropriate for weight.
- □ 4. Notify the HCP since this child likely has an acute otitis media.

11. Which of the following provide the most reliable information about the desired outcome of care for a client with fluid volume excess?
- □ 1. Weight.
- □ 2. Serum electrolyte levels.
- □ 3. Potassium levels.
- □ 4. Urinalysis.

12. The nurse evaluates the drug nitroprusside (Nipride) as effective in an older adult client with shock when the BP is:

- □ 1. 70/40.
- □ 2. 80/60.
- □ 3. 100/70.
- □ 4. 160/110.

13. Three hours after tonsillectomy a client vomits 300 ml of brown emesis. The nurse should first:

- □ 1. Continue to monitor the client.
- □ 2. Document the amount and color of emesis.
- □ 3. Report emesis to the surgeon.
- □ 4. Administer an antiemetic as ordered.

14. The nurse is assisting a primipara and infant to successfully breast-feed. The nurse should emphasize which of the following?

- □ 1. Place the entire areola into the infant's mouth.
- □ 2. Hold the infant below the breast for gravity flow.
- □ 3. Hold the infant on his side, facing the mother's breast.
- □ 4. Assure the infant is making a clicking sound when sucking.

15. A child is being evaluated for autism. Which is a common behavior of the autistic child?

- □ 1. Child clings toward his mother.
- □ 2. Child develops language early.
- □ 3. Child is indifferent to being held.
- □ 4. Child demonstrates cooperative play at early age.

16. AF The nurse is assessing a client who has had a myocardial infarction, and reviewing the ECG strip below.

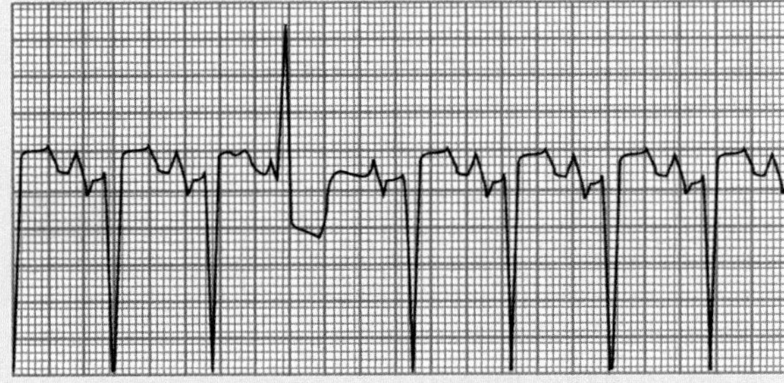

Identify the premature ventricular contraction on this cardiac rhythm strip.

17. The nurse is recording blood loss on a client with placenta previa. The LPN did not obtain a dry weight on the perineal pad before placing it on the client. Which of the following interventions should the nurse perform to ensure an accurate measurement of blood loss?

- □ 1. Chart approximate blood loss using inspection.
- □ 2. Chart lack of output total for this pad.
- □ 3. Weigh another dry pad and use this weight as the base.
- □ 4. Weigh the saturated pad anyway and record this total.

18. When a client with schizophrenia becomes violent and aggressive, which approach should the nurse institute first?

- □ 1. Ask the client to use a punching bag to relieve tension.
- □ 2. Call for sufficient help to safely control the situation.
- □ 3. Administer an antipsychotic medication to the client.
- □ 4. Tell the client that the behavior is not acceptable and will not be permitted on this unit.

19. A client who is at 35 weeks' gestation is admitted with a diagnosis of abruptio placentae. The nurse is completing the admission assessment and receives the following orders. For which order should the nurse seek further clarification?

- □ 1. Anchor an indwelling urinary catheter.
- □ 2. Draw blood for fibrinogen level.
- □ 3. Maintain supine position.
- □ 4. Type and cross-match 2 units of PRBCs.

20. When administering an initial dose of a narcotic analgesic to an alert client with postoperative pain, the most important nursing action is to:

- □ 1. Avoid disturbing the client for the next 4 hr.
- □ 2. Document nonverbal indications of pain.
- □ 3. Administer the next dose of narcotic analgesic in 4 hr.
- □ 4. Reassess client pain within 30 min.

21. AF The nurse is conducting a focused assessment for a client with heart failure who is being admitted to the hospital with shortness of breath. Which of the following questions initially would be most helpful for planning care? Select all that apply.

- □ 1. When did you first notice feeling short of breath?
- □ 2. Do you have a cough?
- □ 3. How long have you had chest pain?
- □ 4. How much caffeine have you had today?
- □ 5. Do you ever wake up during the night feeling short of breath?
- □ 6. How many pillows are you sleeping on?

22. The nurse is giving directions to an unlicensed assistant for collecting a urine specimen from an indwelling catheter. Which of the following statements indicates that the assistant understands the instructions?

- □ 1. "I should collect urine from the catheter drainage bag at the end of the shift and place it in the specimen container."
- □ 2. "I will disconnect the drainage tube from the catheter and let urine run from the catheter into the specimen container."

- ☐ 3. "I will empty the catheter drainage bag, have the client drink some water, and an hour later collect the urine that drains into the bag."
- ☐ 4. "I will get a sterile syringe and remove urine from the catheter through the collection port to place in the specimen container."

23. A client with an abdominal-perineal resection and colostomy had an NG tube inserted during surgery. The nurse is assessing the client's readiness to have the NG tube removed. The NG tube will most likely be removed when the client demonstrates which of the following?

- ☐ 1. A decrease in nausea and vomiting.
- ☐ 2. A flat, soft abdomen on palpation.
- ☐ 3. Passage of flatus from the colostomy.
- ☐ 4. Less than 200 ml gastric drainage in 24 hr.

24. The nurse is planning care for a client with COPD. Which of the following is the most effective indicator for determining the client's need for supplemental oxygen?

- ☐ 1. Client's request to use oxygen.
- ☐ 2. Client's level of fatigue.
- ☐ 3. Oxygen saturation.
- ☐ 4. Hemoglobin level.

25. A client's Pap smear report states, "evidence of altered cell characteristics due to inflammation." The nurse should tell the client:

- ☐ 1. She needs a repeat Pap smear within 1 week.
- ☐ 2. The altered cell characteristics require a colposcopy.
- ☐ 3. The Pap smear is negative and no intervention is necessary.
- ☐ 4. Treatment will be started for the infection and the Pap smear will need to be repeated in 3 months.

26. A client who is 52 years of age has complaints of dyspareunia. Her last menstrual cycle was 4 years ago. The client denies bleeding, discharge, or pruritus. The nurse should:

- ☐ 1. Discuss benefits of hormone-replacement therapy.
- ☐ 2. Recommend using a water-soluble lubricant for intercourse.
- ☐ 3. Refer the client for psychologic counseling.
- ☐ 4. Obtain a urine specimen for culture and sensitivity.

27. A client is to receive 100 mg of chlorpromazine (Thorazine) STAT and then 50 mg twice a day with 2 mg of benztropine mesylate (Cogentin) twice a day PRN. The order for the Cogentin would be given for which of the following manifestations by this client?

- ☐ 1. Shuffling gait and drooling.
- ☐ 2. Photophobia and photosensitivity.
- ☐ 3. Leukopenia and elevated liver enzymes.
- ☐ 4. Complaints of constipation and nausea.

28. An adolescent is hospitalized with a spinal cord injury. Two weeks after the accident, the UAP reports to the nurse that while bathing the client his leg has moved twice. The nurse should:

- ☐ 1. Ask the client if he felt the movement.
- ☐ 2. Notify the physician.
- ☐ 3. Administer a muscle relaxant.
- ☐ 4. Tell the UAP to continue bathing the client.

29. A primigravida is at 18 weeks' gestation. The physician orders an amniocentesis to rule out neural tube defect. In preparing the client for this procedure the nurse should instruct the client to:

- ☐ 1. Drink 2 liters of fluid.
- ☐ 2. Lie on her left side.
- ☐ 3. Swallow her preoperative medicines with 30 ml of water.
- ☐ 4. Take a shower with pHisoHex.

30. A client is admitted with the diagnosis of dementia, Alzheimer type, and has disturbances in cognition and orientation. The nurse should assess the client for:

- ☐ 1. Hearing.
- ☐ 2. Coordination.
- ☐ 3. Appetite.
- ☐ 4. Personality changes.

31. The nurse is providing teaching about safety procedures to parents of a child with autism. What typical behavior of children with autism requires the parents to perform special care to maintain child safety?

- ☐ 1. Fascination with bright colors.
- ☐ 2. Insensitivity to pain.
- ☐ 3. Craving for salt.
- ☐ 4. Loss of hearing for high frequencies.

32. Which of the following instructions should the nurse provide for parents of a child with encopresis?

- ☐ 1. Do not punish the child for encopresis.
- ☐ 2. Clean the child immediately after an accident occurs.
- ☐ 3. Give 4 to 6 tablespoons of bismuth subsalicylate (Kaopectate) per day.
- ☐ 4. Keep the child close to bathroom facilities at all times.

33. A primigravid client at 16 weeks' gestation is HIV-positive, but remains asymptomatic. She is concerned about what her HIV status will do to her unborn infant. The nurse should tell the client:

□ 1. An amniocentesis can be done to rule out the infection.
□ 2. Maternal antibodies cross the placenta and provide immunity to the fetus.
□ 3. A drug can be administered to reduce risk for transmission of HIV to the unborn infant.
□ 4. There is nothing that can be done until after the infant is born.

34. The nurse is providing teaching to the parents of a child with a behavioral disorder. The nurse should instruct the parents that management of children with behavioral disorders is primarily aimed toward:

□ 1. Instituting strict disciplinary action for misbehavior.
□ 2. Protecting family members from the disruptive behavior.
□ 3. Changing the home environment to one that is more consistent.
□ 4. Placing the child in an open-structure school environment.

35. A new mother tells the nurse, "I'm going to quit breast-feeding. My nipples are so sore!" Which of the following questions should the nurse ask the client?

□ 1. "Are your nipples cracked yet?"
□ 2. "Are your nipples everted or inverted?"
□ 3. "Do you want pain medication?"
□ 4. "Have you been using the hand pump to express milk?"

36. A teenage girl is admitted to the emergency department because she has been raped. Which of the following statements by the nurse would be most therapeutic?

□ 1. "Try not to think more about what happened."
□ 2. "Rape is a terrible crime. I'm sorry this happened."
□ 3. "Tell me about what happened to you."
□ 4. "Don't feel guilty. You didn't provoke the attack."

37. The nurse manager on the oncology unit is conducting a staff-development program about documenting the effectiveness of the pain medication within 30 min after administration. Which of the following should the nurse manager do first?

□ 1. Change the policy of documentation to 45 min.
□ 2. Consult with the pharmacist.
□ 3. Consult with the nurses on the evening shift where documentation of analgesia is the greatest problem.
□ 4. Complete a brief quality-improvement study and chart audit to document the rate of adherence to policy and the pattern of documentation over shifts.

38. The nurse is assessing an infant who is 3 months of age and had surgery to repair a pyloric stenosis. To assess pain in an infant the nurse should:

□ 1. Pinch the toe and observe for grimace.
□ 2. Ask the parents if the child is having pain.
□ 3. Observe the infant's facial and body actions.
□ 4. Note crying that lasts for longer than 1 min.

39. A client with schizophrenia is admitted to the inpatient psychiatric unit. The nurse formulates the nursing diagnosis as Altered Thought Processes related to paranoia. The nurse should instruct the staff to:

□ 1. Encourage client to socialize with peers.
□ 2. Have client sign a no self-harm contract.
□ 3. Avoid whispering or laughing in front of the client.
□ 4. Instruct client about the discharge options in his home community.

40. AF A neonate who is tolerating oral feedings would display which of the following? Select all that apply.

□ 1. Abdominal distention.
□ 2. Presence of suck and swallow reflexes.
□ 3. Gastric residual of 1 ml or less before feeding.
□ 4. Presence of bowel sounds.
□ 5. Temperature in normal range.
□ 6. Presence of bowel loops.
□ 7. Presence of Moro reflex.

41. AF The nurse is teaching a disaster preparedness course to community members. Which of the following instructions is true to prevent lightening injury in the event of a thunderstorm with significant lightening? Select all that apply.

□ 1. Stay off the telephone.
□ 2. Seek shelter under a tall tree.
□ 3. Get out of the bathtub immediately.
□ 4. Turn off computers.
□ 5. Seek shelter in a building or vehicle.

42. AF A client who is 2 years of age is admitted to the emergency department with acute epiglottis. The child has a temperature of 101°F, is drooling, and complains of a sore throat. The parents are anxious and upsetting the child. The priorities for care for this child are to do which of the following? Place in order of first to last.

_____ 1. Manage the high fever.
_____ 2. Manage the airway.

_____ 3. Calm the parents.
_____ 4. Administer IV fluids.

43. AF The nurse is planning care for an adult who is hospitalized for diarrhea and dehydration. The client is receiving IV fluids, but continues to have watery stools. The nurse reviews the intake output record for the last 24 hr:

INTAKE/OUTPUT

Intake					Output		
Date	Time	Oral	IV	Total	Urine	Other (stool)	Total
4/14/09	0700	300	1000	1300	1000	700	1700
	1500	300	1000	1300	2030	300	2330
	2300	250	1000	1250	1200	200	1400
4/15/09	0700	300	1000	1300	1800	100	1900

The nurse should plan to do which of the following?

- ☐ 1. Restrict fluids.
- ☐ 2. Increase fluids.
- ☐ 3. Administer stool softener.
- ☐ 4. Administer antiemetic.

44. A client with gross, painless hematuria is being evaluated for bladder cancer. The client asks, "Why do I have to have a cystoscopy? I've already had an IV pyelogram (IVP) and an ultrasound." The nurse should tell the client:

- ☐ 1. "Gross, painless hematuria is the most common clinical finding of bladder cancer; however, the presence of cancer is confirmed by cystoscopy and biopsy."
- ☐ 2. "Bladder cancer can be detected by IVP or ultrasound."
- ☐ 3. "The staging of bladder cancer is determined by visualization by the physician."
- ☐ 4. "Bladder cancers are not easily located."

45. An infant who is 3 months of age is hospitalized with pneumonia. The nurse observes that the UAP is propping a baby's bottle at bedtime to help her fall asleep. The nurse should:

- ☐ 1. Remove the bottle and explain that feeding this way will promote tooth decay.
- ☐ 2. Ask the UAP to apply moisture cream to the baby's face to prevent a rash.
- ☐ 3. Encourage the UAP to continue to offer the baby as many fluids as possible.
- ☐ 4. Tell the UAP to wash the baby after feeding.

46. The RN is making assignments on the oncology unit and assigns the client with Kaposi sarcoma and HIV to the LVN/LPN. The LVN/LPN states she does not want to take care of this client. Which of the following would be an appropriate response by the RN?

- ☐ 1. "I will assign this client to another nurse."
- ☐ 2. "I will help you take care of this client so you are confident with his care."
- ☐ 3. "You seem worried about this assignment."
- ☐ 4. "I will review blood and body fluid precautions with you."

47. The nurse is teaching a woman who just delivered her first baby how to strengthen her pelvic floor muscles. Which of the following exercises will be most effective?

- ☐ 1. Aerobics classes.
- ☐ 2. Kegel exercises.
- ☐ 3. Swimming 3 times a week.
- ☐ 4. Walking 20 min daily.

48. The client is unable to talk, but can nod yes and no. The client is wearing an id bracelet. The client is known to be confused at times. Which is the best approach for the nurse to take when giving the client medications?

- ☐ 1. Not give the medications and inform the physician.
- ☐ 2. Say the client's name and if the client nods yes, administer the medications.
- ☐ 3. Verify the client's identification with a family member and then give the medications.
- ☐ 4. See if the chart by the door has the correct name, and if it does, give the medications.

49. After the physician makes an initial diagnosis of paranoid schizophrenia, the client's mother approaches the nurse angrily and states, "You people are wrong; my son cannot have this condition! You just want him to have to stay here!" The nurse should respond by saying:

- ☐ 1. "You seem very upset by this."
- ☐ 2. "Why would you say that we would want him to stay?"
- ☐ 3. "Your son's doctor would not give you wrong information."
- ☐ 4. "Blaming is really not helpful. What else do you think could be done?"

50. Which of the following nursing activities best illustrates a nurse in the advocacy role?

- ☐ 1. Nurse develops teaching-learning materials for the preoperative phase of a liver transplant.
- ☐ 2. Nurse recommends changes in agency policy that resulted in cost reduction for low-income pregnant clients.
- ☐ 3. Nurse instructs client to ask HCP if the diagnostic test is the most appropriate for the problem.

☐ 4. Nurse contacts local law officials regarding the high crime rate in a low socioeconomic area.

51. AF The nurse is assessing a client who has returned to the nursing unit following a cardiac catheterization 2 hr ago. The left femoral artery was the entry point for the catheterization. The nurse should report which of the following to the physician? Select all that apply.
☐ 1. Time of cardiac catheterization.
☐ 2. Absence of left pedal pulse.
☐ 3. Vital signs.
☐ 4. Recommendation for physician to assess the client.
☐ 5. Client has had 240 ml of water.

52. A woman is found wandering around her neighborhood in the early morning hours in a disheveled and confused state. When questioned, the woman does not know who she is. When brought to the emergency department, it is determined that the client has been given drugs in a drink and was raped. The nursing diagnosis for this client is:
☐ 1. Social Isolation related to being raped.
☐ 2. Disturbed Thought Processes related to alcohol abuse.
☐ 3. Disturbed Personal Identity related to being confused.
☐ 4. Ineffective Coping related to being raped.

53. A client who is 16 years of age and living with her parents is scheduled for surgery. The client's state of residence establishes 16 years of age as the age of maturity in which the client can sign her own surgical permits. Which one of the following individuals should sign the surgical consent form?
☐ 1. The client.
☐ 2. Her parents.
☐ 3. Her husband.
☐ 4. A lawyer.

54. The most significant complication in the immediate postoperative period of a client who has undergone a tonsillectomy is:
☐ 1. Laryngitis.
☐ 2. Acute pain.
☐ 3. Infection.
☐ 4. Hemorrhage.

55. A primigravida who is 15 years of age is in labor and has had no prenatal care. Her support person is her girlfriend who is 16 years of age. Which of the following is the best example of autonomous nursing care?
☐ 1. Explain to the client the labor process and how long it typically lasts.
☐ 2. Administer pain medication because the client did not learn breathing techniques.
☐ 3. Tell the client everything will be alright because she can have an epidural.
☐ 4. Direct the client about what she has to do to get through labor.

56. A client has colorectal cancer. The tumor is classified as stage C and the client has positive lymph nodes. The client is scheduled for radiation and chemotherapy following colon resection. Which of the following are expected outcomes of using surgery, radiation, and chemotherapy for this client?
☐ 1. Both radiation and chemotherapy can be used as palliative treatments.
☐ 2. Radiation is always used as supplemental therapy following surgery.
☐ 3. Chemotherapy cures colorectal cancer.
☐ 4. Radiation decreases the side effects of chemotherapy.

57. While providing client and family teaching about Addison disease, the spouse asks, "How long does my spouse need to take this corticosteroid medicine?" The nurse should tell the spouse:
☐ 1. "Corticosteroids will be required for the remainder of your spouse's life."
☐ 2. "Corticosteroids will no longer be needed when your spouse learns how to manage stress."
☐ 3. "If your spouse participates in indoor activity and stays out of the sun, corticosteroids will not be necessary."
☐ 4. "Corticosteroids are needed only when your spouse has a physician or dental visit."

58. AF The nurse is conducting the initial assessment for a construction worker who is 45 years of age and being admitted to the hospital with low back pain. In which order of priority should the nurse collect data for the care plan? Place in order from first to last.
_____ 1. Take vital signs including pain level.
_____ 2. Assess gait and sensory loss.
_____ 3. Obtain the history of the low back pain.
_____ 4. Determine range of motion and muscle strength.

59. A client is 20 weeks' pregnant and wants to breast-feed her infant after birth. She is concerned that her nipples are inverted and that she will not be able to breast-feed. The nurse should encourage the client to:
☐ 1. Gently pull on each nipple everyday.
☐ 2. Roll the nipples between her fingers 2 to 3 times a day.

□ 3. Roll the nipples each night with a rough bath towel.
□ 4. Wear breast shells the last few months of her pregnancy.

60. Which of the following is a priority assessment for a client immediately following surgery?
□ 1. Level of consciousness.
□ 2. Intensity of pain.
□ 3. Amount IV fluid remaining.
□ 4. Airway patency.

61. When a narcotic analgesic and a nonsteroidal anti-inflammatory drug are administered together, the expected outcome is:
□ 1. Decreased chance of respiratory depression from the narcotic analgesic.
□ 2. Decreased need for medication during the night.
□ 3. Ability to wean the client from the narcotic analgesic.
□ 4. Sustained pain relief.

62. A nurse is providing client teaching about taking atenolol (Tenormin). Which statement indicates the teaching was effective?
□ 1. "The pills should be taken with milk for better absorption."
□ 2. "I will take a pill as soon as I begin to feel chest pain."
□ 3. "I should avoid soaking in my hot tub after consuming alcohol."
□ 4. "The best diet for me is one rich in vitamins and antioxidants."

63. A client is scheduled to take an antilipidemic drug, a beta-blocker, and a multivitamin. The nurse should perform which of the following assessments prior to administering the medications?
□ 1. Ask about the client's urinary frequency.
□ 2. Listen to the client's lung sounds.
□ 3. Determine the client's heart rate.
□ 4. Check for peripheral pulses.

64. To help prevent falls, the nurse should instruct a client who is 80 years of age with orthostatic hypotension to:
□ 1. Drink adequate fluids.
□ 2. Eat high-protein, low-fat foods.
□ 3. Exercise for short periods daily.
□ 4. Rise slowly when standing after lying or sitting.

65. When planning care for an older adult client diagnosed with Alzheimer disease, the nurse should:
□ 1. Allow the client to plan his own day.
□ 2. Encourage outside diversional activities.
□ 3. Limit the client's caloric intake.
□ 4. Provide a calm, predictable environment.

66. A primigravida client at 38 weeks' gestation is concerned that her fetus has stopped growing because the fetus is not as high in her abdomen as last week. Fetal heart rate is 156 and fetal movements were present during fetal monitoring. The nurse should do which of the following?
□ 1. Prepare for an external rotation because the fetus is breech.
□ 2. Admit the client to the labor room because labor has begun.
□ 3. Tell the mother lightening has taken place and the fetus is fine.
□ 4. Have the client weigh herself daily to monitor unexplained weight loss.

67. The nurse is planning care for a group of clients on a medical-surgical unit. Which one of the following clients is at risk for fluid volume deficit?
□ 1. Client who vomited more than 2,000 ml in the last 48 hr and cannot tolerate oral fluids.
□ 2. Client with heart failure who has rales and peripheral edema.
□ 3. Client who has an elevated BUN and creatinine and a diagnosis of acute renal failure.
□ 4. Client with severe indigestion who has been consuming large amounts of calcium carbonate.

68. The nurse is providing client teaching to a father about feeding his newborn infant. Which action, once the father completes the feeding, indicates he understood the nurse's teaching? The father places the newborn in the crib:
□ 1. Prone.
□ 2. Supine.
□ 3. On the left side.
□ 4. On the right side.

69. When administering potassium supplements IV the nurse should:
□ 1. Administer potassium with normal saline solutions.
□ 2. Administer potassium using an intravenous infusion pump.
□ 3. Administer potassium over an 8-hr period of time.
□ 4. Administer potassium through a central IV line.

70. Which one of the following clients is at greatest risk for respiratory alkalosis?
□ 1. Client with hypoxemia.
□ 2. Client who is oversedated.
□ 3. Client with chronic obstructive pulmonary disease.
□ 4. Client with hyponatremia.

71. In choosing a site for peripheral IV therapy the nurse should consider:
- □ 1. Cost of the various types of catheters.
- □ 2. Client's level of consciousness.
- □ 3. Type of fluid to be administered.
- □ 4. Expected duration of IV therapy.

72. Which of the following conditions places a client at risk for fluid-volume deficit?
- □ 1. Constipation.
- □ 2. GI suction.
- □ 3. Sodium excess.
- □ 4. Renal failure.

73. The lactation nurse is teaching a woman how to breast-feed. The nurse assesses teaching effectiveness regarding choosing alternate positions for breast-feeding when the client states:
- □ 1. "I want to prevent sore nipples, so I'll change positions every time."
- □ 2. "I'll try all the best positions, then use the one I like."
- □ 3. "My milk will come in faster if I change positions each time."
- □ 4. "Using different positions will be less tiring for me."

74. On admission to a health care facility, which of the following is a primary goal for the client with paranoid schizophrenia?
- □ 1. Promote increased interactions with other clients.
- □ 2. Decrease anxiety and increase trust.
- □ 3. Improve relationship with family of origin.
- □ 4. Encourage participation in nursing unit government.

75. Nursing actions to minimize fluid-volume deficit due to dehydration in a client who is 65 years of age include:
- □ 1. Ordering a high-protein diet.
- □ 2. Keeping the client warm.
- □ 3. Assuring fluid intake of 60 ml/hr.
- □ 4. Administering gastric tube feedings of 80 ml/hr.

76. A client with catatonic stupor is found lying on the bed curled in the fetal position. The most appropriate nursing intervention for this client would be to:
- □ 1. Ask direct questions of the client to encourage communication.
- □ 2. Sit beside the client in silence asking occasional open-ended questions.
- □ 3. Leave the client alone and have the staff check on her at least hourly.
- □ 4. Take the client to the dayroom so she can watch other clients.

77. A client with dementia has difficulty sleeping and wanders most of the night shift. Which nursing intervention would best promote sleep for this client?
- □ 1. Have the client drink a cup of tea with honey at bedtime.
- □ 2. Ensure the client gets regular exercise during the day.
- □ 3. Make certain the client gets an afternoon nap, so as to not be overtired at bedtime.
- □ 4. Ask the primary HCP to prescribe a hypnotic medication such as flurazepam (Dalmane).

78. AF A child with spastic-type cerebral palsy is admitted to the pediatric unit for a "test dose" of intrathecal baclofen. The nurse will provide close monitoring for side effects during the procedure. Which of the following are potential side effects of baclofen? Select all that apply.
- □ 1. Hypertonia.
- □ 2. Drowsiness.
- □ 3. Seizures.
- □ 4. Rapid respirations.
- □ 5. Nausea and vomiting.
- □ 6. Agitation.

79. A child who is 7 years of age is experiencing pain after an appendectomy. Which data collection tool should the nurse use to assess the child's pain?
- □ 1. Visual analogue scale.
- □ 2. Short-Form McGill questionnaire.
- □ 3. Numeric scale.
- □ 4. Faces pain rating scale.

80. A client admitted with paranoid schizophrenia is experiencing command hallucinations to injure his family members. The nurse should first:
- □ 1. Place the client in restraints.
- □ 2. Administer an injection of clozapine (Clozaril).
- □ 3. Order a high-protein diet.
- □ 4. Ensure the environment is safe for this client and others on the unit.

81. A female client who is 16 years of age enters the clinic and confides in the nurse that she knows she is pregnant and she wants an abortion. Prior to counseling the client about her options, the nurse should first determine:
- □ 1. If there is a partner involved.
- □ 2. The client's menstrual history.
- □ 3. The client's problem-solving strategies.
- □ 4. The gestation of the pregnancy.

82. When a client with schizophrenia attends a family group with members of his family, which of the following is the primary focus of the group?
- □ 1. Inform family members that they are not the only family with this problem.

- □ 2. Inform family of the most current therapies for clients with schizophrenia.
- □ 3. Increase understanding of schizophrenia and to promote interaction with the family.
- □ 4. Discuss adaptive behaviors for stress relief and problem-solving techniques.

83. The family of a client admitted for vascular dementia asks the nurse if one of the client's children can get this condition. The nurse should tell the family that vascular dementia occurs with:

- □ 1. Multiple small strokes.
- □ 2. History of Alzheimer disease.
- □ 3. Advanced age.
- □ 4. History of schizophrenia.

84. AF The nurse is completing the intake and output record for an infant following a pyloromyotomy. The infant has had the following intake and output during the shift:

Intake:

09 00 – ½ ounce expressed breast milk.

10 00 – 1 ounce expressed breast milk.

11 00 – ½ ounce expressed breast milk.

12 00 – 1 ounce expressed breast milk.

13 00 – 2 ounces expressed breast milk.

Output:

10 15 – emesis of ~ 1 ounce.

11 30 – 50 ml of urine.

12 30 – 60 ml of urine mixed with stool.

How many milliliters should the nurse document as the infant's intake? _______ ml.

85. AF A child who is 4 years of age with attention-deficit hyperactive disorder (ADHD) is admitted to the hospital. The nurse should do which of the following? Select all that apply.

- □ 1. Provide an environment as free from distractions as possible.
- □ 2. Encourage one-on-one interactions.
- □ 3. Provide instructions in "chunks" of information.
- □ 4. Engage the child's attention before giving instructions.
- □ 5. Take the child to the playroom to play with other children.

86. A client recently lost her husband and is experiencing difficulty sleeping, anxiety attacks, and weight loss. The physician has diagnosed her as having an adjustment disorder. The nurse should teach the client to:

- □ 1. Relieve symptoms by techniques such as relaxation techniques and journal writing.
- □ 2. Develop new coping mechanism as there are no support systems.
- □ 3. Learn to manage for the rest of her life with this disorder.
- □ 4. Spend time alone to work through the grief process.

87. The nurse has been providing care for a client in a program for eating disorders. Which of the following is the best indicator that the care has been effective?

- □ 1. Client states she is accepting of her body.
- □ 2. Client has maintained her target weight for 4 years.
- □ 3. Client has moved away from her parents' home.
- □ 4. Client visits with her peers while waiting for group therapy sessions.

88. According to Erickson, which of the following is true of child growth and development?

- □ 1. Successful development occurs when the child has mastered the skills of each previous stage of development.
- □ 2. Children move through four broad stages of cognitive development.
- □ 3. A child is well adjusted once he or she receives gratification of sexual and aggressive drives.
- □ 4. Children learn their respective cultures through interactions with the respective cultures.

89. A female child who is 7 years of age with leukemia was hospitalized for chemotherapy treatments. On her return home, the mother reports that she is withdrawn, experiences nightmares, and has begun sucking her thumb again at night. This child is experiencing:

- □ 1. Generalized anxiety disorder.
- □ 2. Dysthymia.
- □ 3. Adjustment disorder.
- □ 4. Oppositional defiant disorder.

90. The nurse is teaching a primigravida about nutrition during pregnancy. Which of the following is an outcome that indicates the client is obtaining sufficient nutrition?

- □ 1. Active fetal movement.
- □ 2. Appropriate maternal weight gain.
- □ 3. Ingestion of daily caloric requirements.
- □ 4. Negative glucose tolerance test.

91. Childhood depression is commonly undiagnosed in adolescents and children because:

- □ 1. Many health care workers think childhood depression does not exist.
- □ 2. Adolescents and children may exhibit acting-out behaviors instead of being able to describe their depressed feelings.
- □ 3. Short periods of being depressed are normal experiences of childhood.

☐ 4. Adolescents and children will mask their true depressed feelings.

92. A child is seen in the outpatient clinic after being diagnosed with ADHD. When the parents complain to the nurse that their child cannot pay attention to school activities for longer than "a moment's time," what can the nurse inform them regarding the treatment plan for this child?

☐ 1. "The medications can be very helpful in improving your child's ability to focus on activities."

☐ 2. "When your child is not paying attention in school, we will teach him a system of negative responses that will increase his ability to focus."

☐ 3. "The social skills training that we have planned will help him to be able to do his schoolwork."

☐ 4. "I wouldn't worry about that. Once we provide rewards, he will start to pay more attention to his school work."

93. The nurse is observing a new father provide a formula feeding to his newborn for the first time. Which of the following behaviors indicates the father is demonstrating correct feeding techniques?

☐ 1. Heating the bottle in the microwave for 30 s.

☐ 2. Keeping the nipple filled with formula.

☐ 3. Placing the infant in a supine position to feed.

☐ 4. Using bottle-propping supported by a blanket.

94. A client diagnosed with bipolar disorder is prescribed lithium carbonate (Lithium) 300 mg PO, 3 times a day. After 4 days of medication treatment, the client states she is experiencing mild shaking of her hands. What is the best response by the nurse?

☐ 1. "Mild, fine tremors of the hands are an expected early effect of Lithium therapy; this effect usually improves after a few weeks of being on the medication."

☐ 2. "This is a side effect you will have for as long as you are on the medication."

☐ 3. "Mild hand tremors are a very serious sign of toxicity. We will need to stop the medication."

☐ 4. "Even if you have a tremor, you will still need to attend group therapy. You cannot avoid any of the parts of your treatment plan."

95. AF Tobramycin sulfate (Nebcin) is prescribed for a client with pyelonephritis. The client is to receive 4 mg/kg/day; the client weighs 185 pounds. How many grams of tobramycin sulfate (Nebcin) is the client to receive per 24 hr? ________ g/24 hr.

96. A client requests help with breast-feeding. She asks the nurse, "What is the best way to prevent sore nipples?" The nurse should instruct the client to:

☐ 1. Apply a lanolin-based cream to the nipples before each feeding.

☐ 2. Position the infant slightly differently for each feeding.

☐ 3. Wash the breasts daily with an antibacterial soap and rinse well.

☐ 4. Wear plastic-lined nursing pads to prevent bacterial growth.

97. The nurse has completed teaching a client about his somatization disorder. Which statement by the client to his wife indicates the teaching was effective?

☐ 1. "There is no treatment available for my illness."

☐ 2. "I have been faking my symptoms."

☐ 3. "Once I complete physical therapy, my symptoms will be better."

☐ 4. "If I learn to cope better with my stress, I will feel better."

98. An older adult client is brought to the emergency department. He has a history of atrial fibrillation, type 2 diabetes, and is in the beginning stages of Alzheimer disease. He is cared for by his middle-aged son at home. The client is unkempt, thirsty, weak, and dehydrated. He has a decubitus ulcer on his coccyx. He cannot answer all the questions the nurse asks in the admission assessment. Which is the most likely explanation for the client's status?

☐ 1. Physical abuse.

☐ 2. Underlying mental and physical condition.

☐ 3. Physical neglect.

☐ 4. The client's age and weakness.

99. The nurse is assessing a client who was raped and beaten by her ex-husband. She has several fractures and lacerations on her face. The client says, "He has done this before." The client does not appear upset and is very cooperative. Which of these descriptions explains the client's affect?

☐ 1. The client is able to handle what happened to her.

☐ 2. The client is not normal and her behavior suggests serious psychologic concerns.

☐ 3. The client is more concerned about physical injuries at this time.

☐ 4. The affect of the client is a normal reaction and she may be making an effort to regain control.

100. The nurse is assigned to care for four postpartum clients today. Which client should receive priority assessment by the nurse?

- □ 1. Client who is 2 days postpartum and had a urinary output of 2,400 ml during the last 24 hr.
- □ 2. Client who has afterpains at the 6 a.m. breast-feeding session today.
- □ 3. Client who is 3 days postpartum and has an oral temperature of 101°F.
- □ 4. Client who is 16 years of age who had a cesarean section yesterday and placed her infant up for adoption.

Answers and Rationales

1. 2 The umbilical clamp may be defective. The nurse places another clamp on the cord stump to aid in controlling bleeding. Umbilical cord clamps are kept on the infant for at least 24 hr. There is no need to notify the physician. Removing the present umbilical clamp would cause increased bleeding. The nurse can not administer another vitamin K injection without a physician's order. (M)

2. 1, 3, 6 Diarrhea, seizures, and lethargy are all signs of lithium toxicity. Cardiovascular signs are typical of tricyclic antidepressant adverse effects. (D)

3. 4 Absent lung sounds suggest the presence of potentially life-threatening oxygen deprivation. Lung injuries are commonly associated with thoracic trauma from motor vehicle accidents. When triaging accident victims, airway and breathing hold the highest priority for assessments. Evaluating for cardiac rhythm, temperature, and urinary bleeding are also important, but are not the first priority in the primary survey of a trauma victim. (A)

4. 4 All women who received general anesthetic must be observed closely for uterine relaxation, leading to uterine atony and postpartal hemorrhage. Some clients may complain of sore throat from the insertion of an endotracheal tube; sipping cold liquids or sucking on ice chips may help relieve the discomfort. Flatus is a common complaint after surgery; ambulation assists in reducing flatus. Gastric reflux is a greater risk during the surgery because the client is prone and there is increased stomach pressure from the weight of the uterus. (R)

5. 2 Procedures are often best taught to the cognitively impaired child if the procedure can be broken down into steps. Because cognitively impaired children are concrete learners, they need to see the procedure actually performed. The other teaching strategies are not appropriate for this child. (H)

6. 1 When an adolescent changes or loses former friends, it is indicative that the peer group has changed. The nurse discusses new friendships with the child to determine what has prompted the change. Family history may put the adolescent at greater risk, but is not as great a risk for alcoholism as the loss of friends. Rapid mood swings and acting-out behaviors may suggest a mood disorder or a conduct disorder. Avoiding contact with unfamiliar people is indicative of a social phobia. (P)

7. 4 Local edema may cause pressure on the urethra, resulting in difficulty to void. Paralytic ileus, pneumonia, and thromboembolism are potential complications that tend to occur in the extended postoperative period (at least 1 to 4 days after surgery). Paralytic ileus is related to anesthetics, analgesics, immobility, and bowel manipulation. Pneumonia is related to ineffective airway clearance. Thromboembolism is related to immobility, injury, or vascular manipulation. (A)

8. 4 Criteria for determining if an infant is receiving adequate nutrition with breastfeeding are voiding 6 to 8 times a day and weight gain. The presence of bowel movements is not used to assess nutritional status. Increased maternal caloric intake assists in milk production, but is not considered in infant hydration. Asking about how long the infant feeds at each breast is not helpful in determining the quality of nutritional hydration for the infant. (M)

9. 2 Electrolyte imbalances may cause disorientation and amnesia; these are reversible when the imbalance is corrected. Vascular dementia is caused by an interruption of the brain's blood flow. Cognitive changes in HIV dementia is a late AIDS complication that is also permanent. Multiple sclerosis is a chronic condition in which some permanent cognitive changes may occur. When cognitive deterioration occurs, the condition is permanent and progressive. (P)

10. 2 An immobile tympanic membrane with a splayed light reflex and an orange-discolored membrane indicates otitis media with effusion (OME). Usually absent from OME is acute ear pain, fever, and an inflamed and bulging yellow or red tympanic membrane; these are symptoms of acute otitis media (AOM). Antibiotics are not required for initial treatment of OME because OME usually resolves spontaneously; antibiotics may be indicated for children with a persistent effusion for more than 3 months. It has been estimated that avoiding unnecessary treatment of OME with antibiotics could save millions of courses of antibiotics each year. (M)

11. 1 Daily weight taken at the same time and under the same condition is the most reliable way to analyze fluid-volume excess. Serum electrolyte levels and potassium levels can help in diagnosing electrolyte imbalances related to the fluid excess, but are not the most reliable information. Urinalysis can provide information about the hydration status of this client but are not as specific as daily weight. (A)

12. 3 The goal of administering nitroprusside (a potent vasodilator) is to decrease the systolic BP to approximately 100/70. BPs of 70/40 and 80/60 are too low to maintain appropriate cerebral perfusion pressures; a BP of 160/110 is elevated while on therapy, indicating the need for medication to be titrated in order to lower BP to an acceptable level. (D)

13. 3 Brown emesis is produced when a client is bleeding and the blood runs down the back of the throat and into the stomach and then reacts with stomach acid. This client is vomiting a large amount of brown emesis, signifying a significant hemorrhage and the need to immediately notify the physician. (M)

14. 3 Holding the infant's chest onto the mother's chest places the breast directly into the infant's face and eliminates the infant having to turn the head to gain access. The mother places as much of the areola as possible into the infant's mouth, not the entire areola. Holding the infant below the breast places the infant at risk for being dropped. If a clicking sound is heard, the infant must be removed from the breast and restarted; clicking indicates that the infant is not properly "latched on." (H)

15. 3 The child with autism does not relate to peers or parents. The child is not clingy towards a parent, does not develop language skills early, and does not play easily with other children. (P)

16. The client is having one premature ventricular contraction on this ECG. (A)

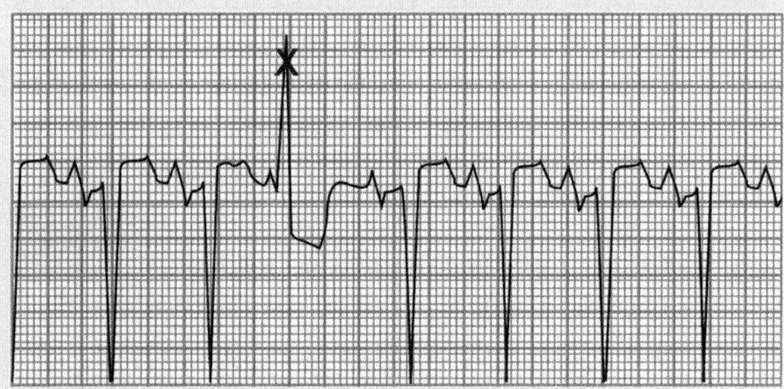

17. 3 To maintain accurate intake and output, the nurse weighs another dry pad of same style and deducts the weight of the pad from the total weight of the saturated pad. Charting blood loss by inspection is guessing. Not including this pad and weighing the saturated pad creates an inaccurate assessment of the client's output. (M)

18. 2 Calling for the sufficient amount of help to handle the incident safely is within the scope of a nurse's role. When a client is aggressive and violent, asking him to hit a punching bag may not alleviate the situation. The client may receive a dose of an antipsychotic medication, but it must be ordered first and then given in the most safe environment. The client who is psychotic and becomes out of control may not be receptive to the instructions of the nurse; therefore, having enough help before giving this directive is the priority. (P)

19. 3 The client is kept in a lateral position to prevent pressure on the vena cava, thus decreasing the chance of interference with fetal circulation. The catheter is anchored to keep the client's bladder empty and to keep the client from having to get up from bed. Fibrinogen level labs and type and cross-match for two units of PRBCs are appropriate to prepare for the need for PRBCs to manage potential complications associated with abruptio placentae. Fibrinogen levels will help detect impending disseminated intravascular coagulation (DIC). Blood typing and cross-matching is done in case of hemorrhaging. (R)

20. 4 Reassessing the clients' pain allows the nurse to determine the effectiveness of the administered medication. Not disturbing the client for the next 4 hr can be detrimental to the client's well-being and safety as adverse effects of pain medication could go undetected. Documenting nonverbal indications of pain is appropriate, but not the most important action. Administering the next dose in 4 hr may be unnecessary as the client may not require it at that time. (D)

21. 1, 2, 5, 6 Because the client has shortness of breath, the nurse should anticipate fluid overload. The heart muscle is not adequately pumping, causing a decrease in the stroke volume and increasing the systemic vascular resistance. Obtaining information about when the client first noticed the shortness of breath provides data about the onset of the fluid buildup. Questioning about a cough provides information about fluid accumulation in the lungs. Asking if the client wakes up at night feeling short of breath, and about the number of pillows used, provides information about the degree and severity of the fluid accumulation in the lungs. The client is not experiencing chest pain; when conducting a complete history, the nurse can ask if the client has had chest pain. Asking about caffeine intake may be helpful for clues related to dietary habits, but this is not immediately helpful when assessing the client's shortness of breath; however, caffeine intake may be a contributing factor to irregularities in heart rhythm such as palpitations. (A)

22. 4 When obtaining a urine specimen from an indwelling catheter, a sterile syringe and needle are used to access the catheter port that allows removal of urine from the closed system. This technique preserves sterility of the system and the urine specimen. Urine cannot be collected from the drainage bag because it would not be a fresh specimen. Disconnecting the tube from the catheter cab could introduce organisms into the urinary system, causing a urinary tract infection. Urine cannot be collected from the drainage bag because it would not be a fresh specimen. (R)

23. 3 A client's colostomy is ready to function when peristalsis returns, as indicated by the passage of flatus and presence of bowel sounds; gastric suction is discontinued and the client is started on fluids and food orally. A decrease in nausea and vomiting is not a criterion for determining whether or not the gastric suction should be discontinued. A flat, soft abdomen is an indication that abdominal distention has not developed, but is not an indicator for removal of the NG tube. Gastric drainage is not a criterion for determining whether or not the gastric suction should be discontinued. (A)

24. 3 A pulse oximeter, which measures oxygen saturation, is the most effective way to determine a client's need for oxygen therapy. Although the client may feel the need for oxygen during periods of dyspnea, this is not a reliable way of determining the client's need. Fatigue may be due to other factors besides oxygenation levels. Evaluating the client's hemoglobin level can provide an indication that the client may have less oxygen-carrying capacity but is not a reliable indicator of oxygen need. (A)

25. 4 Cells are inflamed because of infection. The client needs to be treated and reexamined in 3 months. Repeating the Pap smear in 1 week will not allow time for the infection to heal. Precancerous cells require colposcopy as treatment. The Pap smear would be negative if normal cells were found. (A)

26. 2 Dyspareunia is painful intercourse; decreasing estrogen levels cause vaginal dryness, a common complaint of women entering menopause. Although the client may consider hormone-replacement therapy, it is not a plan of care for everyone and she should discuss options with her HCP. There is no indication that this client needs a referral for counseling. It is not necessary to obtain a urine specimen unless the client has symptoms of a urinary track infection. (H)

27. 1 Benztropine mesylate (Cogentin) is an anti-Parkinson medication ordered for symptoms of a shuffling gait and persistent drooling (extrapyramidal symptoms). Photosensitivity, photophobia, leukopenia, altered liver enzymes, and constipation and nausea are all side effects of the chlorpromazine, but are not treated with the anti-Parkinson medication. (D)

28. 4 Although functional ability to lower extremities may be lost with spinal cord injury, reflex responses may remain. The nurse avoids drawing the client's attention to the muscle movement. The physician does not need to be notified. Muscle relaxants are not needed. (M)

29. 1 To enhance ultrasound visualization, the client's bladder needs to be full. The client is instructed to not void after drinking the fluids. The client will be placed supine for the procedure. It is not necessary for the client to have preop medications or to shower with pHisoHex prior to the procedure. (M)

30. 4 With Alzheimer, the client may exhibit personality changes. Difficulties with coordination, appetite, and hearing are not associated with the diagnosis of Alzheimer disease. (P)

31. 2 A number of children with autism demonstrate poor sensation of pain and thus bite their hands or bang their heads repeatedly. The other behaviors are not typical of children with autism. (H)

32. 1 Encopresis (inappropriate soiling of stool) is a symptom of an underlying stress or disease. The child does not have control over the stooling and, therefore, should not be punished. The parents are instructed to keep the rectal area clean and dry. Bismuth subsalicylate (Kaopectate) will not control the encopresis. The parents are advised to encourage normal activities to the extent possible. (H)

33. 3 Women who are identified as HIV-positive are usually advised not to get pregnant; however, HIV status is often not discovered until after a pregnancy is achieved. Protease inhibitor drugs are available to reduce the transmission of HIV between mother and infant. An amniocentesis increases the risk of maternal-infant blood exchange and is avoided. Maternal antibodies alone will not be effective to protect the client or unborn infant. The HIV virus crosses the placenta early in the first trimester and is found in breast milk. Every precaution will be taken to limit fetal exposure *in utero*; follow-up testing of the newborn will be in order. (R)

34. 3 Children with conduct/behavioral disorders may be reacting to a high level of stress due to life events. Increasing consistency can be helpful; the nurse must consider all family members in the plan of care, including teaching them how to contribute to a consistent environment. Strict disciplinary action may cause the child to become more disruptive. An open-structure school will not have an environment that provides enough limits for this child. (H)

35. 4 The nurse instructs the client who is having difficulty breast-feeding to not use a hand breast pump with sore nipples because the pressure may cause fissures to worsen. An electric or battery-operated pump exerts less pressure on the nipples. Asking if the nipples are cracked yet or if they are everted or inverted does not address the issue of the sore nipples. Using the closed-ended questions about pain medication is not a therapeutic approach. (H)

36. 3 Approaching the client with an open-ended question allows her to disclose information in her own way and time. The other comments are opinions of the nurse and do not facilitate communication and information gathering. (P)

37. 4 To determine the cause of this problem, a quality-improvement study is conducted. Before implementing solutions to a problem, the precise issues in the hospital system must be observed and documented. Consulting with the evening nurses may be helpful, but this is a systems issue and involves all nurses who administer pain medication. It is most effective to determine the cause of a problem before initiating a change. The Joint Commission requirements mandate documentation of the effectiveness of analgesia within 30 min after administration. (M)

38. 3 Because infants are preverbal, observation is the best method to evaluate pain; this includes both facial and body actions. Pinching the toe may illicit a pain response, but the pain will not be related to the surgery. While the parents can likely recognize pain in their child, the nurse must observe the child on a regular basis in order to recognize the presence or absence of pain; it is the nurse's responsibility to rate, prevent, and manage pain. Not all infants with pain express the pain by crying; crying may also indicate hunger or other discomforts, and thus is not a reliable indicator of pain. The nurse must observe the infant along with assessing other physical signs. (C)

39. 3 Laughter and whispering may be interpreted by the client with paranoid schizophrenia as being about himself. Socialization with peers is not a priority for the paranoid client. The client is not demonstrating self-harm behaviors and does not need to sign a contract at this time. Releasing information and discussing postdischarge options are not the priority education needs at admission for this client. (P)

40. 2, 3, 4, 5 The presence of the suck-and-swallow reflex and bowel sounds, lack of gastric residual, and normal temperature are signs of well-being and normal findings of a healthy neonate. Abdominal distention, respiratory distress, and presence of bowel loops are indications of distress and need to be considered carefully before going ahead with oral feeding. The presence of a Moro reflex is a normal finding that does not directly influence feeding. (A)

41. 1, 3, 4, 5 Lightening injuries can be fatal. It is important that the nurse instruct clients to observe the following precautions to prevent injury: Stay off the telephone and turn off nearby computers as electricity can travel through the phone line and computer outlets; get out of the bathtub as water is a conductor of electricity; and seek shelter in a building or vehicle. Seeking shelter under a tall tree is a poor idea as the tree will act as a conductor of the electricity in the lightening. (M)

42. 2, 3, 4, 1 Acute epiglottis is a medical emergency. The first priority is to assure an airway. The nurse then calms the parents to keep the child from becoming agitated as this could precipitate a complete airway obstruction; the parents can hold the child in an upright position for comfort and to ease the child's breathing. Next, the nurse administers IV fluids to prevent dehydration and then administers antipyretic and antibiotics as ordered to manage the high fever. (R)

43. 2 The client's intake and output record indicate the client's output exceeds intake. The goal is to restore fluid balance by increasing fluid intake. The client will likely receive IV fluids with electrolytes. The nurse does not restrict fluids. If the client is having diarrhea, the HCP may order an antidiarrheal drug, not a stool softener. There is no indication that the client is loosing fluids from vomiting; the nurse does not administer an antiemetic. (A)

44. 1 Gross, painless hematuria is the most common clinical finding of bladder cancer. Bladder cancers can be detected using IVP, ultrasound, CT, or MRI; however, the presence of cancer is confirmed by cystoscopy and biopsy. The clinical staging of carcinoma of the bladder is determined by the depth of invasion of the bladder wall and surrounding tissue. Pathologic grading systems are used to classify the malignant potential of tumor cells, indicating a scale from well-differentiated to anaplastic categories. Low-stage, low-grade bladder cancers are the most responsive to treatment and are more easily cured. (A)

45. 1 Falling asleep with a bottle of formula allows formula to remain in contact with teeth for an extended time, which leads to "baby-bottle syndrome," or tooth decay. The nurse intervenes and then also takes the opportunity to explain the rationale for not propping the bottle. The other actions are not appropriate or safe for the baby. (M)

46. 3 The RN making assignments should first give the LVN/LPN the opportunity to explore the concerns and fears about caring for a client with HIV. The other options do not address the present concern or create an environment that will generate useful knowledge regarding future assignments. (M)

47. 2 Kegel exercises are used to alleviate perineal discomfort and to strengthen the muscles of the pelvic floor. The client can begin these exercises on the third postpartum day. The nurse instructs the client to tighten and relax her perineal muscles 10 to 25 times in succession as if she were trying to stop voiding. Aerobic classes, swimming, and walking are also good exercises to incorporate after she progresses through her postpartum period, but do not target the muscles of the pelvic floor. (M)

48. 3 The client's identification must be verified with a family member or another individual who is acquainted with the client. It is not appropriate to rely on a head nod for identification from a client with confusion, nor is the chart by the door an adequate source for verification. Calling the physician will not assist in the process of identifying the client and administering the ordered medications. (S)

49. 1 Reflecting the feeling to the mother elicits further discussion. Asking "why" questions may make the family member more defensive. Comments about the physician indicate to the mother that her opinion is not important, and the blaming comment is accusatory. (P)

50. 3 The focus of the advocacy role is to assist clients in solving health concerns where traditions may interfere with the clients' rights. Developing teaching materials is aligned with the educator role. Recommending changes in agency policy is aligned with the manager role. Contacting local officials about crime rates is aligned with the political activist role. (M)

51. 1, 2, 3, 4 The client is experiencing arterial insufficiency distal to the insertion site and requires follow up by the physician. Using the guidelines of SBAR (situation, background, assessment, recommendation), the nurse reports to the physician the situation (absence of left pedal pulse), background (time of cardiac catheterization), assessment (vital signs), and recommendation (for the physician to assess the client). The client is not NPO following the procedure. (R)

52. 3 The client who does not know who she is has a personal identity disturbance. The assessment information do not support social isolation, disturbances in thought processes, nor ineffective coping. (P)

53. 1 This client's state establishes 16 years of age as the age of maturity in which an individual can sign his or her own surgical permit. It is important, however, for parents to be present during the preoperative period to be an advocate for the client. The other selections would not be appropriate in this case to sign the permit for the client. (M)

54. 4 Laryngitis, acute pain, and infection are all problems related to the client who has undergone a tonsillectomy, but the most significant complication in the immediate postoperative period is hemorrhage. A client who develops a postoperative hemorrhage is at high risk for aspiration, which can be fatal. (R)

55. 1 Explaining and educating the client about the labor process will help reduce fear and tensions and increase understanding of the process. Medicating the client is not allowing her to make choices and learn. Telling the client that everything will be alright once she receives the epidural is planting unrealistic ideas and is not being honest with the client. Being directive is not being a client advocate and does not allow the client to assume any responsibility. (M)

56. 1 The prognosis and treatment of colorectal cancer correlate with pathologic staging of the disease. Several methods of staging are used; the most widely known is Dukes classification. Surgical removal of the primary lesion is the treatment for Dukes stages A, B, and C. Chemotherapy is recommended when a client has positive lymph nodes at the time of surgery or has metastatic disease. Chemotherapy is used both as an adjuvant therapy following colon resection, and as primary treatment for nonresectable colorectal cancer. Radiation may be used postoperatively as an adjuvant to colon resection and chemotherapy or as a palliative measure for patients with advanced lesions. Radiation does not decrease the side effects of chemotherapy. (A)

57. 1 In Addison disease, there is a need for lifelong corticosteroid replacement therapy. Because the client with Addison disease is unable to tolerate physical or emotional stress without additional exogenous corticosteroids, long-term care revolves around recognizing the need for extra medication and techniques for stress management. The need for corticosteroid hormone is proportional to stress levels. A client who cannot produce endogenous hormone must adjust the dose of exogenous hormone to the stress level. Examples of situations requiring corticosteroid adjustment are extraction of teeth and rigorous physical activity such as being outdoors on a hot day. When in doubt, it is better for the client to err on the side of overreplacement. Overall, the client who takes medications consistently can anticipate a normal life expectancy. (H)

58. 3, 2, 4, 1 The initial step is obtaining a history of the injury: when, where, and how the pain started and the precipitating factors. Assessing the neurologic system is the second step in a nursing assessment. After the neurologic system is assessed, then the nurse performs a musculoskeletal assessment including range of motion, strength, and tone. Last, the nurse assesses vital signs and pain level; assessing heart rate and BP may help with assessing the amount of pain the client is having. (P)

59. 4 A plastic shell (nipple cup) can help the nipples become more protuberant. Gently pulling on the nipples, rolling the nipples with fingers, or rolling the nipples with a bath towel can cause uterine contractions and could lead to preterm labor. (H)

60. 4 While a client is in the postanesthesia care unit, priority care includes monitoring and management of respiratory and circulatory function, pain, temperature, and surgical site. Assessment begins with evaluation of a client's airway, breathing, and circulation status. Level of consciousness, pain intensity, and status of IV fluid therapy do need to be assessed, but are not priority. (R)

61. 4 Narcotic analgesics provide rapid and shorter duration pain relief, while nonsteroidal anti-inflammatory drugs provide longer-acting anti-inflammatory effects. These medications work together to provide longer-acting pain relief. The same risk is present for respiratory depression due to narcotic administration. The need for medication is irrelevant to the time of day, and weaning is not achieved any faster when combining the two classifications of medications. (D)

62. 3 Beta-blockers in combination with alcohol and hot water can cause vasodilation, hypotension, and a risk of fainting or injury. Milk does not increase beta-blocker absorption. Although a diet rich in vitamins and antioxidants may be beneficial, it is not required for a client because of beta-blocker therapy. Atenolol is used for long-term management of various conditions and is not indicated for immediate relief of acute chest pain. (D)

63. 3 Beta-blockers can cause significant bradycardia and hypotension. Assessing the client's heart rate and BP prior to administering beta-blocking drugs is required for safe drug administration. Other assessments, such as urinary frequency, lung sounds, and peripheral pulses provide data, but are not routinely required prior to administration of a beta-blocking drug. (D)

64. 4 Orthostatic hypotension, which is a drop in BP caused by an erect position, is prevented by rising slowly from lying down to a sitting position and from a sitting position to standing. Hypotension presents risk for falls, especially in the older adult client. Drinking adequate fluids, eating low-protein, low-fat foods, and exercising for short periods daily do not prevent orthostatic hypotension. (S)

65. 4 A calm, predictable environment aids in keeping client oriented, as interruption of their routine contributes to confusion. The client is usually not capable of planning his own day. Outside diversional activities can overwhelm the client and contribute to confusion. Limiting the client's caloric intake would be of no benefit. (M)

66. 3 Lightening is the process of the fetal head settling into the pelvis to prepare for birth; this process also makes breathing much easier for the pregnant client. There is no indication that the fetus is breech and needs to be turned. Lightening is a precursor to labor, but does not mean that labor has begun. There is no indication that the client is experiencing unexplained weight loss. (M)

67. 1 The client who is experiencing profuse vomiting and is unable to retain oral fluids is at risk for fluid-volume deficit. The client with heart failure and the client with acute renal failure are at risk for fluid overload. The client with indigestion is at risk for hypercalcemia. (M)

68. 4 To facilitate gastric-emptying and peristalsis, the infant must be supported at the back and turned to the right after feeding. Prone position is discouraged. Supine position is used for sleep. Placing the infant on the left side does not assist with gastric-emptying. (H)

69. 2 IV potassium must always be infused using an IV infusion pump at a rate of no more than 10 mEq/L per hour to prevent cardiac dysrhythmias. Potassium is compatible with IV solutions other than normal saline, but the rate is dose-dependent. A central line is not required for infusing intravenous potassium. (D)

70. 1 The client with hypoxemia will increase the rate of breathing in an effort to increase oxygen supply, which places this client at risk for respiratory alkalosis. The client who is oversedated will have a slow respiratory rate and will be at risk for respiratory acidosis. The client with COPD will be at risk for respiratory acidosis due to carbon dioxide retention. Hyponatremia is not related to respiratory alkalosis. (A)

71. 3 Some IV solutions such as blood and blood products require at least an 18-gauge catheter to prevent breakdown of the molecules being infused, and are inserted in a large vein such as the antecubital vein. The cost of the catheter does not affect site selection. The client's level of consciousness and expected duration of therapy have no bearing on site selection. (D)

72. 2 A client with GI suction is most likely to experience a fluid-volume deficit as this removes water from the GI tract. A fluid-volume deficit problem causes constipation. A client with sodium excess will retain water, as will the client with renal failure who will have poor urine output. (A)

73. 1 Rotation to slightly different positions prevents the same area of the areola from receiving constant pulling and pressure. Using different positions is for the comfort of both mother and infant. Milk production is not affected by position changes. Breast-feeding should not tire the mother. (M)

74. 2 The primary goal for the newly admitted client with paranoid schizophrenia is to decrease the level of anxiety and begin to develop trust in the treatment team. With hallucinations or delusions, the client is not ready to interact with the other clients on the acute psychiatric unit. The goal is to deal with the psychotic symptoms, thereby making the relationship with the family of origin not as important as decreased anxiety and trust development. The involvement of the paranoid client in ward government is not the primary goal at this time. (P)

75. 3 Assuring fluid intake of 60 ml/hr of fluid will help to meet the client's fluid requirements and minimize dehydration. Ordering a high-protein diet and keeping the client warm will not have an effect on fluid requirements. Tube feedings are not administered to provide fluid volume to clients with fluid-volume deficits. (C)

76. 2 Repeated approaches by the nurse assists in developing interpersonal contact with the client who is withdrawn. Direct questions are not therapeutic. Leaving the client alone does not establish communication. Having the client watch other clients implies she is ready to learn behavior from the other clients. (P)

77. 2 Regular exercise will help the client sleep at night. Tea contains caffeine and is counterproductive to sleeping at night. An afternoon nap will most likely make the client more awake at night. Sleeping medications frequently result in dependency. (P)

78. 2, 3, 5, 6 The client with cerebral palsy is screened before pump placement by the infusion of a "test dose" of intrathecal baclofen delivered via a lumbar puncture. The nurse monitors the client closely for side effects of excessive hypotonia (goal of therapy is to relieve spasticity), drowsiness, seizures, nausea, vomiting, headache, agitation, and catheter- or pump-related problems. Respiratory depression, not increased respirations, is also an untoward effect of baclofen. (D)

79. 4 The nurse uses the FACES pain rating scale for children or cognitively impaired clients because pain is more easily described through pictures. The visual analogue scale and numeric scale are reserved for adults. The Short-Form McGill questionnaire allows the client to give simple descriptions of pain by sensation and perception and is not necessary for the child who will have short-term pain. (A)

80. 4 The client with paranoid schizophrenia can be violent and is also suspicious of others. Ensuring the environment is safe for this client and the others on the unit is a priority nursing intervention on admission. The client's behavior has not warranted placing the client into restraints. The nurse cannot give a dose of clozapine (Clozaril) without an order from the primary care provider. A high-protein diet is not the priority that safety is for the client and the others on the unit. (M)

81. 4 Abortions are legal in all states as long as the pregnancy is less than 12 weeks. Individual states can regulate abortion in the second trimester. To be able to counsel the client properly, the nurse needs to know the gestation of the pregnancy. Knowledge regarding partner involvement does not play into the situation at this time. There is no need to assess menstrual history at this point, but this information will be helpful for prescribing contraceptives later on. The client's psychologic needs are important and will need to be addressed if she is eligible to have this procedure performed. (M)

82. 3 The nurse provides teaching to the family of the client with schizophrenia about the condition. It is also very important for the family to be able to interact with the team member(s) involved in their family member's care. Telling the family they are not the only family with a member with schizophrenia minimizes the importance of their situation and is not therapeutic. The most current therapies for the client with schizophrenia may or may not work for their family member and is not the primary focus of family therapy groups. Adaptive behaviors for stress relief may be discussed in family group but is definitely not the primary focus of the group. (P)

83. 1 Vascular dementia can occur after the client experiences small strokes. A history of Alzheimer disease and/or schizophrenia does not preclude vascular dementia. In advanced age, while vascular changes may occur, these do not mean the client will develop vascular dementia. (A)

84. 150 ml. There are 30 ml in every ounce of fluid. There was a total of 5 ounces of expressed breast milk consumed. (H)

85. 1, 2, 4 For the preschooler with ADHD, the nurse develops an environment that is as free from distractions as possible. The nurse interacts with the client on a one-on-one basis and engages the child's attention before giving instructions. The nurse refrains from providing instructions in "chunks" and instead separates complex tasks into small steps. Activities in the playroom may cause the child to become distracted; the nurse can provide games or movies that the child can enjoy alone. (P)

86. 1 The nurse provides client teaching about different relaxation techniques to promote coping with clinically significant behavioral symptoms. Adjustment disorders are transient episodes and, if dealt with, the client will not have these symptoms for the rest of her life. The client is unable to develop her own coping mechanisms, so informing her she will have to develop new coping mechanisms is nontherapeutic. The nurse advises the client to not spend time alone during the adjustment disorder. (P)

87. 2 The best indicator of effective care is the client maintaining her target weight for a period of time. The client saying she is accepting of her body is a subjective finding. The client moving away from her parents' home is also important, but is not as reliable of an indicator that the client will not return to previous habits. While interacting with peers is important, it is not the objective indicator of success that the weight maintenance is for this client. (P)

88. 1 Erickson's stages include opposing psychosocial states. On mastery of a stage's positive psychosocial state or task, the child is ready to move to the next stage. Piaget's theory focuses on four stages of development of cognition. Freud's theory encompasses sexual and aggressive drives. Acquiring culturally relevant skills from the mature members of a society is a component of Vygotsky's theory. (P)

89. 3 The child who has started chemotherapy treatments and is experiencing withdrawal, nightmares, and regressive behaviors is experiencing an adjustment disorder. These symptoms are not indicative of generalized anxiety disorder, as the child is not experiencing excessive worry. Oppositional defiant disorder is characterized by hostile defiant and uncooperative behaviors. Dysthymia is characterized by mild depression that lasts for 1 year or longer. (P)

90. 2 To ensure adequate fetal growth, the nurse advises the client to avoid dieting and weight loss during pregnancy. The client must eat adequately to supply enough nutrients to the growing fetus. Fetal movement is desired and viewed as essential for fetal well-being and maturation, but does not necessarily indicate the mother is obtaining sufficient nutrition. The client could consume the required daily caloric intake and still not eat a balanced diet, which leads to poor maternal nutritional intake. The glucose tolerance test checks maternal blood sugar levels; although an important assessment, by itself, the test does not indicate adequate nutrition and appropriate weight gain. (H)

91. 2 Children and adolescents may exhibit acting-out behaviors instead of describing their true feelings of depression. The health care workers often miss the diagnosis, but they do not necessarily believe it is not a condition. Periods of depression are not a normal developmental phase. Adolescents and children will not purposely cover up their feelings of depression. (P)

92. 1 Stimulant medications are the most helpful therapy for children with ADHD. Neither positive nor negative reinforcements are helpful for the ADHD child's attention span. Social skills training would not be as beneficial as medications for the child with ADHD. (D)

93. 2 The nurse assures the nipple of the bottle is kept filled with formula so that the baby is sucking milk and not air. The nurse discourages parents from heating bottles in the microwave because hot spots can be created in the center of the milk within the bottle. Infants are placed on the back or tilted to the right side after eating, with support at the back. There is risk of aspiration if an infant is left alone with a propped bottle. (H)

94. 1 Early therapy with lithium carbonate (Lithium) can result in fine hand tremors as the levels stabilize in the client. This tremor should improve with ongoing treatment. Coarse hand tremors and muscle twitching are signs of toxicity. While tremors do not keep a client from attending group therapy, this response belittles the client's concern. (D)

95. <u>0.3</u> g/day. (D)
1 kg = 2.2 pounds.
185 pounds ÷ 2.2 = <u>84.1 kg.</u>
4 mg × 84.1 kg = <u>336.4 mg.</u>
336.4 mg = <u>0.3364</u> g per 24 hr.
336.4 mg ÷ 1000 = <u>0.34</u> g per 24 hr.
<u>0.3</u> g per 24 hours.

96. 2 Slightly different positioning for each feeding will help prevent the same area of the areola from receiving the majority of pressure. Applying vitamin E lotion after air exposure may toughen the nipples and prevent further irritation. The nurse instructs the client to use water to wipe lotion off before each feeding; washing the breasts with soap will dry the nipple and lead to increased risk for soreness. A plastic-lined nursing pad prevents air from circulating around the breasts. (M)

97. 4 Somatization disorders are a response to stress and anxiety; learning alternate ways to decrease and manage stress will decrease the occurrence of somatic symptoms. Anxiety reduction and learning coping skills are very effective treatments for somatization disorder. The symptoms are psychologically induced, but are not consciously created by the client. Physical therapy will not improve conditions that are psychologically induced and will not address the underlying anxiety that is the cause of the symptoms. (H)

98. 3 The client is not receiving sufficient care. His age and weakness may make caring for the client difficult. His physical condition may predispose him to pressure ulcers; his unkempt appearance and dehydrated appearance suggest neglect. If physical abuse had occurred, the nurse would have seen the injuries. (P)

99. 4 The client who acts calm after the rape and is very cooperative is experiencing a normal reaction to the traumatic experience. She may be making an effort to regain control of her emotions. The fact that she appears emotionally unaffected by the trauma does not mean that the client is handling what happened to her. (P)

100. 3 Presence of an oral temperature of more than 100.4°F, excluding the first 24-hr postpartum period, is considered to be febrile and a postpartum infection may be present. The client with a urinary output of 2,400 ml is responding as expected with diuresis and fluid shifts naturally occurring during the postpartum period. Afterpains are common discomforts associated with breast-feeding. The client who is 16 years of age may need a great deal of psychosocial support after making her decision regarding adoption. (S)

Comprehensive Practice Test 3

1. The nurse is planning infection control procedures for infants and children younger than 24 months of age with chronic lung disease (CLD). What measure is most effective in protecting these clients prior to the start of respiratory syncytial virus (RSV) season?
- ☐ 1. Consistent hand hygiene practices.
- ☐ 2. Contact precautions (gloves, gowns, masks, and goggles).
- ☐ 3. Room assignments that group clients with RSV together.
- ☐ 4. Monthly injection of the monoclonal antibody, palivizumab (Synagis).

2. AF The nurse is providing care for a client with a spinal cord injury. The client has a urinary catheter in place. The nurse finds the client in a recumbent position with a rapid increase in the BP; he is damp from sweating and reports that he is having a pounding headache. The nurse should do which of the following in priority order? Place in order from first to last.
- _____ 1. Notify the HCP.
- _____ 2. Loosen clothing.
- _____ 3. Place client in sitting position.
- _____ 4. Check urinary catheter for kinks.

3. Which of the following provides the most reliable data when monitoring a client for complications of shock?
- ☐ 1. Urine output.
- ☐ 2. Serum sodium.
- ☐ 3. Serum glucose.
- ☐ 4. Radial pulse.

4. A newly delivered mother is breast-feeding her infant. The nurse determines the client understands how to remove the infant from the breast when the client:
- ☐ 1. Gently pulls on the nipple until the infant lets go.
- ☐ 2. Induces crying by tapping the infant on the feet.
- ☐ 3. Inserts a finger into the corner of the infant's mouth.
- ☐ 4. Obstructs the infant's nares so the infant will breathe through the mouth.

5. The nurse is admitting an adolescent with a newly diagnosed seizure disorder. The nurse should delegate which of the following to the LPN?
- ☐ 1. Complete the admission assessment.
- ☐ 2. Set up the suction and oxygen equipment.
- ☐ 3. Tape a padded tongue blade to the head of the bed.
- ☐ 4. Pad the side rails before the child arrives.

6. The nurse is providing client teaching to a mother whose infant has been prescribed supplemental iron for iron deficiency anemia. The nurse should instruct the mother that:
- ☐ 1. Oral iron should be administered for 1 month.
- ☐ 2. The physician should be notified if stools turn black.
- ☐ 3. The supplement should be given with milk to avoid stomach upset.
- ☐ 4. The supplement can be given with vitamin C to aid absorption.

7. A client calls the clinic and tells the nurse she is 24 weeks' pregnant, had sexual intercourse last night, and has noticed some spotting this morning. The nurse should:
- ☐ 1. Tell the client to lie down for 1 hr to see if the spotting stops.
- ☐ 2. Ask the client if she has ever had this happen before.
- ☐ 3. Tell the client to avoid sexual intercourse until after delivery.
- ☐ 4. Tell the client to come to the clinic to be evaluated.

8. A client has been diagnosed with trichomoniasis and is taking metronidazole (Flagyl). The nurse should instruct the client to:
- ☐ 1. Have liver function studies.
- ☐ 2. Expect orange-colored urine.
- ☐ 3. Abstain from alcohol.
- ☐ 4. Report increased urination.

9. A client in hard labor suddenly sits upright, grabs her chest, and complains of intense pain and shortness of breath. The nurse should do which of the following first?
- ☐ 1. Administer a drug to stop uterine contractions.
- ☐ 2. Place a central line catheter.
- ☐ 3. Restrict IV fluids.
- ☐ 4. Start 100% oxygen.

10. The quality-improvement goal on a surgical unit is to reduce the number of clients experiencing septic shock. Evidence for best practice indicates the nurses on this unit should:
- ☐ 1. Maintain hydration in clients.
- ☐ 2. Enforce frequent hand hygiene.
- ☐ 3. Perform appropriate pulmonary toileting.
- ☐ 4. Monitor older adult clients for subtle signs of infection.

11. AF A child is diagnosed with a blood lead level of 45 mcg/dl. The nurse is assessing the child's environment for risk factors. Which of the following presents risks for lead poisoning? Select all that apply.

- □ 1. The child lives in a home built in 1970.
- □ 2. The water supply comes from a well.
- □ 3. The mother uses a wet mop to clean the wood floors.
- □ 4. Food is stored in open cans in the refrigerator.
- □ 5. Orange juice is stored in a plastic pitcher.
- □ 6. The child eats four meals a day.

12. A client has the following arterial blood gas values: pH = 7.30; PCO_2 = 35 mmHg; HCO_3 mEq/L = 16. The nurse should develop a care plan based on the fact that the client has:

- □ 1. Respiratory alkalosis.
- □ 2. Respiratory acidosis.
- □ 3. Metabolic alkalosis.
- □ 4. Metabolic acidosis.

13. A client has just learned she is 8 weeks' pregnant. The nurse has completed obtaining the client's health history and drawn the ordered laboratory tests. Which of the following data requires the nurse's immediate intervention?

- □ 1. Blood type O Rh-negative.
- □ 2. History of premature labor.
- □ 3. Inadequate nutritional intake.
- □ 4. The woman drinks two to three beers a day.

14. A 39-week G1P0 client tells the nurse she has noticed an increase in vaginal mucus discharge that also has a small amount of blood in it. The nurse explains to the client that:

- □ 1. Cervical effacement and dilation are now complete.
- □ 2. She needs to be tested for vaginal infection.
- □ 3. There is a risk of hemorrhage and she should rest in bed.
- □ 4. This is from rupture of small cervical capillaries.

15. A nurse is making a home visit to a client who has been discharged from the hospital. The nurse is reconciling the client's medication with the client's medications at home and those ordered by the physician. The most effective way to reconcile the medication list is for the nurse to:

- □ 1. Read the list of medications the physician has ordered and have the client confirm he is taking them.
- □ 2. Have the client read the list of medications he takes to the nurse.
- □ 3. Look at the client's medications and compare them to the physician's orders.
- □ 4. Ask the client to identify the medications while the nurse compares them to the physician's orders.

16. A young adult client with depression consistently verbalizes negative statements about herself. What strategy should the nurse use to teach the client to promote a more positive sense of self?

- □ 1. Discuss ways to overcome deficits in physical health.
- □ 2. Invite conversation about past experiences that promoted feelings of self-worth.
- □ 3. Address ways to stop or control bad habits and impulses.
- □ 4. Establish how positive learning can occur from dysfunctional family situations.

17. While assessing a toddler's tympanic membrane, the nurse identifies that the membrane is dull orange in color and immobile. The child is afebrile. During the Play Audiometry Exam the child correctly identified 4 of 10 sounds. The child's speech is 50% understandable and has an expressive vocabulary of two to three words. These assessment findings most likely reveal:

- □ 1. An otitis media with effusion (OME).
- □ 2. An acute otitis media (AOM).
- □ 3. A perforation of the tympanic membrane (PTM).
- □ 4. A coloboma of the tympanic membrane (CTM).

18. The nurse is planning care for a client in the fourth stage of labor. The nurse should develop a plan to:

- □ 1. Promote parent-infant bonding.
- □ 2. Begin discharge teaching.
- □ 3. Give the newborn the first bath.
- □ 4. Teach the mother about newborn care.

19. A priority nursing goal for the client with multisystem organ dysfunction (MODS) is to:

- □ 1. Eliminate sepsis.
- □ 2. Promote perfusion of organs.
- □ 3. Enhance overall well-being.
- □ 4. Replace fluid-volume losses.

20. A client is being discharged on daily phenobarbital (Luminal). What should the nurse teach the client about this drug?

- □ 1. "Do not take aspirin while taking this drug."
- □ 2. "Monitor for elevation in BP."
- □ 3. "Do not drink alcohol while on this drug."
- □ 4. "Make sure to stay out of the sun while taking this drug."

21. A child has been diagnosed with autism. The nurse is instructing the parents how to approach the child who is refusing to eat lunch. Which of the following will be most effective for this child?

- ☐ 1. Allow the child to choose which foods to eat first.
- ☐ 2. Use an authoritarian manner to gain control.
- ☐ 3. Hide the spoon to approach his mouth.
- ☐ 4. Encourage repetitive movements of eating finger foods.

22. To decrease the risk of pressure ulcers in a client confined to bed, the nurse should:

- ☐ 1. Elevate the head of the bed to 45 degrees.
- ☐ 2. Encourage dietary intake of protein.
- ☐ 3. Massage the reddened areas every 2 hr.
- ☐ 4. Wash the buttocks daily with an antibacterial soap.

23. AF The nurse is caring for a client receiving nasal oxygen. Where should the nurse inspect the client for signs of pressure from the tubing?

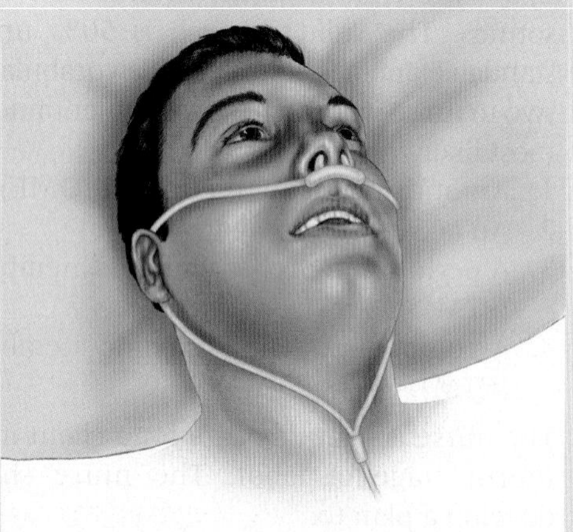

24. Which of the following is an appropriate goal for a client participating in a bowel-training program? The client will:

- ☐ 1. Drink 1,500 ml of fluids daily.
- ☐ 2. Have a normal bowel movement every other day.
- ☐ 3. Request the bedpan frequently.
- ☐ 4. Take milk of magnesia less than twice a week.

25. During a preoperative assessment of a client, the nurse learns that the client has been on long-term corticosteroid therapy. The nurse notifies the surgeon and the surgeon tells the nurse "not to worry." The nurse is concerned because sudden termination of steroids may cause the client to develop:

- ☐ 1. An electrolyte imbalance.
- ☐ 2. Seizure activity.
- ☐ 3. Cardiovascular collapse.
- ☐ 4. Respiratory failure.

26. The charge nurse is making assignments on the acute psychiatric care unit. Which of the following clients must be assigned to an RN?

- ☐ 1. Client with schizophrenia who is experiencing a fever of 103.6°F, BP of 180/110, diaphoresis, and pallor.
- ☐ 2. Client with schizophrenia who is having delusions that his food is being poisoned.
- ☐ 3. Client with depression who wants to spend the entire day in his room.
- ☐ 4. Client with mania who has not slept for three nights and spends much of the day pacing in the dayroom.

27. The laboring client has just received an epidural for pain management. To ensure adequate uteroplacental perfusion, the nurse should maintain maternal systolic BP above:

- ☐ 1. 90 mmHg.
- ☐ 2. 100 mmHg.
- ☐ 3. 110 mmHg.
- ☐ 4. 120 mmHg.

28. Prior to surgery, the nurse teaches a client how to cough and deep breathe effectively. Which one of the following statements would indicate that the client has correctly understood the nurse's instructions?

- ☐ 1. "Taking deep breaths will decrease my incisional pain."
- ☐ 2. "My coughing will be most effective if I lie on my back while coughing."
- ☐ 3. "If I cough and deep breathe, I will be less likely to develop pneumonia."
- ☐ 4. "It is important that I cough three times before I take deep breaths."

29. Following removal of a brain tumor, the client is experiencing "dull, constant, aching pain." The surgeon has left orders for medication for pain. The nurse should question which of the following orders?

- ☐ 1. Acetaminophen (Tylenol) 10 grains PO every 3 to 4 hr PRN pain.
- ☐ 2. Morphine sulfate 1 mg every 3 to 4 hr PRN pain.
- ☐ 3. Ketorolac (Toradol) 15 mg IM every 6 hr PRN pain.
- ☐ 4. Acetaminophen elixir 1 to 2 teaspoons every 4 hr PRN pain.

30. After receiving the preanesthetic medication, the client tells the nurse, "I need to go to the bathroom." The nurse should:

- ☐ 1. Help the client to the bathroom.
- ☐ 2. Ask the client to wait to be catheterized in the operating room.
- ☐ 3. Provide the client with a bedside commode.
- ☐ 4. Give the client a bedpan or urinal.

31. A client who is 18 years of age delivered a 7-pound infant 4 hr ago. An intrathecal morphine injection was used for pain management during labor. The nurse should assess the client for which of the following during the first 24 hr?

- □ 1. Bleeding at the catheter site.
- □ 2. Increased respiratory rate.
- □ 3. Elevated BP.
- □ 4. Pruritus.

32. AF The nurse is assessing a client following surgery. During the immediate postoperative period in the recovery room, the client's vital signs were stable. On admission to the medical-surgical nursing unit at 1030 the client's pulse was 115 and blood pressure was 110/50. The nurse is reviewing the vital signs record of the last 20 min.

VITAL SIGNS

Date	Time	Pulse	Respirations	Blood Pressure
5/20/09	1000	90	20	134/64
	1010	92	20	130/60
	1020	110	22	128/54

The nurse should:

- □ 1. Elevate the head of the bed and encourage deep breathing.
- □ 2. Take vital signs again; the client is most likely still under the influence of the anesthesia.
- □ 3. Increase oxygen flow rate from 2 liters to 3 liters per nasal cannula.
- □ 4. Report vital signs to the surgeon.

33. A young adult male is experiencing withdrawal symptoms from heroin and is brought to the emergency department. As the nurse starts an IV infusion with normal saline, the client asks why the IV is needed and tells the nurse it is not necessary. What explanation should the nurse give the client about the need for IV fluids?

- □ 1. "The fluids will help prevent you from becoming dehydrated."
- □ 2. "You need these fluids since you could have a seizure."
- □ 3. "Because you are groggy I am giving you fluids instead of food."
- □ 4. "There is a need to give you insulin medication through the fluids."

34. The nurse is caring for a client who had abdominal surgery and has had a nasogastric (NG) tube inserted. A priority nursing goal for the care of this client is to:

- □ 1. Maintain client's fluid and electrolyte balance.
- □ 2. Provide a clear liquid diet for the client.
- □ 3. Administer stool softeners as needed.
- □ 4. Help the client stay on complete bed rest.

35. A client who had abdominal surgery 3 days ago is reluctant to ambulate. The nurse notes that the client has developed a nonproductive cough, has a temperature of 100°F, and hears crackles at the base of his lungs. The nurse should first:

- □ 1. Encourage the client to cough.
- □ 2. Remind the client about the importance of ambulation.
- □ 3. Notify the client's HCP.
- □ 4. Chart the assessments in the progress notes.

36. The nurse is preparing to ambulate a postoperative client for the first time since surgery. In order to decrease the risk for falling, the nurse should have the client:

- □ 1. Stand at the bedside for 5 min before walking.
- □ 2. Transfer directly from the bed to a bedside chair.
- □ 3. Elevate the head of the bed before sitting on the bedside.
- □ 4. Avoid taking any narcotics for 30 min before ambulating.

37. The nurse is teaching a client how to change an abdominal dressing and care for the incision. Which of the following responses indicates that the client understands the instructions about wound care?

- □ 1. "I should change my dressing only if I notice a foul odor."
- □ 2. "It is normal for the edges of my wound to look slightly raised."
- □ 3. "It will be normal for me to have an elevated temperature until my wound is healed."
- □ 4. "I should expect my incision to feel warm to touch."

38. AF A client is to receive meperidine (Demerol) 75 mg and atropine 0.7 mg (intramuscularly) on call to the operating room. The vial of atropine is marked 1/120 grain/ml (0.5 mg/ml). How much atropine should the nurse administer? ________ ml

39. The nurse is assessing a client who had a thoracentesis with removal of 300 ml of fluid 2 hr ago. Which of the following findings should the nurse report to the physician?

- □ 1. Symmetric respiratory excursion.
- □ 2. Pain at needle insertion site.
- □ 3. Uncontrollable coughing.
- □ 4. Auscultation of crackles.

40. A client with traits of a dependent personality disorder who is experiencing anxiety is working with the nurse on the problem of

social isolation. Which problem should the nurse and client discuss during their therapeutic interaction?
- ☐ 1. Client's tendency to withdraw from social opportunities.
- ☐ 2. Client's feeling of being in a dreamlike state.
- ☐ 3. Client's frequent and spontaneous travels away from home.
- ☐ 4. Client's misinterpretation of common environmental stimuli.

41. A client with pharyngitis is instructed to take an antibiotic for 10 days. After 3 days of treatment the client reports to the nurse that her symptoms have resolved and she wants to stop taking the antibiotic because she has nausea. An appropriate response for the nurse to make would be:
- ☐ 1. "Stop taking the medication and ask your HCP if you can have a prescription of another antibiotic."
- ☐ 2. "If your symptoms are gone, it is okay for you to stop taking the antibiotics."
- ☐ 3. "Stop the medication for now, but if your symptoms return, start taking the antibiotics again."
- ☐ 4. "Try taking the medication with some food. Your nausea will subside in a few days. It is important to take all of the medication."

42. A client had a laryngectomy 2 days ago. The client is restless and slightly confused and has a respiratory rate of 24 breaths per minute. The nurse should first:
- ☐ 1. Offer the client pain medication.
- ☐ 2. Suction the client.
- ☐ 3. Assess the client.
- ☐ 4. Orient the client.

43. The client with tachycardia is experiencing all of the following clinical manifestations. Which of the following requires the nurse's immediate intervention?
- ☐ 1. Chest pain.
- ☐ 2. Increased urine output.
- ☐ 3. Mild orthostatic hypotension.
- ☐ 4. ECG tracing with P wave touching the T wave.

44. AF A client is admitted with a temperature of 103°F, dyspnea, and a productive cough. The physician's admitting orders include:

Bed rest.
Oxygen at 2 liters/nasal cannula.
Amoxicillin 500 mg IV every 8 hr.
Acetaminophen (Tylenol), two tablets.
Blood culture stat.

In which order of priority should the nurse implement these orders? Place in order from first to last.

_____ 1. Start the oxygen.
_____ 2. Administer the amoxicillin.
_____ 3. Administer the Tylenol.
_____ 4. Obtain the blood culture.

45. A client has a chest tube in place. There is continuous bubbling of the fluid in the water-seal chamber. This is an indication that:
- ☐ 1. Tube has an air leak.
- ☐ 2. Drainage system is blocked.
- ☐ 3. Lung has collapsed.
- ☐ 4. Water needs to be replaced.

46. After a myocardial infarction, an older adult client may experience increased complications related to tissue perfusion because:
- ☐ 1. Peripheral vascular resistance is increased.
- ☐ 2. Aging arteries are more elastic.
- ☐ 3. Increased blood clotting may occur.
- ☐ 4. Older adult clients respond less readily to cardiac medications.

47. A client is receiving thrombolytic therapy with tPA (tissue plasminogen activator) for an acute anterior myocardial infarction. The nurse evaluates the therapy as being effective when:
- ☐ 1. Client's serum cardiac enzymes return to normal.
- ☐ 2. Client's ST segment returns to baseline.
- ☐ 3. Client's chest pain is completely resolved.
- ☐ 4. Client can ambulate the length of the hall.

48. The laboring client has been in a Fowler position for 2 hr. Contractions palpate moderate intensity. The nurse repositions the client to a left lateral side-lying position. An expected outcome is to:
- ☐ 1. Decrease fetal heart rate.
- ☐ 2. Increase contraction frequency.
- ☐ 3. Increase maternal BP.
- ☐ 4. Increase uterine blood flow.

49. AF A client is admitted with an infected finger of 2 days' duration. Which of the following indicates that the client may be experiencing septic shock? Select all that apply.
- ☐ 1. Systolic BP of 70/42.
- ☐ 2. Pulmonary artery wedge pressure of 4 mmHg.
- ☐ 3. Respiratory rate of 18 breaths/min.
- ☐ 4. Heart rate of 60 beats/min.
- ☐ 5. Oral temperature of 98.8°F.
- ☐ 6. Flushed, warm skin.

50. AF A client is admitted to the hospital with an exacerbation of multiple sclerosis (MS). Which of the following indicate the client is at risk for impaired gas exchange? Select all that apply.
- ☐ 1. Blurred vision.
- ☐ 2. Muscle weakness.
- ☐ 3. Slurred speech.
- ☐ 4. Loss of sensation.
- ☐ 5. Numbness.
- ☐ 6. Partial paralysis.

51. A child was revived with rescue breathing following a near-drowning incident in a swimming pool. The nurse should advise the parents to do which of the following next?
- □ 1. Have the child sleep with the head elevated on pillows.
- □ 2. Monitor the child for any respiratory complications.
- □ 3. Wake the child every 2 hr during the night to assess consciousness.
- □ 4. Bring the child to the hospital.

52. A client with newly diagnosed Guillain-Barré syndrome is admitted to the hospital. The nurse should place which of the following at the client's bedside?
- □ 1. Lumbar puncture tray.
- □ 2. Intubation equipment.
- □ 3. Gauze bandage.
- □ 4. Scissors.

53. AF A client who weighs 90 kg and had a 50% burn injury at 1000 is admitted to the hospital at 1200. He is to receive 18,000 ml of fluid during the first 24 hr after his injury. According to the Parkland formula, at what rate should the nurse infuse the fluid when the IV is started at noon?

_______________ ml/hr

54. A nurse is administering enoxaparin (Lovenox) with a 0.5-inch, 25-gauge needle. At what angle should the nurse administer this medication?
- □ 1. 90 degrees.
- □ 2. 60 degrees.
- □ 3. 45 degrees.
- □ 4. 15 degrees.

55. AF A nurse is administering metoprolol succinate (Toprol-XL) 50 mg PO. The nurse on the night shift reported that the client has been wheezing. Prior to administering the drug, the nurse checks the client's BP and heart rate for the last 24 hr.

VITAL SIGNS

Date	Time	Blood Pressure	Pulse
7/19/09	0700	120/80	72
	1100	110/70	65
	1500	110/65	68
	1900	110/70	60
	2300	104/68	54
7/20/09	0300	104/68	48
	0700	110/70	48

At 0800 on 7/20/09 the nurse should:
- □ 1. Arouse the client to increase the BP and heart rate.
- □ 2. Withhold the medication and notify the physician.
- □ 3. Administer the tablet and instruct the client to chew the tablet before swallowing.
- □ 4. Instruct the client to take deep breaths to manage the wheezing.

56. A child has been admitted with a history of frequent absence seizures. The nurse should assess this client for which of the following?
- □ 1. Violent jerking movements of the arms and legs.
- □ 2. Complex auditory or visual hallucinations.
- □ 3. Purposeless automatisms such as running, kicking, or laughing.
- □ 4. Brief losses of consciousness that are often mistaken for daydreaming.

57. Which of the following school-aged children should have an annual tuberculin skin test (TST)?
- □ 1. Child who in the past had confirmed contact with TB-infected person.
- □ 2. Child who has had clinical findings suggesting TB disease.
- □ 3. Child who is infected with human immunodeficiency virus (HIV).
- □ 4. Child who has a history of travel to an endemic country.

58. Which medication listed on a client's home medication sheet prompts the nurse to question this client further about a history of prostate enlargement?
- □ 1. Tamsulosin hydrochloride (Flomax).
- □ 2. Albuterol (Proventil).
- □ 3. Metoprolol succinate (Toprol-XL).
- □ 4. Omeprazole (Prilosec).

59. A client returns to the nursing unit following placement of an endoluminal stent to treat an abdominal aortic aneurysm. The nurse is assessing the operative sites. The nurse should inspect which of the following sites?
- □ 1. Right and left antecubital arteries.
- □ 2. Right and left carotid arteries.
- □ 3. Right and left femoral arteries.
- □ 4. Right and left popliteal arteries.

60. Which of the following findings suggests a potential hearing impairment for an infant?
- □ 1. Persistence of the Moro reflex.
- □ 2. Babbling sounds that disappear at 7 months of age.
- □ 3. Speaking the first words at 14 months of age.
- □ 4. Gesturing to indicate wants at 15 months of age.

61. A client delivered a 10-pound baby 2 hr ago. She has an IV of lactated Ringer solution with 20 units oxytocin (Pitocin). The nurse concludes the medication is providing the desired effect when the client demonstrates which of the following?
- □ 1. BP is 120/70.
- □ 2. Lochia is rubra in color.
- □ 3. Pain is decreased.
- □ 4. Uterus is firm.

62. After receiving a change of shift report at 0700 which of these clients should the nurse assess first?
- □ 1. Toddler with a history of tonic-clonic seizures who seized yesterday.
- □ 2. Preschooler who was started on a ketogenic diet 48 hr ago.
- □ 3. Infant with an open anterior fontanel that is bulging and tense.
- □ 4. School-aged child who is scheduled for a ventriculoperitoneal shunt revision in 1 hr.

63. Which of the following nonpharmacologic pain interventions does the nurse instruct for a child with juvenile idiopathic arthritis (JIA)?
- □ 1. A bath towel, wrung out after being heated in a microwave.
- □ 2. An ice pack covered by a pillowcase or towel.
- □ 3. Immersing painful feet in pans filled with cold water.
- □ 4. Hand massages provided by parents.

64. The nurse is teaching a client who is 72 years of age and newly diagnosed with Parkinson disease. Which of the following instructions does the nurse provide for the client to maintain mobility and independence?
- □ 1. Take warm baths and receive massages.
- □ 2. Use assistive devices such as cane or walker.
- □ 3. Use ice packs to prevent spasticity before stretching.
- □ 4. Use a narrow-based gait.

65. The nurse is assessing a client with a pyloric stenosis who is vomiting and is at risk for developing metabolic alkalosis. The nurse should monitor which of the following laboratory results as indicators of impending metabolic alkalosis?
- □ 1. Elevated serum levels of sodium and potassium.
- □ 2. Elevated serum chloride levels and decreased pH and bicarbonate.
- □ 3. Decreased serum levels of sodium and potassium.
- □ 4. Decreased serum chloride levels and increased pH and bicarbonate.

66. A client has type 1 diabetes mellitus. Which of the following provides the best evidence that the client is managing the disease appropriately?
- □ 1. Client correctly injects insulin.
- □ 2. Wounds on the client's feet are healing.
- □ 3. Glycosylated hemoglobin A1c has decreased from 10 to 6.
- □ 4. Client has lost 10 pounds by following the diet.

67. A child is using prescribed griseofulvin for a ringworm infection on his arms and legs. Which of the following statements by the parents demonstrates the need for further education about the medication?
- □ 1. "I will gradually decrease the medication dose as the infection clears."
- □ 2. "I will make a note to remind us of the blood tests in a couple months."
- □ 3. "I will need to buy some foods high in fat to help the medication absorb."
- □ 4. "I hope my child doesn't get a headache from the medication."

68. A client with angina is taking nitroglycerin sublingually to alleviate chest pain. The medication is effective if chest pain stops in:
- □ 1. 3 min.
- □ 2. 10 min.
- □ 3. 30 min.
- □ 4. 60 min.

69. **AF** The nurse is providing care for an adult client who had a gastric resection yesterday. At 1700, the client is requesting pain medication. The client has an order for meperidine (Demerol) 75 to 100 mg every 3 to 4 hr. The nurse is reviewing the progress notes below.

PROGRESS NOTES

Date	Time	Progress Notes
11/04/2009	1900	The client is alert and oriented following surgery. Bowel sounds are 2–4 per minute. Received Demerol 75 mg IM at 1800. Pain is 3 on scale of 1 to 10. ~Debbie Schwartz, RN
11/05/2009	0900	Client ambulated to chair. Received Demerol IM at 0800; pain is 4 on scale of 1 to 10. Bowel sounds are 4 to 6 per minute. ~Brittany Ragon, RN
11/05/2009	1530	Client resting after ambulating in the hallway. Bowel sounds are 2 to 4 per minute. Client received Demerol 75 mg IM at 1400. ~Debbie Schwartz, RN

The nurse should do which of the following first?

- □ 1. Report the bowel sounds to the physician before administering pain medication.
- □ 2. Administer the pain medication as requested.
- □ 3. Assist the client to ambulate before administering the pain medication.
- □ 4. Tell the client to listen to music until he can have the pain medication at 1800.

70. A young adult client has a full-thickness burn of the right arm caused by an exploding gas can. While evaluating the extremity, the nurse is unable to palpate the radial pulse. The nurse should first:

- □ 1. Call the physician.
- □ 2. Use a Doppler.
- □ 3. Document the finding.
- □ 4. Elevate the arm above the heart.

71. Prior to the discharge of a client with depression from an inpatient mental health setting, the nurse evaluates the teaching about the value of sustaining healthy interpersonal relationships. Which statement by the client indicates understanding of the nurse's teaching?

- □ 1. "It is easy for me to blend into groups."
- □ 2. "I talk to at least two people each day."
- □ 3. "Now I can tell people about my weaknesses."
- □ 4. "I said thank you to the store clerk today."

72. Immediately following surgery, a client complains of nausea. The nurse should first:

- □ 1. Apply a cold wash cloth to the client's forehead.
- □ 2. Turn the client to one side.
- □ 3. Offer ice chips.
- □ 4. Administer an antiemetic.

73. The nurse is teaching the mother of a child with impetigo around the face and neck. Which of the following statements indicates the mother understands the teaching?

- □ 1. "I am so glad that my child will not be left with scars."
- □ 2. "I am going to contact a plastic surgeon to help eliminate the scars."
- □ 3. "I am so relieved that this infection isn't contagious."
- □ 4. "She needs to keep her hands clean in case she scratches herself."

74. The nurse is planning care for a client who is in denial about use of illegal substances. Which of the following goals is a priority?

- □ 1. Promote independent behaviors in the family and on the job.
- □ 2. Verbalize negative feelings related to anticipatory loss.
- □ 3. Discuss the relationship between personal problems and substance use.
- □ 4. Identify how distorted thinking causes problematic behavior.

75. AF Which of the following laboratory results indicate that a child with diabetes insipidus is responding favorably to medical therapy?

LABORATORY RESULTS

Test	Result
Urine specific gravity	1.015
24-hour urine output	1750 ml
WBC	Few WBC in the urine
Glucose	Negative

- □ 1. Specific gravity.
- □ 2. 24-hr urine output.
- □ 3. WBC in urine.
- □ 4. Glucose.

76. The client tells the nurse that he believes his abdominal incision has "ruptured." The nurse assesses the incision and notes that the wound has eviscerated. The nurse should first:

- □ 1. Apply an abdominal binder to support the wound.
- □ 2. Apply pressure to the wound.
- □ 3. Cover the wound with a sterile saline dressing.
- □ 4. Place the client in a supine position with legs extended.

77. Following delivery of an 8-pound baby, the client tells the nurse, "Since I delivered, I cannot get enough to drink." The nurse recognizes this is a physiologic response resulting from:

- □ 1. Excessive hormone fluctuations.
- □ 2. Fluid shifts associated with diuresis.
- □ 3. Increasing blood volume.
- □ 4. Slowed GI function.

78. A client with a substance-abuse disorder tells the nurse, "I have stopped using prescription drugs; I don't need to attend group therapy sessions." What additional information does the nurse need to obtain?

- □ 1. Parental and sibling substance abuse.
- □ 2. Negative behavior and self-injury.
- □ 3. Social and financial resources.
- □ 4. Daily habits and lifestyle.

79. The nurse observes that a hospitalized client is having difficulty accepting the authority of the unit staff and is unable to form relationships with peers. Based on this information, what other assessment data should the nurse collect to determine if the client may have symptoms of a paranoid personality disorder?

□ 1. Feeling entitled or self-centered.
□ 2. Demonstrating anger and adult temper tantrums.
□ 3. Being guarded and hypersensitive around others.
□ 4. Acting aggressive and destroying property.

80. A client with a borderline personality disorder is struggling to learn to express angry feelings in nondestructive ways. Which nursing intervention will assist the client to learn how to express feelings appropriately?

□ 1. Help the client explore feelings about family functioning.
□ 2. Discuss ways for the client to identify and handle frustrations.
□ 3. Teach the client to develop meaningful interpretations of stressors.
□ 4. Determine how compulsive behaviors can lead to acting out behaviors.

81. When administering methylergonovine (Methergine) IV to a woman in labor, an adverse side effect the nurse would recognize is:

□ 1. Headache.
□ 2. Hypertension.
□ 3. Tachycardia.
□ 4. Uterine cramping.

82. The nurse is making a room assignment for a child whose laboratory testing indicates pancytopenia. Which one of the following clients will be the most appropriate roommate for this child?

□ 1. Child with digoxin toxicity.
□ 2. Child with a viral pneumonia.
□ 3. Child with varicella.
□ 4. Child with cellulitis.

83. A client is admitted to the psychiatric unit with a diagnosis of schizophrenia, disorganized type. What initial intervention should the nurse undertake to facilitate the client's comfort and feelings of security?

□ 1. Teach client stress-management skills to decrease the high anxiety level.
□ 2. Assist client to identify actual and perceived losses recently experienced.
□ 3. Speak calmly and directly about unit expectations and procedures.
□ 4. Encourage involvement in unit activities rather than daytime napping.

84. Which one of the following clients is at risk for disseminated intravascular coagulation (DIC)?

□ 1. Client who is HIV-positive.
□ 2. Client with a brain tumor.
□ 3. Client with bacterial sepsis.
□ 4. Client who is pregnant with triplets.

85. A primigravid client is admitted for an induction of labor. She is receiving IV oxytocin (Pitocin) at 3 mU/hr. The latest vaginal exam revealed 2-cm dilation, 70% effacement, and minus 2 station. An epidural was placed 3 hr ago, and she is experiencing no discomfort and is resting quietly. The nurse should first:

□ 1. Assess bladder fullness.
□ 2. Discontinue Pitocin.
□ 3. Discontinue epidural infusion.
□ 4. Rupture amniotic membrane.

86. The nurse administers clozapine (Clozaril) to a male client who is 30 years of age with a long-standing history of schizophrenia. The nurse should withhold the medication and consult the HCP if the client tells the nurse:

□ 1. He might not take this medication after discharge.
□ 2. He feels like he is coming down with the flu.
□ 3. He started smoking cigarettes again.
□ 4. His stomach becomes upset after taking the drug.

87. An infant weighing 7 kg was prescribed 150 mg of acetaminophen (Tylenol) to be given every 4 hr PRN for temperatures more than 38°C. The therapeutic range for Tylenol is 10 to 15 mg/kg/dose. The infant's temperature is now 38.2°C. What should the nurse do next?

□ 1. Give the medication.
□ 2. Call the HCP to check the order.
□ 3. Recheck the medication using the "five rights."
□ 4. Confirm the medication with another RN.

88. AF The nurse is suctioning a client's tracheobronchial tree. Where should the nurse place the catheter?

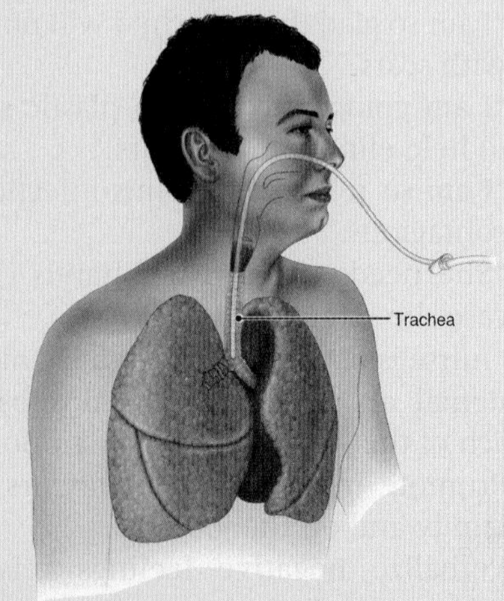

89. The nurse is assessing the lab results of a client with bipolar disorder who takes clonazepam (Klonopin) and carbamazepine (Tegretol). The client has had drug serum levels drawn. Which finding on the lab report would the nurse bring to the attention of the HCP?

- □ 1. Increased carbamazepine level.
- □ 2. Decreased carbamazepine level.
- □ 3. Increased clonazepam level.
- □ 4. Decreased clonazepam level.

90. AF A child who is 8 years of age is diagnosed with acute lymphocytic leukemia (ALL) and admitted for a round of chemotherapy. The nurse is reviewing the results of the child's laboratory tests:

LABORATORY RESULTS

Test	Result
White blood cell count	1,500/mm^3
Hemoglobin	8.5g/dl
Hematocrit	23%
Platelets	85,000/mm^3
Creatinine	0.7 mg/dl

Which laboratory value requires an immediate nursing action?

- □ 1. Creatinine.
- □ 2. Platelets.
- □ 3. Hemoglobin.
- □ 4. WBC count.

91. A toddler in respiratory distress was just brought to the emergency department. The nurse obtains the following initial vital signs:

BP	118/74
Pulse	124
Respirations	36
Temperature	39.2°C
Oxygen saturation	86%

Based on the initial vital signs, which of these physician orders should the nurse implement first?

- □ 1. Place on cardiac monitor.
- □ 2. Administer acetaminophen (Tylenol) for temperatures more than 38°C.
- □ 3. Start oxygen and titrate to maintain oxygen saturation more than 92%.
- □ 4. Administer nebulized albuterol.

92. A client is admitted to the hospital experiencing a manic episode. She has not slept for the past three nights, and has not been eating or drinking. The nurse informs her it is time for dinner. The client says she has too much to do to eat. What action should the nurse take next?

- □ 1. Remind the client that it is a hospital rule that all clients must come to the dining room for meals.
- □ 2. Return with a tray of food to the dayroom and feed the client.
- □ 3. Leave a tray of finger food in the dayroom within the client's reach, and monitor from a distance.
- □ 4. Ask the client if she would prefer to have a snack at bedtime, when she is not so busy.

93. A client who is 55 years of age is being admitted to an inpatient mental health unit. The client stops at the doorway and seems unable to walk in. The nurse asks the client to place his things on the bed. He replies, "Is that a good bed? What about the other one?" When the nurse returns, he is moving his suitcase from one bed to the other. The nurse recognizes that the client is so ambivalent that even when he appears to agree, he continues to be undecided. What is the best action for the nurse?

- □ 1. Move the vacant bed into the storage room because there are no private rooms available.
- □ 2. Turn down the covers on one bed and place his suitcase at the foot.
- □ 3. Give the client the bed by the door so that he will not feel so confined.
- □ 4. Tell the client that if he doesn't make up his mind he will have to sleep in the dayroom.

94. Which of the following indicates to the nurse that a client has recovered from the effects of spinal anesthesia?

- □ 1. Return of spontaneous breathing.
- □ 2. Stabilization of BP.
- □ 3. Resolution of back pain.
- □ 4. Complete return of sensation in toes.

95. A client who is at 32 weeks' gestation is admitted to labor and delivery with preterm labor. She reported using cocaine 20 min prior to admission. The nurse should first:

- □ 1. Apply supplemental oxygen.
- □ 2. Institute seizure precautions.
- □ 3. Monitor fetal heart tones and uterine contractions.
- □ 4. Place the woman in a supine position.

96. A client has been pacing all day. The nurse recognizes that the client is frightened by auditory hallucinations and is also suffering from the delusion that he is being stalked by members of organized crime. What is the best style of interaction for the nurse to initiate with the client?

- □ 1. Decisive action.
- □ 2. Ignore behavior.
- □ 3. Minimally intrusive.
- □ 4. Eager and enthusiastic.

97. A preschooler has periodic, colicky abdominal pain and has been vomiting off and on for the past 12 hr. The child's stools now resemble currant jelly. The nurse should:

- □ 1. Recommend a BRAT diet.
- □ 2. Notify the HCP.
- □ 3. Increase fluids to offset the fluid loss.
- □ 4. Place the child on a full liquid diet.

98. AF The nurse is providing teaching to a client about preparation for a colonoscopy that will take place in 2 days. The nurse should instruct the client to do which of the following prior to surgery? Place in order from first to last.

_____ 1. Drink the ordered bowel preparation.

_____ 2. Follow a clear liquid diet.

_____ 3. Drink one bottle of citrate of magnesia.

_____ 4. Remain NPO.

99. A client's agitation is increasing and the nurse decides to lead him to the quiet room to decrease stimulation. The nurse should make which of the following statements to the client?

- □ 1. "You are out of control and you must go to the quiet room at once."
- □ 2. "Come walk with me to the quiet room where you will be safe."
- □ 3. "You are upsetting everyone around you. It's time to go to the quiet room."
- □ 4. "I will give you 15 min to quiet down and then I am going for help."

100. A child is admitted with bilateral Legg-Calvé-Perthes disease. The nurse should place this child in which of the following positions?

- □ 1. Both legs adducted.
- □ 2. Supine with the spine straight.
- □ 3. Both legs abducted.
- □ 4. Low Fowler with both legs straight.

Answers and Rationales

1. 4 The monoclonal antibody, palivizumab (Synagis) can be given monthly in an intramuscular injection. The drug has been licensed for prevention of RSV disease. The American Academy of Pediatrics, Committee on Infectious Diseases (2003) recommends that RSV prophylaxis be considered for infants born at 32 weeks' gestation or earlier or if they have CLD. Hand hygiene, contact precautions, and structured assignments will all be helpful in preventing the nosocomial spread of RSV between hospitalized clients. (S)

2. 1, 3, 2, 4 The client is having autonomic dysreflexia. The nurse's first action is to notify the HCP, and then to place the client in a sitting position. Next, the nurse loosens clothing and anything that might be constricting the client. Autonomic dysreflexia is often caused by obstruction in a catheter, pressure on the back from lying on an object, or from an impaction. Last, the nurse checks the catheter for an obstruction and, if necessary, for other potential sources of pressure. (M)

3. 1 The most reliable data when monitoring a client for complications of shock is adequate urine output, which indicates adequate fluid status. Serum sodium and glucose do not indicate whether or not a client is experiencing complications of shock. A radial pulse alone is not the most reliable indicator of shock, but when elevated along with respirations and dropping BP provides data about the progression of shock. (A)

4. 3 Suction is broken when the mother inserts a finger into the corner of the infant's mouth. Pulling on the nipple will cause trauma and soreness to the nipple. Causing the infant to cry and obstructing the nares of the infant are unnecessary and dangerous. (H)

5. 2 It is within the scope of practice for the LPN to set up the suction and oxygen equipment. The RN performs the complete initial assessment. Padded side rails are controversial in their ability to protect a child from injury and can cause embarrassment for an adolescent in particular. Tongue blades are not kept at the bedside; nothing is placed inside the mouth of a child during a seizure. (S)

6. 4 Ascorbic acid (vitamin C) appears to facilitate absorption of iron and may be given as vitamin C-enriched foods and juices with the iron preparation. Iron supplementation is typically prescribed for 3 months. Stools will normally turn black with iron supplementations, and is not a concern to report to the physician. Milk will impair absorption of the iron through the gastric mucosa. (D)

7. 4 A woman must report vaginal bleeding, no matter how slight, to the HCP for further evaluation. At 24 weeks' gestation this woman could be experiencing ectopic pregnancy, hydatidiform mole, or premature cervical dilation. Having the client lie down will not stop the bleeding if there is a health problem. The client does not need to abstain from sexual intercourse unless a health problem indicates this is necessary. While the nurse can obtain additional information about the client's health history, spotting is serious and the client needs further evaluation. (R)

8. 3 The nurse instructs the client to avoid alcohol while taking metronidazole because alcohol interacts with the drug to cause flushing, nausea, and vomiting. The client does not need liver studies because the use of the drug is short term. The drug does not cause a change in color of urine. Typically, the drug does not cause a change in urinary patterns, but the client should increase fluid intake and the client may experience increased urination, which would not be unusual. (D)

9. 4 The client is experiencing an amniotic fluid embolism, which occurs when amniotic fluid is forced into an open uterine blood sinus, and is more than likely to occur during hard labor. The immediate nursing management is to administer oxygen for the pulmonary constriction. Death can occur in minutes. The nurse must focus on maintaining blood circulation to the client. Giving medicine to stop uterine contractions and placing a central line catheter require physician orders. IV fluids are increased to support circulating blood volume. (A)

10. 2 Because hand hygiene limits the number of micro-organisms that can be transmitted, it is the most effective method to reduce incidence of septic shock. Because adequate hydration and pulmonary toileting increases the client's resistance to infection, the impact on infection control is indirect. Older adult clients are more prone to infection and present with subtle signs and symptoms, but this option is limited to one population and the goal is to reduce infection for all clients. (M)

11. 1, 4 Homes built before 1978 are at greatest risk for lead poisoning. Canned food and food stored in open cans are also a risk for lead poisoning, particularly if cans are imported. The nurse can also instruct this family that risk for lead poising can increase during remodeling of older homes, and to be sure that children and pregnant women are not in the home until the process is completed. The risk to the water is from old pipes, not from the fact that the water comes from a well. Drinking water must be run until it becomes cold because hot water dissolves lead more quickly than cold water and thus contains higher levels of lead. Wet mopping helps contain allergens, but is not a risk for lead poisoning. Foods that need to be stored after opening should be stored in a plastic container. Lead is absorbed on an empty stomach, and the nurse can encourage the family to continue to eat regular meals. (H)

12. 4 The client has metabolic acidosis. The pH is acidic; the PCO_2 is normal; the HCO_3 is low. The nurse should contact the HCP. (A)

13. 4 Any substance abuse or use during pregnancy places the mother and fetus in jeopardy. The nurse offers the client information on community resources to help her with her substance abuse. The Rh-negative client will need to receive an immune globulin (RhoGAM) injection at 28 weeks' gestation. The history of preterm labor is not an urgent topic at this time; however, there could be a correlation between preterm labor and substance abuse, which would warrant further investigation. Inadequate nutritional intake at this time in the gestation could be considered a normal variance of pregnancy. (R)

14. 4 As the cervix softens and ripens, the cervical canal mucus plug is expelled. The cervical capillaries seep blood as a result of pressure exerted by the fetus. The blood, mixed with mucus, takes on a pink tinge and is referred to as "bloody show." Cervical effacement and dilation is a process of labor; when complete, the cervix is 100% effaced and dilation is 10 cm. There is no indication the client has an infection, nor is this an indication of hemorrhage. (M)

15. 4 The most effective way to ascertain that the client is taking the medications the physician has ordered is to have the client identify them while the nurse checks them against the physician orders. Having the nurse or client read the list and compare them or having the nurse look at the medications does not confirm that the client knows the medications he is taking and that he is taking all that are ordered. (D)

16. 2 The nurse focuses on the client's past positive experiences to facilitate positive feelings and self-validation. Any conversation that focuses on a person's deficits will only reinforce negative thoughts and feelings. Talking to a depressed client about bad habits or impulses can lead the client to focus on negative thoughts and feelings. Talking to depressed clients about learning from her dysfunctional family will only reinforce her negative thoughts and feelings. (P)

17. 1 An immobile tympanic membrane and an orange-discolored membrane indicate OME. Acute ear pain, fever, and a bulging yellow or red tympanic membrane are characteristic of acute otitis media (AOM). Antibiotics are not required for initial treatment of OME, but may be indicated for children with a persistent effusion for more than 3 months. (A)

18. 1 The nurse encourages parent-infant bonding during the fourth stage of labor. This may be an especially challenging task for the nurse if the mother has experienced a prolonged or difficult labor. Infants are in a quiet alert stage for approximately 2 hr postdelivery. This is an excellent time for parent-infant bonding. Discharge teaching and teaching the mother about newborn care will be tasks for the following day. The newborn can be given the first bath after the immediate 2-hr recovery period. (M)

19. 2 The priority goal of nursing care for the client with MODS is to promote perfusion of vital organs to prevent organ failure. MODS is characterized by the failure of three or more organs and carries a high mortality rate. The client may develop organ failure independent of sepsis. Enhancing overall well-being and replacing fluid-volume losses are not the priority goal for the client with MODS. (A)

20. 3 When phenobarbital is used with other CNS depressants such as alcohol there are additive effects that increase CNS depression. The nurse instructs the client to avoid alcohol while on this drug. Aspirin is not known to interact with phenobarbital, and photosensitivity is not a reported side effect. Phenobarbital can cause hypotension, not hypertension. (D)

21. 4 Children with autism typically enjoy repetitive movements or the same action over and over, so the parents can help the child eat by allowing him to use repetitive movements. The child with autism does not easily make choices, and is not able to respond to authority. Hiding the spoon does not foster trust. (H)

22. 2 Pressure ulcer risk reduction centers on the encouragement of dietary intake of proteins to keep the skin healthy and prevent breakdown. Elevating the head of the bed and washing the buttocks daily with antibacterial soap will not reduce the risk of pressure ulcers. It is recommended that the client be repositioned at least every 2 hr, preferably more often. Massaging reddened areas can contribute to skin breakdown and pressure ulcers. (R)

23. The oxygen tubing is most likely to cause irritation of the nares. The nurse can use a lubricant to prevent friction. (C)

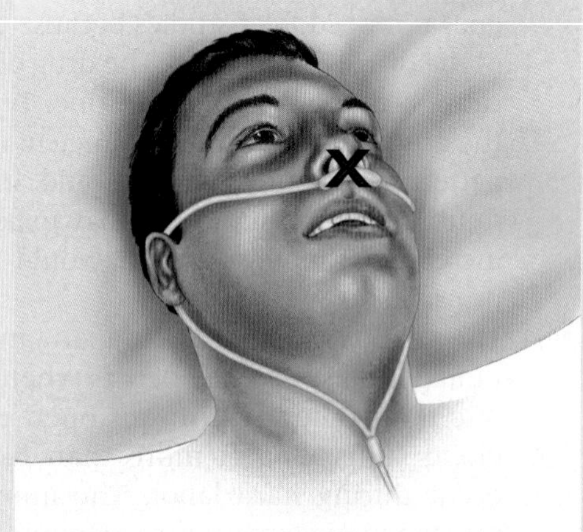

24. 2 Having a normal bowel movement every other day is an appropriate goal in a bowel-training program. Drinking fluids and requesting the bedpan frequently are interventions for a bowel-training program; taking milk of magnesia less than twice a week is not an appropriate goal of a bowel-training program and could contribute to constipation. (H)

25. 3 Sudden withdrawal of long-term corticosteroid therapy in a client can produce symptoms of cardiovascular collapse such as bradycardia and hypotension. Electrolyte imbalance, seizure activity, and respiratory failure are not problems associated with corticosteroid withdrawal. The nurse continues to communicate the concerns to the surgeon. (D)

26. 1 The client with schizophrenia with the high fever, the elevated BP, diaphoresis, and pallor is experiencing neuroleptic malignant syndrome (NMS), which can be fatal. This client requires close assessment and observation, making it imperative to have an RN assigned to this client. The paranoid schizophrenia client who feels that his food is poisoned needs to be observed, but could be assigned to an LPN. The priority is to observe the client with NMS. The depressed client and the client with mania may receive care from an LPN or a UAP. (M)

27. 2 Systolic BP should not fall to less than 100 mmHg or decrease by 20 mmHg or more in a hypertensive woman; a drop greater than this could be life-threatening to a fetus. The nurse must provide frequent monitoring of vital signs. (A)

28. 3 Coughing and deep breathing following surgery decrease the likelihood of the client developing postoperative pneumonia. Taking deep breaths will not decrease incisional pain, and may increase it. Coughing will be most effective if the client splints the incision while coughing. Deep breathing is preferred before coughing to expand lung diameter and volume, which improves cough effectiveness. (H)

29. 2 A client who is at risk of having increased intracranial pressure should not receive opioids such as morphine sulfate because these drugs can mask the signs of an altered mental state, a key indicator of increasing intracranial pressure. The client will likely receive pain relief with acetaminophen or ketorolac. The nurse evaluates effectiveness of the pain medications and collaborates with the surgeon as needed to assure pain management for this client. (A)

30. 4 The most appropriate nursing action is to give the client a bedpan or urinal. The client may be weak and groggy from the effects of the preanesthetic medication, and getting up out of bed may be difficult and unsafe for the client. Asking the client to wait to be catheterized may make the client uncomfortable. (S)

31. 4 Possible side effects of intrathecal morphine are intense pruritus, nausea, and vomiting. IV diphenhydramine (Benadryl) can be administered to reduce the pruritus. There is a low risk for bleeding at the catheter site. Depressed respiratory rate and hypotension may occur immediately following narcotic administration. (A)

32. 4 The client's vital signs are not stable: BP is dropping and the heart rate is increasing, which are signs of shock that could indicate postoperative hemorrhage. These findings need to be reported to the surgeon immediately. The other actions will not cause the vital signs to improve. (M)

33. 1 A client suffering from serious withdrawal symptoms from heroin is at risk for dehydration. The typical symptoms of heroin withdrawal are nausea, vomiting, abdominal cramps, perspiration, lacrimation, and rhinorrhea. Seizures do not tend to be a symptom of heroin withdrawal. Seizures do occur when withdrawing from drugs such as phencyclidine (PCP), sedatives, hypnotics, and anxiolytics. IV fluids are not a substitute for nutritional needs of the client experiencing withdrawal symptoms. IV insulin is not the standard treatment given to a client experiencing heroin withdrawal. (D)

34. 1 NG suction removes gastric secretions, which decreases fluid volume in the postoperative client. NG secretions also contain many electrolytes and the client is at risk for fluid and electrolyte imbalance. These imbalances can lead to complications that are life-threatening. Providing a clear liquid diet and administering stool softeners are appropriate interventions for postoperative care of a client without a NG tube. Maintaining the client on complete bed rest could lead to postoperative complications such as pneumonia or DVT. (A)

35. 3 This client is at risk for postoperative pneumonia due to immobility. The findings indicate a problem that could be consistent with postoperative pneumonia and need to be reported to the HCP. The other actions are appropriate, but the nurse's first action is to notify the HCP. (M)

36. 3 Elevating the head of the bed diverts blood flow from the upper torso and head, helping to prevent the potential for orthostatic hypotension. Standing at the bedside and transferring directly from the bed to a bedside chair will contribute to orthostatic hypotension and increase the risk for falling. Narcotics can cause hypotension, but the avoidance of narcotics will not decrease the potential for orthostatic hypotension. (R)

37. 2 Normal appearance of the edges of a wound should be slightly raised. A foul odor and elevated temperature are not normal findings in a wound and could signify an infection. The incision may feel warm to touch, but the client is instructed to contact the HCP if the incision becomes warmer and also inflamed. (M)

38. 1.4 ml. (D)
Atropine 1/120 grain = 0.5 mg.
0.5 mg:1 ml = 0.7 mg:xml.
0.5x = 0.7.
x = 1.4 ml.

39. 3 Uncontrolled coughing in a client following a thoracentesis could indicate irritation of the diaphragm, which can be a medical emergency. The nurse reports this to the physician immediately. Symmetric respiratory excursion pain at the needle insertion site, and auscultation of crackles are expected findings. (S)

40. 1 The client with a dependent personality disorder who suffers from anxiety usually has a strong tendency to withdraw from opportunities for social contact. The feeling of being in a dreamlike state is a characteristic of a depersonalization disorder and is not a trait associated with dependent personality disorder. The client with a dependent personality disorder does not travel away from the home setting and familiar surroundings; she needs guidance and reassurance, and would not be able to make the decision to travel. The client with a dependent personality disorder does not focus on or misinterpret environmental stimuli and will be preoccupied with the fear of being left alone or abandoned. (P)

41. 4 The nurse encourages the client to continue to take the antibiotic until the full dose of medication is complete. This is the only way to assure full effectiveness of the medication. Nausea is an adverse affect of the drug and may be averted by taking the antibiotic with food, unless otherwise contraindicated; this should be the first approach to managing the nausea. Since the client is not vomiting, loosing fluids, or having an allergic reaction, it is not necessary to contact the HCP for an order for another antibiotic. Nausea is a common side effect of most antibiotics, but most clients can manage the nausea by taking the medication with food. Antibiotics are only effective when the entire dose is completed; stopping and restarting the drug will not provide the necessary therapeutic effects. The HCP must make the decision to stop or change the prescription. (D)

42. 3 Restlessness, confusion, and an elevated respiratory rate are signs of hypoxia. The nurse first assesses the client to determine why he is exhibiting these findings. Offering the client pain medication may mask the signs of hypoxia. Suctioning the client would be performed if, after the assessment, secretions in the airway were found to be the reason for hypoxia. Orienting the client is not the priority at this time. (M)

43. 1 Chest pain is an ominous sign of cardiac ischemia, placing this client at high risk for developing a myocardial infarction. This symptom needs to be reported to the HCP and intervention taken immediately. The other clinical manifestations need to be addressed, but are not the priority at this time. (M)

44. 1, 4, 3, 2 The nurse first starts the oxygen by nasal cannula as the client is having difficulty breathing. The nurse then obtains the blood culture prior to administering any medication to determine the causative organism; administering IV antibiotics will alter the results. Next the nurse can administer the antibiotic, and then give the acetaminophen (Tylenol). (A)

45. 1 Continuous bubbling of the fluid in the water-seal chamber of the chest tube means that the client is experiencing an air leak in the chest tube; this is immediately reported to the HCP. This is not indicative of a collapsed lung or a need to fill the water chamber. The client would show signs of respiratory distress if the tubing from the chest tube was disconnected. The amount of water in the suction control chamber of the chest drainage system regulates the amount of suction to the client. (M)

46. 1 An increase in peripheral vascular resistance is common in the aging client. This may increase the chance of complications in the older adult client, especially after a myocardial infarction, as the aging heart must work harder in pumping against this resistance. This can increase cardiac workload and BP. Aging arteries are less elastic. Blood clotting is not affected by age. The older adult client is more sensitive to medications. (M)

47. 2 Resolution of ST segment elevation to baseline is the most reliable indicator that thrombolytic therapy has been effective in the client who has had an MI. Serum cardiac enzymes do not return to baseline until approximately 1 to 2 weeks because the effects of cardiac enzyme washout from thrombolytic therapy. Relief of chest pain is not a reliable indicator of effective therapy as the relief could have been provided via other medications that were administered. Thrombolytic therapy will have no effect on the client's ability to ambulate. (D)

48. 4 The left lateral side-lying position causes the heavy uterus to tip forward, away from the vena cave, allowing free blood return from the lower extremities and adequate placental filling and circulation. Assuming this position also promotes decreased maternal BP. Positioning the client is a comfort measure. Contraction frequency, increasing BP, and decreasing fetal heart rate are not goals of positioning. (C)

49. 1, 2, 6 Septic shock is characterized by a low systolic BP and a low pulmonary artery wedge pressure (PCWP) due to circulating endotoxins producing vascular leakage into the interstitial space. In the hyperdynamic or "warm phase" of septic shock the skin is also warm and flushed. Other signs include tachycardia, tachypnea, and hypo- or hyperthermia. (M)

50. 2, 3, 6 MS is a disease characterized by an inflammatory response that results in patchy areas of plaque within the white matter of the brain and the spinal cord. Blurred vision, numbness, and loss of sensations are all early indicators of MS and often mimic other diseases. As the disease progresses, the nurse monitors the client for muscle weakness, slurred speech, and paralysis, all of which could indicate weakness of the muscles of respiration, putting the client at risk for aspiration and/or respiratory complications. (M)

51. 4 Children who have a near-drowning experience should be admitted to the hospital for observation. Aspiration pneumonia is a frequent complication that occurs about 48 to 72 hr after a near-drowning episode. Other complications are bronchospasm, abscess formation, and acute respiratory distress syndrome. (R)

52. 2 Guillain-Barré syndrome is an acute autoimmune disorder characterized by varying degrees of motor weakness and paralysis. The nurse places intubation equipment at the bedside as the client with Guillain-Barré syndrome often develops facial muscle paralysis, making breathing impossible. (M)

53. 1,500 ml/hr. According to the Parkland formula for burn resuscitation, half of the fluid requirements must be given in the first 8 hr after the burn occurred. One half of 18,000 ml = 9,000 ml. The client was burned at 1000 but the IV fluid is not being initiated until 1200. In order to catch up and give the 9,000 ml in the first 8 hr, the nurse must divide 9,000 by 6 hr, which equals 1,500 ml/hr. The remaining fluid is administered over the next 16 hr. (D)

54. 1 Subcutaneous enoxaparin (Lovenox) should be administered at a 90-degree angle into a fold of skin. Because the needle length is relatively short, the other angles mentioned would result in too shallow of depth. (D)

55. 2 Metoprolol succinate (Toprol-XL) is a beta-adrenergic blocker that reduces BP and heart rate. Beta-blockers are held and the physician is notified if the pulse rate is less than 50 beats/min or if hypotension occurs. Because the XL indicates this is a long-acting formulation, attempting to crush or chew the medication is not recommended. An adverse effect of beta-blockers is wheezing; it will not reduce wheezing and may contribute to its occurrence. (D)

56. 4 Absence seizures are characterized by brief losses of consciousness, which are often mistaken for inattentiveness or daydreaming. Complex auditory or visual hallucinations and automatisms are characteristic of complex partial seizures. Violent jerking movements of the arms and legs are characteristic of tonic-clonic seizures. (A)

57. 3 Children infected with HIV and incarcerated adolescents should have an annual TST. The other children should have had an initial TST, but do not require annual screenings after the initial incident. (H)

58. 1 Tamsulosin hydrochloride (Flomax) is an alpha-adrenergic blocker that relaxes muscles in the bladder neck and prostate to promote urination in men with benign prostatic hypertrophy. Recognizing that this client has this condition may assist the nurse in the early detection of urinary retention. Albuterol is a bronchodilator. Metoprolol is used to reduce heart and BP. Omeprazole is used to reduce gastric acid production. (D)

59. 3 Endoluminal stents of the abdominal aorta involve deployment of an endoluminal stent via a femoral artery insertion site. The nurse inspects the operative site in both groin areas (femoral arteries) because of bifurcation of the aorta as they become the iliac and femoral arteries. The antecubital and carotid sites would not be used for any type of abdominal aneurysm repair. An abdominal incision is required if there is open or direct repair of the aneurysm. The nurse assesses the popliteal and pedal pulses for adequate blood flow, but the operative site is in the femoral artery. (A)

60. 2 An estimated 2 in 1,000 infants are born with permanent hearing loss. Clinical manifestations of hearing impairment include lack of a startle (Moro) or blink reflex to a loud sound, failure to localize a source of sound by 6 months of age, general indifference to sound, and an absence or disappearance of babble or inflections in voice by 7 months of age. (H)

61. 4 Oxytocin (Pitocin) is used to stimulate uterine contractions, decreasing the risk for postpartum bleeding. Pitocin is not effective in controlling BP or lochia color, or in decreasing pain. (D)

62. 3 The nurse assesses the infant with the bulging and tense anterior fontanel first because these are signs that the infant is experiencing increased ICP. The preschooler started on the ketogenic diet will face issues of hypoglycemia and nausea due to the high fat content of the diet; yet after 48 hr would already be adjusting to the diet. The toddler who had a tonic-clonic seizure will warrant close observation. The school-aged child with the VP shunt revision will have preoperative preparation, which is very important, but neither will take priority over a client with an increased ICP. (S)

63. 1 Heat has been shown to be very beneficial to children with JIA. Moist heat is best for relieving pain and stiffness, and the most efficient and practical method is in the bathtub with warm water. The nurse instructs the client to use a bath towel wrung out after being immersed in hot water or heated in a microwave oven, and then to cover the towel with plastic and apply to the area for 20 min. In the hospital setting, the nurse can apply hot packs. Cold (ice pack, cold water) is not as effective in relieving joint pain and stiffness. Massage increases circulation and may provide comfort, but is not effective in relieving joint pain. (C)

64. 1 Deficiency of dopamine in Parkinson disease results in tremor, bradykinesis, rigidity, and postural changes; therefore, warm baths and massages can help relax the rigid muscles and maintain or improve mobility for a newly diagnosed client. The nurse also instructs the client to participate in regular aerobic and anaerobic exercise programs to maintain muscle endurance and strength. Assistive devices are used in the later stages of the disease process. The use of ice packs to prevent spasticity before stretching is appropriate for clients with multiple sclerosis. Clients with Parkinson disease are taught to use a broad base, heel-toe gait, and increase the width of stride. (H)

65. 4 Laboratory findings reflect the metabolic alterations created by severe depletion of both fluid and electrolytes from extensive vomiting. There are decreased serum levels of both sodium and potassium, although these may be masked by the hemoconcentration from extracellular fluid depletion. Of greater diagnostic value is a decrease in serum chloride levels and increases in pH and bicarbonate characteristic of metabolic alkalosis. (A)

66. 3 Decrease in A1c is the best evidence as this indicates that the serum glucose level was lower during the last 3 months. The other behaviors contribute to this outcome. (A)

67. 1 Treatment with griseofulvin frequently occurs for weeks or months, and because some symptoms subside, children or parents may be tempted to decrease or discontinue the medication. For children who take the drug over many months, testing is required to monitor liver and renal dysfunction. Taking the medication with high-fat foods aids absorption. The nurse instructs the parents about possible drug side effects such as headache, GI upset, fatigue, insomnia, and photosensitivity. (D)

68. 1 Sublingual nitroglycerin works very quickly, with its onset being approximately 1 to 3 min. The client should start to feel relief from chest pain in 3 min and, if not, another dose of nitroglycerin can be repeated in 5 min for a total of three doses. (D)

69. 2 The nurse administers pain medication as requested. The client can have the pain medication every 3 to 4 hr as ordered. It is not necessary to ask the client to use diversional strategies while waiting to receive pain medication. The few bowel sounds are normal during the first 2 to 3 days after abdominal surgery and the nurse does not need to report them to the physician. (M)

70. 2 If unable to palpate a pulse, the nurse uses a Doppler to ascertain the presence of circulation and pulse. If the pulse is lost, an escharotomy by the physician may be necessary to relieve the edema causing pressure on blood vessels and restore adequate circulation. (M)

71. 2 By speaking to people each day, the client practices a social skill, which in turn helps to improve and sustain interpersonal relationships. Blending into groups is not actively developing or participating in daily interpersonal relationships. The purpose of interacting with people is to build social skills and relationships, not to tell others about one's personal weaknesses. Although this client's brief interaction with a clerk is positive, it did not address if the client understands the need to develop and sustain interpersonal relationships. (H)

72. 2 The nurse turns the client completely to one side to protect the airway and prevent aspiration in the event the client vomits. The other interventions are appropriate for nausea, but would not be the nurse's first intervention. (C)

73. 1 Impetigo contagiosa tends to heal without scarring unless a secondary infection occurs. Impetigo is very contagious for other children. Children can also autoinoculate themselves through scratching affected areas and then touching other areas of their bodies; thus, it is imperative to trim children's nails and keep them short. Washing the hands is not sufficient to prevent spread of the disease. (H)

74. 3 The client is using denial as a coping strategy. A discussion focused on the relationship between drug use and personal problems may allow the client to recognize reality. Promoting independent behavior at the client's home and place of employment will not be an effective strategy to help the client accept responsibility for drug use and the unhealthy behavior that accompanies it. Verbalizing feelings related to loss is a goal that the nurse and the client address after the client recognizes how the influence of the substance-abuse problem affects current functioning. A substance-abuse client often experiences distorted thinking, but the most appropriate approach is to help the client identify the relationship between the drug use and personal problems. (P)

75. A normal urine specific gravity (1.003 to 1.030) is assurance that urine concentration is taking place. The 24-hr urine output exceeds normal output. White cells in the urine do not indicate outcome of medical therapy. Glucose is normal. (A)

76. 3 Evisceration refers to a total separation of the layers of a wound with extrusion of the internal organs or viscera through the open wound. It is imperative that the wound be covered with a sterile saline dressing to prevent infection and/or peritonitis of the wound and the affected organs. Applying an abdominal binder may cause injury to the wound or internal organs, as would applying direct pressure to the wound. The nurse can place the client in a supine position to apply the sterile saline dressing, but this position will not solve the problem of evisceration. (S)

77. 2 The rapid diuresis and diaphoresis that occur during the second to fifth postpartal days result in a weight loss of approximately 5 pounds. The client often feels thirsty during this period and wants additional fluid. Although there will be hormone fluctuations after delivery, they will not have an effect on the client's thirst. Blood volume will decrease (not increase) after delivery, and the GI function will return to normal activity within several days. (A)

78. 4 It is important for the client to attend group therapy sessions to learn about how people, places, and situations relate to lifestyle affect recovery. Simply stopping use of a drug is not enough to sustain sobriety; the nurse must also assess the client's lifestyle and habits. Although a family history of substance abuse is important background information, assessment data about habits and lifestyle provides information essential for treatment. Finding out information on negative behavior and self-injury, and information on social and financial resources does not provide the nurse with insight into the client's resistance to attending group therapy. (P)

79. 3 A classic manifestation exhibited by a client with a paranoid personality disorder is the tendency to be guarded for dangers perceived to be in the environment, as well as being hypersensitive. The client who feels entitled and self-centered is demonstrating characteristics of a narcissistic personality disorder. Anger expressed as temper tantrums or other impulsive behavior is characteristic of a borderline personality disorder. Aggressive behaviors and frequent abuse of others' property is characteristic of antisocial personality disorder. (P)

80. 2 The client requires assistance that focuses on developing strategies for identifying feelings and implementing skills to effectively handle frustrations. Without such skills, the client is likely to engage in destructive behaviors to relieve the distress. Exploring feelings about family functioning is not an effective strategy for learning to express angry feelings. Teaching the client to develop meaningful interpretations of stressors does not provide the coping skills needed to manage feelings of anger. Compulsive behaviors are not characteristic of the client with borderline personality disorder. (P)

81. 2 Severe hypertensive episodes, bradycardia, and nausea and vomiting can result after giving methylergonovine (Methergine). There is no indication that headache is associated with receiving Methergine. Uterine cramping is a desired effect. (D)

82. 1 Children with pancytopenia are a higher risk for infection. The child with digoxin toxicity presents the least risk of spreading infection. The children with viral pneumonia, varicella, and cellulites have communicable diseases and would put the child with pancytopenia at risk for infection. (S)

83. 3 To facilitate the client's feelings of security and trust, the nurse explains all unit and care procedures and rules. Consistent expectations and well-defined procedures and rules will enhance the client's trust for staff and increase the level of personal comfort. Although stress-management skills are helpful to teach clients, this action would not be an initial action taken by the nurse. Discussion about the client's actual and perceived losses might be an effective nursing action after the nurse and client have established a trusting and consistent relationship. Only after the nurse provides orientation to the unit, demonstrates consistent, caring behavior, and explains all unit rules and activities to the client, will the client be more comfortable engaging in unit activities. (P)

84. 3 DIC is caused by abnormal activation of the clotting cascade, resulting in clotting in small vessels; when the clotting factors are used, bleeding occurs. Persons at risk for DIC are those with overwhelming infection such as bacterial sepsis or massive tissue injury. The nurse assesses these clients when they are hospitalized because DIC usually has a sudden onset. HIV typically does not precipitate DIC. While lung, colon, and stomach cancers may be associated with DIC, brain tumors are not. While obstetric complications such as abruptio placenta or eclampsia can precipitate DIC, pregnancies with multiple fetuses do not precipitate DIC. (A)

85. 1 A full bladder can impede fetal descent. The nurse's first action is to encourage the client to void every 2 to 4 hr. If the client cannot void and the bladder becomes distended, she may need to be catheterized. Oxytocin (Pitocin) is used to cause labor contractions, leading to delivery of the infant. The epidural infusion relaxes the client and may cause the uterine contractions to fade, necessitating the use of Pitocin to keep the contractions continuing. Rupturing amniotic fluid is not within the scope of the practice for the nurse. (D)

86. 2 If the client reports flulike symptoms, the nurse withholds the medication, collects more data, and discusses findings with the HCP because this might indicate that the client is experiencing agranulocytosis. If the client tells the nurse he may not take the medication after discharge, the nurse can administer the drug now and then discuss further with the client about approaches to medication compliance. The nurse also discusses with the HCP the fact that the client resumed smoking cigarettes because cigarette smoking causes a decrease in the serum level of the drug, requiring that the dose be increased; but the nurse should not withhold the medication. If the client tells the nurse he has an upset stomach, the nurse can advise the client to eat something prior to taking this drug, as food does not hinder the absorption of the drug. (D)

87. 2 A dose of 150 mg of acetaminophen (Tylenol) is an overdose and could potentially cause lethal harm for this infant. The range of safe dosages for Tylenol is 70 to 105 mg. The RN must call the HCP to verify the order. (D)

88. To suction the tracheobronchial tree the nurse inserts the catheter deep in the trachea. (M)

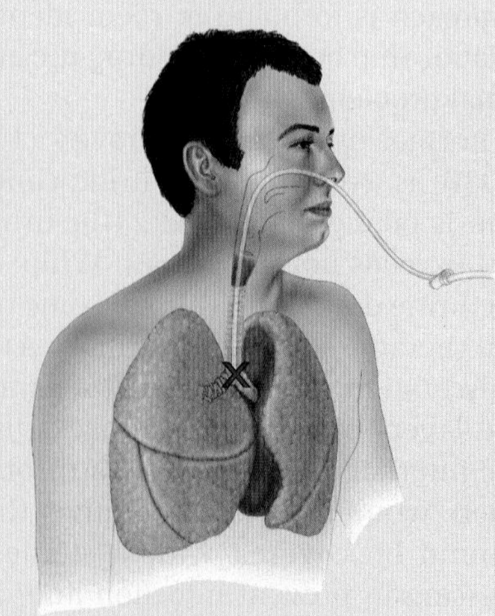

89. 1 When a client is taking clonazepam (Klonopin) and carbamazepine (Tegretol), the interaction of the two drugs often causes clonazepam (Klonopin) to increase the carbamazepine serum level. The clonazepam (Klonopin) serum level is not affected by the carbamazepine (Tegretol). (D)

90. 4 This child is most likely neutropenic since the WBC count is so low (normal is 4.5 to 13.5 × 1,000 cells/mm^3). The child is placed on neutropenic precautions to help prevent an infection. The platelets and creatinine are within normal limits for a school-aged child. The hemoglobin and hematocrit are low, but can be monitored; the child would more likely be transfused after the hemoglobin dropped to less than 8.0 g/dl. (S)

91. 3 The oxygen saturation indicates the child is hypoxic (despite increased respiratory rate). Because this will affect all other body systems, the hypoxia is treated immediately. The other orders are rapidly implemented, but do not require action as urgently as the low oxygen saturation. (M)

92. 3 Bringing finger foods to the client allows her to eat while still moving. Monitoring too closely may agitate the client. A manic client is often disruptive and may be inappropriate in the dining room at this time. It is unlikely the client will sit long enough to eat, and feeding the client is inappropriate if she can feed herself. Waiting to give the client food does not meet her nutritional needs, and the client is not yet stable enough to not continue to be "busy" at bedtime. (P)

93. 1 Limiting the number of choices the client must make will decrease his stress. Leaving both beds in the room will remain as a conflict for the client. Telling the client he will have to sleep in the dayroom if he does not make a decision is punitive and stressful for the client. (P)

94. 4 Spinal anesthesia provides anesthesia from the waist down. Complete return of sensation in the toes signifies to the nurse that the effects of spinal anesthesia have worn off. Lack of spontaneous breathing is not an effect of spinal anesthesia. BP fluctuations usually occur with general anesthesia. Resolution of back pain is not an indicator of recovery from spinal anesthesia. (A)

95. 3 Cocaine causes vasoconstriction and can place the fetus in distress as well as cause hyperstimulation of uterine contractions. Precipitous deliveries occur more frequently in clients who use cocaine. Although supplemental oxygen may be an appropriate intervention, it is not priority. There is low risk of seizure activity. The lateral recumbent position increases blood flow to the fetus and is encouraged. (M)

96. 3 Recognizing the concept of territoriality is important, but basic assessments for safety need to be completed in a nonthreatening manner. Decisiveness can be interpreted as aggressiveness by the client, and threaten sense of safety. Ignoring the client does not meet safety needs. Being enthusiastic will confuse and be threatening to the client. (P)

97. 2 The findings indicate a possible intussusception of the bowel, which, if not treated may lead to a necrosis of the bowel. The nurse must notify the HCP. Intussusception is most common between 3 months and 3 years of age; for a preschooler, intussusception may also suggest a non-Hodgkin lymphoma (abdominal tumor obstructing the bowel). The abdominal tumors found in Hodgkin lymphoma grow relatively quickly, causing an abdominal obstruction, which can lead to an intussusception. (A)

98. 2, 3, 1, 4 The nurse instructs the client who is preparing to have a colonoscopy to follow a clear-liquid diet for the entire day before the procedure. At 8 a.m. the client should drink one bottle (10 ounces) of citrate of magnesia. At 3 p.m. the client should start drinking one gallon of bowel preparation as prescribed over a 2-hr period. The client should remain NPO after midnight. (M)

99. 2 Offering reassurance ("you will be safe") and giving concrete guidance ("walk with me...") will lessen the client's anxiety in a nonthreatening way. Giving orders to the client will often result in defensive, aggressive behavior. The client may not have the insight to understand how her behaviors affect others. Threatening the client with a loss of control will often escalate behavior. (P)

100. 3 Since deformity occurs early in the disease, treatment aims at keeping the femoral heads in the acetabulum, which is done by abducting the legs. This serves as a mold to maintain the spherical shape of the head and to maintain a full range of motion. The other positions will not support the femoral head in the optimal position. (R)

Appendix: State and Territorial Boards of Nursing

Alabama
Alabama Board of Nursing
770 Washington Ave.
RSA Plaza, Suite 250
Montgomery, AL 36130-3900
Phone: 334-242-4060
Fax: 334-242-4360
Web site: www.abn.state.al.us

Alaska
Alaska Board of Nursing
550 W. 7th Ave., Suite 1500
Anchorage, AK 99501-3567
Phone: 907-269-8161
Fax: 907-269-8196
Web site: www.dced.state.ak.us/occ/pnur.htm

Arizona
Arizona State Board of Nursing
4747 N. 7th St., Suite 200
Phoenix, AZ 85014
Phone: 602-889-5150
Fax: 602-889-5155
Web site: www.azbn.gov

Arkansas
Arkansas State Board of Nursing
University Tower Building
1123 S. University, Suite 800
Little Rock, AR 72204-1619
Phone: 501-686-2700
Fax: 501-686-2714
Web site: www.arsbn.org

California
California Board of Registered Nursing
1625 N. Market Blvd., Suite N-217
Sacramento, CA 95834-1924
Phone: 916-322-3350
Fax: 916-574-8637
Web site: www.rn.ca.gov

Colorado
Colorado Board of Nursing
1560 Broadway, Suite 1370
Denver, CO 80202
Phone: 303-894-2430
Fax: 303-894-2821
Web site: www.dora.state.co.us/nursing

Connecticut
Connecticut Board of Examiners for Nursing
Department of Public Health
410 Capitol Ave., MS# 13PHO
P.O. Box 340308
Hartford, CT 06134-0328
Phone: 860-509-7624
Fax: 860-509-7553
Web site: www.state.ct.us/dph

Delaware
Delaware Board of Nursing
861 Silver Lake Blvd.
Cannon Building, Suite 203
Dover, DE 19904
Phone: 302-739-4522
Fax: 302-739-2711
Web site: www.professionallicensing.state.de.us/boards/nursing/index.shtml

District of Columbia
District of Columbia Board of Nursing
Department of Health
Health Professional Licensing Administration
District of Columbia Board of Nursing
717 14th St., NW, Suite 600
Washington, DC 20005
Phone: 877-672-2174
Fax: 202-727-8471
Web site: www.hpla.doh.dc.gov

Florida
Florida Board of Nursing
Capital Circle Officer Center
4052 Bald Cypress Way BIN C02
Tallahassee, FL 32399-3252
Phone: 850-245-4125
Fax: 850-245-4172
Web site: www.doh.state.fl.us/mqa

Georgia
Georgia Board of Nursing
237 Coliseum Dr.
Macon,GA 31217-3858
Phone: 478-207-2440
Fax: 478-207-1354
Web site: www.sos.state.ga.us/plb/rn

Hawaii
Hawaii Board of Nursing
King Kalakaua Bldg., 3rd floor
335 Merchant St.
Honolulu, HI 96813
Phone: 808-586-3000
Fax: 808-586-2689
Web site: www.hawaii.gov/dcca/areas/pvl/boards/nursing

Idaho
Idaho Board of Nursing
280 N. 8th St., Suite 210
P.O. Box 83720
Boise, ID 83720-0061
Phone: 208-334-3110
Fax: 208-334-3262
Web site: www2.state.id.us/lbn

Illinois
Illinois Department of Professional Regulation
James R. Thompson Center
100 W. Randolph, Suite 9-300
Chicago, IL 60601
Phone: 312-814-2715
Fax: 312-814-3145
Web site: www.dpr.state.il.us

Indiana
Indiana State Board of Nursing
Professional Licensing Agency
402 W. Washington St., Room W072
Indianapolis, IN 46204
Phone: 317-234-2043
Fax: 317-233-4236
Web site: www.in.gov/pla

Iowa
Iowa Board of Nursing
RiverPoint Business Park
400 S.W. 8th St., Suite B
Des Moines, IA 50309-4685
Phone: 515-281-3255
Fax: 515-281-4825
Web site: www.state.ia.us/government/nursing

Kansas
Kansas State Board of Nursing
Landon State Office Bldg.
900 S.W. Jackson, Suite 1051
Topeka, KS 66612-1230
Phone: 785-296-4929
Fax: 785-296-3929
Web site: www.ksbn.org

Kentucky
Kentucky Board of Nursing
312 Whittington Parkway, Suite 300
Louisville, KY 40222-5172
Phone: 502-429-3300
Fax: 502-429-3311
Web site: www.kbn.ky.gov

Louisiana
Louisiana State Board of Nursing
5207 Essen Lane, Suite 6
Baton Rouge, LA 70809
Phone: 225-763-3570
Fax: 225-763-3580
Web site: www.lsbn.state.la.us

Maine
Maine State Board of Nursing
#158 State House Station
Augusta, ME 04333
Phone: 207-287-1133
Fax: 207-287-1149
Web site: www.maine.gov/boardofnursing

Maryland
Maryland Board of Nursing
4140 Patterson Ave.
Baltimore, MD 21215-2254
Phone: 410-585-1900
Fax: 410-358-3530
Web site: www.mbon.org

Massachusetts
Massachusetts Board of Registration in Nursing
Commonwealth of Massachusetts
239 Causeway St., 2nd floor
Boston, MA 02114
Phone: 617-973-0800
Fax: 617-973-0984
Web site: www.mass.gov/dpl/boards/rn

Michigan
Michigan/DCH/Bureau of Health Services
Ottawa Towers North
611 W. Ottawa, 1st floor
Lansing, MI 48933
Phone: 517-335-0918
Fax: 517-373-2179
Web site: www.michigan.gov/healthlicense

Minnesota
Minnesota Board of Nursing
2829 University Ave. SE, Suite 200
Minneapolis, MN 55414
Phone: 612-617-2770
Fax: 612-617-2190
Web site: www.nursingboard.state.mn.us

Mississippi
Mississippi Board of Nursing
1935 Lakeland Dr., Suite B
Jackson, MS 39216-5014
Phone: 601-987-4188
Fax: 601-364-2352
Web site: www.msbn.state.ms.us

Missouri
Missouri State Board of Nursing
3605 Missouri Blvd.
P.O. Box 656
Jefferson City, MO 65102-0656
Phone: 573-751-0681
Fax: 573-751-0075
Web site: www.pr.mo.gov/nursing.asp

Montana
Montana State Board of Nursing
301 South Park
P.O. Box 200513
Helena, MT 59620-0513
Phone: 406-841-2345
Fax: 406-841-2305
Web site: www.nurse.mt.gov

Nebraska
Nebraska Dept. of Health and Human Services
Regulations and Licensure
Nursing and Nursing Support
301 Centennial Mall South
Lincoln, NE 68509-4986
Phone: 402-471-4376
Fax: 402-471-1066
Web site: www.hhs.state.ne.us/crl/nursing/nursingindex.htm

Nevada
Nevada State Board of Nursing
5011 Meadowood Mall Way, Suite 300
Reno, NV 89502
Phone: 775-688-2620
Fax: 775-688-2628
Web site: www.nursingboard.state.nv.us

New Hampshire
New Hampshire Board of Nursing
21 S. Fruit St., Suite 16
Concord, NH 03301-2341
Phone: 603-271-2323
Fax: 603-271-6605
Web site: www.state.nh.us/nursing

New Jersey
New Jersey Board of Nursing
P.O. Box 45010
124 Halsey St., 6th floor
Newark, NJ 07101
Phone: 973-504-6430
Fax: 973-648-3481
Web site: www.state.nj.us/lps/ca/medical/nursing.htm

New Mexico
New Mexico Board of Nursing
6301 Indian School NE, Suite 710
Albuquerque, NM 87110
Phone: 505-841-8340
Fax: 505-841-8347
Web site: www.bon.state.nm.us/index.html

New York
New York State Board of Nursing Education Bldg.
89 Washington Ave., 2nd floor, West Wing
Albany, NY 12234
Phone: 518-474-3817, ext. 280
Fax: 518-474-3706
Web site: www.nysed.gov/prof/nurse.htm

North Carolina
North Carolina Board of Nursing
3724 National Dr., Suite 201
Raleigh, NC 27602
Phone: 919-782-3211
Fax: 919-781-9461
Web site: www.ncbon.com

North Dakota
North Dakota Board of Nursing
919 S. 7th St., Suite 504
Bismarck, ND 58504-5881
Phone: 701-328-9777
Fax: 701-328-9785
Web site: www.ndbon.org

Ohio
Ohio Board of Nursing
17 S. High St., Suite 400
Columbus, OH 43215-3413
Phone: 614-466-3947
Fax: 614-466-0388
Web site: www.nursing.ohio.gov

Oklahoma
Oklahoma Board of Nursing
2915 N. Classen Blvd., Suite 524
Oklahoma City, OK 73106
Phone: 405-962-1800
Fax: 405-962-1821
Web site: www.youroklahoma.com/nursing

Oregon
Oregon State Board of Nursing
800 N.E. Oregon St., Suite 465, Box 25
Portland, OR 97232-2162
Phone: 971-673-0685
Fax: 971-673-0684
Web site: www.osbn.state.or.us

Pennsylvania
Pennsylvania State Board of Nursing
P.O. Box 2649
Harrisburg, PA 17105-2649
Phone: 717-783-7142
Fax: 717-783-0822
Web site: www.dos.state.pa.us/bpoa/cwp

Rhode Island
Rhode Island Board of Nurse Registration and Nursing Education
105 Cannon Building
3 Capitol Hill
Providence, RI 02908
Phone: 401-222-5700
Fax: 401-222-3352
Web site: www.healthri.org/hsr/professions/nurses.htm

South Carolina
South Carolina State Board of Nursing
P.O. Box 2367
Columbia, SC 29211
Phone: 803-896-4550
Fax: 803-896-4525
Web site: www.llr.state.sc.us/pol/nursing

South Dakota
South Dakota Board of Nursing
4305 S. Louise Ave., Suite 201
Sioux Falls, SD 57106-3115
Phone: 605-362-2760
Fax: 605-362-2768
Web site: www.state.sd.us/doh/nursing

Tennessee
Tennessee State Board of Nursing
227 French Landing, Suite 300
Nashville, TN 37243
Phone: 615-532-3202
Fax: 615-741-7899
Web site: www.tennessee.gov/health

Texas
Texas Board of Nurse Examiners
333 Guadalupe, Suite 3-460
Austin, TX 78701
Phone: 512-305-7400
Fax: 512-305-7401
Web site: www.bne.state.tx.us

Utah
Utah State Board of Nursing
Heber M. Wells Bldg., 4th floor
160 E. 300 South
Salt Lake City, UT 84111
Phone: 801-530-6628
Fax: 801-530-6511
Web site: www.doplutah.gov/licensing/nurse.html

Vermont
Vermont State Board of Nursing
81 River Rd., Heritage Bldg.
Montpelier, VT 05609-1106
Phone: 802-828-2396
Fax: 802-828-2484
Web site: www.vtprofessionals.org/opr1/nurses

Virginia
Virginia Board of Nursing
6603 W. Broad St., 5th floor
Richmond, VA 23230-1712
Phone: 804-662-9909
Fax: 804-662-9512
Web site: www.dhp.virginia.gov/nursing/

Washington
Washington State Nursing Care Quality Assurance Commission
Department of Health, HPQA#6
310 Israel Rd. SE
Tumwater, WA 98501-7864
Phone: 360-236-4700
Fax: 360-236-4738
Web site: fortress.wa.gov/doh/hpqa1/hps6/nursing/default.htm

West Virginia
West Virginia Board of Examiners for Registered Professional Nurses
101 Dee Dr.
Charleston, WV 25311-1620
Phone: 304-558-3596
Fax: 304-558-3666
Web site: www.wvrnboard.com

Wisconsin
Wisconsin Department of Regulation and Licensing
1400 E. Washington Ave., Rm. 173
Madison, WI 53708
Phone: 608-266-0145
Fax: 608-261-7083
Web site: www.drl.state.wi.us

Wyoming
Wyoming State Board of Nursing
1810 Pioneer Ave.
Cheyenne, WY 82002
Phone: 307-777-7601
Fax: 307-777-3519
Web site: nursing.state.wy.us

Index

Note: Page numbers followed by f indicate figure, and t indicate table.